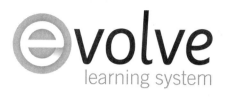
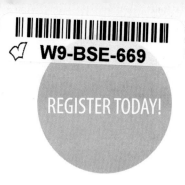

# ESSENTIALS OF

# Cardiopulmonary Physical Therapy

## THIRD EDITION

ELLEN HILLEGASS, PT, EdD, CCS, FAACVPR
Associate Professor
Department of Physical Therapy
North Georgia College & State University
Dahlonega, Georgia

ELSEVIER
SAUNDERS

3251 Riverport Lane
St. Louis, Missouri 63043

ISBN: 978-1-437-70381-8

Executive Editor: Kathy Falk
Developmental Editor: Megan Fennell
Publishing Services Manager: Julie Eddy
Project Manager: Marquita Parker
Design Direction: Paula Catalano

Printed in the United States of America

Last digit is the print number:   9   8   7   6   5   4

*This book is dedicated to my beloved family for all their love and support as well as their understanding during my endless hours of working on this edition:*

*To my husband Dan, who is my rock and my constant support whom I couldn't live without;*

*To my three wonderful children: Patrick, Jamie and Christi who give me moral support, make me laugh, and who constantly try to keep me up to date on all the modern technologies that have helped me communicate with them, communicate with my colleagues, and write this book. They keep me young with their ideas and assistance; they constantly have a "joie de vivre";*

*To my three dogs: Mac, Sparky and Bear who kept my feet warm while I sat for hours at the computer working on this edition but demanded daily play, and provided a wonderful mental break from writing; and*

*To my parents, John and Norma, who keep me busy but are always proud of everything I do.*


*In addition, I dedicate this edition:*

*To my colleagues who keep me informed, give me moral and intellectual support and who keep me inspired to maintain my passion for the field of cardiovascular and pulmonary physical therapy. I especially rely on the support and inspiration of some very dear friends/colleagues including Dianne Jewell, Andrew Ries, Claire Rice and Joanne Watchie.*

*And finally, I can never forget my very special friends/mentors to whom I am forever grateful and whose memories and teachings are with me always: Michael Pollock (1937–1998), Linda Crane (1951–1999), and Gary Dudley (1952–2006).*

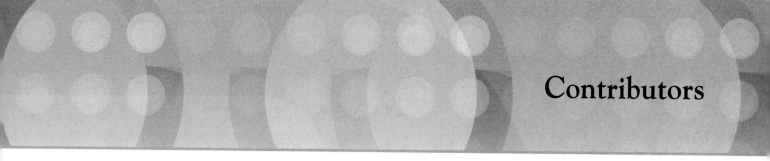

# Contributors

**Tamara L. Burlis, PT, DPT, CCS**
Associate Director of Clinical Education, Assistant Professor, Program in Physical Therapy and Internal Medicine, Washington University, St. Louis, Missouri

**Lawrence P. Cahalin, PhD, MA**
Clinical Professor, Department of Physical Therapy Northeastern University, Boston, Massachusetts

**Rohini K. Chandrashekar, PT, MS, CCS**
Guest Lecturer, Physical Therapy, Texas Woman's University, Houston, Texas
Physical Therapist, Rehabilitation, Triumph Hospital Clear Lake, Webster, Texas

**Peggy Clough, MA, PT**
Supervisor, Physical Therapy Division, University of Michigan Health System, University Hospital, Ann Arbor, Michigan

**Meryl Cohen, DPT, MS, CCS**
Assistant Professor, Department of Physical Therapy, Miller School of Medicine, University of Miami, Coral Gables, Florida
Adjunct Instructor, Massachusetts General Hospital, Institute of Health Professions, Boston, Massachusetts

**Kelley Crawford, DPT**
Level III Clinician, Rehabilitation, Medicine, Maine Medical Center, Portland, Maine

**Rebecca Crouch, PT, DPT, CCS**
Adjunct Faculty, Doctoral Program in Physical Therapy, Duke University, Durham, North Carolina
Coordinator of Pulmonary Rehabilitation, PT/OT, Duke University Medical Center, Durham, North Carolina

**Konrad J. Dias, PT, DPT, CCS**
Associate Professor, Physical Therapy Program, Maryville University, St. Louis, Missouri

**Christen DiPerna, PT, DPT**
Physical Therapist, Indiana University Health Methodist Hospital, Indianapolis, Indiana

**Anne Mejia Downs, PT, CCS**
Assistant Professor, Krannert School of Physical Therapy, University of Indianapolis, Indianapolis, Indiana
Physical Therapist, Department of Rehabilitation Services, Clarian Health Partners, Indianapolis, Indiana

**Jennifer Edelschick, PT, DPT**
Coordinator of Pediatric Acute PT/OT Services, Physical and Occupational Therapy, Duke Medicine, Durham, North Carolina

**Susan L. Garritan, PT, PhD, CCS**
Clinical Assistant Professor of Rehabilitation Medicine, Acute Care Physical Therapy Coordinator, Tisch Hospital, New York University Langone Medical Center, New York, New York

**Kate Grimes, MS, PT, CCS**
Clinical Assistant Professor, Massachusetts General Hospital Institute of Health Professions, Boston, Massachusetts

**Kristin M. Lefebvre, PT, PhD, CCS**
Assistant Professor, Institute for Physical Therapy Education, Widener University, Chester Pennsylvania

**Ana Lotshaw, PT, PhD, CCS**
Rehabilitation Supervisor, Physical Medicine and Rehabilitation, Baylor University Medical Center, Dallas, Texas

**Eugene McColgon, PT**
Program Director, Cardiac Rehabilitation, James A. Haley Veterans Hospital, Tampa, Florida

**Susan Butler McNamara, MMSc, PT, CCS**
Team Leader, Division of Rehabilitation Medicine, Maine Medical Center, Portland, Maine

**Harold Merriman, PT, PhD, CLT**
Assistant Professor, General Medicine Coordinator, Doctor of Physical Therapy Program, Department of Health and Sports Science, University of Dayton, Dayton, Ohio

**Amy Pawlik, PT, DPT, CCS**
Program Coordinator, Cardiopulmonary Rehabilitation Therapy Services, The University of Chicago Hospitals, Chicago, Illinois

**Christiane Perme, PT, CCS**
Senior Physical Therapist, Physical Therapy and
Occupational Therapy Department, The Methodist
Hospital, Houston, Texas

**H. Steven Sadowsky, MS, RRT, PT, CCS**
Assistant Professor, Associate Chair for Professional
Education, Department of Physical Therapy and
Human Movement Sciences, Northwestern University,
Chicago, Illinois

**Alexandra Sciaky, PT, DPT, MS, CCS**
Adjunct Faculty, Department of Physical Therapy,
University of Michigan-Flint, Flint, Michigan
Senior Physical Therapist, Coordinator of Clinical
Education, Physical Medicine and Rehabilitation,
Physical Therapy Section, Veterans Affairs Ann Arbor
Healthcare System, Ann Arbor, Michigan

**Debra Seal, PT, DPT**
Senior Pediatric Physical Therapist, Acute Therapy,
Cedars-Sinai Medical Center, Los Angeles, California

**William C. Temes, PT, MS, OCS, FAAOMPT**
Director of Interactive Mentorship, Therapeutic Associates,
Inc., Eugene, Oregon

**Wolfgang Vogel, MS, PhD**
Professor Emeritus, Department of Pharmacology, Jefferson
Medical College, Thomas Jefferson University,
Philadelphia, Pennsylvania

**Joanne Watchie, MA, PT, CCS**
Owner, Joanne's Wellness Ways, Pasadena, California

# Preface

Originally this text was developed to meet the needs of the physical therapy community, as cardiopulmonary was identified as one of the four clinical science components in a physical therapy education program as well as in clinical practice. Those aspects of physical therapy commonly referred to as "cardiopulmonary physical therapy" are recognized as fundamental components of the knowledge base and practice base of all entry-level physical therapists. Although intended primarily for physical therapists, this text has been useful to practitioners in various disciplines who teach students or who work with patients who suffer from primary and secondary cardiopulmonary dysfunction. This third edition can also be used by all practitioners including those who both teach and work with patients.

This third edition has gone through major revision. The same six sections exist: *Anatomy and Physiology; Pathophysiology; Diagnostic Tests and Procedures; Surgical Interventions, Invasive and Noninvasive Monitoring and Support; Pharmacology;* and *Cardiopulmonary Assessment and Intervention.* The six sections were kept as they facilitate the progression of understanding of the material in order to be able to perform a thorough assessment and provide an optimal intervention. However, an addition was made to the last section to examine special population considerations; specifically, pediatric cardiopulmonary issues and lymphedema. These are two new chapters included to address the great need for this information by practitioners and the fact that these are practice patterns from the *Guide* that were not covered in any depth in the previous edition.

The revisions you should notice include both major and minor changes. All chapters have been revised as well as supplemented with many figures and tables to help the learner visualize the written information. Additional figures, case studies, and resource material can also be found on the Evolve website which accompanies this text. The number of clinical notes was increased to help clinicians and students understand certain clinical findings and help them relate them to the pathophysiology of cardiovascular and pulmonary disease. All chapters discuss the information in each chapter as it relates to the *Guide to Physical Therapist Practice* and present the practice patterns in tables that are appropriate for those specific chapters. And, finally, all chapters were updated with new information, technology and research.

Each chapter had specific revisions that should be highlighted. Chapters 1 and 2, which explain anatomy and physiology, went through major revision to help the learner relate the pathophysiology to the normal anatomy and physiology. In addition, the developmental and maturational anatomy was moved to the pediatrics chapter (Chapter 20) to help the learner compare the pathophysiology to the normal in this population. Chapter 3, *Ischemic Cardiovascular Conditions and Other Vascular Pathologies,* underwent revision as noted by the new title. Material throughout the book was reorganized and taken out of some chapters and transferred here. New material was added, so that you will now find hypertension, peripheral arterial disease, cerebrovascular disease, renal disease and aortic aneurysm is found in this chapter, in addition to ischemic disease. Chapter 4, *Cardiac Muscle Dysfunction and Failure,* was restructured and revised to improve the flow and understanding of this important pathologic condition.

Due to the complexities and number of conditions of restrictive lung dysfunction many more tables were created in Chapter 5 to separate the material and assist the learner to identify key information quickly. Chapter 6, *Obstructive Lung Dysfunction,* was updated and revised due to the increase in the importance of this disease and the fact that COPD is the fourth leading cause of death. Revisions in Chapter 7, *Cardiopulmonary Implications of Specific Diseases,* emphasize information on obesity, diabetes, and metabolic syndrome, as well as cancer and neuromuscular diseases.

New technologies and advancements in diagnostic tests and surgical procedures were added to Chapters 8, 9, 10 and 11. The advances in transplantation were discussed in Chapter 12 and *Invasive and Noninvasive Monitoring and Life Support Equipment* (Chapter 13) was revised to increase the depth of information on ventilators as well as other monitoring equipment.

As advances in health care and diagnostics occur, so do improvements and changes in medications, so both *Cardiovascular Pharmacology* (Chapter 14) and *Pulmonary Pharmacology* (Chapter 15) required updating and were further reviewed by a wonderful pharmacist, Dr. Wolfgang Vogel.

Chapter 16 (*Examination and Assessment Procedures*) had some revision, but the chapters following assessment had the most revision. Acute care, pulmonary rehabilitation and therapeutic interventions all had major updating and revision, new clinical notes and many new figures and tables. *Pediatric Cardiopulmonary Physical Therapy* and *Lymphedema* were two wonderful additions to the third edition of *Cardiopulmonary Physical Therapy.* And, finally, the text ends with the outcomes chapter which was totally revamped and provides great information for measurement of improvement in the cardiopulmonary patient population.

Whenever possible, case studies are provided to exemplify the material being presented. Additional case studies are found on Evolve.

No matter how well you understand the material in this book, it will not make you a master clinician, skilled in the assessment and treatment of cardiovascular and pulmonary disorders. To become even a minimally competent clinician, you will have to practice physical therapy under the tutelage of an experienced clinician. *Essentials of Cardiopulmonary Physical Therapy* cannot provide you with everything there is to know about the assessment and treatment of cardiovascular and pulmonary disorders. It will provide the essentials as the title indicates. Learning is a continuous process, and technology and treatment are forever improving; therefore, this text provides clinicians as well as educators with the most current information at the time of publication.

It is my true hope that you appreciate this edition and are able to learn from all the wealth of information provided by such wonderful contributors. Without heart and breath there is no therapy!

# Acknowledgments

"Change is good and change equals opportunity!" This statement explains how I have approached each edition, but most especially this edition! Hopefully you will gain knowledge and insight from all the changes as there are many excellent contributions from my colleagues, who are THE experts in cardiovascular and pulmonary physical therapy and who poured their passion into their chapters.

During the publication phase of the first edition of the *Essentials of Cardiopulmonary Physical Therapy* I was always worried about new developments in the field of Cardiovascular and Pulmonary diagnosis and treatment that were not going to be covered in the book. My very first editor, Margaret Biblis kept saying "that's what the next edition is for" and that is how I approached the second edition and again the third edition. I have saved comments and suggestions along the way as well as attended conferences regularly to stay current with new developments in the field. And, with the age of the internet, you will now have access to the new Evolve site that my wonderful colleague and friend, Dawn Hayes, has developed to accompany this text. Instructional material including PowerPoint presentations and a test bank are available to instructors in the course, as well as updated information.

So, I would like to thank all the amazing experts who have helped with this third edition, including each of the wonderful contributors as well as all those clinicians, students and faculty members who provided feedback on previous editions and who continue to use this book in their courses and their every day practice. I would like to especially thank the contributors for their ability to work under my constant nagging to achieve their deadlines and for providing great material including figures, tables and clinical notes. One special contributor who needs acknowledgement is Dr. Wolfgang Vogel, a pharmacist who reviewed and revised information in the pharmacology chapters to be consistent with the practice of pharmacists. I would also like to acknowledge and thank Meryl Cohen who kept pressing me to get this edition going as it was her comments that pushed me to finally initiate the third edition.

Of course my family and my dogs need to be acknowledged for all the time I spent at the computer working on this edition instead of spending time with them.

Lastly, this edition truly would not be published were it not for my wonderful editor, Megan Fennell, who called me weekly and pushed this edition to a timely completion. She has become a close friend and the best editor ever! Thanks Megan!

# Contents

## CHAPTER 1

# Anatomy of the Cardiovascular and Pulmonary Systems

*Konrad Dias*

## Chapter Outline

This chapter describes the anatomy of the cardiovascular and pulmonary systems as it is relevant to the physical therapist. Knowledge of the anatomy of these systems provides clinicians with the foundation to perform the appropriate examination and provide optimal treatment interventions for individuals with cardiopulmonary dysfunction. An effective understanding of cardiovascular and pulmonary anatomy allows for comprehension of function and an appreciation of the central components of oxygen and nutrient transport to peripheral tissue. A fundamental assumption is made; namely, that the reader already possesses some knowledge of anatomical terms and cardiopulmonary anatomy.

## Thorax

The bony thorax covers and protects the major organs of the cardiopulmonary system. Within the thoracic cavity exist the heart, housed within the mediastinum centrally, while laterally are two lungs. The bony thorax provides a skeletal framework for the attachment of the muscles of ventilation.

The thoracic cage (Fig. 1-1) is conical at both its superior and inferior aspects and somewhat kidney-shaped in its transverse aspect. The skeletal boundaries of the thorax are the 12 thoracic vertebrae dorsally, the ribs laterally, and the sternum ventrally.

## Sternum

The sternum or breastbone is a flat bone with three major parts: *manubrium*, *body*, and *xiphoid process* (see Fig. 1-1). Superiorly located within the sternum, the manubrium is the thickest component articulating with the clavicles, first and second ribs. A palpable jugular notch or suprasternal notch is found at the superior border of the manubrium of the sternum. Inferior to the manubrium lies the body of the sternum articulating laterally with ribs three to seven. The sternal angle or "angle of Louis" is the anterior angle formed by the junction of the manubrium and the body of the sternum. This easily palpated structure is in level with the second costal cartilage anteriorly and thoracic vertebrae T4 and T5 posteriorly. The most caudal aspect of the sternum is the xiphoid process, a plate of hyaline cartilage that ossifies later in life.

The sternal angle marks the level of bifurcation of the trachea into the right and left main stem bronchi as well as provides for the pump handle action of the sternal body during inspiration.[1]

Pectus excavatum is a common congenital deformity of the anterior wall of the chest, in which several ribs and the sternum grow abnormally (see Fig. 5-19). This produces a caved-in or sunken appearance of the chest. It is present at birth but rapidly progresses during the years of bone growth

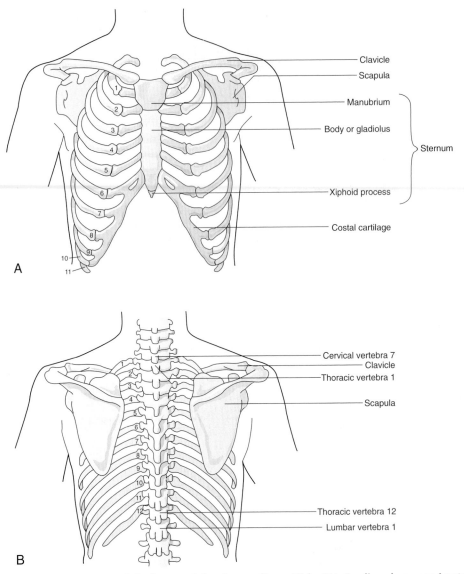

**Figure 1-1** A, Anterior. B, Posterior views of the bones of the thorax. (From Hicks GH. Cardiopulmonary Anatomy and Physiology. Philadelphia, 2000, Saunders.)

in the early teenage years. These patients have several pulmonary complications including shortness of breath caused by altered mechanics of the inspiratory muscles on the caved-in sternum and ribs, and often have cardiac complications caused by the restriction (compression) of the heart.[2]

To gain access to the thoracic cavity for surgery, including coronary artery bypass grafting, the sternum is spit in the median plane and retracted. This procedure is known as a median sternotomy. Flexibility of the ribs and cartilage allow for separation of the two ends of the sternum to expose the thoracic cavity.[3]

## Ribs

The ribs, although considered "flat" bones, curve forward and downward from their posterior vertebral attachments toward their costal cartilages. The first seven ribs attach via their costal cartilages to the sternum and are called the true ribs

(also known as the vertebrosternal ribs); the lower five ribs are termed the false ribs—the eight, ninth, and tenth ribs attach to the rib above by their costal cartilages (the vertebrochondral ribs), and the eleventh and twelfth ribs end freely (the vertebral ribs see Fig. 1-1). The true ribs increase in length from above downward, while the false ribs decrease in length from above downward.

Each rib typically has a vertebral end separated from a sternal end by the body or shaft of the rib. The head of the rib (at its vertebral end) is distinguished by a twin-faceted surface for articulation with the facets on the bodies of two adjacent thoracic vertebrae. The cranial facet is smaller than the caudal, and a crest between these permits attachment of the interarticular ligament.

Figure 1-2 displays the components of typical ribs three to nine, each with common characteristics including a head, neck, tubercle, and body. The neck is the 1-inch long portion of the rib extending laterally from the head; it provides

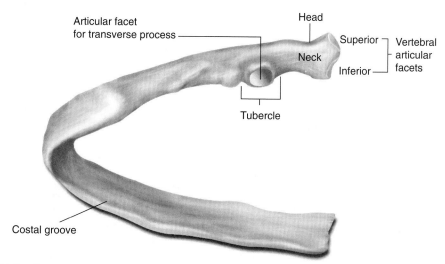

**Figure 1-2** Typical middle rib as viewed from the posterior. The head end articulates with the vertebral bones and the distal end is attached to the costal cartilage of the sternum. (From Wilkins RL. Egan's Fundamentals of Respiratory Care ed 9. St. Louis, 2009, Mosby.)

attachment for the anterior costotransverse ligament along its cranial border. The tubercle at the junction of the neck and the body of the rib consists of an articular and a non-articular portion. The articular part of the tubercle (the more medial and inferior of the two) has a facet for articulation with the transverse process of the inferior most vertebra to which the head is connected. The nonarticular part of the tubercle provides attachment for the ligament of the tubercle.

The shaft or body of the rib is simultaneously bent in two directions and twisted about its long axis, presenting two surfaces (internal and external) and two borders (superior and inferior). A costal groove, for the intercostal vessels and nerve, extends along the inferior border dorsally but changes to the internal surface at the angle of the rib. The sternal end of the rib terminates in an oval depression into which the costal cartilage makes its attachment.

Although rib fractures may occur in various locations, they are more common in the weakest area where the shaft of the ribs bend—the area just anterior to its angle. The first rib does not usually fracture as it is protected posteroinferiorly by the clavicle. When it is injured, the brachial plexus of nerves and subclavian vessel injury may occur.[4] Lower rib fractures may cause trauma to the diaphragm resulting in a diaphragmatic hernia. Rib fractures are extremely painful because of their profound nerve supply. It is important for all therapists to recommend breathing, splinting and coughing strategies for patients with rib fractures. Paradoxical breathing patterns and a flail chest may also need to be evaluated in light of multiple rib fractures in adjacent ribs.[3]

Chest tubes are inserted above the ribs to avoid trauma to vessels and nerves found within the costal grove. A chest tube insertion involves the surgical placement of a hollow, flexible drainage tube into the chest. This tube is used to drain blood, air, or fluid around the lungs and effectively allow the lung to expand. The tube is placed between the ribs and into the space between the inner lining and the outer lining of the lung (pleural space).

The first, second, tenth, eleventh, and twelfth ribs are unlike the other, more typical ribs (Fig. 1-3). The first rib is the shortest and most curved of all the ribs. Its head is small and rounded and has only one facet for articulation with the body of the first thoracic vertebra. The sternal end of the first rib is larger and thicker than it is in any of the other ribs. The second rib, although longer than the first, is similarly curved. The body is not twisted. There is a short costal groove on its internal surface posteriorly. The tenth through twelfth ribs each have only one articular facet on their heads. The eleventh and twelfth ribs (floating ribs) have no necks or tubercles and are narrowed at their free anterior ends. The twelfth rib sometimes is shorter than the first rib.

## The Respiratory System

The respiratory system includes the bony thorax, the muscles of ventilation, the upper and the lower airways, and the pulmonary circulation. The many functions of the respiratory system include gas exchange, fluid exchange, maintenance of a relatively low-volume blood reservoir, filtration, and metabolism, and they necessitate an intimate and exquisite interaction of these various components. Because the thorax has already been discussed, this section deals with the muscles of ventilation, the upper and lower airways, and the pulmonary circulation.

### Muscles of Ventilation

Ventilation or breathing involves the processes of inspiration and expiration. For air to enter the lungs during inspiration, muscles of the thoracic cage and abdomen must move the bony thorax to create changes in volume within the thorax

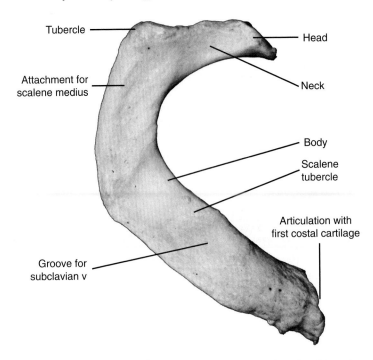

Tubercle

Head

Attachment for
scalene medius

Neck

Body

Scalene
tubercle

Articulation with
first costal cartilage

Groove for
subclavian v

**Figure 1-3** Superior view of the first right rib. (From Liebgott B. The Anatomical Basis of Dentistry ed 2. St. Louis, 2002, Mosby.)

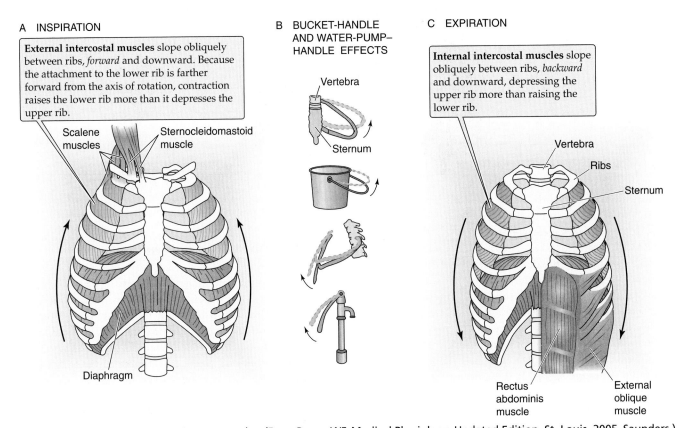

A  INSPIRATION

**External intercostal muscles** slope obliquely between ribs, *forward* and downward. Because the attachment to the lower rib is farther forward from the axis of rotation, contraction raises the lower rib more than it depresses the upper rib.

Scalene
muscles

Sternocleidomastoid
muscle

Diaphragm

B  BUCKET-HANDLE
AND WATER-PUMP–
HANDLE  EFFECTS

Vertebra

Sternum

C  EXPIRATION

**Internal intercostal muscles** slope obliquely between ribs, *backward* and downward, depressing the upper rib more than raising the lower rib.

Vertebra

Ribs

Sternum

Rectus
abdominis
muscle

External
oblique
muscle

**Figure 1-4** Actions of major respiratory muscles. (From Boron WF. Medical Physiology. Updated Edition. St. Louis, 2005, Saunders.)

and cause a concomitant reduction in the intrathoracic pressure. Inspiratory muscles increase the volume of the thoracic cavity by producing bucket handle and pump handle movements of the ribs and sternum depicted in Figure 1-4. The resultant reduced intrathoracic pressure generated is below atmospheric pressure, forcing air into the lungs to help normalize pressure differences. The essential muscles to achieve the active process of inspiration at rest are the diaphragm and internal intercostals. To create a more forceful inspiration during exercise or cardiopulmonary distress, accessory

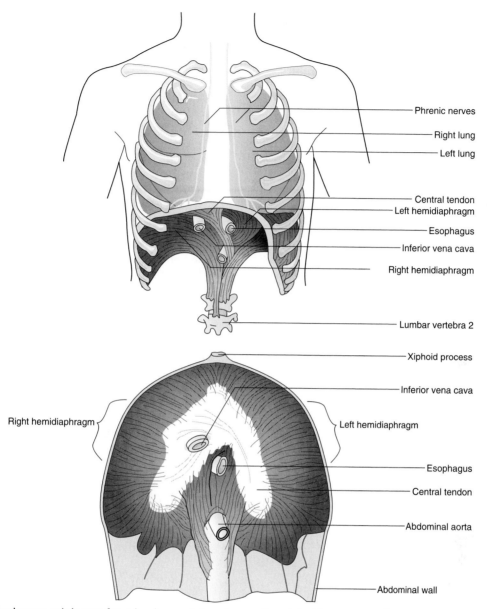

**Figure 1-5** The diaphragm originates from lumbar vertebra, lower ribs, xiphoid process, and abdominal wall and converges in a central tendon. Note the locations of the phrenic nerves and openings for the inferior vena cava, esophagus, and abdominal aorta. (From Hicks GH. Cardiopulmonary Anatomy and Physiology. Philadelphia, 2000, Saunders.)

muscles assist with the inspiration. The accessory muscles include the sternocleidomastoid, scalenes, serratus anterior, pectoralis major and minor, trapezius, and erector spinae muscles.

## Diaphragm

The diaphragm is the major muscle of inspiration. It is a musculotendinous dome that forms the floor of the thorax and separates the thoracic and abdominal cavities (Fig. 1-5). The diaphragm is divided into right and left hemidiaphragms. Both hemidiaphragms are visible on radiographic studies from the front or back. The right hemidiaphragm is protected by the liver and is stronger than the left. The left hemidiaphragm is more often subject to rupture and hernia, usually because of weaknesses at the points of embryologic fusion.

Each hemidiaphragm is composed of three musculoskeletal components, including the sternal, costal, and lumbar portions that converge into the central tendon. The central tendon of the diaphragm is a thin but strong layer of tendons (aponeurosis) situated anteriorly and immediately below the pericardium. There are three major openings to enable various vessels to traverse the diaphragm. These include the vena caval opening for the inferior vena cava, the esophageal opening for the esophagus and gastric vessels and the aortic opening containing the aorta, thoracic duct and azygous veins. The phrenic nerve arises from the third, fourth, and fifth cervical spinal nerves (C3 to C5) and is involved in contraction of the diaphragm.

The resting position of the diaphragm is an arched position high in the thorax. The level of the diaphragm and the amount of movement during inspiration vary as a result of factors such as body position, obesity, and size of various gastrointestinal organs present below the diaphragm. During normal ventilation or breathing, the diaphragm contracts to pull the central tendon down and forward. In doing so, the resting dome shape of the diaphragm is reversed to a flatting of the diaphragm. Contraction of this muscle increases the dimensions of the thorax in a cephalocaudal, anterior posterior, and lateral direction.[1] The increase in volume decreases pressure in the thoracic cavity and simultaneously causes a decrease in volume and an increase in pressure within the abdominal cavity. The domed shape of the diaphragm is largely maintained until the abdominal muscles end their extensibility, halting the downward displacement of the abdominal viscera, essentially forming a fixed platform beneath the central tendon. The central tendon then becomes a fixed point against which the muscular fibers of the diaphragm contract to elevate the lower ribs and thereby push the sternum and upper ribs forward. The right hemidiaphragm meets more resistance than the left (because the liver underlies the right hemidiaphragm; the stomach underlies the left) during its descent; it is therefore more substantial than the left.

In patients with chronic obstructive pulmonary disease there is compromised ability to expire. This results in a flattening of the diaphragm as a result of the presence of hyperinflated lungs.[1,5] It is essential for therapists to reverse hyperinflation and restore the normal resting arched position of the diaphragm prior to any using any exercise aimed at strengthening the diaphragm muscle. A flat and rigid diaphragm cannot be strengthened and will cause an automatic firing of the accessory muscles to trigger inspiration.

Body position in supine, upright or side lying alters the resting position of the diaphragm, resulting in concomitant changes in lung volumes.[6] In the supine position, without the effects of gravity, the level of the diaphragm in the thoracic cavity rises. This allows for a relatively greater excursion of the diaphragm. Despite a greater range of movement of the diaphragm, lung volumes are low as a consequence of the elevated position of the abdominal organs within the thoracic cavity. In an upright position, the dome of the diaphragm is pulled down because of the effects of gravity. The respiratory excursion is less in this position; however, the lung volumes are larger. In the side-lying position, the hemidiaphragms are unequal in their positions: The uppermost side drops to a lower level and has less excursion than that in the sitting position; the lowermost side rises higher in the thorax and has a greater excursion than in the sitting position. In quiet breathing, the diaphragm normally moves about two-thirds

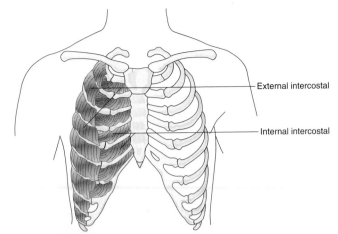

**Figure 1-6** The external intercostal muscles lift the inferior ribs and enlarge the thoracic cavity. The internal intercostal muscles compresses the thoracic cavity by pulling together the ribs. (From Hicks GH. Cardiopulmonary Anatomy and Physiology. Philadelphia, 2000, Saunders.)

of an inch; with maximal ventilatory effort the diaphragm may move from 2.5 to 4 inches.[5]

## External Intercostal Muscles

The external intercostal muscles originate from the lower borders of the ribs and attach to the upper border of the ribs below (Fig. 1-6). There are 11 external intercostal muscles on each side of the sternum. Contraction of these muscles pull the lower rib up and out toward the upper rib thereby elevating the ribs and expanding the chest.

## Accessory Muscles

Figure 1-7 explains the anatomy of the accessory muscles.

### Sternocleidomastoid Muscle

The sternocleidomastoid arises by two heads (sternal and clavicular, from the medial part of the clavicle), which unite to extend obliquely upward and laterally across the neck to the mastoid process. For this muscle to facilitate inspiration, the head and neck must be held stable by the neck flexors and extensors. This muscle is a primary accessory muscle and elevates the sternum, increasing the anterior-posterior diameter of the chest.

### Scalene Muscle

The scalene muscles lie deep to the sternocleidomastoid, but may be palpated in the posterior triangle of the neck. These muscles function as a unit to elevate and fix the first and second ribs.

- The *anterior* scalene muscle passes from the anterior tubercles of the transverse processes of the third or fourth to the sixth cervical vertebrae, attaching by tendinous insertion into the first rib.
- The *middle* scalene muscle arises from the transverse processes of all the cervical vertebrae to insert onto the first rib (posteromedially to the anterior scalene

---

**Clinical Tip**
Stomach fullness, obesity with presence of a large pannus, ascites with increased fluid in the peritoneal space from liver disease, and pregnancy are additional factors affecting the normal excursion of the diaphragm during inspiration.

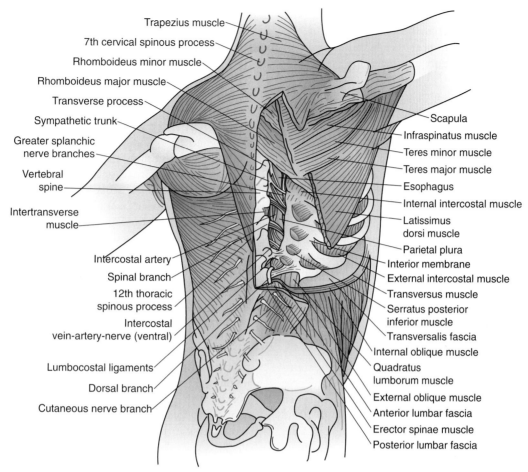

Trapezius muscle
7th cervical spinous process
Rhomboideus minor muscle
Rhomboideus major muscle
Transverse process
Sympathetic trunk
Greater splanchic nerve branches
Vertebral spine
Intertransverse muscle
Intercostal artery
Spinal branch
12th thoracic spinous process
Intercostal vein-artery-nerve (ventral)
Lumbocostal ligaments
Dorsal branch
Cutaneous nerve branch

Scapula
Infraspinatus muscle
Teres minor muscle
Teres major muscle
Esophagus
Internal intercostal muscle
Latissimus dorsi muscle
Parietal plura
Interior membrane
External intercostal muscle
Transversus muscle
Serratus posterior inferior muscle
Transversalis fascia
Internal oblique muscle
Quadratus lumborum muscle
External oblique muscle
Anterior lumbar fascia
Erector spinae muscle
Posterior lumbar fascia

**Figure 1-7** Musculature of the chest wall. (From Ravitch MM, Steichen FM. Atlas of General Thoracic Surgery. Philadelphia, 1988, Saunders.)

the brachial plexus and subclavian artery pass between anterior scalene and middle scalene).

- The *posterior* scalene muscle arises from the posterior tubercles of the transverse processes of the fifth and sixth cervical vertebrae, passing between the middle scalene and levator scapulae, to attach onto the second or third rib.

### Upper Trapezius

The trapezius (upper fibers) muscle arises from the medial part of the superior nuchal line on the occiput and the ligamentum nuchae (from the vertebral spinous processes between the skull and the seventh cervical vertebra) to insert onto the distal third of the clavicle. This muscle assists with ventilation by helping to elevate the thoracic cage.

### Pectoralis Major and Minor

The pectoralis major arises from the medial third of the clavicle, from the lateral part of the anterior surface of the manubrium and body of the sternum, and from the costal cartilages of the first six ribs to insert upon the lateral lip of the crest of the greater tubercle of the humerus. When the arms and shoulders are fixed, by leaning on the elbows or grasping onto a table, the pectoralis major can use its

insertion as its origin and pull on the anterior chest wall, lifting the ribs and sternum and facilitate an increase in the anteroposterior diameter of the thorax.

The pectoralis minor arises from the second to fifth or the third to sixth ribs upward to insert into the medial side of the coracoid process close to the tip. This muscle assists in forced inspiration by raising the ribs and increasing intrathoracic volume.

### Serratus Anterior and Rhomboids

The serratus anterior arises from the outer surfaces of the upper eight or nine ribs to attach along the costal aspect of the medial border of the scapula. The primary action of the serratus is to abduct, rotate the scapula, and hold the medial border firmly over the rib cage. The serratus can only be utilized as an accessory muscle in ventilation, when the rhomboids stabilize the scapula in adduction.[7] The action of the rhomboids fixes the insertion, allowing the serratus to expand the rib cage by pulling the origin toward the insertion.

### Latissimus Dorsi

The latissimus dorsi arises from the spinous processes of the lower six thoracic, the lumbar, and the upper sacral vertebrae, from the posterior aspect of the iliac crest, and slips from the lower three or four ribs to attach to the intertubercular groove of the humerus.[7] The posterior fibers of this muscle assist in inspiration as they pull the trunk into extension.

### Serratus Posterior Superior
The serratus posterior superior passes from the lower part of the ligamentum nuchae and the spinous processes of the seventh cervical and first two or three thoracic vertebrae downward into the upper borders of the second to fourth or fifth ribs. This muscle assists in inspiration by raising the ribs to which it is attached and expanding the chest.

### Thoracic Erector Spinae Muscles
The erector spinae is a large muscle group extending from the sacrum to the skull. The thoracic erector spinae muscles extend the thoracic spine and raise the rib cage to allow greater expansion of the thorax.

## Muscles of Expiration

### Abdominal Muscles
The abdominal muscles include the rectus abdominis, transversus abdominis, and internal and external obliques. These muscles work to raise intraabdominal pressure when a sudden expulsion of air is required in maneuvers such as huffing and coughing. Pressure generated within the abdominal cavity is transmitted to the thoracic cage to assist in emptying the lungs.

### Internal Intercostal Muscles
Eleven internal intercostal muscles exist on each side of the sternum. These muscles arise on the inner surfaces of the ribs and costal cartilages and insert on the upper borders of the adjacent ribs below (see Fig. 1-6). The posterior aspect on the internal intercostal muscles is termed the interosseus portion and depresses the ribs to aid in a forceful expiration. The intercartilaginous portion of the internal intercostals elevates the ribs and assists in inspiration.

## Pulmonary Ventilation
Pulmonary ventilation, commonly referred to as breathing, is the process in which air is moved in and out of the lungs. Inspiration, an active process at rest and during exercise, involves contraction of the diaphragm and external intercostal muscles. The muscle that contracts first is the diaphragm, with a caudal movement and resultant increase within the volume of the thoracic cavity. The diaphragm eventually meets resistance against the abdominal viscera causing the costal fibers of the diaphragm to contract and pull the lower ribs up and out—*the bucket handle movement*. The outward movement is also facilitated by the external intercostal muscles. In addition, a pump handle movement of the upper ribs is achieved through contraction of the external intercostals and the intercartilaginous portion of the internal intercostal muscles. The actions of the inspiratory muscles expand

the dimensions of the thoracic cavity and concomitantly reduce the pressure in the lungs (intrathoracic pressure) below the air pressure outside the body. With the respiratory tract being open to the atmosphere, air rushes into the lungs to normalize the pressure difference, allowing inspiration to occur and the lungs to fill with air.

During forced or labored breathing, additional accessory muscles need to be used to increase the inspiratory maneuver. The accessory muscles raise the ribs to a greater extent and promote extension of the thoracic spine. These changes facilitate a further increase in the volume within the thoracic cavity and a subsequent drop in the intrathoracic pressure beyond that caused by the contraction of the diaphragm and external intercostals. This relatively lower intrathoracic pressure will promote a larger volume of air entering the lung.

At rest, expiration is a passive process and achieved through the elastic recoil of the lung and relaxation of the external intercostal and diaphragm muscle. As the external intercostals relax, the rib drops to its preinspiratory position and the diaphragm returns to its elevated dome position high in the thorax. To achieve a forceful expiration additional muscle can be used, including the abdominals and internal intercostal muscles. The internal intercostals actively pull the ribs down to help expel air out of the lungs. The abdominals contract to force the viscera upward against the diaphragm, accelerating its return to the dome position.

---

**Clinical Tip**
The changes in intraabdominal and intrathoracic pressure that occur with forced breathing assist with venous return of blood back to the heart. The drop in pressure allows for a filling of the veins, while the changing pressure within the abdomen and thorax cause a milking effect to help return blood back to the heart.

---

## Pleurae
Two serous membranes or pleurae exist that cover each lung (Fig. 1-8). The pleura covering the outer surface of each lung is the visceral pleura and is inseparable from the tissue of the lung. The pleura covering the inner surface of the chest wall, diaphragm and mediastinum is called the parietal pleura. The parietal pleura is frequently described with reference to the anatomic surfaces it covers: the portion lining the ribs and vertebrae is named the costovertebral pleura; the portion over the diaphragm is the diaphragmatic pleura; the portion covering the uppermost aspect of the lung in the neck is the cervical pleura; and that overlying the mediastinum is called the mediastinal pleura.[8] Parietal and visceral pleurae blend with one another where they come together to enclose the root of the lung. Normally the pleurae are in intimate contact during all phases of the ventilatory cycle, being separated only by a thin serous film. There exists a potential space between the pleurae called the pleural space or pleural cavity. A constant negative pressure within this space maintains lung inflation. The serous

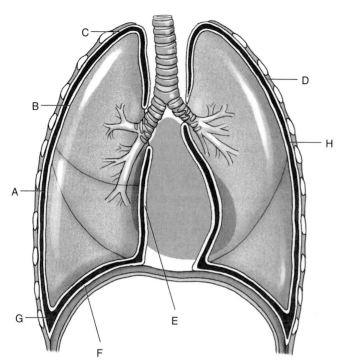

**Figure 1-8** Pleurae of the lungs. **A,** Pleural space. **B,** Visceral pleura. **C,** Cervical parietal pleura. **D,** Costal parietal pleura. **E,** Mediastinal parietal pleura. **F,** Diaphragmatic parietal pleura. **G,** Costodiaphragmatic recess. **H,** Parietal pleura. (From Applegate E. The Sectional Anatomy Learning System: Concepts/Applications ed 3. St. Louis, 2010, Saunders.)

fluid within the pleural space serves to hold the pleural layers together during ventilation and reduce friction between the lungs and the thoracic wall.[6,8]

The parietal pleura receives its vascular supply from the intercostal, internal thoracic, and musculophrenic arteries. Venous drainage is accomplished by way of the systemic veins in the adjacent parts of the chest wall. The bronchial vessels supply the visceral pleura. There exists no innervation to the visceral pleura and therefore no sensation.[5] The phrenic nerve innervates the parietal pleura of the mediastinum and central diaphragm, whereas the intercostal nerves innervate the parietal pleura of the costal region and peripheral diaphragm.

Irritation of the intercostally innervated pleura may result in the referral of pain to the thoracic or abdominal walls, and irritation of the phrenic supplied pleura can result in referred pain in the lower neck and shoulder.[9]

Several complications can affect pleural integrity. Infection with resultant inflammatory response within the pleura is termed pleuritis or pleurisy and is best appreciated through the presence of pleural chest pain, and an abnormal pleural friction rub on auscultation.[9] A pleural effusion refers to a buildup of fluid in the pleural space commonly seen following cardiothoracic surgery or with cancer. This is evidenced by diminished or absent breath sounds in the area of the effusion, more likely to be in gravity dependant areas and accompanied by reduced lung volumes. Blood in the pleural space is termed a hemothorax, whereas air in the pleural space from

a collapsed lung is termed a pneumothorax. Finally, a bacterial infection with resultant pus in the pleural space is referred to as empyema.

Management for several of these complications of the pleural space is achieved through insertion of a chest tube into the pleural space to drain pleural secretions or to restore a negative pressure within the space and allow for lung inflation. A needle aspiration of fluid from the space, a thoracocentesis, may be performed for patients with large pleural effusions.

## Lungs

The lungs are located on either side of the thoracic cavity, separated by the mediastinum. Each lung lies freely within its corresponding pleural cavity, except where it is attached to the heart and trachea by the root and pulmonary ligament. The substance of the lung—the parenchyma—is normally porous and spongy in nature. The surfaces of the lungs are marked by numerous intersecting lines that indicate the polyhedral (secondary) lobules of the lung. The lungs are basically cone shaped and are described as having an apex, a base, three borders (anterior, inferior, posterior), and three surfaces (costal, medial, and diaphragmatic).

The apex of each lung is situated in the root of the neck, its highest point being approximately 1 inch above the middle third of each clavicle. The base of each lung is concave, resting on the convex surface of the diaphragm. The inferior border of the lung separates the base of the lung from its costal surface; the posterior border separates the costal surface from the vertebral aspect of the mediastinal surface; the anterior border of each lung is thin and overlaps the front of the pericardium. Additionally, the anterior border of the left lung presents a cardiac notch. The costal surface of each lung conforms to the shape of the overlying chest wall. The medial surface of each lung may be divided into vertebral and mediastinal aspects. The vertebral aspect contacts the respective sides of the thoracic vertebrae and their intervertebral disks, the posterior intercostal vessels, and nerves. The mediastinal aspect is notable for the cardiac impression; this concavity is larger on the left than on the right lung to accommodate the projection of the apex of the heart toward the left. Just posterior to the cardiac impression is the hilus, where the structures forming the root of the lung enter and exit the parenchyma. The extension of the pleural covering below and behind the hilus from the root of the lung forms the pulmonary ligament.

### Hila and Roots

The point at which the nerves, vessels, and primary bronchi penetrate the parenchyma of each lung is called the hilus. The structures entering the hila of the lungs and forming the roots of each of the lungs are the principal bronchus, the pulmonary artery, the pulmonary veins, the bronchial arteries and veins, the pulmonary nerve plexus, and the lymph vessels (Fig. 1-9). They lie next to the vertebral bodies of the fifth, sixth, and seventh thoracic vertebrae. The right root lies behind the superior vena cava and a portion of the right

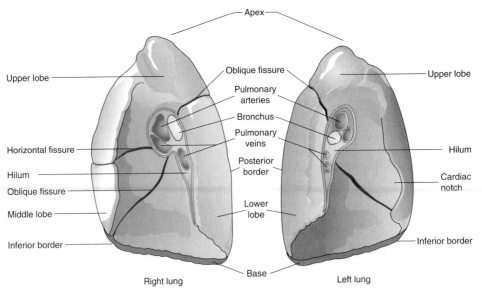

**Figure 1-9** The medial surfaces of the lungs. (From Hicks GH. Cardiopulmonary Anatomy and Physiology. Philadelphia, 2000, Saunders.)

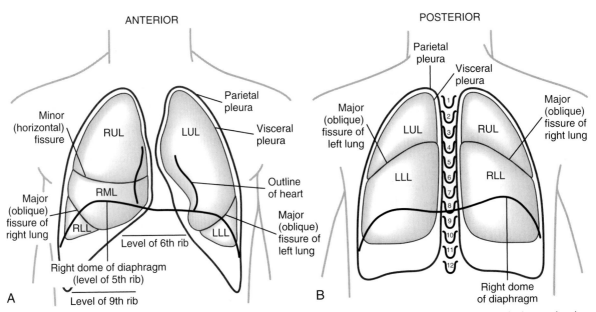

**Figure 1-10** Anterior (**A**) and posterior (**B**) views of the fissures of the lungs and the extent of the parietal pleura. (Redrawn from Kersten LD. Comprehensive Respiratory Nursing: A Decision Making Approach. Philadelphia, 1989, Saunders.)

atrium, below the end of the azygos vein; the left root lies below the arch of the aorta and in front of the descending thoracic aorta. The pulmonary ligament lies below the root; the phrenic nerve and the anterior pulmonary plexus lie in front of the root; the vagus nerve and posterior pulmonary plexus lie behind the root.

### Lobes, Fissures, and Segments
The right lung consists of three lobes including the right upper lobe (RUL), right middle lobe (RML), and right lower lobe (RLL). Two fissures separate these three lobes from one another. The upper and middle lobes of the right lung are separated from the lower lobe by the oblique (major) fissure

(see Fig. 1-9 and Fig. 1-10). Starting on the medial surface of the right lung at the upper posterior aspect of the hilus, the oblique fissure runs upward and backward to the posterior border at about the level of the fourth thoracic vertebra; it then descends anteroinferiorly across the anterior costal surface to intersect the lower border of the lung approximately 5 inches from the median plane, and then passes posterosuperiorly to rejoin the hilus just behind and beneath the upper pulmonary vein. The RML is separated from the RUL by the horizontal (minor) fissure that joins the oblique fissure at the midaxillary line at about the level of the fourth rib and runs horizontally across the costal surface of the lung to about the level of the fourth costal cartilage; on the medial surface, it passes backward to join the hilus near the upper right pulmonary vein.

Each lobe of the right lung is further subdivided into segments. The RUL has three segments, including the apical, posterior, and anterior segments. This lobe extends to the level of the fourth rib anteriorly, and is adjacent to ribs three to five posteriorly. The RML is subdivided into the lateral and medial lobes. This lobe is the smallest of the three lobes. Its inferior border is adjacent to the fifth rib laterally and sixth rib medially. The lowermost lobe, the RLL consist of four segments (anterior basal, superior basal, lateral basal, and posterior basal). The superior border of the RLL is at the level of the sixth thoracic vertebrae and extends inferiorly down to the diaphragm. During maximal inspiration, the inferior border of the RLL may extend to the second lumbar vertebrae and superimpose over the superior aspects of the kidney.

The left lung is relatively smaller than the right lung and has only two lobes including the left upper lobe (LUL) and left lower lobe (LLL). The left lung is divided into upper and lower lobes by the oblique fissure, which is somewhat more vertically oriented than that of the right lung; there is no horizontal fissure. The portion of the left lung that corresponds to the right lung is termed the lingular segment and is a part of the LUL. Posteriorly, the inferior border of the LUL is at the level of the sixth rib, while the LLL is at the level of the eleventh rib.

Table 1-1 describes the topographic boundaries for the bronchopulmonary segments of each lung.

> **Clinical Tip**
> An understanding of the various lobes and segments and their anatomical orientation is essential for appropriate positioning and removal of secretions from various aspects of the lung during bronchopulmonary hygiene procedures.

### Upper Respiratory Tract

**Nose.** The nose is a conglomerate of bone and hyaline cartilage. The nasal bones (right and left), the frontal processes of the maxillae, and the nasal part of the frontal bone combine to form the bony framework of the nose. The septal, lateral, and major and minor alar cartilages combine to form the cartilaginous framework of the nose. The periosteal and perichondral membranes blend to connect the bones and cartilages to one another.

Three major muscles assist with movement of the bony framework of the nose. The procerus muscle wrinkles the skin of the nose. The nasalis muscle has two parts, including the transverse and alar portions, and assists in flaring the anterior nasal aperture.[8] Finally, the depressor septi muscle works with the nasalis muscle to flare the nostrils.[8] Skin covers the external nose.

The nasal cavity is a wedge-shaped passageway, divided vertically into right and left halves by the nasal septum and compartmentalized by the paranasal sinuses (Fig. 1-11). Opening anteriorly via the nares (nostrils) to the external environment, the nasal cavity blends posteriorly with the nasopharynx. The two halves are essentially identical, having a floor, medial and lateral walls, and a roof divided into three regions: the vestibule, the olfactory region, and the respiratory region.

The primary respiratory functions of the nasal cavity include air conduction, filtration, humidification, and temperature control; it also plays a role in the olfactory process. Three nasal conchae project into the nasal cavity from the lateral wall toward the medial wall; they are named the superior, middle, and inferior conchae. The conchae serve to increase the respiratory surface area of the nasal mucous membrane for greater contact with inspired air. The vestibule of the nasal cavity is lined with skin containing many coarse hairs and sebaceous and sweat glands. Mucous membrane lines the remainder of the nasal cavity. Figure 1-12 depicts examples of some selected types of mucosal coverings in the upper and lower respiratory tracts.

The olfactory region of the nasal cavity is distinguished by specialized mucosa. This pseudostratified olfactory epithelium is composed of ciliated receptor cells, nonciliated sustentacular cells, and basal cells that help to provide a sense of smell.[8] Sniffing increases the volume of inspired air entering the olfactory region, allowing the individual to smell something specific.[4]

The respiratory region is lined with a mixture of columnar or pseudostratified ciliated epithelial cells, goblet cells, nonciliated columnar cells with microvilli, and basal cells. Serous and mucous glands, which open to the surface via branched ducts, underlie the basal lamina of the respiratory epithelium.[10] The submucosal glands and goblet cells secrete an abundant quantity of mucus over the mucosa of the nasal cavity, making it moist and sticky. Turbulent airflow, created by the conchae, causes inhaled dust and other particulate matter, larger than approximately 10 μm, to "rain out" onto this sticky layer, which is then moved by ciliary action backward and downward out of the nasal cavity into the nasopharynx at an average rate of about 6 mm per minute.[11,12]

> **Clinical Tip**
> Nasotracheal suctioning must be performed with caution in individuals with low platelet counts because of the likelihood of trauma and bleeding to superficial nasal conchae and cells within the nasal cavity. The placement of a nasopharyngeal airway or nasal trumpet may reduce trauma with recurrent blind suctioning procedures in these patients.

Individuals with seasonal allergies who are prone to developing sinus infections are also prone to developing bronchitis if the infection leaves the sinus cavities and drops down the throat to the bronchioles.

**Pharynx.** The pharynx is a musculomembranous tube approximately 5 to 6 inches long and located posterior to the nasal cavity. It extends from the base of the skull to the esophagus that corresponds with a line extending from the sixth cervical vertebra to the lower border of the cricoid

## Table 1-1 Topographic Boundaries for the Bronchopulmonary Lung Segments

| Lobe | Segment | Borders |
|------|---------|---------|
| Upper Lobe | Anterior segment (right or left) | Upper border: clavicle<br>Lower border: a horizontal line at the level of the third intercostal space (ICS), or fourth rib, anteriorly |
| | Apical segment (R) or apical aspect, apicoposterior segment (L) | Anteroinferior border: clavicle<br>Posteroinferior border: a horizontal line at the level of the upper lateral border of the spine of the scapula |
| | Posterior segment (R) or posterior aspect, apicoposterior segment (L) | Upper border: a horizontal line at the level of the upper lateral border of the spine of the scapula<br>Lower border: a horizontal line at, or approximately 1 inch below, the inferomedial aspect of the spine of the scapula |
| Middle Lobe (R) or Lingula (L) | | Upper border: a horizontal line at the level of the third ICS, or fourth rib, anteriorly<br>Lower and lateral borders: the oblique fissure (a horizontal line at the level of the sixth rib anteriorly) extending to the anterior axillary line; from the anterior axillary line, angling upward to approximately the fourth rib at the posterior axillary line<br>The midclavicular line separates the medial and lateral segments of the right middle lobe<br>A horizontal line at the level of the fifth rib, anteriorly, separates the superior and inferior lingular segments |
| Lower Lobe | Superior (basal) segment (right or left) | Upper border: a horizontal line at, or approximately 1 inch below, the inferomedial aspect of the spine of the scapula<br>Lower border: a horizontal line at, or approximately 1 inch above, the inferior angle of the scapula |
| | Posterior (basal) segment (right or left) | Upper border: a horizontal line at, or approximately 1 inch above, the inferior angle of the scapula<br>Lateral border: a "plumb line" bisecting the inferior angle of the scapula<br>Lower border: a horizontal line at the level of the tenth ICS, posteriorly |
| | Lateral (basal) segment (right or left) | Upper border: a horizontal line at, or approximately 1 inch above, the inferior angle of the scapula<br>Medial border: a "plumb line" bisecting the inferior angle of the scapula<br>Lateral border: the midaxillary line<br>Lower border: a horizontal line at the level of the tenth ICS, posteriorly |
| | Anterior (basal) segment (R) or anterior aspect, anteromedial (basal) segment (L) | Upper border: the oblique fissure (a horizontal line at the level of the sixth rib anteriorly, extending to the anterior axillary line; from the anterior axillary line, angling upward to approximately the fifth rib at the midaxillary line<br>Lateral border: the midaxillary line |

cartilage. The pharynx consists of three parts: the nasopharynx, the oropharynx, and the laryngopharynx.

Nasopharynx. The nasopharynx is a continuation of the nasal cavity, beginning at the posterior nasal apertures and continuing backward and downward. Its roof and posterior wall are continuous; its lateral walls are formed by the openings of the eustachian tubes; and its floor is formed by the soft palate anteriorly and the pharyngeal isthmus (the space between the free edge of the soft palate and the posterior wall of the pharynx), which marks the transition to the oropharynx. The epithelium of the nasopharynx is composed of ciliated columnar cells.

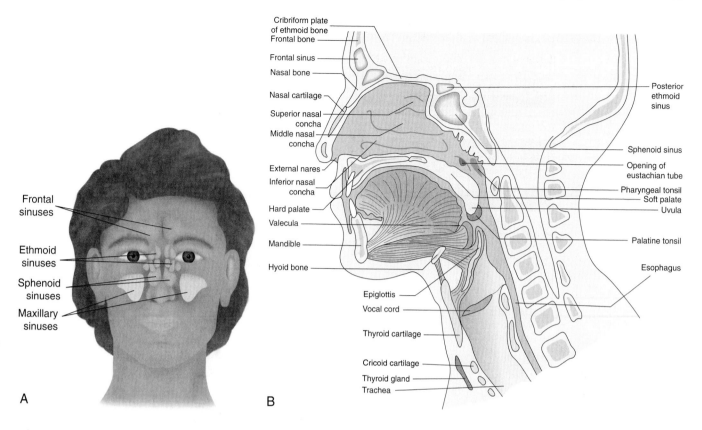

**Figure 1-11 A,** Positions of the frontal, maxillary, sphenoid, and ethmoid sinuses; the nasal sinuses are named for the bones in which they occur. **B,** Midsagittal section through the upper airway. (From Wilkins R. Egan's Fundamentals of Respiratory Care, ed 9. St. Louis, 2009, Mosby.)

OROPHARYNX. The oropharynx extends from the soft palate and pharyngeal isthmus superiorly to the upper border of the epiglottis inferiorly. Anteriorly, it is bounded by the oropharyngeal isthmus (which opens into the mouth) and the pharyngeal part of the tongue. The posterior aspect of the oropharynx is at the level of the body of the second cervical vertebra and upper portion of the body of the third cervical vertebra. The epithelium in the oropharynx is composed of stratified squamous cells.

LARYNGOPHARYNX. The laryngopharynx extends from the upper border of the epiglottis to the inferior border of the cricoid cartilage and the esophagus. The laryngeal orifice and the posterior surfaces of the arytenoid and cricoid cartilages form the anterior aspect of the laryngopharynx. The posterior aspect is at the level of the lower portion of the third, the bodies of the fourth and fifth, and the upper portion of the body of the sixth cervical vertebrae. The epithelium in the laryngopharynx is composed of stratified squamous cells.

**Larynx.** The larynx or voice box is a complex structure made up of several cartilages and forms a connection between the pharynx and the trachea. The position of the larynx depends upon the age and sex of the individual, being opposite the third to sixth cervical vertebrae in the adult male and somewhat higher in adult females and children.

The larynx consists of the endolarynx and its surrounding cartilaginous structures. The endolarynx is made of two sets

of folds including the false vocal cords (supraglottis) and true vocal cords.[8] Between the true cords are slit-shaped spaces that form the glottis. A space exists above the false vocal cords and is termed the vestibule. Six supporting cartilages, including three large (epiglottis, thyroid, cricoid) and three smaller (arytenoid, corniculate, cuneiform), prevent food, liquids, and foreign objects from entering the airway. Two sets of laryngeal muscles (internal and external) play important roles in swallowing, ventilation and vocalization. The larynx controls airflow and closes to increase intrathoracic pressure to generate an effective cough. Sounds with speech are created as expired air vibrates over the contracting vocal cords.

> **Clinical Tip**
> Endotracheal intubation may cause damage to structures within the larynx, producing an inflammatory response—laryngitis—where patients present with hoarseness and pain during speech.

### Lower Respiratory Tract

The lower respiratory tract extends from the level of the true vocal cords in the larynx to the alveoli within the lungs. Generally, the lower respiratory tract may be divided into two parts: the tracheobronchial tree, or conducting airways, and the acinar or terminal respiratory units.

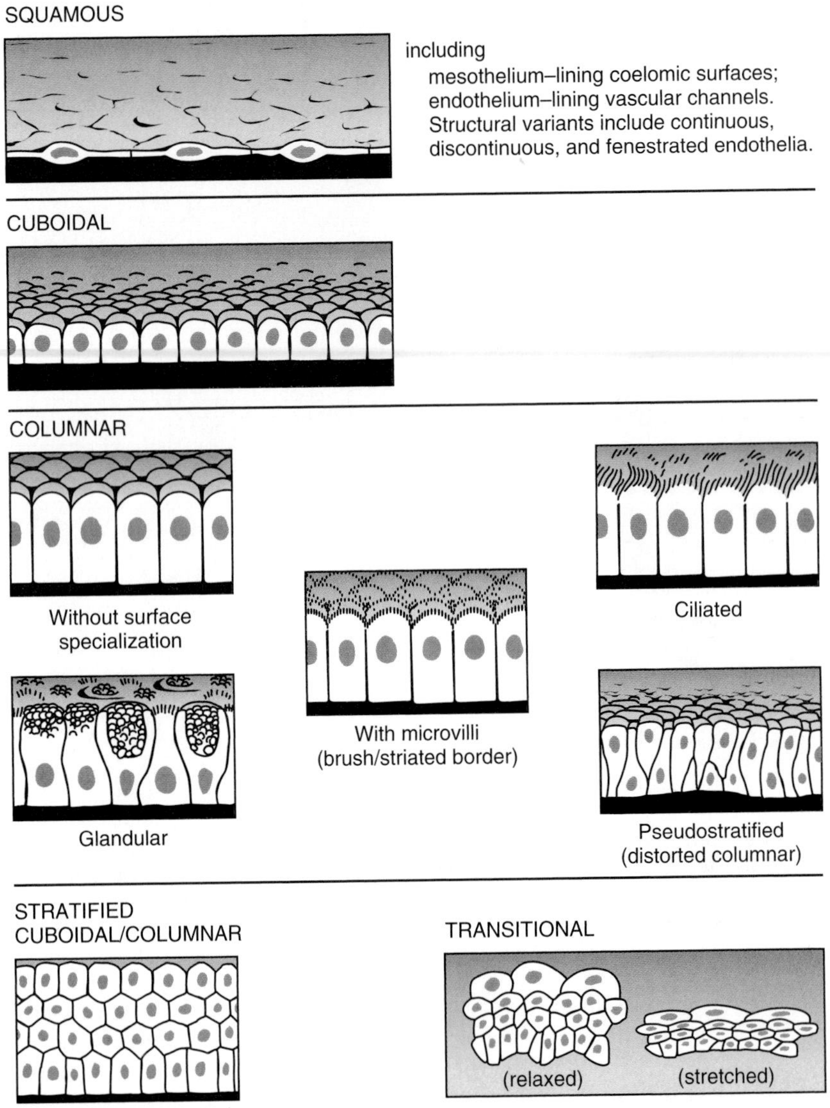

SQUAMOUS

including
mesothelium—lining coelomic surfaces;
endothelium—lining vascular channels.
Structural variants include continuous,
discontinuous, and fenestrated endothelia.

CUBOIDAL

COLUMNAR

Without surface
specialization

With microvilli
(brush/striated border)

Ciliated

Glandular

Pseudostratified
(distorted columnar)

STRATIFIED
CUBOIDAL/COLUMNAR

TRANSITIONAL

(relaxed)        (stretched)

**Figure 1-12** Types of cells composing the mucosal lining of the upper and lower respiratory tracts. (Modified from Williams PL, Warwick R, Dyson M, et al. eds. Gray's Anatomy, ed 37. New York, 1989, Churchill Livingstone.)

**Tracheobronchial tree—conducting airways.** The conducting airways are not directly involved in the exchange of gases in the lungs. They simply conduct air to and from the respiratory units. Airway diameter progressively decreases with each succeeding generation of branching, starting at approximately 1 inch in diameter at the trachea and reaching 1 mm or less at the terminal bronchioles. The cartilaginous rings of the larger airways give way to irregular cartilaginous plates, which become smaller and more widely spaced with each generation of branching, until they disappear at the bronchiolar level.[13] There may be as many as 16 generations of branching in the conducting airways from the mainstem bronchi to the terminal bronchioles (Fig. 1-13).[14]

**Trachea.** The trachea is a tube approximately 4 to 4.5 inches long and approximately 1 inch in diameter, extending downward along the midline of the neck, ventral to the esophagus. As it enters the thorax, it passes behind the left brachiocephalic vein and artery and the arch of the aorta. At its distal end, the trachea deviates slightly to the right of midline before bifurcating into right and left mainstem bronchi. Between 16 and 20 incomplete rings of two or more hyaline cartilages are often joined together along the anterior two-thirds of the tracheal circumference, forming a framework for the trachea. Fibrous and elastic tissues and smooth muscle fibers complete the ring posteriorly. The first and last tracheal cartilages differ somewhat from the others: The first is broader and is attached by the cricotracheal ligament to the lower border of the cricoid cartilage of the larynx. The last is thicker and broader at its middle, where it projects a hook-shaped process downward and backward from its lower border—the carina—between the two main stem bronchi. The carina is located at the fifth thoracic vertebrae or sternal notch and represents the cartilaginous

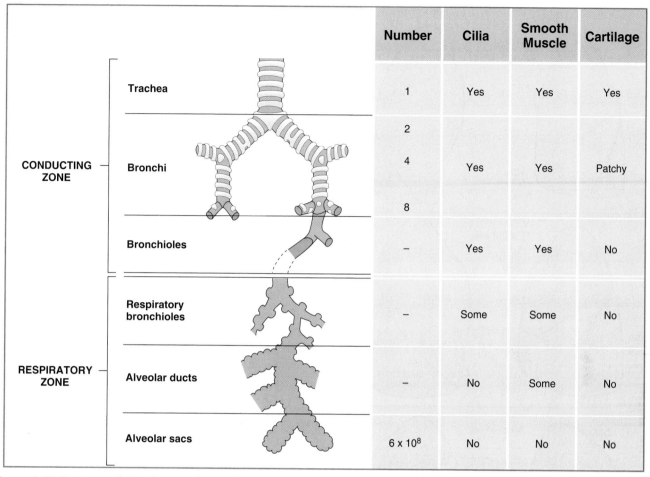

| | Number | Cilia | Smooth Muscle | Cartilage |
|---|---|---|---|---|
| **CONDUCTING ZONE** | | | | |
| Trachea | 1 | Yes | Yes | Yes |
| Bronchi | 2<br>4<br>8 | Yes | Yes | Patchy |
| Bronchioles | – | Yes | Yes | No |
| **RESPIRATORY ZONE** | | | | |
| Respiratory bronchioles | – | Some | Some | No |
| Alveolar ducts | – | No | Some | No |
| Alveolar sacs | $6 \times 10^8$ | No | No | No |

**Figure 1-13** Structure of the airways. The number of the various structures is reported for two lungs. (From Costanzo LS. Physiology, ed 3. St. Louis, 2007, Saunders.)

wedge at the bifurcation of the trachea into the right and left main stem bronchi.

> **Clinical Tip**
> During suctioning procedures, the catheter is inserted to the level of the carina. When the catheter is in contact with the carina, a cough ensues along with a strong parasympathetic response. Therapists must monitor for adverse responses in heart rate and provide supplemental oxygen as needed.

**Main stem and lobar bronchi.** The right main stem bronchus is wider and shorter than its left counterpart, and it diverges at approximately a 25-degree angle from the trachea. It passes laterally downward behind the superior vena cava for approximately 1 inch before giving off its first branch—the upper lobe bronchus—and entering the root of the right lung. Approximately 1 inch farther, it gives off its second branch—the middle lobe bronchus—from within the oblique fissure. Thereafter, the remnant of the main stem bronchus continues as the lower lobe bronchus.

The left main stem bronchus leaves the trachea at an angle of approximately 40 to 60 degrees and passes below the arch of the aorta and behind the left pulmonary artery, proceeding for a little more than 2 inches before it enters the root of the left lung, giving off the upper lobe bronchus and continuing on as the lower lobe bronchus. The left lung has no middle lobe, which is a major distinguishing feature in the general architecture of lungs.

> **Clinical Tip**
> The angulation of the right main stem bronchus relative to the position of the trachea predisposes foreign objects, food, and fluids to enter the right lung. Consequently, aspiration is relatively more common in the right lung compared to the left lung.

**Segmental and subsegmental bronchi.** Each of the lobar bronchi gives off two or more segmental bronchi; an understanding of their anatomy is essential to the appropriate assessment and treatment of pulmonary disorders (Fig. 1-14). The RUL bronchus divides into three segmental bronchi about 0.5 inches from its own origin: the first—the apical segmental bronchus—passes superolaterally toward its distribution in the apex of the lung; the second—the posterior segmental bronchus—proceeds slightly upward and

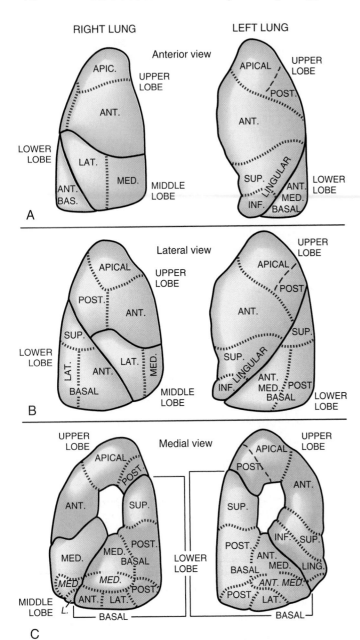

**Figure 1-14** Anterior (**A**), lateral (**B**), and medial (**C**) views of the bronchopulmonary segments as seen projected to the surface of the lungs. (Redrawn from Waldhausen JA, Pierce WS, eds. Johnson's Surgery of the Chest, ed 4. Chicago, 1985, Year Book Medical Publishers.)

bronchus yields the medial basal segmental bronchus (distributed to a small area below the hilus) from its anteromedial surface. The next offshoots from the lower lobe bronchus are the anterior basal segmental bronchus, which continues its descent anteriorly, and a very small trunk that almost immediately splits into the lateral basal segmental bronchus (distributed to the lower lateral area of the lower lobe) and the posterior basal segmental bronchus (distributed to the lower posterior area of the lower lobe).

The LUL bronchus extends laterally from the anterolateral aspect of the left mainstem bronchus before dividing into correlates of the right upper and middle lobar bronchi. However, these two branches remain within the LUL because there is no left middle lobe. The uppermost branch ascends for approximately one-third inch before yielding the anterior segmental bronchus, then continues its upward path as the apicoposterior segmental bronchus before subdividing further into its subsegmental distribution. The caudal branch descends anterolaterally to its distribution in the anteroinferior area of the LUL, a region called the lingula. This lingular bronchus divides into the superior lingular and inferior lingular segmental bronchi.

The LLL bronchus descends posterolaterally for approximately one-third inch before giving off the superior segmental bronchus from its posterior surface (its distribution is similar to that of the RLL superior segmental bronchus). After another one-half to two-thirds inch, the lower lobe bronchus splits in two: the anteromedial division is called the anteromedial basal segmental bronchus, and the posterolateral division immediately branches into the lateral basal and posterior basal segmental bronchi. The distributions of these segmental bronchi are similar to those of their right lung counterparts.

The epithelium of the upper regions of the conducting airways is pseudostratified and, for the most part, ciliated. The epithelium of the terminal and respiratory bronchioles is single-layered and more cuboidal in shape, and many of the cells are nonciliated. The lamina propria, to which the epithelial basal lamina is attached, contains, throughout the length of the tracheobronchial tree, longitudinal bands of elastin that spread into the elastin network of the terminal respiratory units. The framework thus created is responsible for much of the elastic recoil of the lungs during expiration.

The most abundant types of cells in the bronchial epithelium are the ciliated cells. Ciliated cells are found in all levels of the tracheobronchial tree down to the level of the respiratory bronchioles. The cilia projecting from their luminal surfaces are intimately involved in the removal of inhaled particulate matter from the airways via the "mucociliary escalator" mechanism.

Two of the bronchial epithelial cells are mucus-secreting: the mucous cells and serous cells.[15] Mucous cells, formerly called goblet cells, are normally more numerous in the trachea and large airways, becoming less numerous with distal progression until they are infrequently found in the bronchioles. Serous cells are much less numerous than mucous cells and

posterolaterally to its distribution in the posteroinferior aspect of the upper lobe; the third—the anterior segmental bronchus—runs anteroinferiorly to its distribution in the remainder of the upper lobe. The RML bronchus divides into a lateral segmental bronchus, which is distributed to the lateral aspect of the middle lobe, and a medial segmental bronchus to the medial aspect. The RLL bronchus first gives off a branch from its posterior surface—the superior segmental bronchus—which passes posterosuperiorly to its distribution in the upper portion of the lower lobe. Then, after continuing to descend posterolaterally, the lower lobe

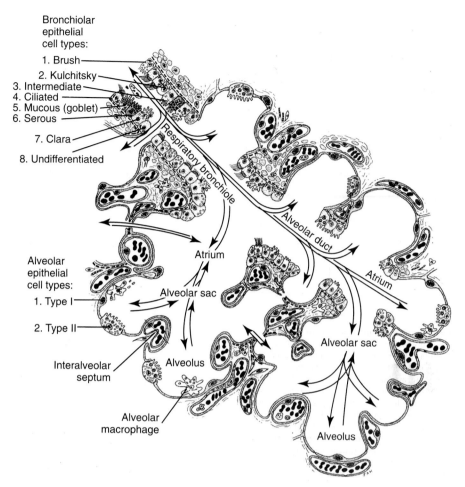

Bronchiolar
epithelial
cell types:
1. Brush
2. Kulchitsky
3. Intermediate
4. Ciliated
5. Mucous (goblet)
6. Serous
7. Clara
8. Undifferentiated

Respiratory bronchiole

Alveolar duct

Atrium

Atrium

Alveolar
epithelial
cell types:
1. Type I
2. Type II

Alveolar sac

Alveolar sac

Interalveolar
septum

Alveolus

Alveolus

Alveolar
macrophage

**Figure 1-15** A cross-sectional view of the terminal respiratory unit showing the bronchiolar and alveolar epithelial cell types. (From Williams PL. Warwick R. Dyson M, et al., eds. Gray's Anatomy, ed 37. New York, 1989, Churchill Livingstone.)

are confined predominantly to the extrapulmonary bronchi. Both types of cells are nonciliated, although both exhibit filamentous surface projections.

> **Clinical Tip**
> Smoking paralyzes ciliated epithelial cells. These cilia will be paralyzed for 1 to 3 hours after smoking a cigarette, or will be permanently paralyzed in chronic smokers.[16] The inability of the mucociliary escalator to work increases the individual's risk for developing respiratory infections.

**Terminal respiratory (acinar) units.** The conducting airways terminate in gas-exchange airways made up of respiratory bronchioles, alveolar ducts, and alveoli (Fig. 1-15). These structures together are termed the *acinus* and participate in gas exchange. The functional unit of the lung is the alveoli where gas exchange occurs. The acinus is connected to the interstitium through a dense network of fibers. Two major types of epithelial cells exist along the alveolar wall. Squamous pneumocytes (type I) cells are flat and thin and cover approximately 93% of the alveolar surface. Granular pneumocytes (type II) cells are thick, cuboidal shaped, cover 7% of the alveolar wall, and involved in the

production of surfactant.[13] Surfactant is a lipoprotein that lowers alveolar surface tension at end expiration and thereby prevents the lung from collapsing. The alveoli, like the bronchi contain cellular components of inflammation and immunity. The alveolar macrophage engulfs and ingests foreign material in the alveoli and provides a protective function against disease.

Capillaries composed of a single layer of endothelial cells deliver blood in close proximity to the alveoli. Capillaries can distend and accommodate to the volume of blood being delivered to the lung. The alveolar capillary interface is where exchange of gases occurs. The thickness of the alveolar capillary membrane is between 0.5 and 1.0 μm.

### Innervation of the Lungs

The lungs are invested with a rich supply of afferent and efferent nerve fibers and specialized receptors. Parasympathetic fibers are supplied, by preganglionic fibers from the vagal nuclei via the vagus nerves, to ganglia around the bronchi and blood vessels. Postganglionic fibers innervate the bronchial and vascular smooth muscle, as well as the mucous cells and submucosal bronchial glands. The parasympathetic postganglionic fibers from thoracic sympathetic ganglia innervate essentially the same structures. Posterior

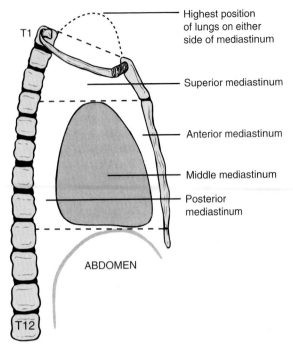

**Figure 1-16** Divisions of mediastinum. (From Liebgott B. The Anatomical Basis of Dentistry ed 2. St. Louis, 2002, Mosby.)

and anterior pulmonary plexuses are formed by contributions from the postganglionic sympathetic and parasympathetic fibers at the roots of the lungs. Generally, stimulation of the vagus nerve results in bronchial constriction, dilation of pulmonary arterial smooth muscle, and increased glandular secretion.[17] Stimulation of the sympathetic nerves causes bronchial relaxation, constriction of pulmonary arterial smooth muscle, and decreased glandular secretion.[17]

Bronchodilators enhance sympathetic stimulation to the lungs to cause relaxation of bronchial smooth muscle cells and reduce secretions.

## The Cardiovascular System

### Mediastinum

The mediastinum lies between the right and left pleura of the lungs and near the median sagittal plane of the chest (Fig. 1-16). From an anterior-posterior perspective, it extends from the sternum in front to the vertebral column behind, and contains all the thoracic viscera except the lungs.[8] It is surrounded by the chest wall anteriorly, the lungs laterally, and the spine posteriorly. It is continuous with the loose connective tissue of the neck and extends inferiorly onto the diaphragm. It is the central compartment of the thoracic cavity and contains the heart, the great vessels of the heart, esophagus, trachea, phrenic nerve, cardiac nerve, thoracic duct, thymus, and lymph nodes of the central chest.[8,13]

A shifting of the structures within the mediastinum (mediastinal shift) is appropriate to consider and examine on the chest radiograph in patients who have air trapped in the pleural space (pneumothorax) or following removal of a lung (pneumonectomy).[3] In a tension pneumothorax or pneumonectomy, the mediastinum shift away from the affected or operated side.

## Heart

The heart is the primary pump that circulates blood through the entire vascular system. It is closely related to the size of the body and is roughly the size of the individual's closed fist. It lies obliquely (diagonally) in the mediastinum, with two-thirds lying left of the midsagittal plane. The superior portion of the heart formed by the two atria is termed the base of the heart. It is broad and exists at the level of the second intercostal space in adults. The apex of the heart defined by the tip of the left ventricle projects into the fifth intercostal space at the midclavicular line.

The heart moves freely and changes its position during its contraction and relaxation phase as well as during breathing. As the heart contracts, the heart moves anteriorly and collides with the chest wall. The portion of the heart that strikes the chest wall is the apex of the heart and is termed the point of maximum impulse.[1] Normally, this point is evidenced at the anatomical landmark of the apex, which is the fifth intercostal space at the midclavicular line. In regards to ventilation, quiet resting breathing does not alter the point of maximum impulse because of minimal excursion of the diaphragm. However, with deep inspiration, there is more significant inferior depression of the diaphragm causing the heart to descend and rotate to the right, displacing the point of maximum impulse away from the normal palpable position.[1]

> **Clinical Tip**
> The point of maximum impulse is relatively more lateral in patients with left ventricular hypertrophy caused by an increase in left ventricular mass. Also, patients with a pneumothorax and resultant mediastinal shift will demonstrate an altered point of maximum impulse away from the normal anatomical position of the apex of the heart.

### Tissue Layers
#### Pericardium

The heart wall is made up of three tissue layers (Fig. 1-17). The outermost layer of the heart is a double-walled sac termed the pericardium, anchored to the diaphragm inferiorly and connective tissue of the great vessels superiorly. The two layers of the pericardium include an outer parietal pericardium and an inner visceral pericardium also referred to as the epicardium.[8] The parietal pericardium is a tough fibrous layer of dense irregular connective tissue, whereas the visceral pericardium is a thin smooth and moist serous layer. Between the two layers of the pericardium is a closed space termed the pericardial space or pericardial cavity filled with approximately 10 to 20 mL of clear pericardial fluid.[18]

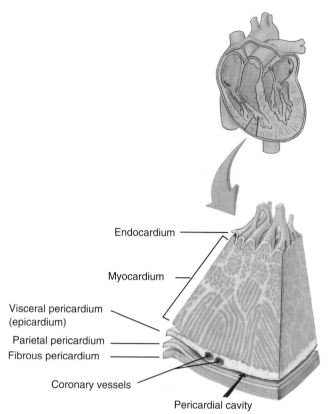

**Figure 1-17** Layers of the heart wall. (From Applegate E. The Anatomy and Physiology Learning System ed 3. St. Louis, 2007, Saunders.)

Labels in figure:
- Endocardium
- Myocardium
- Visceral pericardium (epicardium)
- Parietal pericardium
- Fibrous pericardium
- Coronary vessels
- Pericardial cavity

This fluid separates the two layers and minimizes friction during cardiac contraction.

In patients with inflammation of the pericardium, fluid may accumulate in the closed pericardial space producing cardiac tamponade; evidenced as compromised cardiac function and contractility caused by build up of fluid in the pericardial space. Finally, pericarditis is also commonly noted following a coronary artery bypass grafting procedure.

### Myocardium

The middle layer of the heart is termed the myocardium. It is the layer of the heart that facilitates the pumping action of the heart as a result of the presence of contractile elements. Myocardial cells are unique as they demonstrate three important traits: automaticity—the ability to contract in the absence of stimuli, rhythmicity—the ability to contract in a rhythmic manner; and conductivity—the ability to transmit nerve impulses.[17] Myocardial cells may be categorized into two groups based on their function: mechanical cells contributing to mechanical contraction and conductive cells contributing to electrical conduction.[1,17] Mechanical cells, also termed myocytes, are large cells containing a larger number of actin and myosin myofilaments enabling a grater capacity for mechanical shortening needed for pump action. In addition, these cells have a large number of mitochondria (25% of cellular volume) to provide sufficient energy in the form of adenosine triphosphate (ATP) to the heart, an organ that

can never rest.[5,17] The conducting myocardial cells are joined by intercalated disks forming a structure known as a syncytium. A syncytium characterizes a group of cells in which the protoplasm of one cell is continuous with that of adjacent cells.[8] Intercalated disks contain two junctions: desmosomes attaching one cell to another and connexins that allow the electrical flow to spread from one cell to another. These two junctions work together to move the impulse through a low resistance pathway.

> **Clinical Tip**
> Injured myocardial cells cannot be replaced, as the myocardium is unable to undergo mitotic activity. Thus, death of cells from an infarction or a cardiomyopathy may result in a significant reduction in contractile function.

### Endocardium

The innermost layer of the heart is termed the endocardium. This layer consists of simple squamous endothelium overlying a thin areolar tissue layer.[18] The tissue of the endocardium forms the inner lining of the chambers of the heart and is continuous with the tissue of the valves and the endothelium of the blood vessel.

As the endocardium and valves share similar tissue, patients with endocarditis, must be ruled out for valvular dysfunction. Endocardial infections can spread into valvular tissue developing vegetations on the valve.[19] Bronchopulmonary hygiene procedures, including percussions and vibrations, are contraindicated for patients with unstable vegetations as they may dislodge, move as emboli, and cause an embolic stroke.

## Chambers of the Heart

The heart is divided into right and left halves by a longitudinal septum. The right side of the heart receives deoxygenated venous blood (returning from the body), while the left side of the heart receives oxygenated blood (returning from the lungs). Each half of the heart is made up of two chambers: superiorly the atria and inferiorly the ventricles. Thus the four chambers of the heart include the right atrium (Fig. 1-18A), right ventricle (Fig. 1-18A), left atrium (Fig. 1-18B), and left ventricle (Fig. 1-18B). The atria receive blood from the systemic and pulmonary veins and eject blood into the ventricles. The ventricles eject blood that is received from the atria into arteries that deliver blood to the lungs and the systemic circulation.

### Right Atrium

The chamber of the right atrium (see Fig. 1-18A) consists of a smooth posterior and medial inner wall. Anteriorly and laterally exist parallel muscle bundles known as pectinate muscles. Both right and left atria have small earlike extensions called auricles that help to increase volume within the chambers. The right atrium receives deoxygenated blood from three major vessels. The superior vena cava collects venous blood from the head and upper extremities; the

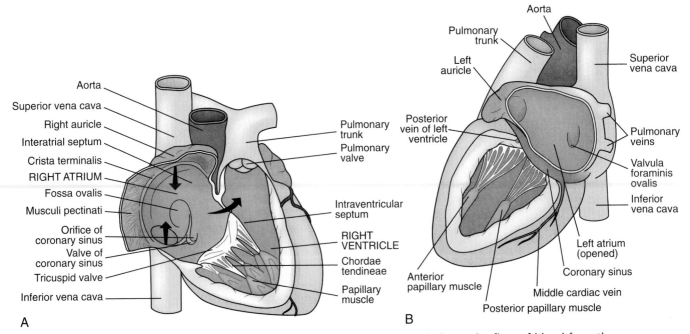

**Figure 1-18** Schematic of the heart. **A,** Right atrium and ventricle. The arrows indicate the flow of blood from the venae cavae to the right atrium and from the right atrium to the right ventricle. **B,** Left atrium and ventricle. The blood flows from the pulmonary veins to the left atrium, through the mitral valve into the left ventricle, and from there into the systemic circulation. (From Snopek AM. Fundamentals of Special Radiographic Procedures ed 5. St. Louis, 2007, Saunders.)

inferior vena cava collects blood from the trunk and lower extremities; and the coronary sinus collects venous blood specifically from the heart. The coronary sinus empties into the right atrium above the tricuspid valve. Normal diastolic pressures to enable filling are 0 to 8 mm Hg and is clinically referred to as the central venous pressure.

The effective contraction of the pectinate muscles of the atria account for approximately 15 to 20% of cardiac output—the atrial kick.[19] In patients with abnormal electrical conduction causing a quivering of the atria (atrial fibrillation), the mechanical contractile ability of the pectinate muscles is reduced, resulting in a low atrial kick and compromised cardiac output.[1,5]

### Right Ventricle

The right ventricle is shaped like a crescent or triangle, enabling it to eject large volumes of blood through a small valve into a low-pressure pulmonary system. Blood within the right ventricle is received from the right atrium through a one-way valve present between the atrium and ventricle termed the tricuspid atrioventricular valve. It ejects blood to the lungs via the pulmonic semilunar valve into pulmonary artery. The right ventricle (see Fig. 1-18A), like the right atrium, may be considered in two parts: (a) a posteroinferior inflow tract, termed the body, which contains the tricuspid valve, chordae tendineae, papillary muscles, and trabeculated myocardium, and (b) an anterosuperior outflow tract, called the infundibulum from which the pulmonary trunk arises.[8] There exist four muscular bands that separate the inflow and outflow portions of the right ventricle, including the

infundibular septum, the parietal band, the septal band, and moderator band. Pressures within the right ventricle are relatively lower compared to the left ventricle, with diastolic pressures ranging from 0 to 8 mm Hg and systolic pressures ranging from 15 to 30 mm Hg.[17]

Patients with chronic lung pathologies including chronic obstructive pulmonary disease (COPD) and pulmonary fibrosis, during periods of exacerbation, often present with hypoxemia and increased pressure within the pulmonary vasculature, termed pulmonary artery hypertension, caused by compromised perfusion capacity to the lung.[19,20] The increase pressure within the pulmonary artery increases the workload on the right ventricle, causing cor pulmonale or right ventricular hypertrophy and resultant right ventricular failure.

### Left Atrium

The left atrium is divided from the right atrium by an interatrial septum. It has a relatively thicker wall compared to the right atrium to adapt to higher pressures of blood entering the chamber from the lung. Oxygenated blood from the lungs enters the left atrium posteriorly via the pulmonary veins. These vessels have no valves; instead, pectinate muscles extend from the atria into the pulmonary veins and exert a sphincter-like action to prevent backflow of blood during contraction of the atria. The normal filling pressure of the left ventricle is between 4 and 12 mm Hg. Oxygenated blood is ejected out of the left atrium through the mitral atrioventricular (bicuspid) valve to enter the left ventricle.

Regurgitation or insufficiency of the mitral valve causes blood to accumulate in the left atrium and elevate left atrial pressures. These chronically elevated pressures alter the integrity of the atrial wall and predispose the individual to developing a quivering of the atria wall (atrial fibrillation) and potential blood clots within the left atrium.

### Left Ventricle

The almost conical left ventricle (see Fig. 1-18B) is longer and narrower than the right ventricle. The walls of the left ventricle are approximately three times thicker than those of the right, and the transverse aspect of the cavity is almost circular. In contrast to the inflow and outflow orifices of the right ventricle, those of the left are located adjacent to one another, being separated only by the anterior leaflet of the mitral valve and the common fibrous ridge to which it and the left and posterior cusps of the aortic valve are attached. The interventricular septum forms the medial wall of the left ventricle and creates a separation between the left and right ventricle.

This chamber receives oxygenated blood from the left atrium via the mitral valve and ejects blood through the aortic valve and into the aorta to the peripheral systemic vasculature. Normal systolic pressures within the left ventricle are 80 to 120 mm Hg, while diastolic pressures are 4 to 12 mm Hg. Because of the elevated pressures within this chamber, the wall thickness of the left ventricle is the greatest compared to the three other chambers of the heart.

Pathologic thickening of the left ventricular wall is evidenced in patients with various cardiovascular complications, including, but not limited to, hypertension, aortic stenosis, and heart failure as a consequence of an increase in the afterload. This pathologic thickening alters the contractile ability of the ventricle and reduces the filling capacity of the ventricle, causing a reduction in the cardiac output.

## Heart Valves

Four heart valves (Fig. 1-19) ensure one-way blood flow through the heart. Two atrioventricular valves exist between the atria and ventricle, including the tricuspid valve on the right and mitral or bicuspid valve on the left between the left atrium and ventricle. The semilunar valves lie between the ventricles and arteries and are named based on their corresponding vessels: pulmonic valve on the right in association with the pulmonary artery and aortic valve on the left relating to the aorta.

Flaps of tissue called leaflets or cusps guard the heart valve openings. The right atrioventricular valve has three cusps and therefore is termed tricuspid, whereas the left atrioventricular valve has only two cusps and hence is termed bicuspid. These leaflets are attached to the papillary muscles of the myocardium by chordae tendineae. The primary function of the atrioventricular valves is to prevent backflow of blood into the atria during ventricular contraction or systole, while the semilunar valves prevent backflow of blood from the aorta and pulmonary artery into the ventricles during diastole. Opening and closing of each valve depends on pressure gradient changes within the heart created during each cardiac cycle.

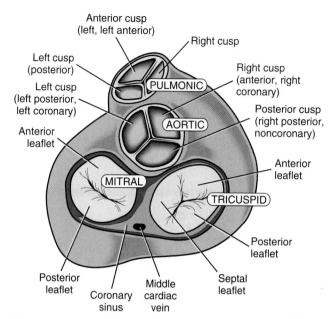

**Figure 1-19** Nomenclature for the leaflets and cusps of the principal valves of the heart.

An initial disturbance of valvular function may be picked by through auscultation of the heart sounds and evidenced by variety of murmurs. It must be noted that the identification of a murmur would warrant the need for additional testing, including echocardiography to accurately diagnose pathology within a particular valve.

## Conduction System

In a normal conduction system (Fig. 1-20), electrical impulses arise in the sinoatrial (SA) or sinus node. The SA node is located at the junction of the right atrium and superior vena cava. The P cells of the SA node are the sites for impulse generation; consequently, the SA node is termed the pacemaker of the heart as it makes or creates the impulses that pace the heart.[8] The normal pacing ability of the SA node is between 60 and 100 beats per minute (bpm) at rest. The impulse generated at the SA node, travels down one of three internodal tracts to the atrioventricular (AV) node. The three conduction pathways that exist between the SA and AV node include an anterior tract of Bachman, a middle tract of Wenckebach, and a posterior tract of Thorel.[8]

The AV node is located at the inferior aspect of the right atrium, near the opening of the coronary sinus and above the tricuspid valve. Posterior to the AV node are several parasympathetic autonomic ganglia that serve as receptors for the vagus nerve and cause slowing of the cardiac cycle. The major function of the AV node during each cardiac cycle is to slow down the cardiac impulse to mechanically allow time for the ventricles to fill.

Conducting fibers from the AV node converge to form the bundle of His to carry the impulse into the ventricles. The bundle of His appears as a triangle of nerve fibers within the posterior border of the interventricular septum. The bundle bifurcates to give rise to the right and left bundle

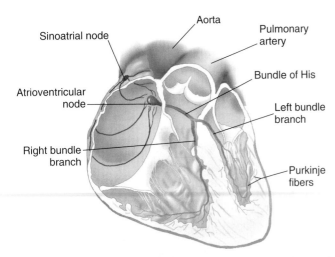

**Figure 1-20** Conduction system of the heart. The electrical impulse originates in the heart, and contraction of the heart's chambers is coordinated by specialized heart tissues. (From Leonard PC. Building a Medical Vocabulary: With Spanish Translations ed 7. St. Louis, 2009, Saunders.)

branches carrying the impulse to the right and left ventricles, respectively. The right bundle branch (RBB) is thin, with relatively fewer branches proceeding inferiorly to the apex of the right ventricle. The left bundle branch (LBB) arises perpendicularly and divides into two branches or fascicles.[8] The left anterior bundle branch crosses the left anterior papillary muscle and proceeds along the base of the left ventricle toward the aortic valve. The left posterior bundle branch advances posteriorly through the posterior papillary muscle toward the posterior inferior left ventricular wall.

Both bundles terminate into a network of nerve fibers called the Purkinje fibers. These fibers extend from the apex of each ventricle and penetrate the heart wall to the outer myocardium. Electrical stimulation of the Purkinje fibers causes mechanical contraction of the ventricles. It may be important to appreciate that normal electrical conduction through the heart allows for appropriate mechanical activity and maintenance of cardiac output to sustain activity. An alteration in the conduction pathway subsequently alters the mechanical activity of the heart and reduces cardiac output.

> **Clinical Tip**
> An evaluation of electrocardiographic (ECG) changes is necessary to help a clinician recognize and differentially diagnose reduced exercise tolerance caused from an electrical disturbance producing mechanical alterations that reduce cardiac output and exercise tolerance and not a true mechanical problem within the heart.

## Innervation

Although the SA node and conduction pathway have an intrinsic rate of depolarization causing contraction of the myocardium, the autonomic nervous system influences the rate of impulse generation, contraction, relaxation, and strength of contraction.[6,17] Thus autonomic neural transmis-

sion creates changes in the heart rate and contractility to allow adjustments in cardiac output to meet metabolic demands. A cardiac plexus contains both sympathetic and parasympathetic nerve fibers and is located anterior to the tracheal bifurcation.

The cardiac plexus receives its parasympathetic input from the right and left vagus nerve.[17] Subsequently nerves branch off the plexus, follow the coronary vessels, and innervate the SA node and other components of the conduction system. There is relatively less parasympathetic innervation to the ventricles resulting in a sympathetic dominance on ventricular function. Vagal stimulation is inhibitory on the cardiovascular system and is evidenced by decreased heart rate and blood pressure.[6] The neurohormone involved with parasympathetic stimulation is acetylcholine.

The sympathetic input to the plexus arises from the sympathetic trunk in the neck. Cardiac nerves from the cervical and upper four to five thoracic ganglia feed into the cardiac plexus.[6,17] Sympathetic stimulation releases catecholamines (epinephrine and norepinephrine) that interact with β-adrenergic receptors on the cardiac cell membrane, causing an excitation of the cardiovascular system. This is evidenced by an increase in heart rate, contractility through greater influx of calcium into myocytes, blood pressure, a shortening of the conduction time through the AV node, and an increase in rhythmicity of the AV pacemaker fibers.

Sympathetic nervous system stimulation is cardioexcitatory and increases heart rate and contractility—the fight of flight response. Conversely, parasympathetic stimulation is cardioinhibitory and slows down heart rate and contractility.

## Cardiac and Pulmonary Vessels

### Aorta

The ascending aorta begins at the base of the left ventricle and is approximately 2 inches long. From the lower border of the third costal cartilage at the left of the sternum, it passes upward and forward toward the right as high as the second right costal cartilage. The aorta exhibits three dilations above the attached margins of the cusps of the aortic valve at the root of the aorta—the aortic sinuses (of Valsalva). The coronary arteries (Fig. 1-21) open near these aortic sinuses of Valsalva. Three branches typically arise from the upper aspect of the arch of the aorta: the brachiocephalic trunk (innominate artery), the left common carotid artery, and the left subclavian artery. The openings of the coronary arteries are blocked from blood entering into the arteries when the aortic valve is open (during systole). Therefore, the part of the cardiac cycle when the coronary arteries receive their blood is during diastole when the aortic valves are closed.

### Right Coronary Artery

The right coronary artery arises from the right anterolateral surface of the aorta and passes between the auricular appendage of the right atrium and the pulmonary trunk, typically

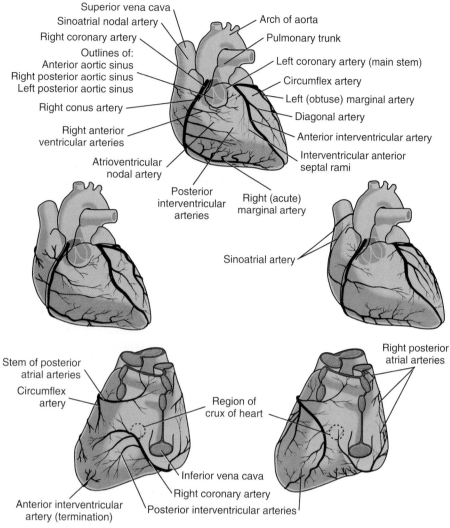

**Figure 1-21** Typical distributions of the right and left coronary arteries. (Redrawn from Williams PL, Warwick R, Dyson M, et al., eds. Gray's Anatomy, ed 37. New York, 1989, Churchill Livingstone.)

giving off a branch to the sinus node and yielding two or three right anterior ventricular rami as it descends into the coronary sulcus to come around the right (acute) margin of the heart into the posterior aspect of the sulcus. As the right coronary artery crosses the right margin of the heart, it gives off the right (acute) marginal artery before continuing as far as the posterior interventricular sulcus, where it usually turns to supply the diaphragmatic surfaces of the ventricles as the posterior interventricular (posterior descending) artery. In approximately 70% of hearts, an atrioventricular nodal artery is given off just before the posterior interventricular artery.[21]

## Left Coronary Artery

The left coronary artery originates from the left anterolateral aspect of the aorta and splits into two major branches: the anterior interventricular and circumflex arteries. The anterior interventricular or left anterior descending artery (LAD) traverses the anterior interventricular groove to supply sternocostal aspects of both ventricles. In its course, the anterior interventricular artery gives off right and left anterior ventricular and anterior septal branches. The larger left anterior ventricular branches vary in number from two to nine, the first being designated the diagonal artery. Approximately 70% of the left ventricle is fed by the LAD artery. The circumflex artery runs in the coronary sulcus between the left atrium and ventricle, crosses the left margin of the heart, and usually continues to its termination, just short of the junction of the right coronary and the posterior interventricular arteries. In many instances, as the circumflex artery crosses the left margin of the heart it gives off a large branch that supplies this area—the left marginal (obtuse) artery.

> **Clinical Tip**
> Occlusion of the left main coronary artery results in a large myocardial infarction and often is termed the widow maker.

The right coronary artery is the primary supply route for blood to the majority of the right ventricle as well as the inferior and posterior portions of the left ventricle. In addition, specialized conduction tissue within the right atrium including the SA node and AV node are nourished by the right coronary artery. The LAD supplies blood to the anterior and septal aspects of the left ventricle, while the circumflex artery supplies blood to the lateral aspect of the left ventricle.

Occlusion of a coronary artery produces an infarction in a defined region within the heart. Right coronary artery occlusions cause inferior or posterior infarctions and also affect the functioning of the SA node in the right atrium. LAD occlusions produce anterior septal infarctions, also termed the widow maker, whereas circumflex occlusions are responsible for generating lateral infarctions.

Distribution of blood supply within the heart is variable from one individual to another because of the presence of collateral circulation involving the formation of new blood vessels (angiogenesis) in areas of the heart that are partially occluded.

## Pulmonary Artery

The pulmonary trunk runs upward and backward (first in front of, and then to the left of the ascending aorta) from the base of the right ventricle; it is approximately 2 inches in length. At the level of the fifth thoracic vertebra, it splits into right and left pulmonary arteries. The right pulmonary artery runs behind the ascending aorta, superior vena cava, and upper pulmonary vein, but in front of the esophagus and right primary bronchus to the root of the lung. The left pulmonary artery runs in front of the descending aorta and the left primary bronchus to the root of the left lung. It is attached to the arch of the aorta by the ligamentum arteriosum.

---

**Clinical Tip**

A saddle embolus is life-threatening and involves an embolus dislodged at the bifurcation of the right and left pulmonary artery.

---

## Pulmonary Veins

The pulmonary veins, unlike the systemic veins, have no valves. They originate in the capillary networks and join together to ultimately form two veins—a superior and an inferior pulmonary vein—from each lung, which open separately into the left atrium.

## Vena Cava and Cardiac Veins

The superior vena cava is approximately 3 inches long from its termination in the upper part of the right atrium opposite the third right costal cartilage to the junction of the two brachiocephalic veins. The inferior vena cava extends from the junction of the two common iliac veins, in front of the fifth lumbar vertebra, passing through the diaphragm to open into the lower portion of the right atrium. The vena cavae have no valves.

The cardiac veins (Fig. 1-22) will be considered as three groups: the coronary sinus and its supplying veins, the anterior cardiac veins, and the thebesian veins. Most of the veins of the heart drain into the coronary sinus, which runs in the posterior aspect of the coronary sulcus and empties through the valve of the coronary sinus, a semilunar flap, into the right atrium between the opening of the inferior vena cava and the tricuspid valve. As Figure 1-22 shows, the small and middle cardiac veins, the posterior vein of the left ventricle, the left marginal vein, and the great cardiac vein feed the coronary sinus.

The anterior cardiac veins are fed from the anterior part of the right ventricle. They originate in the subepicardial tissue, crossing the coronary sulcus as they terminate directly into the right atrium. The right marginal vein runs along the right border of the heart and usually opens directly into the right atrium. Occasionally, it may join the small cardiac vein.

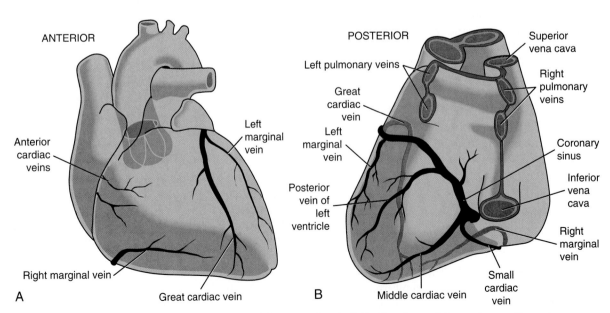

**Figure 1-22** Anterior (**A**) and posterior (**B**) views of typical distributions of the major cardiac veins.

The thebesian veins (venae cordis minimae) vary greatly in their number and size. These tiny veins open into all the cavities of the heart, but are most numerous in the right atrium and ventricle, occasional in the left atrium, and rare in the left ventricle.

## Systemic Circulation

Oxygenated blood ejected out of the heart flows through the aorta into systemic arteries. These arteries branch into smaller vessels called arterioles, which further branch into the smallest vessels, the capillaries primarily involved in the exchange of nutrients and gases. Deoxygenated blood from the capillaries, enters venules that join together to form larger veins that return blood back to the right heart and lungs. Blood vessels have three layers: the innermost tunica intima, middle tunica media, and outermost tunica adventitia.

### Arteries

The wall of the artery is composed of elastic and fibrous connective tissue and smooth muscle. Anatomically, arteries can be categorized into two types depending on the structural components along their wall. Elastic arteries, including the aorta and pulmonary trunk, have a thick tunica media with more elastic fibers than smooth muscle cells, allowing for a greater stretch as blood is ejected out of the heart. During diastole, the elasticity of the vessel promotes recoil of the artery and maintains blood pressure within the vessel. Muscular arteries are present in medium and small arteries and contain more smooth muscle cells within the middle tunica media layer. These arteries have the ability of vasoconstriction and vasodilation as a result of the presence of smooth muscles cells to control the amount of blood flow to periphery.[6] These smooth muscle cells are under autonomic nervous system influence through the presence of α-receptors. The more distal the artery, a greater amount of smooth muscle is evidenced. Arterioles have primarily smooth muscle along their wall enabling their diameter to alter significantly as needed. Arterioles empty into capillary beds. The density of capillaries within a capillary bed is greater in active tissue, including the muscle. Exchange of nutrients and gases occur within the capillary bed. Figure 1-23 depicts the major arterial tree within the human body.

### Endothelium

Endothelial cells form the endothelium or endothelial lining of the blood vessel. These cells have the ability to adjust their number and arrangement to accommodate local requirements. Endothelial cells serve several important functions, including filtration and permeability, vasomotion, clotting, and inflammation.[19] Atherosclerosis is initiated through endothelial dysfunction evidenced by endothelial cells that are extensively permeable to fat cells and white blood cells.

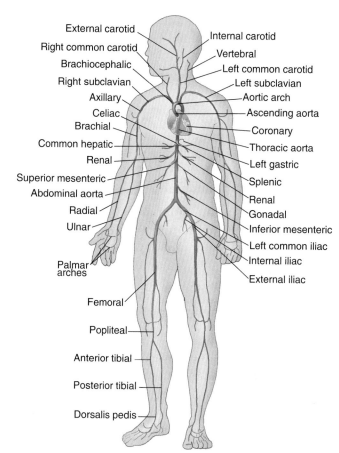

**Figure 1-23** Anterior view of the aorta and its principal arterial branches. Labels for the ascending, arch, thoracic, and abdominal aorta and their corresponding arteries are shown. (From Leonard PC. Building a Medical Vocabulary: With Spanish Translations, ed 7. St. Louis, 2009, Saunders.)

### Veins

Compared to arteries, veins have thinner walls and a larger diameter. Veins also have less elastic tissue and hence are not as distensible. In the lower extremity, veins have valves to assist with unidirectional flow of blood back to the heart. Blood is transferred back to the heart through muscle pump activity, which causes a milking effect on the veins.

Patients with incompetent valves in their veins develop varicosities in their lower extremity. Also, patients on prolonged bed rest are likely to develop deep vein thrombosis, from a lack of muscle activity resulting in a pooling of blood and clot formation within the venous vasculature.

## Summary

This chapter provides the reader with an understanding of the anatomy of the cardiovascular and pulmonary systems and its relevance for the therapist. This content provides the basis for an understanding of the pathophysiology of these systems as well as lays a foundation for development of relevant examination and treatment strategies to use when managing patients with cardiopulmonary dysfunction. A comprehensive understanding of anatomy is fundamental to the knowledge base of the therapist in understanding the central components involved in the delivery of oxygen and nutrients to peripheral tissue.

## References

1. DeTurk W, Cahalin L. Cardiovascular and Pulmonary Physical Therapy: An Evidenced-Based Approach. New York, 2004, McGraw-Hill.
2. Townsend CM, Beauchamp RD, Evers BM, et al. Sabiston Textbook of Surgery. ed 18. Philadelphia, 2008, Saunders.
3. Paz J, West M. Acute Care Handbook for Physical Therapists, ed 3. Philadelphia, 2009, Saunders.
4. Ganong, WF. Review of Medical Physiology. ed 21. New York, 2003, McGraw-Hill.
5. Frownfelter D, Dean E. Cardiovascular and Pulmonary Physical Therapy: Evidence and Practice, ed 4. St. Louis, 2006, Mosby.
6. Fox S. Human Physiology, ed 11. Boston, 2009, McGraw-Hill.
7. Kendall FP, McCreary EP, Provance PG, et al. Muscles: Testing and Function, ed 5. Baltimore, 2005, Lippincott Williams and Wilkins.
8. Gray H, Bannister LH, Berry MM, et al. Gray's Anatomy: The Anatomical Basis of Medicine and Surgery, ed 38. New York, 1996, Churchill Livingstone.
9. Goodman C, Fuller K. Pathology: Implications for the Physical Therapist, ed 3. St. Louis, 2009, Saunders.
10. Lund VJ. Nasal physiology: Neurochemical receptors, nasal cycle and ciliary action. Allergy Asthma Proc 17(4):179–84, 1996.
11. Richerson HB. Lung defense mechanisms. Allergy Proc 11(2):59–60, 1990.
12. Janson-Bjerklie S. Defense mechanisms: Protecting the healthy lung. Heart Lung 12(6):643–9, 1983.
13. Moore K, Dalley A. Clinically Oriented Anatomy, ed 5. Baltimore, 2006, Lippincott, Williams and Wilkins.
14. Berend N, Woolcock AJ, Marlin GE. Relationship between bronchial and arterial diameters in normal human lungs. Thorax 34(3):354–8, 1979.
15. Mason RJ, Broaddus VC, Murray JF, et al. Textbook of Respiratory Medicine, ed 4 Philadelphia, 2006, Saunders.
16. Heuther SE, McCance KL. Understanding Pathophysiology, ed 3. St. Louis, 2004, Mosby.
17. Guyton AC, Hall JE. Textbook of Medical Physiology, ed 11. Philadelphia, 2006, Saunders.
18. Moore K, Dalley A. Clinically Oriented Anatomy, ed 5. Baltimore, 2006, Lippincott, Williams and Wilkins.
19. Cheitlin MD. Clinical Cardiology, ed 7. Stamford, CT, 2004, Appleton & Lange.
20. Berne RM, Levy MN. Cardiovascular Physiology, ed 8. Philadelphia, 2002, Mosby.
21. Abuin G, Nieponice A. New findings on the origin of the blood supply to the atrioventricular node. Clinical and surgical significance. Tex Heart Inst J 25(2):113–17, 1998.

## CHAPTER 2

# Physiology of the Cardiovascular and Pulmonary Systems

*Konrad Dias*

This chapter reviews concepts relating to the physiology of the cardiovascular and pulmonary systems and its relevance in physical therapy practice. The cardiopulmonary systems not only share a close spatial relationship in the thoracic cavity, but also have a close functional relationship to maintain homeostasis. Physiologically, these systems must work collaboratively to provide oxygen required for energy production and assist in removing carbon dioxide manufactured as a waste product. A disorder affecting the lungs has a direct effect on the heart and vice versa. An understanding of normal physiology helps the reader better appreciate pathophysiologic changes associated with diseases and dysfunction of these systems that will be discussed in subsequent chapters.

## The Pulmonary System

The pulmonary system has several important functions. The most important function of the pulmonary system is to exchange oxygen and carbon dioxide between the environment, blood and tissue. Oxygen is necessary for the production of energy. If a cell has oxygen, a single molecule of glucose can undergo aerobic metabolism and produce 36 ATP. However, if a cell is devoid of oxygen, each molecule of glucose undergoes anaerobic metabolism yielding only 2 ATP. Thus, pathology of the pulmonary system will result in reduced energy production because of decreased oxygen within the tissue and a concomitant reduction in the exercise tolerance of the individual. Carbon dioxide is another gas that must be effectively exchanged at the level of the lung. Through the release of carbon dioxide from the body, the pulmonary system plays an important role in regulating acid

base balance and maintaining normal blood pH. The second function of the pulmonary system is temperature homeostasis, which is achieved through evaporative heat loss from the lungs. Finally, the pulmonary system helps to filter and metabolize toxic substances, as it is the only organ that receives all blood coming from the heart.

To facilitate a comprehension of the physiology of the pulmonary system, three major physiologic components are discussed in this chapter, including (a) the process of ventilation or breathing, (b) the process of gas exchange or respiration, and (c) the transport of gases to peripheral tissue.

### Ventilation

Ventilation or breathing, often misnamed respiration, involves the mechanical movement of gases into and out of the lungs.[1] At rest, an adult breathes at a rate of 10 to 15 breaths/minute, termed the ventilatory rate or respiratory rate. Approximately 350 to 500 mL of air is inhaled or exhaled at rest with each breath, and is termed the tidal volume. The amount of effective ventilation, termed the minute ventilation, expressed in liters/minute, is calculated by multiplying the ventilatory rate and tidal volume. The minute ventilation represents the total volume of air that is inhaled or exhaled in one minute. At rest the minute ventilation is approximately 5 L/min, while at maximum exercise it increases to a level between 70 and 125 L/min.[2]

### Additional Lung Volumes

Before considering the mechanical properties of the lungs during ventilation or breathing, it is helpful to consider the static volumes of the lungs measured via spirometry studies

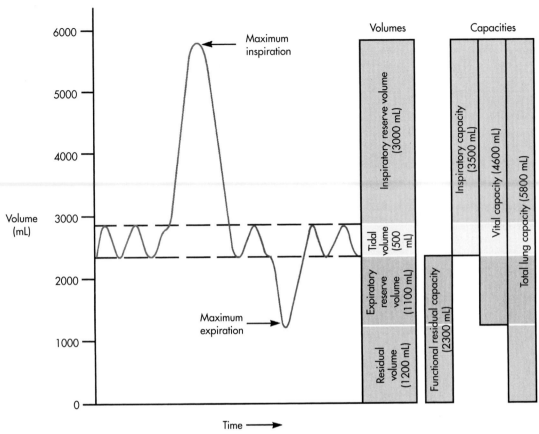

**Figure 2-1** Lung volumes and capacities as displayed by a time versus volume spirogram. Values are approximate. The tidal volume is measured under resting conditions. (From Seeley RR, Stephens TD, Tate P. Anatomy & Physiology, ed 3, New York, 1995, McGraw-Hill.)

(Fig. 2-1).[2-4] As mentioned earlier, the volume of air normally inhaled and exhaled with each breath during quiet breathing is called the tidal volume (VT). The additional volume of air that can be taken into the lungs beyond the normal tidal inhalation is called the inspiratory reserve volume (IRV). The additional volume of air that can be let out beyond the normal tidal exhalation is called the expiratory reserve volume (ERV). The volume of air that remains in the lungs after a forceful expiratory effort is called the residual volume (RV). The inspiratory capacity (IC) is the sum of the tidal and inspiratory reserve volumes; it is the maximum amount of air that can be inhaled after a normal tidal exhalation. The functional residual capacity (FRC) is the sum of the expiratory reserve and RV; it is the amount of air remaining in the lungs at the end of a normal tidal exhalation. The importance of FRC cannot be overstated; it represents the point at which the forces tending to collapse the lungs are balanced against the forces tending to expand the chest wall. The vital capacity (VC) is the sum of the inspiratory reserve, tidal, and expiratory reserve volumes; it is the maximum amount of air that can be exhaled following a maximum inhalation. The total lung capacity (TLC) is the maximum volume to which the lungs can be expanded; it is the sum of all the pulmonary volumes.

## Control of Ventilation

Breathing requires repetitive stimulation from the brain, as skeletal muscles required for ventilation are unable to contract without nervous stimulation.[5] Although breathing usually occurs automatically and involuntarily, there are circumstances when individuals hold their breath, take deep breaths or change ventilation, such as when singing or laughing. In light of this, it is important to review the mechanisms involved in helping to control breathing.

This section describes the neural mechanisms that regulate ventilation. Neurons in parts of the brainstem, including the medulla oblongata and pons, provide control for automatic breathing and adjust ventilatory rate and tidal volume for normal gas exchange (Fig. 2-2).[5] The medulla oblongata contains inspiratory neurons that produce inspiration and expiratory neurons that are triggered with forced expiration. Inspiratory neurons are located in the inspiratory center or dorsal respiratory group of the medulla. An enhanced frequency of firing of these neurons increases the motor units recruited and results in a deeper breath.[6] An elongation in the time of firing prolongs each breath and results in a slower respiratory rate.[6] A cessation of neural stimulation of these neurons causes elastic recoil of the lungs and passive expiration.

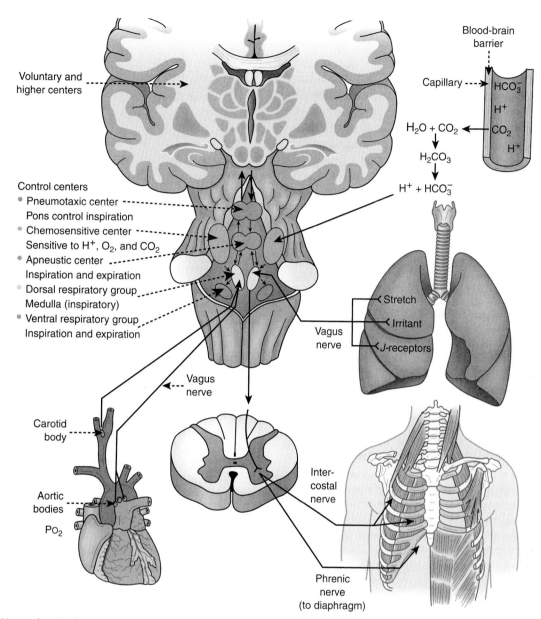

**Figure 2-2** Neurochemical respiratory control system. (From McCance KL, Huether SE, Brashers VL, et al. (eds.) Pathophysiology: The Biologic Basis for Disease in Adults and Children, ed 6. St. Louis, 2010, Mosby.)

The expiratory center or ventral respiratory group in the medulla contains inspiratory neurons in the midregion and expiratory neurons in the anterior and posterior zones. Neural stimulation of the expiratory neurons causes inhibition of the inspiratory center when a deeper expiration is warranted.

The pons has two major centers that assist with ventilation, including the pneumotaxic center in the upper pons and apneustic center in the lower pons.[5] The pneumotaxic center maintains rhythm of ventilation, balancing the time periods of inspiration and expiration by inhibiting the apneustic center or the inspiratory center of the medulla. The apneustic center facilitates apneustic or prolonged breathing patterns when it is uninhibited from the pneumotaxic center.

Breathing concerning a conscious change in pattern, involves control from the motor cortex of the frontal lobe of

the cerebrum.[6] Here impulses are sent directly down to the corticospinal tracts to the respiratory neurons in the spinal cord, bypassing the respiratory centers in the brainstem to trigger changes in ventilation.

## Afferent Connections to the Brainstem

The respiratory centers of the brainstem receive afferent input from various locations, including the limbic system, hypothalamus, chemoreceptors, and lungs.[5]

### Hypothalamic and Limbic Influence

Sensations of pain and alterations in emotion alter ventilation through input coming to the brainstem from the limbic system and hypothalamus.[7] For example, anxiety triggers hyperventilation and a concomitant reduction in carbon dioxide levels in blood, as the rate of carbon dioxide elimination out of the lungs exceeds the rate of carbon dioxide production in the body.

> **Clinical Tip**
> Patients with injuries within the central nervous system from an acute brain injury or stroke demonstrate altered ventilatory patterns following neurologic insult. These patients lose the normal response to breathing, resulting in altered ventilatory rates and volumes.

### Chemoreceptors

Chemoreceptors are located in the brainstem and peripheral arteries. These receptors are responsible for sensing alterations in blood pH, carbon dioxide, and oxygen levels.[7] There primarily exist two types of chemoreceptors, including central and peripheral chemoreceptors. The receptors found along the anterior lateral surfaces of the upper medulla of the brainstem are called central chemoreceptors. These receptors are stimulated when carbon dioxide concentrations rise in the cerebrospinal fluid. Central chemoreceptors facilitate an increased depth and rate of ventilation so as to restore normal carbon dioxide levels and pH in the body.[5,7] Peripheral chemoreceptors are found within the carotid artery and aortic arch. These receptors help to increase ventilation in response to increasing levels of carbon dioxide in blood (hypercapnia) as well as low oxygen levels in blood (hypoxia).[5,7]

In a small percentage of patients, with chronically high carbon dioxide levels in blood, such as in patients with severe chronic obstructive lung disease (COPD), the body begins to rely more on oxygen receptors and less on carbon dioxide receptors to regulate breathing. This is termed the hypoxic drive to breathe and is a form of respiratory drive in which the body uses oxygen receptors instead of carbon dioxide receptors to regulate the respiratory cycle.[8] Normal ventilation is driven mostly by the levels of carbon dioxide in the arteries, which are detected by peripheral chemoreceptors, and very little by oxygen levels. An increase in carbon dioxide triggers the chemoreceptors and causes a resultant increase in ventilatory rate. In these few patients with COPD who demonstrate the hypoxic drive, oxygen receptors serve as the primary means of regulating breathing rate. For these patients, oxygen supplementation must be prudently administered, as an increase in oxygen within blood (hyperoxemia) suppresses the hypoxic drive and results in a reduced drive to breathe.[8]

### Lung Receptors

There exist three types of receptors on the lung that send signals to the respiratory centers within the brainstem.

1. *Irritant receptors:* These receptors are found within the epithelial layer of the conducting airways and respond to various noxious gases, particulate matter and irritants causing them to initiate a cough reflex. When stimulated, these receptors also cause bronchial constriction and increase ventilatory rate.[5]

2. *Stretch receptors:* These receptors are located along the smooth muscles lining of the airways and are sensitive to increasing size and volume within the lung.[6] Hering and Breuer discovered, that ventilatory rate and volume was reduced following distention of anesthetized animal lungs. This stimulation of the ventilatory changes in response to increased volume and size is termed the Hering-Breuer reflex and is more active in newborns. In adults, this reflex is only active with large increases in the tidal volume, which is especially seen during exercise, and protects the lung from excessive inflation.[6]

3. *J receptor:* The juxtapulmonary receptors are located near the pulmonary capillaries and are sensitive to increased pulmonary capillary pressures. On stimulation, these receptors initiate a rapid, shallow breathing pattern.[7] Additionally, the interstitial J receptors produce a cough reflex with fluid accumulation within the lung in patients with pulmonary edema and pleural effusions.

> **Clinical Tip**
> In patients with acute left-side congestive heart failure and resultant pulmonary edema, the interstitial J receptors within the lung are stimulated. The firing of these receptors causes the patient to breathe in a shallow, tachypneic pattern. This breathing pattern causes a milking the lymphatic vasculature to facilitate a removal of fluid out of the lungs.[9]

### Joint and Muscle Receptors

Receptors within peripheral joints and muscles of the extremities respond to changes in movement and increase ventilation. During exercise a twofold increase in minute ventilation is noted—an initial abrupt increase in ventilation followed by a secondary gradual increase in ventilation (Fig. 2-3).[10] The initial abrupt increase in ventilation is a result of sensory

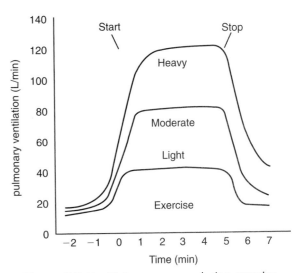

**Figure 2-3** Ventilatory response during exercise.

input conveyed from receptors within peripheral joints and muscles, whereas the secondary gradual increase in ventilation a result of to changes in pH within blood caused by increased lactic acid production. This is conveyed to the brainstem by the chemoreceptors.

## Mechanics of Breathing

Movement of air into and out of the lungs occurs as a result of pressure differences between the two ends of the airway. Airflow through conducting airway is directly proportional to the pressure difference created between the ends of the airway and inversely proportional to the resistance within the airway. In addition, ventilation is affected by various physical properties of the lungs including compliance, elasticity, and surface tension. This section focuses on pressure changes that allow breathing to occur, as well as explains how lung compliance, elasticity, and surface tension affect breathing. The physiologic importance for pulmonary surfactant is also discussed.

### Intrapulmonary and Atmospheric Pressures

Inspiration is always an active process and involves contraction of the respiratory muscles. When the diaphragm and external intercostals contract, they increase the volume of the thoracic cavity and lung. This in turn causes a concomitant reduction in the intrapulmonary pressure or pressure within the lung (Fig. 2-4).[11] The pressure within the lung is reduced in accordance with Boyle's Law, which states that the pressure of a given quantity of gas is inversely proportional to its volume. During inspiration, an increase in lung volume within the thoracic cavity decreases intrapulmonary pressures below atmospheric levels. This is termed a subatmospheric or negative intrapulmonary pressure. This difference in pressure between the atmosphere and the lungs facilitates the flow of air into the lungs to normalize pressure differences. Conversely, expiration occurs when the intrapulmonary pressure exceeds the atmospheric pressure, allowing the lungs to recoil inward and expel air into the atmosphere.

There exists a primary difference between normal ventilation and mechanical ventilation. In normal ventilation, air is pulled into the lungs because of a negative pressure created through activation of the respiratory muscles. Patients placed on mechanical ventilation lack the ability to generate an effective negative or subatmospheric pressure. In light of this, the mechanical ventilator forces air into the lungs through creation of a positive pressure greater than the atmospheric pressure that exists within the lung.

It is also important to note that patients on mechanical ventilation often demonstrate reduced strength of the inspiratory muscles (including the diaphragm), as the ventilator assists with breathing. These patients may benefit from breathing exercises, positioning and the use of an inspiratory muscle trainer to improve functioning of the inspiratory muscles.

### Intrapleural and Transmural Pressures

There exist two layers that cover each lung, including the outer parietal pleura and inner visceral pleura, separated by

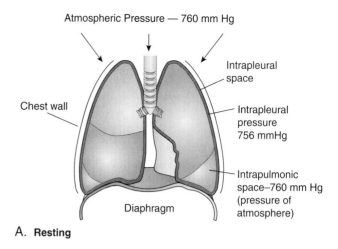

A. **Resting**

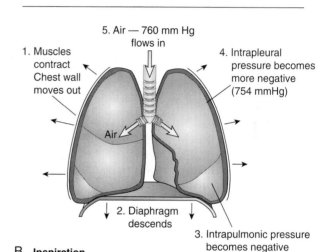

B. **Inspiration**

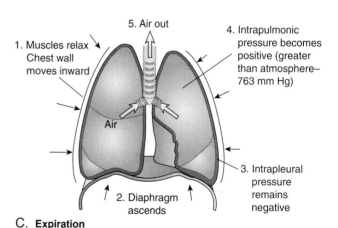

C. **Expiration**

**Figure 2-4** Ventilation: Changes in pressure with inspiration and expiration. (From Gould BE. Pathophysiology for the Health Professions, ed 3. St. Louis, 2007, Saunders.)

an intrapleural space containing a thin layer of viscous fluid. A small amount of viscous fluid within the intrapleural space serves as a lubricant and allows for the lungs to slide relative to the chest during breathing. With ventilation, there exist two opposing forces, including an inward pull from the elastic tension of the lung tissue trying to collapse the lung, and an outward pull of the thoracic wall trying to expand the lungs.[1,2,5] These two opposing forces give rise to a subatmospheric (negative) pressure within the intrapleural space, termed the intrapleural pressure. This intrapleural pressure is normally lower than the intrapulmonary pressure developed during both inspiration and expiration. In light of these two pressure differences, a transpulmonary or transmural pressure is developed across the wall of the lung.[1,2,5] The transmural pressure considers the difference between the intrapulmonary and intrapleural pressure. The inner intrapulmonary pressure is relatively greater than the outer intrapleural pressure, allowing the difference in pressure (the transmural pressure) to maintain the lung near the chest wall. It is the transmural or transpulmonary pressure that allows changes in lung volume to parallel changes in thoracic excursion during inspiration and expiration.

When changes in lung volume do not parallel the normal outward and inward pull during inspiration and expiration, respectively, and are in fact opposite, the breathing pattern is said to be paradoxical. This breathing pattern is often seen in patients with multiple rib fractures and a resultant flail chest.

### Physical Properties of Lungs

The processes of inspiration and expiration are facilitated by three physical properties of lung tissue. Compliance allows lung tissue to stretch during inspiration, the elastic recoil of the lung allows passive expiration to occur, and surface tension forces with the alveoli allow the lung to get smaller during expiration.

**Compliance.** The lung can be compared to a balloon during inspiration, where there exists a tendency to collapse or recoil while inflated. To maintain inflation, the transmural pressure or pressure difference between the intrapulmonary pressure and intrapleural pressure must be maintained. A distending force is needed to overcome the inward recoil forces of the lung. This outward force is provided by the elastic properties of the lung and through the action of the inspiratory muscles.

*Compliance* describes the distensibility of lung tissue. It is defined as the change in lung volume per change in transmural or transpulmonary pressure, expressed symbolically as $\Delta V/\Delta P$ (Fig. 2-5).[12] In other words, a given transpulmonary pressure, will cause a greater or lesser degree of lung expansion, depending on the distensibility or compliance of the lung. The compliance of the lung is reduced by factors that produce a resistance to distension. Also, the compliance is reduced as the lung approaches its TLC, where it becomes relatively stiffer and less distensible.

In patients with emphysema, the chronicity of the disease leads to progressive destruction of the elastic recoil, making

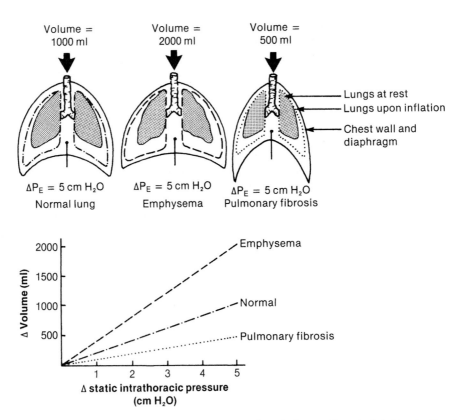

**Figure 2-5** Lung compliance changes associated with disease. (From Cherniack RM, Cherniack L. *Respiration in Health and Disease*, ed 2 Philadelphia, 1972, Saunders.)

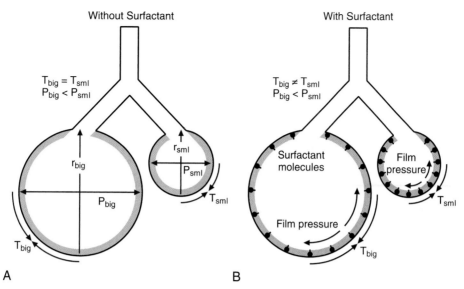

**Figure 2-6** Two pairs of unequally filled alveoli arranged in parallel illustrate the effect of a surface-active agent. One pair of alveoli is shown without surfactant (**A**) and the other is shown with surfactant (**B**). In the alveoli without surfactant, if Tsml were the same as Tbig, Psml would have to be many times greater than Pbig; otherwise, the smaller alveolus would empty into the larger one. In the alveoli with surfactant, Tsml is reduced in proportion to the radius of the alveolus, which permits Psml to equal Pbig. Thus, alveoli of different radii can coexist. Refer to the text for details.

the compliance high.[13] A reduced inward pull from low recoil allows small changes in transmural pressure to cause large changes in lung volumes and resultant hyperinflation of the lung. The changes seen in individuals with emphysema include a barrel chest and flattened diaphragms. These negative sequelae result in less diaphragm use with breathing, more accessory muscle, and an increase in the work of breathing.

In patients with pulmonary fibrosis, the lung is fibrotic and stiff, and thereby reducing compliance.[13] In these patients, despite large changes in transmural pressure, only small changes in lung volume will occur as a result of the stiffness or lack of distensibility of lung tissue. Consequently, clinically one sees individuals with increased respiratory rates and accessory muscle use because of decreased lung volumes. The work of breathing with activity is greatly increased as a consequence of the inability to increase lung volumes.

**Elasticity.** *Elasticity* refers to the tendency of a structure to return to its initial size after being distended. A network of elastin and collagen fibers within the alveolar wall and surrounding bronchi and pulmonary capillaries provides for the elastic properties of the lung.

**Surface tension.** Although the elastic characteristics of the lung tissue itself play a role in resisting lung distension or compliance, the surface tension at the air–liquid interface on the alveolar surface has a greater influence. Anyone who has ever attempted to separate two wet microscope slides by lifting (not sliding) the top slide from the bottom has first-hand experience with the forces of surface tension. In the lung, a thin film of fluid on the alveolus has a surface tension, which is caused by water molecules at the surface being relatively more attracted to other water molecules than to air.

This surface tension acts to collapse the alveolus and increase the pressure of air within the alveolus. The Law of Laplace states that the pressure created within the alveolus is directly proportional to the surface tension and inversely proportional to the radius of the alveolus.

For example, consider two alveoli of different sizes, one at either end of a bifurcated respiratory bronchiole (Fig. 2-6); because of the size difference, the smaller alveolus must have a higher pressure than the larger alveolus if the surface tension of each is the same. To keep the air in the smaller alveolus from emptying into the larger, a surface-active agent is needed to decrease the overall surface tension of the alveoli so as to lower wall tension in proportion to the radius of the alveolus (see Fig. 2-6). Moreover, it must do so almost in anticipation of diminishing alveolar size. Only if such a surface-active agent were present could alveoli with different radii coexist in the lungs.

The surface-active agent in the human lung that performs this function is called surfactant.[14,15] Pulmonary surfactant is not composed of a single class of molecules but, rather, is a collection of interrelated macromolecular lipoprotein complexes that differ in composition, structure, and function.[14,15] Nonetheless, the principal active ingredient of surfactant is dipalmitoyl phosphatidylcholine (DPPC). The structure of the surfactant molecule is such that it presents a nonpolar end of fatty acids (two palmitate residues) that is insoluble in water, and a smaller, polar end (a phosphatidylcholine group) that dissolves readily in water. Thus, surfactant orients itself perpendicularly to the surface in the alveolar fluid layer; its nonpolar end projecting toward the lumen. If surfactant were uniformly dispersed throughout the alveoli, its concentration at the air–fluid interface would vary in accordance with the surface area of any individual alveolus. Thus, the molecules would be compressed in the smaller alveoli, as depicted in Figure 2-6. Compressing the surfactant molecules increases their density and builds up a film pressure that counteracts much of the surface tension at the air–fluid interface. The rate of change in the surface tension resulting from compression of the surfactant molecules, as the alveolus gets smaller is faster than the rate of change of the decreasing alveolar radius so that a point is rapidly reached in which the pressure in the small alveolus equals the pressure in the big alveolus.

Surfactant begins to develop in late fetal life. Premature babies may be born with less surfactant, resulting in collapsed alveoli and respiratory distress. In an effort to reduce complications in women likely to go into premature labor (<7 months' gestation), the fetus is injected with amniotic fluid from the placenta of an infant born through cesarean section to mature the fetus' lungs. It is important to note that even under normal circumstances, the first breath of life is more challenging, as the newborn must overcome greater surface tension forces in order to inflate its partially collapsed alveoli.

**Resistance to airflow.** The ability to inflate the lungs with air depends on pressure differences and resistance to flow within the airways.[2,5] Poiseuille's law states that flow through a vessel or airway is directly proportional to the pressure difference and radius and inversely proportional to the length of the airway and viscosity of the gas. In addition, it is important to note that the radius is raised to the fourth power and so small changes in the radius account for large changes in airflow through the airway.[5,7]

The upper airways are responsible for most of the airway resistance. Relatively, the lower airways play a much smaller role in influencing airway resistance because of the irregularity of the branching patterns as well as variations in the diameter of the lumen of the distal airway.[6] In addition, resistance in smaller airways is lower because flow is laminar. This involves only slight resistance between the sides of the airway and resistance caused by collision of air molecules. In the upper airway airflow is relatively highly turbulent involving increased resistance as a result of frequent molecular collisions in addition to the resistance along the sides of the tube (Fig. 2-7).

Resistance to airflow is also affected by the diameter of the airway, which is influenced by changes in the transmural pressure within the lung during ventilation. With inspiration, the pressure outside the airway within the lung (transmural pressure) is relatively more negative than the airway pressure, thereby increasing the radius of the airway and reducing resistance to airflow. Conversely, with expiration, the transmural pressure is greater than the airway pressure, reducing the radius and increasing airway resistance.[2]

Finally, resistance to airflow may also be affected by autonomic nervous system control. Increases in parasympathetic nervous system activation cause constriction of the smooth muscle cells of the bronchi and increase airway resistance, whereas sympathetic influence decreases airway resistance. Also, mucus and edema in the airway as a consequence of inflammation increase airway resistance and reduce airflow.[1,2]

Status asthmaticus, an acute asthma attack is marked by severe airway resistance caused by constriction of bronchial smooth muscle cells and mucus production within the airway (Fig. 2-8). These patients use accessory muscles to increase transmural pressures to increase airway radius. In addition, they benefit from bronchodilators to relieve smooth muscle cell constriction and from steroids to reduce the inflammatory process and mucus production.

## Respiration

Respiration refers to the process of gas exchange in the lungs facilitated through the process of simple diffusion. This process serves two major functions, including the replenishment of the blood's oxygen supply used for oxidative energy production, and the removal of carbon dioxide returning from venous blood manufactures as a waste product. For diffusion to occur, there are two requirements: air bringing in oxygen into the lungs (alveolar ventilation) and blood to receive the oxygen and give up carbon dioxide (pulmonary perfusion). Air is delivered to the distal alveolus for gas exchange via the process of pulmonary ventilation; blood is brought to the lungs from the right side of the heart through the pulmonary artery and branching pulmonary capillaries. Gas exchange or respiration between the alveoli and pulmonary capillary occurs across the semipermeable

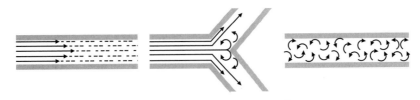

| A    Laminar Flow | B  Turbulence at Bifurcation | C    Turbulent Flow |

**Figure 2-7** Laminar and turbulent airflow in the airways. **A,** At low flow rates, air flows in a laminar pattern and the resistance to airflow is proportional to the flow rate. **B,** At airway bifurcation, eddy formation creates a transitional flow pattern. **C,** At high flow rates, when a great deal of turbulence is created, the resistance to airflow is proportional to the square of the flow rate. (Redrawn from West JB. Respiratory Physiology: The Essentials, ed 2. Baltimore, 1979, Lippincott Williams & Wilkins.)

alveolar–capillary membrane, also referred to as the respiratory membrane.

## Partial Pressures of Gases

The air delivered to distal alveoli is a mixture of gases. It is important to understand that each gas exerts its own pressure in a proportion to its concentration in the gas mixture. The amount of individual pressure exerted by each gas within the mixture is termed the partial pressure of that individual gas. According to Dalton's Law, the total pressure of a mixture of gases equals the sum of the individual gases within the mixture. Atmospheric air is a mixture of gases containing 79.04% nitrogen, 20.93% oxygen, and 0.03% carbon dioxide.[7]

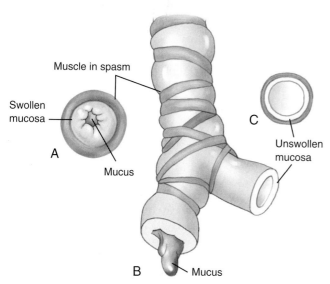

**Muscle in spasm**

**Swollen mucosa**

**A**

**Mucus**

**C**

**Unswollen mucosa**

**B**   **Mucus**

**Figure 2-8** Factors causing expiratory obstruction in asthma. **A,** Cross-section of a bronchiole occluded by muscle spasm, swollen mucosa, and mucus. **B,** Longitudinal section of an obstructed bronchiole. **C,** Cross-section of a clear bronchiole. (From Shiland BJ. Mastering Healthcare Terminology, ed 3. St. Louis, 2010, Mosby.)

At sea level, the barometric or atmospheric pressure is 760 mm Hg. This is considered the total pressure of the mixture of the three gases present in the atmosphere. Therefore, the partial pressure of nitrogen in the atmosphere is 600 mm Hg (79.04% of 760), oxygen is 159 mm Hg (20.83% of 760) and carbon dioxide atmospheric pressure is 0.2 mm Hg (0.03% of 760). Once gases enter the body, Henry's Law explains how gases in the body are dissolved in fluids. According to this law, gases dissolve in liquids in proportion to their partial pressure (Fig. 2-9).[16]

## Diffusion

To allow for effective gas exchange to occur between the alveoli and pulmonary capillary, different partial pressures of oxygen and carbon dioxide must exist in each of the two areas. The differences in partial pressure of each gas within the alveoli and pulmonary capillary create a pressure gradient across the alveolar capillary interface. This gradient will enable gases to diffuse from area of high concentration to areas of low concentration across the semipermeable respiratory membrane.

---

***Clinical Tip***

The diffusing capacity of lung for carbon monoxide (DLCO) is a test of the integrity of the alveolar–capillary surface area for gas transfer.[13] It may be reduced in disorders that damage the alveolar walls (septa), such as emphysema, leading to a loss of effective surface area. The DLCO is also reduced in disorders that thicken or damage the alveolar walls, such as pulmonary fibrosis.

---

## Perfusion

Perfusion refers to blood flow to the lungs available for gas exchange. The driving pressure in the pulmonary circulation is much less than the systemic circulation, yet flow rates in both circulation systems are similar because of reduced vascular resistance within the pulmonary circulation. Thus the

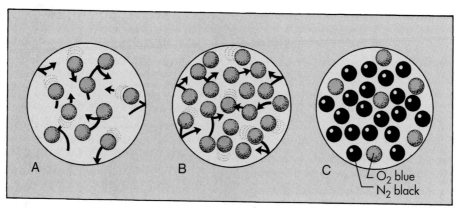

**A**   **B**   **C**   $O_2$ blue   $N_2$ black

**Figure 2-9** Relationship between number of gas molecules and pressure exerted by the gas in an enclosed space. **A,** Theoretically 10 molecules of the same gas exert a total pressure of 10 within the space. **B,** If the number of molecules is increased to 20, total pressure is 20. **C,** If there are different gases in the space, each gas exerts a partial pressure: here the partial pressure of nitrogen ($N_2$) is 18, that of oxygen ($O_2$) is 6, and total pressure is 24. (From McCance KL, Huether SE, Brashers VL, et al. (eds.). Pathophysiology: The Biologic Basis for Disease in Adults and Children, ed 6. St. Louis, 2010, Mosby.)

pulmonary circulation system is termed a low resistance, low-pressure pathway. The low pressure allows for relatively lower filtration pressures compared to the systemic vascular system thereby protecting the lung from pulmonary edema, a dangerous condition where fluid accumulates in the lung, hindering alveolar ventilation and gas exchange.

In addition, perfusion of the lung is affected by alterations in the partial pressures of oxygen within the alveoli.[16] Pulmonary arterioles constrict when partial pressures of oxygen in alveoli are low, and dilate when alveolar partial pressures for oxygen increase. These vasomotor changes of the pulmonary and systemic vasculature help to reduce blood flow to areas in the lung that are poorly ventilated and increase blood flow to peripheral tissue that needs more oxygen. The vasoconstriction of the pulmonary vasculature to low oxygen levels is automatic and improves the ability for gas exchange. This phenomenon prevents blood from poorly ventilated alveoli (with low partial pressures of oxygen) from mixing with blood from well-ventilated alveoli (with relatively higher partial pressures of oxygen). If blood did have to mix, then the overall oxygen concentration for blood leaving the lungs and returning to the heart would be lower because of the dilution effect.

Finally, alterations in the pH of blood affect vasomotor tone of the pulmonary vasculature, thereby affecting perfusion required for gas exchange.[6] A low pH, or acidemia causes pulmonary vasoconstriction. The lung is significantly involved in regulating acid–base balance in blood. When the pH of blood is reduced as a result of lung pathology, vasoconstriction of the pulmonary vessels is potentiated in response to the altered pH, which, in turn, affects the gas exchange and exacerbates the problem to a higher degree.

## Ventilation and Perfusion Matching

For optimal respiration or gas exchange to occur, the distribution of gas (ventilation, abbreviated V) and blood (perfusion, abbreviated Q) at the level of the alveolar capillary interface must be matched. Position plays a vital role in the distribution of ventilation and perfusion to different aspects of the lung. In the upright position, gravity allows for a greater amount of blood flow or perfusion to the base of the lung relative to the apices.[16] In addition, alveoli in the upper portions or apices of the lung have greater RV of gas and are subsequently larger.[16] The larger alveoli have greater surface tension and have relatively more difficulty inflating because of less compliance than the smaller alveoli toward the base of the lung. In light of this, ventilation and perfusion are relatively greater toward the base of the lung, favoring better matching and resultant respiration or gas exchange.[16] A change in the position of the patient changes areas of ventilation and perfusion. Generally, greater ventilation and perfusion occur in gravity dependant areas, thereby allowing better respiration to occur in the dependant lung when an individual is in the side-lying position (Fig. 2-10).

Often ventilation and perfusion ratios are not uniform within the lung, which compromises gas exchange. Regions of the lung with relatively greater amounts of perfusion compared to ventilation act as shunts. Conversely, regions of the lung with relatively greater amounts of ventilation compared to perfusion act as dead space. Alterations in the ventilation–perfusion matching lead to hypoxia and reduced oxygen to peripheral tissue.

An effective noninvasive tool to measure respiration is the pulse oximeter. It is important for clinicians to monitor pulse oximeter readings and observe for signs of distress when changing patient positions that alter the V/Q matching. Abnormal V/Q ratios cause concomitant reductions in pulse oximetry are noted in patients with pneumonia, pulmonary embolus, edema, emphysema, bronchitis and other pulmonary disorders.

## Transport of Oxygen and Carbon Dioxide

Following the previous discussions of how air is brought into the lungs through the process of pulmonary ventilation, and exchanged within the lungs via respiration, it is important to consider the mechanisms for the delivery of oxygen to peripheral tissue and the removal of carbon dioxide that the tissue produces as a waste product. This section reviews transport of each gas individually.

### Transport of Oxygen

A majority of oxygen (98%) is transported to the peripheral tissue bound to hemoglobin within red blood cells of blood. A very small portion of oxygen (<2%) is dissolved in plasma within blood.

### Hemoglobin

A hemoglobin molecule consists of four protein chains called globins and four iron-containing organic molecules called hemes.[2,5] The protein component of the molecule contains two identical $\alpha$ and two identical $\beta$ protein chains. The $\alpha$ chains contain 141 amino acids and the $\beta$ chains contain 146 amino acids.[7] The four-polypeptide chains are connected to each heme molecule. Each heme molecule has a central iron atom that can combine with a single molecule of oxygen. Consequently, as a result of the presence of four heme molecules, one hemoglobin has the ability to carry four oxygen molecules to the peripheral tissue.

Hemoglobin molecules within blood can exist in one of four conditions, depending on the molecule that binds to, unloads from, or is unable to bind to the iron atom within heme. Oxyhemoglobin represents a hemoglobin molecule bound to oxygen, because iron in heme is in its reduced state. Deoxyhemoglobin refers to the oxyhemoglobin molecule that has released its oxygen molecule to peripheral tissue. Because methemoglobin has iron in its oxidized state, it is unable to bind to oxygen and participate in oxygen transport. Blood contains a very small amount of this molecule. Carboxyhemoglobin is another abnormal form of hemoglobin; it involves the binding of heme to carbon monoxide instead of oxygen. Because the bond with carbon monoxide is 210 times stronger than oxygen, it displaces oxygen and inhibits oxygen's binding capacity.

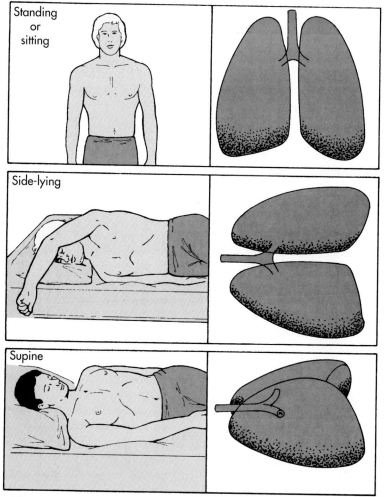

**Figure 2-10** Pulmonary blood flow and gravity. The greatest volume of pulmonary blood flow will normally occur in the gravity-dependent areas of the lungs. Body position has a significant effect on the distribution of pulmonary blood flow. (From McCance KL, Huether SE, Brashers VL, et al. (eds.). Pathophysiology: The Biologic Basis for Disease in Adults and Children, ed 6. St. Louis, 2010, Mosby.)

> *Clinical Tip*
> Carbon monoxide poisoning results from smoke inhalation and suicide attempts in its severe form and is treated by placing patients in a hyperbaric oxygen environment. This strategy enables the patient to breathe 100% oxygen at 2 to 3 atmospheres pressure. In a milder form, carboxyhemoglobin is generated in blood from breathing smoggy air and through chronic cigarette smoking.

The oxygen-carrying capacity of the body is determined by the concentration of hemoglobin. Normal levels of hemoglobin are between 12 and 16 g/dL for women and 13 and 18 g/dL for men.[17] A below-normal level of hemoglobin occurs with anemia and compromises the ability to carry oxygen. Conversely, an increase in hemoglobin concentrations, a condition called polycythemia, increases oxygen-carrying capacity within the system.

> *Clinical Tip*
> In patients with chronic lung disease, there may be a compensatory increase in red blood cells, termed secondary polycythemia, to compensate for chronically low levels of oxygen in blood.

The percent of oxyhemoglobin to total hemoglobin provides an indication of how well the blood has been oxygenated by the lungs. This is termed the percent oxyhemoglobin saturation. In the systemic arteries, at a partial pressure of 100 mm Hg, the percent hemoglobin is 97%, indicating that 97% of hemoglobin molecules in blood are bound to oxygen. The remaining 3% reflects deoxyhemoglobin, methemoglobin, and carboxyhemoglobin concentrations. The gold standard for measuring oxyhemoglobin saturation is through an analysis of arterial blood gases. However, pulse oximeter can also be used to obtain this number.

### Oxyhemoglobin Dissociation Curve

The oxyhemoglobin dissociation curve (Fig. 2-11) describes the relationship between the amount of $O_2$ bound to hemoglobin (Hb), clinically, referred to as the percentage of saturation of hemoglobin and the partial pressure of $O_2$ ($PO_2$)

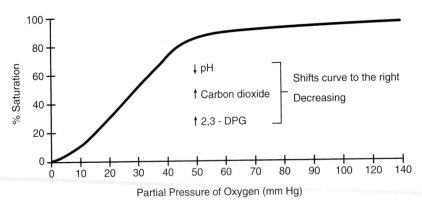

**Figure 2-11** The oxyhemoglobin dissociation curve. Note that in the "flat" portion of the curve (80 mm Hg and above), a change in the partial pressure of arterial oxygen (PaO$_2$) of as much as 20 mm Hg does not appreciably alter the hemoglobin saturation. However, in the "steep" portion of the curve (below 60 mm Hg), relatively small changes in saturation result in large changes in the PaO$_2$. pH, The logarithm of the reciprocal of hydrogen ion concentration; DPG, diphosphoglycerate.

with which the Hb is in equilibrium.[18-20] Under ideal conditions (blood pH = 7.4, body temperature = 37° C, Hb = 147 g · L−1), less than 10% of the O$_2$ dissociates from the Hb as PO$_2$ falls 40 mm Hg, from 100 to 60 mm Hg. However, nearly 60% of the O$_2$ is dissociated from the Hb as PO$_2$ falls another 40 mm Hg, from 60 to 20 mm Hg. Decreasing the pH (increasing acidemia) of the blood from the normal value of 7.40 to 7.30 shifts the hemoglobin dissociation curve downward and to the right an average of 7 to 8%; in contrast, alkalemia shifts the curve to the left. Increasing the concentration of CO$_2$ in the tissue capillary beds displaces oxygen from the hemoglobin, delivering the O$_2$ to the tissues at a higher PO$_2$ than would otherwise occur. In conditions of prolonged hypoxemia (lasting longer than a few hours), the amount of 2,3-diphosphoglycerate in the blood is increased, resulting in a rightward shift in the hemoglobin dissociation curve. 2,3-Bisphosphoglycerate is present in human red blood cells and binds with greater affinity to deoxygenated hemoglobin than it does to oxygenated hemoglobin. In bonding to partially deoxygenated hemoglobin, it allosterically upregulates the release of the remaining oxygen molecules bound to the hemoglobin, thus enhancing the ability of red blood cells to release oxygen near tissues that need it most. Furthermore, increasing the temperature of the tissue, as happens normally in exercising muscle, also results in a shift of the hemoglobin dissociation curve to the right. The result of these rightward shifts is a decreased hemoglobin affinity for oxygen. Although a rightward shift in the hemoglobin dissociation curve can be beneficial, the reader is cautioned that the range of variability normally tolerated by the body is relatively narrow: rapid fluctuations in pH or core temperature are not at all well tolerated.

### Carbon Dioxide Transport

Carbon dioxide released from metabolically active cells, is carried by blood in one of three ways:

- Dissolved in plasma
- Bound to the protein component of hemoglobin (carbaminohemoglobin)
- As bicarbonate ion

**Dissolved carbon dioxide.** Carbon dioxide released from tissue may get dissolved in blood plasma and transported through the system. A very small percentage of carbon dioxide, approximately only 7 to 10%, is transported is this manner.

**Carbaminohemoglobin.** Carbon dioxide can also be transported by binding to the hemoglobin molecule in blood. The carbon dioxide molecule binds to the protein chains rather than the heme component of the hemoglobin molecule. The complex formed from the binding of carbon dioxide and hemoglobin is termed carbaminohemoglobin. About one-fifth of the total blood carbon dioxide is carried in this manner.

**Bicarbonate Ions and the chloride and reverse chloride shifts.** The majority of carbon dioxide combines with water to form a compound called carbonic acid. This reaction is facilitated through the action of the carbonic anhydrase enzyme under conditions of high partial pressure of carbon dioxide at the level of the tissue.[2,7] This enzyme is confined to the red blood cell, thereby allowing most of the carbonic acid to be produced within the red blood cell. A small amount of carbonic acid is also produced spontaneously within the plasma of blood.

$$CO_2 + H_2O - carbonic\ anhydrase \rightarrow H_2CO_3$$

Carbonic acid that is built up within the red blood cell dissociates into positively charged hydrogen ions (protons) and negatively charged bicarbonate ions.

$$H_2CO_3 \rightarrow H^+ + HCO_3^-$$

The hydrogen ions released from carbonic acid combines with deoxyhemoglobin molecules within red blood cells. As a result, fewer hydrogen ions move out of red blood cells, causing the negatively charged bicarbonate ions to leak out of the blood cell into plasma. The trapping of hydrogen ions within the red blood cell results in a net positive charge within the blood cell and a compensatory shift of negative chloride ions into the red blood cell as bicarbonate moves out. This exchange of anions as blood travels through tissue capillaries is termed the chloride shift (Fig. 2-12).

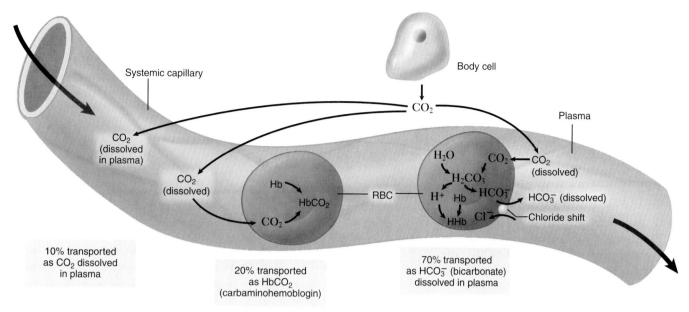

**Figure 2-12** Transport of carbon dioxide and the chloride shift.

It is important to appreciate that deoxyhemoglobin bonds more strongly to hydrogen ions than to oxyhemoglobin. In light of this, the unloading of oxygen to peripheral tissue is increased (the Bohr effect) as more hydrogen ions are released from carbonic acid to produce a greater amount of deoxyhemoglobin for the hydrogen ions to bind to. In summary, increased carbon dioxide production increases oxygen unloading into the tissue, which, in turn, improves carbon dioxide transport out of the tissue.

At the level of the lung, deoxyhemoglobin is converted to oxyhemoglobin. As mentioned earlier, oxyhemoglobin has a weaker affinity for hydrogen ions. With the partial pressure of oxygen being high at the level of the lung, free hydrogen ions are released from hemoglobin within the red blood cell. The free hydrogen ions attract bicarbonate ions from the plasma and join to form carbonic acid.

$$H^+ + HCO_3^- \rightarrow H_2CO_3$$

Under conditions of low partial pressures of carbon dioxide within the lung, carbonic anhydrase facilitates the breakdown of carbonic acid into carbon dioxide and water. The carbon dioxide is then released from the lungs through the process of expiration.

$$H_2CO_3 - \text{carbonic anhydrase} \rightarrow CO_2 + H_2O$$

A reverse chloride shift occurs at the level of the lungs to facilitate the entry of bicarbonate into the red blood cell. As bicarbonate ion leaves the plasma to enter the blood cell, chloride ions shift out of the red blood cell and enter the plasma. These processes are vital in maintaining acid–base regulation and normal pH of blood.

## Acid–Base Balance

Metabolically produced acids are largely eliminated from the body via the lungs in the form of $CO_2$ because the major blood acid, carbonic acid ($H_2CO_3$), is volatile; that is, it can chemically vary between a liquid and gaseous state. The other blood acids (dietary acids, lactic acids, and ketoacids) are regulated by the kidneys and the liver. The measurement of arterial oxygen or carbon dioxide tension and hydrogen ion concentration for assessment of acid–base balance and oxygenation status are commonly accomplished by means of laboratory analysis of arterial blood gases (ABGs). Generally, an ABG report contains the pH, the $PaCO_2$, the $PaO_2$, and the $HCO_3^-$, and base excess (BE) values for the sample analyzed. Chapter 10 provides a detailed discussion of acid–base balance and arterial blood gases.

## The Cardiovascular System

The primary function of the cardiovascular (circulatory) system is the transportation and distribution of essential substances to the tissues of the body and the removal of the by-products of cellular metabolism (Fig. 2-13). The heart provides the principal force that pushes blood through the vessels of the pulmonary and systemic circuits. In the case of the systemic circuit, the forward movement of blood is also facilitated by to the recoil of the arterial walls during diastole, skeletal muscle compression of veins during exercise, and negative thoracic pressure during inspiration. The pulmonary circuit receives the entire output of the right ventricle with each cardiac cycle.

## The Cardiac Cycle

The period from the beginning of one heartbeat to the beginning of the next is called the cardiac cycle. Figures 2-14 and 2-15 depict selected events during the cardiac cycle. Beginning with an action potential in the sinoatrial (SA) node, a depolarization wave is spread through both atria, to the atrioventricular (AV) node, and then, through the His-Purkinje

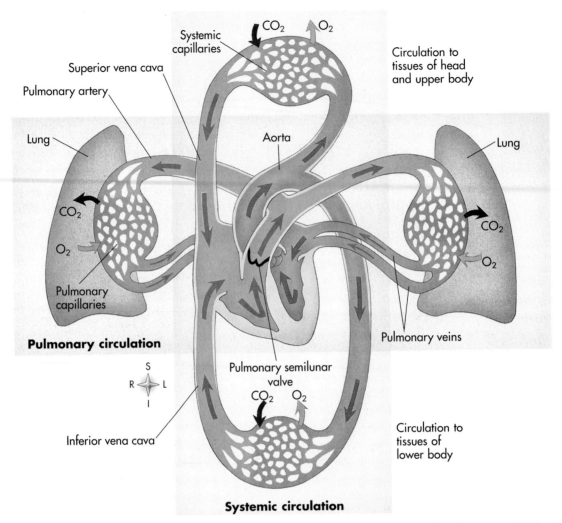

**Figure 2-13** Blood flow through the circulatory system. In the pulmonary circulatory route, blood is pumped from the right side of the heart to the gas-exchange tissues of the lungs. In the systemic circulation, blood is pumped from the left side of the heart to all other tissues of the body. (From Thibodeau GA. The Human Body in Health & Disease ed 4. St. Louis, 2006, Mosby.)

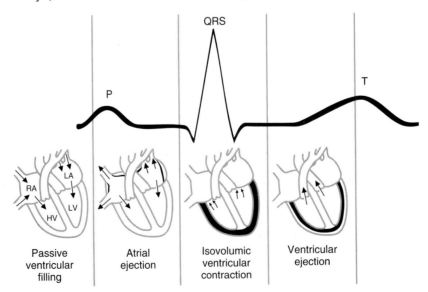

**Figure 2-14** The mechanical events of the cardiac cycle shown in relation to the electrical events of the electrocardiogram. In late diastole, just prior to the P wave, the ventricles fill passively. At about the time that the P wave ends, the atria contract to eject up to 30% of the end-diastolic ventricular volume. A period of isovolumic ventricular contraction begins very shortly after the onset of the QRS complex. Ventricular ejection coincides with the early portion of the ST segment.

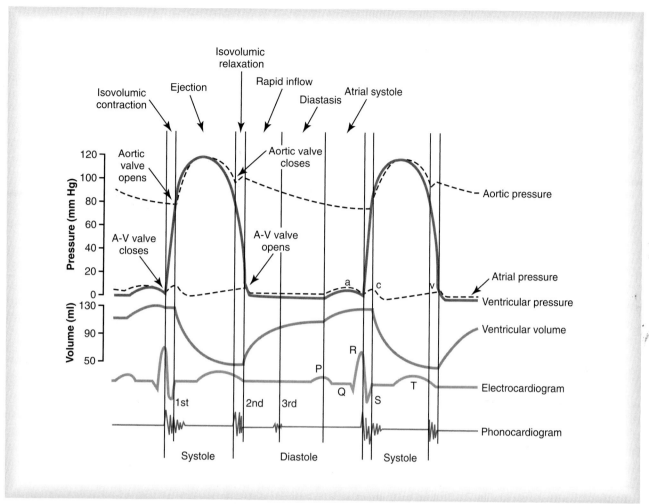

**Figure 2-15** Events of the cardiac cycle for left ventricular function, showing changes in left atrial pressure, left ventricular pressure, aortic pressure, ventricular volume, the electrocardiogram, and the phonocardiogram. (From Guyton AC, Hall JE. Textbook of Medical Physiology. ed 11. St. Louis, 2006, Saunders.)

complex, into the ventricles. However, because of the nature of the specialized conduction system, the impulse is delayed for about 0.1 second in the upper two-thirds of the AV node. This allows the atria to contract (a result of excitation–contraction coupling) and pump an additional volume of blood into the ventricles—an atrial "kick."[21] The ventricles provide the primary force to move blood through the vascular system.

> ### Clinical Tip
> In patients with atrial fibrillation, and a resultant quivering of the atria, the atrial kick is lost, losing 15 to 20% of the cardiac output, especially when the heart rate increases.[22] When managing patients with atrial fibrillation and rapid ventricular rates, signs and symptoms of compromised cardiac output must be continually assessed during treatment.

The cardiac cycle may be further divided into two periods: systole and diastole. Systole is the period of ventricular contraction; diastole is the period of ventricular relaxation.

Figure 2-15 illustrates left-sided pressure and volume, electrocardiogram (ECG), and phonocardiographic events associated with the cardiac cycle. Closure of the tricuspid and mitral valves generates the first heart sound ($S_1$), signaling the onset of ventricular systole, and is shown on the phonocardiographic tracing just after the peak of the R wave on the ECG tracing. In early ventricular systole, the ventricular volume remains unchanged despite a rapid rise in ventricular pressure. This isovolumic contraction occurs until the aortic valve opens, at which time the ventricular ejection phase begins. The retrograde bulging of the mitral valve into the left atrium is responsible for the rise in atrial pressure seen during the isovolumic ventricular contraction, the c wave. Ventricular ejection continues until the aortic valve closes, terminating systole and generating the second heart sound ($S_2$). Immediately following aortic valve closure, there is a phase of isovolumic relaxation that continues until the mitral valve opens when ventricular pressure falls below atrial pressure. The rise in atrial pressure indicated by the v wave of the atrial pressure tracing is probably brought about by the relative negative pressure resulting from ventricular relaxation.

Once the mitral valve opens, ventricular volume begins rising as the ventricle passively fills during the rapid-filling phase. Immediately following the rapid-filling phase is the slow-filling phase, also called diastasis, which continues until atrial systole. Atrial systole is indicated on the atrial pressure tracing as the a wave. These same events are essentially mirrored on the right side of the heart.

## Physiology of Cardiac Output

The previous section outlines the sequence of events to allow the heart to function as an efficient pump, with the end product being an ejection of blood out of the heart. An adequate volume of blood must be ejected out of the heart to sustain life and activity. The cardiac output reflects the volume of blood ejected out of the left ventricle into the systemic vasculature per minute. It is a function of the number of heartbeats per minute (heart rate) and the volume of blood ejected per beat (stroke volume). On average, the cardiac output at rest is between 4 and 6 L/min to allow for sufficient tissue perfusion.

## Cardiac Output = Heart Rate × Stroke Volume

It is also interesting to note that the average total blood volume is approximately 5.5 liters.[7] This indicates that the ventricle pumps an amount of blood equivalent to the total blood volume each minute. Therefore, it takes approximately 1 minute for a given volume of blood (a drop of blood) to complete the systemic and pulmonary circuits. With exercise, an increase in cardiac output is warranted, to meet the metabolic needs of the working muscles. To allow for this increase in cardiac output, an increase in blood volume must also exist. The following section reviews factors that regulate heart rate and stroke volume to accomplish an increase in blood volume and cardiac output.

## Regulation of Heart Rate

As mentioned in Chapter 1, the heart continues to beat automatically between 60 and 100 beats per minute (bpm) as long as myocardial cells are alive as a consequence of spontaneous depolarization of the pacemaker cells in the SA node. Sympathetic and parasympathetic nerve fibers to the heart are activated to alter this intrinsic pacing rate of the SA node.[23] Epinephrine from the adrenal medulla of the adrenal gland and norepinephrine from the sympathetic axons open channels of the pacemaker cells of the SA node and increase the rate of depolarizations resulting in an increase in heart rate.[1,5,7] Conversely, parasympathetic influence is achieved through the release of acetylcholine released by vagus nerve endings that bind to acetylcholine receptors, slowing down the rate of action potential production at the level of the SA node, thereby depressing heart rate.[1,5,7] It is important to understand that the actual pacing rate of the SA node is because of the net effect of these antagonistic influences. Mechanisms that alter the cardiac rate are said to have chronotropic effect. Influences that increase heart rate are said to have a positive chronotropic effect, whereas those that decrease heart rate are said to produce negative chronotropic effects.

Autonomic nervous system influences not only affect the firing of the SA node, but also affect sympathetic endings (β-adrenergic receptors) in the myocardial wall of the atria and ventricles.[2,5] Sympathetic stimulation vasodilates coronary arteries to increase blood flow to the heart and also increases myocardial contraction. On the other hand, parasympathetic influence vasoconstricts coronary arteries, reducing blood flow to the myocardium and depressing myocardial contractility.[2,5] Mechanisms that affect the contractility of the myocardium are said to have an ionotropic effect. Those that increase contractility have a positive ionotropic effect, whereas those that reduce contractility have a negative ionotropic effect.

---

**Clinical Tip**

A common goal in the pharmacologic management of patients with heart failure is to provide medications that cause a positive ionotropic effect, to increase the pumping ability of the failing heart. These medications include phosphodiesterase inhibitors and dobutamine that allow the heart to pump stronger and increase cardiac output.

---

A bout of aerobic exercise causes a linear increase in heart rate with increasing intensity as a result of decreased vagus nerve inhibition and increased sympathetic nerve stimulation. In addition, the slow resting heart rate or bradycardic responses seen in endurance-trained athletes continues to be controversial, but is often thought to occur as a consequence of enhanced parasympathetic input to the heart.

Patients on β blockers have a blunted heart rate response during exercise, as β receptors on the myocardial wall are unable to respond to sympathetic stimulation and appropriately increase heart rate. In light of this, it is effective to use a subjective assessment of intensity (Borg rate of perceived exertion), as objective measures of intensity examined through heart rate responses will be inaccurate.

## Regulation of Stroke Volume

The stroke volume or volume of blood ejected out of the heart per beat is affected by three variables:
- Preload
- Contractility
- Afterload

### Preload

The preload is a reflection of the volume of blood returning to the heart. It is often correlated with the end-diastolic volume (EDV), which is the maximum amount of blood that can be in the ventricles immediately prior to contraction. In normal cardiovascular physiology, the preload is directly proportional to the stroke volume. In other words, as more blood returns to the heart, a greater volume of blood leaves the heart with every contraction. Two physiologists, Otto Frank and Ernst Starling, demonstrated an intrinsic property of heart muscle to increase stroke volume based on the precontractile myocardial cell length. Within physiologic limits, the strength of ventricular contraction resulting in increased stroke volume varies proportionally to its precontraction length.[6,12] This length is influenced by the volume of blood in the ventricles prior to contraction. This is termed the Frank Starling mechanism and in summary explains how a greater volume of blood is ejected out of the ventricles when a greater volume of blood is returned to the heart (Fig. 2-16). Clinically the term preload, directly influenced by the EDV, refers to the amount of stretch on the myocardial wall prior to contraction. In other words, it refers to the load (stretch) on the myocardial wall prior to or precontraction.

It is interesting to note that in patients with congestive heart failure and a resultant failing heart, an increase in the EDV does not produce an increase in the preload and subsequent increase in stroke volume through the Frank Starling mechanism. In fact, an increase in the preload puts additional stress on the failing heart. Therefore, a variety of treatments are geared at reducing the preload or stretch on the myocardial wall. One such intervention appropriate in physical therapy practice is appropriate positioning to help adjust the preload in patients with left-sided heart failure. These patients will often not tolerate a supine or recumbent position, when the effects of gravity are minimized and a greater volume of blood returns to the heart. This increased volume puts greater load or stretch on a heart causing blood to back up into the lungs and exacerbate signs and symptoms. Conversely, these patients tolerate the upright position better, as the effects of gravity are maximized, allowing less blood to return to the heart and relatively less stress on the failing heart.

### Contractility

Myocardial contractility is influenced by intrinsic and extrinsic factors. The intrinsic control of contraction strength is as a result of the degree of myocardial stretch caused by changes in the end-diastolic volume.[12,13] This is discussed more comprehensively in the preceding section. In addition, force–frequency relationships cause an increase in myocardial contractility when heart rate increases. Physiologically, at higher heart rates (>120 bpm) an increased availability of calcium ions allows for excitation–contraction coupling and a resultant stronger contraction.[13]

The extrinsic control of contractility depends on the activity of the sympathoadrenal system (Fig. 2-17). Epinephrine from the adrenal medulla and norepinephrine from the sympathetic nerve endings produce a positive ionotropic

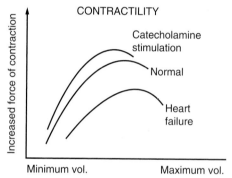

**Figure 2-16** Contractility. (From Irwin S, Tecklin SJ. Cardiopulmonary Physical Therapy: A Guide to Practice. ed 4. St. Louis, 2005, Mosby.)

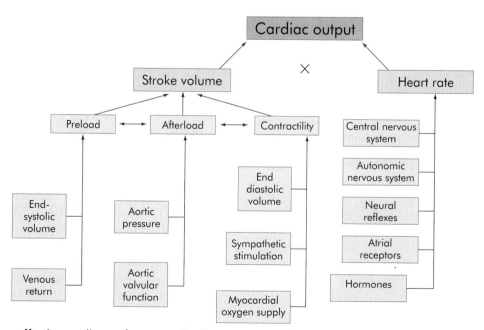

**Figure 2-17** Factors affecting cardiac performance. Cardiac output, which is the amount of blood (in liters) ejected by the heart per minute, depends on heart rate (beats per minute) and stroke volume (milliliters of blood ejected during ventricular systole). (From McCance KL, Huether SE, Brashers VL, et al. (eds.). Pathophysiology: The Biologic Basis for Disease in Adults and Children, ed 6. St. Louis, 2010, Mosby.)

effect, or increase myocardial contractility by promoting an influx of calcium available to the sarcomeres of the myocardial cells. Conversely, a reduction in sympathetic stimulation as well as reduction in heart rate results in reduced myocardial contractility.

### Afterload

Blood flows from areas of high pressure to areas of low pressure. Therefore, to enable blood to be ejected out of the ventricle into the aorta, the pressure generated within the ventricle must exceed the pressure within the systemic vasculature.[24] The pressure within the arterial system, during the diastolic phase of the cardiac cycle, while the heart is filling, is a function of the total peripheral resistance. An increase in the total peripheral resistance increases the pressure within the systemic vasculature. The afterload is a reflection of the pressure against which the heart has to contract to pump blood into the aorta. The total peripheral resistance presents a hindrance to the ejection of blood from the ventricles or represents an afterload on the ventricular wall after contraction has begun (Fig. 2-18). The afterload is inversely proportional to the stroke volume. Thus, an increase in the afterload or total peripheral resistance reduces the amount of blood ejected with each contraction. It is valuable to note that a reduced stroke volume from an increased afterload triggers compensatory mechanisms to maintain the cardiac output at a normal level of approximately 5.5 L/min. Initially, as blood has greater difficulty being ejected because of an increase in the afterload, a greater volume of blood builds within the ventricle, triggering the Frank Starling mechanism and a resultant greater myocardial contraction to help increase the stroke volume. An inability of the heart to compensate in this way leads to congestive heart failure and a compensatory increase in the heart rate to maintain the cardiac output at a normal level of approximately 5.5 L/min.

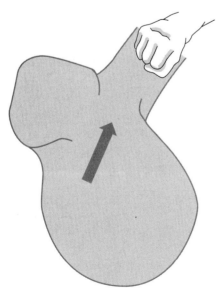

**Figure 2-18** Afterload. (From Irwin S, Tecklin SJ. Cardiopulmonary Physical Therapy: A Guide to Practice, ed 4. St. Louis, 2005, Mosby.)

### Ejection Fraction

The ejection fraction is the best indicator of cardiac function and represents a ratio or percentage of the volume of blood ejected out of the ventricles relative to the volume of blood received by the ventricles before contraction.[10] In other words, the ventricles receive a certain volume of blood during the diastolic phase, then contract and surge out a certain volume of blood. The ejection fraction reflects the ratio of the volume of ejected relative to what was received prior to systole or contraction of the ventricles. This can be mathematically presented as systolic volume (SV)/EDV. The normal ejection fraction is 60 to 70%. This means that for every 100 mL of blood poured into the ventricles during relaxation, 60 to 70 mL of blood is ejected per contraction. The volume of blood that remains in the ventricle following contracting is termed the end-systolic volume (ESV), and is approximately 30% of the EDV. There must exist a certain volume of blood remaining within the ventricles at the end of contraction to maintain a certain degree of stretch within muscle fibers of the myocardial cells.[25]

In patients with systolic heart failure, the ejection fraction is compromised as evidenced by a ratio less than 40%. This means that for every 100 mL of blood brought into the ventricles, less than 40 mL of blood is ejected per contraction caused by a failing heart. Thus blood that cannot be ejected backs up into the ventricle and causes an array of complications. These consequences are more comprehensively discussed in subsequent chapters.

### Venous Return

Venous return represents the return of blood to the right side of the heart via the veins. There are two factors that dictate the rate at which the right atrium fills with venous blood. These include the total blood volume and the pressure within the venous vasculature. Blood returned to the heart is primarily returned because of venous pressure. The mean venous pressure through the venous vasculature is approximately 2 mm Hg and is very different from mean arterial pressure, which is 90 to 100 mm Hg. This pressure is highest in the distal venules (approximately 10 mm Hg) and lowest at the junction of the vena cava with the right atrium (0 mm Hg). This pressure difference is the driving force of blood back to the heart. In addition, return is aided by the muscle pump activity, whereby the squeezing of peripheral muscles milk veins and assist with venous return. Also, sympathetic nerve fibers stimulate smooth muscle cell contraction in veins. Finally, pressure differences between the thoracic and abdominal cavities promote flow back to the heart. This phenomenon may be facilitated by active deep diaphragmatic inspiratory maneuvers. During contraction of the diaphragm, the central tendon contract and pulls the two hemidiaphragms caudally. This creates an increase in the abdominal pressure and a partial vacuum in the thoracic cavity, driving blood from the abdominal cavity into the thoracic cavity.

It is also noteworthy that veins have very thin walls and are less muscular compared to arteries. This increases their compliance and they can distend much more with any given amount of pressure. In light of this, veins have an ability to hold large volumes of blood and are often referred to as capacitance vessels, being similar to electrical capacitors that store electrical charges. Approximately two-thirds of total blood volume is stored within the venous vasculature.

It is often thought that the Trendelenburg position (elevation of the pelvis and lower extremities above the horizontal plane in the supine position) is effective for assisting with venous return in patients who are dehydrated or hypovolemic. The Trendelenburg position is not likely to augment cardiac output because of the high capacitance of veins.[26] The high capacitance of veins acts as a volume reservoir and counteracts any changes in the pressure gradient between peripheral and central veins. The venous system is more likely to transmit pressure when the veins are overloaded and less distensible. Therefore, the Trendelenburg position is more likely to assist with venous return when the patient has excess volume and not during episodes of volume depletion. Thus using the Trendelenburg position with patients in hypovolemia is not recommended.

## Coronary Blood Flow

The coronary arteries, discussed in Chapter 1, have a multitude of capillaries that help to perfuse myocardial tissue. It is interesting to note that the capillary density in myocardial tissue ranges from 2500 to 4000 capillaries per cubic millimeter of myocardial tissue in contrast to skeletal muscle tissue where the capillary density is only 300 to 400 capillaries per cubic millimeter of muscle tissue.[27] The heart is a muscle that survives through constant aerobic respiration, both at rest and during heavy exercise. Thus it is imperative that adequate amounts of blood and oxygen be constantly perfused to myocardial tissue.

During systole, or contraction of the myocardium, coronary arteries are squeezed, reducing perfusion of blood. Consequently, coronary perfusion to the myocardium occurs more during the diastolic or relaxation phase of each cardiac cycle. To provide a continuous supply of oxygen to myocardial cells despite the temporary reduction in the flow of blood during systole, the myocardium contains a large amount of molecules called myoglobin. These structures are similar to the hemoglobin found in red blood cells and have the ability to store oxygen during diastole and release the stored oxygen during systole to myocardial cells.

Coronary blood flow is regulated by autonomic nervous system influence. The fight-or-flight response triggers the sympathetic hormone epinephrine that affects the β-adrenergic receptors on the coronary arteries producing vasodilatation.[28] Therefore, to fight or flight during a stressful state, a surge of blood is perfused to the myocardium because of vasodilation to excite myocardial tissue and increase cardiac output.

## Blood Flow to Muscles during Exercise

As the body transitions from rest to exercise, blood flow patterns change markedly as a consequence of actions of the sympathetic nervous system.[10] Systemic vessels contain both α and β receptors that cause peripheral vasoconstriction and vasodilation, respectively. Through the action of the sympathetic nervous system, blood can be redirected from certain organs and shunted to working muscles to provide oxygen and energy and sustain activity. The shift in blood flow to muscle tissue is accomplished primarily by reducing blood to the kidneys, intestines, liver, and stomach.

During exercise, when the active muscles experience a need for additional blood, norepinephrine released by sympathetic nerve fibers stimulate the α-adrenergic receptors along the blood vessels of the digestive organs and kidneys. Stimulation of these receptors raises vascular resistance through vasoconstriction of the vessels, thereby diverting blood to skeletal muscles. At the level of the working muscles, epinephrine released by the adrenal medulla stimulates the β-adrenergic receptors within the blood vessel of the muscle, to produce vasodilation and increase blood flow to the active muscles.[10]

During exercise, alterations in autonomic nervous system stimulation also influence coronary blood flow by directly affecting heart rate and force of contraction—the two primary determinants of the myocardium's metabolic rate. The rate pressure product or double product is a clinically useful tool to estimate the myocardial oxygen demand and is calculated by multiplying heart rate by systolic blood pressure.

---

> ### Clinical Tip
> During aerobic exercise, heart rate and systolic blood pressure are the two main factors determining the workload on the heart. If these factors increase, the heart has to work harder, and will require more oxygen and nutrients to keep going requiring greater myocardial blood flow.

---

## Aging and Cardiovascular Physiology

Normal aging alters functioning of the cardiovascular system. In addition, chronic illnesses and comorbidities, seen more in the geriatric population, further affect functioning of the system. This section addresses normal cardiac system changes that occur with aging. It is important to note, however, that because exercise has positive physiologic effects on aging, the changes mentioned may not be evidenced in all older individuals.

With increasing age, left ventricular wall thickness increases as a consequence of increased collagen and enhanced size of myocardial cells.[6] Also, increased vascular thickness and vascular intimal thickness are additional changes noted in older individuals. The diastolic or filling properties of the heart are negatively influenced with reduced rate of ventricular filling and prolonged period of isovolumic myocardial relaxation, which is the time between aortic valve closure and the opening of the mitral valve.[6]

Maximal oxygen uptake ($VO_2max$) and cardiac output also reduce with increasing age. Reduced exercise performance and increased body weight collectively contribute to reductions in the relative oxygen consumption. Additionally, central and peripheral factors, including decreased maximum heart rate, reduced stroke volume, and compromised arteriovenous oxygen uptake, have been documented as factors contributing toward the decline in the $VO_2$max.[24] Finally, cardiac output during exercise reduces with increasing age as a result of low exercise heart rate and stroke volume values.

## Summary

This chapter reviews the basic physiology of the cardiovascular and pulmonary systems and its clinical relevance for the practitioner. The physiologic principles of ventilation, respiration, and transport of gases provide the clinician with an understanding of the mechanisms involved in getting oxygen to the peripheral tissue and removal of waste products generated through metabolic processes. In addition, the physiologic principles involved within each cardiac cycle, both electrical and mechanical, that enable the delivery of oxygen to vital organs to sustain life and activity are discussed. Finally, factors influencing cardiac output, blood flow to peripheral tissue, and venous return provide a basis for understanding possible pathophysiologic processes that can occur with disease.

## References

1. West JB. Respiratory Physiology: The Essentials, ed 7. Baltimore, 2004, Lippincott Williams & Wilkins.
2. Beachy W. Respiratory Care Anatomy and Physiology: Foundations of Clinical Practice, ed 2. St. Louis, 2008, Mosby.
3. Kendrick AH. Comparison of methods of measuring static lung volumes. Monaldi Arch Chest Dis 51(5):431–9, 1996.
4. Baydur A, Sassoon CS, Carlson M. Measurement of lung mechanics at different lung volumes and esophageal levels in normal subjects: Effects of posture change. Lung 174:139–51, 1996.
5. Fox S. Human Physiology, ed 11. Boston, 2009, McGraw-Hill.
6. Frownfelter D, Dean E. Cardiovascular and Pulmonary Physical Therapy: Evidence and Practice, ed 4. St. Louis, 2006, Mosby.
7. Guyton AC, Hall JE. Textbook of Medical Physiology, ed 11. Philadelphia, 2006, Saunders.
8. Kim V, Benditt JO, Wise RA, et al. Oxygen therapy in chronic obstructive pulmonary disease. Proc Am Thorac Soc 5(4):513–18, 2008.
9. Cahalin LP. Heart failure. Phys Ther 76:516–33, 1996.
10. Wilmore JH, Costill DL. Physiology of Sport and Exercise, ed 2. Champaign, IL, 2000, Human Kinetics.
11. Gould BE. Pathophysiology for the Health Professions, ed 3. St. Louis, 2007, Saunders.
12. Irwin S, Tecklin J. Cardiopulmonary Physical Therapy: A Guide to Practice, ed 4. St. Louis, 2005, Mosby.
13. DeTurk W, Cahalin L. Cardiovascular and Pulmonary Physical Therapy: An Evidence-Based Approach. New York, 2004, McGraw-Hill.
14. Lacaze-Masmonteil T. Pulmonary surfactant proteins. Crit Care Med 21:S376–79, 1993.
15. Johansson J, Curstedt T. Molecular structure and interactions of pulmonary surfactant components. Eur J Biochem 244(3):675–93, 1993.
16. Heuther S, McCance KL. Understanding Pathophysiology, ed 3. St. Louis, 2004, Mosby.
17. Goodman C, Fuller K. Pathology: Implications for the Physical Therapist, ed 3. St. Louis, 2009, Saunders.
18. Goodfellow LM. Application of pulse oximetry and the oxyhemoglobin dissociation curve in respiratory management. Crit Care Nurs Q 20(2):22–7, 1997.
19. Sims J. Making sense of pulse oximetry and oxygen dissociation curve. Nurs Times 92(1):34–5, 1996.
20. Dickson SL. Understanding the oxyhemoglobin dissociation curve. Crit Care Nurse 15(5):54–8, 1995.
21. Berne RM, Levy MN. Cardiovascular Physiology, ed 8. Philadelphia, 2000, Mosby.
22. Cheitlin MD. Clinical Cardiology, ed 7. Stamford, CT, 2004, Appleton & Lange.
23. Dubin D. Rapid Interpretation of EKGs: A Programmed Course, ed 6. Tampa, FL, 2006, Cover Publishing.
24. Ehrman JK, Gordon PM, Visich PS, et al. Clinical Exercise Physiology. Champaign, IL, 2003, Human Kinetics.
25. Ganong WF. Review of Medical Physiology, ed 21. New York, 2003, McGraw-Hill.
26. Marino P: The ICU Book, ed 2. Philadelphia, 1998, Lippincott Williams and Wilkins.
27. Moore K, Dalley A. Clinically Oriented Anatomy, ed 5. Baltimore, 2006, Lippincott, Williams and Wilkins.
28. Paz J, West M. Acute Care Handbook for Physical Therapists. ed 3. St. Louis, 2009, Saunders.

## CHAPTER 3

# Ischemic Cardiovascular Conditions and Other Vascular Pathologies

*Ellen Hillegass, Joanne Watchie, Eugene McColgon*

## Chapter Outline

The current estimate is that at least 80 million Americans have one or more forms of cardiovascular disease.[1] Cardiovascular disease is, in reality, many diseases. The American Heart Association (AHA) considers ischemic (coronary) heart disease, hypertension, heart failure, and cerebrovascular disease (stroke) to be the major cardiovascular diseases. Of the leading causes of death in the United States in 2006, heart disease continued to rank first. Heart disease was responsible for 35.3% of all deaths in 2006, which represents a 9.6% decline in the mortality rate from 1995, with cardiovascular disease responsible for 56% of total deaths.[1]

This chapter presents a detailed description of the anatomy and physiology of normal myocardial perfusion, a discussion of the pathologic changes that occur in coronary arteries as the result of coronary artery disease (CAD), and common cardiovascular diseases that are linked to the same process called atherosclerosis, including hypertension, cerebrovascular disease, peripheral arterial disease and other vascular disorders such as vascular aneurysms. The risk factors associated with the development of atherosclerosis are presented along with the major patterns of clinical presentation for CAD—chronic stable angina, and acute coronary syndrome (unstable angina, sudden cardiac death, and acute myocardial infarction).

The clinical presentation of the patient with CAD, the clinical signs and symptoms caused when the myocardium becomes ischemic, was first described by Heberden[2] in his lecture on "Disorders of the Breast" in 1772:

> There is a disorder of the breast, marked with strong and peculiar symptoms considerable for the kind of danger belonging to it, and not extremely rare, of which I do not recollect any mention among medical authors. The seat of it, and sense of strangling and anxiety, with which it is attended, may make it not improperly be called angina pectoris. Those, who are afflicted with it, are seized while they are walking and most particularly when they walk soon after eating, with a painful and most disagreeable sensation in the breast, which seems as if it would take their life away, if it were to increase or to continue; the moment they stand still, all this uneasiness vanishes.

The prevalence of CAD and its surprising presence in seemingly healthy young men was not fully appreciated until 1953, when Enos and colleagues[3] published the results of the autopsies they performed on soldiers killed in the Korean conflict. The investigation found that 77.3% of the 300 soldiers examined (mean age: 22.1 years) had observable blockages of their coronary arteries.[4] In 10 of the men, complete obstruction of one or more coronary arteries was found. As a direct result of the work of Enos and coworkers,[3] the medical community now distinguishes CAD (the presence of an obstruction that limits coronary blood flow but does not significantly inhibit heart muscle function) from coronary heart disease (CHD—the presence of an obstruction that causes permanent damage to heart muscle fibers downstream, thus inhibiting heart muscle function).

Enos' report[3] was followed by the now famous Framingham Heart Study in which 5209 apparently healthy men and women between the ages of 30 and 62 years were followed for 20 years.[5] During that period, the subjects were seen for biennial examinations, which consisted of questionnaires on activity and smoking history, blood chemistry studies, blood pressure measurement, and a resting 12-lead electrocardiogram (ECG). Although no one specific cause of CAD could be identified in the Framingham cohort, several major and minor risk factors for its development were discovered and are discussed later in this chapter.

> **Clinical Tip**
> The Framingham Heart Study provided landmark epidemiologic research that has led to the public and professional acceptance of the role of risk factors in the development and progression of cardiovascular disease.[5]

## Anatomy of the Coronary Arteries

Although the anatomy of the coronary arteries has been well understood for several years, to fully understand what is known about the coronary atherosclerotic process, a presentation of the normal triple-layered structure of arteries is necessary.[6]

### Outer Layer

The outer layer of an artery (adventitia) consists chiefly of collagenous fibers, mostly fibroblasts, and provides the basic support structure for the artery (Fig. 3-1). This portion of the artery also houses the vessels that furnish the middle layer of the artery with its blood supply—the *vasa vasorum*.

### Middle Layer

The middle layer (media) of all arteries (of which the coronary arteries are considered medium-size) consists of multiple layers of smooth muscle cells separated from the inner and outer layers by a prominent elastic membrane, or lamina. Through alterations in vasomotor tone, as demands for

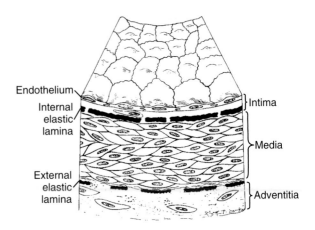

**Figure 3-1** Structure of the normal arterial wall, consisting of the adventitia (outer), the media (middle), and the intima (inner) layers. (From Ross R, Glomset J. The pathogenesis of atherosclerosis. N Engl J Med 295(8):420–5, 1976.)

changes in blood flow to the myocardium are perceived, this muscular layer is responsible for making adjustments to the luminal diameter. These smooth muscle cells are also capable of synthesizing collagen, elastin, and glycosaminoglycans, especially when they react to different physical and chemical stimuli.

### Inner Layer

The inner layer (intima) consists of an endothelial layer, the basement membrane, and variable amounts of isolated smooth muscle cells, as well as collagen and elastin fibers. The boundary of the intima and media is marked by the internal elastic lamina.

The two inner layers of the artery wall have received the most attention with regard to the development of the processes that lead to myocardial ischemia. The arterial endothelium is selectively permeable to macromolecules of the size of a low-density lipoprotein (LDL). The concentration of LDL in the lymph of the arterial wall has been found to be approximately one-tenth of that in the bloodstream.[7] Although many plasma proteins can enter the artery wall in this concentration, lipoproteins and fibrinogen are particularly likely to accumulate in the intima.[8]

## Myocardial Perfusion

Before discussing the particulars of myocardial perfusion, it is important to review two basic rules of fluid dynamics. First, all fluids flow according to a pressure gradient, that is, from an area of higher pressure to an area of lower pressure. Second, all fluids follow the path of least resistance. Consequently, if an obstruction is encountered, fluid tends to follow the less-resistant path, thereby reducing the fluid volume across the obstruction and decreasing the pressure that would drive the fluid farther down the path beyond the obstruction.

As with all muscle beds, myocardial perfusion occurs primarily during periods of muscle relaxation, in this case, during

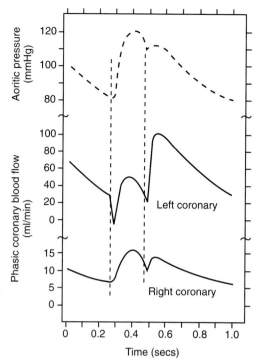

**Figure 3-2** The relationship between blood pressure in the aorta (top) and blood flow in the left (middle) and right (bottom) coronary arteries. The first vertical dotted line is the beginning of systole, and the second dotted line is the beginning of diastole. (From Boucek R, Morales A, Romanelli R, et al. Coronary Artery Disease: Pathologic and Clinical Assessment. Baltimore, 1984, Williams & Wilkins.)

diastole.[9,10] Figure 3-2 shows the relationship between mean aortic pressure and blood flow in the coronary arteries. Blood flow increases in both the right and left coronary arteries at the onset of systole (first vertical dotted line). When the aortic valve is closed, aortic diastolic pressure is transmitted through the dilated Valsalva sinuses to the openings of the coronary arteries themselves. Throughout diastole the sinuses act as miniature reservoirs, facilitating maintenance of relatively uniform coronary inflow. The pressure generated by the right ventricle during systole is in the range of 15 to 20 mm Hg, whereas the left ventricle produces pressures of 120 mm Hg or higher. Consequently, the occlusive pressure on the right coronary artery terminal vessel is less than that on the left vessel during systole, so there is less difference in blood flow in the right coronary artery between systole and diastole.

Just as with any other arteries, the coronary arteries distend when blood is forced back into them by the contracting muscle. Inasmuch as the pressure within the coronary arteries is less than that in the aorta, the coronary arteries themselves

---

**Clinical Tip**

The coronary arteries receive their blood supply during diastole because the aortic valve leaflets are closed. One mechanism to optimize the filling of the coronary arteries in individuals with disease is to place patients on β-blocking medications that lower the resting and exercise heart rates and increase diastolic filling time.

---

**Box 3-1**

**Myocardial Blood Flow Relationship**

| | |
|---|---|
| F | = DBP + VMT − R − LVEDP |
| F | = flow of blood to the myocardium |
| DBP | = diastolic blood pressure |
| VMT | = vasomotor tone (additive if the vessel is in a dilated state and subtractive if constricted) |
| R | = the resistance to flow offered by an obstructive lesion |
| LVEDP | = left ventricular end-diastolic pressure |

---

become reservoirs for the storage of blood. The resultant engorgement provides the initial "pressure head" that drives blood into the myocardium once intramyocardial pressure drops following systole.

An especially important difference between the coronary vascular bed and most others is the presence of anastomotic connections that lack intervening capillary beds (known as collateral vessels). In human hearts, the distribution and extent of collateral vessels is quite variable.[11] Under normal conditions, such vessels are generally less than 40 μm in diameter and appear to have little or no functional role. However, when myocardial perfusion is compromised by obstructions that affect major vessels, these collateral vessels enlarge over several weeks, and blood flow through them increases.[12,13] Given the time to make this adaptation, perfusion via collateral vessels may equal or exceed perfusion via the obstructed vessel.

## Major Determinants of Myocardial Blood Flow

- Diastolic blood pressure (DBP) is the primary driving force moving blood into the myocardial tissue.
- Vasomotor tone (VMT) plays a major role in determining the volume of blood passed along to the tissue by regulating the caliber of the artery. VMT is usually uniform throughout the coronary vascular tree. It aids or opposes DBP.
- Resistance to flow (R) is most commonly caused by atherosclerosis. A significant increase in the size and number of collateral vessels decreases total resistance to flow by providing an alternative route for the blood to take around an obstruction.
- Left ventricular end-diastolic pressure (LVEDP) is the pressure within the ventricle at end diastole; it causes an occlusive force on the capillary beds of the muscle closest to the pumping chamber, the endocardium.
- Myocardial blood flow relationship (Box 3-1).

## Atherosclerosis

The development of atherosclerosis is a complex process dependent on the interaction of several risk factors and the sensitivity of the individual to these factors. Atherosclerotic

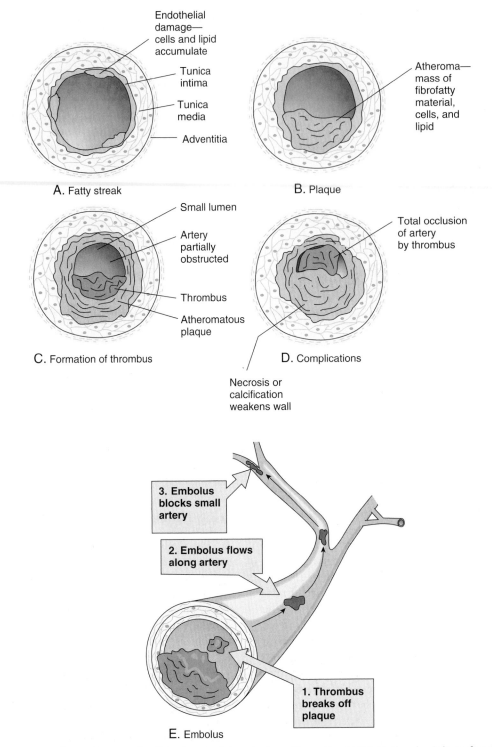

A. Fatty streak
- Endothelial damage— cells and lipid accumulate
- Tunica intima
- Tunica media
- Adventitia

B. Plaque
- Atheroma— mass of fibrofatty material, cells, and lipid

C. Formation of thrombus
- Small lumen
- Artery partially obstructed
- Thrombus
- Atheromatous plaque

D. Complications
- Total occlusion of artery by thrombus
- Necrosis or calcification weakens wall

E. Embolus
- 3. Embolus blocks small artery
- 2. Embolus flows along artery
- 1. Thrombus breaks off plaque

**Figure 3-3** Development of an atheroma leading to arterial occlusion. (From Gould BE. Pathophysiology for the Health Professions, ed 3. St. Louis, 2007, Saunders.)

plaques are composed of lipid and thrombus; the relative concentration of each varies widely from individual to individual (Fig. 3-3) In an effort to clarify this process, atherosclerosis is presented here as two processes—"atherosis" and "sclerosis"—that occur within the intima and endothelium of arterial walls. Undoubtedly, one of these components is more prominent than the other in each person who develops this disease. However, in very rare cases (homozygous familial

hypercholesterolemia), atherosis is the only cause of the obstructive lesion.

## Pathophysiology

### Atherosis

The first detectable lesion of atherosclerosis is the often discussed fatty streak, which consists of lipid-laden macrophages and smooth muscle cells. Fatty streaks have been found in the arteries of patients as young as 10 years of age, at the sites where major lesions appear later in life (see Fig. 3-3A).[14,15]

The development and progression of the fatty streak in humans can be inferred from the findings of animal studies. In such studies, fatty streaks have been found in the lining of the aorta within 12 days of the initiation of a high-fat, high-cholesterol diet. Clusters of monocytes have been found in junctional areas, between endothelial cells, where they accumulate lipid and are known as foam cells.[15,16] The subendothelial accumulation of these macrophages constitutes the first stage of fatty streak development. After several months, accumulations of lipid-laden macrophages grow so large that the endothelium is stretched and begins to separate over them (see Fig. 3-3B). Such endothelial separation exposes the intima-based lesion and the underlying connective tissue to the circulation. Consequently, platelets aggregate and thrombus forms at these locations, a hallmark characteristic of the "sclerotic" phase of atherosclerosis (see Fig. 3-3C).

## Sclerosis

The sclerotic components of the lesions of atherosclerosis are responsible for a reduction of blood vessel compliance. Atherosclerotic intimal lesions that produce symptoms or end-organ damage (ischemia or infarction in the organs fed by the vessel involved) invariably have a major fibrous component. Increased lesion collagen and destruction of medial elastin, in addition to changes in the composition of these fibrous proteins, are important mechanisms underlying sclerosis in atherosclerosis.[17,18] Pure atherosis (lipid deposition alone), such as that in fatty streaks, does not produce end-organ damage (except with homozygous familial hypercholesterolemia) but may contribute to sclerosis. The exposure of subendothelial structures to the raw material of thrombus formation and the subsequent effect of such exposure on endogenous factors such as endothelium-derived relaxation factor contribute to the process of sclerosis.

One of the long-standing theories of the development of the atherosclerotic lesion is that of encrustation, that is, the formation of an organized "fibrous cap" of thrombi over advanced plaques that have developed on the endothelial lining.[6,19,20] Although this theory has never adequately accounted for the exact origin of the lesions, it has always been considered an important part of the process because of findings of extensive thrombus formation on microscopic examination of these plaques. A "response-to-injury" hypothesis has been postulated in an effort to define the initial stages of development of the atherosclerotic plaque (see Fig. 3-3).[21,22]

Although the response-to-injury hypothesis does not identify the agent or process responsible for it, investigations of vasospasm have provided some clues to the origin.[23–27] Platelet-derived growth factor (PDGF) contributes to lesion formation in two ways. First, as the name implies, PDGF stimulates the replication of connective tissue cells in the areas in which it is released. Second, PDGF is a chemoattractant; when released from tissues at the site of endothelial injury, it attracts smooth muscle cells so that they migrate from the media into the intima.[28–30]

When examining patients who are diagnosed with atherosclerosis in one organ, one should keep in mind that atherosclerosis occurs throughout the body in large as well as small arteries based upon the disease process. Therefore, patients may have undiagnosed disease in other arteries because of a lack of presenting symptoms.

## Vasospasm

At the beginning of this century, Sir William Osler was the first to suggest that a basic abnormality existed in the smooth muscle of coronary arteries that were affected by atherosclerosis when he reported to the Royal College of Physicians: "We have, I think, evidence that sclerotic arteries are specially prone to spasm."[31] For the next 50 years, coronary vasospasm was considered only a minor factor in the myocardial blood flow equation. Prinzmetal and colleagues[32] first identified the connection between vasospasm and what they called "variant angina." Variant angina differs from "typical angina," as first described by Heberden,[2] in that it is associated with ST-segment elevation instead of depression, occurs at rest (typically in the early morning) instead of during a predictable level of activity, and is not associated with any preceding increase in myocardial oxygen demand. This syndrome, which became known as Prinzmetal angina, was similar to typical angina in that it was promptly relieved with nitroglycerin and other vasodilators. Subsequent investigators found that this syndrome was considerably more widespread than had been previously believed, and by 1976, the "proved hypothesis" of a vasospastic nonlesion cause for angina was widely accepted.[33]

It has long been known that hyperplasia of intimal smooth muscle cells is a hallmark of advanced atherosclerosis.[21,22,34] It should not be surprising, therefore, that coronary arteries so afflicted would be prone to spasm. Experiments have shown that if the endothelium of the coronary artery is damaged, the intimal smooth muscle constricts instead of relaxing when stimulated.[35,36] Although exactly what triggers this process continues to be inadequately understood, recent investigations have focused on the interactions of endothelial-derived relaxation factor (EDRF), endothelium-derived hyperpolarizing factor (EDHF), and endothelium-derived contracting factor (EDCF).[37–39]

## Risk Factors

The Framingham study[5] was the first to test relationships between genetic and behavioral factors and their contribution to the development of coronary atherosclerosis and CHD in a long-term, large-scale epidemiologic trial. As a result of the original Framingham study and subsequently many other studies, the AHA has identified several risk factors for coronary heart disease; some of these factors can be changed, although others cannot (Box 3-2).[1] Vita and colleagues[40] suggested that in addition to accelerating the disease process once it is established, risk factors may

## Box 3-2

### Risk Factors of Heart Disease

- Hypertension
- Smoking
- Elevated serum total cholesterol
  - Elevated LDL
  - Decreased high-density lipoprotein (HDL)
- Physical inactivity
- Family history
- Diabetes
- Stress
  - Personality factors of anger and hostility
- Obesity
- Age
- Sex
  - Male risk is higher until females reach menopause, then risk is equal

themselves constitute the "injury" in the response-to-injury hypothesis of Ross and Glomset.[21,22] Although the presence or absence of significant CAD cannot be determined by any simple arithmetic formula, there is considerable evidence to support the contention that the greater the number of risk factors present, the greater the likelihood that CAD, and ultimately CHD, will be present.[41–45] In addition to being risk factors of CAD, these are also the risk factors of the other vascular diseases that are discussed later in this chapter (carotid and vertebral disease, peripheral arterial disease).

## Major Risk Factors

The four modifiable major risk factors for coronary heart disease are cigarette/tobacco smoking, high blood pressure (hypertension), high blood cholesterol levels (hypercholesterolemia), and physical inactivity.[1] The three nonmodifiable risk factors are heredity, male sex, and increased age. Each of these risk factors not only has an additive effect on the ability of the other factors to contribute to the development of CAD and to subsequent CHD, but also exerts a multiplicative effect. Consequently, although each modifiable risk factor is discussed individually, it is critical to remember that these factors exist individually only in the isolation of the scientist's laboratory.

### Cigarette Smoking

One-fifth of all deaths related to heart disease are a result of cigarette smoking.[1,46] Cigarette smoking has been associated with increased risk of cardiovascular disease since 1958.[47] Although no one component of cigarette smoke has been identified as the causative agent for this association, a number of studies have shown how cigarette smoking has a deleterious effect on other known factors involved in the development of atherosclerosis.[48–51] As few as four cigarettes a day increases a smoker's risk of developing CAD and CHD above that of a nonsmoker or an ex-smoker.[52,53] In comparison to nonsmokers, smokers have been shown to manifest

leukocytosis, lower serum high-density lipoprotein (HDL) levels, elevated fibrinogen and plasma catecholamine levels, and increased blood pressure.[54,55] That similar alterations in the risk factor profiles of the preadolescent children of smoking parents have also been observed suggests that cigarette smoking increases the risk of developing CHD in both the smoker and the nonsmoking family members.[56,57]

### Hypertension

Hypertension, or high blood pressure, is known to be one of the most prevalent disease states in America, estimated to be present in 61 million people.[58–60] Hypertension, both systolic (over 140 mm Hg) and diastolic (over 90 mm Hg), is believed to be an independent risk factor for the development of CAD and peripheral and cerebral vascular disease.[61–63] So far, efforts to lower the morbidity and mortality rates associated with hypertension have proved better at reducing stroke than heart attack.[64,65] Such findings have led some investigators to believe that high blood pressure and coronary vascular disease merely coexist instead of influencing one another in a causal relationship.[66] Nonetheless, the epidemiologic evidence still overwhelmingly points to hypertension as a significant risk factor for the development of CAD.[1,67,68]

### Elevated Cholesterol

Since the first published results of the Framingham study, the direct link between abnormal levels of cholesterol and the development of CHD has been well established.[69,70] Several forms of cholesterol have been shown to play a role in atherogenesis: very-low-density lipoprotein (VLDL), intermediate-density lipoprotein (IDL), LDL, and lipoprotein a (LpA).[71–73] Direct dietary intake of cholesterol is not the principal influence on the level of cholesterol in the blood; instead, intake of saturated fat does influence the lipoproteins.[74–78] The cholesterol-to-saturated fat index (CSI) has proved to be a valuable clinical education tool because it clearly shows the discrepancy between dietary and serum levels of cholesterol.[79–81]

From the CSI formula (CSI = [1.01 × g saturated fat] + [0.05 × mg cholesterol]) it is clear that the contribution of saturated fat in any particular food item is about 20 times more atherogenic than its cholesterol content.

Other studies have documented the importance of HDL as an independent predictor of CHD risk.[82–84] Although the exact mechanism by which increased levels of HDL provide protection from coronary disease is poorly understood, several theories have been proposed. The concept of "reverse cholesterol transport"—bringing free cholesterol from the tissues back to the liver for safe storage—is most often cited.[85–92] The best predictor of risk for developing cholesterol-related blockages in an artery is the ratio of total cholesterol-to-HDL (CHOL/HDL); a ratio of greater than 4.5 increases an individual's risk of developing atherosclerosis.[93–95] Elevated triglycerides have also become a marker for the development of coronary atherosclerosis (>150 mg/dL), particularly when they are associated with low levels of HDL (<35 mg/dL).[96–98] Therefore, current consensus recommendations call for the following: in the absence of CAD and with fewer than two risk factors, target levels for LDL cholesterol should be 160 mg/dL; with more than two risk factors, 130 mg/dL; in the presence of CAD, 100 mg/dL. In individuals with hypertriglyceridemia the target level for triglycerides is 200 mg/dL.[74,99–101] In 2004 the National Cholesterol Education Program (NCEP) published treatment goals and intervention strategies for cholesterol testing and management and endorsed the use of the Framingham risk scoring (FRS) for identifying 10 year CHD risk (Fig. 3-4).[102] The risk factors used in this estimation of 10-year risk include age, total cholesterol, systolic blood pressure, HDL, and smoking.[103]

### Physical Inactivity

The role of exercise in the management of CHD has been acknowledged since Morris[104] reported a decreased incidence of myocardial infarction in conductors of British double-decker buses, when compared with drivers. Physical inactivity remains a significant risk factor for developing CHD and is comparable to that observed for high cholesterol, high blood pressure, or cigarette smoking.[1] The Centers for Disease Control and Prevention reported that lack of adequate exercise is the most prevalent risk factor for CHD and that more than 60% of adult Americans do not perform the minimum recommended amount of physical activity.[105–107] In addition, the prevalence of sedentary lifestyle in the United States was higher among women as compared to men, and higher among diabetics versus nondiabetics.[108]

There is more than ample evidence that regular aerobic exercise has a beneficial impact on many CHD risk factors.[109–114] The effects of regular aerobic exercise training on lipids and lipoproteins have been reviewed in several metaanalyses, yet controversy exists as to the amount of change that occurs in lipids as a result of exercise training. Kelley performed a metaanalysis on aerobic exercise and lipid changes and found that changes were equivalent to improvements of 2% for total cholesterol (TC) and HDL cholesterol (HDL-C), 3% of LDL cholesterol (LDL-C), and 9% for triglycerides (TG).[115] Carroll and Dudfield reported that regular aerobic exercise was effective in reducing TG (−18.7 mg/dL, −12%) and increasing HDL-C (1.6 mg/dL, +4.1%) in overweight and obese, sedentary adults with dyslipidemia.[116] Katzel and coworkers[117] showed that aerobic exercise coupled with weight training can yield reductions in plasma TG of 17% and LDL-C of 8%, in addition to increasing HDL-C by 11% (3.7 mg/dL). Although the amount of change may vary depending on the type of activity, evidence exists to conclude that activity does improve the lipid profile whether it is resistive, aerobic, or both.[118]

Some of the lesser-known benefits of long-term endurance training are an increase in fibrinolysis and red blood cell deformability, as well as a decrease in platelet aggregability,[119–124] which may be beneficial in preventing initial or subsequent coronary ischemic events. It has been shown that exercise of adequate intensity, duration, and frequency is beneficial in preventing cardiovascular disease and increasing longevity in the healthy population.[114,121,125–129]

## Contributing Risk Factors

The contributing risk factors are not independently significant in predicting the likelihood of an individual's developing CHD. As their name implies, however, they do play a role in its establishment and growth.

### Diabetes

Nonenzymatic glycosylation, or the chemical attachment of glucose to proteins without the involvement of enzymes, is known to affect fibrinogen, collagen, antithrombin III, HDL, and LDL, all of which are involved in the evolution of CAD.[130–132] The attachment of glucose to these molecules renders them less sensitive to the enzymes and other substances with which they interact. For example, antithrombin III activity, which normally inhibits excessive blood coagulation, is decreased when it undergoes glycosylation, and fibrinogen is less likely to perform its function of degrading fibrin when so affected. In both these cases, thrombus formation is enhanced. This process may even be the principal cause of basement membrane thickening, long known to be a major tissue change associated with prolonged diabetes (see Chapter 7).

The Adult Treatment Panel (ATP) III guidelines identified diabetes as a high-risk condition based upon the evidence demonstrating patients with diabetes have a relatively high 10-year risk for developing cardiovascular disease.[102] In addition, the Heart Protective Study (HPS) studied individuals who had both diabetes and cardiovascular disease and discovered that these individuals were at very high risk for future cardiovascular events, warranting intensive lipid-lowering therapy (goal of LDL < 70 mg dL).[133]

### Obesity

Several studies have associated obesity (body mass index [BMI] $\geq$ 30 kg/m$^2$) with the development of CHD.[134–136] This relationship appears to be more significant if the excess body fat is concentrated in the abdomen (central obesity) as opposed to being more evenly distributed throughout the body.[137,138] Nonetheless, it is difficult to prove that obesity is an independent risk factor for CAD because it is associated with so many other risk factors, such as hypertension, diabetes, and sedentary lifestyle.

### Family History

Family history of CHD, defined as its presence in a parent or sibling, has been shown to be a minor risk factor for the development of CAD.[139–142] With the exception of the

**Framingham Point Scores by Age Group**

| Age | Points | |
|---|---|---|
| | Male | Female |
| 20-34 | −9 | −7 |
| 35-39 | −4 | −3 |
| 40-44 | 0 | 0 |
| 45-49 | 3 | 3 |
| 50-54 | 6 | 6 |
| 55-59 | 8 | 8 |
| 60-64 | 10 | 10 |
| 65-69 | 11 | 12 |
| 70-74 | 12 | 14 |
| 75-79 | 13 | 16 |

**Framingham Point Scores by Age Group and Total Cholesterol**

| Total cholesterol, mg/dL | 20-39 years | | 40-49 years | | 50-59 years | | 60-69 years | | 70-79 years | |
|---|---|---|---|---|---|---|---|---|---|---|
| | M | F | M | F | M | F | M | F | M | F |
| <160 | 0 | 0 | 0 | 0 | 0 | 0 | 0 | 0 | 0 | 0 |
| 160-199 | 4 | 4 | 3 | 3 | 2 | 2 | 1 | 1 | 0 | 1 |
| 200-239 | 7 | 8 | 5 | 6 | 3 | 4 | 1 | 2 | 0 | 1 |
| 240-279 | 9 | 11 | 6 | 8 | 4 | 5 | 2 | 3 | 1 | 2 |
| 280+ | 11 | 13 | 8 | 10 | 5 | 7 | 3 | 4 | 1 | 2 |

M, Male; F, Female

**Framingham Point Scores by Age and Smoking Status**

| | 20-39 years | | 40-49 years | | 50-59 years | | 60-69 years | | 70-79 years | |
|---|---|---|---|---|---|---|---|---|---|---|
| | M | F | M | F | M | F | M | F | M | F |
| Nonsmoker | 0 | 0 | 0 | 0 | 0 | 0 | 0 | 0 | 0 | 0 |
| Smoker | 8 | 9 | 5 | 7 | 3 | 4 | 1 | 2 | 1 | 1 |

M, Male; F, Female

**Framingham Point Scores by HDL Level**

| HDL | Points | |
|---|---|---|
| | Male | Female |
| 60+ | −1 | −1 |
| 50-59 | 0 | 0 |
| 40-49 | 1 | 1 |
| <40 | 2 | 2 |

**Framingham Point Scores by Systolic Blood Pressure and Treatment Status**

| Systolic BP | Untreated | | Treated | |
|---|---|---|---|---|
| | Male | Female | Male | Female |
| <120 | 0 | 0 | 0 | 0 |
| 120-129 | 0 | 1 | 1 | 3 |
| 130-139 | 1 | 2 | 2 | 4 |
| 140-159 | 1 | 3 | 2 | 5 |
| 160+ | 2 | 4 | 3 | 6 |

**10-Year Risk by Total Framingham Point Scores**

| Male | | Female | |
|---|---|---|---|
| Point Total | 10-Year Risk | Point Total | 10-Year Risk |
| <0 | < 1% | < 9 | < 1% |
| 0 | 1% | 9 | 1% |
| 1 | 1% | 10 | 1% |
| 2 | 1% | 11 | 1% |
| 3 | 1% | 12 | 1% |
| 4 | 1% | 13 | 2% |
| 5 | 2% | 14 | 2% |
| 6 | 2% | 15 | 3% |
| 7 | 3% | 16 | 4% |
| 8 | 4% | 17 | 5% |
| 9 | 5% | 18 | 6% |
| 10 | 6% | 19 | 8% |
| 11 | 8% | 20 | 11% |
| 12 | 10% | 21 | 14% |
| 13 | 12% | 22 | 17% |
| 14 | 16% | 23 | 22% |
| 15 | 20% | 24 | 27% |
| 16 | 25% | 25 or more | ≥30% |
| 17 or more | ≥30% | | |

From National Cholesterol Education Program(NCEP). Executive summary of the third report of the Expert Panel on Detection, Evaluation and Treatment of High Cholesterol in Adults (Adult Treatment Panel III). JAMA 2001; 285:2486-2497.

**Figure 3-4** Estimate of 10-year risk for men and women based upon Framingham study. (From National Cholesterol Education Program (NCEP). Executive summary of the third report of the Expert Panel on Detection, Evaluation and Treatment of High Cholesterol in Adults (Adult Treatment Panel III). JAMA 285:2486–2497, 2001.)

familial hypercholesterolemias, no genetic link has been established for CHD; like obesity, the atherogenic contribution of family history is not entirely genetic. Fortunately, the modification of risk factors in subjects with a strong family history of premature coronary disease provides a reduction in overall risk of developing subsequent disease.[143,144] Premature or early coronary disease is defined as men younger than age 50 years and women younger than age 60 years, but the AHA defines family history as significant if either parent (genetic linked parents) had a diagnosis of heart disease (first event of myocardial infarction [MI], angina, coronary artery bypass graft [CABG] or percutaneous transluminal coronary angioplasty [PTCA]) at an age younger than 60 years. Although the Framingham Score (see Fig. 3-4) does not take into account family history, most experts report a premature or early family history of heart disease doubles one's risk for cardiovascular disease.[145,146]

Although scientific literature has not established a genetic link with HDL cholesterol specifically, there appear to be findings of lower HDL and higher total CHOL/HDL ratios in offspring of individuals with CHD. Another genetic theory involves a possible inheritance of platelet stickiness in individuals with CHD. The current theory is to recommend aspirin use on a long-term basis in offspring with a strong family CHD history, as well as to monitor C reactive protein levels (an antiinflammatory marker) in individuals with a positive family history.[145-148]

### Age

Increased age (older than 65 years) is known to be a risk factor for CHD.[149] Whether older age is an independent pathologic process or simply a consequence of prolonged exposure to the risk factors is less clear. Studies show that interventions on other risk factors have proved to be beneficial in older subsets of patients and have resulted in the reduction of clinical end points, for example, MI and symptoms.[150,151] Also, both patients and subjects without known disease in the young-old and middle-old age groups (ages 67 to 76 years) have responded to the same extent as young subjects to attempts at risk factor reduction.[152-154]

Although biochemical changes are known to occur as people age—for example, decreased nerve conduction velocity and decreased aerobic enzyme activity—the functional significance of these changes appears to be negligible if they are not complicated by preexisting disease.[155,156]

### Gender

It is a common perception that premenopausal women are "immune" from CHD. Men are six times more likely than women to experience a MI before age 55 years,[83,157-159] and the overall onset of clinically significant coronary heart disease in women lags 10 years behind that in men.[160-162]

Although it is true that, in general, women experience lower CHD morbidity and mortality rates than men do, this disease still represents a significant health risk to women. Coronary heart disease is the second leading cause of death in all women younger than age 45 years; it is the leading cause

of death in black women younger than 45 years, an age when the majority are still premenopausal.[160,163-166] In terms of age group, the largest "gain" in either sex during which the greatest increase in CHD occurs is in women ages 55 to 64 years.[167-169] Once a MI occurs, women of all age groups have a higher mortality rate than men. Slightly more women have unrecognized or "silent" MIs than men (34% vs. 27%), but interestingly, the initial clinical event in women is most often angina, whereas in men it is an acute MI. Women who have diabetes are more susceptible to developing CHD than are men.[170-172] Because the gap between CHD incidence in men and women closes between the fifth and sixth decades, it has been argued that menopause plays some nonspecific role in regulating this disease process. It has been found, however, that the risk of developing CHD is no different in women who had natural menopause, were premenopausal, or had "surgical" menopause and were undergoing estrogen replacement therapy. Estrogen is a factor, however, for it was noted that women who had surgical menopause but did not take estrogen replacement therapy did have a significant increase in the incidence of CHD.[163,173] Females who develop preeclampsia during pregnancy are also identified at increased risk of cardiovascular disease (CVD), as they are more likely to develop hypertension and cerebrovascular disease.[174] Women who also develop placental problems during pregnancy and who have traditional cardiovascular risk factors, including prepregnancy hypertension, diabetes mellitus, obesity, dyslipidemia, or metabolic syndrome, are also defined as elevated risk for CVD.[174]

In the absence of a family history of breast cancer, estrogen replacement is recommended in all younger peri- and postmenopausal (age at menopause: <55 years) women with a family history of CHD. Hormone therapy (HT) reduces the risk of CHD events in younger postmenopausal women (age at menopause: <55 years). In older women, HT increases risk in first year, then decreases risk after 2 years.[175-179] The AHA guidelines for hormone replacement report that hormone therapy and selective estrogen-receptor modulators (SERMs) should not be used for the primary or secondary prevention of CVD.[180]

### Stress

Although the pathogenesis may not have been defined, Friedman and Rosenman[181] related the sense of time urgency and easily aroused hostility to a sevenfold increase in prevalence of CHD—what they termed type A behavior. Therefore, the personality characteristics of hostility and anger may be more descriptive than the traditional term "type A behavior." The identification of what has been termed type A behavior, as an independent risk factor for CHD, is still being debated.[182-184] The exact mechanism by which this predominantly psychological trait increases the risk for the tissue changes of CHD is believed to be related to platelet activation. This contribution to the sclerotic component of CHD is known to be related to increases in levels of catecholamine and platelet-secreted proteins, which have been found in subjects undergoing emotional stress.[185,186] It is known also that alterations in this type A behavior can reduce morbidity and mortality rates for post-MI patients.[91]

> **Clinical Tip**
> Psychosocial distress is also associated with increased mortality and morbidity rates after MI. In addition, social isolation and depression are associated with a poor prognosis after MI. These findings should emphasize the importance of identifying this risk factor prior to rehabilitation to ensure it is addressed in the total rehabilitation of the patient.

## Emerging Risk Factors

Additional risk factors for atherosclerotic disease that may or may not have a role in thrombus development or initiation of atherosclerosis include the following:[187–190]

- Lipoprotein a (Lp[a]),
- LDL subclasses,
- Oxidized LDL,
- Homocysteine,
- Hematologic factors (primarily fibrinogen, factor VII, and tissue plasminogen activator [tPA]),
- Inflammatory markers such as C-reactive protein (CRP), and
- Infective agents such as *Chlamydia pneumoniae*.

Each of these risk factors are discussed is greater detail in Chapter 8 in the clinical laboratory section. Lp(a) appears to have an atherogenic and prothrombic effect that interferes with plasminogen and tPA binding to fibrin. Lp(a) levels are thought to be genetic in origin, and were found in 50% of the offspring of patients with CAD in the Framingham study.[187] Increased Lp(a) levels are associated with a threefold increase in the risk of a primary CAD event.[187] In addition to Lp(a), the presence of an elevated amount of small dense LDL particle subtype (phenotype B) is also associated with an elevated risk for CAD (threefold increased risk).[187,188] Small dense LDL is also associated with elevated triglyceride levels.

Homocysteine, which is a type of amino acid found in the blood, has been linked to increased risk of development of cardiovascular diseases when the levels in the blood are elevated.[189,190]

Individuals with elevated CRP levels, especially those in the highest quartile, might benefit from more aggressive long-term dietary, lifestyle, and coronary risk factor modification than would be the standard of care in a primary prevention population. and resulting fibrosis could predispose an individual to sudden cardiac death.[191]

## Clinical Course

The clinical presentation of the patient with CHD typically occurs in one of four ways:
- Sudden cardiac death
- Chronic stable angina
- Acute coronary syndrome (ACS), an umbrella term used to define acute myocardial ischemia that is further divided into three components:

> **Box 3-3**
>
> **Risk Factors Associated with Sudden Death**
>
> | **Undiagnosed CHD Population** | **Diagnosed CHD Population** |
> |---|---|
> | Age | Decreased left ventricular ejection fraction (LVEF) (<35%) |
> | Systolic Blood pressure (elevated) | |
> | Left ventricular hypertrophy | |
> | Intraventricular block on ECG | |
> | Nonspecific ECG abnormalities | |
> | Serum Cholesterol (elevated) | |
> | Heart rate (elevated resting HR) | |
> | Vital capacity (low, especially a factor in females) | |
> | Cigarettes consumed daily | |
> | Relative weight | |

The ventricular fibrillation (VF) sudden cardiac arrest survival rate is only 2 to 5% if defibrillation is provided more than 12 minutes after collapse.[1] Early cardiopulmonary resuscitation (CPR) and rapid defibrillation combined with early advanced care can produce high long-term survival rates for witnessed cardiac arrest. In some cities with public access defibrillation or "community AED programs," when bystanders provide immediate CPR and the first shock is delivered within 3 to 5 minutes, the reported survival rates from VF sudden cardiac arrest are as high as 48% to 74%.[1]

- Unstable angina
- ST-segment elevation myocardial infarction (STEMI)
- Non-STEMI
- Cardiac muscle dysfunction (see Chapter 4)

## Sudden Cardiac Death

In 40% of patients with CHD, sudden cardiac death (SCD; death within 1 hour of onset of symptoms) is the initial presenting syndrome.[192] Of all SCDs, 50% occur among the 10% of the population with the highest number of risk factors. Ventricular tachycardia and ventricular fibrillation, leading to cessation of cardiac output, are the usual cause of death. Box 3-3 lists the risk factors for SCD. For these patients, prompt delivery of bystander cardiopulmonary resuscitation with an automatic external defibrillator (AED) and entry into the emergency medical system within 10 minutes is their only chance of survival.[1,193,194]

## Angina

The majority of patients with CHD first seek medical attention because of angina (an Old English term meaning "strangling") pectoris. This sensation, most commonly described as a substernal pressure, can occur anywhere from the epigastric area to the jaw and is described as squeezing, tightness, or crushing (Fig. 3-5). It is now known to be caused by an imbalance in supply and demand of myocardial oxygen. Table 3-1 lists the types of chest discomfort.

## Chronic Stable Angina

Chronic stable angina, as its name implies, usually has a well-established level of onset and is the result of not enough blood supply to meet the metabolic demand (Fig. 3-6). Patients are able to predict reliably those activities that

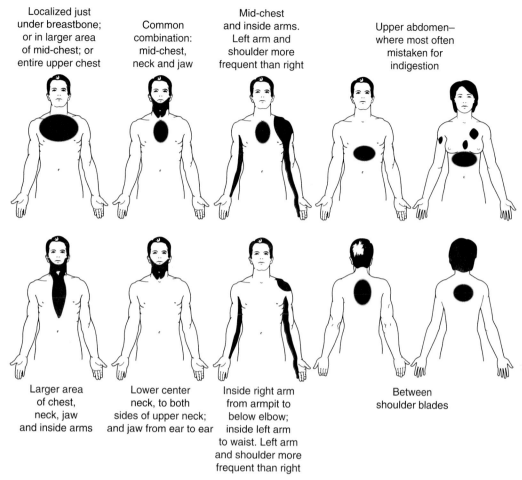

Localized just under breastbone; or in larger area of mid-chest; or entire upper chest

Common combination: mid-chest, neck and jaw

Mid-chest and inside arms. Left arm and shoulder more frequent than right

Upper abdomen– where most often mistaken for indigestion

Larger area of chest, neck, jaw and inside arms

Lower center neck, to both sides of upper neck; and jaw from ear to ear

Inside right arm from armpit to below elbow; inside left arm to waist. Left arm and shoulder more frequent than right

Between shoulder blades

**Most common warning signs of heart attack**

- Uncomfortable pressure, fullness, squeezing or pain in the center of the chest (prolonged)
- Pain that spreads to the throat, neck, back, jaw, shoulders, or arms
- Chest discomfort with lightheadedness, dizziness, sweating, pallor, nausea, or shortness of breath
- Prolonged symptoms unrelieved by antacids, nitroglycerin, or rest

**Atypical, less common warning signs (especially women)**

- Unusual chest pain (quality, location, e.g., burning, heaviness; left chest), stomach or abdominal pain
- Continuous midthoracic or interscapular pain
- Continuous neck or shoulder pain
- Isolated right biceps pain
- Pain relieved by antacids; pain unrelieved by rest or nitroglycerin
- Nausea and vomiting; flu-like manifestation without chest pain/discomfort
- Unexplained intense anxiety, weakness, or fatigue
- Breathlessness, dizziness

**Figure 3-5** Early warning signs of a heart attack. Multiple segmental nerve innervation shown in accounts for the varied pain patterns possible. A woman can experience any of the various patterns described but is more likely to develop atypical symptoms of pain as depicted here. (From Goodman CC. Pathology: Implications for the Physical Therapists, ed 3. St. Louis, 2009, Saunders.)

provoke their discomfort; this condition is usually associated with a set level of myocardial oxygen demand. As mentioned earlier, myocardial oxygen demand is closely related to heart rate and systolic blood pressure. By multiplying these values, the so-called double product or rate pressure product (RPP), an index that is useful in correlating functional activities with myocardial capabilities, can be obtained. Wall stress, the third determinant of the myocardial oxygen consumption ($MVO_2$) rate, can be accurately measured only with invasive monitoring and is therefore not usually available to the patient performing routine activities.

Patients with stable angina are usually able to bring their symptoms under control by reducing slightly the intensity of the exercise they are performing or by taking sublingual nitroglycerin. Patients have some variability in their tolerance for activity—that is, they have "good days and bad days"—which is probably related to variations in coronary vascular tone, but overall, stable angina is a predictable syndrome.

## Acute Coronary Syndrome

The term *acute coronary syndrome* is increasingly used to describe patients who present with either unstable angina (UA) or acute myocardial infarction (AMI). UA is chest discomfort that is accelerating in frequency or severity and may occur while at rest but does not result in myocardial necrosis. The discomfort may be more severe and prolonged

## Table 3-1 Types of Angina and Other Chest Pain

| Types | Descriptors |
|---|---|
| Classic stable angina | Described as tightness, pressure, indigestion anywhere above waist (substernum, neck, left arm, right arm, cervical, between shoulder blades) that develops with exertional activity and diminishes with rest or nitroglycerin (NTG). |
| | Women typically complain of nausea, indigestion, discomfort between shoulder blades, or excessive fatigue. |
| | Individuals with diabetes often complain of shortness of breath. |
| Unstable angina (UA) | Chest discomfort that is accelerating in frequency or severity and may occur while at rest but does not result in myocardial necrosis. The discomfort may be more severe and prolonged than typical angina pain or may be the first time a person has angina pain. |
| Prinzmetal angina | Chest discomfort associated with ST-segment elevation instead of depression, occurs at rest (typically in the early morning) instead of during a predictable level of activity, and is not associated with any preceding increase in myocardial oxygen demand. |
| Pericarditis | Pain at rest, may worsen with activity, but is not relieved with rest or NTG. Responds to antiinflammatory medications. |
| | Common in post-CABG patients. |
| Chest wall pain (musculoskeletal) | Pain/discomfort that is increased with palpation over chest wall. |
| Pulmonary/pleuritic | Pain/discomfort that changes with breathing. |
| Bronchospasm | Exertionally related or induced by cold, extreme difficulty breathing, relieved with bronchodilator or stopping of activity. |

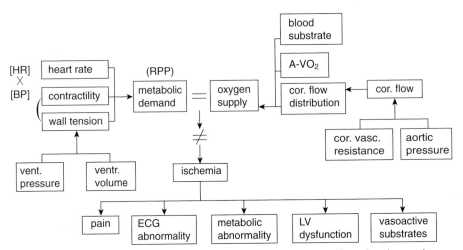

**Figure 3-6** Factors that affect the supply of blood to the heart and factors that affect the demand or workload on the heart muscle. Ischemia results when there is an imbalance in supply and demand and an individual will often perceive symptoms of angina.

than typical angina pain or may be the first time a person has angina pain. UA and AMI share common pathophysiologic origins related to coronary plaque progression, instability, or rupture with or without luminal thrombosis and vasospasm.).[1]

Decisions about medical and interventional treatments are based on specific findings noted when a patient presents with ACS. Such patients are classified clinically into one of three categories, according to the presence or absence of ST-segment elevation on the presenting ECG and abnormal

("positive") elevations of myocardial biomarkers such as troponins as follows:

- UA
- STEMI and
- Non-STEMI

UA, can be defined as the presence of signs or symptoms of an inadequate blood supply to the myocardium in the absence of the demands that usually provoke such an imbalance (usually at rest, often waking an individual in the middle of the night). The patient who presents with UA or has

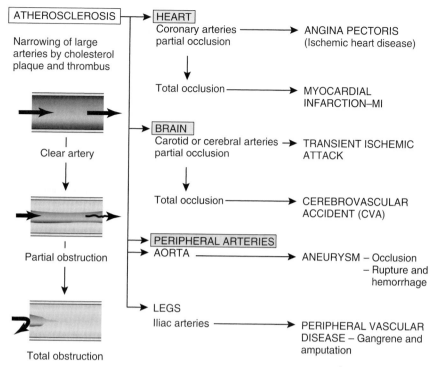

**Figure 3-7** Possible consequences of atherosclerosis. (From Gould BE. Pathophysiology for the Health Professions, ed 3. St. Louis, 2007, Saunders.)

chronic stable angina that develops an unstable pattern (see later discussion) requires quick recognition and referral for treatment. Although the allied health professional is not responsible for making the diagnosis of UA, he or she may be the person who first detects its presence while following a patient in a cardiac rehabilitation program. It is therefore important for such professionals to have a basic understanding of the mechanisms of UA and know how to detect it.

Patients who have UA are known to have increased morbidity and mortality rates when compared with those who have stable angina, even though the absolute amount of coronary atherosclerosis in both groups is not significantly different.[195,196] The major physiologic difference between unstable and chronic stable angina is the absence of an increase in myocardial oxygen demand to provoke the syndrome. Chierchia and colleagues proved that imbalances in myocardial blood flow could be related to a primary reduction in oxygen supply without an increase in demand.[197] They were able to show that a fall in cardiac vein oxygen saturation always preceded the electrocardiographic or hemodynamic indicators of ischemia in 137 patients who experienced angina while at rest.

### Factors That Contribute to Unstable Angina

Several factors have been implicated as contributors to this syndrome. Circadian variations in catecholamine levels (e.g., epinephrine), which increase heart rate and blood pressure; increases in plasma viscosity, known to occur in the first 4 hours of awakening; increases in platelet activation; and pathologic changes in the atherosclerotic plaques themselves all have been proposed as triggers of UA.[198–200]

The atherosclerotic plaque is known to undergo physical changes when a patient is experiencing UA (Fig. 3-7). There are distinct differences in the morphology of atherosclerotic lesions of persons who are experiencing UA compared with that of persons who have stable angina.[201,202] Recent developments in fiberoptic technology have allowed direct visual inspection of coronary atherosclerotic lesions, thus permitting differentiation of plaques by their appearance.

Because coronary plaque is a dynamic entity and not just a mound of debris, the stability of the disease can be altered quickly. Several clinical clues to the development of UA should alert the health professional to notify a patient's physician:

- Angina at rest
- Occurrence of the patient's typical angina at a significantly lower level of activity than usual
- Deterioration of a previously stable pattern, for example, discomfort occurring several times a day compared with several times a week
- Evidence of loss of previously present myocardial reserve, such as a drop in blood pressure or increase in heart rate with levels of activity previously well tolerated

UA should be distinguished from Prinzmetal or vasospastic angina (see Table 3-1). Both are most likely to occur in the first few hours of rising, but vasospastic discomfort is usually not as severe and is often relieved with minor activity, whereas UA is not. Patients with vasospastic angina are able to perform high levels of work later in the day without discomfort, but patients with UA are unable to increase their cardiac output significantly without provoking further discomfort, even if their earlier pain has waned.

Up to this point, consideration has been given only to primary prevention schemes. The reader must not lose sight of the fact that although the number of Americans dying from heart disease is decreasing, the number of those living with heart disease is increasing. Primary health care providers must realize that those risk factor modification interventions that have proved so effective for the primary prevention of CAD and CHD are also applicable to secondary prevention and should be incorporated into the plan of care (see Chapter 18).

### Other Acute Coronary Syndrome: STEMI and Non-STEMI

ACS refers to symptoms that signify acute myocardial ischemia and/ or infarction as a result of insufficient supply to the heart muscle. Individuals with symptoms of insufficient blood supply to the myocardium will be given an ECG to look for STEMI or other ECG changes indicative of ischemia or infarction (non-STEMI or UA). A STEMI develops a Q wave on the ECG in the subsequent 24 to 48 hours and these previously were defined as Q wave or transmural (full or near-full thickness) infarctions. Thirty-two percent of ACSs are STEMI.[1] A STEMI with transmural injury occurs distal to a totally occluded coronary artery that has become occluded secondary to a thrombus that occluded an area of plaque or ruptured plaque. However, other factors may affect the extent of injury, including whether or not collateral flow exists in the area, and whether or not vasospasm also occurred to complete the blockage of the area with plaque and thrombus. A non-STEMI does not develop a Q wave on the ECG and has been referred to as a non–Q-wave infarction or subendocardial (nontransmural or affecting only the subendocardial region) infarction. Current studies using magnetic resonance imaging actually show that the development of a Q wave on the ECG is caused by the size of the infarct and not the depth of the mural involvement (see Figs. 3-3D and 3-3E).[203]

The actual progression of atherosclerosis may be gradual, or may be sudden. In the case of sudden change in plaque, the plaque may disrupt and promote platelet aggregation, thrombus generation and thrombus formation. The thrombus may interrupt blood flow temporarily by becoming lodged in a soft lipid-laden or hard plaque-laden area of a coronary artery, which, in turn, interrupts supply of oxygen to the myocardium and possibly myocardial necrosis. If the blood flow interruption is less than 30 minutes the patient may experience symptoms of UA with myocardial ischemia, and demonstrate reversible changes in the myocardial tissue, therefore leading to a non-STEMI. Non-STEMIs often occur when coronary arteries are not completely blocked but have severely narrowed diameters and are at risk of becoming completely blocked (Fig. 3-8).[204] Identification of the location of the injury/infarction is made on the 12-lead ECG based upon the leads that demonstrate the ST elevation (for STEMIs) or ST depression or T-wave changes (in non-STEMIs) (Table 3-2).

When reperfusion of myocardium undergoing the evolutionary changes from ischemia to infarction occurs sufficiently early (i.e., within 15 to 20 minutes), it can suc-

cessfully prevent necrosis from developing. Beyond this early stage, the number of salvaged myocytes and therefore the amount of salvaged myocardial tissue (area of necrosis/area at risk) relates directly to the length of time of total coronary artery occlusion, the level of myocardial oxygen consumption, and the collateral blood flow (Fig. 3-9). Typically reperfused infarcts show a mixture of necrosis, hemorrhage within zones of irreversibly injured myocytes, coagulative necrosis with contraction bands, and distorted architecture of the cells in the reperfused zone. After reperfusion, when areas have become necrotic, mitochondria may develop deposits of calcium phosphate. Reperfusion of infarcted myocardium also promotes removal of intracellular proteins, resulting in an exaggerated and early peak value of substances such as creatine kinase-myocardial bound (CK-MB) and cardiac-specific troponin T and I. Table 3-3 describes changes that occur in first few hours to weeks.

For the nonatherosclerotic causes of MI see Table 3-4. Pathologic processes other than atherosclerosis can result in STEMI (see Table 3-4). These processes include embolization, inflammatory processes, infection, radiation, and vasospasm.[204] Cocaine abuse has become one of the more frequent causes of vasospastic-induced MI in patients with and without coronary artery disease.

### Medical Management of Acute Coronary Syndrome

The primary concern for management of the ACS is to reperfuse the area of the heart not receiving enough blood and oxygen, as well as to control for cardiac pain, limit any amount of necrosis, and prevent complications. Early reperfusion is accomplished with fibrinolysis (thrombolytic agents) and PTCA if the individual enters into the emergency room or receives emergency care with an ambulance or emergency medical technician within 3 hours of the onset of intense chest pain (the earlier the reperfusion, the less the necrosis and the better the prognosis). The other general treatment measures include:[204]

- Aspirin
- Control of cardiac pain
  - Use of nitrates
  - Use of morphine
  - Use of β blockers
- Improve oxygenation
  - Use of oxygen
- Limitation of infarct size
  - Early reperfusion
- Prophylaxis for arrhythmias
  - Use of lidocaine or amiodarone
- Control of other complications
  - Treatment for heart block with temporary or permanent pacemaker
  - Treatment of left ventricular dysfunction

### Complications with STEMI and Non-STEMI

Upon interruption of flow in an epicardial coronary artery, the zone of myocardium supplied by that vessel (Fig. 3-10) immediately loses its ability to shorten and perform

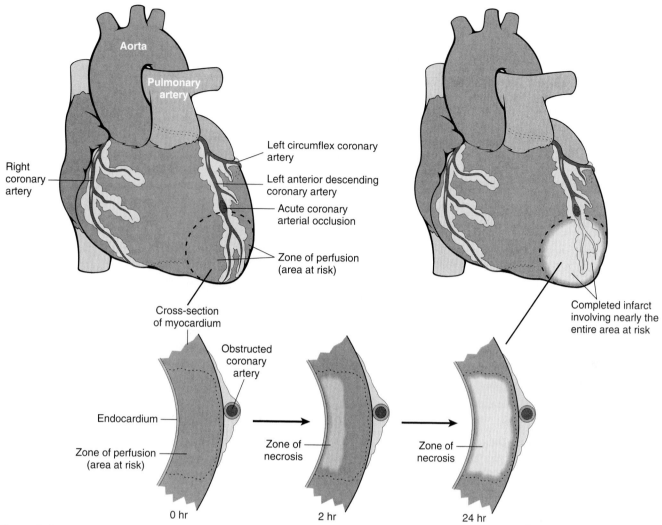

**Figure 3-8** Progression of myocardial necrosis after coronary artery occlusion. Necrosis begins in a small zone of the myocardium beneath the endocardial surface in the center of the ischemic zone. The area that depends on the occluded vessel for perfusion is the "at risk" myocardium (shaded). Note that a very narrow zone of myocardium immediately beneath the endocardium is spared from necrosis because it can be oxygenated by diffusion from the ventricle. (From Kumar V, Abbas AK, Fausto N, et al. (eds.). Robbins and Cotran Pathologic Basis of Disease, ed 8. St. Louis, 2010, Saunders.)

## Table 3-2  Coronary Anatomy and Location of Infarction

| Anatomy | Location of Infarct | ECG Changes | Common Complications |
|---|---|---|---|
| Right coronary artery | Inferior | II, III, aVF | ↑ Risk of atrioventricular block and/or arrhythmias |
| | | | 50% have right ventricular infarct |
| Left main | Anterior and lateral | V1-V6, I, aVL | Pump dysfunction or failure |
| Left anterior descending (LAD) | Anterior | V1-V4 | Pump dysfunction or failure |
| Circumflex | Lateral | V5, V6, aVL, I | None specific |

contractile work. Four abnormal contraction patterns develop in sequence: (1) dyssynchrony, that is, dissociation in the time course of contraction of adjacent segments; (2) hypokinesis, reduction in the extent of shortening; (3) akinesis, cessation of shortening; and (4) dyskinesis, paradoxical expansion, and systolic bulging.[205,206] Hyperkinesis of the

remaining normal myocardium initially accompanies dysfunction of the infarcting segment. The early hyperkinesis of the noninfarcted zones likely results from acute compensations including increased activity of the sympathetic nervous system and the Frank-Starling mechanism.[204] When the abnormally contracting segment exceeds 15%, the stroke

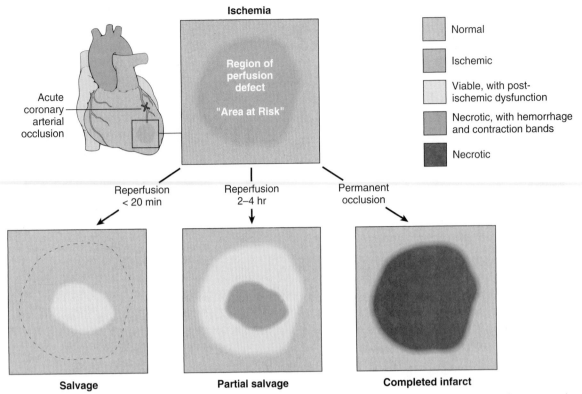

**Figure 3-9** Schematic illustration of the progression of myocardial ischemic injury and its modification by restoration of flow (reperfusion). Hearts suffering brief periods of ischemia of longer than 20 minutes followed by reperfusion do not develop necrosis (reversible injury). Brief ischemia followed by reperfusion results in stunning. If coronary occlusion is extended beyond 20 minutes' duration, a wavefront of necrosis progresses from subendocardium to subepicardium over time. Reperfusion before 3 to 6 hours of ischemia salvages ischemic but viable tissue. This salvaged tissue may also demonstrate stunning. Reperfusion beyond 6 hours does not appreciably reduce myocardial infarct size. (From Kumar V, Abbas AK, Fausto N, et al. (eds.). Robbins and Cotran Pathologic Basis of Disease, ed 8. St. Louis, 2010, Saunders.)

## Table 3-3 Progression of STEMI

| Timeline | Pathophysiologic Changes |
|---|---|
| First hours | Myocardial injury is potentially reversible for the first 30 min after onset |
| | Progressive loss of viable tissue from 30 min up to 6 to 12 hrs post onset |
| | Zones of necrosis identified as early as 2 to 3 hrs post-MI |
| First days | Affected myocardium is pale and swollen |
| | 18 to 36 hrs post-MI erythrocytes are trapped |
| | 48 hrs post-MI neutrophils infiltrate |
| First weeks | 8 to 10 days post-MI thickness of infracted cardiac wall ↓ |
| | Mononuclear cells remove necrotic muscle |
| | From 3 wks to 3 to 4 mons infracted area converts to shrunken thin firm scar |

volume may decline, reflected in a decline in ejection fraction (EF) and elevations of LVEDP and volume (LVEDV) occur.[204] A lower stroke volume will also lower the aortic pressure and subsequently reduce coronary perfusion pressure that may ultimately intensify myocardial ischemia, thereby initiating a vicious circle. The risk of developing physical signs and symptoms of left ventricular failure also increase proportionally to increasing areas of abnormal left ventricular wall motion.[206] Clinical heart failure accompanies areas of abnormal contraction exceeding 25%, and cardiogenic shock, often fatal, accompanies loss of more than 40% of the left ventricular myocardium.

Over several weeks, end-diastolic volume increases and diastolic pressure begins to fall toward normal. As with impairment of systolic function, the magnitude of the diastolic abnormality appears to relate to the size of the infarct. Regardless of the age of the infarct, patients who continue to demonstrate abnormal wall motion of 20% to 25% of the left ventricle will likely demonstrate hemodynamic signs of left ventricular failure, and as a result will have a poor prognosis for long-term survival.[204]

Other common complications that occur with STEMIs include persistent angina and arrhythmias due to persistent ischemia possibly in other coronary arteries. Table 3-5 has a

## Table 3-4 Nonatherosclerotic Causes of Acute Myocardial Infarction

| Cause of MI | Etiology of Cause |
|---|---|
| Embolization | Infective endocarditis |
| | Nonbacterial thrombotic endocarditis |
| | Mural thrombi |
| | Prosthetic valves |
| | Neoplasm |
| | Air secondary to cardiac surgery |
| | Calcium deposits from calcified valves during surgery |
| Thrombosis | From chest wall trauma |
| Inflammatory process | Viral infections (Coxsackie B Virus) |
| | Syphilitic aortitis |
| | Takayasu arteritis |
| | Necrotizing arteritis |
| | Polyarteritis nodosa |
| | Kawasaki disease |
| | Systemic lupus erythematosus (SLE) |
| Mediastinal radiation | |
| Amyloidosis | |
| Homocystinuria | |
| Hurler syndrome | |
| Severe vasospasm | Cocaine abuse |

From American Heart Association, Emergency Cardiac Care Committee and Subcommittees. Guidelines for cardiopulmonary resuscitation and emergency cardiac care. Part IX. Ensuring effectiveness of communitywide emergency cardiac care. JAMA 268:2289–2295, 1992.

full list of complications that may occur in other organs with STEMI. Knowing the complications the individual might have or has demonstrated as a result of the STEMI will affect hospital course and prognosis. Criteria for a complicated post-MI hospital course was defined by McNeer and coworkers and includes the following (complications should have occurred within first 24 to 48 hours):[207]

• Ventricular tachycardia and fibrillation
• Atrial flutter or fibrillation
• Second- or third-degree atrioventricular (AV) block
• Persistent sinus tachycardia (above 100 beats per minute)
• Persistent systolic hypotension (below 90 mm Hg)
• Pulmonary edema
• Cardiogenic shock
• Persistent angina or extension of infarction

Patients who were characterized as "uncomplicated" had significantly lower morbidity and mortality rates following their initial cardiac events. A prolonged or complicated

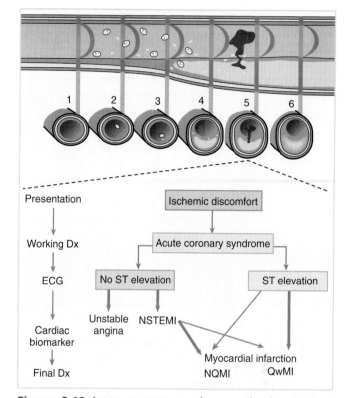

**Figure 3-10** Acute coronary syndromes. The longitudinal section of an artery depicts the "timeline" of atherogenesis from (1) a normal artery, to (2) lesion initiation and accumulation of extracellular lipid in the intima, to (3) the evolution to the fibrofatty stage, to (4) lesion progression with procoagulant expression and weakening of the fibrous cap. An acute coronary syndrome develops when the vulnerable or high-risk plaque undergoes disruption of the fibrous cap (5); disruption of the plaque is the stimulus for thrombogenesis. Thrombus resorption may be followed by collagen accumulation and smooth muscle cell growth (6). CK-MB, MB isoenzyme of creatine kinase; Dx, diagnosis; NQMI, non–Q-wave myocardial infarction; QwMI, Q-wave myocardial infarction. (Modified from Libby P. Current concepts of the pathogenesis of the acute coronary syndromes. Circulation 104(3):365–72, 2001; Hamm CW, Bertrand M, Braunwald E. Acute coronary syndrome without ST elevation: Implementation of new guidelines. Lancet 358(9292):1533–8, 2001; Davies MJ. The pathophysiology of acute coronary syndromes. Heart 83(3):361–6, 2000; and Antman EM, Anbe DT, Armstrong PW, et al. ACC/AHA guidelines for the management of patients with ST-elevation myocardial infarction—executive summary: A report of the American College of Cardiology/American Heart Association Task Force on Practice Guidelines (Writing Committee to Revise the 1999 Guidelines for the Management of Patients With Acute Myocardial Infarction). Circulation 110(5):588–636, 2004. In Libby P, Bonow RO, Mann DL, et al. Braunwald's Heart Disease, ed 8. Philadelphia, 2008, Saunders.)

hospital course affected an individual's activity progression owing to the effects of inactivity or bedrest.

## Ventricular Remodeling

With STEMI there is a change in shape, size and thickness of the myocardium as a result of both infracted and

## Table 3-5 Postmyocardial Infarction Complications

| System/Hormones | Complications |
| --- | --- |
| Pulmonary | Problems with gas exchange, ventilation and perfusion |
| | Interstitial edema/pulmonary edema |
| | Hypoxemia, ↓ vital capacity |
| Circulation | ↓ Affinity of hemoglobin for $O_2$ |
| | Platelets: hyperaggregable, ↑ aggregation, release vasoactive substances |
| Endocrine | Impaired glucose tolerance |
| | Hyperglycemia/Insulin resistance |
| | Excessive secretion of catecholamines |
| Renin-angiotensin-aldosterone (RAS) system | Activation of RAS with ↑ angiotensin II production |
| | May get vasoconstriction, impaired fibrinolysis, ↑ Na retention |
| Natriuretic peptides | Released early, peak at 16 hrs |
| | Elevated levels 6 hrs after onset of symptoms have ↑ in mortality |
| Adrenal cortex | Rise in cortisol (correlates with infarct size and mortality) |
| | Rise in aldosterone, ketosteroids, and hydroxycorticosteroids |
| Renal | Prerenal azotemia and acute renal failure can occur as a result of ↓ CO |

Data from Libby P, Bonow RO, Mann DL, et al. Braunwald's Heart Disease: A Textbook of Cardiovascular Medicine, ed 8. Philadelphia, 2007, Saunders.

noninfarcted areas. This is called *ventricular remodeling* and includes areas of ventricular dilation as well as ventricular hypertrophy. Factors that affect remodeling include:
- Size of infarct
- Ventricular load (increased pressure or increased volume will increase the load)
- Patency of the artery that was infarcted.

When there is an increased infarction size, an increased ventricular load, or poor blood supply to the area infracted, there will be decreased remodeling, possibly increased infarction expansion, and higher risk of complications and increased mortality. With a decrease in infarction size, decreased ventricular load or increase in blood supply to the infracted area, there will be increase in scar formation and improved remodeling.[204]

## Prognosis

An individual's prognosis post-MI is related to the complications, infarction size, presence of disease in other coronary arteries and most importantly left ventricular function.[204] Therefore, monitoring an individual post-MI is extremely important, especially in individuals with complicated post-MI.

## Natural History of Coronary Disease

Although many population and longitudinal studies have been carried out that document the relative importance of single factors or combinations of risk factors, still little is known about the natural history of CHD as it applies to an individual patient.[208,209] Knowledge of risk factors has allowed the establishment of a model from which relative risk can be approximated, but such tools decrease in value for those who are at either end of the normal distribution of the population. The only "guarantee" that can be offered to the patient with known CHD is that if the factors that caused the disease to be present in the first place remain unchanged, it will progress.

There is some evidence that the progression of atherosclerotic CHD is not inevitable and, in fact, that it is reversible.[18,210–212] More than 50 randomized trials have documented the efficacy and safety of aspirin as an antiplatelet agent and a cardiovascular drug. For patients with ischemic heart disease the range recommended for the prevention of a secondary event, based on strong clinical evidence, is 75 to 160 mg aspirin per day for men and 75 to 325 mg per day for women older than 65 years of age and at high risk.[213,214] In addition, the strict control of diabetes also appears to decrease atherosclerotic changes in endothelial and intimal elastin, contributing to beneficial decreases in vessel wall compliance.

Since the Cholesterol Lowering in Atherosclerosis Study,[215,216] the importance of treating patients pharmacologically to lower cholesterol levels and lessen the risk of developing atherosclerosis is well accepted. There is also clear evidence that aggressive lifestyle modification can elicit significant results without the use of medication (Box 3-4).[212] Nonetheless, many general practitioners do not have an aggressive attitude toward the prescription of lipid-lowering interventions, especially when older patients with atherosclerotic lesions are concerned.[217] Perhaps physical therapists should seize the opportunity to incorporate secondary prevention measures for cardiovascular disease into their clinical practices. Chapter 18 provides a full discussion of secondary prevention as an intervention. The establishment of secondary prevention clinics in England resulted in reduced hospital admissions for participants.[218]

## Hypertension

Hypertension (HTN) is diagnosed when DBP equals or exceeds 90 mm Hg or when systolic blood pressure (SBP) is

## Box 3-4

### Secondary Prevention Methods to Reduce the Risk Factors of CHD

- Maintaining a normal blood pressure
- Smoking cessation
- Maintaining normal total cholesterol, lowering LDLs and raising HDLs
- Reducing stress, anger, and hostility
- Maintaining normal blood glucose levels and glycosylated hemoglobin (HbA1c)
- Maintaining normal BMI and weight
- Performing physical activity 5 to 7 days/week

### Table 3-6  Blood Pressure Levels for Adults*

| Category | | Systolic (mm Hg) | Diastolic (mm Hg) |
|---|---|---|---|
| Normal | | <120 | <80 |
| High normal/ prehypertension | | 120–139 | 80–89 |
| Hypertension | Stage 1 | 140–159 | 90–99 |
| | Stage 2 | >159 | >99 |

*These values are for adults ages 18 years and older who are not taking antihypertensive medications and are not acutely ill.*
*From Rosendorff C, Black HR, Cannon CP, et al. Treatment of hypertension in the prevention and management of ischemic heart disease: A scientific statement from the American Heart Association Council for High Blood Pressure Research and the Councils on Clinical Cardiology and Epidemiology and Prevention [published correction appears in Circulation 116(5):e121, 2007]. Circulation 115(21):2762, 2007.*

The major determinants of arterial BP are cardiac output and total peripheral resistance. If either one, or both, of these factors becomes elevated, BP will rise. However, both cardiac output and total peripheral resistance are determined by a number of other factors (Fig. 3-11). Cardiac output is the product of heart rate and stroke volume; yet, each of those factors has several determinants, as described in Chapter 2. Similarly, total peripheral resistance (TPR) is affected by several variables, including the caliber of the arteriolar bed, the viscosity of the blood, the elasticity of the arterial walls, and sympathetic influence and activity.

Consequently, there are many physiologic pathways where abnormal function can result in high BP, and many of these share a number of common features, as shown in Figure 3-11. Furthermore, it is probable that the mechanisms that are responsible for initiating HTN differ from those that serve to maintain it. For example, there is evidence that many individuals with labile or early mild HTN have increased cardiac output, probably related to enhanced activity of the sympathetic nervous system and apparently normal peripheral resistance.[222,223] However, later when HTN becomes established, the classic findings of elevated TPR and normal or decreased cardiac output are found.[223]

### Clinical Tip

It is important for the clinician to keep in mind that HTN often goes undetected for many years. Labile hypertension can be particularly difficult to identify because multiple BP measurements must be made to diagnose HTN. Mild to moderate elevations in BP are usually not symptomatic. Consequently, standards of physical therapy practice should include the assessment of resting BP and activity BP during an initial examination (as part of the Systems Review).

The consequences of HTN are directly related to the level of BP, even within the accepted normal range. Actuarial data reveal that persons with diastolic BPs of 88 to 92 mm Hg have a 32% to 36% higher mortality rate over 20 years of followup than those with diastolic pressures less than 80 mm Hg.[224] Higher systolic BP levels at any given level of DBP also are associated with an increased morbidity rate in both men and women.[221,225-227] The most common complications of HTN include atherosclerotic heart disease, congestive heart failure, cerebrovascular accidents, renal failure, dissecting aneurysm, peripheral vascular disease, and retinopathy (Fig. 3-12).

### Hypertensive Heart Disease

Regardless of its etiology and pathophysiologic mechanisms, HTN produces a pressure overload on the left ventricle (LV), which is compensated for by left ventricular hypertrophy (LVH).[228] Initially, normal systolic LV function is maintained by the hypertrophied LV. However diastolic dysfunction with impairment of LV relaxation develops early in the course of

consistently higher than 140 mm Hg, with values of 130 to 139/85 to 89 mm Hg being considered high normal (prehypertension), as shown in Table 3-6.[219] Labile HTN refers to blood pressure (BP) that fluctuates between hypertensive and normal values. Usually individuals with HTN have elevated levels of both systolic and diastolic BP; however, isolated systolic hypertension (ISH), which occurs when SBP exceeds 140 mm Hg but DBP remains within the normal range, becomes increasingly more common in the elderly.[220,221] Approximately 90% to 95% of individuals with HTN have no discernible cause for their disease and are said to have primary or essential hypertension. The remainder have secondary hypertension resulting from another identifiable medical problem, such as renovascular or endocrine disease.

Despite much research, the etiology of essential HTN continues to be unknown. Both genetic and environmental factors, such as dietary sodium excess, stress, obesity, and alcohol consumption, have been implicated. Regardless of the underlying cause(s), the result is a failure of one or more of the control mechanisms that are responsible for lowering BP when it becomes elevated.

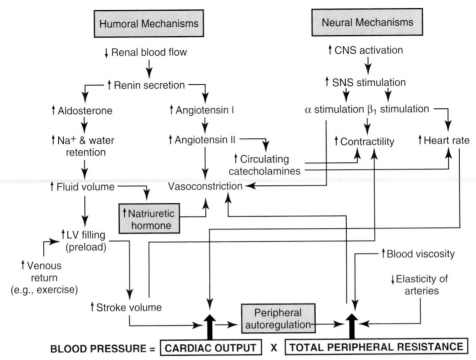

**Figure 3-11** Factors contributing to elevated blood pressure. Because blood pressure is a product of cardiac output and peripheral resistance, any influence that increases either of these factors results in a rise in blood pressure. The enclosed boxes identify some of the proposed mechanisms involved in the pathogenesis of essential hypertension. Note the number of interrelationships among the different mechanisms. CNS, central nervous system; LV, left ventricle; SNS, sympathetic nervous system; ↑, increased; ↓, decreased.

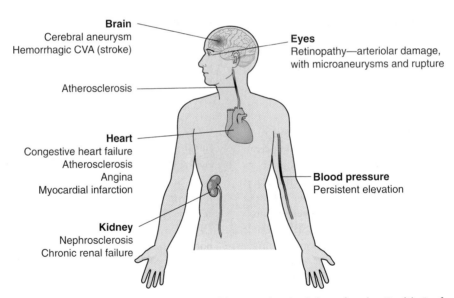

**Figure 3-12** Effects of uncontrolled hypertension. (From Gould BE. Pathophysiology for the Health Professions, ed 3. St. Louis, 2007, Saunders.)

essential HTN (Box 3-5).[229–232] The combination of LVH and diastolic dysfunction leads to reduced LV compliance (i.e., a stiffer LV), which creates a greater load on the left atrium and resultant left atrial enlargement. In addition, LVH alters the equilibrium between the oxygen supply and demand of the myocardium. Coronary reserve is reduced in patients with HTN and LVH, even in the absence of any coronary artery stenosis.[230,233] Thus, there is a predisposition toward myocardial ischemia and ventricular dysrhythmias. Superimposed is the role of HTN as a major risk factor for atherosclerotic heart disease (ASHD), as previously discussed. This interaction makes it difficult to differentiate between the ischemic effects of ASHD and hypertensive heart disease.

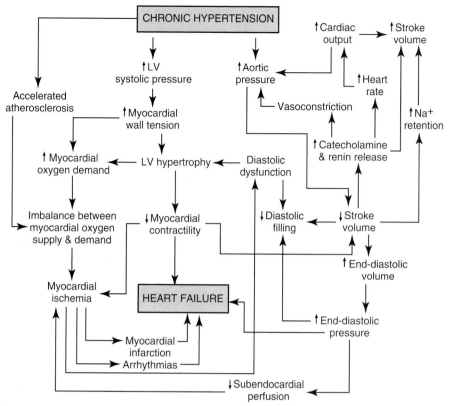

**Figure 3-13** Some of the mechanisms and interrelationships in hypertension that may lead to the development of left ventricle (LV) failure. Repeating cycles tend to aggravate the problem. ↑, Increased; ↓, decreased.

---

**Box 3-5**

**Systolic vs. Diastolic Dysfunction**

**Systolic Dysfunction**
An impairment in ventricular contraction, resulting in decrease in stroke volume and decrease in ejection fraction. An increase in end systolic volume will also occur.

**Diastolic Dysfunction**
Changes in ventricular diastolic properties that lead to an impairment in ventricular filling (reduction in ventricular compliance) and an impairment in ventricular relaxation. A consequence of diastolic dysfunction is the rise in end diastolic pressure.

---

If adequate LV filling volume is not achieved, either because of reduced filling times associated with higher heart rates or arrhythmias in which active atrial contraction is missing (e.g., atrial fibrillation, nodal rhythm, frequent premature ventricular beats), stroke volume will diminish. Thus, symptoms of inadequate cardiac output, such as lightheadedness or dizziness, dyspnea, and impaired exercise tolerance, can result from diastolic dysfunction rather than impaired systolic function.[234,235] However, as HTN becomes more

severe or prolonged, impairment of systolic function may also develop, appearing as subnormal LV functional reserve initially during exercise and later at rest.[236–239]

Although normal cardiac output may be maintained for some time at the expense of pulmonary congestion, the ultimate consequence of progressive LVH is the development of left ventricular failure, as shown in Figure 3-13. A number of factors, such as further elevation of BP, increased venous return, or impaired contractile function, may precipitate decompensation and overt LV failure.

**Treatment of Hypertension**

The goals of antihypertensive therapy are to normalize BP both at rest and during exertion and to reverse LVH and the myocardial dysfunction it creates.[1,240–243] Pharmacologic therapy is the most commonly prescribed intervention in the management of HTN. However, the latest medical guidelines recommend beginning with lifestyle modifications in most patients diagnosed with HTN (Table 3-7).[219] The most effective modifications have proved to be weight reduction, sodium restriction, moderation of alcohol intake, and regular aerobic exercise.[244,245] Although these interventions may not eliminate the need for antihypertensive medications in most patients, they often permit a lower dosage of medications to be used, thus reducing the potential for adverse side effects. In addition, because HTN tends to cluster with other

## Table 3-7 Treatment Guidelines for Hypertension

| Category | Blood Pressure Range | Treatment |
|---|---|---|
| Prehypertension | 120–139 systolic<br>80–89 diastolic | Lifestyle modification |
| Stage 1 hypertension | 140–159 systolic<br>90–99 diastolic | Thiazide diuretics<br>May consider angiotensin-converting enzyme (ACE) inhibitor<br>β Blocker, calcium channel blocker |
| Stage 2 hypertension | >160 systolic<br>>100 diastolic | 2-Drug combination<br>Thiazide and ACE or other |

*From Rosendorff C, Black HR, Cannon CP, et al. Treatment of hypertension in the prevention and management of ischemic heart disease: a scientific statement from the American Heart Association Council for High Blood Pressure Research and the Councils on Clinical Cardiology and Epidemiology and Prevention [published correction appears in Circulation 116(5):e121, 2007]. Circulation 115(21):2762, 2007.*

coronary risk factors, such as dyslipidemia, insulin resistance, glucose intolerance, and obesity,[221] some of the interventions, such as aerobic exercise and weight reduction, by virtue of their effect on more than one factor, may significantly reduce the risk of cardiovascular disease and death.

The medications used to treat HTN fall into the following major categories: diuretics, β-adrenergic blockers, α-adrenergic blockers, vasodilators, centrally acting adrenergic antagonists, calcium-channel blockers, and angiotensin-converting enzyme (ACE) inhibitors.[246-249] Many of these drugs have additional cardiovascular effects and side effects and may be used to treat other clinical problems. In addition, there are several new classes of antihypertensive agents, such as renin inhibitors and angiotensin II antagonists, that are currently under investigation.[28] Chapter 14 has more complete information on these drugs.

## Hypertension and Exercise

Research involving hypertensive individuals has revealed that exercise capacity is reduced by 15% to 30%, even in those who are asymptomatic, when compared with age- and fitness-matched control subjects.[237,250,251] Stroke volume increases subnormally and peak heart rate is lower; therefore, cardiac output is decreased. There is some evidence that these changes may be as a result of diastolic dysfunction and impaired coronary flow reserve.[233,237] In addition, exercise time and anaerobic threshold are also reduced.

Treatment of HTN with medications may modify the physiologic responses to exercise. Antihypertensive medications lower resting BP, but many do not maintain the same degree of effectiveness during exertion, especially with isometric activities.[236,252-254] Thus, patients on antihypertensive medications may have acceptable BP levels at rest but display exaggerated responses to exercise. Furthermore, some of the drugs have side effects that are affected by or have an effect upon exercise. Of particular concern is the hypokalemia that can be induced by diuretic therapy using the thiazides and loop diuretics. When combined with the systemic demands of exercise, hypokalemia can precipitate dangerous

arrhythmias, skeletal muscle fatigue and cramps, weakness, and occasionally other problems. The potassium-sparing diuretics and β blockers are associated with a greater risk of hyperkalemia, which can also cause arrhythmias.

A great deal of research has been directed at assessing the efficacy of exercise training for the treatment of HTN. Although the data are not consistent, the general consensus is that reductions of approximately 10 mm Hg in both systolic and diastolic BP can be achieved through exercise training in the hypertensive population. These reductions are significant enough to allow some patients to avoid or discontinue drug treatment and many others to reduce their drug dosages.[252,255-259] In addition, exercise training has been demonstrated to cause a significant regression of LVH.[260]

> **Clinical Tip**
> The problem with exercise training as a treatment for hypertension is the high percentage of dropouts from exercise programs, or noncompliance. The effects of exercise training on BP are maintained only as long as the individual remains compliant with the exercise program.

## Implications for Physical Therapy Intervention

According to some estimates, approximately 40 to 50 million Americans, including nearly a third of all black adults and more than half of all adults older than age 60 years, have high BP, and a third of this population does not even know they have it.[261,262] The prevalence of HTN increases with age. Therefore, the percentage of patients referred to physical therapy (PT) who may have recognized or unrecognized HTN is very high. Patients with any of the following diagnoses are particularly likely to have HTN: stroke, diabetes, coronary artery disease, aortic aneurysm, peripheral vascular disease, obesity, renal failure, and alcoholism. In addition, patients with chronic pain syndromes and those in high-stress occupations, such as air traffic controllers, firefighters, and middle-level and upper-level managers, may be at higher risk for HTN.

With the growing trend toward independent practice, PT may represent the mode of entry into the medical care system for a number of adults. This fact, combined with the prevalence of HTN, supports the need for inclusion of BP monitoring during the PT evaluation and treatment of all adults older than age 35 years. In addition to the valuable information this might provide for both the client and the physician, the positive professional image created could improve acceptance by the medical community of the PT position as an independent healthcare provider. Furthermore, when a client with diagnosed HTN is seen for PT, the clinician should question the client about prescribed treatments, determine the level of compliance, and reinforce the importance of strict adherence. If the client complains of unpleasant side effects of a particular medication, the client should be encouraged to discuss the side effects with the physician so that a different medication can be prescribed. With so many antihypertensive agents available, most patients can receive comfortable and effective treatment.

Because BP values vary considerably during the day, it is beneficial to include monitoring during two to three different treatment sessions. Also, inasmuch as BP can be normal or borderline at rest but become excessively elevated during exertion, it is important to monitor BP during exercise as well as at rest.

---

**Clinical Tip**

Proper technique for monitoring of BP is important. Proper cuff size is essential to accuracy: A cuff that is too narrow will produce a reading that is falsely elevated and one that is too wide will yield a reading that is erroneously low. The arm should be relaxed and supported at the level of the heart. If the arm is lower than the heart or if the arm muscles are not relaxed, the BP readings, both systolic and diastolic, will be erroneously high.

---

If the resting BP is excessively high (SBP >200 mm Hg or DBP >100 mm Hg), physician clearance should be obtained before continuing with the PT evaluation or treatment. Furthermore, any evidence of target organ damage secondary to HTN, such as retinopathy, renal disease, or LVH, necessitates that BP be controlled both at rest and during exercise prior to PT intervention. Exercise should be terminated if BP becomes excessively high (SBP >250 mm Hg or DBP >110 mm Hg).[246] The risk of myocardial ischemia during exercise is enhanced in individuals with HTN, especially those with evidence of LVH, and angina may occur. Furthermore, if LV function is impaired, LV end-diastolic volume and

---

**Clinical Tip**

Orthostatic hypotension is defined as a drop in systolic (and often diastolic) BP when assuming an upright position, which often renders the individual symptomatic (dizzy, lightheaded, and sometimes passing out). It is not the same as a hypotensive BP response to activity.

---

**Box 3-6**

**Guidelines for Exercise in Individuals with Hypertension**

- If resting BP excessively elevated (>200 mm Hg systolic or >100 mm Hg diastolic) obtain physician clearance preexercise
- Discontinue exercise if systolic >250 mm Hg, diastolic >110 mm Hg
- Consider side effects of medications
  - Particularly watch for hypotension with:
    - Change of position
    - Postexercise
    - Long-term standing
    - When in warm whirlpools or hot tubs
- Avoid breath hold and Valsalva, especially with resistive exercises
- Encourage low weights and high repetitions to avoid excessive BP responses
- Endurance training should be a part of comprehensive management

From American College of Sports Medicine. Guidelines for Exercise Testing and Prescription. 3rd ed. Baltimore, Williams & Wilkins, 2009.

pressure, and therefore intrapulmonary pressures, will rise during exercise, resulting in shortness of breath (Box 3-6).

## Cerebrovascular Disease

Approximately 700,000 individuals experience a cerebral vascular accident (stroke) in the United States each year, and more than half result from extracranial atherosclerotic carotid artery disease.[1] The resultant symptoms that develop with a stroke are mostly caused by embolic events and only a minority of ischemic strokes are caused by thrombotic occlusion.[204] Stroke is the leading cause of disability and the third leading cause of death after coronary artery disease and cancer in the United States.[1] Figure 3-14 shows the actual anatomy of the vascular supply to the brain, demonstrating two internal carotid arteries and two vertebral arteries that come together at the base of the skull to form the circle of Willis. There is a vast amount of individual variability in the circle of Willis, and some individuals do not even have a complete circle.

A cerebrovascular event is defined as a transient ischemic attack (TIA) if symptoms resolve completely within 24 hours, and as a stroke if deficit results after 24 hours. Patients with a TIA have a 1 in 20 (5%) chance of stroke within 30 days, and almost 25% will have a recurrent cerebrovascular event within 1 year. Individuals who have involvement of a single carotid will have contralateral hemiparesis or hemiparesthesia and possibly aphasia and/or ipsilateral blindness, which are defined as hemispheric symptoms. Individuals who have more than a single carotid or have circle of Willis involvement have what are known as nonhemispheric symptoms,

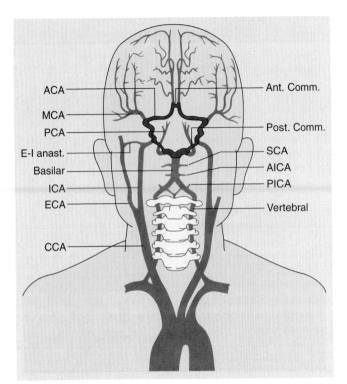

**Figure 3-14** Extracranial and intracranial arterial supply to the brain. Vessels forming the circle of Willis are highlighted. ACA, anterior cerebral artery; AICA, anterior inferior cerebellar artery; Ant. Comm., anterior communicating artery; CCA, common carotid artery; ECA, external carotid artery; E-I anast., extracranial–intracranial anastomosis; ICA, internal carotid artery; MCA, middle cerebral artery; PCA, posterior cerebral artery; PICA, posterior inferior cerebellar artery; Post. Comm., posterior communicating artery; SCA, superior cerebellar artery. (Modified from Lord K. Surgery of the Occlusive Cerebrovascular Disease St. Louis, 1986, Mosby. In Goodman CC: Pathology: Implications for the Physical Therapist, ed 3. St. Louis, 2009, Saunders.)

which include dysarthria, diplopia, vertigo, syncope, and/or transient confusion.[204]

Many of the risk factors for stroke are the same as those of cardiac and peripheral vascular disease, yet stroke presents with a variety of different conditions and pathophysiologic processes. The treatment interventions for stroke are too numerous to present in this chapter, but the interventions for stroke prevention as outlined by the American Stroke Association/American Heart Association are presented in the following sections.[1,263–266]

### Treatment for Stroke Prevention: Primary and Secondary Prevention

According to the American Stroke Association, primary and secondary prevention includes risk factor reduction and medical management. Medical management includes platelet antiaggregants (primarily aspirin), anticoagulants (aspirin, warfarin or Coumadin), lipid-lowering medications, and antihypertensive medications.[263,264] The benefit of the use of aspirin outweighs the risk of bleeding in all individuals who are at moderate to high risk of stroke based upon risk factors, especially women. Women who were defined as having a moderate to high risk of stroke demonstrated a 17% reduction in risk with the inclusion of aspirin in their daily regime as defined in the Women's Health Study.[267] Aspirin in combination with sustained-release dipyrimidole was found to reduce risk of second stroke by 37%.[264,268] Anticoagulation (warfarin/ Coumadin) has been used for years to reduce the risk of a first event of embolism due to conditions like mechanical heart valves, atrial fibrillation, and cardiomyopathy; however, the Warfarin-Aspirin Recurrent Stroke Study (WARSS) found a slight advantage with the use of aspirin as compared to warfarin for prevention of a second stroke because of the risk of bleeding complications with warfarin and the need for additional monitoring.[269]

The role of statins is well documented in the management of patients with coronary artery disease and is also well documented in the primary prevention of stroke. The HPS was the first large study to document the use of statin for secondary prevention of stroke.[133] Those with a prior history of stroke showed a 20% reduction in frequency of major vascular events (MI, stroke, revascularization procedure, or vascular death) with the use of statins.

Finally, the American Stroke Association and the *Seventh Report of the Joint National Committee on Prevention, Detection, Evaluation, and Treatment of High Blood Pressure* (JNC 7) agree that the reduction in blood pressure is far more important than the actual medications used to achieve the reduction and that with a reduction in blood pressure, risk for stroke is reduced between 28% and 35%.[219,263] Therefore, a combination of aspirin, lipid-lowering medication, and antihypertensive medication may be the optimal regimen for primary and secondary prevention of stroke in addition to risk factor modification. Chapter 11 discusses other treatments for those with documented carotid disease in greater detail.

### Implications for Physical Therapy Intervention

Because of the incidence of atherosclerotic disease in this patient population, patients with a diagnosis of carotid or vertebral disease should have their BP monitored at rest and with all new activities, should be educated about primary or secondary prevention of stroke (medical management as outlined above), and taught the symptoms of instability (signs of TIAs) and the need for immediate medical treatment should these symptoms appear. The earlier a patient receives emergency medical management for an impending stroke, the lower the risk of permanent brain injury.

### Peripheral Arterial Disease

Peripheral arterial disease (PAD), or more specifically atherosclerotic occlusive disease (AOD), involves atheromatous

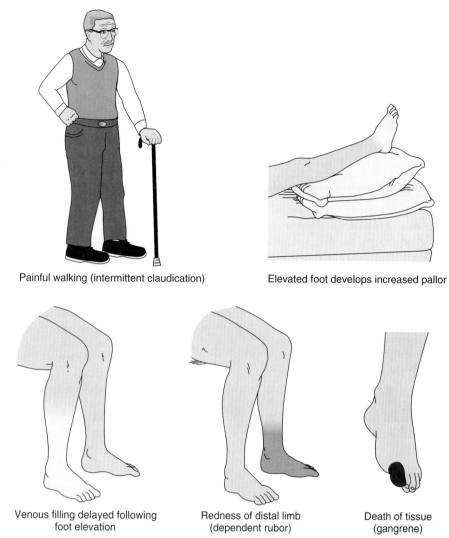

Painful walking (intermittent claudication)

Elevated foot develops increased pallor

Venous filling delayed following foot elevation

Redness of distal limb (dependent rubor)

Death of tissue (gangrene)

**Figure 3-15** Signs and symptoms of arterial insufficiency. (From Goodman CC. Pathology: Implications for the Physical Therapists, ed 3. St. Louis, 2009, Saunders.)

plaque obstruction of the large- or medium-size arteries supplying blood to one or more of the extremities (usually lower). AOD results from the same atherosclerotic process previously described and becomes symptomatic when the atheroma becomes so enlarged that it interferes with blood flow to the distal tissues, it ruptures and extrudes its contents into the bloodstream or obstructs the arterial lumen, or it encroaches on the media, causing weakness of that layer and aneurysmal dilation of the arterial wall. The hemodynamic significance of the disease depends upon the location and number of lesions in an artery, the rapidity with which the atherosclerotic process progresses, and the presence and extent of any collateral arterial system. When blood flow is not adequate to meet the demand of the peripheral tissues (i.e., during activity), the patient may experience symptoms of ischemia, such as intermittent claudication of a lower extremity. As the disease progresses, the patient experiences more severe symptoms, such as

rest pain and skin changes. Complete obstruction to flow will cause tissue necrosis and possibly loss of the limb (Fig. 3-15).

Individuals with lower-extremity PAD should be assumed to have ASHD, which is the main cause of higher morbidity and mortality rates in these individuals.[270] One study noted that coronary atherosclerosis may be present in at least 90% of patients hospitalized for PAD.[271] Individuals with asymptomatic disease appear to have the same increased risk of cardiovascular events and death found in those with symptoms of claudication.[272]

## Exercise and Peripheral Arterial Disease

Individuals with PAD are unable to produce the normal increases in peripheral blood flow essential for enhanced oxygen supply to exercising muscles. If the oxygen supply is inadequate to meet the increasing demand of the exercising muscles, ischemia develops and leads to the production of lactic acid. When excessive lactic acid accumulates in the muscle, pain is experienced (this symptom is known as intermittent claudication); and when it reaches the central circulation, respiration is further stimulated and patients may experience shortness of breath.

Patients with intermittent claudication have moderate to severe impairment in walking ability. Their peak exercise capacity during graded treadmill exercise is severely limited, allowing for only light to very-light activities[273–275]; the energy requirements of many leisure and work-related activities usually exceed their capacity. Metabolic measurements during exercise testing reveal that maximal oxygen consumption and anaerobic threshold are reduced in patients with AOD.[273,275] Yet, even though the anaerobic threshold may be so low that it cannot be detected, evidence of systemic lactic acidosis may be minimal because of the reduced muscle perfusion.

Several studies have documented the efficacy of exercise training in the management of patients with AOD. Increases in both pain-free and maximal walking tolerance on level ground and during constant-load treadmill exercise achieved during exercise testing have been reported.[276–284] Studies even have concluded that greater symptomatic relief and functional improvement in patients with mild to moderate claudication not requiring immediate therapeutic interventions is achieved through supervised exercise therapy rather than percutaneous transluminal angioplasty.[277,285] Some studies have demonstrated the benefit of exercise for patients with rest pain.[286] Several mechanisms have been postulated to account for these improvements: increased walking efficiency, increased peripheral blood flow through changes in the collateral circulation, reduced blood viscosity, regression of atherosclerotic disease, raising of the pain threshold, and improvements in skeletal muscle metabolism. There is evidence that periods of brief repetitive walking can successfully increase oxygenation in the feet of limbs with more severe arterial obstruction.[287]

### Implications for Physical Therapy Intervention

Because of the high prevalence of ASHD in patients with PAD, all patients should receive heart rate and BP monitoring during PT evaluation and initial treatment. Such monitoring is especially needed when working with patients who have undergone amputation, which implies severe disease. Notably, patients with PAD may exhibit precipitous rises in BP during exercise owing to their atherosclerosis and diminished vascular bed.

Including a subjective gradation of pain for expressing claudication discomfort, as described in Table 3-8, is extremely useful during exercise.[246] Patients should exercise to levels of maximal tolerable pain, that is to grade III discomfort, in order to obtain optimal symptomatic benefit over time, possibly through enhanced collateral circulation or increased muscular efficiency.[246,287,288] Box 3-7 provides additional exercise recommendations.

**Table 3-8 Subjective Gradation of Claudication Discomfort**

| Grade | Pain Description |
|-------|-----------------|
| I | Initial discomfort (established, but minimal) |
| II | Moderate discomfort but attention can be diverted |
| III | Intense pain (attention cannot be diverted) |
| IV | Excruciating and unbearable pain |

*From American College of Sports Medicine. Guidelines for Exercise Testing and Prescription, ed 3. Baltimore, 2009, Williams & Wilkins.*

**Box 3-7**

**Exercise Recommendations for Individuals with Peripheral Arterial Disease**

- Perform exercise in intervals as short as 1 to 5 minutes, alternating with rest periods.
- Progress the length of exercise intervals and decrease the length of rest periods.
- Most convenient and functional mode is walking.
- Non–weight-bearing activities may allow for longer duration and higher intensities, but progressive walking should be encouraged.
- Longer warmup time required in colder environments because of peripheral vasoconstriction.
- Sensory examination should be performed prior to providing an exercise prescription because of the possibility of peripheral neuropathy.
- Footwear and foot hygiene should be emphasized.

## Other Vascular Disorders

### Renal Artery Disease

Renal artery stenosis (RAS) results from atherosclerosis of the renal artery and is associated with increased cardiovascular events and mortality. The prevalence of RAS is approximately 20% to 30% in the high-risk population.[289] RAS is a progressive disease that is associated with loss of renal mass, progressing to renal insufficiency, refractory hypertension, and renal failure. Approximately 20% of individuals older than 50 years of age who begin renal dialysis have atherosclerotic RAS as the cause of their renal failure. Renal dialysis patients with RAS have a 56% 2-year survival rate, 18% 5-year survival and 5% 10-year survival.[290] Clearly, the early diagnosis of RAS and the prevention of end-stage renal disease (ESRD) are important goals.

### Aortic Aneurysm

An aortic aneurysm is a pathologic permanent dilation of the aortic wall involving any number of segments of the aorta of

## Table 3-9  Risk Factors of Aneurysms

| Risk Factors | Complications |
|---|---|
| Smoking | Duration of smoking is significant, not amount |
| Age | Incidence of abdominal aortic aneurysm rises rapidly after age 55 years in men, age 70 years in women |
| Gender | 5 to 10× higher incidence in men than in women |
| | Women with aneurysm have a higher risk of rupture |
| Family history | First-degree relative has an increased risk |
| | Siblings have a 19% higher risk |
| Hypertension | |
| Hyperlipidemia | |
| Atherosclerosis | |

*Data from Isselbacher EM. Diseases of the Aorta. In Libby P, Bonow RO, Mann DL, et al. Braunwald's Heart Disease: A Textbook of Cardiovascular Medicine, ed 8. Philadelphia, 2007, Saunders.*

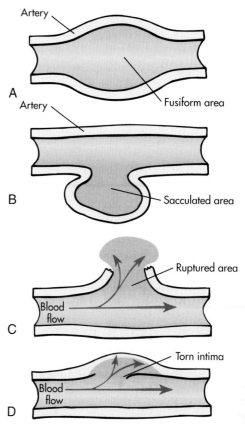

**Figure 3-16 A,** True fusiform abdominal aortic aneurysm. **B,** True saccular aortic aneurysm. **C,** Aortic dissection. **D,** False aneurysm or pseudoaneurysm. (From Lewis SM. Medical-Surgical Nursing: Assessment and Management of Clinical Problems, ed 7. St. Louis, 2008, Mosby.)

at least 1.5 times the expected normal diameter.[204] Aneurysms are usually described in terms of their location, size, morphologic appearance, and origin. An aortic aneurysm is usually uniform in shape, although some aneurysms form a sac or outpouching of a portion of the aorta. Many individuals have multiple aneurysms, with 25% of those with thoracic aneurysms also having abdominal aneurysms (Table 3-9).[204] The large majority of abdominal aortic aneurysms arise below the renal arteries and are known as infrarenal aneurysms. Only a small minority, known as suprarenal aneurysms, arise between the level of the diaphragm and the renal arteries.

As a result of flow disturbance through the aneurysmal aortic segment, blood may stagnate along the walls, allowing the formation of mural thrombus. Thrombi, as well as atherosclerotic debris, may embolize and compromise the circulation of distal arteries. However, rupture is the major risk of abdominal aortic aneurysms. When rupture does occur, 80% rupture into the retroperitoneum, which may contain the rupture, whereas most of the remainder rupture into the peritoneal cavity and cause uncontrolled hemorrhage and rapid circulatory collapse.[204] Because 80% of abdominal aortic aneurysms expand over time, with as many as 15% to 20% expanding rapidly (>0.5 cm/yr), the risk of rupture may concomitantly increase with time. A rapid rate of expansion apparently also predicts aneurysm rupture, especially abdominal aneurysms 5.0 cm or greater in diameter (Fig. 3-16).[204]

### Implications for Physical Therapy

Although not all aortic aneurysms will have signs or symptoms, the most common signs/symptoms include:

- Pulsating tumor/mass in abdominal area
- Bruit heard over swollen area in abdomen
- Pressure on surrounding parts such as low back, thoracic area
- Leg pain/claudication pain
- Numbness in the lower extremities
- Excessive fatigue, especially with walking
- Poor distal pulses, especially the dorsalis pedis
- Low back pain with elevated pressure that may indicate renal artery aneurysm

Blood pressures should be higher in the lower extremities; if the upper-extremity BPs are higher than the lower-extremity blood pressures one should suspect vascular disease.

During the initial assessment, the therapist should identify risk factors for aneurysm, especially age (>60 years) and immediate family history (see Table 3-9).

### Summary

- Coronary heart disease is the most common disease in the industrialized world.
- The presence of coronary heart disease in a given individual is dependent on the presence of any of the following 10 risk factors for the disease and the susceptibility of the individual to those factors.

- Cigarette smoking
- Hypertension
- Elevated cholesterol levels
- Physical inactivity
- Diabetes
- Obesity
- Family history
- Age
- Gender
- Stress
- The risk factors of coronary artery disease are the same risk factors of PAD, carotid and vertebral vascular disease, and other vascular diseases. Therefore, individuals with any of these diseases should be examined for all other diseases.
- The plaques that obstruct the coronary arteries are a combination of atheroma and thrombus, and they begin to form early in life, probably in the second decade.
- Coronary artery disease remains undetected until it occludes approximately 70% of the original coronary lumen.
- The majority of the risk factors for CAD are modifiable.
- Through control of these risk factors, the progress of CAD can be arrested and in some cases reversed.
- Patients with diabetes have a relatively high 10-year risk for developing cardiovascular disease.
- Premature or early coronary disease is defined as men older than age 50 years and women older than age 60 years, but the AHA defines family history as significant if either parent (genetic linked parents) had a diagnosis of heart disease (first event of MI, angina, CABG or PTCA) at an age earlier than 60 years.
- HT reduces the risk of CHD events in younger postmenopausal women (age at menopause <55 years). In older women, HT increases risk in first year, then decreases risk after 2 years.
- Psychosocial distress is also associated with increased mortality and morbidity rates after MI. In addition, social isolation and depression are associated with a poor prognosis after MI.
- Individuals with elevated CRP levels might benefit from more aggressive long-term dietary, lifestyle, and coronary risk factor modification than would be the standard of care in a primary prevention population.
- In 40% of patients with CHD, SCD (death within 1 hour of onset of symptoms) is the initial presenting syndrome.
- The term *acute coronary syndrome* is increasingly used to describe patients who present with either UA or AMI, which includes STEMI and non-STEMI.

- An STEMI develops a Q wave on the ECG in the subsequent 24 to 48 hours and these previously were defined as Q-wave or transmural (full or near-full thickness) infarctions.
- When reperfusion of myocardium undergoing the evolutionary changes from ischemia to infarction occurs sufficiently early (i.e., within 15 to 20 minutes), it can successfully prevent necrosis from developing. Beyond this early stage, the number of salvaged myocytes and therefore the amount of salvaged myocardial tissue (area of necrosis/area at risk) relates directly to the length of time of total coronary artery occlusion, the level of myocardial oxygen consumption, and the collateral blood flow.
- When there is an increased infarction size, an increased ventricular load, or poor blood supply to the area infracted, there will be decreased remodeling, possibly increased infarction expansion and higher risk of complications and increased mortality.
- An individual's prognosis post-MI is related to the complications, infarction size, presence of disease in other coronary arteries, and, most importantly, LV function.
- Standards of PT practice should include the assessment of resting BP and activity BP during an initial examination (as part of the Systems Review).
- Systolic dysfunction refers to an impairment in ventricular contraction, resulting in decrease in stroke volume and decrease in EF. Diastolic dysfunction refers to changes in ventricular diastolic properties that lead to an impairment in ventricular filling (reduction in ventricular compliance) and an impairment in ventricular relaxation.
- A cerebrovascular event is defined as a TIA if symptoms resolve completely within 24 hours, and as a stroke if deficit results after 24 hours.
- Medical management includes platelet antiaggregants (primarily aspirin), anticoagulants (aspirin, warfarin, or Coumadin), lipid-lowering medications, and antihypertensive medications.
- Coronary atherosclerosis may be present in at least 90% of patients hospitalized for PAD.
- RAS results from atherosclerosis of the renal artery and is associated with increased cardiovascular events and mortality.
- An aortic aneurysm is a pathologic permanent dilation of the aortic wall involving any number of segments of the aorta of at least 1.5 times the expected normal diameter. Aneurysms are usually described in terms of their location, size, morphologic appearance, and origin.

## CASE STUDY 3-1

Mr. H is a 38-year-old white male who, at the age of 30 years, was experiencing angina with low levels of exertion and was found to have severe obstructions of his left anterior descending (LAD), first diagonal (DI), circumflex (CIRC), first obtuse marginal (OMI), and right coronary (RCA) arteries. He underwent five-vessel coronary artery bypass grafting, which relieved his angina. He now has a 2-year history of chronic stable angina, which in the past month has become more frequent, occurring with minimal exertion and occasionally while at rest. Mr. H was admitted to the hospital.

He underwent a repeat cardiac catheterization, which revealed total obstructions of his native proximal LAD, mid-CIRC, and RCA. His venous bypass grafts to his LAD and DI were also 100% occluded, whereas the grafts to his OMI and distal RCA were patent.

He has a 20 pack/year (number of packs per day multiplied by the number of years smoked) history of smoking, which he stopped at the time of his bypass surgery. He has a 12-year history of

hypertension, which is controlled by medication. He is 67 inches tall and weighs 270 pounds, which is 50 pounds more than he weighed at the time of his bypass surgery. His current blood lipids are: TC = 188 mg/dL, triglycerides = 147 mg/dL, HDL = 27 mg/dL, and CHOL/HDL = 6.96 mg/dL. He had been employed as an accountant but stated that he had to quit his job because he was experiencing frequent angina during stressful situations at work. He has never engaged in an organized exercise program.

### Study Questions

What is this patient's admitting diagnosis?

Why did this patient's angina return less than 5 years after bypass surgery?

Which risk factors did Mr. H modify after his bypass surgery?

Which risk factors did he not modify after his surgery?

What lifestyle changes should this patient make to keep his remaining grafts patent?

## References

1. Lloyd-Jones D, Adams R, Carnethon M, et al. Heart Disease and Stroke Statistics 2009 Update: A Report from the American Heart Association Statistics Committee and Stroke Statistics Subcommittee. Circulation 119:e21–181, 2009.
2. Heberden E. William Heberden the elder (1710–1801): aspects of his London practice. Med Hist Jul;30(3):303–21, 1986.
3. Enos W, Holmes R, Beyer J. Coronary disease among United States soldiers killed in action in Korea. JAMA 152(12):1090–3, 1953.
4. Strong JP. Landmark perspective: Coronary atherosclerosis in soldiers. A clue to the natural history of atherosclerosis in the young. JAMA 256(20):2863–6, 1986.
5. Kannel WB, Castelli WP, Gordon T, et al. Serum cholesterol, lipoproteins, and the risk of coronary heart disease. The Framingham study. Ann Intern Med 74(1):1–12, 1971.
6. Wissler R. Principles of the pathogenesis of atherosclerosis. In Braunwald E (ed.). Heart Disease: A Textbook of Cardiovascular Medicine, ed 2. Philadelphia, 1984, WB Saunders.
7. Reichl D. Lipoproteins of human peripheral lymph. Eur Heart J 11(Suppl E):230–6, 1990.
8. Haberland ME, Fless GM, Scanu AM, et al. Malondialdehyde modification of lipoprotein(a) produces avid uptake by human monocyte-macrophages. J Biol Chem 25;267(6):4143–51, 1992.
9. Gorlin R. Coronary anatomy. Major Probl Intern Med 11:40–58, 1976.
10. Ambrose JA, Tannenbaum MA, Alexopoulos D, et al. Angiographic progression of coronary artery disease and the development of myocardial infarction. J Am Coll Cardiol 12(1):56–62, 1988.
11. Fulton WFM. Coronary Arteries: Arteriography, Microanatomy, and Pathogenesis of Obliterative Coronary Artery Disease. Springfield, IL, 1965, Charles C Thomas.
12. Allwork SP: The applied anatomy of the arterial blood supply to the heart in man. J Anat 153:1–16, 1987.
13. Schaper W. The physiology of the collateral circulation in the normal and hypoxic myocardium. Ergeb Physiol 63:102–45, 1971.
14. Tracy RE, Newman 3rd WP, Wattigney WA, et al. Risk factors and atherosclerosis in youth autopsy findings of the Bogalusa Heart Study. Am J Med Sci 310(Suppl 1):S37–41, 1995.
15. Stary HC. Evolution and progression of atherosclerotic lesions in coronary arteries of children and young adults. Arteriosclerosis 9(1 Suppl):I19–32, 1989.
16. Srinivasan SR, Radhakrishnamurthy B, Vijayagopal P, et al. Proteoglycans, lipoproteins, and atherosclerosis. Adv Exp Med Biol 285:373–81, 1991.
17. Hässig A, Wen-Xi L, Stampfli K. The pathogenesis and prevention of atherosclerosis. Med Hypotheses 47(5):409–12, 1996.
18. Blankenhorn DH, Kramsch DM. Reversal of atherosis and sclerosis. The two components of atherosclerosis. Circulation 79(1):1–7, 1989.
19. Campbell JH, Campbell GR. Cell biology of atherosclerosis. J Hypertens Suppl 12(10):S129–32, 1994.
20. Kinlay S, Ganz P. Role of endothelial dysfunction in coronary artery disease and implications for therapy. Am J Cardiol 57:791–804, 1997.
21. Ross R, Glomset JA. The pathogenesis of atherosclerosis (second of two parts). N Engl J Med 295:420–5, 1976.
22. Ross R, Glomset JA. The pathogenesis of atherosclerosis (first of two parts). N Engl J Med 295:369–77, 1976.
23. DiCorleto PE. Cellular mechanisms of atherogenesis. Am J Hypertens 6:314S–18S, 1993.
24. Forstermann U, Mugge A, Alheid U, et al. Selective attenuation of endothelium-mediated vasodilation in atherosclerotic human coronary arteries. Circ Res 62:185–90, 1988.
25. Ludmer PL, Selwyn AP, Shook TL, et al. Paradoxical vasoconstriction induced by acetylcholine in atherosclerotic coronary arteries. N Engl J Med 315:1046–51, 1986.
26. Marmur JD, Poon M, Rossikhina M, et al. Induction of PDGF-responsive genes in vascular smooth muscle. Implications for

the early response to vessel injury. Circulation 86:III53–III60, 1992.

27. Nilsson J, Volk-Jovinge S, Svensson J, et al. Association between high levels of growth factors in plasma and progression of coronary atherosclerosis. J Intern Med 232:397–404, 1992.

28. Grotendorst GR, Chang T, Seppa HE, et al. Platelet-derived growth factor is a chemoattractant for vascular smooth muscle cells. J Cell Physiol 113:261–6, 1982.

29. Krettek A, Fager G, Lindmark H, et al. Effect of phenotype on the transcription of the genes for platelet-derived growth factor (PDGF) isoforms in human smooth muscle cells, monocyte-derived macrophages, and endothelial cells in vitro. Arterioscler Thromb Vasc Biol 17:2897–903, 1997.

30. Marumo T, Schini-Kerth VB, Fisslthaler B, et al. Platelet-derived growth factor-stimulated superoxide anion production modulates activation of transcription factor NF-kappa B and expression of monocyte chemoattractant protein 1 in human aortic smooth muscle cells. Circulation 96:2361–7, 1997.

31. Osler W. Second Lumleian lecture on angina pectoris. Lancet March 26:839–44, 1910.

32. Prinzmetal M, Ekemecki A, Kennamer R, et al. Angina pectoris. 1. A variant form of angina pectoris. Am J Med 27:375–88, 1959.

33. Meller J, Pichard A, Dack S. Coronary arterial spasm in Prinzmetal's angina: A proved hypothesis. Am J Cardiol 37, 1976, 938–40.

34. Haudenschild CC. Pathogenesis of atherosclerosis: State of the art. Cardiovasc Drugs Ther 4(Suppl 5):993–1004, 1990.

35. Yasue H, Matsuyama K, Matsuyama K, et al. Responses of angiographically normal human coronary arteries to intracoronary injection of acetylcholine by age and segment. Possible role of early coronary atherosclerosis. Circulation 81:482–90, 1990.

36. Okumura K, Yasue H, Matsuyama K, et al. Diffuse disorder of coronary artery vasomotility in patients with coronary spastic angina. Hyperreactivity to the constrictor effects of acetylcholine and the dilator effects of nitroglycerin. J Am Coll Cardiol 27:45–52, 1996.

37. Das UN. Can free radicals induce coronary vasospasm and acute myocardial infarction? Med Hypotheses 39:90–4, 1992.

38. Abrams J. Role of endothelial dysfunction in coronary artery disease. Am J Cardiol 79:2–9, 1997.

39. Vanhoutte PM. Endothelial dysfunction and atherosclerosis. Eur Heart J 18(Suppl E):E19–E29, 1997.

40. Vita JA, Treasure CB, Nabel EG, et al. Coronary vasomotor response to acetylcholine relates to risk factors for coronary artery disease. Circulation 81:491–7, 1990.

41. Kannel WB. Some lessons in cardiovascular epidemiology from Framingham. Am J Cardiol 37:269–82, 1976.

42. Kannel WB. Contributions of the Framingham Study to the conquest of coronary artery disease. Am J Cardiol 62:1109–12, 1988.

43. Mancia G. The need to manage risk factors of coronary heart disease. Am Heart J 115:240–2, 1988.

44. Battegay E, Gasche A, Zimmerli L, et al. Risk factor control and perceptions of risk factors in patients with coronary heart disease. Blood Press Suppl 1:17–22, 1997.

45. Goble A, Jackson B, Phillips P, et al. The family atherosclerosis risk intervention study (FARIS): Risk factor profiles of patients and their relatives following an acute cardiac event. Aust N Z J Med 27:568–77, 1997.

46. Chronic Disease Notes and Reports. In National Center for Chronic Disease Prevention and Health Promotion, Centers for Disease Control and Prevention, U.S. Department of Health and Human Services, 1–36, 1997.

47. Hammond EC, Horn D. Landmark article, March 15, 1958: Smoking and death rates—Report on forty-four months of follow-up of 187,783 men. JAMA 251:2840–53, 1984.

48. Heitzer T, Yla-Herttuala S, Luoma J, et al. Cigarette smoking potentiates endothelial dysfunction of forearm resistance vessels in patients with hypercholesterolemia. Role of oxidized LDL. Circulation 93:1346–53, 1996.

49. Lin SJ. Risk factors, endothelial cell turnover and lipid transport in atherogenesis. Zhonghua Yi Xue Za Zhi (Taipei) 58:309–16, 1996.

50. Vogel RA. Coronary risk factors, endothelial function, and atherosclerosis: A review. Clin Cardiol 20:426–32, 1997.

51. Veyssier Belot C. [Tobacco smoking and cardiovascular risk]. Rev Med Interne 18:702–8, 1997.

52. Rosengren A, Wilhelmsen L, Wedel H. Coronary heart disease, cancer and mortality in male middle-aged light smokers. J Intern Med 231:357–62, 1992.

53. Wilhelmsen L. Coronary heart disease: Epidemiology of smoking and intervention studies of smoking. Am Heart J 115:242–9, 1988.

54. Simon JA, Fong J, Bernert Jr JT, Browner WS. Relation of smoking and alcohol consumption to serum fatty acids. Am J Epidemiol 144:325–34, 1996.

55. van de Vijver LP, van Poppel G, van Houwelingen A, et al. Trans-unsaturated fatty acids in plasma phospholipids and coronary heart disease: A case-control study. Atherosclerosis 126:155–61, 1996.

56. He Y, Lam TH, Li LS, et al. The number of stenotic coronary arteries and passive smoking exposure from husband in lifelong non-smoking women in Xi'an, China. Atherosclerosis 127:229–38, 1996.

57. Moskowitz WB, Mosteller M, Schieken RM, et al. Lipoprotein and oxygen transport alterations in passive smoking preadolescent children. The MCV Twin Study. Circulation 81:586–92, 1990.

58. Marwick C. NHANES III health data relevant for aging nation. JAMA 277:100–2, 1997.

59. Gillum RF. Coronary heart disease, stroke, and hypertension in a U.S. national cohort: The NHANES I epidemiologic follow-up study. Ann Epidemiol 6:259–62, 1996.

60. Sorel JE, Heiss G, Tyroler HA, et al. Black-white differences in blood pressure among participants in NHANES II: The contribution of blood lead. Epidemiology 2:348–52, 1991.

61. Redon J, Campos C, Narciso ML, et al. Prognostic value of ambulatory blood pressure monitoring in refractory hypertension: A prospective study. Hypertension 31:712–18, 1998.

62. Nielsen WB, Lindenstrom E, Vestbo J, Jensen GB. Is diastolic hypertension an independent risk factor for stroke in the presence of normal systolic blood pressure in the middle-aged and elderly? Am J Hypertens 10:634–9, 1997.

63. Rutan GH, Kuller LH, Neaton JD, et al. Mortality associated with diastolic hypertension and isolated systolic hypertension among men screened for the Multiple Risk Factor Intervention Trial. Circulation 77:504–14, 1988.

64. Black HR. The coronary artery disease paradox. Am J Hypertens 9:2S–10S, 1996.

65. Borhani NO. Risk management in stroke prevention: Major clinical trials in hypertension. Health Rep 6:76–86, 1994.

66. Doyle AE. Does hypertension predispose to coronary disease? Conflicting epidemiological and experimental evidence. Am J Hypertens 1:319–24, 1988.

67. Waters D, Craven TE, Lesperance J. Prognostic significance of progression of coronary atherosclerosis. Circulation 87:1067–75, 1993.

68. Assmann G, Schulte H. The Prospective Cardiovascular Münster Study: Prevalence and prognostic significance of hyperlipidemia in men with systemic hypertension. Am J Cardiol 59:9G–17G, 1987.

69. Olson RE. Discovery of the lipoproteins, their role in fat transport and their significance as risk factors. J Nutr 128:439S–43S, 1998.

70. Pekkanen J, Linn S, Heiss G, et al. Ten-year mortality from cardiovascular disease in relation to cholesterol level among men with and without preexisting cardiovascular disease. N Engl J Med 322:1700–7, 1990.

71. Shoji T, Nishizawa Y, Kawagishi T, et al. Atherogenic lipoprotein changes in the absence of hyperlipidemia in patients with chronic renal failure treated by hemodialysis. Atherosclerosis 131:229–36, 1997.

72. Chapman MJ, Guerin M, Bruckert E. Atherogenic, dense low-density lipoproteins. Pathophysiology, and new therapeutic approaches. Eur Heart J 19(Suppl A):A24–30, 1998.

73. Frost PH, Havel RJ. Rationale for use of non-high-density lipoprotein cholesterol rather than low-density lipoprotein cholesterol as a tool for lipoprotein cholesterol screening and assessment of risk and therapy. Am J Cardiol 81:26B–31B, 1998.

74. Grundy SM, Balady GJ, Criqui MH, et al. When to start cholesterol-lowering therapy in patients with coronary heart disease. A statement for healthcare professionals from the American Heart Association Task Force on Risk Reduction. Circulation 95:1683–5, 1997.

75. Kris-Etherton PM, Krummel D, Russell ME, et al. The effect of diet on plasma lipids, lipoproteins, and coronary heart disease. J Am Diet Assoc 88:1373–400, 1988.

76. Kris-Etherton PM, Krummel D. Role of nutrition in the prevention and treatment of coronary heart disease in women. J Am Diet Assoc 93:987–93, 1993.

77. Smith-Schneider LM, Sigman-Grant MJ, Kris-Etherton PM. Dietary fat reduction strategies. J Am Diet Assoc 92:34–8, 1992.

78. Srinath U, Jonnalagadda SS, Naglak MC, et al. Diet in the prevention and treatment of atherosclerosis. A perspective for the elderly. Clin Geriatr Med 11:591–611, 1995.

79. Connor SL, Gustafson JR, Artaud-Wild SM, et al. The cholesterol/saturated-fat index: An indication of the hypercholesterolaemic and atherogenic potential of food. Lancet 1:1229–32, 1986.

80. Connor SL, Gustafson JR, Artaud-Wild SM, et al. The cholesterol-saturated fat index for coronary prevention: Background, use, and a comprehensive table of foods. J Am Diet Assoc 89:807–16, 1989.

81. Artaud-Wild SM, Connor SL, Sexton G, Connor WE. Differences in coronary mortality can be explained by differences in cholesterol and saturated fat intakes in 40 countries but not in France and Finland. A paradox. Circulation 88:2771–9, 1993.

82. Gordon DJ, Probstfield JL, Garrison RJ, et al. High-density lipoprotein cholesterol and cardiovascular disease. Four prospective American studies. Circulation 79:8–15, 1989.

83. Miller M, Mead LA, Kwiterovich Jr PO, Pearson TA. Dyslipidemias with desirable plasma total cholesterol levels and angiographically demonstrated coronary artery disease. Am J Cardiol 65:1–5, 1990.

84. Drexel H, Amann FW, Beran J, et al. Plasma triglycerides and three lipoprotein cholesterol fractions are independent predictors of the extent of coronary atherosclerosis. Circulation 90:2230–5, 1994.

85. Verdery RB. Reverse cholesterol transport from fibroblasts to high density lipoproteins: Computer solutions of a kinetic model. Can J Biochem 59:586–92, 1981.

86. Berger GM. High-density lipoproteins, reverse cholesterol transport and atherosclerosis—Recent developments. S Afr Med J 65:503–6, 1984.

87. Miller NE, La Ville A, Crook D. Direct evidence that reverse cholesterol transport is mediated by high-density lipoprotein in rabbit. Nature 314:109–11, 1985.

88. Gwynne JT. High-density lipoprotein cholesterol levels as a marker of reverse cholesterol transport. Am J Cardiol 64:10G–17G, 1989.

89. Schmitz G, Bruning T, Williamson E, Nowicka G. The role of HDL in reverse cholesterol transport and its disturbances in Tangier disease and HDL deficiency with xanthomas. Eur Heart J 11(Suppl E):197–211, 1990.

90. Pieters MN, Schouten D, Van Berkel TJ. In vitro and in vivo evidence for the role of HDL in reverse cholesterol transport. Biochim Biophys Acta 1225:125–34, 1994.

91. Assmann G, Schulte H, von Eckardstein A, Huang Y. High density lipoprotein cholesterol as a predictor of coronary heart disease risk. The PROCAM experience and pathophysiological implications for reverse cholesterol transport. Atherosclerosis 124(Suppl):S11–S20, 1996.

92. Hill SA, McQueen MJ. Reverse cholesterol transport—A review of the process and its clinical implications. Clin Biochem 30:517–25, 1997.

93. Kannel WB. Hazards, risks, and threats of heart disease from the early stages to symptomatic coronary heart disease and cardiac failure. Cardiovasc Drugs Ther 11(Suppl 1):199–212, 1997.

94. Chennell A, Sullivan DR, Penberthy LA, Hensley WJ. Comparability of lipoprotein measurements, total HDL cholesterol ratio and other coronary risk functions within and between laboratories in Australia. Pathology 26:471–6, 1994.

95. Castelli WP, Anderson K. A population at risk. Prevalence of high cholesterol levels in hypertensive patients in the Framingham Study. Am J Med 80:23–32, 1986.

96. Krauss RM. Atherogenicity of triglyceride-rich lipoproteins. Am J Cardiol 81:13B–17B, 1998.

97. Hodis HN, Mack WJ. Triglyceride-rich lipoproteins and progression of atherosclerosis. Eur Heart J 19(Suppl A):A40–4, 1998.

98. Castelli WP. The triglyceride issue: A view from Framingham. Am Heart J 112:432–7, 1986.

99. McNicoll S, Latour Y, Rondeau C, et al. Cardiovascular risk factors and lipoprotein profile in French Canadians with premature CAD: Impact of the National Cholesterol Education Program II. Can J Cardiol 11:109–16, 1995.

100. Stein Y. Comparison of European and USA guidelines for prevention of coronary heart disease. Atherosclerosis 110 (Suppl):S41–4, 1994.

101. Schaefer EJ. New recommendations for the diagnosis and treatment of plasma lipid abnormalities. Nutr Rev 51:246–53, 1993.

102. Grundy SMN, Cleeman JI, Merez NB, et al. ATP guidelines: Implications of recent clinical trials for the National Cholesterol Education Program Adult Treatment Panel III Guidelines. J Am Coll Cardiol 44:720–32, 2004.

103. Ashen MD, Blumenthal RS: Clinical practice: Low HDL cholesterol levels. N Engl J Med 353:1251–60, 2005.

104. Morris JN, Kagan A, Pattison DC, Gardner MJ. Incidence and prediction of ischaemic heart-disease in London busmen. Lancet 2:553–9, 1966.

105. Health risk factor surveys of commercial plan- and Medicaid-enrolled members of health-maintenance organizations: Michigan, 1995. MMWR Morb Mortal Wkly Rep 46:923–6, 1997.

106. Prevalence of physical inactivity during leisure time among overweight persons: Behavioral Risk Factor Surveillance System, 1994. MMWR Morb Mortal Wkly Rep 45:185–8, 1996.

107. Prevalence of sedentary lifestyle—behavioral risk factor surveillance system, United States, 1991 MMWR Morb Mortal Wkly Rep 42:576–9, 1993.

108. Cheng YJ, Gregg EW, Narayan KMV, et al. Secular trend in sedentary lifestyle among US adults with and without diabetes 1997–2004. Med Sci Sports Exerc 38(5):S94, 2006.

109. Berg MH, Franz I, Keul J. Physical activity and lipoprotein metabolism: Epidemiological evidence and clinical trials. Eur J Med Res 2:259–64, 1997.

110. Fonong T, Toth MJ, Ades PA, et al. Relationship between physical activity and HDL-cholesterol in healthy older men and women: A cross-sectional and exercise intervention study. Atherosclerosis 127:177–83, 1996.

111. Leon AS, Casal D, Jacobs Jr D. Effects of 2000 kcal per week of walking and stair climbing on physical fitness and risk factors for coronary heart disease. J Cardiopulm Rehabil 16:183–92, 1996.

112. Manninen V, Elo MO, Frick MH, et al. Lipid alterations and decline in the incidence of coronary heart disease in the Helsinki Heart Study. JAMA 260:641–51, 1988.

113. Wood PD. Physical activity, diet, and health: Independent and interactive effects. Med Sci Sports Exerc 26:838–43, 1994.

114. Young DR, Haskell WL, Jatulis DE, Fortmann SP. Associations between changes in physical activity and risk factors for coronary heart disease in a community-based sample of men and women: The Stanford Five-City Project. Am J Epidemiol 138:205–16, 1993.

115. Kelley GA, Kelley KS, Vu Tran Z. Aerobic exercise, lipids and lipoproteins in overweight and obese adults: a meta-analysis of randomized controlled trials. Int J Obes (Lond) 29(8):881–93, 2005.

116. Carroll S, Dudfield M. What is the relationship between exercise and metabolic abnormalities? A review of the metabolic syndrome. Sports Med 34(6):371–418, 2004.

117. Katzel LI, Bleecker ER, Rogus EM, Goldberg AP. Sequential effects of aerobic exercise training and weight loss on risk factors for coronary disease in healthy, obese middle-aged and older men. Metabolism 46:1441–7, 1997.

118. Katcher HI, Hill AM, Lanford JL, Yoo JS, Kris-Etherton PM. Lifestyle approaches and dietary strategies to lower LDL-cholesterol and triglycerides and raise HDL-cholesterol. Endocrinol Metab Clin North Am 38(1):45–78, 2009.

119. Huonker M, Halle M, Keul J. Structural and functional adaptations of the cardiovascular system by training. Int J Sports Med 17(Suppl 3):S164–72, 1996.

120. Kvernmo HD, Osterud B. The effect of physical conditioning suggests adaptation in procoagulant and fibrinolytic potential. Thromb Res 87:559–69, 1997.

121. Ponjee GA, Janssen EM, Hermans J, van Wersch JW. Regular physical activity and changes in risk factors for coronary heart disease: A nine month prospective study. Eur J Clin Chem Clin Biochem 34:477–83, 1996.

122. Sasaki Y, Morimoto A, Ishii I, et al. Preventive effect of long-term aerobic exercise on thrombus formation in rat cerebral vessels. Haemostasis 25:212–17, 1995.

123. Drygas WK. Changes in blood platelet function, coagulation, and fibrinolytic activity in response to moderate, exhaustive, and prolonged exercise. Int J Sports Med 9:67–72, 1988.

124. De JA Paz, Lasierra J, Villa JG, et al. Changes in the fibrinolytic system associated with physical conditioning. Eur J Appl Physiol 65:388–93, 1992.

125. Tanaka K, Nakanishi T. Obesity as a risk factor for various diseases: necessity of lifestyle changes for healthy aging. Appl Human Sci 15:139–48, 1996.

126. Jako P. [The role of physical activity in the prevention of certain internal diseases]. Orv Hetil 136:2379–83, 1995.

127. Nolte LJ, Nowson CA, Dyke AC. Effect of dietary fat reduction and increased aerobic exercise on cardiovascular risk factors. Clin Exp Pharmacol Physiol 24:901–3, 1997.

128. Haskell WL. J.B. Wolffe Memorial Lecture. Health consequences of physical activity: Understanding and challenges regarding dose-response. Med Sci Sports Exerc 26:649–60, 1994.

129. Larson EB, Bruce RA. Health benefits of exercise in an aging society. Arch Intern Med 147:353–6, 1987.

130. Brownlee M. The pathological implications of protein glycation. Clin Invest Med 18:275–81, 1995.

131. Giugliano D, Ceriello A, Paolisso G. Diabetes mellitus, hypertension, and cardiovascular disease: Which role for oxidative stress? Metabolism 44:363–8, 1995.

132. Duncan BB, Heiss G. Nonenzymatic glycosylation of proteins—A new tool for assessment of cumulative hyperglycemia in epidemiologic studies, past and future. Am J Epidemiol 120:169–89, 1984.

133. Heart Protection Study Collaborative Group. MRC/BHF Heart Protection Study of cholesterol lowering with simvastatin in 20,536 high-risk individuals: A randomised placebo-controlled trial. Lancet 360:7–22, 2002.

134. Bao W, Srinivasan SR, Valdez R, et al. Longitudinal changes in cardiovascular risks from childhood to young adulthood in offspring of parent with coronary artery disease: The Bogalusa Heart Study. JAMA 278:1749–54, 1997.

135. Colombel A, Charbonnel B. Weight gain and cardiovascular risk factors in the post-menopausal woman. Hum Reprod 12(Suppl 1):134–45, 1997.

136. Gensini GF, Comeglio M, Colella A. Classical risk factors and emerging elements in the risk profile for coronary artery disease. Eur Heart J 19(Suppl A):A53–61, 1998.

137. Anderssen SA, Holme I, Urdal P, Hjermann I. Associations between central obesity and indexes of hemostatic,

carbohydrate and lipid metabolism. Results of a 1-year intervention from the Oslo Diet and Exercise Study. Scand J Med Sci Sports 8:109–15, 1998.

138. Shaper AG. Obesity and cardiovascular disease. Ciba Found Symp 201:90–103, 1996.

139. Akimova EV, Bogmat LF. Premature coronary heart disease: The influence of positive family history on platelet activity in vivo in children and adolescents (family study). J Cardiovasc Risk 4:13–18, 1997.

140. Saito T, Nanri S, Saito I, et al. A novel approach to assessing family history in the prevention of coronary heart disease. J Epidemiol 7:85–92, 1997.

141. Allen JK, Blumenthal RS. Risk factors in the offspring of women with premature coronary heart disease. Am Heart J 135:428–34, 1998.

142. Pohjola-Sintonen S, Rissanen A, Liskola P, Luomanmaki K. Family history as a risk factor of coronary heart disease in patients under 60 years of age. Eur Heart J 19:235–9, 1998.

143. Khaw KT, Barrett-Connor E. Family history of heart attack: A modifiable risk factor? Circulation 74:239–44, 1986.

144. Barrett-Connor E, Khaw K. Family history of heart attack as an independent predictor of death due to cardiovascular disease. Circulation 69:1065–9, 1984.

145. De Backer G, Ambrosioni E, Borch-Johnsen K, et al. European guidelines on cardiovascular disease prevention in clinical practice. Third Joint Task Force of European and Other Societies on Cardiovascular Disease Prevention in Clinical Practice. Eur Heart J 24:1601–10, 2003.

146. McPherson R, Frohlich J, Fodor G, et al. Canadian Cardiovascular Society position statement—Recommendations for the diagnosis and treatment of dyslipidemia and prevention of cardiovascular disease. Can J Cardiol 22:913–27, 2006.

147. Taraboanta C, Wu E, Lear S, et al. Subclinical atherosclerosis in subjects with family history of premature coronary artery disease. Am Heart J 155(6):1020–6, 2008.

148. Centers for Disease Control and Prevention (CDC). Awareness of family health history as a risk factor for disease: United States, 2004. MMWR Morb Mortal Wkly Rep 53:1044–7, 2004.

149. Neaton JD, Wentworth D. Serum cholesterol, blood pressure, cigarette smoking, and death from coronary heart disease. Overall findings and differences by age for 316,099 white men. Multiple Risk Factor Intervention Trial Research Group. Arch Intern Med 152:56–64, 1992.

150. Smith Jr SC. Risk reduction therapies for patients with coronary artery disease: A call for increased implementation. Am J Med 104:23S–6S, 1998.

151. Grundy SM, Balady GJ, Criqui MH, et al. Primary prevention of coronary heart disease: Guidance from Framingham: A statement for healthcare professionals from the AHA task force on risk reduction. Circulation 97:1876–87, 1998.

152. Haskell WL, Alderman EL, Fair JM, et al. Effects of intensive multiple risk factor reduction on coronary atherosclerosis and clinical cardiac events in men and women with coronary artery disease. The Stanford Coronary Risk Intervention Project (SCRIP). Circulation 89:975–90, 1994.

153. Williams MA. Cardiovascular risk-factor reduction in elderly patients with cardiac disease. Phys Ther 76:469–80, 1996.

154. McCann TJ, Criqui MH, Kashani IA, et al. A randomized trial of cardiovascular risk factor reduction: Patterns of attrition after randomization and during follow-up. J Cardiovasc Risk 4:41–6, 1997.

155. Morley JE, Reese SS. Clinical implications of the aging heart. Am J Med 86:77–86, 1989.

156. Rodeheffer RJ, Gerstenblith G, Beard E, et al. Postural changes in cardiac volumes in men in relation to adult age. Exp Gerontol 21:367–78, 1986.

157. Dahlberg ST. Gender difference in the risk factors for sudden cardiac death. Cardiology 77:31–40, 1990.

158. Orchard TJ. The impact of gender and general risk factors on the occurrence of atherosclerotic vascular disease in non-insulin-dependent diabetes mellitus. Ann Med 28:323–33, 1996.

159. Motro M, Shemesh J. Prevalence of coronary calcification in relation to age, gender and risk factor profile in the insight population. Br J Clin Pract Suppl 88:1–5, 1997.

160. Villablanca AC. Coronary heart disease in women. Gender differences and effects of menopause. Postgrad Med 100:191–6, 201–202, 1996.

161. Rao AV. Coronary heart disease risk factors in women: Focus on gender differences. J La State Med Soc 150:67–72, 1998.

162. Kitler ME. Coronary disease: Are there gender differences? Eur Heart J 15:409–17, 1994.

163. Gorcdeski GI. Impact of the menopause on the epidemiology and risk factors of coronary artery heart disease in women. Exp Gerontol 29:357–75, 1994.

164. Wister AV, Gee EM. Age at death due to ischemic heart disease: Gender differences. Soc Biol 41:110–26, 1994.

165. Adams Jr KF, Dunlap SH, Sueta CA, et al. Relation between gender, etiology and survival in patients with symptomatic heart failure. J Am Coll Cardiol 28:1781–8, 1996.

166. Roger VL, Jacobsen SJ, Pellikka PA, et al. Gender differences in use of stress testing and coronary heart disease mortality: A population-based study in Olmsted County, Minnesota. J Am Coll Cardiol 32:345–52, 1998.

167. Shumaker SA, Brooks MM, Schron EB, et al. Gender differences in health-related quality of life among postmyocardial infarction patients: Brief report. CAST Investigators. Cardiac Arrhythmia Suppression Trials. Womens Health 3:53–60, 1997.

168. Kambara H, Kinoshita M, Nakagawa M, Kawai C. Gender difference in long-term prognosis after myocardial infarction—Clinical characteristics in 1000 patients. The Kyoto and Shiga Myocardial Infarction (KYSMI) Study Group. Jpn Circ J 59:1–10, 1995.

169. Behar S, Zion M, Reicher-Reiss H, et al. Short- and long-term prognosis of patients with a first acute myocardial infarction with concomitant peripheral vascular disease. SPRINT Study Group. Am J Med 96:15–19, 1994.

170. Brochier ML, Arwidson P. Coronary heart disease risk factors in women. Eur Heart J 19(Suppl A):A45–52, 1998.

171. Lunetta M, Barbagallo A, Attardo T, et al. Coronary heart disease in type 2 diabetic patients: Common and different risk factors in men and women. Diabetes Metab 23:230–1, 1997.

172. Frost PH, Davis BR, Burlando AJ, et al. Coronary heart disease risk factors in men and women aged 60 years and older: Findings from the systolic hypertension in the elderly program. Circulation 94:26–34, 1996.

173. Dallongeville J, Marecaux N, Isorez D, et al. Multiple coronary heart disease risk factors are associated with menopause and influenced by substitutive hormonal therapy in a cohort of French women. Atherosclerosis 118:123–33, 1995.

174. Bellamy L, Casas J-P, Hingorani AD, Williams DJ. Pre-eclampsia and risk of cardiovascular disease and cancer in later life: Systematic review and meta-analysis. BMJ 335:974, 2007.

175. Salpeter SR, Walsh JME, Greyber E, Salpeter EE. Coronary heart disease events associated with therapy in younger and older women; a meta-analysis. J Gen Intern Med 21(4):363–6, 2006.

176. Grodstein F, Stampfer MJ, Manson JE, et al. Postmenopausal estrogen and progestin use and the risk of cardiovascular disease. N Engl J Med 335:453–61, 1996.

177. Rossouw JE, Anderson GL, Prentice RL, et al. Risks and benefits of estrogen plus progestin in healthy postmenopausal women: principal results from the Women's Health Initiative randomized controlled trial. JAMA 288:321–33, 2002.

178. Anderson GL, Limacher M, Assaf AR, et al. Effects of conjugated equine estrogen in postmenopausal women with hysterectomy: The Women's Health Initiative randomized controlled trial. JAMA 291:1701–12, 2004.

179. Salpeter SR, Walsh JM, Greyber E, Ormiston TM, Salpeter EE. Mortality associated with hormone replacement therapy in younger and older women: A meta-analysis. J Gen Intern Med 19:791–804, 2004.

180. Mosca L, Banka CL, Benjamin EJ, et al. Evidence-based guidelines for cardiovascular disease prevention in women: 2007 Update. Circulation 115(15):e407, 2007.

181. Friedman M, Rosenman RH. Association of specific overt behavior pattern with blood and cardiovascular findings. JAMA 169:1286–96, 1959.

182. Lachar BL. Coronary-prone behavior. Type A behavior revisited. Tex Heart Inst J 20:143–51, 1993.

183. Keltikangas-Jarvinen L, Raikkonen K, Hautanen A, Adlercreutz H. Vital exhaustion, anger expression, and pituitary and adrenocortical hormones. Implications for the insulin resistance syndrome. Arterioscler Thromb Vasc Biol 16:275–80, 1996.

184. King KB. Psychologic and social aspects of cardiovascular disease. Ann Behav Med 19:264–70, 1997.

185. Grignani G, Pacchiarini L, Zucchella M, et al. Effect of mental stress on platelet function in normal subjects and in patients with coronary artery disease. Haemostasis 22:138–46, 1992.

186. Markovitz JH, Matthews KA. Platelets and coronary heart disease: Potential psychophysiologic mechanisms. Psychosom Med 53:643–68, 1991.

187. Superko HR, Fogelman A. Lipoproteins and atherosclerosis—The role of HDL cholesterol, Lp(a), and LDL particle size. Presented at the American College of Cardiology, 48th Scientific Session, New Orleans, LA, March 7–10, 1999.

188. Cohen J, Wilson WF. Homocysteine, fibrinogen, Lp(a), small dense LDL, oxidative stress, and C. pneumoniae infection: How important are they? Presented at the American College of Cardiology, 48th Scientific Session, New Orleans, LA, March 7–10, 1999.

189. Robinson K, Arheart K, Refsum H, et al. Concentrations: Risk factors for stroke, peripheral vascular disease and coronary artery disease. European Comac Group. Circulation 97(5):437–43, 1998.

190. Glueck CJ, Shaw P, Lang JE, et al. Evidence that homocysteine is an independent risk factor for atherosclerosis in hyperlipidemic patients. Am J Cardiol 75(2):132–6, 1995.

191. Albert CM, Ma J, Rifai N, Stampfer MJ, Ridker PM. Prospective Study of C-reactive protein, homocysteine, and plasma lipid levels as predictors of sudden cardiac death. Circulation 105:2595–9, 2002.

192. Kannel WB, Shatzkin A. Sudden death: Lessons from subsets in population studies. J Am Coll Cardiol 5(Suppl 6):141B, 1985.

193. Guidelines for cardiopulmonary resuscitation and emergency cardiac care. Emergency Cardiac Care Committee and Subcommittees, American Heart Association. Part IX. Ensuring effectiveness of communitywide emergency cardiac care. JAMA 268:2289–95, 1992.

194. White RD. Optimal access to and response by public and voluntary services, including the role of bystanders and family members, in cardiopulmonary resuscitation. New Horiz 5:153–7, 1997.

195. Hilton TC, Chaitman BR. The prognosis in stable and unstable angina. Cardiol Clin 9:27–38, 1991.

196. Brann WM, Tresch DD. Management of stable and unstable angina in elderly patients. Compr Ther 23:49–56, 1997.

197. Chierchia S, Brunelli C, Simonetti I, et al. Sequence of events in angina at rest: primary reduction in coronary flow. Circulation 61:759–68, 1980.

198. Chasen C, Muller JE. Cardiovascular triggers and morning events. Blood Press Monit 3:35–42, 1998.

199. Kristensen SD, Ravn HB, Falk E. Insights into the pathophysiology of unstable coronary artery disease. Am J Cardiol 80:5E–9E, 1997.

200. Osborne JA, Stone PH. Recent advances in the understanding and management of stable and unstable angina pectoris and asymptomatic myocardial ischemia. Curr Opin Cardiol 9:448–56, 1994.

201. Haft JI, Mariano DL, Goldstein J. Comparison of the histopathology of culprit lesions in chronic stable angina, unstable angina, and myocardial infarction. Clin Cardiol 20:651–5, 1997.

202. Thieme T, Wernecke KD, Meyer R, et al. Angioscopic evaluation of atherosclerotic plaques: Validation by histomorphologic analysis and association with stable and unstable coronary syndromes. J Am Coll Cardiol 28:1–6, 1996.

203. Moon JC, De Arenaza DP, Elkington AG, et al. The pathologic basis of Q-wave and non-Q-wave myocardial infarction: A cardiovascular magnetic resonance study. J Am Coll Cardiol 44:554, 2004.

204. Libby P, Bonow RO, Mann DL, et al. Braunwald's Heart Disease: A Textbook of Cardiovascular Medicine, ed 8. Philadelphia, 2007, Saunders.

205. Swan HJ, Forrester JS, Diamond G, et al.. Hemodynamic spectrum of myocardial infarction and cardiogenic shock. A conceptual model. Circulation 45:1097, 1972.

206. Forrester JS, Wyatt HL, Da Luz PL, et al. Functional significance of regional ischemic contraction abnormalities. Circulation 54:64, 1976.

207. McNeer JF, Wallace AG, Wagner GS, et al. The course of acute myocardial infarction. Circulation 51:410, 1975.

208. Rosengren A, Wilhelmsen L, Hagman M, Wedel H. Natural history of myocardial infarction and angina pectoris in a general population sample of middle-aged men: A 16-year follow-up of the Primary Prevention Study, Goteborg, Sweden. J Intern Med 244:495–505, 1998.

209. Lewis CE, Raczynski JM, Oberman A, Cutter GR. Risk factors and the natural history of coronary heart disease in blacks. Cardiovasc Clin 21:29–45, 1991.

210. Kramsch DM, Blankenhorn DH. Regression of atherosclerosis: Which components regress and what influences their reversal. Wien Klin Wochenschr 104:2–9, 1992.

211. Hodis HN. Reversibility of atherosclerosis—Evolving perspectives from two arterial imaging clinical trials: The cholesterol lowering atherosclerosis regression study and the monitored atherosclerosis regression study. J Cardiovasc Pharmacol 25: S25–31, 1995.

212. Ornish D, Scherwitz LW, Billings JH, et al. Intensive lifestyle changes for reversal of coronary heart disease. JAMA 280: 2001–7, 1998.

213. Patrono C. Prevention of myocardial infarction and stroke by aspirin: Different mechanisms? Different dosage? Thromb Res 92:S25–32, 1998.

214. Mosa L, Banka CL, Benjamin EJ, et al. Evidence-based guide for cardiovascular disease prevention in women: 2007 Update. Circulation 115:1481–501, 2007.

215. Azen SP, Mack WJ, Cashin-Hemphill L, et al. Progression of coronary artery disease predicts clinical coronary events. Long-term follow-up from the Cholesterol Lowering Atherosclerosis Study. Circulation 93:34–41, 1996.

216. Blankenhorn DH, Johnson RL, Nessim SA, et al. The Cholesterol Lowering Atherosclerosis Study (CLAS): Design methods, and baseline results. Control Clin Trials 8:356–87, 1987.

217. Strandberg TE, Pitkanen A, Larjo P, et al. Attitude changes of general practitioners towards lowering LDL cholesterol. J Cardiovasc Risk 5:43–6, 1998.

218. Campbell NC, Thain J, Deans HG, et al. Secondary prevention clinics for coronary heart disease: Randomised trial of effect on health. BMJ 316:1434–7, 1998.

219. Chobanian AV, Bakris GL, Black HR, et al. The seventh report of the Joint National Committee on prevention, detection, evaluation, and treatment of high blood pressure: The JNC 7 report. JAMA 289(19):2560–72, 2003.

220. Cushman WC. The clinical significance of systolic hypertension. Am J Hypertens 11:182S–5S, 1998.

221. Kannel WB. Blood pressure as a cardiovascular risk factor: Prevention and treatment. JAMA 275:1571–6, 1996.

222. Cohn JN, Limas CJ, Guiha NH. Hypertension and the heart. Arch Intern Med 133:969–79, 1974.

223. Frohlich ED. The heart in hypertension. In Genest J, Kuchel O, Hamet P, et al. (eds.). Hypertension: Physiopathology and Treatment. New York, 1983, McGraw-Hill.

224. Society of Actuaries & Association of Life Insurance Medical Directors of America. Blood Pressure Study 1979. Chicago, 1980, Society of Actuaries & Association of Life Insurance Medical Directors of America.

225. Kannel WB. Framingham study insights into hypertensive risk of cardiovascular disease. Hypertens Res 18:181–96, 1995.

226. Kannel WB, Wolf PA, Verter J, McNamara PM. Epidemiologic assessment of the role of blood pressure in stroke: The Framingham Study, 1970. JAMA 276:1269–78, 1996.

227. Rutan GH, Kuller LH, Neaton JD, et al. Mortality associated with diastolic hypertension and isolated systolic hypertension among men screened for the Multiple Risk Factor Intervention Trial. Circulation 77:504–14, 1988.

228. Strauer BE. Left ventricular wall stress and hypertrophy. In Messerli FH (ed.). The Heart and Hypertension. New York, 1987, Yorke Medical Books.

229. Graettinger WF, Bryg RJ. Left-ventricular diastolic function and hypertension. Cardiol Clin 13:559–67, 1995.

230. Lopez Sendon J. Regional myocardial ischaemia and diastolic dysfunction in hypertensive heart disease. Eur Heart J 14 (Suppl J):110–13, 1993.

231. Smith V-E, Katz AM. Left ventricular relaxation in hypertension. In Messerli FH (ed.). The Heart and Hypertension. New York, 1987, Yorke Medical Books.

232. Wikstrand J. Diastolic function of the hypertrophied left ventricle. In Messerli FH (ed.). The Heart and Hypertension. New York, 1987, Yorke Medical Books.

233. Kozakova M, Palombo C, Pratali L, et al. Mechanisms of coronary flow reserve impairment in human hypertension. An integrated approach by transthoracic and transesophageal echocardiography. Hypertension 29:551–9, 1997.

234. Iriarte M, Murga N, Sagastagoitia D, et al. Congestive heart failure from left ventricular diastolic dysfunction in systemic hypertension. Am J Cardiol 71:308–12, 1993.

235. Johnson DB, Dell'Italia LJ. Cardiac hypertrophy and failure in hypertension. Curr Opin Nephrol Hypertens 5:186–91, 1996.

236. Borer JS, Jason M, Devereux RB, et al. Function of the hypertrophied left ventricle at rest and during exercise. Hypertension and aortic stenosis. Am J Med 75:34–9, 1983.

237. Lim PO, MacFadyen RJ, Clarkson PB, MacDonald TM. Impaired exercise tolerance in hypertensive patients. Ann Intern Med 124:41–55, 1996.

238. Manolas J, Kyriakidis M, Anastasakis A, et al. Usefulness of noninvasive detection of left ventricular diastolic abnormalities during isometric stress in hypertrophic cardiomyopathy and in athletes. Am J Cardiol 81:306–13, 1998.

239. Tarazi RC. Cardiovascular hypertrophy in hypertension. Arthur C. Corcoran Memorial Lecture. Hypertension 8:II187–90, 1986.

240. Devereux RD, Agabiti-Rosei E, Dahlof B, et al. Regression of left ventricular hypertrophy as a surrogate end-point for morbid events in hypertension treatment trialsc [published erratum appears in J Hypertens 15(1):103, 1997]. J Hypertens Suppl 14:S95–101, 1996.

241. Muiesan ML, Salvetti M, Rizzoni D, et al. Association of change in left ventricular mass with prognosis during long-term antihypertensive treatment. J Hypertens 13:1091–5, 1995.

242. Schulman DS, Flores AR, Tugoen J, et al. Antihypertensive treatment in hypertensive patients with normal left ventricular mass is associated with left ventricular remodeling and improved diastolic function. Am J Cardiol 78:56–60, 1996.

243. Sytkowski PA, D'Agostino RB, Belanger AJ, Kannel WB. Secular trends in long-term sustained hypertension, long-term treatment, and cardiovascular mortality. The Framingham Heart Study 1950 to 1990. Circulation 93:697–703, 1996.

244. Kaplan NM. Long-term effectiveness of nonpharmacological treatment of hypertension. Hypertension 18:I153–60, 1991.

245. Kaplan NM. Treatment of hypertension: Insights from the JNC-VI report. Am Fam Physician 58:1323–30, 1998.

246. American College of Sports Medicine. Guidelines for Exercise Testing and Prescription, ed 8. Baltimore, 2009, Lippincott Williams & Wilkins.

247. Fagard R, Staessen J, Thijs L, Amery A. Influence of antihypertensive drugs on exercise capacity. Drugs 46(Suppl 2):32–6, 1993.

248. Head A. Exercise metabolism and beta-blocker therapy. An update. Sports Med 27:81–96, 1999.

249. Kendrick ZV, Cristal N, Lowenthal DT. Cardiovascular drugs and exercise interactions. Cardiol Clin 5:227–44, 1987.

250. Fagard R, Staessen J, Amery A. Maximal aerobic power in essential hypertension. J Hypertens 6:859–65, 1988.

251. Goodman JM, McLaughlin PR, Plyley MJ, et al. Impaired cardiopulmonary response to exercise in moderate hypertension. Can J Cardiol 8:363–71, 1992.

252. Skinner JS. Exercise Testing and Exercise Prescription for Special Cases—Theoretical Basis and Clinical Application. Philadelphia, 1993, Lea & Febiger.

253. Franz IW. Blood pressure response to exercise in normotensives and hypertensives. Can J Sport Sci 16:296–301, 1991.

254. Nyberg G. Blood pressure and heart rate response to isometric exercise and mental arithmetic in normotensive and hypertensive subjects. Clin Sci Mol Med Suppl 3:681s–5s, 1976.

255. Hagberg JM, Seals DR. Exercise training and hypertension. Acta Med Scand Suppl 711:131–6, 1986.

256. Hagberg JM, Montain SJ, Martin WH, Ehsani AA. Effect of exercise training in 60- to 69-year-old persons with essential hypertension. Am J Cardiol 64:348–53, 1989.

257. Hagberg JM, Brown MD. Does exercise training play a role in the treatment of essential hypertension? J Cardiovasc Risk 2:296–302, 1995.

258. Papademetriou V, Kokkinos PF. The role of exercise in the control of hypertension and cardiovascular risk. Curr Opin Nephrol Hypertens 5:459–62, 1996.

259. Petrella RJ. How effective is exercise training for the treatment of hypertension? Clin J Sport Med 8:224–31, 1998.

260. Kokkinos PF, Narayan P, Colleran JA, et al. Effects of regular exercise on blood pressure and left ventricular hypertrophy in African-American men with severe hypertension. N Engl J Med 333:1462–7, 1995.

261. Burt VL, Whelton P, Roccella EJ, et al. Prevalence of hypertension in the US adult population. Results from the Third National Health and Nutrition Examination Survey, 1988–1991. Hypertension 25:305–13, 1995.

262. Izzo JL, Black HR. Hypertension Primer. Dallas, TX, American Heart Association, 1993.

263. Goldstein LB, Adams R, Alberts MJ, et al. Primary prevention of ischemic stroke: A guideline from the American Heart Association/American Stroke Association Stroke Council. Stroke 37:1583, 2006.

264. Sacco RL, Adams R, Albers G, et al. Guidelines for prevention of stroke in patients with ischemic stroke or transient ischemic attack. A statement for healthcare professionals from the American Heart Association/American Stroke Association Council on Stroke. Stroke 37:577, 2006.

265. Adams HP, Adams RJ, Brott T, et al. Guidelines for the early management of patients with ischemic stroke: A scientific statement from the Stroke Council of the American Stroke Association. Stroke 34:1056, 2003.

266. Adams HP, Adams R, Del Zoppo G, Goldstein LB. Guidelines for the early management of patients with ischemic stroke: 2005 Guidelines update. A scientific statement from the Stroke Council of the American Heart Association/American Stroke Association. Stroke 36:916, 2005.

267. Ridker PM, Cook NR, Lee I-M, et al. A randomized trial of low-dose aspirin in the primary prevention of cardiovascular disease in women. N Engl J Med 352:1293, 2005.

268. Esprit Study Group, Halkes PH, van Gijn J, et al. Aspirin plus dipyridamole versus aspirin alone after cerebral ischaemia of arterial origin (ESPRIT): Randomised controlled trial. Lancet 367:1665, 2006.

269. Mohr JP, Thompson JLP, Lazar RM, et al. A comparison of warfarin and aspirin for the prevention of recurrent ischemic stroke. N Engl J Med 345:1444, 2001.

270. Kallero KS. Mortality and morbidity in patients with intermittent claudication as defined by venous occlusion plethysmography. A ten-year follow-up study. J Chronic Dis 34:455–62, 1981.

271. Hertzer NR, Beven EG, Young JR, et al. Coronary artery disease in peripheral vascular patients. A classification of 1000 coronary angiograms and results of surgical management. Ann Surg 199:223–33, 1984.

272. Leng GC, Lee AJ, Fowkes FG, et al. Incidence, natural history and cardiovascular events in symptomatic and asymptomatic peripheral arterial disease in the general population. Int J Epidemiol 25:1172–81, 1996.

273. Bauer TA, Regensteiner JG, Brass EP, Hiatt WR. Oxygen uptake kinetics during exercise are slowed in patient with peripheral arterial disease. J Appl Physiol 87:809–16, 1999.

274. Eldridge JE, Hossack KF. Patterns of oxygen consumption during exercise testing in peripheral vascular disease. Cardiology 74:236–40, 1987.

275. Hansen JE, Sue DY, Oren A, Wasserman K. Relation of oxygen uptake to work rate in normal men and men with circulatory disorders. Am J Cardiol 59:669–74, 1987.

276. Boyd CE, Bird PJ, Teates CD, et al. Pain free physical training in intermittent claudication. J Sports Med Phys Fitness 24:112–22, 1984.

277. Creasy TS, McMillan PJ, Fletcher EW, et al. Is percutaneous transluminal angioplasty better than exercise for claudication? Preliminary results from a prospective randomised trial. Eur J Vasc Surg 4:135–40, 1990.

278. Dahllof AG, Holm J, Schersten T. Exercise training of patients with intermittent claudication. Scand J Rehabil Med Suppl 9:20–6, 1983.

279. Ernst EE, Matrai A. Intermittent claudication, exercise, and blood rheology. Circulation 76:1110–14, 1987.

280. Hiatt WR, Regensteiner JG, Hargarten ME, et al. Benefit of exercise conditioning for patients with peripheral arterial disease. Circulation 81:602–9, 1990.

281. Hiatt WR, Wolfel EE, Meier RH, Regensteiner JG. Superiority of treadmill walking exercise versus strength training for patients with peripheral arterial disease. Implications for the mechanism of the training response. Circulation 90:1866–74, 1994.

282. Jonason T, Ringqvist I, Oman-Rydberg A. Home-training of patients with intermittent claudication. Scand J Rehabil Med 13:137–41, 1981.

283. Mannarino E, Pasqualini L, Menna M, et al. Effects of physical training on peripheral vascular disease: A controlled study. Angiology 40:5–10, 1989.

284. Ruell PA, Imperial ES, Bonar FJ, et al. Intermittent claudication. The effect of physical training on walking tolerance and venous lactate concentration. Eur J Appl Physiol 52:420–5, 1984.

285. Perkins JM, Collin J, Creasy TS, et al. Exercise training versus angioplasty for stable claudication. Long and medium term results of a prospective, randomised trial. Eur J Vasc Endovasc Surg 11:409–13, 1996.

286. Larsen OA, Lassen NA. Effect of daily muscular exercise in patients with intermittent claudication. Lancet 2:1093–6, 1966.

287. Gardner AW. Peripheral arterial disease. In American College of Sports Medicine. ACSM's Exercise Management for Persons with Chronic Diseases and Disabilities. Champaign, IL, 1997, Human Kinetics.

288. Smith RB, Perdue GD. Diseases of the peripheral arteries and veins. In Alexander RW, Schlant RC, King S, et al. (eds.). Hurst's The Heart, Arteries and Veins, ed 9. New York, 1998, McGraw-Hill.

289. Weber-Mzell D, Kotanko P, Schumacher M, et al. Coronary anatomy predicts presence or absence of renal artery stenosis. A prospective study in patients undergoing cardiac catheterization for suspected coronary artery disease. Eur Heart J 23:1684, 2002.

290. Safian RD, Textor SC. Renal-artery stenosis. N Engl J Med 344:431, 2001.

# CHAPTER 4

# Cardiac Muscle Dysfunction and Failure

*Ellen Hillegass, Lawrence Cahalin*

## Chapter Outline

Cardiac muscle dysfunction (CMD) is a term that has gained popularity in describing an apparently common finding in patients with heart and lung disease.[1-3] CMD effectively, yet very simply, describes the most common cause of congestive heart failure (CHF).[2] CMD develops as a result of some underlying abnormality of cardiac structure or function. Those presenting only with CMD (who are at risk of heart failure) may present without symptoms. As the abnormality progresses, the heart begins to fail to function effectively to meet the demands of the system, and heart failure begins. The syndrome of heart failure is accompanied by symptoms of shortness of breath and fatigue at rest or with activity. It is estimated that 5.7 million or more Americans suffer from CHF and that 670,000 new cases occur yearly, requiring 1.1 million hospitalizations each year.[4] In addition, the lifetime risk of developing heart failure for both men and women at age 40 years is 1 in 5, with the annual rate of developing heart failure of 65.2 at >85 years of age years.[4] Individuals with a wide variety of heart and lung diseases very likely will develop CHF at some time during their lives,[3] frequently manifested as pulmonary congestion or pulmonary edema.[1] This chapter describes the etiology, pathophysiology, clinical manifestations, medical management, prognosis of CMD and CHF, and indications for physical therapy including patient management.

> **Clinical Tip**
> The practice pattern associated with CMD and CHF is Practice Pattern 6-D: Impaired Aerobic Capacity/Endurance Associated with Cardiovascular Pump Dysfunction or Failure.

## Causes and Types of Cardiac Muscle Dysfunction

Most often CMD may not present with symptoms, but many of the signs and symptoms of CHF are the result of a "sequence of events with a resultant increase in fluid in the interstitial spaces of the lungs, liver, subcutaneous tissues, and serous cavities."[5] The etiology of CHF is varied, but it is most commonly the result of CMD.

The varied causes of CMD and subsequently CHF can be best classified according to 11 specific processes/causes, which are described in Table 4-1.[5-7]

## Hypertension

The increased arterial pressure seen in systemic hypertension eventually produces left ventricular hypertrophy. An extremely elevated ventricular and occasionally elevated atrial pressure commonly seen in patients with CMD tend to produce a less-effective pump as the myocardial contractile fibers become overstretched, thus increasing the work of each myocardial fiber in an attempt to maintain an adequate cardiac output.[8,9] Myocardial work continued in this manner eventually produces left ventricular hypertrophy as the contractile fibers adapt to the increased workload.[10,11] The two problems with left ventricular hypertrophy are the increase in afterload and the increased energy expenditure (metabolic cost) required for myocardial contraction because of increased myocardial cell mass.[8,10,12] The increased cell mass without an additional increase in vasculature also affects blood supply to the muscle, resulting in a decreased blood supply to some of the new muscle mass. Medical management of hypertension should begin upon diagnosis after echocardiogram is performed for baseline documentation of ventricular involvement. Medical management usually consists of angiotensin-converting enzyme

## Table 4-1 Etiology of Congestive Heart Failure

| Causes | Description |
|---|---|
| Hypertension | ↑ Arterial pressure leads to left ventricular hypertrophy (↑ myocardial cell mass) and ↑ energy expenditure. |
| Coronary artery disease (myocardial ischemia) | Dysfunction of the left or right ventricle or both as a result of injury. Scar formation and ↓ contractility may occur, as well as reduced relaxation. |
| Cardiac dysrhythmias | Extremely rapid or slow cardiac arrhythmias impair the functioning ventricles. Dysfunction may be reversible if arrhythmia controlled. |
| Renal insufficiency | Causes fluid overload, which frequently progresses to CMD and CHF that may be reversed. |
| Cardiomyopathy | Contraction and relaxation of myocardial muscle fibers are impaired. Primary causes: pathologic processes in the heart muscle itself, which impair the heart's ability to contract. Secondary causes: systemic disease processes. |
| Heart valve abnormality | Valvular stenosis or incompetent valves (valvular insufficiency because of abnormal or poorly functioning valve leaflets), cause myocardial hypertrophy and cause a decrease in ventricular distensibility with mild diastolic dysfunction. |
| Pericardial effusion | Injury to the pericardium can cause acute pericarditis (inflammation of the pericardial sac surrounding the heart) and progress to pericardial effusion and cardiac compression as fluid fills the pericardial sac. May also develop cardiac tamponade. |
| Pulmonary embolism | Severe hypoxemia may result from embolus blocking a moderate to large amount of lung, resulting in elevated pulmonary artery pressures, a ↑ right ventricular work and right heart. |
| Pulmonary hypertension | Elevated pressures in pulmonary artery lead to increased afterload for the right ventricle and subsequently, over time, to right ventricular failure. |
| Spinal cord injury | Transection of the cervical spinal cord prevents the sympathetic-driven changes necessary to maintain cardiac performance. |
| Age-related changes | Aging appears to decrease cardiac output by altered contraction and relaxation of cardiac muscle. The two most common congenital heart defects are nonstenotic bicuspid aortic valve and the leaflet abnormality associated with mitral valve prolapse. |

(ACE) inhibitors, calcium channel blockers, diuretics, or possibly β blockers. Chapter 14 provides detailed information on medications. Exercise training performed regularly has demonstrated changes in systolic pressure of 10 mm Hg and diastolic pressure of 8 mm Hg, but must be maintained throughout an individual's lifetime to maintain benefits.

## Coronary Artery Disease (Myocardial Infarction/Ischemia)

Coronary artery disease is the second most common cause of CMD,[3] which occurs because of dysfunction of the left or right ventricle or both as a result of injury.[13-15] Besides the ischemic injury from disease restricting blood flow to the cardiac muscle, there could be actual injury from infarction resulting in scar formation and decreased contractility, as well as reduced relaxation. In addition, other factors can cause injury, including myocardial damage or "stunning" following coronary angioplasty[16,17] and postperfusion (postpump) syndrome following cardiopulmonary bypass surgery.[18,19] Essentially postpump syndrome results in organ and subsystem dysfunction following abnormal bleeding, inflammation, concomitant renal dysfunction, and peripheral and central vasoconstriction. Box 4-1 lists the actual risk factors associated with postpump syndrome.

## Cardiac Arrhythmias

Cardiac arrhythmias can also cause CMD for reasons similar to those given for myocardial infarction.[5] Extremely rapid or slow cardiac arrhythmias can impair the functioning of the left or right ventricle, or both, and an overall CMD ensues. Prolonged very slow or very fast heart rates are frequently caused by a sick sinus node syndrome or heart block (producing very slow heart rates), prolonged supraventricular tachycardia (i.e., rapid atrial fibrillation or flutter), or ventricular tachycardia (both tachycardias produce very fast heart rates).[20,21] (See Chapter 9 for explanation and pictures.) Very slow heart rates or heart blocks are often an adverse reaction or side effect of a specific medication, but when medications are withheld and slow heart rates or a heart block persists, the implantation of a permanent pacemaker is generally performed.[20] This type of CMD is readily amenable to treatment and quite reversible.

CMD caused by very rapid heart rates is also reversible. Rapid atrial fibrillation or flutter can produce CMD and is often easily treated by the administration of verapamil or digoxin[20] (see Chapter 14). If these drugs fail, electrical cardioversion is usually performed, after which rapid heart rates frequently become much more normal as the cyclic "circus movement" propagating the rapid rhythm is disrupted and the sinoatrial node is allowed to resume control of the heart's rhythm.[20] Ventricular tachycardia and fibrillation are life-threatening cardiac arrhythmias, which, if prolonged, rapid, or both, can also produce CMD and death. The treatment of ventricular tachycardia and fibrillation is dependent on the clinical status of the patient and follows the guidelines set forth by the American Heart Association.[20] The use of implantable cardiac defibrillators (ICDs) has been a treatment of choice for patients with recurrent ventricular tachycardia and fibrillation that is unresponsive to antiarrhythmic medications.[21,22] Ventricular function is intimately related to cardiac rhythm. Any abnormally fast, slow, or unsynchronized rhythm can impair ventricular and atrial function quickly and progress to CHF and even death.[20] Many patients with CMD have preexisting arrhythmias that must be controlled, typically with medication, but sometimes by other methods (e.g., ablation, ICD)[21] to prevent further deterioration of a muscle that is already compromised.

Because antiarrhythmic agents act as cardiodepressants and often have proarrhythmic effects, they are not usually indicated in individuals with CHF.[23]

## Renal Insufficiency

Acute or chronic renal insufficiency tends to produce a fluid overload, which frequently progresses to CMD and CHF that can often be reversed if it is the only underlying pathophysiologic process. However, other pathophysiologic processes may produce the fluid overload that caused CMD.[24] Consequently, CMD is seldom reversed by the correction of fluid volume alone. Nevertheless, the primary treatment is to decrease the reabsorption of fluid from the kidneys so that more fluid is eliminated (in essence, diuresed).[24] The diuretic most commonly used is furosemide (Lasix), which can be given intravenously or orally. In addition to and as a result of the administration of a diuretic, electrolyte levels are carefully monitored, ensuring that potassium and sodium levels are within the normal range to prevent further retention of fluid from high levels of potassium and sodium or the detrimental effects of low levels (e.g., cardiac arrhythmias and muscle weakness). Low-dose aldosterone antagonists are also recommended in individuals with moderately severe heart failure symptoms or with left ventricle (LV) dysfunction after acute coronary syndrome (as long as serum creatinine is <2.5 mg dL).[25]

---

### Box 4-1

**Risk Factors Associated with Postcoronary Bypass Pump Syndrome**

- Duration of cardiopulmonary bypass greater than 90 to 120 minutes for young infants or 150 minutes for adults
- Patient age
- Presence of preoperative cyanosis
- Perfusion flow rate
- Composition of the perfusate
- Oxygenating surface
- Patient temperature during perfusion

From Kirklin JW, Blackstone EH, Kirklin JK. Cardiac surgery. In Braunnwald E (ed.). Heart Disease: A Textbook of Cardiovascular Medicine. Philadelphia, 1988, Saunders.

Severe renal insufficiency, demonstrating advanced azotemia, is best treated by dialysis (peritoneal or hemodialysis), which may remove as much as 1 L of extracellular fluid per hour.[24]

## Cardiomyopathy

Cardiomyopathy is a disease in which the contraction and relaxation of myocardial muscle fibers are impaired.[10] This impaired contractility can result from either primary or secondary causes.[26] The primary causes are the result of pathologic processes in the heart muscle itself, which impair the heart's ability to contract. The secondary causes of cardiomyopathy are the result of a systemic disease processes rather than of pathologic myocardial processes and can be classified according to the systemic disease that subsequently affects myocardial contraction (Table 4-2). They may also be subdivided into tertiary causes to allow for treatment of root causation using the most appropriate protocol available.

Cardiomyopathies are differentiated based on a functional standpoint, emphasizing three basic categories: dilated,

### Table 4-2 Secondary and Tertiary Causes of Cardiomyopathy

| Secondary Causes | Tertiary Causes |
|---|---|
| Inflammation | Viral infection |
| | Bacterial infection |
| Metabolic | Selenium deficiency |
| | Diabetes mellitus |
| Toxic | Alcohol |
| | Bleomycin |
| Infiltrative | Sarcoidosis |
| | Neoplastic |
| Hematologic | Carcinoid fibrosis |
| | Endomyocardial fibrosis |
| Hypersensitivity | Sickle cell anemia |
| | Leukemia |
| Genetic | Cardiac transplant rejection |
| | Methyldopa |
| Miscellaneous acquired | Hypertrophic cardiomyopathy |
| | Duchenne muscular dystrophy |
| Idiopathic | Postpartum cardiomyopathy |
| | Obesity |
| Physical agents | Idiopathic hypertrophic cardiomyopathy |
| | Heat stroke |
| | Hypothermia |
| | Radiation |

*Adapted from Braunwald E. Heart Disease: A Textbook of Cardiovascular Medicine. ed 3. Philadelphia, 1988, Saunders.*

hypertrophic, and restrictive (Table 4-3). Patients often present with a combination of these functional classifications.[10] The cardiomyopathies are distinguished from one another by echocardiographic and myocardial biopsy results.[10]

## Dilated Cardiomyopathies

Dilated cardiomyopathies "probably represent a final common pathway that is the end result of myocardial damage produced by a variety of toxic, metabolic, or infectious agents."[10] Possible causes of dilated cardiomyopathies include the following:[10]

- Long-term alcohol abuse
- Systemic hypertension
- A variety of infections
- Cigarette smoking
- Pregnancy
- Carnitine deficiency

These conditions may not be primarily responsible for dilated cardiomyopathy but may act to lower the threshold for its development. Little is known regarding the further development of dilated cardiomyopathies, but the dilation that occurs in this type of cardiomyopathy, and which sets it apart from hypertrophic cardiomyopathy, appears to be a result of myocardial mitochondrial dysfunction.[10] Dysfunction of myocardial mitochondria leads to a lack of energy necessary for proper cardiac function, causing the heart to be a less-effective pump.[10] Ineffective pumping increases both the left ventricular end-diastolic volume and pressure, which dilate the left ventricle (and frequently the other heart chambers). Because of inappropriate energy sources, the left ventricle is unable to contract properly or to relax individual muscle fibers in response to increased workload, thereby preventing myocardial hypertrophy but producing ineffective systolic (pumping) function. Cardiomyopathy as a consequence of treatment of malignancy with chemotherapy is often related to anthracycline administration. Anthracycline cardiomyopathy is dose related and, depending on the aggressiveness of treatment protocols, can be seen in 5% to 20% of patients receiving these agents.

## Hypertrophic Cardiomyopathy

Hypertrophic cardiomyopathy should be thought of as the opposite of dilated cardiomyopathy, both functionally and etiologically. The hypertrophy associated with hypertrophic cardiomyopathy is inappropriate for the applied hemodynamic load and is associated with proper myocardial mitochondrial function. Furthermore, the dysfunction of hypertrophic cardiomyopathy is one of diastolic dysfunction, which impairs the filling of the ventricles during diastole.[10] This increases the left ventricular end-diastolic pressure and eventually increases left atrial, pulmonary artery, and pulmonary capillary pressures, all of which cause a hypercontractile left ventricle. The hypercontractile myocardial muscle fibers of hypertrophic cardiomyopathy are frequently disorganized and demonstrate a cellular disarray. The greater the disarray, the greater the hypertrophic cardiomyopathy.[10] In addition,

## Table 4-3  Classification of Cardiomyopathy

| Classification | Identifying Characteristics | Causes | Pathologic Results |
|---|---|---|---|
| Dilated | Ventricular dilation<br>Cardiac muscle contractile dysfunction | Long-term alcohol abuse<br>Systemic hypertension<br>A variety of infections<br>Cigarette smoking<br>Pregnancy<br>Carnitine deficiency | Myocardial damage resulting from mitochondrial dysfunction |
| Hypertrophic | Inappropriate and excessive left ventricular hypertrophy<br>Normal or even enhanced cardiac muscle contractile function | Genetic (autosomal dominant trait)<br>Malalignment of myocardial fibers<br>Abnormal sympathetic stimulation<br>Subendocardial ischemia<br>Abnormal calcium ion dynamics | Rapid ventricular emptying<br>High ejection fraction |
| Restrictive | Marked endocardial scarring of the ventricles, with resulting impaired diastolic filling | Myocardial fibrosis<br>Ventricular hypertrophy<br>Infiltration of the cardiac muscle | Diastolic dysfunction with unimpaired contractile function |

*Adapted from Braunwald E. Heart Disease: A Textbook of Cardiovascular Medicine, ed 3. Philadelphia, 1988, Saunders.*

hypertrophic cardiomyopathy has a high risk of sudden cardiac death.[27]

Susceptibility to hypertrophic cardiomyopathy appears to be genetically transmitted as an autosomal dominant trait. It has been suggested that the apparent myocardial isometric contraction of hypertrophic cardiomyopathy is the result of malaligned myocardial muscle fibers[11] or an abnormal configuration of the interventricular septum in response to a genetic influence.[28] Other causes of hypertrophic cardiomyopathy have been suggested, including abnormal sympathetic stimulation, subendocardial ischemia, and abnormal calcium ion dynamics.[10]

The characteristic findings of hypertrophic cardiomyopathy are rapid ventricular emptying and high ejection fraction, which are the opposite of those found in dilated cardiomyopathy but somewhat similar to those found in restrictive cardiomyopathy.[10]

### Restrictive Cardiomyopathy

Restrictive cardiomyopathy, like hypertrophic cardiomyopathy, is a cardiomyopathy of diastolic dysfunction and frequently unimpaired contractile function. Little is known about restrictive cardiomyopathy, but certain pathologic processes, including myocardial fibrosis, hypertrophy, infiltration, or a defect in myocardial relaxation may result in its development.[10]

The specific treatment of cardiomyopathy is dependent on the underlying cause but in general includes physical, nutritional, pharmacologic, mechanical, and surgical intervention.[10] One pharmacologic intervention worth mentioning is β-adrenergic blockade, which appears to improve symptoms and survival through five means:[10]

- Negative chronotropic effect with reduced myocardial oxygen demand,
- Reduced myocardial damage because of decreased catecholamines,
- Improved diastolic relaxation,
- Inhibition of sympathetically mediated vasoconstriction, and
- Increase in myocardial β-adrenoceptor density.

These factors are important because they are the basic mechanisms supporting the use of β blockers for dilated, restrictive, and hypertrophic cardiomyopathies, as well as CHF in general, because "treatment is on the same basis as that for heart failure."[10]

### Heart Valve Abnormalities and Congenital/Acquired Heart Disease

Heart valve abnormalities can also cause CMD, as blocked valves (valvular stenosis) or incompetent valves (valvular insufficiency caused by abnormal or poorly functioning valve leaflets), or both, cause heart muscle to contract more forcefully to expel the cardiac output. This subsequently produces myocardial hypertrophy, which can decrease ventricular distensibility and produce a mild diastolic dysfunction; if untreated and prolonged, this dysfunction can lead to more profound diastolic as well as systolic dysfunction.[29] Incompetent valves are frequently associated with myocardial dilation in addition to hypertrophy, because regurgitant blood fills the atria or ventricles forcefully.[29] Atrial dilation often accompanies mitral and tricuspid insufficiency, whereas ventricular dilation accompanies aortic or pulmonary insufficiency. Aortic insufficiency can dilate the left ventricle, whereas pulmonary insufficiency can dilate the right ventricle. Mitral insufficiency frequently dilates the left atrium, whereas tricuspid insufficiency dilates the right atrium. Such dilation can lengthen individual cardiac muscle fibers in the atria and ventricles to such a degree that myocardial contraction is impaired severely, but frequently the accompanying myocardial hypertrophy prevents such extreme dilation. However, the abnormal hemodynamics from hypertrophy and dilation often produce CMD.[29]

Acute heart valve dysfunction or rupture can cause rapid and life-threatening CMD because a ruptured valve impairs cardiac output and regurgitant blood fills the heart's chambers rather than exiting the aorta.[6] If left untreated, valve rupture ultimately produces pulmonary edema and eventually death.

Heart valve abnormalities that cause CMD appear to be reversible to a point. If the abnormality persists for too long, cardiac function appears to be permanently impaired.[29] Acute problems such as heart valve rupture can affect proper cardiac muscle function profoundly and as mentioned are fatal if not surgically repaired within a relatively short period. The most common valvular surgeries are valvular replacement, valvuloplasty (pressurized reduction of atherosclerotic plaque, similar to angioplasty of the coronary arteries), valvulotomy (incision), and commissurotomy (incision to separate adherent, thickened leaflets).[29]

Other heart valve conditions can be classified as chronic conditions and include the stenotic and regurgitant abnormalities of the aortic, pulmonary, mitral, or tricuspid valves. Prolonged valvular stenosis or regurgitation affects cardiac function and can eventually lead to CMD, but cardiac function is less likely to return to normal after valvuloplasty or surgical repair or replacement of a chronic valvular condition.[29]

## Pericardial Effusion or Myocarditis

Injury to the pericardium of the heart can cause acute pericarditis (inflammation of the pericardial sac surrounding the heart), which may progress to pericardial effusion, possibly resulting in cardiac compression as fluid fills the pericardial sac.[10] Increased fluid accumulation within the pericardial space increases intrapericardial pressure and produces cardiac tamponade. Cardiac tamponade is characterized by elevated intracardiac pressures, progressively limited ventricular diastolic filling, and reduced stroke volume.[10] Thus, the mechanism of CMD, which is primarily a diastolic dysfunction (limited ventricular diastolic filling because of cardiac compression), produces a secondary systolic dysfunction. The same sequence of primary diastolic CMD producing secondary systolic CMD occurs in myocarditis.

The prompt treatment of pericarditis with nonsteroidal antiinflammatory agents (aspirin or indomethacin) or corticosteroids (usually prednisone) frequently prevents pericardial effusion. Treatment of the causative inflammatory process in myocarditis (most commonly viral) should prevent the diastolic and systolic CMD of pericardial effusion and

myocarditis.[10] However, patients who do not respond to this therapy must undergo more extensive treatment, including drainage of fluid from the pericardium (pericardiocentesis) for pericardial effusion; immunosuppressive, antibiotic, and possibly antiviral agents for myocarditis; and aggressive CHF management (digitalization, diuresis, and afterload or preload reduction) for both pericardial effusion and myocarditis.[10]

## Pulmonary Embolism

Cardiac muscle dysfunction from a pulmonary embolism is the result of elevated pulmonary artery pressures that dramatically increase right ventricular work. Right as well as left ventricular failure can occur because of decreased oxygenated coronary blood flow and decreased blood flow to the left ventricle.[30] A similar, but often less extreme, condition occurs in pulmonary hypertension.

An acute pulmonary embolism is also a potentially life-threatening condition. As previously mentioned, the primary CMD resulting from a pulmonary embolism is a result of a very high pulmonary artery pressure (because of damaged lung tissue and less area for proper pulmonary perfusion), which increases the work of the right ventricle and eventually produces right-sided heart failure. Left-sided heart failure may accompany right-sided failure because of decreased blood volume and coronary perfusion to the left ventricle, impairing the pumping ability of the heart.[30]

The treatment of a pulmonary embolism consists of the following[30,31]:
- A rapidly acting fibrinolytic agent (typically heparin) should be administered immediately. Heparin reduces the mortality rate of pulmonary embolism as it slows or prevents clot progression. Two forms of recombinant tissue plasminogen activator (alteplase [TPA] and or reteplase [r-PA]) are commonly used;
- A sedative to decrease the patient's anxiety and pain;
- Oxygen to improve the $PaO_2$ (partial pressure of arterial oxygen) and decrease the pulmonary artery pressure;
- Occasionally an embolectomy.

CMD caused by a pulmonary embolism occasionally can be reversed (especially if treatment is initiated immediately), but quite frequently some degree of CMD ensues because of infarcted lung tissue, which increases the work of the right ventricle.[30] When such a condition exists, the pulmonary artery pressure rises and may produce pulmonary hypertension. Pulmonary hypertension can often produce CMD by increasing right ventricular work, resulting in right ventricular hypertrophy (and inefficient right ventricular performance). This may reduce the right ventricular stroke volume, thereby decreasing the left ventricular stroke volume and cardiac output.

## Pulmonary Hypertension

Pulmonary hypertension is defined by mean pulmonary arterial pressure (mPAP) and is considered abnormal in

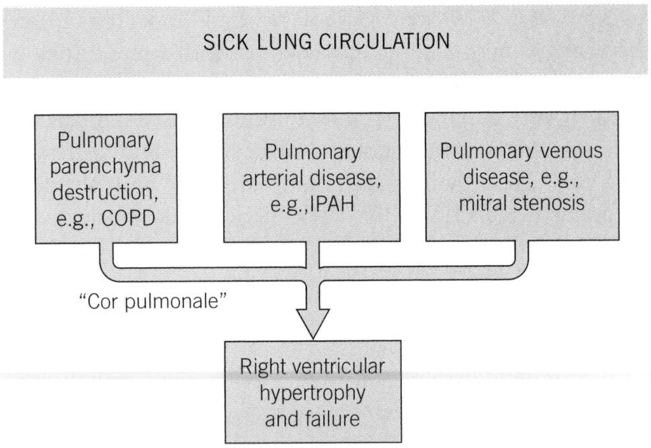

SICK LUNG CIRCULATION

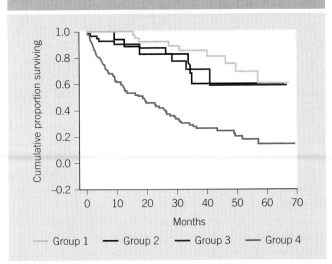

**Figure 4-1** Three categories of diseases leading to an elevated pressure in the pulmonary circulation, right ventricular hypertrophy, and right ventricular failure. The common denominator is a "sick lung circulation." COPD, chronic obstructive pulmonary disease; IPAH, idiopathic pulmonary arterial hypertension. (From Crawford MH, DiMarco JP, Paulus WJ. Cardiology, ed 3. Philadelphia, 2010, Saunders.)

SURVIVAL RATES WITHOUT URGENT HEART TRANSPLANTATION

**Figure 4-2** Survival rates without urgent heart transplantation in patients grouped according to the coupling between mean pulmonary artery pressure (mPAP) and right ventricular ejection fraction (RVEF). Group 1: normal PAP, preserved RVEF ($n = 73$); group 2: normal PAP, low RVEF ($n = 68$); group 3: high PAP, preserved RVEF ($n = 21$); and group 4: high PAP, low RVEF ($n = 215$). (From Ghio S, Gavazzi A, Campana C, et al. Independent and additive prognostic value of right ventricular systolic function and pulmonary artery pressure in patients with chronic heart failure. J Am Coll Cardiol 37(1):183–8, 2001.)

individuals with primary pulmonary hypertension if >25 mm Hg, and abnormal in individuals with chronic obstructive pulmonary disease (COPD) if >20 mm Hg. An elevated mPAP is a predictor of poor prognosis in patients with COPD. The usual suspect accused of the development of pulmonary hypertension in COPD is hypoxia, which is undoubtedly, both acutely and chronically, associated with an increase in pulmonary vascular resistance (PVR). An increase in PVR can increase the work of the right ventricle, and lead to right heart dysfunction and eventually failure. Figure 4-1 shows the three categories of diseases that lead to elevated pressure in pulmonary circulation, right ventricular hypertrophy, and right ventricular failure. In addition, Figure 4-2 shows survival curves for individuals with normal and low right ventricular ejection fractions.

## Spinal Cord Injury

Spinal cord injury also can produce CMD when the cervical spinal cord becomes transected, which "causes an imbalance between parasympathetic and sympathetic control of the cardiovascular system."[32] Several studies have identified neurogenic pulmonary edema as a frequently fatal complication of cervical spinal cord transection.[33-35] Transection of the cervical spinal cord prevents sympathetic nervous system information from reaching the cardiovascular system (heart, lung, arterial and venous systems), thus preventing the sympathetic-driven changes necessary to maintain cardiac performance (i.e., increased heart rate and force of myocardial contraction, constriction of venous capacitance vessels, or arterial constriction). Lacking these cardiovascular adaptations, patients with spinal cord injuries (who frequently are volume-depleted because of fluid loss from multiple injuries) may develop a specific type of CMD that produces neurogenic

pulmonary edema.[32] Because of the possibility of volume depletion, it has been recommended that cardiac filling pressures be monitored, that "cardiac preload be increased by giving fluids,"[32] and that construction of a ventricular function curve may be useful in guiding therapy and treatment for patients with spinal cord injuries that are at risk for neurogenic pulmonary edema.[32] It appears, then, that a slightly elevated pulmonary capillary wedge pressure (not exceeding 18 mm Hg) many facilitate optimal cardiac performance in these patients.

## Age-Related Changes

Although distinctly different processes, congenital or acquired heart diseases and the aging process can produce a similar type of CMD, which is often initially well tolerated but, as the dysfunction persists, may become more symptomatic and troublesome. The adaptability of infants and children to extreme conditions is evident in congenital heart disease, which frequently can be managed for many years with specific medications before surgical intervention becomes necessary.[36,37] The CMD associated with the aging process is initially well tolerated not because of the aged individual's ability to adapt but because the degree of CMD is usually mild. Aging appears to decrease cardiac output by altered contraction and relaxation of cardiac muscle.[38,39] However, heart disease, hypertension, and other pathologic processes can increase CMD substantially and subsequently can impair functional abilities, and these pathologic processes are more prevalent in the older population.[38,39]

## Congenital and Acquired Heart Disease

Congenital heart disease is the result of "altered embryonic development of a normal structure or failure of such a structure to progress beyond an early stage of embryonic or fetal development."[36] Approximately 0.6% of live births but 1.3% live preterm births are complicated by cardiovascular malformations, such as ventricular septal defect, atrial septal defect, patent ductus arteriosus, coarctation of the aorta, and tetralogy of Fallot. The two most common cardiac anomalies are the congenital nonstenotic bicuspid aortic valve and the leaflet abnormality associated with mitral valve prolapse.[36,40]

Acquired heart disease can occur in infancy and childhood as a result of disease processes such as those outlined in Box 4-2. Although the disease processes are different in acquired and congenital heart disease, the resultant pathophysiologic processes are not unlike those seen in adults with CMD because it is dysfunctional cardiac muscle that eventually produces the clinical signs and symptoms.[36]

## Age-Associated Changes in Cardiac Performance

The aging process involves several interrelated pathophysiologic processes, all of which have the potential to impair physical performance, including cardiac function. Although several earlier studies have revealed a reduced cardiac output in the elderly (at rest and with exercise),[41-43] a study that excluded subjects with ischemic heart disease demonstrated no "age effect" on cardiac performance.[44] In this study, the heart rates of the elderly were lower at most workloads, but increased stroke volume apparently compensated for the decreased heart rates and thus maintained cardiac output (cardiac output = heart rate × stroke volume).[44]

> **Clinical Tip**
> - ↑ Systolic arterial pressure because of ↓ distensibility of arteries
> - ↓ Aortic distensibility
> - May develop left ventricular hypertrophy if pressure not treated; will subsequently develop diastolic dysfunction
> - Other changes are caused by disease and not by the aging process

However, other age-associated changes, such as increased systolic arterial pressure and decreased aortic distensibility, probably contribute to the mild to moderate left ventricular hypertrophy commonly found in the elderly.[45] This hypertrophy preserves left ventricular systolic function but impairs left ventricular diastolic function. Diastolic dysfunction delays left ventricular filling, which is more profound in the presence of hypertension, coronary artery disease, and higher heart rates.[46] Additionally, increased norepinephrine levels (probably because of decreased catecholamine sensitivity) and decreased baroreceptor sensitivity and plasma renin concentrations have been reported in elderly subjects.[38]

These pathophysiologic processes, as well as other confounding variables such as coronary artery disease, exposure to environmental toxins (cigarette smoking, radiation), malnutrition, and other lifestyle habits, must be considered to accurately document the effects of aging on cardiac and exercise performance. Nonetheless, the consensus regarding the cardiovascular aging process is as follows:[39]

- After neonatal development, the number of myocardial cells in the heart does not increase.
- There is moderate hypertrophy of left ventricular myocardium, probably in response to increased arterial vascular stiffness and dropout of myocytes.

---

### Box 4-2

**Disease Processes of Congenital vs. Acquired Heart Disease and the Primary Manifestations of Both**

| Disease Processes | | Primary Manifestations |
|---|---|---|
| Congenital | "Altered embryonic development of a normal structure or failure of such a structure to progress beyond an early stage of embryonic or fetal development."[36] | Congestive heart failure |
| Acquired | Rheumatic heart disease | Cyanosis |
| | Connective tissue disorders | Hepatomegaly |
| | Mucopolysaccharidoses | Acid–base imbalances |
| | Hyperlipidemia | Impaired growth |
| | Nonrheumatic inflammatory diseases (infective myocarditis, infective pericarditis, and postpericardiotomy syndrome) | Pulmonary hypertension |
| | Primary (endocardial fibroelastosis) and secondary cardiomyopathies (caused by glycogen storage disease, neonatal thyrotoxicosis, infantile beriberi, protein-calorie malnutrition, tropical endomyocardial fibrosis, anthracycline toxicity, Kawasaki disease, and diabetes in mothers)[36] | Chest pain / Syncope / Arrhythmias |

Data from Friedman WF. Congenital heart disease in infancy and childhood. In Braunwald E (ed.). Heart Disease: A Textbook of Cardiovascular Medicine. Philadelphia, 1988, Saunders.

- When myocardial hypertrophy occurs, it is disproportionate to capillary and vascular growth. The ability of the myocardium to generate tension is well maintained as a result of prolonged duration of contraction and greater stiffness despite a modest decrease in the velocity of shortening of cardiac muscle.
- There is a selective decrease in β-adrenergic receptor-mediated inotropic, chronotropic, and vasodilating cardiovascular responses with aging.
- Increased pericardial and myocardial stiffness and delayed relaxation during aging may limit left ventricular filling during stress.

The primary cause of the changes associated with aging has been attributed to one or a combination of three theories: the genome, the physiologic, and the organ theories.[39] The genome theories are based on the programming of genes for aging, death, or both, whereas the physiologic theories (cross-linkage theory) are dependent on specific pathophysiologic processes. The organ theories (primarily immunologic and neuroendocrine) may be the most encompassing because immunologic and neurohormonal dysfunction is hypothesized to produce both general and specific aging effects.[39] Table 4-4 provides a useful overview of the effects of aging.

## Cardiac Muscle

Animal studies reveal that the contraction and relaxation times of cardiac muscle are prolonged in aged rats.[47–50] This prolongation "can be attributed to alterations in mechanisms that govern excitation–contraction coupling in the heart,"[39] primarily the increase and decrease of cytosolic calcium in the myofilaments. The rate that the sarcoplasmic reticulum pumps calcium is reduced in hearts of older animals and "appears to be a major contributor to the prolonged transient and prolonged time course of cardiac muscle relaxation."[39] The diminished ability of the sarcoplasmic reticulum to pump calcium may also be responsible for the following changes observed in elderly animals:

- Prolonged time to peak force and half relaxation time of peak stiffness.[51–53]
- Lower muscular twitch force at higher stimulation rates.[54]

## Pathophysiology

The interdependence and interrelationship between the cardiac and pulmonary systems are demonstrated in the clinical manifestations of heart failure. One of the most common clinical manifestations is pulmonary edema which is primarily a result of increased pulmonary capillary pressure, although other factors may contribute to its origin (Table 4-5). Left ventricular failure is the most common cause of such increased pulmonary capillary pressure, which produces the congestion of CHF. Consequently, the term CMD accurately describes the primary cause of pulmonary edema as well as the

### Table 4-4 Changes and Effects of Aging

| Change | Effect |
|---|---|
| Decreased vascular elasticity | Increased blood pressure |
| Left ventricular hypertrophy | Decreased ventricular compliance |
| Decreased adrenergic responsiveness | Decreased exercise heart rate |
| Decreased rate of calcium pumped by the sarcoplasmic reticulum | Prolonged time for cardiac muscle relaxation |
| Prolonged time to peak force of cardiac muscle | Prolonged contraction time of cardiac muscle |
| Decreased cardiac muscle twitch force | Reduction in the velocity of the cardiac muscle shortening |
| Decreased rate of adenosine triphosphate (ATP) hydrolysis | Reduction in the velocity of the cardiac muscle shortening |
| Decreased myosin adenosine triphosphatase (ATPase) activity | Reduction in the velocity of the cardiac muscle shortening |
| Diastolic dysfunction | Impaired ventricular filling with potential to increase cardiac preload and congestive heart failure |
| Decreased lean body mass | Decreased muscle strength and peak oxygen consumption |

### Table 4-5 Mechanisms Responsible for Pulmonary Edema

| Mechanisms | Examples |
|---|---|
| Increased pulmonary capillary pressure | Left ventricular failure |
| Decreased plasma oncotic pressure | Hypoalbuminemia secondary to multisystem dysfunction |
| Increased negativity of interstitial pressure | Asthma |
| Altered alveolar–capillary membrane permeability | Aspiration of acidic gastric contents or infectious pneumonia |
| Lymphatic insufficiency | After lung transplant |
| Unknown or incompletely understood | High altitude, after cardiopulmonary bypass |

underlying pathophysiology of CHF because CMD essentially impairs the heart's ability to pump blood or the left ventricle's ability to accept blood.[5]

The heart's ability to accept and pump blood depends upon a number of factors of which the primary variables include total blood volume, body position, intrathoracic pressure, atrial contributions to ventricular filling, pumping action of the skeletal muscle, venous tone, and intrapericardial pressure. Many of these factors are responsible for CMD and CHF. Conversely, many of them can be used to treat the pathophysiology of CMD and CHF. Examples of this include providing supplemental oxygen to decrease myocardial ischemia, and subsequently improve myocardial contraction or using different body positions to either increase or decrease the return of blood to the heart (such as supine versus sitting positions, respectively). Increased return of blood to the heart as a result of a supine body position could worsen CMD and CHF in a person with existing CHF and an increased volume of blood in the ventricles, but the same body position might be beneficial for a person with CHF and decreased volume of blood in the ventricles because of aggressive diuresis to remove fluid from the lungs and various parts of the body.[5]

This apparent ambiguity can be better understood by further discussing Figure 4-3B in which the volume of blood in the ventricle of the heart (ventricular end-diastolic volume [VEDV]) is plotted against ventricular performance. Excessive VEDV decreases ventricular performance (if extreme, shock can ensue), but lower levels of VEDV tend to improve ventricular performance. However, if the VEDV is inadequate because of decreased body fluid and blood volume or change in body position (both of which may decrease the return of blood to the heart), ventricular performance can worsen. A person with CHF typically has increased VEDV (because of a poorly contracting heart), which can increase further from the increased venous return of a supine position. Other mechanisms can also increase venous return such as

increasing venous tone and the pumping action of skeletal muscle. Even a slight increase in the VEDV of a person with CHF may worsen the CMD and CHF.[5]

CHF is often described as a syndrome with many pathophysiologic and compensatory mechanisms that occur in an attempt to maintain an adequate ejection of blood from the ventricle each minute (cardiac output) to the organs and tissues of the body (cardiac index). The following sections help clarify the pathophysiology.

## Congestive Heart Failure Descriptions

CHF is described in numerous ways based upon the pathophysiology associated with it (Table 4-6). Right-sided or left-sided CHF simply describes which side of the heart is failing, as well as the side that is initially affected and behind which fluid tends to localize. For example, left-sided heart failure is frequently the result of left ventricular insult (e.g., myocardial infarction, hypertension, aortic valve disease), which causes fluid to accumulate behind the left ventricle (left atrium, pulmonary veins, pulmonary capillaries, lungs). If the

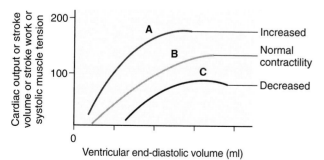

**Figure 4-3** Frank-Starling law of the heart. Relationship between length and tension in the heart. End-diastolic volume determines end-diastolic length of ventricular muscle fibers and is proportional to tension generated during systole, as well as to cardiac output, stroke volume, and stroke work. A change in myocardial contractility causes the heart to perform on a different length-tension curve. **A,** Increased contractility; **B,** normal contractility; **C,** heart failure or decreased contractility. (From McCance KL. Pathophysiology: The Biologic Basis for Disease in Adults and Children, ed 6. St. Louis, 2010, Mosby.)

**Table 4-6 Descriptors of Heart Failure**

| Heart Failure Classification | Descriptions |
|---|---|
| Right heart failure vs. left heart failure vs. bilateral | Right: Right ventricle fails to pump effectively with backup into right atrium and then into periphery |
| | Left: Left ventricle fails to pump effectively with back up into lungs |
| | Biventricular: Left ventricle fails to pump effectively with back up into lungs; with too much back up in lungs; pressures in pulmonary artery rise, increasing resistance for right ventricle, and it, too, fails |
| Low-output vs. high-output failure | Low output: Low cardiac output at rest or with exertion |
| | High output: Results from fluid overload on heart with decreased contractility |
| Systolic vs. diastolic dysfunction | Systolic dysfunction: impaired contractility of ventricles causes low stroke volume and low ejection fraction |
| | Diastolic dysfunction: Inability of ventricles to accept blood from atria during rest or with activity |

left-sided failure is severe, there is progressive accumulation beyond the lungs, manifesting itself as right-sided failure.[5] Thus, right-sided CHF may occur because of left-sided CHF or because of right ventricular failure (e.g., secondary to pulmonary hypertension, pulmonary embolus, right ventricular infarction). In either case, fluid backs up behind the right ventricle and produces the accumulation of fluid in the liver, abdomen, and bilateral ankles and hands.

Low-output CHF is the description most frequently associated with heart failure and is the result of a low cardiac output at rest or during exertion. High-output CHF usually results from a volume overload, as may occur in pregnancy, thyrotoxicosis (overactivity of the thyroid gland, such as in Graves disease), and renal insufficiency.[5–7,55,56] It is important to note that although the term high-output implies a greater cardiac output, it nonetheless is still lower than it was before CHF developed.

Systolic versus diastolic heart failure is perhaps the most informative and useful distinction in CHF because optimal cardiac performance is dependent on both proper systolic and diastolic functioning. The impaired contraction of the ventricles during systole that produces an inefficient expulsion of blood (low stroke volume) is termed systolic heart failure. Diastolic heart failure is associated with an inability of the ventricles to accept the blood ejected from the atria during rest or diastole. Both types are very important in the overall scheme of CHF and often occur simultaneously, as in the patient who suffers a massive anterior myocardial infarction (loss of contracting myocardium, producing systolic heart failure) with subsequent replacement of the infarcted area with nondistensible fibrous scar tissue (which does not readily or adequately accept the blood ejected into the left ventricle from the left atria and produces diastolic heart failure). Despite the various descriptions of CHF just presented, the primary cause of CHF is CMD.

## Specific Pathophysiologic Conditions Associated with Congestive Heart Failure

The pathophysiologic conditions associated with CMD appear to involve eight independent, yet interrelated, systems and one process (nutritional/biochemical), which are found in Table 4-7. The remainder of this section describes and explains each of these factors as they relate to CHF in CMD. Figure 4-4 provides an overview of the specific pathophysiologic areas affected by CHF.

### Cardiovascular Function

The pathophysiology of CHF can be understood best by describing the Frank-Starling mechanism. The Frank-Starling mechanism was one of the earliest efforts to better understand cardiac muscle relaxation and contraction or, in essence, "the relation between ventricular filling pressure (or end-diastolic volume) and ventricular mechanical activity,"[57] expressed as

**Table 4-7  Pathophysiologic Conditions Associated with Congestive Heart Failure**

| Pathologic Site | Effects |
| --- | --- |
| Cardiovascular | Decreased myocardial performance with subsequent peripheral vascular constriction to increase venous return (attempting to increase stroke volume and cardiac output) |
| Neurochemical | Increased sympathetic stimulation that eventually desensitizes the heart to $\beta_1$-adrenergic receptor stimulation, thus decreasing the heart's inotropic effect |
| Renal | Water retention because of decreased cardiac output |
| Pulmonary | Pulmonary edema because of a "backup" of blood as a result of poor cardiac performance and fluid overload |
| Hepatic | Possible cirrhosis from hypoperfusion because of inadequate cardiac output or hepatic venous congestion |
| Hematologic | Possible polycythemia, anemia, and hemostatic abnormalities because of a reduction in oxygen transport, accompanying liver disease, or stagnant blood flow in the heart's chambers because of poor cardiac contraction |
| Pancreatic | Possible impaired insulin secretion and glucose tolerance as well as the source of a possible myocardial depressant factor |
| Nutritional/ biochemical | Anorexia that leads to malnutrition (protein-calorie and vitamin deficiencies) and cachexia |
| Musculoskeletal | Skeletal muscle wasting and possible skeletal muscle myopathies as well as osteoporosis from inactivity or other accompanying diseases |

the volume output of the heart or the stroke volume (cardiac output divided by heart rate because $CO = HR \times SV$).

In the early 1900s, Frank and Starling discovered that the stroke volume is dependent on both diastolic cardiac muscle fiber length and myocardial contractility (force of contraction and heart rate).[58] This relationship can be better understood by studying Figure 4-5, in which left ventricular

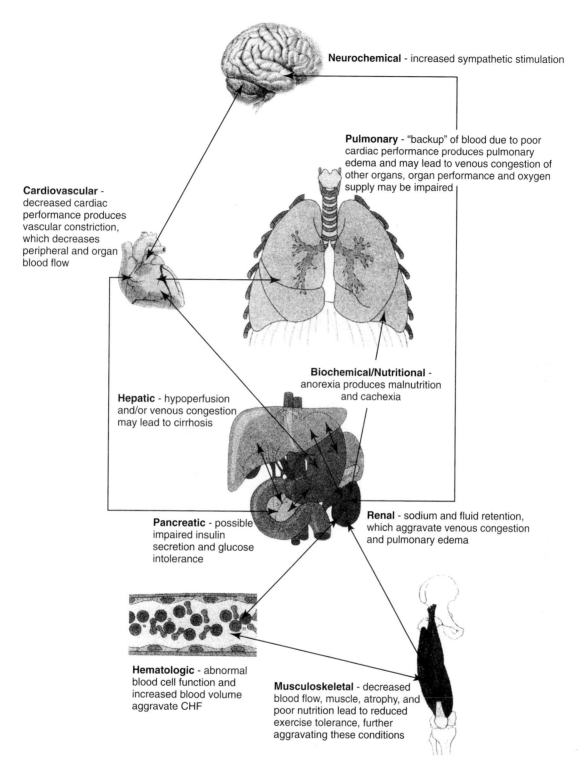

**Neurochemical** - increased sympathetic stimulation

**Pulmonary** - "backup" of blood due to poor cardiac performance produces pulmonary edema and may lead to venous congestion of other organs, organ performance and oxygen supply may be impaired

**Cardiovascular** - decreased cardiac performance produces vascular constriction, which decreases peripheral and organ blood flow

**Biochemical/Nutritional** - anorexia produces malnutrition and cachexia

**Hepatic** - hypoperfusion and/or venous congestion may lead to cirrhosis

**Pancreatic** - possible impaired insulin secretion and glucose intolerance

**Renal** - sodium and fluid retention, which aggravate venous congestion and pulmonary edema

**Hematologic** - abnormal blood cell function and increased blood volume aggravate CHF

**Musculoskeletal** - decreased blood flow, muscle, atrophy, and poor nutrition lead to reduced exercise tolerance, further aggravating these conditions

**Figure 4-4** The compensatory and pathophysiologic interrelationships among organs and organ systems affected by congestive heart failure (CHF). (From Cahalin LP. Heart failure. Phys Ther 76(5):516, 1996.)

stroke work is plotted against left ventricular filling pressure. The figure shows that an optimal range of left ventricular filling pressures exists that, when exceeded, decreases left ventricular stroke work considerably.[9,57] As the left ventricular filling pressure increases, so does the stretch on cardiac muscle fiber during diastole. Taken a step further, the left ventricular filling pressure is representative of the left VEDV, which determines the degree of stretch on the myocardium.[57,58] This is apparent in Figure 4-3, which also demonstrates that an optimal range of ventricular end-diastolic volume (or filling pressure) exists, which, if exceeded or insignificant, decreases ventricular performance. In summary,

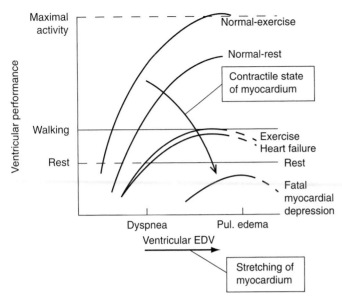

**Figure 4-5** Illustration showing a number of ventricular function curves, which depict the relationship between ventricular end-diastolic volume (EDV) through stretching of the myocardium (i.e., the Frank-Starling law of the heart), and the effects of various states of contractility. Sympathetic stimulation, as normally occurs during exercise, increases stroke volume at a given level of ventricular filling, whereas heart failure results in lower stroke volume at a given level of ventricular filling, which may or may not increase during exercise. The *dashed* lines are the descending limbs of the ventricular performance curves, which are seen only rarely in patients. Levels of ventricular EDV associated with filling pressures that induce dyspnea and pulmonary edema are indicated, along with levels of ventricular performance required during rest, walking, and maximal activity. (Modified from Braunwald E, Ross Jr J, Sonnenblick EH. Mechanisms of Contraction of the Normal and Failing Heart, ed 2. Boston, 1976, Little, Brown. In Watchie Cardiovascular and Pulmonary Physical Therapy: A Clinical Manual, ed 2. St. Louis, 2010, Saunders.)

the following major influences that determine the degree of myocardial stretch should be considered when examining patients with CHF and when developing interventions:[9]
- Atrial contribution to ventricular filling,
- Total blood volume,
- Body position,
- Intrathoracic pressure,
- Intrapericardial pressure,
- Venous tone, and
- Pumping action of skeletal muscle.

Stroke volume is the result of the degree of myocardial stretch as well as that of myocardial contractility. Myocardial contractility is influenced by many variables; Table 4-8 lists the major ones.

Despite these major influences, without adequate diastolic filling (and the necessary degree of myocardial stretch), stroke volume remains unchanged. The importance of diastolic filling of the ventricles is apparent in patients who have pericardial effusion (i.e., cardiac tamponade) or myocarditis, who are unable to attain adequate diastolic filling. This situation results in a decreased stroke volume that can be

**Table 4-8 Factors Affecting Myocardial Contractility**

| | Increase | Decrease |
|---|---|---|
| Force-frequency relations | ↑ | ↓ |
| Circulating catecholamines | ↑ | |
| Sympathetic nerve impulses | ↑ | |
| Intrinsic depression | | ↓ |
| Loss of myocardium | | ↓ |
| Pharmacologic depressants | | ↓ |
| Inotropic agents such as digitalis and Lanoxin | ↑ | |
| Anoxia | | ↓ |
| Hypercapnia | | ↓ |
| Acidosis | | ↓ |

*Data from Braunwald E, Sonnenblick EH, Ross Jr J. Mechanisms of cardiac contraction and relaxation. In Braunwald E (ed.). Heart Disease: A Textbook of Cardiovascular Medicine. Philadelphia, 1988, Saunders.*

hemodynamically significant, producing a hypoadaptive systolic blood pressure response to exercise (decrease in systolic blood pressure with increased heart rate).

The left ventricular end-diastolic pressure is often referred to as the preload. This filling pressure (the pressure in the left ventricle before the ejection of the stroke volume) is analogous to the pulling backward on the rubber band of a slingshot before releasing the rubber band to eject an object. The afterload is the resistance that the stroke volume encounters after it is ejected from the left ventricle. The resistance (or afterload), therefore, is essentially the peripheral vascular resistance. Much of the treatment for CMD involves lowering both the preload and afterload of the cardiovascular system.

The left ventricular filling pressure discussed earlier can be closely approximated by the pulmonary capillary wedge pressure, which is frequently monitored in patients in coronary care or intensive care units.[59] Left ventricular systolic performance is deteriorating when the pulmonary capillary wedge pressure is greater than 15 to 20 mm Hg.

## Biochemical Markers: Natriuretic Peptides Released by Cardiac Muscle

The natriuretic peptides are structurally related but genetically distinct peptides.[60] Atrial natriuretic peptide (ANP) was identified in granules in atria and discovered to also be secreted by endothelial cells. Brain natriuretic peptide (BNP) and its amino-terminal fragment N-terminal pro-B-type natriuretic peptide NT-proBNP. The peptide is stored as proBNP, and then cleaved into the inactive N-terminal proBNP (NT-proBNP). It was first identified in brain tissue but has now been recognized to be produced by cardiac tissue. *Dendroaspis* natriuretic peptide (DNP) is another peptide that

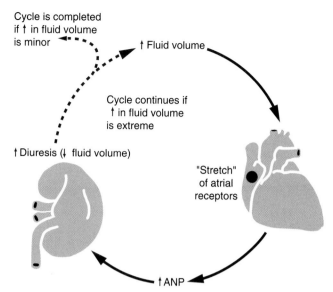

**Figure 4-6** Atrial natriuretic peptide (ANP). Elevated vascular volume releases ANP, which increases the glomerular filtration rate (GFR) and facilitates natriuresis and diuresis.

can be measured in human blood; it is elevated with CHF and causes relaxation of isolated arteries.[61–63]

ANP and BNP are released from arterial and cardiac myocytes, respectively, in response to increased stretch resulting from high filling pressure, high arterial pressure, or cardiac dilation (Fig. 4-6). Once released, both ANP and BNP bind to receptors in target tissues, such as the aorta, vascular smooth muscle, renal cortex and medulla, and adrenal zona glomerulosa.[24] Both ANP and BNP act to reduce the adverse stimulus of stretch by causing arterio- and venodilation, reduction in blood volume through natriuresis, and suppression of secretions of renin and aldosterone. Although the peptides produce these effects to reduce fluid volume, they are only minor forces, which, unfortunately, are no match for the profound fluid retention produced by the kidneys. Therefore, the cause-and-effect relationship between stretch and release of ANP and BNP represents a classical physiologic negative-feedback regulatory system. In general, the natriuretic peptides cause relaxation of vascular smooth muscle but the potency varies depending on the peptide and the anatomic origin of the blood vessel.[64]

Clinicians are increasingly using biochemical markers to diagnose and manage disease states. Levels of plasma BNP are increased in patients with various forms of heart disease, especially those with heart failure.[65] Levels of plasma BNP are also increased in patients with acute coronary syndrome, where it correlates with the degree of left ventricular systolic dysfunction and survival. Although echocardiography is the most widely used method for the confirmation of the clinical diagnosis of heart failure, BNP is rapidly emerging as a very sensitive and specific adjunctive diagnostic marker.[65] It may also be an important prognostic marker, and can be used as a rapid screening test in the urgent care setting.[64,65] Greater levels of ANP and BNP also are associated with higher morbidity and mortality rates.[66,67] Plasma BNP, although consistently increased in patients with heart failure caused by systolic dysfunction, is also increased in some patients with aortic stenosis, chronic mitral regurgitation, diastolic heart failure, and hypertrophic cardiomyopathy.

When fluid volume that typically produces increased left VEDV "backs up" into the left atrium, producing elevated atrial pressure, the elevated atrial pressure stimulates the release of a specific regulatory hormone, ANP. ANP is released from atrial myocyte granules when atrial pressure or volume exceeds an unknown value (see Fig. 4-6).[24]

## Renal Function

The subtle, yet devastating, effects of the renal system in CHF can be appreciated best in Figure 4-7, which outlines the five major steps for the initiation and maintenance of renal sodium retention. As previously mentioned, sodium (and ultimately water) is retained in CHF because of inadequate cardiac output.[8,12] The arterial system of the body senses, via renal and extrarenal sensors, that the arterial blood flow is inadequate, often because of a poor cardiac output, and initiates a process to retain fluid (to increase arterial blood flow), which is identical to that initiated in hypovolemic states.[24] In effect, the kidneys in CHF act like those in an individual with a reduced volume of body fluid.

The subsequent retention of sodium and water is a result of several factors:[24]

- Augmented α-adrenergic neural activity;
- Circulating catecholamines (e.g., epinephrine, norepinephrine); and
- Increased circulating and locally produced angiotensin II, which results in renal vasoconstriction, thus decreasing the glomerular filtration rate (GFR) as well as renal blood flow.

These effects increase the renal filtration fraction (the ratio of GFR to renal blood flow), which increases the protein concentration in the peritubular capillaries and results in an increased quantity of sodium reabsorbed in the proximal tubule.[68,69] Figure 4-8 illustrates the reabsorption process and provides a thorough overview of renal function in CHF. Laboratory findings suggestive of impaired renal function in CHF include increases in blood urea nitrogen (BUN) or other nitrogenous bodies (azotemia), as well as increased blood creatinine levels. This prerenal azotemia is the result of enhanced water reabsorption in the collecting duct, which becomes more pronounced with increased antidiuretic hormone levels and which augments the passive reabsorption of urea (the rate of which can be increased with an acute myocardial infarction and by the catabolic state of CHF).[24] An increase in urea production, a decrease in excretion of urine, and an increased BUN may occur even before a

---

*Clinical Tip*
Laboratory findings of impaired renal function: increased BUN and increased blood creatinine levels.

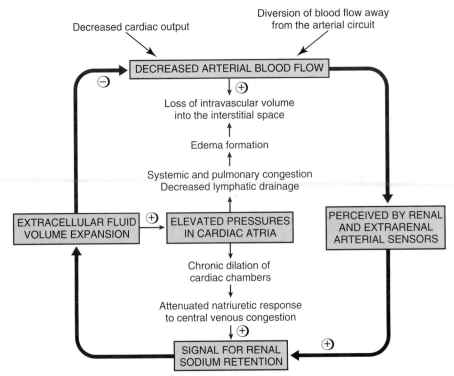

**Figure 4-7** Mechanisms of congestive heart failure. Cardiac muscle dysfunction decreases the cardiac output and resultant arterial blood flow, which initiates the cycle illustrated. (From Skorecki KL, Breuner BM. Body fluid homeostasis in congestive heart failure and cirrhosis with ascites. Am J Med 72(2):323-38, 1982.)

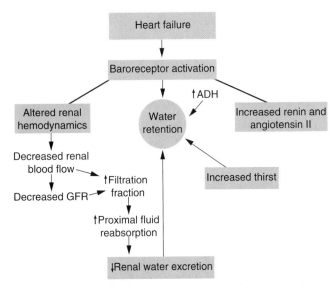

**Figure 4-8** Physiologic effects of myocardial failure. Heart failure produces a variety of altered responses that lead to retention of water and often to congestive heart failure.

decrease in GFR. A decreased GFR is the primary reason for the increased BUN and serum creatinine levels commonly seen in patients with CHF.[24]

## Pulmonary Function

Pulmonary edema can be cardiogenic (hemodynamic) or noncardiogenic (caused by alterations in the pulmonary capillary membrane) in origin.[5] The differential diagnosis can be made by history, physical examination, and laboratory examination, as shown in Table 4-5. Despite the different origins of pulmonary edema, the sequence of liquid accumulation is similar for both and appears to consist of three distinct stages (Fig. 4-9):

- **Stage 1 (Fig. 4-9A).** Difficult to detect or quantify because it seems to represent "increased lymph flow without net gain of interstitial liquid."[70] The edema associated with the increased lymph flow may actually improve gas exchange in the lung as more of the small pulmonary vessels are distended. However, if lymph flow continues, pulmonary edema increases, and the airways and vessels become filled with increased amounts of liquid, particularly in the gravity-dependent portions of the lung.[70]
- **Stage 2 (Fig. 4-9B).** Accumulation of liquid compromises the small airway lumina, resulting in a mismatch between ventilation and perfusion, which produces hypoxemia and wasted ventilation. Tachypnea of CHF often ensues.[70] In addition, the degree of hypoxemia appears to be correlated to the degree of elevation of the pulmonary capillary wedge pressure.[71]
- **Stage 3 (Fig. 4-9C).** As lymph flow continues, pulmonary edema increases, increasing the pulmonary capillary wedge pressure and eventually flooding the alveoli known as pulmonary edema, which significantly compromises gas exchange, producing severe hypoxemia and hypercapnia.[70] In addition, severe

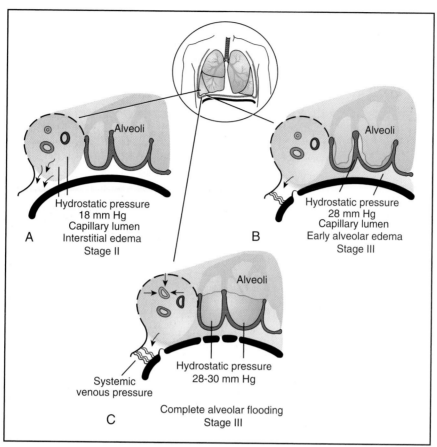

**Figure 4-9** Pulmonary edema resulting from left-sided cardiac muscle failure may present in different stages. **A,** In stage II, interstitial edema results from an elevated capillary pressure (18 mm Hg), which forces fluid (plasma) into the interstitial area. **B,** Early alveolar edema occurs when the capillary hydrostatic pressure is significantly elevated (18 to 28 mm Hg), causing fluid to move from the capillary, invade the interstitium, and cross the alveolar membrane. **C,** Complete alveolar flooding occurs when the capillary hydrostatic pressure is severely elevated (>28 mm Hg), causing fluid to flood the alveoli and possibly invade the large airways.

alveolar flooding can produce the following: (1) filling of the large airways with blood-tinged foam, which can be expectorated; (2) reductions in most lung volumes (e.g., vital capacity); (3) a right-to-left intrapulmonary shunt; and (4) hypercapnia with acute respiratory acidosis.[70]

Perhaps the most important principle regarding pulmonary edema is that of maintaining pulmonary capillary pressures at the lowest possible levels.[70] Pulmonary edema can be decreased by more than 50% when pulmonary capillary wedge pressures are decreased from 12 to 6 mm Hg.

The effect of repeated bouts of pulmonary edema (which is common in CHF) upon pulmonary function appears to be profound. More advanced CHF may produce a "global respiratory impairment" that is associated with varying degrees of obstructive and restrictive lung disease.[72,73]

## Neurohumoral Effects

The neurohumoral system profoundly affects heart function in physiologic (fight-or-flight mechanism) and pathologic states (CMD). In general, the neural effects are much more rapid, whereas humoral effects are slower because the information sent by the autonomic nervous system via efferent nerves travels faster than the information traveling through the vascular system.[74]

## Normal Cardiac Neurohumoral Function

Neurohumoral signals to the heart are perceived, interpreted, and augmented by the transmembrane signal transduction systems in myocardial cells.[74] The primary signaling system in the heart appears to be the receptor-G-protein-adenylate cyclase (RGC) complex as it regulates myocardial contractility. Figure 4-10 illustrates the complexity of this system, which consists of (1) membrane receptors; (2) guanine nucleotide-binding regulatory proteins (the G proteins, which transmit stimulatory or inhibitory signals); and (3) adenylate cyclase, which converts adenosine triphosphate (ATP) to cyclic adenosine monophosphate (cAMP). Adenylate cyclase is an effector enzyme activated by a receptor agonist, thus enhancing cAMP synthesis. The lower portion of Figure 4-10 shows that increased cAMP synthesis ultimately increases the force of myocardial contraction (the inotropic effect).[74]

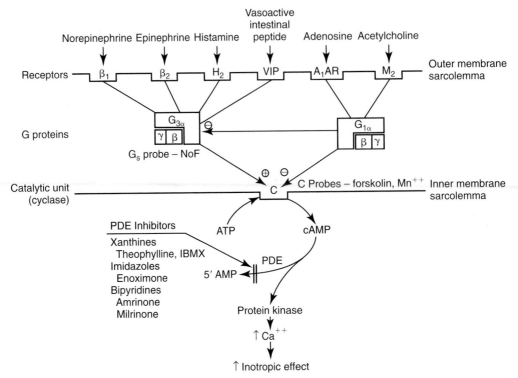

**Figure 4-10** Neural control of cardiopulmonary function. The receptor-G-protein-adenylate cyclase complex and other important receptors, all of which affect the inotropic state of the heart. ATP, adenosine triphosphate; cAMP, cyclic adenosine monophosphate; Gs, G-stimulatory protein; G1, G-inhibitory protein; IBMX, isobutyl methylxanthine; PDE, phosphodiesterase.

The top portion of Figure 4-10 shows the receptor agonists responsible for the initial activation of the RGC complex. These agents include norepinephrine, epinephrine, histamine, vasoactive intestinal peptide, adenosine, and acetylcholine.

Although Figure 4-10 shows the complete system, it does not reveal the degree of influence each receptor agonist has on cardiac function. In general, the most influential receptor agonists are the sympathetic neurotransmitters norepinephrine and epinephrine, as they relay excitatory autonomic nervous system stimuli to both postsynaptic α- and β-adrenergic receptors (primarily β for norepinephrine) in the myocardium.[74] Inhibitory autonomic nervous system stimuli are transmitted by the parasympathetic nervous system via the vagus nerve and the neurotransmitter acetylcholine. The adrenergic receptors ($\alpha_1$, $\alpha_2$, $\beta_1$, and $\beta_2$) are discussed briefly in the next paragraphs so that Figure 4-10 can be appreciated fully, as are the neurohumoral changes that accompany CMD.

### α-Adrenergic Receptors

Stimulation of $\alpha_1$-adrenergic receptors appears to activate the phosphodiesterase transmembrane signaling system,[75,76] which increases phosphodiesterase and activates protein kinase, thus marginally increasing the inotropic effect.[77] Conversely, stimulation of $\alpha_2$-adrenergic receptors activates the inhibitory G protein and inhibits adenylate cyclase, which decreases the inotropic effect.[78]

### β-Adrenergic Receptors

The importance of the β-adrenergic pathway cannot be overemphasized because it has been proposed that the heart is a β-adrenergic organ.[79] Two β-adrenergic receptors have been identified, $\beta_1$ and $\beta_2$, which are "distinguished by their differing affinities for the agonists epinephrine and norepinephrine." The $\beta_2$-adrenergic receptor has a 30-fold greater affinity for epinephrine than for norepinephrine.[80] In brief, $\beta_2$-adrenergic receptor stimulation promotes vasodilation of the capillary beds and muscle relaxation in the bronchial tracts, whereas $\beta_1$-adrenergic receptor stimulation increases heart rate and myocardial force of contraction.[74]

### Guanine Nucleotide-Binding Regulatory Proteins

As briefly discussed, the G proteins transmit stimulatory (Gs) or inhibitory (G1) signals to the catalytic unit (inner membrane sarcolemma) of myocardial contractile tissue. The stimulatory and inhibiting signals are dependent on a very complex, and only partially understood, mechanism of receptor-mediated activation.

### Catalytic Unit of Adenylate Cyclase

The activation of adenylate cyclase (and subsequent increase in myocardial force of contraction) is, unfortunately, poorly understood but has been observed to be decreased in patients with CHF. This decrease is the result of "a paradoxical diminution in the function of the RGC complex,"[74] which alters the receptor–effector coupling and "limits the ability of both endogenous and exogenous adrenergic agonists to augment cardiac contractility."[74] The inability of endogenous (produced in the body) or exogenous (medications) adrenergic agonists to increase the force of myocardial contraction is frequently seen in patients with CHF, and may be a contributing factor in CMD.[74,81]

## Neurohumoral Alterations in the Failing Human Heart

### Abnormalities in Sympathetic Neural Function

The sympathetic neural function of the heart is profoundly affected in CHF. The effects are primarily caused by abnormal RGC complex function, despite increased concentrations of norepinephrine in interstitial (in the interspaces of the myocardium), intrasynaptic, and systemwide.[74]

The abnormal RGC complex function in CHF appears to be associated with the insensitivity of the failing heart to β-adrenergic stimulation.[74] This insensitivity to β-adrenergic stimulation is apparently the result of a decrease in $\beta_1$-adrenergic receptor density[74] and is very important because the heart contains a ratio of $3.3:1.0$ $\beta_1$- to $\beta_2$-adrenergic receptor.[74] In CHF, the ratio decreases to approximately $1.5:1.0$, producing a 62% decrease in the $\beta_1$-adrenergic receptors and no significant increase in $\beta_2$ density.[82,83] Although the number of $\beta_2$ receptors does not appear to change in CHF, the $\beta_2$ receptor "is partially 'uncoupled' from the effector enzyme adenylate cyclase."[81,84] This uncoupling only mildly desensitizes the $\beta_2$-adrenergic receptors, which initially are able to compensate for the decreased number of $\beta_1$ receptors by providing substantial inotropic support.[85] The duration of inotropic support appears to be short-lived, and myocardial failure becomes more pronounced.[74]

> **Clinical Tip**
> Excessive sympathetic nervous system stimulation occurs in CHF, and because of abnormalities in particular parts of the neurohumoral system, the heart becomes insensitive to β-adrenergic stimulation, which results in a decreased force of myocardial contraction and an inability to attain higher heart rates during physical exertion. This is where the role of β blockers play a major part in treatment of CHF.

## Hepatic Function

The fluid overload associated with CHF affects practically all organs and body systems, including liver function. Increased fluid volume eventually leads to hepatic venous congestion,

> **Clinical Tip**
> Hepatomegaly, or liver enlargement, is frequently associated with CHF and can be identified readily as tenderness in the right upper quadrant of the abdomen. Patients with long-standing CHF, however, are generally not tender to palpation, although hepatomegaly is frequently present. Lab values showing liver involvement include abnormal aspartate aminotransferase (AST), bilirubin, lactate dehydrogenase (LDH-5).

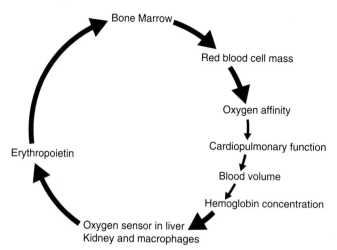

**Figure 4-11** Mechanisms of hematologic function. Hematologic function is occasionally disrupted in congestive heart failure and can further impair cardiopulmonary function and patient status.

which prevents adequate perfusion of oxygen to hepatic tissues. Subsequent hypoxemia from the hypoperfusion produces a cardiac cirrhosis, which is characterized histologically by central lobular necrosis, atrophy, extensive fibrosis, and occasionally sclerosis of the hepatic veins.[10]

## Hematologic Function

The normal morphology of the blood and blood-forming tissues is frequently disrupted in CHF. The most common abnormality is a secondary polycythemia (excess of red corpuscles in the blood), which is a result of either a reduction in oxygen transport or an increase in erythropoietin production.[86] Erythropoietin is an $\alpha_2$-globulin responsible for red blood cell production, and its important role is demonstrated in Figure 4-11. This figure shows that the hypoxia occasionally observed in patients with CHF may stimulate erythropoietin production, which increases not only red blood cell mass, but also blood volume in an already compromised cardiopulmonary system (partly because of fluid volume overload). This potentially vicious circle can progress and cause cardiopulmonary function to deteriorate further.

Clinically, anemia (low hemoglobin and hematocrit), which may be present in some patients with CHF, is a paradox, for when it is severe it can cause CHF independently, but when it precedes CHF, anemia may actually allow for a more efficient and effective cardiac function.[86] Improved cardiac output may occur because blood viscosity is reduced in patients with anemia, which subsequently decreases systemic vascular resistance. Consequently, anemia acts as an afterload reducer and may promote an increased cardiac output but at the cost of lower arterial oxygen and oxygen saturation levels as well as increased work for the heart.[86] A term that is frequently applied when such a condition (and others) exists is "a shift in the oxyhemoglobin curve." The curve can be shifted to the right or left but normally

## Table 4-9 Relationship of PaO$_2$ to SpO$_2$

| | Oxygen Saturation | | |
|---|---|---|---|
| PaO$_2$ (mm Hg) (partial pressure of arterial oxygen) | 40% | 50% | 60% |
| SpO$_2$ (%) (oxygen saturation measured by pulse oximetry) | 70% | 80% | 90% |

follows the pattern depicted in Figure 4-11, which represents a specific percentage of oxygen saturation for a given concentration of arterial oxygen. Oxygen saturation remains relatively stable, with arterial oxygen concentrations greater than 60 mm Hg, but below this level the oxygen saturation drops dramatically. Table 4-9 shows the oxygen saturation levels when arterial oxygen concentrations are less than 60 mm Hg.

Various conditions move this normal curve to the right or left, and these changes subsequently affect the respective oxygen saturation. For example, anemia shifts the curve to the right, representing a lower concentration of arterial oxygen, which moves the critical point of oxygen saturation to 70 mm Hg (therefore, to the right). This means that at levels of less than 70 mm Hg, the level of oxygen saturation decreases dramatically compared with the normal level of 60 mm Hg. Thus, patients with anemia have less reserve before their oxygen stores desaturate.[86]

> **Clinical Tip**
> Treatment for severe anemia often involves blood transfusion, however, a blood transfusion may increase the heart's work because of the increase in volume and subsequently increased preload on a weak heart. The patient with a poor performing heart should be monitored carefully after blood transfusions, including heart rate, dyspnea, SpO$_2$ (oxygen saturation measured by pulse oximetry), blood pressure, and other symptoms.

Also of concern for patients with advanced CMD (or CHF in general) is the state of hemostasis (the mechanical and biochemical aspects of platelet function and coagulation), which is frequently disrupted as a result of accompanying liver disease.[5] Inhibition of platelet function to the point at which the platelet count drops below 150,000 cells/μL is termed *thrombocytopenia* and is caused by hereditary factors or drugs, or often is acquired from systemic disease.[87] Inherited thrombocytopenia is uncommon; however, thrombocytopenia caused by drugs is much more common and frequently is an adverse reaction associated with use of aspirin, corticosteroids, antimicrobial agents (penicillins and cephalothins), phosphodiesterase inhibitors (dipyridamole), caffeine, sympathetic blocking agents (β antagonists), and heparin.[87] Acquired disorders of platelet function are a common complication of renal failure. This is usually corrected by renal dialysis, but patients with chronic CHF may demonstrate a mild-to-moderate level of platelet dysfunction.[87]

> **Clinical Tip**
> Hematologic impairments in CHF consists of the following: possible polycythemia, possible anemia (if present, oxygen saturation should be monitored), and possible hemostasis abnormalities such as thrombocytopenia (monitoring laboratory blood values is recommended).

### Skeletal Muscle Function

Skeletal muscle myopathy has been identified in patients with CHF and in those with CHF and preexisting cardiomyopathy.[88,89] Skeletal muscle function with CHF alone is different than when CHF is present as a result of a cardiomyopathy and thus is presented separately.[88,89]

### Skeletal Muscle Activity in Congestive Heart Failure Without Cardiomyopathy

Skeletal muscle dysfunction in patients with CHF has been studied far less in patients without cardiomyopathy than in patients with cardiomyopathy. However, two studies have evaluated skeletal muscle activity in the presence of CHF without preexisting cardiomyopathy.[88,89] Shafiq and colleagues found no abnormalities in the normal subjects but found a decrease in the average diameters of the type I and type II fibers in the patients with CHF but without cardiomyopathy. The patients with CHF and cardiomyopathy were found to have three distinct skeletal muscle abnormalities (selective atrophy of type II fibers, pronounced nonselective myopathy, and hypotrophy of type I fibers).[88] Patients with diseases known to affect skeletal muscle (diabetes, collagen vascular disease, and alcoholism) were excluded from the study. In addition, Lipkin and associates identified decreased isometric maximal voluntary contraction of the quadriceps (only 55% [range: 31% to 75%] of the predicted value for weight) in individuals with CHF and no evidence of cardiomyopathy.[90] The biopsies revealed increased intracellular acid phosphatase activity, increased intracellular lipid accumulation and atrophy of type I and type II muscle fibers.[89] Skeletal muscle fatigue in patients with CHF was associated with intracellular acidosis and phosphocreatine depletion(as identified by nuclear magnetic resonance),[91] which if prolonged may predispose to myopathic processes.

### Skeletal Muscle Activity in Congestive Heart Failure with Cardiomyopathy

Skeletal muscle abnormalities caused by dilated and hypertrophic cardiomyopathies have been reported previously and have consistently revealed type I and type II muscle fiber atrophy.[92–99] Electromyographic studies revealed abnormalities typical of myogenic myopathy in nine patients (five dilated, four hypertrophic), but none of the patients showed signs of neurogenic alteration (i.e., a reduction of nerve conduction velocities or an increase in single motor unit potential duration).[100] Muscle biopsies consistently detected pathologic changes (primarily mitochondrial abnormalities) in the type I (slow-twitch) fibers in all nine patients from whom a biopsy was obtained; eight of the biopsies demonstrated increases of atrophy factors. No alteration of type II fibers was observed in any patient.[100]

Isometric maximal muscle strength of persons with CHF appears to be reduced to nearly 50% of the value for age-, sex-, and weight-matched control subjects. Loss of muscle strength will result in each muscle fiber operating nearer to its maximal capacity for a given absolute power output. Consequently, the changes in skeletal muscle metabolism that are associated with fatigue might be expected to occur at lower absolute workloads and hence to limit maximal exercise capacity in these patients.[89]

## Pancreatic Function

Severe CMD can potentially reduce blood flow to the pancreas "as a consequence of splanchnic visceral vasoconstriction, which accompanies severe left ventricular failure."[101] The reduction in blood flow to the pancreas impairs insulin secretion and glucose tolerance, which are further impaired by increased sympathetic nervous system activity and augmented circulatory catecholamines (inhibiting insulin secretion) that stimulate glycogenolysis and elevate blood sugar levels.[102]

Reduced secretion of insulin is of paramount importance because hypoxic and dysfunctional heart muscle depends a great deal on the energy from the metabolism of glucose, which is reduced significantly if insulin secretion is impaired.[101] Ultimately, there is further deterioration of left ventricular function, creating a vicious circle.

Normally, when oxygen is available, the heart obtains 60% to 90% of its energy requirements from the oxidation of free fatty acids, which inhibits glucose uptake, glycolytic flux, and glycogenolysis.[103] The oxidation of free fatty acids increases the production of acetylcoenzyme A (acetyl-CoA), which inhibits pyruvate dehydrogenase and limits carbohydrate metabolism.[103] However, as previously noted, myocardial ischemia (because of the limited supply of oxygen) inhibits the oxidation of free fatty acids and long-chain acylcarnitine palmitoyl transferase enzyme activity, thus preventing the transport of cytosolic acyl-coenzyme A (acyl-CoA) to the mitochondria for oxidation. "Accordingly, intracellular concentrations of acyl-CoA increase and acetyl-CoA content declines."[104]

Increased levels of acyl-CoA produce several deleterious effects on proper cardiac function:

- Increased synthesis of triglycerides, which accumulate in the myocardium;
- Inhibition of further formation of coenzyme A esters of fatty acids, limiting oxidation of free fatty acids; and
- Inhibition of adenine nucleotide translocase, which is important for myocardial energy metabolism because it transports ATP synthesized in the mitochondria to the cytosol.[103]

This final inhibition of adenine nucleotide translocase may be a key factor contributing to myocardial dysfunction.[103]

Finally, CMD and CHF is common in persons with diabetes and is an important risk factor for the development of a cardiomyopathy. Such a relationship clearly identifies the important role nutrition and proper biochemical function have in cardiovascular disease.

## Nutritional and Biochemical Aspects

Nutritional concerns are very important when assessing and treating patients with CMD. Stomach and intestinal abnormalities are not uncommon in these patients, who frequently receive many medications with profound side effects.[105] In addition, the interrelated disease processes occurring in other organs because of CMD and CHF frequently produce anorexia, which leads ultimately to malnutrition. The primary malnutrition is a protein-calorie deficiency, but vitamin deficiencies have also been observed (folic acid, thiamine, and hypocalcemia-accompanied vitamin D deficiency).[105] These deficient states may simply be the result of decreased intake, but "abnormal intestinal absorption and increased rates of excretion may also contribute."[105]

Protein-calorie deficiency is common in chronic CHF because of cellular hypoxia and hypermetabolism that frequently produces cachexia (malnutrition and wasting).[105] A catabolic state may also develop, yielding an excess of urea or other nitrogenous compounds in the blood (azotemia). This, as with most organ dysfunction associated with CHF, causes a vicious circle, which, because of gastrointestinal hypoxia and decreased appetite (anorexia) and protein intake, produces cardiac atrophy and more pronounced CMD.[105]

One particular area of concern is thiamine deficiency because of improper nutrition, which can affect this population dramatically. The force of myocardial contraction and cardiac performance in general appear to be dependent on the level of thiamine, and it has been suggested that "the possibility of thiamine deficiency should be considered in many patients with heart failure of obscure origin."[55] In addition, patients undergoing prolonged treatment with furosemide (Lasix; the first drug of choice in the treatment of CHF) have demonstrated significant thiamine deficiency, which may improve with replacement.[106]

Two other nutritional concerns include carnitine deficiency and coenzyme Q10. Skeletal muscle carnitine deficiency has been observed in a small population of patients with hypertrophic cardiomyopathy. When carnitine was replenished, cardiac symptoms and echocardiographic parameters apparently improved.[107] In addition, substantial literature supports the supplementation of coenzyme Q10 in persons with CHF deficient of this apparently important biochemical component, which appears to have a role in the essential function of mitochondria, antioxidation of heart muscle, and cardiostimulation.[108–112]

Individuals with CHF and renal dysfunction may also demonstrate:

- Decreased production of erythropoietin (a hormone synthesized in the kidney that is an important precursor of red blood cell production in bone marrow), causing anemia and possibly less free fatty acid oxidation[113,114];
- Decreased synthesis of 1,25-dihydroxycholecalciferol, which may lead to decreased calcium absorption from the gastrointestinal tract,[115] as well as the development of hyperparathyroidism[116]; and
- Impaired intermediary metabolism (impaired gluconeogenesis and lipid metabolism, as well as degradation of several peptides, proteins, and peptide hormones including insulin, glucagon, growth hormone, and parathyroid hormone).[117]

Individuals with CHF may benefit from enteral or parenteral products to improve nutrition and the biochemical profile.

---

**Clinical Tip**

There are several nutritional and biochemical aspects of CHF, including malnutrition (this may occur), thiamine and carnitine deficiency (this should be considered in patients with CHF of obscure origin), and a deficiency of coenzyme Q10 (supplementation appears to improve myocardial performance and functional status).

---

## Clinical Manifestations of Congestive Heart Failure

Heart failure is commonly associated with several characteristic signs and symptoms (Box 4-3).

### Symptoms of Congestive Heart Failure

#### Dyspnea

Dyspnea (breathlessness or air hunger) is probably the most common finding associated with CHF and is frequently the result of poor gas transport between the lungs and the cells

---

**Box 4-3**

**Characteristic Signs and Symptoms of Heart Failure**

- Dyspnea
- Tachypnea
- Paroxysmal nocturnal dyspnea (PND)
- Orthopnea
- Peripheral edema
- Cold, pale, and possibly cyanotic extremities
- Weight gain
- Hepatomegaly
- Jugular venous distension
- Rales (crackles)
- Tubular breath sounds and consolidation
- Presence of an $S_3$ heart sound
- Sinus tachycardia
- Decreased exercise tolerance or physical work capacity

---

of the body. The cause of poor transport at the lungs is often excessive blood and extracellular fluid in the alveoli and interstitium, interfering with diffusion and causing a reduction in vital capacity.[5] However, the cause of poor transport at the cellular level may be less apparent. Inadequate oxygen supply either at rest or during muscular activity increases the frequency of breathing (respiratory rate) or the amount of air exchanged (tidal volume) or both.[118] For this reason, subjects with CHF characteristically complain of easily provoked dyspnea or, in severe cases of CHF, dyspnea at rest.

### Paroxysmal Nocturnal Dyspnea

Another common complaint of individuals suffering from CHF is paroxysmal nocturnal dyspnea (PND), in which sudden, unexplained episodes of shortness of breath occur as patients with CHF assume a more supine position to sleep.[5] After a period of time in a supine position, excessive fluid fills the lungs. Earlier in the day, this fluid is shunted to the lower extremities and the lower portions of the lungs because upright positions and activities permit more effective minute ventilation (V) and perfusion (Q) of the lungs (correcting the V/Q mismatch) and the effects of gravity keep the lungs relatively fluid-free. Individuals who suffer from PND frequently place the head of the bed on blocks or sleep with more than two pillows. Patients with marked CHF often assume a sitting position to sleep and are sometimes found sleeping in a recliner instead of a bed.[5]

### Orthopnea

The term *orthopnea* describes the development of dyspnea in the recumbent position.[5] Sleeping with two or more pillows elevates the upper body to a more upright position and enables gravity to draw excess fluid from the lungs to the more distal parts of the body. The severity of CHF can sometimes be inferred from the number of pillows used to prevent orthopnea. Thus, the terms two-, three-, four-, or more pillow orthopnea indirectly allude to the severity of CHF (e.g., four-pillow orthopnea suggests more severe CHF than two-pillow orthopnea).

### Signs Associated with Congestive Heart Failure

#### Breathing Patterns

A rapid respiratory rate at rest, characterized by quick and shallow breaths, is common in patients with CHF. Such tachypnea is apparently not caused by hypoxemia (which may or may not be of sufficient magnitude) but rather to stimulation of interstitial J-type receptors (stretch receptors in the interstitium stimulated by increased pressure/fluid). The quick, shallow breathing of tachypnea may assist the pumping action of the lymphatic vessels, thus minimizing or delaying the increase in interstitial liquid.[70]

A clinical finding observed in many patients with CMD is extreme dyspnea after a change in position, most frequently from sitting to standing. This response appears to be occasionally but inconsistently associated with orthostatic hypotension and increased heart rate activity. The orthostatic hypotension and dyspnea (tachypnea) may be the result of (a) lower-extremity muscle deconditioning, producing a pooling of blood in the lower extremities when standing, with a subsequent decrease in blood flow to the heart and lungs, which may result in marked dyspnea and increased heart rates; or (b) attenuation of the natriuretic peptide factor (ANP/BNP), which may suggest advanced atrial distension and poor left ventricular function.[119] It appears that the more pronounced the dyspnea, the more severe the CMD, and vice versa. This pattern of breathing, therefore, is another clinical finding that can be timed (time for the dyspnea to subside) and occasionally measured (blood pressure and heart rate) to document progress or deterioration in patient status.

In addition, frequently associated with CHF is a breathing pattern characterized by waxing and waning depths of respiration with recurring periods of apnea. Although the Scottish physician John Cheyne and the Irish physician William Stokes first observed this breathing pattern in asthmatics and thus coined the term Cheyne-Stokes respiration, it has been observed in individuals who are suffering central nervous system damage (particularly those in comas) and in individuals with CMD.[5]

---

> **Clinical Tip**
> Patients with CHF often demonstrate breathing impairments including tachypnea, resting dyspnea, dyspnea with exertion, occasional dyspnea with positional change (with or without orthostatic hypotension), and/or waxing and waning depth of breathing (Cheyne-Stokes respiration).

---

### Rales (Crackles)

Pulmonary rales, sometimes referred to as crackles, are abnormal breath sounds that, if associated with CHF, occur during inspiration and represent the movement of fluid in the alveoli and subsequent opening of alveoli that previously were closed because of excessive fluid.[5] This sound is produced in the body with the opening of alveoli and airways that previously had no air; after the sound associated with such an opening is transmitted through the tissues overlying the lungs, the characteristic sound of rales is identical to that of hair near the ears being rubbed between two fingers. Rales are frequently heard at both lung bases in individuals with CHF but may extend upward, depending on the patient's position, the severity of CHF, or both. Therefore, auscultation of all lobes should be performed in a systematic manner, allowing for bilateral comparison.

The importance of the presence and magnitude of rales was addressed in 1967 and provided data for the Killip and Kimball classification of patients with acute myocardial infarction.[120] Table 4-10 defines classes I through III, each of which is associated with an approximate mortality rate. Individuals with rales extending over more than 50% of the lung fields were observed to have a very poor prognosis.

**Table 4-10 Killip Classification of Patients with Acute Myocardial Infarction and Approximate Mortality Rate**

| | Definition | Approximate Mortality Rate (%) |
|---|---|---|
| Class I | Absence of rales and $S_3$ heart sound | 8 |
| Class II | Presence of $S_3$ heart sound or rales in 50% or less of the lung fields | 30 |
| Class III | Rales extending over more than 50% of the lung fields | 44 |

### Heart Sounds

Heart sounds can provide a great deal of information regarding cardiopulmonary status but unfortunately are ignored in most physical therapy examinations. The normal heart sounds include a first heart sound ($S_1$), which represents closure of the mitral and tricuspid valves, and a second sound ($S_2$), which represents closure of the aortic and pulmonary valves. The most common abnormal heart sounds are the third ($S_3$) and fourth ($S_4$), which occur at specific times in the cardiac cycle as a result of abnormal cardiac mechanics. An $S_3$ heart sound may be normal in children and young adults and is termed a *physiologic normal S3*.[121] An $S_4$ is presystolic (heard before $S_1$), and $S_3$ occurs during early diastole (after $S_2$). The presence of an $S_3$ indicates a noncompliant left ventricle and occurs as blood passively fills a poorly relaxing left ventricle that appears to make contact with the chest wall during early diastole.[121] The presence of an $S_3$ is considered the hallmark of CHF.[122] There are several reasons why the left ventricle may be noncompliant, of which fluid overload and myocardial scarring (via myocardial infarction or cardiomyopathy) appear to be the most common.

The presence of an $S_4$, represents "vibrations of the ventricular wall during the rapid influx of blood during atrial contraction" from an exaggerated atrial contraction (atrial "kick").[121] It is commonly heard in patients with hypertension, left ventricular hypertrophy, increased left ventricular end-diastolic pressure, pulmonary hypertension, and pulmonary stenosis.[121]

Auscultation of the heart (Fig. 4-12) may also reveal adventitious (additional) sounds, most frequently murmurs. Murmurs not only are common in patients with CMD but also appear to be of great clinical significance. Stevenson and coworkers demonstrated that the systolic murmur of secondary mitral regurgitation was an important marker in the treatment of a subgroup of patients with congestive cardiomyopathy.[123] The patients who benefited from afterload (the resistance to ventricular ejection or peripheral vascular resistance) reduction were those with a very large left

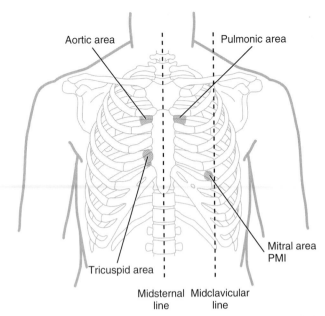

**Figure 4-12** Primary auscultatory areas. Auscultation of the heart is performed in a systematic fashion using both the bell and diaphragm of the stethoscope at the indicated sites.

ventricle (left ventricular end-diastolic dimension >60 cm) and a resultant systolic murmur.[123] This study demonstrated the importance of auscultation of the heart at rest and immediately after exercise in persons with CHF to gain insight into the dynamics of myocardial activity.

### Peripheral Edema

Peripheral edema frequently accompanies CHF, but in some clinical situations it may be absent when, in fact, a patient has significant CHF.[5] In CHF, fluid is retained and not excreted because the pressoreceptors of the body sense a decreased volume of blood as a result of the heart's inability to pump an adequate amount of blood. The pressoreceptors subsequently relay a message to the kidneys to retain fluid so that a greater volume of blood can be ejected from the heart to the peripheral tissue.[68] Unfortunately, this compounds the problem and makes the heart work even harder, which further decreases its pumping ability. The retained fluid commonly accumulates bilaterally in the dependent extracellular spaces of the periphery.[5] Dependent spaces, such as the ankles and pretibial areas, tend to accumulate the majority of fluid and can be measured by applying firm pressure to the pretibial area for 10 to 20 seconds, then measuring the resultant indentation in the skin (pitting edema). This is frequently graded as mild, moderate, or severe, or it is given a numerical value, depending on the measured scale (Table 4-11). Peripheral edema can also accumulate in the sacral area (the shape of which resembles the popular fanny packs) or in the abdominal area (ascites). By using the pitting edema scale to determine the severity and location of peripheral edema (pretibial or sacral, distal or proximal) and obtaining girth measurements of the lower extremities and the abdomen, important information regarding patient status can be obtained.

**Table 4-11 Pitting Edema Scale**

| Edema Characteristics | Score |
| --- | --- |
| Barely perceptible depression (pit) | 1+ |
| Easily identified depression (EID) (skin rebounds to its original contour within 15 sec) | 2+ |
| EID (skin rebounds to its original contour within 15–30 sec) | 3+ |
| EID (rebound >30 sec) | 4+ |

However, it should be noted that peripheral edema is a sign that is associated with many other pathologies and does not by itself imply CHF.

### Jugular Venous Distention

Jugular venous distension also results from fluid overload. As fluid is retained and the heart's ability to pump is further compromised, the retained fluid "backs up," not only into the lungs but also into the venous system, of which the jugular veins are the simplest to identify and evaluate. The external jugular vein lies medial to the external jugular artery, and with an individual in a 45-degree semirecumbent position, it can be readily measured for signs of distension. Although individuals with marked CHF may demonstrate jugular venous distension in all positions (supine, semisupine, and erect), typically jugular venous distension is measured when the head of the bed is elevated to 45 degrees.[59,121] The degree of elevation should be noted as well as the magnitude of distension (mild, moderate, severe). Normally, the level is less than 3 to 5 cm above the sternal angle of Louis. Measurements of the internal jugular vein may be more reliable than those of the external jugular vein. Nonetheless, the highest point of visible pulsation is determined as the trunk and head are elevated and the vertical distance between this level and the level of the sternal angle of Louis is recorded (Fig. 4-13).[70,121]

Evaluation of the jugular waveforms can also be performed in this position, but catheterization of the pulmonary artery for assessment of pulmonary arterial pressures provides the greatest amount of information. A tremendous amount of information can be projected to a hemodynamic monitor, where the pulmonary artery pressure can be assessed and specific waveforms may be observed. The A wave of venous distension from right atrial systole, occurring just before $S_1$, and the V wave, frequently indicating a regurgitant tricuspid valve, are two such examples and are displayed in Figure 4-14.[70,121] Although the assessment of hemodynamic function via pulmonary artery pressure monitoring is considered an advanced skill, it is relatively simple to interpret the typical intensive care unit monitor and thus obtain important hemodynamic information. Perhaps the most important aspect of such monitoring is identifying the pulmonary artery pressure, which is schematized in Figure 4-14. A mean pulmonary artery pressure greater than 25 mm Hg is the definition of pulmonary hypertension and appears to be associated with a variety of pathophysiologic phenomena (hypoxia, cardiac arrhythmias, and pulmonary abnormalities).[59,121]

## Pulsus Alternans

Pulsus alternans (mechanical alteration of the femoral or radial pulse characterized by a regular rhythm and alternating strong and weak pulses) can frequently identify severely depressed myocardial function and CHF in general. This is performed using light pressure at the radial pulse with the patient's breath held in midexpiration (to avoid the superimposition of respiratory variation on the amplitude of the pulse).[121] Sphygmomanometry can more readily recognize this phenomenon, which commonly demonstrates 20 mm Hg

or greater alternating systolic blood pressure. Characteristically, if pulsus alternans exists, a 20 mm Hg or greater decrease in systolic blood pressure occurs during breath holding because of increased resistance to left ventricular ejection. It should be noted that a difference exists between pulsus alternans and pulsus paradoxus, which is characterized by a marked reduction of both systolic blood pressure (−20 mm Hg) and strength of the arterial pulse during inspiration. Pulsus paradoxus can also be detected by sphygmomanometry[121] and is occasionally seen in CHF. However, it is associated more frequently with cardiac tamponade and constrictive pericarditis primarily because of increased venous return and volume to the right side of the heart, which bulges the interventricular septum into the left ventricle, thus decreasing the amount of blood present in the left ventricle and the amount of blood ejected from it (because of decreased left ventricular volume and opposition to stroke volume from the bulging septum).[121]

## Changes in the Extremities

Occasionally, the extremities of persons with CHF will be cold and appear pale and cyanotic. This abnormal sensation and appearance are a result of the increased sympathetic nervous system activation of CHF, which increases peripheral vascular vasoconstriction and decreases peripheral blood flow.[124,125]

## Weight Gain

As fluid is retained, total body fluid volume increases, as does total body weight. Fluctuations of a few pounds from day to day are usually considered normal, but increases of several pounds per day (more than 3 lbs) are suggestive of CHF in a patient with CMD.[5] Body weight should always be measured from the same scale at approximately the same time of day with similar clothing and before exercise is started.

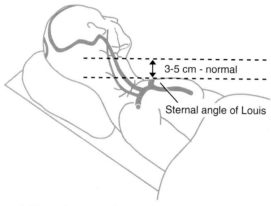

**Figure 4-13** Evaluation of venous pressure. Elevated venous pressure frequently represents right-sided and left-sided heart failure, which is characterized by pulmonary congestion and distension of the external jugular vein that is greater than 3 to 5 cm above the sternal angle of Louis.

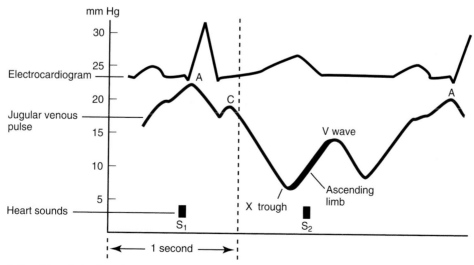

**Figure 4-14** The relationship of the jugular venous pulse to the electrocardiogram and heart sounds. The jugular venous pulse (and its various component wave patterns, C, V, and A waves) can be observed in the external jugular vein or via intensive care monitoring (which is often accompanied by an electrocardiogram). The physiologic and mechanical events producing the above wave patterns can be better analyzed by assessing the heart sounds and their respective location in the cardiac and venous pulse cycles.

## Sinus Tachycardia

Sinus tachycardia or other tachyarrhythmias may occur in CHF as the pressoreceptors and chemoreceptors of the body detect decreased fluid volume and decreased oxygen levels, respectively.[5] The body attempts (via increased heart rate) to increase the delivery of fluid and oxygen to the peripheral tissues where it is needed. Unfortunately, this only compounds the problem and makes the heart work even harder, which further impairs its ability to pump.

## Decreased Exercise Tolerance

Decreased exercise tolerance is ultimately the culmination of all of the preceding pathophysiologies that produce the characteristic signs and symptoms just discussed. It is apparent that as individuals at rest become short of breath, gain weight, and develop a faster resting heart rate, their ability to exercise is dramatically decreased. This effect has been observed repeatedly in patients with CHF and is the result of the interrelationships among the pathophysiologies briefly discussed.[5]

Individuals with heart failure demonstrate early onset anaerobic metabolism as a result from abnormalities in the skeletal muscle. The other changes in the skeletal muscle include fiber atrophy, loss of oxidative type I fibers and an increase in glycolytic type IIB fibers.[126,127]

The methods of measuring exercise tolerance in patients with CHF have improved significantly in the past few years, but many investigators still use the criteria set forth by the New York Heart Association in 1964.[128] These criteria categorize patients into one of four classes, depending on the development of symptoms and the amount of effort required to provoke them. In short, patients in class I have no limitations in ordinary physical activity, whereas patients in class IV are unable to carry on any physical activity without discomfort. Patients in classes II and III are characterized by slight limitation and marked limitation in physical activities, respectively (Table 4-12).

A great deal of investigation has been done on measuring exercise tolerance, functional capacity, and survival in persons with CHF.[128–140] Peak oxygen consumption measurements have traditionally been used to categorize persons with CHF and numerous studies have shown that persons with lower levels of peak oxygen consumption have poorer exercise tolerance, functional capacity, and survival than persons with greater levels of peak oxygen consumption (Table 4-13).[128–135] A peak oxygen consumption threshold range of 10 to 14 mL/kg/min appears to exist, below which patients have been observed to have poorer survival.[130–135] In fact, a peak oxygen consumption below this range is frequently used to list patients for cardiac transplantation.[135]

Measurement of the anaerobic threshold (or ventilatory threshold) and the "slope of the rate of $CO_2$ output from aerobic metabolism plus the rate of $CO_2$, generated from buffering of lactic acid, as a function of the $VO_2$," as well as the change in oxygen consumption to change in work rate above the anaerobic threshold, appear to be useful and relatively reliable in determining exercise tolerance in patients with CHF (Fig. 4-15).[136–140]

Unfortunately, most physical therapists do not have access to equipment (or training in its use) to measure respiratory gases. However, simple but thorough exercise assessments that evaluate symptoms, heart rate, blood pressure, heart rhythm via electrocardiogram, oxygen saturation via oximetry, and respiratory rate at specific workloads can provide important and useful information to compare patient response from day to day. Examples of such an assessment include

---

### Table 4-12 New York Heart Association (NYHA) Functional Classification

| Functional Capacity | Objective Assessment |
| --- | --- |
| Class I. Patients with cardiac disease but without resulting limitation of physical activity. Ordinary physical activity does not cause undue fatigue, palpitation, dyspnea, or anginal pain. | A. No objective evidence of cardiovascular disease. |
| Class II. Patients with cardiac disease resulting in slight limitation of physical activity. They are comfortable at rest. Ordinary physical activity results in fatigue, palpitation, dyspnea, or anginal pain. | B. Objective evidence of minimal cardiovascular disease. |
| Class III. Patients with cardiac disease resulting in marked limitation of physical activity. They are comfortable at rest. Less-than-ordinary activity causes fatigue, palpitation, dyspnea, or anginal pain. | C. Objective evidence of moderately severe cardiovascular disease. |
| Class IV. Patients with cardiac disease resulting in inability to carry on any physical activity without discomfort. Symptoms of heart failure or the anginal syndrome may be present even at rest. If any physical activity is undertaken, discomfort is increased. | D. Objective evidence of severe cardiovascular disease. |

*From Hunt SA, Baker DW, Chin MH, et al. ACC/AHA Guidelines for the Evaluation and Management of Chronic Heart Failure in the Adult: Executive Summary A Report of the American College of Cardiology/American Heart Association Task Force on Practice Guidelines (Committee to Revise the 1995 Guidelines for the Evaluation and Management of Heart Failure): Developed in Collaboration With the International Society for Heart and Lung Transplantation; Endorsed by the Heart Failure Society of America. J Am Coll Cardiol 104(24):2996–3007, 2001.*

treadmill ambulation, bicycle ergometry, hallway ambulation, and gentle calisthenic or strength training. Through this type of assessment, progress or deterioration can be documented and appropriate therapy implemented.

The 6-minute walk test (6MWT) is a valuable tool when assessing patients with CHF.[141] It provides an insight into the functional status, exercise tolerance, oxygen consumption, and survival of persons with CHF. Although the exercise performed during the 6MWT is considered submaximal, it nonetheless closely approximates the maximal exercise of persons with CHF and is correlated to peak oxygen consumption.[141,142] Information obtained from the 6MWT has been used to predict peak oxygen consumption (unfortunately with a modest degree of error) and survival in persons with advanced CHF awaiting cardiac transplantation (Table 4-14). Figure 4-16 demonstrates that patients unable to

### Table 4-13 Weber Classification of Functional Impairment in Aerobic Capacity and Anaerobic Threshold as Measured During Incremental Exercise Testing

| Class | Degree of Impairment | VO₂max (mL/min/kg) | Anaerobic Threshold (mL/min/kg) |
|---|---|---|---|
| A | None to mild | >20 | >14 |
| B | Mild to moderate | 16–20 | 11–14 |
| C | Moderate to severe | 10–16 | 8–11 |
| D | Severe | 6–10 | 5–8 |
| E | Very severe | <6 | ≤4 |

VO₂max, peak exercise oxygen consumption.
From Mann DL. Heart Failure: A Companion to Braunwald's Heart Disease. Philadelphia, 2004, Saunders.

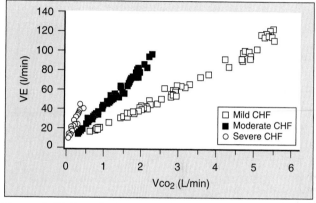

**Figure 4-15** Plot of minute ventilation (VE) versus the rate of carbon dioxide production (VCO₂) in patients with different degrees of severity of chronic heart failure. (Data from Coats AJ. Heart failure: What causes the symptoms of heart failure? Heart 86(5):574–8, 2001.)

### Table 4-14 Multivariate Equations for the Prediction of Peak Oxygen Uptake (VO₂)

| | Variants | Equation Outline | Equation Sample | |
|---|---|---|---|---|
| 1 | Distance | Distance + 3.98 | [0.03 × distance (m)] | r = 0.64; r² = 0.42; p < 0.0001; SEE = 3.32 |
| 2 | Distance, Age, Weight, Height, RPP | Distance – Age – Weight + Height + RPP + 2.45 | [0.02 × distance (m)] – [0.191 × age (yr)] – [0.07 × wt (kg)] + [0.09 × height (cm)] + [0.26 × RPP (×10⁻³)] + 2.45 | r = 0.81; r² = 0.65; p < 0.0001; SEE = 2.68 |
| 3 | Distance, Age, Weight, Height, RPP, FEV1, FVC | Distance – Age – Weight + Height + RPP + FEV1 + FVC + 7.77 | [0.02 × distance (m)] – [0.14 × age (yr)] – [0.07 × wt (kg)] + [0.03 × height (cm)] + [0.23 × RPP (×10⁻³)] + [0.10 × FEV1(L)] + [1.19 × FVC (L)] + 7.77 | r = 0.83; r² = 0.69; p < 0.0001; SEE = 2.59 |
| 4 | Distance, Age, Weight, Height, RPP, LVEF, PAP, CI | Distance – Age – Weight + Height + RPP + LVEF – PAP + CI + 8.43 | [0.02 × distance (m)] – [0.15 × age (yr)] – [0.05 × wt (kg)] + [0.04 × height (cm)] + [0.17 × RPP (×10⁻³)] + [0.03 × LVEF (%)] – [0.04 × PAP (mm Hg)] + [0.31 × CI (mL/min/m²)] + 8.43 | r = 0.85; r² = 0.72; p = 0.001; SEE = 2.06 |

CI = Cardiac index; LVEF = left ventricular ejection fraction; PAP = pulmonary artery pressure; r = correlation coefficient; r² = coefficient of determination; RPP = rate-pressure product; SEE = standard error of the estimate.

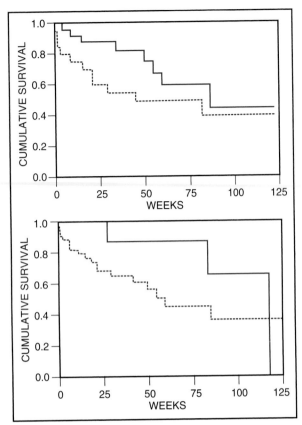

**Figure 4-16** Survival curves from 6-minute walk test distance ambulated.

**Box 4-4**

### Responses Observed During Submaximal and Maximal Exercise Testing in Patients with CMD

- A more rapid heart rate rise during submaximal workloads.
- A lower peak oxygen consumption and oxygen pulse (an indirect measure of stroke volume obtained by dividing the heart rate into oxygen consumption) during submaximal and maximal work.
- A flat, blunted, and occasionally hypoadaptive (decrease) systolic blood pressure response to exercise.
- A possible increase in diastolic blood pressure.
- Electrocardiographic signs of myocardial ischemia (ST depression and/or T-wave inversion).
- More easily provoked dyspnea and fatigue, often accompanied by angina.
- Lower maximal workloads when compared with those of subjects without heart disease.
- A chronotropic (increased heart rate response) and possibly an inotropic (force of myocardial contraction) incompetence (resulting in an inability to increase the heart rate or force of myocardial contraction) during exercise in patients with severe coronary artery disease and multisystem disease that may be partially caused by an autonomic nervous system dysfunction.

Data from Braunwald E. Clinical manifestations of heart failure. In Braunwald E. (ed.). Heart Disease: A Textbook of Cardiovascular Medicine. Philadelphia, 1988, Saunders, and Wasserman K, Beaver WL, Whipp BJ. Gas exchange theory, and the lactic acidosis (anaerobic) threshold. Circulation 81(1 Suppl):II14–30, 1990.

ambulate greater than 300 m during the 6MWT had poorer short-term survival but did not find a relationship with long term survival. However, Bittner and colleagues[143] found patients unable to ambulate greater than 300 m had poorer long-term survival. Therefore, not only can the cardiopulmonary response and exercise tolerance of a person with CHF be evaluated with the 6MWT, but a distance of 300 m appears to be important in determining short- and long-term survival. Several important responses observed during submaximal and maximal exercise testing in patients with CMD are also important factors of prognosis and are found in Box 4-4.

## Quality of Life in Congestive Heart Failure

Very little research has been performed in the area of quality of life in CHF. Early attempts to understand quality of life issues used instruments to measure quality of life that were less than comprehensive, such as dyspnea indices and exercise tolerance.[144–146] More comprehensive instruments have been designed and consist primarily of questionnaires that measure specific attributes of life such as socioeconomic factors, psychological status, and function.

One of the earliest such questionnaires was designed by Rector and associates and is titled the Minnesota Living with Heart Failure Questionnaire.[147] This questionnaire (Table 4-15) consists of 21 questions that the patient answers to the best of the patient's ability. This self-administered questionnaire appears to be more accurate and reliable with a modest degree of supervision. The Minnesota Living with Heart Failure Questionnaire has been used in several recent studies investigating the effects of various pharmacologic agents in persons with CHF as well as exercise training in CHF, and appears useful for measuring quality of life and changes in the quality of life.[148–150] These areas are two very important issues for clinical practice and research, and the information provided by this questionnaire is therefore highly desirable. Other similar questionnaires have been developed, but none have been used as extensively as the Minnesota Living with Heart Failure Questionnaire.

The Minnesota Living with Heart Failure Questionnaire was used to investigate which variables were of greatest importance in determining the quality of life of elderly persons with CHF. In two separate studies, significant correlates to the quality of life of elderly persons with CHF were identified.[151,152] In one study, the most powerful predictor of quality of life was quadriceps muscle strength. In this study of 30 elderly persons with CHF (mean age: 72 ± 10 years) poorer quadriceps muscle strength was associated with better quality of life, and persons with greater quadriceps muscle strength had a poorer quality of life.[151] In the second study,

## Table 4-15 The Minnesota Living with Heart Failure Questionnaire

These questions concern how your heart failure (heart condition) has prevented you from living as you wanted during the past month. The items listed here describe different ways some people are affected. If you are sure an item does not apply to you or is not related to your heart failure, then circle 0 (No) and go on to the next item. If an item does apply to you, then circle the number rating of how much it prevented you from living as you wanted. Remember to think about ONLY THE PAST MONTH. Did your heart failure prevent you from living as you wanted during the last month by

|  | No | Very Little |  |  | Very Much |  |
|---|---|---|---|---|---|---|
| 1. Causing swelling in your ankles, legs, etc? | 0 | 1 | 2 | 3 | 4 | 5 |
| 2. Making your working around the house or yard difficult? | 0 | 1 | 2 | 3 | 4 | 5 |
| 3. Making your relating to or doing things with your friends or family difficult? | 0 | 1 | 2 | 3 | 4 | 5 |
| 4. Making you sit or lie down to rest during the day? | 0 | 1 | 2 | 3 | 4 | 5 |
| 5. Making you tired, fatigued, or low on energy? | 0 | 1 | 2 | 3 | 4 | 5 |
| 6. Making your working to earn a living difficult? | 0 | 1 | 2 | 3 | 4 | 5 |
| 7. Making your walking about or climbing stairs difficult? | 0 | 1 | 2 | 3 | 4 | 5 |
| 8. Making you short of breath? | 0 | 1 | 2 | 3 | 4 | 5 |
| 9. Making your sleeping well at night difficult? | 0 | 1 | 2 | 3 | 4 | 5 |
| 10. Making you eat less of the foods you like? | 0 | 1 | 2 | 3 | 4 | 5 |
| 11. Making your going places away from home difficult? | 0 | 1 | 2 | 3 | 4 | 5 |
| 12. Making your sexual activities difficult? | 0 | 1 | 2 | 3 | 4 | 5 |
| 13. Making your recreational pastimes, sports, or hobbies difficult | 0 | 1 | 2 | 3 | 4 | 5 |
| 14. Making it difficult for you to concentrate or remember things? | 0 | 1 | 2 | 3 | 4 | 5 |
| 15. Giving you side effects from medications? | 0 | 1 | 2 | 3 | 4 | 5 |
| 16. Making you worry? | 0 | 1 | 2 | 3 | 4 | 5 |
| 17. Making you feel depressed? | 0 | 1 | 2 | 3 | 4 | 5 |
| 18. Costing you money for medical care? | 0 | 1 | 2 | 3 | 4 | 5 |
| 19. Making you feel a loss of self-control in your life? | 0 | 1 | 2 | 3 | 4 | 5 |
| 20. Making you stay in a hospital? | 0 | 1 | 2 | 3 | 4 | 5 |
| 21. Making you feel you are a burden to your family or friends? | 0 | 1 | 2 | 3 | 4 | 5 |

*Median responses from 83 patients are underlined for each item.*
*Spearman rank-order correlation between sum of items 1 to 21 and each item.*
*From Rector TS, Cohn JN. Assessment of patient outcome with the Minnesota Living with Heart Failure Questionnaire: Reliability and validity during a randomized, double-blind, placebo-controlled trial of pimobendan. Pimobendan Multicenter Research Group. Am Heart J 124(4):1017–25, 1992.*

body weight was the most powerful predictor of quality of life in elderly persons with CHF (mean age: 72 ± 9 years).[152] Patients with lower body weight had better quality of life scores compared to patients who were heavier.[152]

Significant depression is associated with an increased risk of functional decline as well as increased morbidity and mortality independent of severity of disease.[153–156] Significant depression also is associated with more than a double increase in mortality at 3 months and with triple the rate of rehospitalization in 1 year.[153]

### Radiologic Findings in Congestive Heart Failure

Identification of several of the signs and symptoms frequently suggests the presence of CHF, but radiologic and occasionally laboratory findings usually confirm the diagnosis and provide

a baseline from which to evaluate therapy.[5] Radiologic evidence of CHF is dependent on the size and shape of the cardiac silhouette (evaluating left VEDV) as well as the presence of interstitial, perivascular, and alveolar edema (evaluating fluid in the lungs).[5] Interstitial, perivascular, and alveolar edema form the radiologic hallmark of CHF and generally occur when pulmonary capillary pressures (which reflect the left ventricular end-diastolic pressure) exceed 20 to 25 mm Hg.[5] Pleural effusions (parenchymal fluid accumulations) and atelectasis (collapsed lung segments) may also be present.

### Laboratory Findings in Congestive Heart Failure

Proteinuria; elevated urine specific gravity, BUN, and creatinine levels; and decreased erythrocyte sedimentation rates

## Box 4-5

### Lab Findings in CHF

- ↑ BNP or NT-proBNP
- ↑ Protein in urine
- ↑ Urine specific gravity
- ↑ BUN
- ↑ Creatinine
- ↓ Erythrocyte sedimentation rates
- ↓ $PaO_2$
- ↓ $SpO_2$
- ↑ $PaCO_2$
- ↑ AST
- ↑ Alkaline phosphatase
- ↑ Bilirubin
- ↓ Na+
- ↑ or ↓ K+

## Box 4-6

### Common Precipitating Factors in Decompensated Heart Failure

- Medicine and dietary noncompliance
- Cardiac causes
- Ischemia
- Arrhythmia
- Uncontrolled hypertension
- Noncardiac causes
- Infection (pneumonia with or without hypoxia)
- Exacerbation of comorbidity (chronic obstructive pulmonary disease)
- Pulmonary embolus
- Toxins (nonsteroidal antiinflammatory drugs)
- Volume overload

(because of decreased fibrinogen concentrations resulting from impaired fibrinogen synthesis) are associated with CHF.[5] Frequently, but not consistently, $PaO_2$ and oxygen saturation levels are reduced and $PaCO_2$ levels elevated.[91] Liver enzymes, such as AST and alkaline phosphatase, are often elevated, and hyperbilirubinemia commonly occurs, resulting in subsequent jaundice.[5] Serum electrolytes are generally normal, but individuals with chronic CHF may demonstrate hyponatremia (decreased Na+) during rigid sodium restriction and diuretic therapy, or hypokalemia (decreased K+), which also may be the result of diuretic therapy.[1] Hyperkalemia can occur for several reasons, but most commonly is caused by a marked reduction in the GFR (especially if individuals are receiving a potassium-retaining diuretic) or overzealous potassium supplementation (when a non–potassium-retaining diuretic is used) (Box 4-5).[5]

BNP and its amino-terminal fragment NT-proBNP have an established role in the diagnosis of patients presenting with dyspnea of uncertain etiology and possibly in determining decompensation in CHF.[65]

### Echocardiography

Echocardiography(including Doppler flow studies) is the most useful diagnostic test for evaluation of anatomy, possible etiology, and severity of heart failure. The following three major concerns regarding heart failure can be answered with echocardiography:

- Is the left ventricular ejection fraction (EF) preserved or reduced?
- What is the structure of the LV (hypertrophy, dilated, normal)?
- Are other structural abnormalities present (pericardial, Valvular functioning, right ventricle) that would affect LV functioning?[23]

The echocardiography report should include EF, ventricular dimensions, ventricular volume, wall thickness measurement, chamber geometry, and regional wall motion.[23]

## Medical Management

The treatment of CHF, in general, is directed at the underlying cause or causes. The fundamental treatment for CHF involves controlling the pathophysiologic mechanisms responsible for its existence. By improving the heart's ability to pump and reducing the workload and controlling sodium intake and water retention, CHF can be relatively well controlled.[157] Table 4-16 outlines these measures. In addition, Box 4-6 defines common predisposing factors causing decompensated heart failure.

The specific treatments for CHF include the restriction of sodium intake, use of medications (diuretics, digitalis and other positive inotropic agents, dopamine, dobutamine, amrinone, vasodilator therapy, venodilators, angiotensin-converting enzyme inhibitors, and β-adrenergic blockers), other special measures, and properly prescribed physical activity. Figure 4-17 outlines these treatments and a brief discussion of each reveals how the pathophysiology of CHF is affected with each of the following measures.

### Dietary Changes and Nutritional Supplementation

Because of the associated dietary and nutritional deficiencies, supplementation of vitamins, minerals, and amino acids is often provided to persons with CHF. Vitamins C and E as well as various minerals have shown some promise as important supplements to the diet of persons with CHF.[158–161]

Dietary changes are also important for persons with CHF and include decreasing sodium intake, fluid restrictions, and eating heart-healthy foods that are low in cholesterol and fat. Such changes have been observed to decrease hospital readmissions in persons with CHF. Also, dietary counseling alone has been found to produce similar reductions in hospital readmissions and to improve patient outcomes.[162,163]

### Pharmacologic Treatment

See Chapter 14 for detailed description of the following medications.

## Table 4-16 Outline of Treatment of Chronic Congestive Heart Failure

| | |
|---|---|
| Proper prescription of physical activity | Decrease or discontinue exhaustive activities |
| | Decrease or discontinue full-time work or equivalent activity, introducing rest periods during the day |
| | Gradual progressive exercise training that fluctuates frequently from day to day |
| | Exercise intensity determined by level of dyspnea or adverse physiologic effort (i.e., angina or decrease in systolic blood pressure) |
| Restriction of sodium intake | Institute a low-sodium diet |
| Digitalis glycoside and other inotropic agents | Dopamine |
| | Dobutamine |
| | Amrinone |
| Diuretics | Moderate diuretic (thiazide) |
| | Loop diuretic (furosemide) |
| | Loop diuretic plus distal tubular (potassium-sparing) diuretic |
| | Loop diuretic plus thiazide and distal tubular diuretic |
| Aldosterone antagonists | Spironolactone |
| Vasodilators or venodilators | Captopril, enalapril, or combination of hydralazine plus isosorbide dinitrate |
| | Intensification of oral vasodilator regimen |
| | Intravenous nitroprusside |
| Angiotensin-converting enzyme | Captopril—may prevent cardiac dilation |
| | Enalapril maleate |
| | Lisinopril |
| β Blockers | Metoprolol |
| | Bucindolol |
| | Xamoterol |
| Special measures | Dialysis and ultrafiltration |
| | Assisted circulation (intraaortic balloon, left ventricular assist device, artificial heart) |
| | Cardiac transplantation |

The specific medications below are used for the pharmacologic treatment of CHF including diuretics, digitalis and other positive inotropic agents, dopamine, dobutamine, amrinone, vasodilator therapy, venodilators, angiotensin-converting enzyme inhibitors, and β-adrenergic blockers. Three classes of drugs can exacerbate the syndrome of heart failure and should be avoided in most patients including:

- Antiarrhythmic agents, which act as cardiodepressants and often have proarrhythmic effects. Only amiodarone and dofetilide have been shown to not adversely affect survival.
- Calcium channel blockers can lead to worsening heart failure and are associated with increased risk of cardiovascular events.
- Nonsteroid antiinflammatory drugs often increase sodium retention and cause peripheral vasoconstriction.[23]

## Diuretics

Diuretics remain the cornerstone of treatment for CHF.[157] As outlined in Table 4-16, moderate diuretics and loop diuretics are commonly used to reduce the fluid overload of CHF by increasing urine flow. Most of these diuretics act directly on kidney function by inhibiting solute (substances dissolved in a solution) and water reabsorption. As previously discussed, furosemide (Lasix) is the most commonly used diuretic, and its principal site of action is the thick ascending limb of Henle loop, where it inhibits the cotransport of sodium, potassium, and chloride.[157] As a result, individuals on Lasix need to be on K+ supplements.

The major principles of diuretic use are the following:

- Higher doses are required to restore than to maintain optimal volume status.
- Doses should generally be doubled when an increased effect is desired.
- The addition of metolazone or intravenous thiazides frequently resolves apparent "diuretic resistance" but should be reserved for intermittent rather than chronic use.
- Adequacy of oral diuretic dosing should be demonstrated prior to discharge.

With these considerations, furosemide (in bolus or continuous infusion) is generally effective to achieve diuresis, sometimes with the addition of intravenous thiazides.[129]

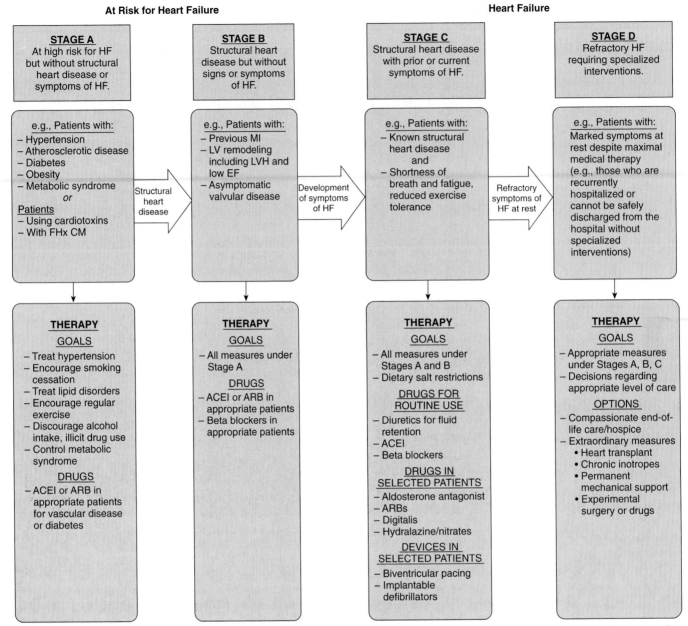

**Figure 4-17** Stages in the development of heart failure (HF) and recommended therapy by stage. ACEI, angiotensin-converting enzyme inhibitor; ARB, angiotensin receptor blocker; EF, ejection fraction; FHx CM, family history of cardiomyopathy; LV, left ventricular; LVH, left ventricular hypertrophy; MI, myocardial infarction. (From Jessup M, Abraham WT, Casey DE, et al. 2009 Focused update: ACCF/AHA Guidelines for the Diagnosis and Management of Heart Failure in Adults: A report of the American College of Cardiology Foundation/American Heart Association Task Force on Practice Guidelines: developed in collaboration with the International Society for Heart and Lung Transplantation. Circulation 119(14):1977–2016, 2009.)

## Aldosterone Antagonists

Aldosterone antagonists (e.g., spironolactone) are often added to the medical regimen of individuals with mild to moderate symptoms of heart failure in addition to other diuretics.[23]

## Digoxin (Lanoxin) and Other Positive Inotropic Agents

Digoxin (digitalis) is one of medicine's oldest drugs, and most of the digitalis drugs in use today are steroid glycosides derived from the leaves of the flowering plant foxglove, or

*Digitalis purpurea.* Despite its long history, there is still controversy over its use in patients with CHF and normal sinus rhythm.[164–166] However, several studies demonstrate favorable hemodynamic and clinical responses in selected patients.[167–171] The most significant clinical observations tend to be related to the positive inotropic (increased force of contraction) effect evidenced by an increased LVEF.[172] In addition, the electrophysiologic effects of digoxin on the heart help control rapid supraventricular arrhythmias (primarily atrial fibrillation or flutter) by increasing the parasympathetic tone in the sinus and atrioventricular nodes, thereby slowing conduction.[172] Current standard treatment recommendations involve the four-drug approach (digoxin, diuretics, ACE inhibitors and β blockers) for all patients with left ventricular dysfunction and symptomatic heart failure regardless of cause.[129]

Results from the Prospective Randomized Study of Ventricular Function and Efficacy of Digoxin (PROVED) and the Randomized Assessment of Digoxin and Inhibitors of Angiotensin-Converting Enzyme (RADIANCE) trials indicate that digoxin increases LVEF more in patients with dilated cardiomyopathy than in patients with ischemic heart disease and that withdrawal of digoxin leads to a significantly greater likelihood of clinical deterioration in patients with dilated cardiomyopathy.[173]

## Dopamine

Dopamine hydrochloride is a chemical precursor of norepinephrine, which stimulates dopaminergic, $\beta_2$-adrenergic, and $\alpha$-adrenergic receptors, as well as the release of norepinephrine. This results in increased cardiac output and, at doses greater than 10 μg/kg/min, markedly increased systemic vascular resistance and preload.[20] For this reason, the primary indication for dopamine is hemodynamically significant hypotension in the absence of hypovolemia.[20] Dopamine is also useful for patients with refractory CHF, in which case it is carefully titrated until urine flow or hemodynamic parameters improve. In such patients, the hemodynamic and renal effects of dopamine can be profound. Frequently, dopamine is infused together with nitroprusside or nitroglycerin to counteract the vasoconstricting action. In addition, dopamine is frequently administered (as are dobutamine and amrinone) during and after cardiac surgery to improve low cardiac output states.[20]

## Dobutamine

Dobutamine is a sympathomimetic amine that stimulates $\beta_1$ receptors in the myocardium, with very little effect on $\alpha$-adrenergic receptors. Dobutamine provides potent inotropic effects, but is only given via intravenous infusion.[174] Like dopamine, dobutamine increases cardiac output and decreases the peripheral resistance; with the use of dopamine, there is a potentially significant increase in peripheral resistance. For this reason dobutamine in addition to a moderate increase in volume is the treatment of choice in patients with hemodynamically significant right ventricular infarction.[20]

## Amrinone/Milrinone

Amrinone and milrinone are phosphodiesterase inhibitors that lead to increased cAMP by preventing its breakdown, thereby producing rapid inotropic and vasodilatory effects. Some of the side effects can include exacerbation of myocardial ischemia if coronary occlusion exists,[175] hypotension as a result of intense vasodilation, elevation in heart rate, and increase in atrial and ventricular tachyarrhythmias. Amrinone can also cause thrombocytopenia in 2% to 3% of patients, as well as a variety of other side effects (e.g.,

gastrointestinal dysfunction, myalgia, fever, hepatic dysfunction, cardiac arrhythmias). Milrinone has a prolonged half-life and its physiologic half-life may be excessive in individuals with renal dysfunction. More has been learned about the long-term effects of milrinone than about the other intravenous inotropic drugs in current use. Mortality from both heart failure and sudden death was increased with chronically administered milrinone compared with placebo without any significant improvement in symptoms.[176] Despite these adverse effects, amrinone is recommended and has proved to be therapeutic for patients with severe CHF that is refractory to diuretics, vasodilators, and other inotropic agents.[177] In addition, an increase in exercise tolerance has been observed with the use of milrinone.[178]

## Vasodilators and Venodilators

Vasodilators (nesiritide, nitroglycerin, nitroprusside) are given to patients with CHF or CMD to relax smooth muscle in peripheral arterioles and to produce peripheral vasodilation that reduces filling pressures, decreases the afterload, lessens the work of the heart, decreases symptoms, and potentially decreases the degree of CMD. These medications include calcium channel blockers as well as $\alpha$ blockers. The clinical management of patients with CHF and CMD frequently combines vasodilators, venodilators, and angiotensin-converting enzyme inhibitors.

## Angiotensin-Converting Enzyme Inhibitors and $\alpha$ Receptor Blockers

The combined use of ACE inhibitors, vasodilators, and venodilators has been demonstrated to be very effective in reducing symptoms and improving exercise tolerance.[188] The primary mechanism of action of these inhibitors is probably via the reduction of angiotensin II, a hormone that causes vasoconstriction,[172] but other less well-defined actions may be responsible for the therapeutic effects of ACE inhibitors in patients with CHF. Other poorly understood mechanisms of such inhibitors include "nonspecific vasodilation with unloading of the ventricle, inhibition of excessive sympathetic drive and perhaps modulation of tissue receptor systems."[172]

A great deal of interest has focused on the "prevention" hypothesis regarding the use of ACE inhibitors and the prevention of progressive CMD (dilation and CHF).[180-183] Notably, captopril may prevent such progressive cardiac dilation.[180,181] Recent studies have focused on the addition of β blockers to ACE inhibitors (and sometimes $\alpha$-receptor blockers) and demonstrated a greater improvement in symptoms and reduction in the risk of death than when ACE inhibitors were used alone and the dosage was increased.[184]

## β-Adrenergic Antagonists and Partial Agonists

Perhaps one of the most confusing groups of medications used in treating CHF and CMD is the β-adrenergic blockers group. One of the many uses of β blockers is to lower blood pressure, primarily via a reduction in cardiac output.[172] This reduction in cardiac output is the result of a decrease in heart rate and stroke volume, which causes an increase in end-diastolic volume and end-diastolic pressure (the slowing of the heart rate allows more time for the ventricles to fill before the next myocardial contraction with more time for the coronary arteries to fill) but somewhat paradoxically reduces the myocardial oxygen requirement.[179] This paradoxical reduction in oxygen requirement probably is the result of a decrease in sympathetic nervous system stimulation because of the blocking of the β receptors. Sympathetic (catecholamine-driven) increases in heart rate, force of myocardial contraction, velocity, and extent of myocardial contraction, as well as systolic blood pressure, are prevented by β blockade.[185,186]

β Blockers interfere with the sustained activation of the nervous system and therefore block the adrenergic effects on the heart.

Although there are a number of potential benefits to blocking all three receptors ($β_1$, $β_2$, and $α$), most of the deleterious effects of sympathetic activation are mediated by the $β_1$-adrenergic receptor. β Blockers are usually prescribed in conjunction with ACE inhibitors and in combination have demonstrated a reversal of the LV remodeling that occurs with injury and long-standing muscle dysfunction, improves symptoms, prevents rehospitalizations, and prolongs life. Consequently, β blockers are indicated for patients with symptomatic or asymptomatic heart failure and a depressed EF of lower than 40%. Three β blockers have been shown to be effective in reducing mortality in patients with chronic heart failure including Toprol (metoprolol succinate), bisoprolol, and carvedilol.[187-190]

In the Metoprolol CR/XL Randomized Intervention Trial in Congestive Heart Failure (MERIT-HF), a 34% reduction in mortality was reported in individuals with mild to moderate heart failure and moderate to severe systolic dysfunction who were taking metoprolol CR/XL when compared to placebo.[191] In addition, metoprolol CR/XL reduced mortality from both sudden death and progressive pump failure.[191]

In patients with dilated cardiomyopathy who were supported with a left ventricular assist device (LVAD) and given a specific pharmacologic regimen consisting of an ACE inhibitor, an angiotensin receptor blocker, an aldosterone antagonist, and a β blocker, followed by treatment with a $β_2$-adrenergic receptor agonist (clenbuterol), improvement in the myocardium resulted in explantation of the LVAD as well as an improvement in quality of life and absence of recurrent heart failure for 1 to 4 years.[192] Thus, β blockers, in addition to other pharmacologic agents like ACE inhibitors, play a significant role in LV remodeling. Recent studies indicate that β blockers can be started as early as during the hospitalization after an acute injury and should be continued for a minimum of 1 year postinjury date to optimize the ventricular remodeling.[187-190]

## Anticoagulation

The patient hospitalized with heart failure is at increased risk for thromboembolic complications and deep venous thrombosis and should receive prophylactic anticoagulation with either intravenous unfractionated heparin or subcutaneous preparations of unfractionated or low-molecular-weight heparin, unless contraindicated.[193]

## Mechanical Management

### ICD Implantation

ICD implantation is recommended in the 2009 American Heart Association guidelines for the treatment of CHF for patients with an EF less than or equal to 35% and mild to moderate symptoms of heart failure and in whom survival with good functional capacity is otherwise anticipated to extend beyond 1 year. ICD implantation should not be considered until medical therapy has been maximized and the patients' EF is measured under the current medical therapy.[23] ICDs are not indicated in patients with refractory symptoms of heart failure (stage D) or in patients with concomitant diseases that would shorten their life expectancy independent of CHF.[23]

### Cardiac Resynchronization Therapy

In individuals with heart failure with abnormalities in the chamber size, ventricular dyssynchrony often exists. The consequences of dyssynchrony include suboptimal ventricular filling, a reduction in the rate of rise of ventricular contractile force or pressure, prolonged duration of mitral regurgitation, and paradoxical septal wall motion.[174,175,177] These same individuals may demonstrate a prolonged QRS on the electrocardiogram (>0.12 seconds). Ventricular dyssynchrony has also been associated with increased mortality in heart failure patients.[149-151] As a result, electrical stimulation (activation) of the right and left ventricles in a synchronized manner can be provided by a biventricular pacemaker device. This approach, called *cardiac resynchronization therapy* (CRT), may improve ventricular contraction and reduce the degree of secondary mitral regurgitation.[57,58,152] In addition, the short-term use of CRT is associated with improvements in cardiac function and hemodynamics without an accompanying increase in oxygen use.[194] When CRT was added to patients on optimal medical therapy who continued to have symptoms, significant improvement was noted in quality of life, functional class, exercise capacity and 6-minute walk distance (6MWD) and EF.[67,68,148] In a metaanalysis of several CRT trials, heart failure hospitalizations were reduced by 32% and all-cause mortality by 25%.[68,195]

### Special Measures

Patients who respond unfavorably to the aforementioned methods of treatment for CHF and CMD and who demonstrate signs and symptoms of severe CHF are frequently managed using several rather extreme methods. As noted in Table 4-14, there are three "special measures" categories for treating CHF and CMD: dialysis and ultrafiltration, assisted circulation, and cardiac transplantation.

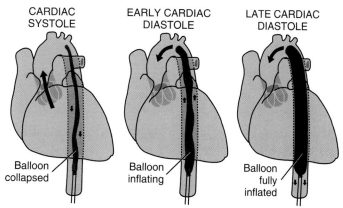

**Figure 4-18** The intraaortic balloon pump. Inflation and deflation of the intraaortic balloon pump improve diastolic and systolic heart function, respectively.

## Dialysis and Ultrafiltration

The mechanical removal of fluid from the pleural and abdominal cavities of patients with CHF is usually unnecessary, but patients unresponsive to diuretic therapy because of severe CHF or insensitivity to diuretics may be in need of peritoneal dialysis or extracorporeal ultrafiltration.[23,157] The mechanical removal of fluid in patients with acute respiratory distress because of large pleural effusions or diaphragms elevated by ascites (both of which compress the lungs) frequently brings rapid relief of dyspnea. However, mechanical removal of fluid (primarily peritoneal dialysis) may be associated with risk of pneumothorax, infection, peritonitis, hypernatremia, hyperglycemia, hyperosmolality, and cardiac arrhythmias.[157,196] Cardiovascular collapse may also occur if too much fluid is removed or if removal takes place too rapidly. It is recommended that no more than 200 mL of fluid per hour be removed and no more than 1500 mL of pleural fluid be removed during dialysis.[157,196]

For these reasons, as well as for simplicity, cost effectiveness, and long-lasting effects, ultrafiltration has become the treatment of choice for patients in need of mechanical fluid removal.[196] Extracorporeal ultrafiltration is a relatively new technique; it removes plasma water and sodium via an ultrafiltrate (a blend of water, electrolytes, and other small molecules with concentrations identical to those in plasma) from the blood by convective transport through a highly permeable membrane. Ultrafiltration can be performed vein-to-vein using an extracorporeal pump or with an arteriovenous approach.[196]

Although hemodynamic side effects (hypotension, organ malperfusion, and hemolysis) are also possible with ultrafiltration, proper monitoring of the rate of blood flow through the filter (rates above 150 mL/min or below 500 mL/hr are tolerated without side effects) as well as right atrial pressure (ultrafiltration should be discontinued when the right atrial pressure falls to 2 or 3 mm Hg)[197] and hematocrit levels (should not exceed 50%) should, for the most part, prevent them.[196]

## Assisted Circulation

Several methods of treatment assist the circulation of blood throughout the body. Perhaps the most widely used is intraaortic balloon counterpulsation via the intraaortic balloon pump (IABP). The IABP catheter is positioned in the thoracic aorta just distal to the left subclavian artery via the right or left femoral artery (Fig. 4-18). Inflation of the balloon occurs at the beginning of ventricular diastole, immediately after closure of the aortic valve. This increases intraaortic pressure as well as diastolic pressure in general and forces blood in the aortic arch to flow in a retrograde direction into the coronary arteries. This mechanism of action is referred to as *diastolic augmentation* and profoundly improves oxygen delivery to the myocardium.[100] In addition to this physiologic assist (greater availability of oxygen for myocardial energy production) to improve cardiac performance, hemodynamic assistance is also obtained as the balloon deflates just before systole, which decreases left ventricular afterload by forcing blood to move from an area of higher pressure to one of lower pressure to fill the space previously occupied by the balloon.[100] Consequently, the intraaortic balloon pump causes "a 10% to 20% increase in cardiac output as well as a reduction in systolic and an increase in diastolic arterial pressure with little change in mean pressure. There is also a diminution of heart rate and an increase in urine output."[100] In addition, intraaortic balloon counterpulsation produces a reduction in myocardial oxygen consumption "and decreased myocardial ischemia and anaerobic metabolism,"[100] all of which are very important in the management of CHF and CMD.

The IABP is occasionally used in conjunction with a slightly different but similar treatment called pulmonary artery balloon counterpulsation (PABC) in the pulmonary artery versus the thoracic aorta, which is helpful in treating right ventricular and biventricular failure unresponsive to inotropic drugs and the IABP alone.[100]

## Ventricular Assist Devices

Patients awaiting heart transplantation, or those in whom ventricular function is expected to return, occasionally benefit from prosthetic devices that consist of a flexible polyurethane blood sac and diaphragm placed within a rigid case outside the body (Fig. 4-19). Pulses of compressed carbon dioxide from a pneumatic drive line are delivered between

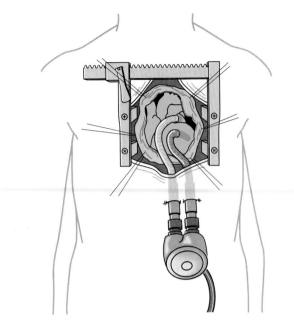

**Figure 4-19** Left ventricular assist device. The left ventricular assist device provides myocardial assistance until heart transplantation or corrective measures are taken.

the rigid case and the diaphragm. This provides the force necessary to eject blood that has traveled to the prosthetic device via a cannula inserted into the left ventricle through a Dacron graft into the ascending aorta and finally to the periphery. This device can handle almost all the output from the left side of the heart,[157] providing rest or assistance to the impaired myocardium. Patients may require a biventricular assist device (BiVAD) if both ventricles are involved. See Chapter 12 for more information on ventricular assist devices.

## Surgical Management

Reparative, reconstructive, excisional, and ablative surgeries are sometimes performed in the treatment of CHF and CMD. Reparative procedures correct cardiac malfunctions such as ventricular septal defect, atrial septal defect, and mitral stenosis, and frequently improve cardiac hemodynamics, resulting in improved cardiac performance. Coronary artery bypass graft surgery is probably the most common reconstructive surgery because myocardial ischemia and infarction are the primary causes of CMD and CHF.[198] Its effects are often profound, improving cardiac muscle function and eliminating CHF. Reconstruction of incompetent heart valves is also common.[18] Excisional procedures, in patients with atrial myxomas (tumors) and large left ventricles, are employed less often. The excision of a tumor or aneurysm is occasionally performed, and the excised area is replaced with Dacron patches.[18] Ablative procedures are also used less frequently, but for patients with persistent and symptomatic Wolff-Parkinson-White syndrome or intractable ventricular tachycardia, ablation (e.g., via laser

or cryotherapy) of the reentry pathways appears to be very therapeutic.[18] The surgical implantation of automatic implantable defibrillators is increasingly common and also appears to be of great therapeutic value for those with ventricular tachycardia that is unresponsive to medications and ablative procedures.[18]

### Left Ventricular Muscle Flaps

Although somewhat unusual, the use of muscle flaps (cardiomyoplasty), usually dissected from the latissimus dorsi or trapezius muscle, may be an alternative treatment for a limited number of patients with severe CMD and CHF.[199] The muscle flap is wrapped around the left ventricle and attached to a pacemaker, which stimulates the flap to contract, thus contracting the left ventricle. Many years of animal research have provided procedural treatment protocols and have resulted in the use of muscle flap techniques in approximately 12 human subjects who apparently "carry on a reasonably normal life with adequate exercise tolerance."[199]

The major problem with the use of muscle flaps is muscle fatigue, because skeletal muscle, unlike cardiac muscle, does not have the ability to contract continuously. However, it has been demonstrated that skeletal muscle, after careful training and conditioning could assume the functions of the cardiac muscle.[199]

### Cardiomyoplasty (Partial Left Ventriculectomy—Batista Procedure)

Several investigations have shown that the removal of dilated, noncontracting myocardium of persons with CHF and subsequent suturing of remaining viable myocardial tissue decrease the left ventricular chamber size and improve myocardial performance. Improvements in myocardial performance appear to improve the functional status and symptoms of CHF.[200–202]

### Cardiac Transplantation

Cardiac transplantation is the last treatment effort for a patient with CHF and CMD because "potential recipients of cardiac transplants must have end-stage heart disease with severe heart failure and a life expectancy of less than 1 year."[157] Heart transplantation can be heterologous (or xenograft, from a nonhuman primate) or more commonly homologous (or allograft, from another human).[157] Orthotopic homologous cardiac transplantation is performed by removing the recipient's heart, leaving the posterior walls of the atria with their venous connections on which the donor's atria are sutured. In heterotopic homologous cardiac transplantation, the recipient's heart is left intact and the donor heart is placed in parallel, with anastomoses between the two right atria, pulmonary arteries, left atria, and aorta. Heterotopic heart transplantation may be preferable to orthotopic transplantation because if the donor heart is rejected (a primary complicating factor, as are infection and

**Box 4-7**

**Framingham Clinical Scoring System for Heart Failure**

| **Major Criteria** | **Minor Criteria** | **Major or Minor Criteria** |
|---|---|---|
| Paroxysmal nocturnal dyspnea or orthopnea<br>Neck-vein distension<br>Rales<br>Cardiomegaly<br>Acute pulmonary edema<br>S$_3$ gallop<br>Increased venous pressure >6 cm H$_2$O<br>Circulation time >25 sec<br>Hepatojugular reflux | Ankle edema, night cough, dyspnea on exertion<br>Hepatomegaly<br>Pleural effusion<br>Vital capacity decreased 50% from maximal capacity<br>Tachycardia (rate >120 bpm) | Weight loss >4.5 kg in 5 days in response to treatment |

Diagnosis of heart failure: two major, or one major and two minor criteria.
From Mosterd A, Deckers JW, Hoes AW, et al. Classification of heart failure in population based research: An assessment of six heart failure scores. Eur J Epidemiol 13(5):491–502, 1997.

nephrotoxicity secondary to vigorous immunosuppression), the presence of the patient's own heart may improve the likelihood of survival.[157] However, orthotopic heart transplantation is most commonly performed.

Chapter 12 provides a more complete description of cardiac transplantation.

## Prognosis

As a result of multivariate analysis of clinical variables, the most significant predictors of survival in individuals with CHF have been identified and include decreasing LVEF; worsening New York Heart Association (NYHA) functional status; degree of hyponatremia; decreasing peak exercise oxygen uptake; decreasing hematocrit; widened QRS on 12-lead electrocardiogram; chronic hypotension; resting tachycardia; renal insufficiency; intolerance to conventional therapy; and refractory volume overload.[203,204] In addition, elevated circulating levels of neurohormonal factors also are associated with high mortality rates, but routine lab assessment of norepinephrine or endothelin is neither practical nor helpful in managing the patient's clinical status. Likewise, elevated BNP (or NT-proBNP) levels predict higher risk of heart failure and other events after myocardial infarction, whereas marked elevation in BNP levels during hospitalization for heart failure may predict rehospitalization and death. However, controversy still exists regarding BNP measurement and its prognostic value.[203,204]

Currently, a few mathematical models exist to help predict outcome in heart failure patients for clinicians managing treatment. Aaronson and colleagues developed a noninvasive risk stratification model based upon clinical findings and peak VO$_2$ that includes seven variables: presence of ischemia, resting heart rate, left ventricular EF, presence of a QRS duration greater than 200 msec, mean resting blood pressure, peak VO$_2$, and serum sodium.[205] A heart failure score was then developed and related to subsequent morbidity and mortality. The model defined low-, medium-, and high-risk groups based upon 1-year event-free survival rates of 93%, 72%, and 43%, respectively. Interestingly, adding invasive data did not improve the prediction. Campana and coworkers developed a model using cause of heart failure, NYHA functional class, presence of an S$_3$ gallop, cardiac output, mean arterial pressure, and either pulmonary artery diastolic pressure or pulmonary capillary wedge pressure.[206] Patients were risk stratified into low-, intermediate-, and high-risk groups for 1-year event-free survival rates of 95%, 75%, and 40% respectively.[206]

For three other clinical scoring systems for evaluation of heart failure (Framingham, Boston, and National Health and Nutritional Examination Surveys [NHANES]), see Box 4-7 and Table 4-17.

## Physical Therapy Assessment

Because of the increase in number of patients with CHF, physical therapists in all practice settings are seeing these individuals and are responsible for assessing functional status and providing optimal treatment to improve the quality of their lives and possibly decrease morbidity and mortality. Although Chapter 16 provides cardiopulmonary assessment in detail and Chapter 18 provides detailed interventions, a brief overview of assessment and interventions for individuals with CHF is provided here.

A thorough assessment includes an interview that should include a series of questions:
- When did the symptoms start?
- Are the symptoms stable or are they getting worse?
- Are symptoms provoked or do they occur at rest?
- Are there accompanying symptoms such as chest pain or calf claudication?
- Is orthopnea or PND present?

## Table 4-17 Boston and NHANES-1 Clinical Scoring Systems for Heart Failure

| Categories | Criteria | | NHANES | Boston |
|---|---|---|---|---|
| History | Dyspnea | At rest | | 4 |
| | | On level ground | 1 | 2 |
| | | On climbing | 1 | 1 |
| | | Stop when walking at own pace or on level ground after 100 yards | 2 | 3 |
| | Orthopnea | | | 4 |
| | Paroxysmal nocturnal dyspnea | | 3 | |
| Physical examination | Heart rate | 91–110 bpm | 1 | 1 |
| | | >110 bpm | 2 | 2 |
| | Jugular venous pressure (>6 cm $H_2O$) | | | |
| | | Alone | 1 | 2 |
| | | Plus hepatomegaly or edema | 2 | 3 |
| | Rales | Basilar crackles | 1 | 1 |
| | Crackles | More than basilar crackles | 2 | 2 |
| | Wheezing | | | 3 |
| | $S_3$ gallop | | | 3 |
| Chest radiography | Alveolar pulmonary edema | | | 4 |
| | Alveolar fluid plus pleural fluid | | 3 | |
| | Interstitial pulmonary edema | | 2 | 3 |
| | Interstitial edema plus pleural fluid | | 3 | |
| | Bilateral pleural effusion | | | 3 |
| | Cardiothoracic ratio > 0.5 (PA projection) | | | 3 |
| | Upper zone flow redistribution | | 1 | 2 |

*Diagnosis of heart failure Boston criteria: Definite (8–12 points); Possible (5–7 points); Unlikely (≤4 points).*
*Diagnosis of heart failure NHANES-1 criteria: ≥3 points.*
*NHANES, National Health and Nutrition Examination Surveys.*
*From Mosterd A, Deckers JW, Hoes AW, et al. Classification of heart failure in population based research: An assessment of six heart failure scores. Eur J Epidemiol 13(5):491–502, 1997.*

- How far can you walk?
- Do you retain fluid?
- Do you restrict sodium in their diet?
- What sorts of activity can you no longer do?
- Are you losing or gaining weight?
- How do you sleep?

Following the interview, a physical examination should involve an assessment of the patient's cardiopulmonary status including:

- Notation of symptoms of CHF (dyspnea, PND, and orthopnea)
- Evaluation of pulse and electrocardiogram to determine heart rate and rhythm
- Evaluation of respiratory rate and breathing pattern
- Auscultation of the heart and lungs with a stethoscope
- Evaluation of radiographic findings to determine the existence and magnitude of pulmonary edema
- Performance of laboratory blood studies to determine the $PaO_2$ and $PaCO_2$ levels

- Evaluation of the oxygen saturation levels via oximetry
- Palpation for fremitus and percussion of the lungs to determine the relative amount of air or solid material in the underlying lung
- Performance of sit-to-stand test to evaluate heart rate and blood pressure (orthostatic hypotension) as well as dyspnea
- Objective measurement of other characteristic signs produced by fluid overload, such as peripheral edema, weight gain, and jugular venous distension
- Assessment of cardiopulmonary response to exercise (e.g., heart rate, blood pressure, electrocardiogram)
- Administration of a questionnaire to measure quality of life

Upon the collection of data and the determination of a treatment diagnosis and prognosis, a plan of care is developed for the patient with CHF that details the interventions that are used to achieve the optimal outcome.

## Table 4-18   Summary of Interventions for CHF

| Intervention | Guidelines |
| --- | --- |
| Exercise training (In general) | Low level, low-impact exercise (e.g., walking) for 5–10 min/day gradually increasing duration to 30 min. Intensity should be monitored via level of dyspnea or perceived exertion. Frequency: 1–2×/day for 5–7 days/wk. |
| Exercise training with intravenous inotropic agents | Progressive increase in low-impact exercise with monitoring of blood pressure response. If patient has an ICD, monitor for ICD firing, especially with exercise. |
| Exercise with LVADs | Progressive increase in exercise; should demonstrate normal responses. May have flow limitations (10 to 12 L/min), or cardiovascular function from the mechanically driven cardiac output, and the effects of a 6-lb mass resting below the diaphragm that may alter ventilatory performance. |
| Exercise with continuous positive airway pressure (CPAP) | CPAP may function to reduce preload and afterload on heart, and decrease the workload on inspiratory muscles which may also increase lung compliance. |
| Breathing exercises | Exercise program set at a specific percentage of the maximal inspiratory pressure or maximal expiratory pressure (similar to aerobic exercise training) with a device that resists either inspiration or expiration. |
| Expiratory muscle training | Performed in a variety of ways; most commonly with weights upon the abdomen and hyperpneic breathing. Results in improved symptoms, functional status, and pulmonary function and reduced pulmonary complications. May also use positive end-expiratory pressure devices. |
| Inspiratory muscle training | One protocol: Threshold inspiratory muscle trainer at 20% of maximal inspiratory pressure, 3 times a day, for 5 to 15 min. |
| Instruction in energy-conservation techniques | Balancing activity and rest, and performing activities in an energy-efficient manner; scheduling activities and rest. |
| Self-management techniques | Incorporate the individual into the management of the disease by making them responsible for their own health. |

## Physical Therapy Interventions

### Exercise Training

Exercise training is a therapeutic modality that should be considered for all patients with ventricular dysfunction (Table 4-18). Patients who are prescribed exercise training and other interventions need to be without any overt signs of decompensated heart failure, and should be monitored during treatment to observe for abnormal responses and symptoms. Increased levels of physical activity do not appear to have adverse effects on subsequent cardiac mortality or on ventricular function in patients with ventricular dysfunction. In addition, these patients derive psychological benefits from participation in exercise training, and the close medical surveillance available in the content of a supervised exercise program may facilitate better clinical decisions concerning pharmacologic therapy, interpretation of symptoms, or the necessity for and timing of operative procedures.[198]

Specific benefits of exercise training for individuals with heart failure include improvement in symptoms, clinical status and exercise duration.[207,208] Other studies have reported improved functional capacity and quality of life, and reduced hospitalizations for heart failure.[209] There also is indication that exercise training may have beneficial effects on ventricular structure and remodeling.[210] The most recent Heart Failure Action Study reported that exercise training was associated with modest significant reductions for both all-cause mortality or hospitalization and cardiovascular mortality or heart failure hospitalization.[211,212]

### Guidelines for Exercise Training

Studies that have demonstrated improvements in exercise tolerance and patient symptoms were all performed using different methodology—varying modes, intensities, durations, and frequencies of exercise. Specific guidelines for exercise training of patients with CHF are difficult to implement because patient status frequently changes. Despite a lack of specific guidelines for exercising persons with CHF, the U.S. Department of Health and Human Services Agency for Health Care Policy and Research outlined the importance of exercise training in treatment of CHF.[211-213] Exercise training was recommended "as an integral component of the symptomatic management" of persons with CHF "to attain functional and symptomatic improvement but with a potentially higher likelihood of adverse events." This recommendation was based upon significant scientific evidence from previously

## Table 4-19 Exercise Training Guidelines for Patients with CHF

| | |
|---|---|
| I. Relative criteria necessary for the initiation of an aerobic exercise training program: compensated CHF | Ability to speak without signs or symptoms of dyspnea (able to speak comfortably with a respiratory rate <30 breaths/min) |
| | <Moderate fatigue |
| | Crackles present in <one-half of the lungs |
| | Resting heart rate <120 bpm |
| | Cardiac index ≥2.0 L/min/m$^2$ (for invasively monitored patients) |
| | Central venous pressure <12 mm Hg (for invasively monitored patients) |
| II. Relative criteria indicating a need to modify or terminate exercise training | Marked dyspnea or fatigue (e.g., Borg rating > 3/10) |
| | Respiratory rate >40 breaths/min during exercise |
| | Development of an S$_3$ heart sound or pulmonary crackles |
| | Increase in pulmonary crackles |
| | Significant increase in the sound of the second component of the second heart sound (P2) |
| | Poor pulse pressure (<10 mm Hg difference between the systolic and diastolic blood pressure) |
| | Decrease in heart rate or blood pressure of >10 bpm or mm Hg, respectively, during continuous (steady state) or progressive (increasing workloads) exercise |
| | Increased supraventricular or ventricular ectopy |
| | Increase of >10 mm Hg in the mean pulmonary artery pressure (for invasively monitored patients) |
| | Increase or decrease of >6 mm Hg in the central venous pressure (for invasively monitored patients) |
| | Diaphoresis, pallor, or confusion |

*From Cahalin LP. Heart failure. Phys Ther 76(5):516, 1996.*

published investigations that were reviewed by experts in the field of cardiac rehabilitation.[213]

Patients with decompensated (uncontrolled) CHF are typically very dyspneic and therefore should not begin aerobic exercise training until the CHF is compensated. Table 4-19 lists specific exercise training guidelines, which include the attainment of a cardiac index of 2.0 L/min/m$^2$ or greater (for invasively monitored patients in the hospital) before aerobic exercise training is implemented and the maintenance of an adequate pulse pressure (not less than a 10 mm Hg difference between the systolic and diastolic blood pressure) during exercise. The development of marked dyspnea and fatigue, S$_3$ heart sound, or crackles during exercise requires the modification or termination of exercise.[214]

Progression of an exercise conditioning program for patients with CHF can be done as outlined in Activity Guidelines for Patients Hospitalized with CHF (Table 4-20). Although this protocol is designed for hospitalized patients, the same methodology and progression can be applied to patients with CHF in outpatient clinics, nursing homes, and their own homes. For most patients, ambulation may be the most effective and functional mode of exercise to administer and prescribe, beginning with frequent short walks and progressing to less frequent, longer bouts of exercise. Occasionally, patients may be so deconditioned that gentle strengthening exercises, restorator cycling, or ventilatory muscle training is the preferred mode of exercise conditioning. As strength and endurance improve, patients can be progressed to upright cycle ergometry or ambulating with a rolling walker.

Because dyspnea is the most common complaint of patients with CHF, the level of dyspnea or Borg rating of perceived exertion appears to be an acceptable method to prescribe and evaluate an exercise program.[198] This is supported by the observation that these subjective indices correlate well with training heart rate ranges in this patient population.[215] Therefore, a basic guideline of increasing the exercise intensity to a level that produces a moderate degree of dyspnea (conversing with modest difficulty, ability to count to 5 without taking a breath, or a Borg rating of 3 on a scale of 10) may be the simplest and most effective method to prescribe exercise for patients with CHF. It also appears to be the most effective method to progress a patient's exercise prescription. The exercise prescription of patients with CHF can be progressed when (1) the cardiopulmonary response to exercise is adaptive (see Table 4-17) and (2) workloads that previously produced moderate dyspnea (e.g., Borg rating of 3/10) produce mild dyspnea (e.g., Borg rating of 2/10 or less). Because an increasing number of patients with CMD and CHF are being prescribed β blockers, which often cause little or no change

## Table 4-20 Activity Guidelines for Patients Hospitalized with CHF*

| Day | Standard Activity Regimen | Gradual Activity Regimen |
| --- | --- | --- |
| 1 | Commode/chair | Bedrest |
| 2 | Room ambulation | Bedrest/gentle active strengthening exercises |
| 3 | Hallway ambulation and cycle ergometry ×2 (1–10 min) MET (metabolic equivalent of task) level goal = 2.0–3.0 | Commode/chair/bathroom/restorator cycling/room ambulation/gentle strengthening exercises |
| 4 | Independent hallway ambulation ×3 (1–15 min) MET level goal = 3.0–4.0; patient adequately ascends/descends two flights of stairs and showers independently Has adequate understanding of home exercise prescription. Outpatient cardiac rehabilitation appointment scheduled. Patient discharged. | Hallway ambulation/restorator or cycle ergometry ×2, exercise duration (1–5 min): MET level goal = 1.0–2.0 strengthening exercises |
| 5 | | Hallway ambulation/restorator or cycle ergometry ×2, exercise duration (1–8 min) MET level goal = 1.5–2.5 strengthening exercises |
| 6 | | Hallway ambulation/restorator or cycle ergometry ×2, exercise duration (1–10 min.) MET level goal = 2.0–3.0 strengthening exercises |
| 7 | | Hallway ambulation ×2, exercise duration (1–15 min) MET level goal = 2.0–4.0 strengthening exercises; patient adequately ascends/descends two flights of stairs and showers independently Has adequate understanding of home exercise prescription. Outpatient cardiac rehabilitation appointment scheduled. Patient discharged. |

*Activity protocol is based upon risk stratification (degree of ventricular dysfunction and signs/symptoms) and upon cardiopulmonary response (heart rate no greater than 20–30 bpm above resting heart rate without hypoadaptive blood pressure response no greater than 10–20 mm Hg decrease) and without significant dysrhythmias or dyspnea.
From Cahalin LP. Heart failure. Phys Ther 76(5):516, 1996.

in resting and exercise heart rates, the Borg rating scale again is a good clinical tool. In addition, instructing patients to increase the respiratory rate to a level that allows one to converse comfortably may be an additional method for prescribing exercise training in patients with CHF ("talk test").[198]

The end result of such exercise assessments and exercise training is an improved quality of life for patients with CHF.

### Exercise Training and Quality of Life

The quality of life of persons with CHF appears to be related to the ability to exercise.[147,149,150,209,216–222] However, only two recent studies have investigated the effects of exercise training upon the quality of life of persons with CHF.[149,219] Kavanagh and associates[149] and Keteyian and associates[219] found significant improvements in exercise capacity, symptoms, and quality of life after 24 and 52 weeks of exercise training, respectively. Therefore, in view of limited data, quality of life does appear to be improved after exercise training in persons with CHF.

### Exercise Training During Continuous Intravenous Dobutamine Infusion

Many patients with severe CHF are hospitalized for prolonged periods, receiving continuous intravenous (IV) dobutamine infusion for inotropic support (to improve cardiac muscle contraction) while awaiting cardiac transplantation.[223] Also, it is becoming common practice for patients with severe CHF to be occasionally hospitalized for IV dobutamine infusion ("dobutamine holiday") to transiently improve myocardial performance.[224] Many patients are also being sent home on portable IV dobutamine pumps; their physical activity is less restricted when the large IV pumps are not used.[225] However, exercise training during continuous IV dobutamine infusion has received little attention.[226]

Individuals receiving inotropic support have only recently been prescribed exercise training programs.[227] Kataoka and associates[226] presented the results of a single case study in which a 53-year-old man with CHF was prescribed an exercise training program while receiving 10 μg/kg/min IV dobutamine (which he had been prescribed for 10 months prior to exercise training). Positive training adaptations were observed without complication and resulted in the patient being weaned from dobutamine.[227] In the ESSENTIAL trial, no adverse effects occurred when exercising patients with heart failure and enoximone, yet clinically significant differences were not reported between the treatment and the placebo groups.[228] The 6MWD was increased in the group with the inotrope support but not statistically significant, and no improvement in other clinical outcomes were reported.[228]

### Exercise Training with Ventricular Assist Devices

Particular adjuncts to exercise conditioning in CHF include mechanical support of severe CMD via IABP and left or right ventricular assist devices. Although individuals with IABP are limited to breathing exercises and gentle exercise with upper extremities and the noncatheterized leg, individuals with ventricular assist devices (VADs) have enjoyed the freedom to exercise with minimal limitation. Improved technology has enabled patients, who otherwise were immobilized because of IABP placement or nonmobile VAD placement, to become mobile and ambulate with a cart or electric belt system that provides left ventricular assistance via portable pumping of the heart.[229-231] Patients using LVADs underwent 1173.6 hours of exercise conditioning without major complication and with only 4 minor complications (3.4 incidents per 1000 patient hours). The four minor complications were quickly corrected and resulted from an acute decrease in pump flow from venous pooling, decreased driveline air volume, and hypovolemia. Improvements in exercise tolerance and functional capacity continued until week 6 of conditioning, after which further improvements were minimal. It has been suggested that delay in cardiac transplantation until 6 weeks of exercise conditioning have been performed may improve postoperative recovery and surgical success.[232]

The reason for a lack of further improvement in exercise tolerance and functional capacity after week 6 was most likely because of the mechanical constraints of the LVAD. Cardiopulmonary exercise testing has demonstrated that LVAD patients demonstrate a modest training effect from chronic exercise training and appear to be limited at maximal exercise by the mechanics of the LVAD.[233] The mechanical constraints of the LVAD appear to prevent maximal levels of exercise from being attained and result in no substantial change in peak oxygen consumption after a mean of 16 weeks of aerobic exercise training. Possible mechanical constraints of the LVAD include flow limitations (10 to 12 L/min), altered cardiovascular function from the mechanically driven cardiac output, and the effects of a 6-lb mass resting below the diaphragm that may alter ventilatory performance. Limited training adaptations may also be a result of the same mechanism, but the reductions in submaximal heart rate and blood pressure as well as increases in exercise duration, ventilation, and oxygen consumption at the ventilatory threshold support the benefits that can be attained by exercising patients on LVAD.[230,231,233]

### Exercise Training During Continuous Positive Airway Pressure Ventilation

Continuous positive airway pressure (CPAP) and bilevel positive airway pressure (BiPAP) have been observed to improve the exercise performance of patients with obstructive lung disease.[234-236] Despite the lack of research on the effect of CPAP or BiPAP upon the exercise performance of patients with CHF, resting myocardial performance has repeatedly been observed to improve with CPAP in patients with CHF[237-239] and patients with CHF and coexistent obstructive or central sleep apnea.[240-242] The beneficial effect of CPAP upon cardiac performance is postulated to be caused by increased intrathoracic pressure, which reduces cardiac preload (by impeding cardiac filling) and afterload (by reducing left ventricular transmural pressure),[237,238,242-244] as well as unloading the inspiratory muscles by providing positive pressure ventilation that may increase lung compliance.[239] The effects of CPAP or BiPAP upon exercise performance in patients with CHF are unknown, but several studies cited here have noted an improvement in dyspnea and functional status and exercise tolerance.[245]

## Ventilation

### Ventilatory Muscle Training

#### Breathing Exercises

Persons with CHF appear to benefit from breathing exercises.[246,247] Breathing exercises can be simple or complex and should be provided after a measurement of breathing strength is obtained. Such measurements include the maximal inspiratory pressure (MIP) and the maximal expiratory pressure (MEP), which are frequently measured with a manometer in centimeters of water. After strength measurements are obtained, patients are provided a breathing exercise program at a specific percentage of the MIP or MEP (similar to aerobic exercise training) with a device that resists either inspiration or expiration. The methods of measuring MIP and MEP and implementing a ventilatory muscle training program are provided.[246,247]

Facilitation of diaphragmatic breathing and inhibition of excessive accessory muscle use may decrease the work of breathing for a person with CHF and in conjunction with pursed-lip breathing may improve respiratory performance and possibly, cardiac performance. Pursed-lip breathing is beneficial for persons with COPD by maintaining airway patency via increased positive end-expiratory pressure (PEEP).[248,249] In view of recent research, the same maintenance of airways from increased PEEP may be helpful for persons with CHF.[250,251] Furthermore, the increased PEEP and associated increase in intrathoracic pressure from varying degrees of pursed-lip breathing may decrease venous return which could possibly decrease the left VEDV and pressure and improve myocardial performance for persons with severe CHF.[252]

*Expiratory Muscle Training*

The majority of studies investigating the effects of expiratory muscle training have involved persons with spinal cord injury or other neurologic disorders. In the majority of these studies, expiratory muscle training (performed in a variety of ways but most commonly with weights on the abdomen and hyperpneic breathing) improved symptoms, functional status, and pulmonary function, and reduced pulmonary complications. There is a recent interest in expiratory muscle training of persons with various forms of COPD using PEEP devices, but very little literature exists. Likewise, there is little literature regarding expiratory muscle training alone in CHF. A study by Mancini and associates evaluated the effects of inspiratory and expiratory muscle training in CHF and found significant improvements in ventilatory muscle force and endurance, submaximal and maximal exercise performance, and dyspnea after 3 months of aggressive ventilatory muscle training in eight patients with chronic CHF.[247]

Despite a lack of research in expiratory muscle training alone in CHF, the observations of Mancini and associates[247] and others suggest that expiratory muscle training may be beneficial for persons with CHF by (1) increasing expiratory muscle strength to improve pulmonary function, (2) increasing PEEP to improve airway compliance, and (3) possibly decreasing venous return and the left VEDV to improve myocardial performance.[252] These changes may improve the exercise tolerance and functional status of persons with CHF. However, further investigation is needed in this area.

*Inspiratory Muscle Training*

Inspiratory muscle training has previously been shown to be helpful for patients with pulmonary disease by increasing ventilatory muscle strength and endurance and by decreasing dyspnea, need for medications, emergency room visits, and number of hospitalizations.[253,254] Individuals with chronic CHF have been found to have poor ventilatory muscle strength,[255–257] yet following inspiratory muscle training demonstrated significant improvements in ventilatory muscle strength and endurance as well as dyspnea.[247,258]

Significant improvements in maximal inspiratory and expiratory pressures and degree of dyspnea were recently observed as soon as 2 weeks after ventilatory muscle training was initiated with the Threshold inspiratory muscle trainer at 20% of MIP, three times a day, for 5 to 15 minutes (Fig. 4-20).[246] The improvement in ventilatory muscle strength was associated with significantly less dyspnea at rest and with exercise. However, the effects of ventilatory muscle training upon ventilatory muscle endurance, which may be the most important effect of ventilatory muscle training in this patient population, were not evaluated. Nonetheless, improvement in ventilatory muscle strength may decrease the dependency, impairment, and possibly even cost associated with chronic CHF. Increased ventilatory muscle strength may also enhance early postoperative recovery in patients undergoing cardiac transplantation or other cardiac surgery.

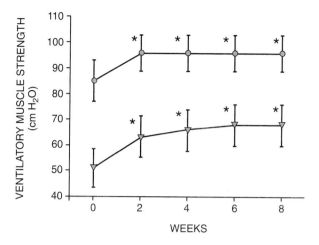

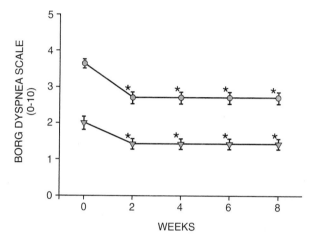

**Figure 4-20** **Top,** Maximal inspiratory pressure (*triangle*) and maximal expiratory pressure (*circle*) throughout the ventilatory muscle training period. **Bottom,** Dyspnea at rest (*triangle*) and during submaximal exercise (*circle*) throughout the ventilatory muscle training period. Asterisks (*) indicate values that are different from baseline values ($p < 0.05$). (From Cahalin LP, Semigran MJ, Dec G. Inspiratory muscle training in patients with chronic heart failure awaiting cardiac transplantation: Results of a pilot clinical trial. Phys Ther 77(8):830–8, 1997.)

## Instruction in Energy Conservation

Energy conservation techniques should be included in the interventions for individuals with heart failure to decrease the workload on the heart without loss of function. An analysis of all the activities an individual performs helps to develop an inventory to set priorities and organize the individual's day. Particular attention should be paid to activities that create fatigue or increased dyspnea. Box 4-8 provides suggestions for conserving energy for patients with heart failure.

## Self-Management Techniques

Chronic disease management programs should identify the patients who are at high risk for morbidity and mortality and incorporate the individual into the management of the disease by making them responsible for their own health. Disease management programs for heart failure should include

## Box 4-8

### Energy Conservation Techniques for Individuals with Heart Failure

- Sit while working whenever possible.
- Before you get tired stop and rest.
- Spread tedious tasks out throughout the week.
- Do the tasks that require the most energy at times that you have the most energy.
- Alternate easy tasks with difficult tasks, and plan a rest period.
- Devote a portion of your day to an activity you enjoy and find relaxing.
- Keep items within easy reach.
- Plan ahead so you don't have to rush or push yourself hard.
- Decide activities that are not necessary for you to do, and delegate to other family members or caregivers/share the work.

components that not only improve the management of the disease, but which also demonstrate improved outcomes and reduction of costs. These components include[259]:

- Individualized, comprehensive patient and family or caregiver education and outpatient counseling
- Optimization of medical therapy
- Vigilant followup
- Increased access to healthcare professionals
- Early attention to fluid overload
- Coordination with other agencies as appropriate
- Physician-directed care (and/or use of nurse coordinators or nurse-managed care)
- Specific content for patient and family education and counseling should include:
  - Discussion of limitation of dietary sodium to 2 to 3 g/day
  - Adherence to medication regimen
  - Regular flu and pneumococcal immunizations
  - Importance of daily weighing and monitoring of symptoms (shortness of breath, dizziness, or swelling)
  - Instruction in signs/symptoms of decompensation (excessive shortness of breath, fatigue, peripheral swelling, waking at night with dyspnea or cough, etc.)
  - Instruction in importance of seeking assistance when necessary
  - Adherence to regular exercise program
  - Limitation of alcohol intake
  - Control of comorbid conditions (diabetes, elevated blood pressure, elevated lipids)

The above educational content is much better received and remembered if given when the patient is in an outpatient versus an inpatient setting. Inpatient education is usually inadequate as well, as individuals do not retain what they are taught in the hospital. Individuals who are in the hospital are usually ill, anxious, distracted, or in poor condition to listen, learn, and retain any instructions. Instruction in

self-management techniques after a critical event resulting in hospitalization results in improved adherence, if the patient is ready and able to learn, and in improved management of the disease.

## Summary

- Causes of CMD include:
  - myocardial infarction or ischemia,
  - cardiomyopathy,
  - cardiac arrhythmias,
  - heart valve abnormalities,
  - pericardial effusion or myocarditis,
  - pulmonary embolus,
  - pulmonary hypertension,
  - renal insufficiency,
  - spinal cord injury,
  - congenital abnormalities, and
  - aging.
- The term *cardiac muscle dysfunction* accurately describes the primary cause of pulmonary edema as well as the underlying pathophysiology, which essentially impairs the heart's ability to pump blood or the left ventricle's ability to accept blood.
- Cardiomyopathy, congenital abnormalities, renal insufficiency, and aging are associated more commonly with chronic heart failure, whereas the other factors tend to cause acute CHF.
- Right-sided or left-sided CHF simply describes which side of the heart is failing, as well as the side initially affected and behind which fluid tends to localize.
- Low-output CHF is the description associated with heart failure and is the result of a low cardiac output at rest or during exertion. High-output CHF usually results from a volume overload.
- The impaired contraction of the ventricles during systole that produces an inefficient expulsion of blood is termed systolic heart failure. Diastolic heart failure is associated with an inability of the ventricles to accept the blood ejected from the atria.
- Hypertension and coronary artery disease are the most common causes of CMD.
- Cardiac arrhythmias and renal insufficiency can also cause CMD for reasons similar to those of myocardial infarction.
- Cardiomyopathies are classified from a functional standpoint, emphasizing three categories: dilated, hypertrophic, and restrictive.
- Heart valve abnormalities can also cause CMD as blocked or incompetent valves, or both, cause heart muscle to contract more forcefully to expel the cardiac output.
- Injury to the pericardium can cause acute pericarditis, which may progress to pericardial effusion.
- CMD from a pulmonary embolus is the result of elevated pulmonary artery pressures, which dramatically increase right ventricular work.

- Spinal cord injury can also produce CMD because of cervical spinal cord transection, which causes an imbalance between sympathetic and parasympathetic control of the cardiovascular system.
- CHF is commonly associated with several characteristic signs and symptoms, including dyspnea, tachypnea, PND, orthopnea, hepatomegaly, peripheral edema, weight gain, jugular venous distension, rales, tubular breath sound and consolidation, presence of an $S_3$ heart sound, sinus tachycardia, and decreased exercise tolerance.
- Proteinuria; elevated urine specific gravity, BNP, BUN, and creatinine levels; and decreased erythrocyte sedimentation rates are associated with CHF.
- Dyspnea is probably the most common finding associated with CHF.
- A rapid respiratory rate at rest, characterized by quick and shallow breaths, is common in patients with CHF.
- The presence of an $S_3$ heart sound indicates a noncompliant left ventricle and occurs as blood passively fills a poorly relaxing left ventricle.
- The retention of sodium and water is caused by (1) augmented $\alpha$-adrenergic neural activity; (2) circulating catecholamines; and (3) increased levels of circulating and locally produced angiotensin II, resulting in renal vasoconstriction.
- Laboratory findings suggestive of impaired renal function in CHF include increases of BUN as well as blood creatinine levels and BNP.
- Pulmonary edema can be cardiogenic or noncardiogenic in origin.
- The most common hematologic abnormality is a secondary polycythemia, which is caused by either a reduction in oxygen transport or an increase in erythropoietin production.
- Skeletal muscle abnormalities caused by dilated and hypertrophic cardiomyopathies have been reported previously and consistently reveal type I and type II fiber atrophy.
- Severe CMD has the potential to reduce blood flow to the pancreas, which impairs insulin secretion and glucose tolerance.
- The primary malnutrition in CHF is a protein-calorie deficiency, but vitamin deficiencies have also been observed.
- The specific treatments for CHF include restriction of sodium intake, use of medications, and self-management techniques.
- Many patients with CHF apparently have lower anaerobic thresholds, and the resultant anaerobic metabolism (because of acidosis) becomes the limiting factor in exercise performance.
- Although echocardiography is the most widely used method for the confirmation of the clinical diagnosis of heart failure, BNP is rapidly emerging as a very sensitive and specific adjunctive diagnostic marker.[65] It may also be an important prognostic marker, and can be used as a rapid screening test in the urgent care setting.[64,65] Greater levels of ANP and BNP have also been found to be associated with higher morbidity and mortality rates.
- Plasma BNP, although consistently increased in patients with heart failure because of systolic dysfunction, is also increased in some patients with aortic stenosis, chronic mitral regurgitation, diastolic heart failure, and hypertrophic cardiomyopathy.
- The most significant predictors of survival in individuals with CHF have been identified and include decreasing LVEF; worsening NYHA functional status; degree of hyponatremia; decreasing peak exercise oxygen uptake; decreasing hematocrit; widened QRS on 12-lead electrocardiogram; chronic hypotension; resting tachycardia; renal insufficiency; intolerance to conventional therapy; and refractory volume overload.

## CASE STUDY 4-1

This 85-year-old woman had a medical history of coronary artery bypass graft surgery in 1992 to the right coronary artery and left anterior diagonal artery, cholecystectomy, hiatal hernia, gastritis, and peptic ulcer disease. She was admitted August 9, 2010 with angina (a myocardial infarction was ruled out) and underwent cardiac catheterization on August 16, 2010, which revealed 99% occlusion of the right coronary artery graft, 85% occlusion of the left anterior diagonal artery graft, 95% stenosis of the circumflex artery, moderate mitral regurgitation, dilated left atrium, inferior hypokinesis, and an EF of approximately 30%. Echocardiographic study revealed severe left ventricular hypertrophy with a small left ventricular chamber size, inferior hypokinesis, calcified mitral valve with moderate mitral regurgitation, abnormal left ventricular compliance (left ventricular stiffness), and a dilated left atrium.

The referral for cardiac rehabilitation was written on August 11, 2010, at which time the patient was assessed and complained of left scapular pain that increased with deep breathing (different from previous angina and altered with breathing pattern). Physical examination revealed normal sinus rhythm and slightly decreased breath sounds in the left lower lobe. The patient ambulated approximately 250 feet with an adaptive heart rate and blood pressure response, without angina. The patient continued with twice-daily cardiac rehabilitation, increasing the distance ambulated to 800 feet, and underwent a thallium treadmill stress test on August 13, 2010. The patient completed 2 minutes 25 seconds of the modified Bruce protocol (attaining a maximal heart rate of 104 bpm, 67% of the age-predicted maximal heart rate), which was terminated because of leg fatigue. The patient experienced no angina and demonstrated no electrocardiographic (ECG) changes consistent with myocardial ischemia. The thallium scan demonstrated moderately severe stress-induced ischemic change in the inferior and septal areas.

*Continued*

## CASE STUDY 4-1—cont'd

Cardiac rehabilitation was performed August 14, 2010 through August 16, 2010, during which the patient walked 5 to 10 minutes (500 to 1000 feet) with adaptive heart rate and blood pressure responses to exercise, without angina. On August 17, 2010, while resting in bed, the patient developed severe angina and dyspnea, which required morphine sulfate, nitroglycerin, and heparin, suggesting impending graft occlusion. In view of these findings, coronary artery bypass graft surgery was repeated on August 20, 2010, after which the patient developed numerous complications, requiring intraaortic balloon pump assistance from which weaning was difficult. In addition, the patient experienced a postoperative anterolateral myocardial infarction as a result of a third-degree heart block that decreased the blood supply to the myocardium, respiratory failure that required full ventilatory support, congestive heart failure, and severe abdominal distension.

The patient's status further deteriorated as she became anemic and was unable to maintain adequate nutritional requirements. However, a radiograph on August 24, 2010 revealed no evidence of CHF, and ventilatory measurements demonstrated improved pulmonary function. In addition, hemoglobin and hematocrit levels were slightly increased (10.7 and 29.4, respectively). The patient was extubated on August 25, 2010 and began ambulation with nursing on August 26, 2010, during which she complained of severe abdominal pain and a feeling of increased abdominal swelling. Because of persistent abdominal pain and distension, an exploratory laparotomy was performed on August 28, 2010, resulting in resection of the small bowel.

The patient remained on bedrest for 3 days, after which she began ambulating with nursing. On September 4, 2010, the patient ambulated 50 feet with physical therapy, during which she complained of severe dyspnea and mild to moderate abdominal discomfort. For this reason, physical therapy discontinued ambulation but continued chest physical therapy and bedside exercise to the upper and lower extremities. However, nursing continued to ambulate the patient approximately four times per day despite her complaints of severe shortness of breath and abdominal discomfort. On September 6, 2010, immediately after walking, she developed severe abdominal discomfort associated with nausea and vomiting. Nonetheless, that evening, the patient was ambulated 200 feet, walking approximately 15 minutes, at which time she complained of severe abdominal pain; her respiratory rate was noted to be in the high 50s. On September 7, 2010, the patient was again walked approximately 75 feet with a walker and maximal assist of three, at which time she became unresponsive. Physician examination at this time revealed severe tachypnea and abdominal distension. On September 10, 2010, the patient's status further deteriorated with effusion and atelectasis of the left lung base, ischemic bowel, possible abdominal infection, anemia, and azotemia. She expired on September 11, 2010.

### Discussion

This case study is an example of an 85-year-old patient who underwent bypass surgery after the following occurred:

1. She remained asymptomatic during prolonged cardiac rehabilitation exercise assessments with adaptive heart rate and blood pressure responses, but somewhat paradoxically developed angina at rest.
2. A thallium treadmill stress test demonstrated moderately severe ischemic change.
3. A cardiac catheterization revealed occluded grafts to the right coronary artery and left anterior diagonal artery and high-grade occlusion of the circumflex artery, inferior hypokinesis, and depressed EF (approximately 30%).

Unfortunately, after bypass surgery was performed, the patient developed numerous complications caused primarily by pump failure and improper exercise training that was not appropriately adjusted to the patient's needs. At no time should a patient be ambulated with moderate to severe pain (whatever the location or cause), as it most likely represents a pathologic process (in this case, ischemia of the small intestine). In addition, inappropriate responses to exercise training, such as a rapid heart rate or respiratory rate with minimal exercise, must be reassessed and treated before subsequent exercise is performed, or at least changes must be made in the type of exercise performed. Sitting lower-extremity exercise would have been much more appropriate for this patient, who demonstrated many interrelated pathophysiologic processes that were exacerbated by improper exercise training and ultimately led to her death.

### References

1. The European "Corwin" Study Group. Xamoterol in mild to moderate heart failure: A subgroup analysis of patients with cardiomegaly but no concomitant angina pectoris. J Clin Pharmacol Suppl 1:67S–9S, 1989.
2. Kannel WB. Epidemiological aspects of heart failure. Cardiol Clin 7(1):1–9, 1989.
3. Kannel WB, Belanger AJ. Epidemiology of heart failure. Am Heart J 121(3 Pt 1):951–7, 1991.
4. Lloyd-Jones D, Adams R, Carnethon M, et al. Heart Disease and Stroke Statistics 2009 Update: A report from the American Heart Association Statistics Committee and Stroke Statistics Subcommittee. Circulation 108;119:e21–181, 2008.
5. Braunwald E. Clinical manifestations of heart failure. In Braunwald E (ed.). Heart Disease: A Textbook of Cardiovascular Medicine. Philadelphia, 1988, Saunders.
6. Cheng TO. Cardiac failure in coronary heart disease. Am Heart J 120(2):396–412, 1990.
7. Hildner FJ. Pulmonary edema associated with low, left ventricular filling pressures. Am J Cardiol 44(7):1410–11, 1979.
8. Auchincloss JH, Gilbert R, Morales R, et al. Reduction of trial and error in the equilibrium rebreathing cardiac output method. J Cardiopulm Rehab 9(2):85, 1989.
9. Braunwald E, Sonnenblick EH, Ross Jr J. Mechanisms of cardiac contraction and relaxation. In Braunwald E (ed.). Heart Disease: A Textbook of Cardiovascular Medicine. Philadelphia, 1988, Saunders.

10. Wynne J, Braunwald E. The cardiomyopathies and myocarditides. In Braunwald E (ed.). Heart Disease: A Textbook of Cardiovascular Medicine. Philadelphia, 1988, Saunders.

11. Perloff JK. Pathogenesis of hypertrophic cardiomyopathy: Hypothesis and speculation. Am Heart 101:219, 1981.

12. Braunwald E. Pathophysiology of heart failure. In Braunwald E (ed.). Heart Disease: A Textbook of Cardiovascular Medicine. Philadelphia, 1988, Saunders.

13. Goldberger JJ, Peled HB, Stroh JA, et al. Prognostic factors in acute pulmonary edema. Arch Intern Med 146(3):489–93, 1986.

14. Baigrie RS, Haq A, Morgan CD, et al. The spectrum of right ventricular involvement in inferior wall myocardial infarction. J Am Coll Cardiol 1(6):1396–404, 1983.

15. Cintron GB, Hernandez E, Linares E, et al. Bedside recognition, incidence and clinical course of right ventricular infarction. Am J Cardiol 47(2):224–7, 1981.

16. Klein LW, Kramer BL, Howard E, et al. Incidence and clinical significance of transient creatinine kinase elevations and the diagnosis of non-Q wave myocardial infarction associated with coronary angioplasty. J Am Coll Cardiol 17(3):621–6, 1991.

17. Fischell TA, Derby G, Tse TM, et al. Coronary artery vasoconstriction routinely occurs after percutaneous transluminal coronary angioplasty. A quantitative arteriographic analysis. Circulation 78:1323, 1988.

18. Kirklin JW, Blackstone EH, Kirklin JK. Cardiac surgery. In Braunwald E (ed.). Heart Disease: A Textbook of Cardiovascular Medicine. Philadelphia, 1988, Saunders.

19. Breisblatt WM, Stein KL, Wolfe CJ, et al. Acute myocardial dysfunction and recovery: A common occurrence after coronary bypass surgery. J Am Coll Cardiol 15(6):1261–9, 1990.

20. Zipes DP, Camm AJ, Borggrefe M, et al. ACC/AHA/ESC 2006 guidelines for management of patients with ventricular arrhythmias and the prevention of sudden cardiac death-executive summary: A report of the American College of Cardiology/American Heart Association Task Force and the European Society of Cardiology Committee for Practice Guidelines. Circulation 114(10):1088–132, 2006.

21. Cruz FES, Cheriex EC, Smeets JL, et al. Reversibility of tachycardia-induced cardiomyopathy after cure of incessant supraventricular tachycardia. J Am Coll Cardiol 16(3):739–44, 1990.

22. Epstein AE, DiMarco JP, Ellenbogen KA, et al. ACC/AHA/HRS 2008 guidelines for device-based therapy of cardiac rhythm abnormalities: executive summary. Circulation 117(21):2820–40, 2008.

23. Jessup M, Abraham WT, Casey DE, et al. 2009 Focused update: ACCF/AHA guidelines for the diagnosis and management of heart failure in adults: a report of the American College of Cardiology Foundation/American Heart Association Task Force on practice management of heart failure in adults. Circulation 119(14):1977–2016, 2009.

24. Pastan SO, Braunwald E. Renal disorders and heart disease. In Braunwald E (ed.). Heart Disease: A Textbook of Cardiovascular Medicine. Philadelphia, 1988, Saunders.

25. Pitt B, Williams G, Remme W, et al. The EPHESUS trial: Eplerenone in patients with heart failure due to systolic dysfunction complicating acute myocardial infarction. Eplerenone Post-AMI Heart Failure Efficacy and Survival Study. Cardiovasc Drugs Ther 15(1):79–87, 2001.

26. Abelmann WH. Classification and natural history of primary myocardial disease. Prog Cardiovasc Dis 27(2):73–94, 1984.

27. Maron BJ, Fananapazir L. Sudden cardiac death in hypertrophic cardiomyopathy. Circulation 85(1 Suppl):I57–63, 1992.

28. Silverman KJ, Hutchins GM, Weiss JL, et al. Catenoidal shape of the interventricular septum in idiopathic hypertrophic subaortic stenosis: Two-dimensional echocardiographic confirmation. Am J Cardiol 49(1):27–32, 1982.

29. Braunwald E. Valvular heart disease. In Braunwald E (ed.). Heart Disease: A Textbook of Cardiovascular Medicine. Philadelphia, 1988, Saunders.

30. Goldhaber SZ, Braunwald E. Pulmonary embolism. In Braunwald E (ed.). Heart Disease: A Textbook of Cardiovascular Medicine. Philadelphia, 1988, Saunders.

31. Geerts WH, Bergqvist D, Pineo GF, et al. Prevention of venous thromboembolism: American College of Chest Physicians evidence-based clinical practice guidelines (8th edition). Chest 133(6 Suppl):381S–453S, 2008.

32. MacKenzie CF, Shin B, Krishnaprasad D, et al. Assessment of cardiac and respiratory function during surgery on patients with acute quadriplegia. J Neurosurg 62(6):843–9, 1985.

33. Woolman L. The disturbance of circulation in traumatic paraplegia in acute and late stages. A pathological study. Paraplegia 2:213–26, 1965.

34. Meyer GA, Berman IR, Doty DB, et al. Hemodynamic responses to acute quadriplegia with or without chest trauma. J Neurosurg 34(2 Pt 1):168–77, 1971.

35. Bellamy R, Pitts FW, Stauffer ES. Respiratory complications in traumatic quadriplegia. Analysis of 20 years' experience. J Neurosurg 39(5):596–600, 1973.

36. Friedman WF. Congenital heart disease in infancy and childhood. In Braunwald E (ed.). Heart Disease: A Textbook of Cardiovascular Medicine. Philadelphia, 1988, Saunders.

37. Borow KM, Braunwald E. Congenital heart disease in the adult. In Braunwald E (ed.). Heart Disease: A Textbook of Cardiovascular Medicine. Philadelphia, 1988, Saunders.

38. Moser M. Physiological differences in the elderly. Are they clinically important? Eur Heart J 9(Suppl D):55–61, 1988.

39. Weisfeldt ML, Lakatta KG, Gerstenblith G. Aging and cardiac disease. In Braunwald E (ed.). Heart Disease: A Textbook of Cardiovascular Medicine. Philadelphia, 1988, Saunders.

40. Tanner K, Sabrine N, Wren C. Cardiovascular malformations among preterm infants. Pediatrics 116(6):e833–8, 2005.

41. Brandfonbrener M, Landowne M, Shock NW. Changes in cardiac output with age. Circulation 12(4):557–66, 1955.

42. Strandell T. Circulatory studies on healthy old men. With special reference to the limitation of the maximal physical working capacity. Acta Med Scand 175:1, 1964.

43. Conway I, Wheeler R, Sannerstedt R. Sympathetic nervous activity during exercise in relation to age. Cardiovasc Res 5(4):577–81, 1971.

44. Rodeheffer RJ, Gerstenblith G, Becker LC, et al. Exercise cardiac output is maintained with advancing age in healthy human subjects: Cardiac dilatation and increased stroke volume compensate for a diminished heart rate. Circulation 69(2):203–13, 1984.

45. Sjögren AL. Left ventricular wall thickness determined by ultrasound in 100 subjects without heart disease. Chest 60(4):341–6, 1971.

46. Gerstenblith G, Fleg JL, Becker LC, et al. Maximum left ventricular filling rate in healthy individuals measured by gated blood pool scans: Effect of age. Circulation 68:91–101, 1983.

47. Capasso JM, Malhotra A, Remily R, et al. Effects of age on mechanical and electrical performance of rat myocardium. Am J Physiol 245(1):H72–81, 1983.

48. Lakatta KG, Yin FCP. Myocardial aging: Functional alterations and related cellular mechanisms. Am J Physiol 242(6):H927–41, 1982.

49. Bhatnagar GM, Walford GD, Beard ES, et al. ATPase activity and force production in myofibrils and twitch characteristics in intact muscle from neonatal, adult, and senescent rat myocardium. J Mol Cell Cardiol 16(3):203–18, 1984.

50. Wei JY, Spurgeon HA, Lakatta KG. Excitation-contraction in rat myocardium: Alterations with adult aging. Am J Physiol 246(6 Pt 2):H784–91, 1984.

51. Spurgeon HA, Steinbach MF, Lakatta KG. Chronic exercise prevents characteristic age-related changes in rat cardiac contraction. Am J Physiol 244(4):H513–18, 1983.

52. Spurgeon HA, Thorne PR, Yin FCP, et al. Increased dynamic stiffness of trabeculae carneae from senescent rats. Am J Physiol 232(4):H373–80, 1977.

53. Yin FCP, Spurgeon HA, Weisfeldt ML, et al. Mechanical properties of myocardium from hypertrophied rat hearts. A comparison between hypertrophy induced by senescence and by aortic banding. Circ Res 46(2):292–300, 1980.

54. Orchard CH, Lakatta KG. Intracellular calcium transients and developed tensions in rat heart muscle. A mechanism for the negative interval-strength relationship. J Gen Physiol 86(5):637–51, 1985.

55. Grossman W, Braunwald E. High-cardiac output states. In Braunwald E (ed.). Heart Disease: A Textbook of Cardiovascular Medicine. Philadelphia, 1988, Saunders.

56. Perloff JK. Pregnancy and cardiovascular disease. In Braunwald E (ed.). Heart Disease: A Textbook of Cardiovascular Medicine. Philadelphia, 1988, Saunders.

57. Braunwald E. Assessment of cardiac function. In Braunwald E (ed.). Heart Disease: A Textbook of Cardiovascular Medicine. Philadelphia, 1988, Saunders.

58. Parmley WW. Hemodynamic monitoring in acute ischemic disease. In Fishman AP (ed.). Heart Failure. New York, 1978, McGraw-Hill.

59. Andreoli KG, Fowkes VH, Zipes DP, et al. Comprehensive Cardiac Care, ed 4. St. Louis, 1979, Mosby.

60. D'Souza SP, Davis M, Baxter GF. Autocrine and paracrine actions of natriuretic peptides in the heart. Pharmacol Ther 101(2):113–29, 2004.

61. Collins E, Bracamonte MP, Burnett Jr JC, et al: Mechanism of relaxations to dendroaspis natriuretic peptide in canine coronary arteries. J Cardiovasc Pharmacol 35(4):614–18, 2000.

62. Best PJ, Burnett JC, Wilson SH, et al: Dendroaspis natriuretic peptide relaxes isolated human arteries and veins. Cardiovasc Res 55(2):375–84, 2002.

63. Richards AM, Lainchbury JG, Nicholls MG, et al: Dendroaspis natriuretic peptide: Endogenous or dubious? Lancet 359(9300):5–6, 2002.

64. Creager MA, Dzau V, Loscalzo J. Vascular Medicine. A Companion to Braunwald's Heart Disease Philadelphia, 2006, Saunders.

65. Maisel A. B-type natriuretic peptide levels: A potential novel "white count" for congestive heart failure. J Card Fail 7(2):183–93, 2001.

66. Wallén T, Landahl S, Hedner T, et al. Atrial natriuretic peptides predict mortality in the elderly. J Intern Med 241(4):269–75, 1997.

67. Iivanainen AM, Tikkanen I, Tilvis R, et al. Associations between atrial natriuretic peptides, echocardiographic findings and mortality in an elderly population sample. J Intern Med 241(4):261–8, 1997.

68. Skorecki KL, Brenner BM. Body fluid homeostasis in congestive heart failure and cirrhosis with ascites. Am J Med 72(2):323–38, 1982.

69. Hostetter TH, Pfeffer JM, Pfeffer MA, et al. Cardiorenal hemodynamics and sodium excretion in rats with myocardial infarction. Am J Physiol 245(1):H98–103, 1983.

70. Ingram RH Jr, Braunwald E. Pulmonary edema: Cardiogenic and noncardiogenic. In Braunwald E (ed.). Heart Disease: A Textbook of Cardiovascular Medicine. Philadelphia, 1988, Saunders.

71. Fillmore SJ, Giumaraes AC, Scheidt AC, et al. Blood gas changes and pulmonary hemodynamics following acute myocardial infarction. Circulation 45(3):583–91, 1972.

72. Light RW, George RB. Serial pulmonary function in patients with acute heart failure. Arch Intern Med 143(3):429–33, 1983.

73. Wright RS, Levine S, Bellamy PE, et al. Ventilatory and diffusion abnormalities in potential heart transplant recipients. Chest 98(4):816–20, 1990.

74. Feldman AM, Bristow MR. The beta-adrenergic pathway in the failing human heart: Implications for inotropic therapy. Cardiology 77(Suppl 1):1–32, 1990.

75. Lefkowitz RJ, Caron MG. Adrenergic receptors: Models for the study of receptors coupled to guanine nucleotide regulatory proteins. J Biol Chem 263(11):4993–6, 1988.

76. Exton JH. Molecular mechanisms involved in alpha-adrenergic responses. Mol Cell Endocrinol 23(3):233–64, 1981.

77. Scholz A, Schaefer B, Schmitz W, et al. Alpha-1 adrenoceptor-mediated positive inotropic effect and inositol trisphosphate increase in mammalian heart. J Pharmacol Exp Ther 245(1):327–35, 1988.

78. Gilman AG. G proteins: Transducers of receptor-generated signals. Annu Rev Biochem 56:615–49, 1987.

79. Bristow MR. The beta-adrenergic receptor. Configuration, regulation, mechanism of action. Postgrad Med 29;Spec No:19–26, 1988.

80. Bristow MR, Minobe W, Rasmussen R, et al. Alpha-1 adrenergic receptors in the nonfailing and failing human heart. J Pharmacol Exp Ther 247(3):1039–45, 1989.

81. Feldman MA, Copelas L, Gwathney JK, et al. Deficient production of cyclic AMP. Pharmacologic evidence of an important cause of contractile dysfunction in patients with end-stage heart failure. Circulation 75(2):331–9, 1987.

82. Bristow MR, Ginsburg R, Umans V, et al. Beta1-and beta2-adrenergic-receptor subpopulations in nonfailing and failing human ventricular myocardium: Coupling of both receptor subtypes to muscle contraction and selective beta 1-receptor down-regulation in heart failure. Circ Res 59(3):297–309, 1986.

83. Fowler MB, Laser JA, Hopkins GL, et al. Assessment of the beta-adrenergic receptor pathway in the intact failing human heart: Progressive receptor down-regulation and subsensitivity to agonist response. Circulation 74(6):1290–302, 1986.

84. Bristow MR, Hershberger RE, Port D, et al. Beta 1- and beta 2-adrenergic receptor-mediated adenylate cyclase stimulation

in nonfailing and failing human ventricular myocardium. Mol Pharmacol 35(3):295–303, 1989.

85. Cardellach F, Galofre J, Cusso R, et al. Decline in skeletal muscle mitochondrial respiration chain function with aging [letter]. Lancet 334(8653):44–5, 1989.

86. Rosenthal DS, Braunwald E. Hematological-oncological disorders and heart disease. In Braunwald E (ed.). Heart Disease: A Textbook of Cardiovascular Medicine. Philadelphia, 1988, Saunders.

87. Jandl JH. Blood: Textbook of Hematology. Boston, 1987, Little, Brown.

88. Shafiq SA, Sande MA, Carruthers RR, et al. Skeletal muscle in idiopathic cardiomyopathy. J Neurol Sci 15(3):303–20, 1972.

89. Poole-Wilson PA. The origin of symptoms in patients with chronic heart failure. Eur Heart J 9(Suppl H):49–53, 1988.

90. Lipkin DP, Jones DA, Round JM, et al. Abnormalities of skeletal muscle in patients with chronic heart failure. Int J Cardiol 18(2):187–95, 1988.

91. Wilson JR, Fink L, Maris J, et al. Evaluation of energy metabolism in skeletal muscle of patients with heart failure with gated phosphorus-31 nuclear magnetic resonance. Circulation 71(1):57–62, 1985.

92. Isaacs H, Muncke G. Idiopathic cardiomyopathy and skeletal muscle abnormality. Am Heart J 90(6):767–73, 1975.

93. Dunnigan A, Pierpont ME, Smith SA, et al. Cardiac and skeletal myopathy associated with cardiac dysrhythmias. Am J Cardiol 53(6):731–7, 1984.

94. Dunnigan A, Staley NA, Smith SA, et al. Cardiac and skeletal muscle abnormalities in cardiomyopathy: Comparison of patients with ventricular tachycardia or congestive heart failure. J Am Coll Cardiol 10:608–18, 1987.

95. Smith ER, Heffernan LP, Sangalang VE, et al. Voluntary muscle involvement in hypertrophic cardiomyopathy: A study of 11 patients. Ann Intern Med 85(5):566–72, 1976.

96. Hootsmans WJM, Meerschwam IS. Electromyography in patients with hypertrophic obstructive cardiomyopathy. Neurology 21(8):810–16, 1971.

97. Meerschwam IS, Hootsmans WJM. An electromyographic study in hypertrophic obstructive cardiomyopathy. In Wolstenholme GEW, O'Connor M, London J, Churchill A (eds.). Hypertrophic Obstructive Cardiomyopathy. Ciba Foundation Study Group No. 37. New York, 1971, Wiley.

98. Przybosewki JZ, Hoffman HD, Graff AS, et al. A study of family with inherited disease of cardiac and skeletal muscle. Part 1: Clinical electrocardiographic, echocardiographic, hemodynamic, electrophysiological and electron microscopic studies. S Afr Med J 59(11):363–73, 1981.

99. Lochner A, Hewlett RH, O'Kennedy A, et al. A study of a family with inherited disease of cardiac and skeletal muscle. Part 2: Skeletal muscle morphology and mitochondrial oxidative phosphorylation. S Afr Med J 59(13):453–61, 1981.

100. Poole-Wilson PA, Buller NP, Lipkin DP. Regional blood flow, muscle strength and skeletal muscle histology in severe congestive heart failure. Am J Cardiol 62(8):49E–52E, 1988.

101. Massie B, Conway M, Yonge R, et al. Skeletal muscle metabolism in patients with congestive heart failure: Relation to clinical severity and blood flow. Circulation 76(5):1009–19, 1987.

102. Massie B, Conway M, Yonge R, et al. 31P nuclear magnetic resonance evidence of abnormal skeletal muscle metabolism

in patients with congestive heart failure. Am J Cardiol 60(4):309–15, 1987.

103. Braunwald E, Sobel BE. Coronary blood flow and myocardial ischemia. In Braunwald E (ed.). Heart Disease: A Textbook of Cardiovascular Medicine. Philadelphia, 1988, Saunders.

104. Neely JR, Rovetto MJ, Whitmer JT, et al. Effects of ischemia on ventricular function and metabolism in the isolated working rat heart. Am J Physiol 225(3):651–8, 1973.

105. Williams GH, Braunwald E. Endocrine and nutritional disorders and heart disease. In Braunwald E (ed.). Heart Disease: A Textbook of Cardiovascular Medicine. Philadelphia, 1988, Saunders.

106. Yui Y, Fujiwara H, Mitsui H, et al. Furosemide-induced thiamine deficiency. Jpn Circ J 14(9):537–40, 1978.

107. Bautista J, Rafel E, Marunez A, et al. Familial hypertrophic cardiomyopathy and muscle carnitine deficiency. Muscle Nerve 13(3):192–4, 1990.

108. Folkers K. Heart failure is a dominant deficiency of coenzyme Q10 and challenges for future clinical research on CoQ10. Clin Investig 71(8 Suppl):S51–4, 1993.

109. Lampertico M, Comis S. Italian multicenter study on the efficacy and safety of coenzyme Q10 as adjuvant therapy in heart failure. Clin Investig 71(8 Suppl):S129–33, 1993.

110. Morisco C, Trimarco B, Condorelli M. Effect of coenzyme Q10 therapy in patients with congestive heart failure: A long-term multicenter randomized study. Clin Investig 71(8 Suppl):S134–6, 1993.

111. Jameson S. Statistical data support prediction of death within 6 months on low levels of coenzyme Q10 and other entities. Clin Investig 71(8 Suppl):S137–9, 1993.

112. Langsjoen PH, Folkers K. Isolated diastolic dysfunction of the myocardium and its response to CoQ10 treatment. Clin Investig 71(8 Suppl):S140–4, 1993.

113. Eschbach JW, Adamson JW. Anemia of end-stage renal disease (ESRD). Kidney Int 28(1):1–5, 1985.

114. Eschbach JW, Egrie JC, Downing MR, et al. Correction of the anemia of end-stage renal disease with recombinant human erythropoietin: Results of a combined phase I and II clinical trial. N Engl J Med 316(2):73–8, 1987.

115. Wilson L, Felsenfeld A, Drezner MK, et al. Altered divalent ion metabolism in early renal failure: Role of 1,25(OH)2D. Kidney Int 27(3):565–73, 1985.

116. Madsen S, Olgaard K, Ladefoged J. Suppressive effect of 1,25-dihydroxyvitamin D3 on circulating parathyroid hormone in acute renal failure. J Clin Endocrinol Metab 53(4):823–7, 1981.

117. Klahr S. Nonexcretory functions of the kidney. In Klahr S (ed.). The Kidney and Body Fluids in Health and Disease. New York, 1983, Plenum Medical Publishing.

118. Wasserman K, Hansen JE, Sue DY, et al. Principles of Exercise Testing and Interpretation. Philadelphia, 1987, Lea & Febiger.

119. Moe GW, Canepa-Anson R, Howard RJ, et al. Response of atrial natriuretic factor to postural change in patients with heart failure versus subjects with normal hemodynamics. J Am Coll Cardiol 16(3):599–606, 1990.

120. Killip T, Eimball JT. Treatment of myocardial infarction in a coronary care unit. A two-year experience with 250 patients. Am J Cardiol 20(4):457–64, 1967.

121. Braunwald E. The physical examination. In Braunwald E (ed.). Heart Disease: A Textbook of Cardiovascular Medicine. Philadelphia, 1988, Saunders.

122. Chezner MA. Cardiac auscultation: Heart sounds. Cardiol Pract Sept/Oct:141, 1984.

123. Stevenson LW, Brunken RC, Belil D, et al. Afterload reduction with vasodilators and diuretics decreases mitral regurgitation during upright exercise in advanced heart failure. J Am Coll Cardiol 15:174–80, 1990.

124. Constant J. Bedside Cardiology. Boston, 1985, Brown, Little.

125. Guyton AC. The relationship of cardiac output and arterial pressure control. Circulation 64(6):1079–88, 1981.

126. Sullivan MJ, Green HJ, Cobb FR. Skeletal muscle biochemistry and histology in ambulatory patients with long-term heart failure. Circulation 81(2):518–27, 1990.

127. Drexler H, Riede U, Munzel T, et al: Alterations of skeletal muscle in chronic heart failure. Circulation 85(5):1751–9, 1992.

128. Criteria Committee, New York Heart Association. Diseases of the Heart and Blood Vessels, ed 6. Boston, 1964, Little, Brown.

129. Mann DL. Heart Failure: A Companion to Braunwald's Heart Disease. Philadelphia, 2004, Saunders.

130. Mancini D, Eisen H, Kussmaul W, et al. Value of peak exercise oxygen consumption for optimal timing of cardiac transplantation in ambulatory patients with heart failure. Circulation 83(3):778–86, 1991.

131. Cohn J, Rector T. Prognosis of congestive heart failure and predictors of mortality. Am J Cardiol 62(2):25A–30A, 1988.

132. Slazchic J, Massie B, Kramer B, et al. Correlates and prognostic implication of exercise capacity in chronic congestive heart failure. Am J Cardiol 55(8):1037–42, 1985.

133. Likoff M, Chandler S, Kay H. Clinical determinants of mortality in chronic congestive heart failure secondary to idiopathic dilated or ischemic cardiomyopathy. Am J Cardiol 59(6):634–8, 1987.

134. Cohn J, Johnson G, Shabetai R, et al. Ejection fraction, peak exercise oxygen consumption, cardiothoracic ratio, ventricular arrhythmias, and plasma norepinephrine as determinants of prognosis in heart failure. The V-HeFT VA Cooperative Studies Group. Circulation 87(6 Suppl):VI5–16, 1993.

135. Aaronson KD, Mancini DM. Is percentage of predicted maximal exercise oxygen consumption a better predictor of survival than peak exercise oxygen consumption for patients with severe heart failure? J Heart Lung Transplant 14(5):981–9, 1995.

136. Sullivan MJ, Cobb FR. The anaerobic threshold in chronic heart failure. Relation to blood lactate, ventilatory basis, reproducibility, and response to exercise training. Circulation 81(1 Suppl):II47–58, 1990.

137. Tavazzi L, Gattone M, Corra U, et al. The anaerobic index: Uses and limitations in the assessment of heart failure. Cardiology 76(5):357–67, 1989.

138. Wasserman K, Beaver WL, Whipp BJ. Gas exchange theory, and the lactic acidosis (anaerobic) threshold. Circulation 81(1 Suppl):II14–30, 1990.

139. Koike A, Itoh H, Taniguchi K, et al. Relationship of anaerobic threshold (AT) to AVO$_2$/WR in patients with heart disease [abstract]. Circulation 78(Suppl 11):624, 1988.

140. Wenger NK. Left ventricular dysfunction, exercise capacity and activity recommendations. Eur Heart J 9(Suppl F):63–6, 1988.

141. Cahalin LP, Mathier MA, Semigran MJ, et al. The six-minute walk test predicts peak oxygen uptake and survival in patients with advanced heart failure. Chest 110(2):325–32, 1996.

142. Faggiano P, D'Aloia A, Gualeni A, et al. Assessment of oxygen uptake during the six-minute walk test in patients with heart failure [letter]. Chest 111(4):1146, 1997.

143. Bittner V, Weiner DH, Yusuf S, et al. Prediction of mortality and morbidity with a 6-minute walk test in patients with left ventricular dysfunction. JAMA 270(14):1702–7, 1993.

144. Guyatt GH, Thompson PJ, Berman LB, et al. How should we measure function in patients with chronic heart and lung disease? J Chronic Dis 38(6):517–24, 1985.

145. Goldman L, Hashimoto D, Cook EF. Comparative reproducibility and validity of systems for assessing cardiovascular functional class: Advantages of a new specific activity scale. Circulation 64(6):1227–34, 1981.

146. Blackwood R, Mayou RA, Garnham JC, et al. Exercise capacity and quality of life in the treatment of heart failure. Clin Pharmacol Ther 48(3):325–32, 1990.

147. Rector TS, Kubo SH, Cohn JN. Patients' self-assessment of their congestive heart failure: II. Content, reliability and validity of a new measure—The Minnesota Living with Heart Failure Questionnaire. Heart Fail 3:198, 1987.

148. Kavanagh T, Myers MG, Baigrie RS, et al. Quality of life and cardiorespiratory function in chronic heart failure: Effects of 12 months' aerobic training. Heart 76:42–9, 1996.

149. Tyni-Lenné R, Cordon A, Sylvén C. Improved quality of life in chronic heart failure patients following local endurance training with leg muscles. J Card Fail 2(2):111–17, 1996.

150. GH Guyatt: Measurement of health-related quality of life in heart failure. J Am Coll Cardiol 22(4 Suppl A):185A–91A, 1993.

151. Ball E, Michel T, Cahalin LP. Quality of life in elderly heart failure patients is related to quadriceps muscle performance [abstract]. J Cardiopulm Rehabil 17(5):329, 1997.

152. Cahalin LP, Semigran M, Kacmarek R, et al. Quality of life in elderly heart failure patients is related to lower body weight. Chest 112:95S, 1997.

153. Jiang W, Alexander J, Christopher E, et al. Relationship of depression to increased risk of mortality and rehospitalization in patient with congestive heart failure. Arch Intern Med 161(15):1849–56, 2001.

154. Rumsfeld JS, Havranek E, Masoudi FA, et al. Depressive symptoms are the strongest predictors of short-term declines in health status in patients with heart failure. J Am Coll Cardiol 42(10):1811–17, 2003.

155. Fulop G, Strain HH, Stettin G. Congestive heart failure and depression in older adults: Clinical course and health services use 6 months after hospitalization. Psychosomatics 44(5):367–73, 2003.

156. Havranek EP, Ware MG, Lowes BD. Prevalence of depression in congestive heart failure. Am J Cardiol 84(3):348–50, A9, 1999.

157. Smith TW, Braunwald E, Kelly RA. The management of heart failure. In Braunwald E (ed.). Heart Disease: A Textbook of Cardiovascular Medicine. Philadelphia, 1988, Saunders.

158. Burton KP. Evidence of direct toxic effects of free radicals on the myocardium. Free Radic Biol Med 4(1):15–24, 1988.

159. Padh H. Vitamin C: Newer insights into its biochemical functions. Nutr Rev 49(3):65–70, 1991.

160. Belch JJ, Bridges AB. Oxygen free radicals and congestive heart failure. Br Heart J 65(5): 245–8, 1991.

161. Gaziano JM. Antioxidant vitamins and coronary artery disease risk. Am J Med 97(3A):18S–21S, 1994.

162. Dracup K, Baker DW, Dunbar SB, et al. Management of heart failure. II. Counseling, education, and lifestyle modifications. JAMA 272(18):1442–6, 1994.

163. Fonarow CC, Stevenson LW, Walden JA, et al. Impact of a comprehensive heart failure management program on hospital readmission and functional status of patients with advanced heart failure. J Am Coll Cardiol 30(3):725–32, 1997.

164. Parmley WW. Should digoxin be the drug of first choice after diuretics in chronic congestive heart failure? J Am Coll Cardiol 12(1):265–73, 1988.

165. Pitt B. Clot-specific thrombolytic agents: Is there an advantage? J Am Coll Cardiol 12(3):588, 1988.

166. Mulrow CD, Feussner JR, Velez R. Reevaluation of digitalis efficacy. New light on an old leaf. Ann Intern Med 101(1):113–17, 1984.

167. Arrold SB, Byrd RC, Meister W, et al. Long-term digitalis therapy improves left ventricular function in heart failure. N Engl J Med 303(25):1443–8, 1980.

168. Lee DC-S, Johnson RA, Gingham JB, et al. Heart failure in outpatients. A randomized trial of digoxin versus placebo. N Engl J Med 306(12):699–705, 1982.

169. Gheorghiade M, St. Clair J, St. Clair C, et al. Hemodynamic effects of intravenous digoxin in patients with severe heart failure initially treated with diuretics and vasodilators. J Am Coll Cardiol 9(4):849–57, 1987.

170. Guyatt GH, Sullivan MD, Fallen EL, et al. A controlled trial of digoxin in congestive heart failure. Am J Cardiol 61(4):371–5, 1988.

171. The Captopril-Digoxin Multicenter Research Group. Comparative effects of therapy with captopril and digoxin in patients with mild to moderate heart failure. JAMA 259(4):539–44, 1988.

172. Francis GS. Which drug for what patients with heart failure, and when? Cardiology 76(5):374–83, 1989.

173. Adams Jr K, Gheorghiade M, Uretsky B, et al. Patients with mild heart failure worsen during withdrawal from digoxin therapy. J Am Coll Cardiol 30(1):42–8, 1997.

174. Leier CV. Acute inotropic support. In Leier CV (ed.). Cardiotonic Drugs: A Clinical Survey. New York, 1986, Marcel Dekker.

175. Rude RE, Kloner RA, Maroko PR, et al. Effects of amrinone on experimental acute myocardial ischemic injury. Cardiovasc Res 14(7):419–27, 1980.

176. Packer M, Carver JR, Rodeheffer RJ, et al. Effect of oral milrinone on mortality in severe chronic heart failure. The PROMISE Study Research Group. N Engl J Med 325(21):1468–75, 1991.

177. Taylor SH, Verma SP, Hussain M, et al. Intravenous amrinone in left ventricular failure complicated by acute myocardial infarction. Am J Cardiol 56(3):29B–32B, 1985.

178. DiBianco R, Shabetai R, Kostuk W, et al. Oral milrinone and digoxin in heart failure: Results of a placebo-controlled, prospective trial of each agent and the combination [abstract]. Circulation 76(Suppl IV):IV256, 1978.

179. Massie BM, Packer M, Hanlon JT, et al. Combined captopril and hydralazine for refractory heart failure: A feasible and efficacious regimen. J Am Coll Cardiol 2:338, 1983.

180. Sharpe N, Smith H, Murphy J, et al. Treatment of patients with symptomless left ventricular dysfunction after myocardial infarction. Lancet 1(8580):255–9, 1988.

181. Pfeffer MA, Lamas GA, Vaughan DA, et al. Effect of captopril on progressive ventricular dilatation after anterior myocardial infarction. N Engl J Med 319(2):80–6, 1988.

182. Pfeffer JM, Pfeffer MA, Braunwald E. Hemodynamic benefits and prolonged survival with long-term captopril therapy in rats with myocardial infarction and heart failure. Circulation 75(Suppl 1):1149, 1987.

183. Pfeffer MA, Pfeffer JM. Ventricular enlargement and reduced survival after myocardial infarction. Circulation 75(Suppl IV):93, 1987.

184. Douglas LM. Pathophysiology of heart failure. In Libby P, Bonow RO, Mann DL, et al. Braunwald's Heart Disease: A Textbook of Cardiovascular Medicine, ed 8. Philadelphia, 2008, Saunders.

185. Rutherford JD, Braunwald E, Cohn PF. Chronic ischemic heart disease. In Braunwald E (ed.). Heart Disease: A Textbook of Cardiovascular Medicine. Philadelphia, 1988, Saunders.

186. Cahalin LP. Cardiovascular medications. In Malone T (ed.). Physical and Occupational Therapy: Drug Implications for Practice. Philadelphia, 1989, Lippincott.

187. Packer M, Bristow M, Cohn J, et al. The effect of carvedilol on morbidity and mortality in patients with chronic heart failure. U.S. Carvedilol Heart Failure Study Group. N Engl J Med 334:1349–55, 1996.

188. Gattis WA, O'Connor CM, Gallup DS, et al. Predischarge initiation of carvedilol in patients hospitalized for decompensated heart failure: results of the Initiation Management Predischarge: Process for Assessment of Carvedilol Therapy in Heart Failure (IMPACT-HF) trial. J Am Coll Cardiol 43(9):1534–41, 2004.

189. Costanzo MR, Johannes RS, Pine M, et al. The safety of intravenous diuretics alone versus diuretics plus parenteral vasoactive therapies in hospitalized patients with acutely decompensated heart failure: a propensity score and instrumental variable analysis using the Acutely Decompensated Heart Failure National Registry (ADHERE) database. Am Heart J 154(2):267–77, 2007.

190. Douglas LM. Management of heart failure patients with reduced ejection fraction. In Libby P, Bonow RO, Mann DL, et al. Braunwald's Heart Disease: A Textbook of Cardiovascular Medicine, ed 8. Philadelphia, 2008, Saunders.

191. Hunt SA, Abraham WT, Chin MH, et al. ACC/AHA 2005 guideline update for the diagnosis and management of chronic heart failure in the adult: A report of the American College of Cardiology/American Heart Association Task Force on Practice Guidelines. Circulation 112:e154, 2005.

192. Birks EJ, Tansley PD, Hardy J, et al. Left ventricular assist device and drug therapy for the reversal of heart failure. N Engl J Med 355:1873, 2006.

193. Cullen MJ, Appleyard ST, Bindoff L. Morphologic aspects of muscle breakdown and lysosomal activation. Ann N Y Acad Sci 317:440, 1979.

194. Laragh JH. Atrial natriuretic hormone, the renin-aldosterone axis, and blood pressure-electrolyte homeostasis. N Engl J Med 313:1330, 1985.

195. McAlister FA, Ezekowitz JA, Wiebe N, et al. Systematic review: Cardiac resynchronization in patients with symptomatic heart failure. JAMA 297(22):2502–14, 2007.

196. L'Abbate A, Emdin M, Piacenh M, et al. Ultrafiltration: A rational treatment for heart failure. Cardiology 76:384, 1989.

197. Rimondini A, Cipolla CM, Della Bella P, et al. Hemofiltration as short-term treatment for refractory congestive heart failure. Am J Med 83:43, 1987.

198. William RS. Exercise training of patients with ventricular dysfunction and heart failure. In Wenger NK (ed.). Exercise and the Heart. 2nd ed. Philadelphia, FA Davis, 1985.

199. Cardiac Alert 11:6, 1990.

200. Bocchi EA, Moreira LFP, Bacal F, et al. Left ventricular regional wall motion, ejection fraction, and geometry changes after partial left ventriculectomy. Eur J Cardiothorac Surg 18(4):458–65, 2000.

201. Vijayanagar R, Weston M, Sears N, et al. Partial left ventriculectomy (PLV) for treatment of end-stage heart disease (ESHD): Evaluation of early experience. Chest 112:48S, 1997.

202. Wong J, Garcia MJ, Starling RC, et al. Alterations in left ventricular wall stress after partial left ventriculectomy surgery. Circulation 96:1–344, 1997.

203. Aaronson KD, Schwartz JS, Chen TM, et al. Development and prospective validation of a clinical index to predict survival in ambulatory patients referred for cardiac transplant evaluation. Circulation 95:2660–7, 1997.

204. Levy WC, Mozaffarian D, Linker DT, et al. The Seattle heart failure model: Prediction of survival in heart failure. Circulation 113:1424–33, 2006.

205. Bart BA, Shaw LK, McCants CV, et al. Clinical determinants of mortality in patients with angiographically diagnosed ischemic or nonischemic cardiomyopathy. J Am Coll Cardiol 30:1002–8, 1997.

206. Kellerman JJ, Shemesh J. Exercise training of patients with severe heart failure. J Cardiovasc Pharmacol 10:S172–83, 1987.

207. Keteyian SJ, Levine AB, Brawner CA, et al. Exercise training in patients with heart failure: A randomized, controlled trial. Ann Intern Med 124:1051–7, 1996.

208. Coats AJ. Exercise training for heart failure: Coming of age. Circulation 99:1138–40, 1999.

209. Belardinelli R, Georgiou D, Cianci G, et al. Randomized, controlled trial of long-term moderate exercise training in chronic heart failure: Effects on functional capacity, quality of life, and clinical outcome. Circulation 99:1173–82, 1999.

210. Giannuzzi P, Temporelli PL, Corra U, et al. Antiremodeling effect of long-term exercise training in patients with stable chronic heart failure: Results of the Exercise in Left Ventricular Dysfunction and Chronic Heart Failure (ELVD-CHF) Trial. Circulation 108:554–9, 2003.

211. Whellan DJ, O'Connor CM, Lee KL, et al. HF-ACTION Trial Investigators. Heart failure and a controlled trial investigating outcomes of exercise training (HF-ACTION) design and rationale. Am Heart J 153(2):201–11, 2007.

212. O'Connor CM, Whellan DJ, Lee KL, et al. Efficacy and safety of exercise training in patients with chronic heart failure: HF-ACTION randomized controlled trial. JAMA 301(14):1439–50, 2009.

213. Cardiac Rehabilitation: Clinical Practice Guideline, Number 17. U.S. Department of Health and Human Services. Public Health Service. Washington, DC, Agency for Health Care Policy and Research. National Heart, Lung, and Blood Institute, 1995.

214. Cahalin LP. Heart failure. Phys Ther 76(5):516, 1996.

215. Whaley MH, Brubaker PH, Kaminsky LA, et al. Validity of rating of perceived exertion during graded exercise testing in apparently healthy adults and cardiac patients. J Cardiopulm Rehabil 17(4):261–7, 1997.

216. LP Cahalin, Certo C, LaFiandra M, et al. Exercise training increases the oxygen uptake-work rate relationship in advanced heart failure. Chest 112:49S, 1997.

217. Keteyian SJ, Marks CRC, Brawner CA, et al. Responses to arm exercise in patients with compensated heart failure. J Cardiopulm Rehabil 16:366, 1996.

218. Barlow CW, Qayyum MS, Davey PP, et al. Effect of physical training on exercise-induced hyperkalemia in chronic heart failure: Relation with ventilation and catecholamines. Circulation 89:1144, 1994.

219. Keteyian SJ, Levine TB, Levine AB, et al. Quality of life and exercise training in patients with heart failure: A randomized trial. Circulation 96:1–84, 1997.

220. Franciosa JA, Park M, Levine TB. Lack of correlation between exercise capacity and indexes of resting left ventricular performance in heart failure. Am J Cardiol 47:33, 1981.

221. Franciosa JA, Ziesche S, Wilen M. Functional capacity of patients with chronic left ventricular failure. Am J Med 67:460, 1979.

222. Jafri SM, Lakier JB, Rosman HS, et al. Symptoms and tests of ventricular performance in the evaluation of chronic heart failure. Am Heart J 112(1):194–6, 1986.

223. Pickworth KK. Long-term dobutamine therapy for refractory congestive heart failure. Clin Pharm 11(7):618–24, 1992.

224. Coats AJS, Adamopoulos S. Physical and pharmacological conditioning in chronic heart failure: A proposal for pulsed inotrope therapy. Postgrad Med J 67(Suppl 1):S69–72, 1991.

225. Miller LW. Outpatient dobutamine for refractory congestive heart failure: Advantages, techniques, and results. J Heart Lung Transplant 10(3):482–7, 1991.

226. Kataoka T, Keteyian SJ, Marks CRC, et al. Exercise training in a patient with congestive heart failure on continuous dobutamine. Med Sci Sports Exerc 26(6):678–81, 1994.

227. Applefeld MM, Newman KA, Grove WR, et al. Intermittent, continuous outpatient dobutamine infusion in the management of congestive heart failure. Am J Cardiol 51(3):455–8, 1983.

228. Metra M, Eichhorn E, Abraham WT, et al. Effects of low-dose oral enoximone administration on mortality, morbidity, and exercise capacity in patients with advanced heart failure: the randomized, double-blind placebo-controlled, parallel group Essential trials. Eur Heart J 30(24):3015–26, 2009.

229. McCarthy PM. HeartMate implantable left ventricular assist device: Bridge to transplantation and future applications. Ann Thorac Surg 59(2 Suppl):S46–51, 1995.

230. Kennedy MD, Haykowsky M, Humphrey R. Function, eligibility, outcomes and exercise capacity associated with left ventricular assist devices: Exercise rehabilitation and training for patients with ventricular assist devices. J Cardiopulm Rehabil 23(3):208–17, 2003.

231. Mettauer B, Geny B, Lonsdorfer-Wolf E, et al. Exercise training with a heart device: A hemodynamic, metabolic, and hormonal study. Med Sci Sports Exerc 33(1):2–8, 2001.

232. Morrone T, Buck L, Catanese K, et al. Early progressive mobilization of left ventricular assist device patients is safe and optimizes recovery prior to cardiac transplant. J Heart Lung Transplant 15(5):423–9, 1996.

233. Buck L, Morrone T, Goldsmith R, et al. Exercise training of patients with left ventricular assist devices: A pilot study of physiologic adaptations [abstract]. J Cardiopulm Rehabil 17(5):324, 1997.

234. O'Donnell DE, Sanii R, Younes M. Improvement in exercise endurance in patients with chronic airflow limitation using continuous positive airway pressure. Am Rev Respir Dis 138(6):1510–14, 1988.

235. Henke KG, Regnis JA, Bye PTP. Benefits of continuous positive airway pressure during exercise in cystic fibrosis and relationship to disease severity. Am Rev Respir Dis 148(5):1272–6, 1993.

236. Cahalin LP, Cannan J, Prevost S, et al. Exercise performance during assisted ventilation with bi-level positive airway pressure (BiPAP). J Cardiopulm Rehabil 14(5):323, 1994.

237. Baratz DM, Westbrooke PR, Shah PK, et al. Effect of nasal continuous positive airway pressure on cardiac output and oxygen delivery in patients with congestive heart failure. Chest 102(5):1397–401, 1992.

238. Bradley TD, Holloway RM, McLaughlin PR, et al. Cardiac output responses to continuous positive airway pressure in congestive heart failure. Am Rev Respir Dis 145(2 Pt 1):377–82, 1992.

239. Naughton MT, Rahman MA, Hara K, et al. Effect of continuous positive airway pressure on intrathoracic and left ventricular transmural pressures in patients with congestive heart failure. Circulation 91(6):1725–31, 1995.

240. Malone S, Liu PP, Hollway R, et al. Obstructive sleep apnoea in patients with dilated cardiomyopathy: Effects of continuous positive airway pressure. Lancet 338(8781):1480–4, 1991.

241. Takasaki Y, Orr D, Popkin J, et al. Effect of nasal continuous positive airway pressure on sleep apnea in congestive heart failure. Am Rev Respir Dis 140(6):1578–84, 1989.

242. Naughton MT, Liu PP, Benard DC, et al. Treatment of congestive heart failure and Cheyne-Stokes respiration during sleep by continuous positive airway pressure. Am J Respir Crit Care Med 151(1):92–7, 1995.

243. Pinsky MR, Summer WR, Wise RA, et al. Augmentation of cardiac function by elevation of intrathoracic pressure. J Appl Physiol 84(4):370–5, 1983.

244. Pinsky MR, Summer WR. Cardiac augmentation by phasic high intrathoracic pressure support in man. Chest 84:370, 1983.

245. Cahalin LP, Zambernardi L, Dec GW. Multiple systems assessment during inpatient cardiopulmonary rehabilitation [abstract]. J Cardiopulm Rehabil 13(5):344, 1993.

246. Cahalin LP, Semigran MJ, Dec GW. Inspiratory muscle training in patients with chronic heart failure awaiting cardiac transplantation: Results of a pilot clinical trial. Phys Ther 77(8):830–8, 1997.

247. Mancini DM, Henson D, LaManca J, et al. Benefit of selective respiratory muscle training on exercise capacity in patients with chronic congestive heart failure. Circulation 91(2):320–9, 1995.

248. Barach AL. Physiologic advantages of grunting, groaning, and pursed-lip breathing: Adaptive symptoms related to the development of continuous positive pressure breathing. Bull N Y Acad Med 49(8): 666–73, 1973.

249. Tiep BL, Burns M, Kao D, et al. Pursed lips breathing training using ear oximetry. Chest 90(2):218–21, 1986.

250. Mancini DM, Henson D, LaManca J, et al, Respiratory muscle function and dyspnea in patients with chronic congestive heart failure. Circulation 86(3):909–18, 1992.

251. Mancini DM, LaManca J, Donchez L, et al. The sensation of dyspnea during exercise is not determined by the work of breathing in patients with heart failure. J Am Coll Cardiol 28(2):391–5, 1996.

252. Collins SM, Cahalin LP, Semigran MJ, et al. Strength or Endurance? Phys Ther 77(8):1764–6, 1997.

253. Larson JL, Kim MJ, Sharp JT, et al. Inspiratory muscle training with a pressure threshold breathing device in patients with chronic obstructive pulmonary disease. Am Rev Respir Dis 138(3):689–96, 1988.

254. Weiner P, Azgad Y, Ganam R, et al. Inspiratory muscle training in patients with bronchial asthma. Chest 102(5):1357–61, 1992.

255. McParland C, Krishnan B, Wang E, et al. Inspiratory muscle weakness and dyspnea in congestive heart failure. Am Rev Respir Dis 146(2):467–72, 1992.

256. Aubuer M, Trippenbach T, Rousso C. Respiratory muscle fatigue during cardiogenic shock. J Appl Physiol 51(2):499–508, 1981.

257. Hammond MD, Bauer KA, Sharp JT, et al. Respiratory muscle strength in congestive heart failure. Chest 98(5):1091–4, 1990.

258. Winkelmann ER, Chiappa GR, Lima COC, et al. Addition of inspiratory muscle training to aerobic training improves cardiorespiratory responses to exercise in patients with heart failure and inspiratory muscle weakness. Am Heart J 158(5):768.e1–7, 2009.

259. Ham RJ, Sloane PD, Washaw GA, et al. Primary Care Geriatrics: A Case-Based Approach, ed 5. St. Louis, 2007, Mosby.

# CHAPTER 5

# Restrictive Lung Dysfunction

*Ellen Hillegass, Peggy Clough*

## Chapter Outline

Pulmonary pathology can be organized and discussed in a number of ways. Within this text, pulmonary function abnormalities have been divided into two main categories: obstructive dysfunction and restrictive dysfunction. If the flow of air is impeded, the defect is obstructive. If the volume of air or gas is reduced, the defect is restrictive. Although this organization of pulmonary pathology may in some ways clarify the discussion, it must be remembered that a number of diseases and conditions result in both obstructive and restrictive lung impairment. This chapter discusses those

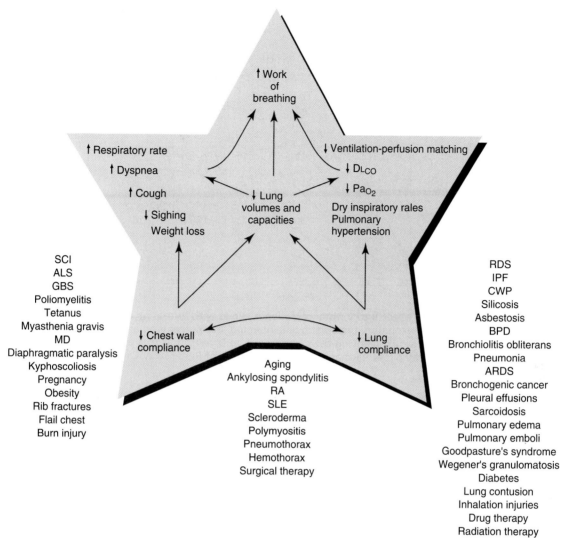

**Figure 5-1** Interactive star diagram in restrictive lung dysfunction. SCI, spinal cord injury; ALS, amyotrophic lateral sclerosis; GBS, Guillain–Barré syndrome; MD, muscular dystrophy; RA, rheumatoid arthritis; SLE, systemic lupus erythematosus; RDS, respiratory distress syndrome; IPF, idiopathic pulmonary fibrosis; CWP, coal workers' pneumoconiosis; BPD, bronchopulmonary dysplasia; ARDS, adult respiratory distress syndrome; DLCO, diffusing capacity of the lungs for carbon monoxide; PaO₂, arterial partial pressure of oxygen.

pathologies and interventions that result in restrictive lung dysfunction.

## Etiology

Restrictive lung dysfunction (RLD) is an abnormal reduction in pulmonary ventilation. Lung expansion is diminished. The volume of air or gas moving in and out of the lungs is decreased.[1]

Restrictive lung dysfunction is not a disease. In fact, this dysfunction may result from many different diseases arising from the pulmonary system or almost any other system in the body. It can also result from trauma or therapeutic interventions, such as radiation therapy, or the use of certain drugs (Fig. 5-1).

## Pathogenesis

Three major aspects of pulmonary ventilation must be considered to understand the pathophysiology of RLD. They are compliance of both the lung and the chest wall, lung volumes and capacities, and the work of breathing.

## Compliance

Pulmonary compliance encompasses both lung and chest wall compliance. It is the physiologic link that establishes a relationship between the pressure exerted by the chest wall or the lungs and the volume of air that can be contained within the lungs.[1] With RLD, chest wall or lung compliance, or both, is decreased.

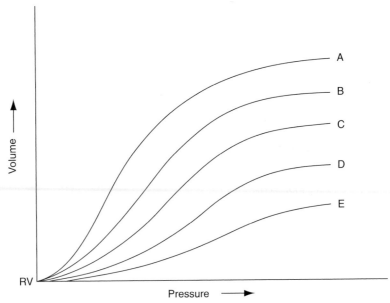

**Figure 5-2 A,** Normal total compliance curve. **B** to **E,** Total compliance curves with increasing acute respiratory distress syndrome (ARDS). The application of positive end-expiratory pressure, by maintaining alveoli recruited and increasing transpulmonary pressure gradients, can alter the compliance curve, moving the curve from **E** to **D** or from **D** to **B** and ideally returning the pressure–volume relationship closer to normal (**A**). (From Kacmarek RM. The Essentials of Respiratory Care, ed 4. St. Louis, 2006, Mosby.)

As discussed in Chapter 2, a decrease in compliance of the lungs indicates that they are becoming stiffer and thus more difficult to expand. It takes a greater transpulmonary pressure to expand the lung to a given volume in a person with decreased lung compliance.[2] If the amount of pressure used to move air into the lungs is constant, the volume of air would be decreased in the person with decreased lung compliance. The pressure–volume or compliance curve is shifted to the right (Fig. 5-2; see also the discussion of compliance in Chapter 2). A chest wall low in compliance limits thoracic expansion and therefore lung inflation even if the lung has normal compliance.

Because pulmonary compliance is decreased in RLD, resistance to lung expansion is increased. In other words, decreased pulmonary compliance requires an increase in pressure just to maintain adequate lung expansion and ventilation. This means the patient has to work harder just to move air into the lungs.

### Lung Volumes

Restrictive lung dysfunction eventually causes all the lung volumes and capacities to become decreased. Because the distensibility of the lung is decreased, the inspiratory reserve volume (IRV) is diminished. Tidal volume (VT) is the volume of air or gas normally moved in and out of the lungs at rest. Although the body tries to preserve the tidal volume in RLD, the compliance gradually decreases and the work of breathing increases; thus the tidal volume decreases. The expiratory reserve volume (ERV) is the volume of air or gas that can be exhaled following a normal exhalation. No matter the etiology, RLD effects a reduction in the ERV; this reduction is particularly pronounced if a decrease in lung compliance is the principal etiologic factor. The residual volume

(RV) is usually decreased, but with some causes of RLD (spinal cord injury, amyotrophic lateral sclerosis, and other neuromuscular disorders) it may be increased. This results in decreasing the dynamic lung volumes. The most marked decreases in lung volumes are seen in the IRV and ERV.

Because all lung volumes are decreased with RLD, all lung capacities are also decreased. Total lung capacity (TLC) and vital capacity (VC) are the two most common spirometric measurements used in the identification of RLD. Decreases in TLC and functional residual capacity (FRC) are a direct result of a decrease in lung compliance. At TLC the force of the inspiratory muscles is balanced by the inward elastic recoil of the lung. Because the recoil pressure is increased if lung compliance is decreased, this balance occurs at a lower volume, and thus the TLC is diminished. At FRC, the outward recoil of the chest wall is balanced by the inward elastic recoil of the lung. Because this elastic recoil is increased, the balance is achieved at a lower lung volume and so the FRC is decreased (Fig. 5-3).[2]

### Work of Breathing

With RLD, the work of breathing is increased. The respiratory system normally fine-tunes the respiratory rate and the VT to minimize the mechanical work of breathing. As previously mentioned, a greater transpulmonary pressure is required to achieve a normal VT. The result is that the patient's work of breathing is increased and a new equilibrium, with a decreased VT and an increased respiratory rate, is sought in an effort to reduce energy expenditure. However, if the respiratory rate is too high, energy is wasted in overcoming airway resistance and in ventilating the anatomic dead space. Furthermore, if the tidal volume is larger than required, energy is wasted overcoming the natural recoil of the lung and in

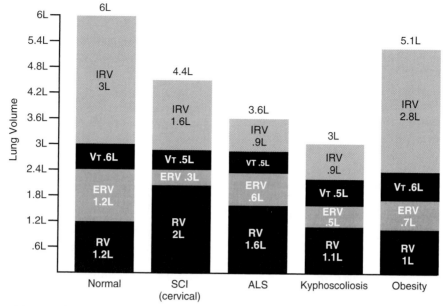

**Figure 5-3** Examples of lung volumes in different restrictive impairments. IRV, inspiratory reserve volume: VT, tidal volume; ERV, expiratory reserve volume; RV, residual volume; SCI, spinal cord injury; ALS, amyotrophic lateral sclerosis.

expanding the chest wall. Anything that increases airway resistance, increases flow rates, or decreases lung or chest wall compliance increases the work of breathing. In RLD, both lung and chest wall compliance and lung volumes may decrease. These changes can significantly change the work of breathing.[3] To overcome the decrease in pulmonary compliance, the respiratory rate is usually increased; the normal inspiratory muscles, especially the diaphragm, work harder; and the accessory muscles of respiration, the scaleni and the sternocleidomastoid (see Chapters 1 and 2), are recruited to assist in expanding the thorax.[4] These additional efforts require additional oxygen ($O_2$) expenditure. In normal persons at rest, the body uses less than 5% of the oxygen consumption per minute ($O_2$), or 3 to 14 mL $O_2 \bullet min^{-1}$, to support the work of breathing.[3,5] With RLD, the percentage of $O_2$ needed to support the work of breathing can reach and exceed 25%.[3,5] This change is usually very insidious as the RLD progresses and is countered by the concurrent decrease in activity seen in these patients. Although the respiratory muscle pump is very resistant to fatigue, these patients can experience respiratory muscle fatigue, overuse, and failure as RLD progresses.

## Clinical Manifestations

There are six classic signs and three classic symptoms that indicate RLD (Box 5-1).

### Signs

Six classic signs often indicate and are always consistent with RLD (see Box 5-1). The first is tachypnea or an increased respiratory rate. Because the inspiratory muscles have to work so hard to overcome the decreased pulmonary compliance,

---

**Box 5-1**

**Signs and Symptoms of Restrictive Lung Dysfunction**

| Signs | Symptoms |
|---|---|
| Tachypnea[a] | Dyspnea[b] |
| Hypoxemia[a] | Cough[b] |
| Decreased breath sounds[a] | Weight loss[b] |
| Decreased lung volumes and capacities[a] | Muscle wasting |
| Decreased diffusing capacity[a] | |
| Cor pulmonale[a] | |
| Altered chest radiograph (often reticulonodular pattern) | |
| Pulmonary hypertension | |

[a]Classic signs of restrictive lung dysfunction.
[b]Classic symptoms of restrictive lung dysfunction.

---

an involuntary adjustment is made to increase the respiratory rate and decrease the volumes so that the minute ventilation is maintained. Early in the course of RLD there may be overcompensation, with the respiratory rate increasing to the point that minute ventilation is increased and alveolar hyperventilation occurs, resulting in greater exhalation of carbon dioxide ($CO_2$).

Ventilation–perfusion mismatching, an invariable finding in RLD, leads to the second classic sign: hypoxemia. This mismatching may be due to changes in the collagenous framework of the lung, scarring of capillary channels, distortion or narrowing of the small airways, compression from tumors within the lung or bony abnormalities of the chest wall, or a variety of other causes. Even if patients are not hypoxemic at rest, they may quickly become hypoxemic with exercise.

The third classic sign of RLD is decreased breath sounds with dry inspiratory rales (Velcro crackles), which are thought to be caused by atelectatic alveoli opening at end-inspiration and are most often heard at the bases of the lungs.

The fourth and fifth classic signs are apparent from pulmonary function testing. The decrease in lung volumes and capacities, determined by spirometry, is the fourth classic sign of RLD. The fifth classic sign is the decreased diffusing capacity (DLCO). This arises as a consequence of a widening of the interstitial spaces as a result of scar tissue, fibrosis of the capillaries, and ventilation–perfusion abnormalities. In RLD, the DLCO has been measured at less than 50% of predicted.[6]

The sixth classic sign usually apparent with RLD is cor pulmonale. This right-sided heart failure is due to hypoxemia, fibrosis, and compression of the pulmonary capillaries, which leads to pulmonary hypertension. The rise in pressure in the pulmonary circulation increases the work of the right ventricle. Because the pulmonary capillary bed is fibrotic, it is also less able to distend to handle the ordinary increase in cardiac output expected with exercise. Therefore, during exercise hypoxemia may occur earlier or be more pronounced. Other signs include a decrease in chest wall expansion and possible cyanosis or clubbing (see Box 5-1).

## Symptoms

Three hallmark symptoms are usually experienced with RLD (see Box 5-1). The first is dyspnea or shortness of breath. This symptom typically manifests itself with exercise, but as RLD progresses, dyspnea at rest may also be experienced. The second symptom and the one that usually brings the patient into the physician's office is an irritating, dry, and nonproductive cough. The third hallmark symptom of RLD is the wasted, emaciated appearance these patients present as the disease progresses. With the work of breathing increased as much as 12-fold over normal, these individuals are using caloric requirements similar to those necessary for running a marathon 24 hours a day.[3] Additionally, because breathing is such hard work and eating makes breathing more difficult, these patients usually are not eager to eat and often report a decrease in appetite. Because their energy expenditure is up and their caloric intake is down, they are very often in a continual weight loss cycle, which becomes more severe as the RLD progresses.

## Treatment

Treatment interventions for RLD are discussed briefly for each disease. Generally, however, if the etiologic factors that are causing RLD are permanent (spinal cord injury) or progressive (idiopathic pulmonary fibrosis), the treatment consists primarily of supportive measures (Box 5-2). Supportive interventions include supplemental oxygen to support the arterial partial pressure of oxygen ($PaO_2$), antibiotic therapy to fight secondary pulmonary infection, measures to promote

---

**Box 5-2**

**Supportive Measures for Treatment of Restrictive Lung Dysfunction**

- Supplemental $O_2$
- Antibiotic therapy for secondary infection
- Interventions to promote adequate ventilation
- Interventions to prevent accumulation of secretions
- Good nutritional support

---

**Box 5-3**

**Preferred Practice Patterns Associated with Patients with Pulmonary Dysfunction**

- 6A: Primary Prevention/Risk Reduction for Cardiovascular/Pulmonary Disorders
- 6B: Impaired Aerobic Capacity/Endurance Associated with Deconditioning
- 6C: Impaired Ventilation, Respiration/Gas Exchange, and Aerobic Capacity/Endurance Associated with Airway Clearance Dysfunction
- 6D: Impaired Aerobic Capacity/Endurance Associated with Cardiovascular Pump Dysfunction or Failure
- 6E: Gas Exchange Associated with Respiratory Failure
- 6F: Impaired Ventilation and Respiration
- 6G: Impaired Ventilation, Respiration/Gas Exchange, and Aerobic Capacity/Endurance Associated with Respiratory Failure in the Neonate

Data from American Physical Therapy Association. Guide to Physical Therapist Practice, ed 2. Phys Ther 81:9–744, 2001.

---

adequate ventilation and prevent the accumulation of pulmonary secretions, and good nutritional support. However, if the changes that are causing the RLD are acute and reversible (pneumothorax) or chronic but reversible (Guillain–Barré syndrome), the treatment consists of specific corrective interventions (e.g., chest tube placement) as well as supportive measures (e.g., temporary mechanical ventilation) to assist the patient to maintain adequate ventilation until the patient is again able to be independent in this activity. Box 5-3 lists the potential practice patterns from the APTA's *Guide to Physical Therapist Practice, Second Edition*, that help to classify patients with the pulmonary dysfunction found in this chapter when approaching physical therapy treatment. Each section discusses the pathology and the practice patterns that would apply to each condition.

## Maturational Causes of Restrictive Lung Dysfunction

### Abnormalities in Fetal Lung Development

- Agenesis is the total absence of the bronchus and the lung parenchyma. Unilateral agenesis is rare.[7]

- Aplasia is the development of a rudimentary bronchus without the development of the normal lung parenchyma. This condition is also rare.[7]
- Hypoplasia is the development of a functioning although not always normal bronchus with the development of reduced amounts of lung parenchyma. This developmental abnormality is much more common and may affect one lung or one lobe of a lung. It is often present in infants born with a large diaphragmatic hernia and displaced abdominal organs.[7]

### Clinical Manifestation

Depending on the amount of lung parenchyma lost, these infants can be asymptomatic or can exhibit severe pulmonary insufficiency. The pulmonary impairment is restrictive in that the volumes are decreased even though the lung compliance may be normal.

### Respiratory Distress Syndrome

Respiratory distress syndrome (RDS), also known as hyaline membrane disease (HMD), is a disorder of prematurity or lack of complete lung maturation in the human fetus. It usually takes 36 weeks of normal gestation to achieve lung maturity in the fetus. Infants born with a gestational age less than 36 weeks often exhibit respiratory distress and may develop the full complement of signs and symptoms associated with RDS.[8]

### Etiology

Insufficient maturation of the lungs is the cause of RDS, and it is usually linked directly to the gestational age of the fetus at birth. The incidence of RDS in infants with a gestational age of 26 to 28 weeks at birth is approximately 75%.[8] In contrast, the incidence of RDS in infants with a gestational age of 36 weeks at birth is less than 5%.[8] Other factors that seem to contribute to the development of RDS are gender, race, and diabetes in the mother. Premature male infants are more at risk to develop RDS than premature female infants. Caucasian premature infants have a greater incidence of RDS than African-American premature infants. Fetal lung maturation is delayed in pregnant women with diabetes, so infants born of diabetic mothers are at increased risk of developing RDS. Worldwide, 1% of infants are affected by RDS.[8] In the United States, RDS is seen in approximately 50,000 infants each year.[9]

### Pathophysiology

RDS is caused primarily by abnormalities in the surfactant system and inadequate surfactant production. Structural abnormalities, such as alveolar septal thickening, within the immature lung may also contribute to the pathophysiology of this syndrome. The surfactant dysfunction causes the overall retractive forces of the lung to be greater than normal, which decreases lung compliance, increases the work of breathing, and leads to progressive diffuse microatelectasis, alveolar collapse, increased ventilation–perfusion mismatching, and impaired gas exchange (Fig. 5-4). In addition, alveolar

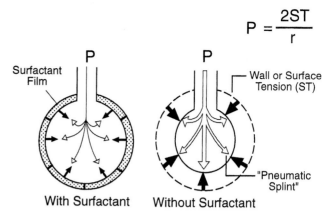

$$P = \frac{2ST}{r}$$

**Figure 5-4** Surfactant abnormalities.

epithelial and endothelial permeability are abnormal in the immature lung. Therefore, when these premature infants are mechanically ventilated without sufficient normal surfactant, the bronchiolar epithelium is disrupted. This leads to pulmonary edema and the generation of hyaline membranes. Further, because the proximal and distal airways in the infant are very compliant and the alveoli may be less compliant owing to atelectasis and the formation of hyaline membrane, the mechanical ventilator pressures used can disrupt, dilate, and deform the airways. Mechanical ventilator pressures can also cause air leaks, tension pneumothorax, and extensive pulmonary interstitial emphysema.

Another cause of decreased gas exchange is the often severe pulmonary hypertension evident in infants with RDS. These infants have hypoxemia and are acidotic, both of which cause vasoconstriction. This response is exaggerated in the infant and causes severe pulmonary hypertension, increased ventilation–perfusion mismatching, and decreased gas exchange. RLD may be complicated further by persistent patency of the ductus arteriosus, resulting in a left-to-right shunt within the infant's heart. The patent ductus arteriosus increases pulmonary pressures and blood flow and could allow plasma proteins to leak into the alveolar space, causing pulmonary edema and further interfering with surfactant function.

Complications common in infants with RDS include intracranial hemorrhage, sepsis, pneumonia, pneumothorax, pulmonary hemorrhage, and pulmonary interstitial emphysema. This syndrome can also result in the development of bronchopulmonary dysplasia. Recovery in RDS is usually preceded by an abrupt unexplained diuresis.[8]

### Clinical Manifestation
The clinical manifestation of RDS can be found in Table 5-1.

### Treatment
Beginning in the late 1980s and early 1990s, surfactant replacement therapy has become the treatment of choice for these infants. Early intervention is extremely important, and the surfactant replacement therapy is most effective when started within the first 2 hours of life. The earlier the

## Table 5-1  Clinical Manifestation of Respiratory Distress Syndrome

|          |                          | Findings |
|----------|--------------------------|----------|
| Signs    | Pulmonary function tests | ↑ RR |
|          |                          | ↓ Lung compliance |
|          |                          | ↓ Lung volumes (FRC, VC) |
|          |                          | ↑ Work of Breathing |
|          | Chest radiograph         | Fine reticulogranular pattern of lung parenchyma (homogeneous ground-glass appearance)[9,10] |
|          |                          | In severe RDS, air bronchograms are prominent |
|          |                          | In severe RDS, cardiothymic silhouette indistinct (diffuse microatelectasis) |
|          | Arterial blood gases     | Marked ↓ in PaO$_2$ |
|          |                          | ↑ PaCO$_2$ |
|          |                          | ↓ pH (acidosis) |
|          |                          | ↑ Dead space ventilation and ↓ alveolar ventilation, with V/Q mismatch |
|          | Breath sounds            | Presence of expiratory grunt |
|          |                          | Possible rales and/or decreased breath sounds due to atelectasis |
|          | Cardiovascular           | Possible bradycardia |
|          |                          | Possible cerebral, pulmonary, or intraventricular hemorrhage |
| Symptoms | Respiratory pattern      | Rapid and labored |
|          |                          | Significant intercostal, sternal, and substernal retractions |
|          | Nasal flaring            | |
|          | Grunting                 | |
|          | Crying: decreased in volume and strength | |
|          | May be cyanotic          | |

*FRC, functional residual capacity; PaCO$_2$, arterial partial pressure of CO$_2$; PaO$_2$, arterial partial pressure of O$_2$; RDS, respiratory distress syndrome; RR, respiratory rate; VC, vital capacity; V/Q, ventilation–perfusion.*

intervention, the shorter and more benign the course of the disease. The artificial surfactant is given as a liquid suspension in saline and delivered to the infant by aerosol via endotracheal intubation. The results of this therapeutic intervention are immediate reduction in oxygen requirements, a major decrease in pulmonary complications such as pneumothoraces or pulmonary interstitial emphysema, and rapid weaning from mechanical ventilation, often within 12 to 24 hours.[9] Death in RSD is now almost entirely limited to infants of 24 to 26 weeks' gestation weighing 500 to 800 g at birth.[9] Although administration of artificial surfactant has proved effective in decreasing the morbidity and mortality rates of RSD, studies are continuing to determine the best surfactant formulation and therapy regimen.

If the infant does not adequately respond to surfactant administration, then the infant, if large enough, may be treated with extracorporeal membrane oxygenation (ECMO) or nitric oxide administration delivered in the inspiratory gas to cause pulmonary vasodilation.[9]

An alternative to treatment of RDS is prevention of the disease by maternal/fetal treatment with corticosteroids. Administration of corticosteroids to the mother before delivery can accelerate fetal lung maturation by stimulating surfactant synthesis, inducing changes in the elastic properties of the fetal lung, stimulating alveolarization, and decreasing the permeability of the airway and alveoli epithelium.[8,9]

For additional therapeutic management see practice pattern 6G (Impaired Ventilation, Respiration/Gas Exchange, and Aerobic Capacity/Endurance Associated with Respiratory Failure in the Neonate).[11]

## Normal Aging

Maturation of the various body systems is a natural process that takes place throughout a lifetime. Normal aging usually refers to physiologic changes that occur with regularity in the majority of the population and can therefore be predicted. Physiologic changes that commonly are considered part of the aging process can begin as early as 20 years of age.[12]

### Etiology

The normal aging process in the pulmonary system is very slow and insidious, and because we have great ventilatory reserves the changes are often not felt functionally until the

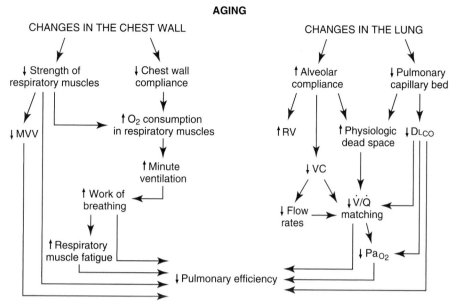

**Figure 5-5** Respiratory changes with aging. MVV, maximum voluntary ventilation; RV, residual volume; VC, vital capacity; V/Q, ventilation–perfusion; PaO₂, arterial partial pressure of oxygen; DLCO, diffusing capacity of the lungs for carbon monoxide.

sixth or seventh decade of life.[13] Universally, the normal aging process in the lungs is complicated by the fact that throughout life the lungs have had to cope with the external environment. Environmental factors that affect the aging process include general pollution, noxious gases, specific occupational exposures, inhaled drug use, and of course cigarette smoking.[12]

## Physiology

The compliance of the pulmonary system starts to decrease at about age 20 and decreases approximately 20% over the next 40 years.[12] Maximum voluntary ventilation decreases by 30% between the ages of 30 and 70.[12] Vital capacity also drops by about 25% between 30 and 70 years of age.[13] However, as stated previously, although some changes start as early as the second and third decades of life, functional status often is not affected until the sixth and seventh decades.

The control of ventilation undergoes significant change (Fig. 5-5). The peripheral chemoreceptors are not as responsive to hypoxia, and the central receptors are not as responsive to acute hypercapnia. These changes mean that the ventilatory response mediated by the central nervous system is significantly depressed.[3,8] The normal PaO₂ in a 70-year-old is 75, a measurement that is not interpreted as hypoxia by the central nervous system.[12]

The thorax undergoes a number of changes, including decalcification of the ribs, calcification of the costal cartilages, arthritic changes in the joints of the ribs and vertebrae, dorsal thoracic kyphosis, and increased anteroposterior diameter of the chest (barrel chest). The effects of these changes combine to decrease the compliance of the chest wall and increase the work of breathing. Oxygen consumption in the respiratory muscles is increased, causing an increase in

the minute ventilation. The strength and endurance of the inspiratory muscles gradually diminishes. This results in a decreased maximal ventilatory effort.[3] The forced expiratory volume in 1 second (FEV1) is reduced by about 40 mL per year.[12]

The lung tissue itself shows enlargement of the air spaces owing to enlargement of the alveolar ducts and terminal bronchioles. The alveolar surface area and the alveolar parenchymal volume are decreased. The alveolar walls become thinner, and the capillary bed incurs considerable loss, with an increase in ventilation–perfusion mismatching. Distribution of inspired air and pulmonary blood flow becomes less homogeneous with age. Diffusing capacity is therefore reduced, and physiologic dead space is increased.[12]

The static elastic recoil of the alveolar tissue decreases, which means that alveolar compliance is increased and the lungs do not empty well. The lung compliance curve is shifted to the left in the elderly. Thus, although TLC may not change with age, RV increases and dynamic volumes therefore decrease.[12,13]

Closing volumes are increased, which results in early closure of the small airways, particularly in the dependent lung regions. By approximately age 55, small airways are closed at or above FRC in the supine position. In the upright position, with the attendant increase in FRC, this change occurs at approximately age 70.[12]

Of course, normal concomitant aging changes take place in the cardiovascular system, including a decrease in maximum heart rate and cardiac output. These changes combine with the decreased oxygen exchange capability of the lungs and result in a decrease in the maximum oxygen uptake with exercise and therefore a decrease in the anaerobic threshold. After 50 years of age, the maximum oxygen uptake usually declines at a rate of 0.45 mL/kg/min for each year.[3,8]

## Table 5-2 Clinical Manifestation of Normal Aging

| | | Findings |
|---|---|---|
| Signs | Pulmonary Function Tests | TLC and airway resistance unchanged<br>↑ RV<br>↓ VC by approximately 25% at age 7–13<br>↓ Flow rates<br>↓ MVV by 30%12<br>↓ DLCO |
| | Chest radiograph | Variety of changes in bony thorax and parenchyma possible:<br>Kyphosis<br>Barrel chest<br>Decalcification of ribs<br>Larger air spaces |
| | Arterial blood gases | ↓ $PaO_2$ (to about 75 mm Hg at age 7–12)<br>Usually $PaCO_2$ normal or slightly elevated |
| | Breath sounds | Slightly diminished |
| | Cardiovascular | ↓ maximal HR<br>↓ stroke volume<br>↓ cardiac output<br>↑ systolic blood pressure |
| Symptoms | Changes in activity patterns | ↓ activity and recreational pursuits<br>↑ symptoms with activity |

HR, heart rate; MVV, maximum voluntary ventilation; $PaCO_2$, arterial partial pressure of $CO_2$; $PaO_2$, arterial partial pressure of $O_2$; RV, residual volume; TLC, total lung capacity; VC, vital capacity.

Ventilation during sleep is altered in the elderly. Electroencephalographic (EEG) studies have shown that total nocturnal sleep time is shorter, with more frequent and longer nocturnal awakenings in the elderly. The pattern of ventilation during sleep is irregular more often in the elderly than in young adults. Repetitive periodic apneas occur in 35% to 40% of the elderly, predominantly in males during sleep stages 1 and 2.[8]

### Clinical Manifestation

The clinical manifestation of normal aging can be found in Table 5-2.

### Treatment

Aging is normal: no treatment is required. Existing evidence, however, supports the need to keep aerobically exercising as well as possibly adding strength training into one's daily regimen.[14–16]

The elderly should be encouraged to remain active and fit. Although even with regular activity about 0.45 mL/kg/min of oxygen consumption is lost each year, the fit elderly person has a greater maximum oxygen consumption than the sedentary person. In addition, a sedentary elderly person beginning regular exercise can improve maximum oxygen consumption by 5% to 25% and can regain the exercise capability that was present as much as 5 to 10 years earlier.[12]

## Pulmonary Causes of Restrictive Lung Dysfunction

### Idiopathic Pulmonary Fibrosis

Idiopathic pulmonary fibrosis (IPF) is an inflammatory process involving all of the components of the alveolar wall that progresses to gross distortion of lung architecture. The components of the alveolar wall include the epithelial cells, the endothelial cells, the cellular and noncellular components of the interstitium, and the capillary network. These components are supported by the connective tissue framework made up of collagen and elastic fibers and containing a milieu of ground substance. Other synonyms used for IPF are cryptogenic fibrosing alveolitis, interstitial pneumonitis, and Hamman–Rich syndrome.[17,18] Prevalence of IPF is approximately 6 to 32 individuals/100,000.

### Etiology

By definition, IPF is of unknown origin. It may be due to viral, genetic, or immune system disorders or a combination of

## Table 5-3 Clinical Manifestation of Idiopathic Pulmonary Fibrosis

| | | Findings |
|---|---|---|
| Signs | Pulmonary function tests | ↓ TLC, ↓ VC, ↓ FRC, ↓ RV |
| | | Normal or ↓ flow rates |
| | | ↓ DLCO |
| | | As disease progresses, VT ↓ and RR ↑ |
| | Chest radiograph | Diffuse reticulonodular patterns throughout both lungs |
| | | Predominance of abnormal markings in lower lung fields |
| | Computed tomography (HRCT) | Areas of inflammation and cellularity: ground-glass appearance with areas of fibrosis and cystic changes[20] |
| | Arterial blood gases | ↓ $PaO_2$ |
| | | $PaCO_2$ normal |
| | | Patients hypoxemic with exercise early in disease, hypoxemic at rest as disease progresses |
| | Breath sounds | Bibasilar end-inspiratory dry rales |
| | | ↓ Breath sounds[10] |
| | Cardiovascular | One third of IPF patients develop pulmonary hypertension[10] |
| | | With pulmonary hypertension, right ventricular dysfunction, and cor pulmonale |
| | | Late in course: cyanosis, clubbing of digits[17] |
| Symptoms | | Dyspnea on exertion progresses to dyspnea at rest in late disease |
| | | Repetitive nonproductive cough (some have mucus hypersecretion and expectoration)[20] |
| | | Weight loss, decrease in appetite |
| | | Fatigue |
| | | Sleep disturbances with loss of rapid eye movement sleep[17,19] |

*DLCO, diffusing capacity of the lungs for carbon monoxide; FRC, functional residual capacity; HR, heart rate; HRCT, high-resolution computed tomography; IPF, idiopathic pulmonary fibrosis; $PaCO_2$, arterial partial pressure of $CO_2$; $PaO_2$, arterial partial pressure of $O_2$; RR, respiratory rate; RV, residual volume; TLC, total lung capacity; VC, vital capacity; VT, tidal volume.*

these disorders.[19] IPF seems to be an immunologically mediated disease set in motion by an initial acute injury or infection.[20] Current evidence points to a number of environmental and occupational exposures that initiate the injury, including six major exposures: smoking exposure, agriculture/farming, livestock, wood dust, metal dust, and stone/sand dust exposure.[21,22]

## Pathophysiology

The lung involvement in IPF often shows patchy focal lesions scattered throughout both lungs. These lesions first show inflammatory changes and then scar and become fibrotic, distorting the alveolar septa and the capillary network. The alveolar spaces become irregular in size and shape. There can be significant progressive destruction of the capillary bed. These changes combine to cause decreased lung compliance; decreased lung volumes; increased ventilation–perfusion mismatching; decreased surface area for gas exchange; decreased diffusing capacity; increased pulmonary arterial pressure, which increases the work of the right ventricle; increased

work of breathing; increased caloric requirements; and decreased functional capacity.[17,19]

The two major pathologic components of IPF are (1) an inflammatory process in the alveolar wall (sometimes called an alveolitis) and (2) a scarring or fibrotic process that is thought to be secondary to the active inflammation. Both of these pathologic processes occur simultaneously within the lung.[17] There is also an increased incidence of lung cancer in IPF patients, as much as 6-fold in women and 14-fold in men.[10,20]

Idiopathic pulmonary fibrosis is a progressive disease with slow and steady decline in lung function. The course includes acute exacerbations characterized by rapid deterioration in lung function not due to infections or heart failure. The acute exacerbations include low-grade fever, worsening dyspnea and cough, worsening gas exchange, and appearance of new opacities on radiology.[22]

## Clinical Manifestation

The clinical manifestation of IPF can be found in Table 5-3.

## Treatment

Corticosteroids (usually prednisone) continue to be the mainstay in the treatment of IPF. However, cytotoxic drugs such as cyclophosphamide and azathioprine have also been used in patients who do not seem to be responsive to corticosteroids. In fact, there is now some evidence that initial treatment with steroids and cyclophosphamide or cyclophosphamide alone may be preferable.[9,20] It is the active alveolitis that seems to have some positive response to these drugs. The progressive fibrosis is nonreversible, and these drugs have no effect on lung tissue that is already fibrotic.

The remaining treatment measures are supportive. They include smoking cessation, maintaining adequate oxygenation and ventilation, good nutrition, and aggressive treatment of infection.[20]

The final therapeutic intervention that can be offered to IPF patients is lung transplantation. Orthotopic single lung transplantation (SLT) is a viable therapeutic option for selected IPF patients.[19] In 1983, the Toronto Group reported the first long-term survival of an IPF patient with an SLT.[20] Idiopathic pulmonary fibrosis is now one of the four primary diagnoses (IPF, emphysema, cystic fibrosis, pulmonary hypertension) for which lung transplantation is performed.[23] However, this surgical therapeutic intervention is not without risks (see Chapter 12), including restrictive lung dysfunction, namely, obliterative bronchiolitis.

For additional therapeutic management see practice pattern 6E (Impaired Ventilation and Respiration/Gas Exchange Associated with Ventilatory Pump Dysfunction or Failure) or 6B (Impaired Aerobic Capacity/Endurance Associated with Deconditioning).[11]

## Coal Workers' Pneumoconiosis

Coal workers' pneumoconiosis (CWP) is an interstitial lung disease, an occupational pneumoconiosis, caused by the inhalation of coal dust. This disease is most commonly divided into simple CWP and complicated CWP.[24]

### Etiology

Coal workers' pneumoconiosis is caused by repeated inhalation of coal dust over a long period of time; usually, 10 to 12 years of underground work exposure is necessary for the development of simple CWP.[25] Complicated CWP, sometimes called progressive massive fibrosis, usually occurs only after even longer exposure to coal dust. Anthracite coal is more hazardous than bituminous in the development of this disease.[26]

Coal workers' pneumoconiosis is not the most common respiratory disease found in this occupational group. Chronic bronchitis is even more common, usually occurs earlier, and often coexists with CWP in coal miners.

### Pathophysiology

The pathologic hallmark of CWP is the coal macule, which is a focal collection of coal dust with little tissue reaction either in terms of cellular infiltration or fibrosis. These coal macules are often located at the division of respiratory bronchioles and are often associated with focal emphysema.[25] Lymph nodes are enlarged and homogeneously pigmented and are firm but not fibrotic. The pleural surface appears black owing to the deposits of coal dust. Simple CWP is a benign disease if complications do not develop. Less than 5% of cases progress to complicated CWP.[27]

The mechanism for the progression of simple CWP to complicated CWP is unknown. It has been suggested that simple CWP may progress when it is combined with infection, silicosis, tuberculosis, or altered immunologic mechanisms. Complicated CWP results in large confluent zones of dense fibrosis that are usually present in apical segments in one or both lungs. These zones are made up of dense, acellular, collagenous, black-pigmented tissue. The normal lung parenchyma can be completely replaced, and the blood vessels in the area then show an obliterative arteritis. These fibrous zones can completely replace the entire upper lobe.[25]

Common complications associated with complicated CWP include emphysema, chronic bronchitis, tuberculosis, cor pulmonale, and pulmonary thromboembolism

### Clinical Manifestation

The clinical manifestation of CWP can be found in Table 5-4.

### Treatment

Complicated CWP with pulmonary fibrosis is nonreversible; there is no cure for it. Supportive treatment includes cessation of exposure to coal dust, good nutrition, interventions to ensure adequate oxygenation and ventilation, and progressive exercise training to maximize the remaining lung function and tolerance to activity.

For additional therapeutic management, see practice pattern 6E (Impaired Ventilation and Respiration/Gas Exchange Associated with Ventilatory Pump Dysfunction or Failure) or 6B (Impaired Aerobic Capacity/Endurance Associated with Deconditioning).[11]

## Silicosis

Silicosis, one of the occupational pneumoconioses, is a fibrotic lung disease caused by the inhalation of the inorganic dust known as free or crystalline silicon dioxide.[24]

### Etiology

The disease as mentioned is caused by the repeated inhalation of free or crystalline silicon dioxide, which is very common and widely distributed in the earth's crust in a variety of forms, including quartz, flint, cristobalite, and tridymite.[25] Industries in which silicon dioxide exposure can occur include mining, tunneling through rock, quarrying, grinding and polishing rock, sandblasting, ship building, and foundry work.[27]

### Pathophysiology

Inhaled silica causes macrophages to enter the area to ingest these particles. But the macrophages are destroyed by the cytotoxic effects of the silica. This process releases lysosomal

## Table 5-4  Clinical manifestation of Coal Workers' Pneumoconiosis (CWP)

|  |  | Findings |
|---|---|---|
| Signs | Pulmonary function tests | Spirometric tests often normal or slight ↓ VC and ↓ RV with ↓ DLCO |
|  |  | Complicated |
|  |  | ↓ TLC, ↓ VC, ↓ FRC, ↓ lung compliance, ↓ DLCO, ↑ RR |
|  | Chest radiograph | Simple |
|  |  | Small discrete densities more nodular than linear |
|  |  | Predominantly in upper regions |
|  |  | Complicated |
|  |  | Coalescent opacities of black fibrous tissue, |
|  |  | Usually in posterior segments of upper lobes or superior segments of lower lobes. Cavities may be present as a result of superimposed TB or secondary to ischemic necrosis |
|  | Arterial blood gases | ↓ PaO₂ |
|  | Breath sounds | Simple |
|  |  | Slightly diminished breath sounds, rhonchi due to concomitant bronchitis |
|  |  | Complicated |
|  |  | Abnormal bronchial breath sounds above compressed atelectatic areas and rhonchi or rales with bronchitis |
|  | Cardiovascular | Complicated |
|  |  | Fibrotic pulmonary hypertension |
|  |  | Cor pulmonale |
| Symptoms |  | Severe dyspnea and cough |
|  |  | Copious amounts of black sputum |
|  |  | Barrel chest |
|  |  | Progressive weight loss |

*DLCO, diffusing capacity of the lungs for carbon monoxide; FRC, functional residual capacity; PaO₂, arterial partial pressure of O₂; RR, respiratory rate; RV, residual volume; TB, tuberculosis; TLC, total lung capacity; VC, vital capacity.*

enzymes that then induce progressive formation of collagen, which eventually becomes fibrotic. Another characteristic of silicosis is the formation of acellular nodules composed of connective tissue called silicotic nodules. Initially these nodules are small and discrete, but as the disease progresses they become larger and coalesce. Silicosis normally affects the upper lobes of the lung more than the lower lobes. Silicosis also seems to predispose the patient to secondary infections by mycobacteria including Mycobacterium tuberculosis. Complicated silicosis follows a steadily deteriorating course that leads to respiratory failure.[2,27]

## Clinical Manifestation

The clinical manifestation of silicosis can be found in Table 5-5.

## Treatment

There is no treatment except to avoid further exposure to silica. Supportive therapy is used to counteract the patient's symptoms and includes measures to provide adequate oxygenation, ventilation, and nutrition. Annual TB screening using PPD skin testing is also recommended.[20]

For additional therapeutic management see practice pattern 6E (Impaired Ventilation, Respiration/Gas Exchange Associated with Ventilatory Pump Dysfunction or Failure).[11]

## Asbestosis

Asbestosis is a diffuse interstitial pulmonary fibrotic disease caused by asbestos exposure.[26] Occupational asbestos exposure is also associated with an increased incidence of primary cancer of the larynx, oropharynx, esophagus, stomach, and colon.[25]

## Etiology

The term *asbestos* is used generically to name a specific group of naturally occurring fibrous silicates. There are four types of commercially significant asbestos. Chrysolite accounts for more than 70% of the asbestos used in the United States and is primarily mined in Canada and the Commonwealth of Independent States. Crocidolite and amosite are mined primarily in South Africa. Anthophyllite comes from Finland.[26]

Asbestos is valued because of its resistance to fire; it has been used widely since the 1930s. Those at most risk for

## Table 5-5 Clinical Manifestation of Silicosis

| | | Findings |
|---|---|---|
| Signs | Pulmonary function tests | ↓ TLC, ↓ VC, ↓ pulmonary compliance, ↓ FEV1 |
| | Chest radiograph | Small rounded opacities or nodules that enlarge over time (more in upper lung fields) |
| | | Hilar lymph nodes enlarged and calcified |
| | Arterial blood gases | ↓ $PaO_2$ with exercise |
| | Breath sounds | Decreased breath sounds in upper lobes |
| | | Rhonchi may be present |
| | Cardiovascular | No specific changes |
| Symptoms | | Shortness of breath and cough (may be productive) |

*FEV1, forced expiratory volume in 1 second; $PaO_2$, arterial partial pressure of $O_2$; TLC, total lung capacity; VC, vital capacity.*

asbestosis are asbestos miners and millers, construction workers, shipbuilders, insulation workers, pipe fitters, steamfitters, sheet metal workers, welders, workers who remove old asbestos insulation, workers employed in building renovation or demolition, and auto mechanics who work on brake linings.

### Pathophysiology

How asbestos causes a fibrotic reaction is not understood. There seems to be a considerable latency period after an initial exposure, which can extend to 15 to 20 years. It is hypothesized that the asbestos fiber causes an alveolitis in the area of the respiratory bronchioles, which then progresses to peribronchiolar fibrosis owing to the release of chemical mediators. Plaques, which are localized fibrous thickenings of the parietal pleura, are common and are usually seen posteriorly, laterally, or on the pleural surface of the diaphragm. Pleural effusions may also occur with asbestosis. Also "asbestos bodies" or ferruginous bodies appear in the lungs and sputum of these patients. These rod-shaped bodies with clubbed ends seem to be an asbestos fiber coated by macrophages with an iron–protein complex.[2,7,25,26]

Studies have shown conclusively that cigarette smoking has a multiplicative effect in the development of primary lung cancer in persons who have been exposed to asbestos. In addition, several studies have shown a dose–response relationship between the amount of cigarette smoking and the degree of fibrotic response to inhaled asbestos.[25] Complica-

tions of asbestosis include bronchiectasis, pleural mesothelioma, and bronchogenic carcinoma.[7]

### Clinical Manifestation

The clinical manifestation of asbestosis can be found in Table 5-6.

### Treatment

There is no curative treatment for asbestosis, and the disease progresses even though exposure to asbestos has ceased. Symptomatic support includes cessation of smoking, good nutrition, exercise conditioning to maximize lung function, and prompt treatment of recurrent pulmonary infections.

For additional therapeutic management, see practice pattern 6E (Impaired Ventilation and Respiration/Gas Exchange Associated with Ventilatory Pump Dysfunction or Failure) or 6B (Impaired Aerobic Capacity/Endurance Associated with Deconditioning).[11]

### Bronchopulmonary Dysplasia

Bronchopulmonary dysplasia (BPD) is a chronic pulmonary syndrome in neonates that occurs in some survivors of RDS who have been ventilated mechanically and have received high concentrations of oxygen over a prolonged period of time. Other names used for this syndrome are pulmonary fibroplasia and ventilator lung.[7,8]

### Etiology

The incidence of BPD following RDS varies from 2% to 68% in different studies.[8] The incidence increases in neonates who had low birth weights (less than 1000 g); required mechanical ventilation, particularly using continuous positive pressure; received inspired oxygen concentrations ($FIO_2$) at 60% or higher; or received supplemental oxygen for more than 50 hours.[7,8] In fact, BPD almost invariably develops in neonates who received oxygen at an $FIO_2$ of 60% or higher for 123 hours or more.[7] See Chapter 6 for more details on BPD.

### Bronchiolitis Obliterans

Bronchiolitis obliterans is a fibrotic lung disease that affects the smaller airways. It can produce restrictive and obstructive lung dysfunction. This syndrome has been known and discussed under a variety of names including bronchiolitis, bronchiolitis obliterans with organizing pneumonia (BOOP), bronchiolitis fibrosa obliterans, follicular bronchiolitis, and bronchiolitis obliterans with diffuse interstitial pneumonia.[17]

### Etiology

Bronchiolitis obliterans was first recognized in children, usually those under the age of 2 years. Pediatric bronchiolitis obliterans is often caused by a viral infection, most commonly by the respiratory syncytial virus, parainfluenza virus, influenza virus, or adenovirus.[26] An adult form of the disease has

## Table 5-6  Clinical Manifestation of Asbestosis

| | | Findings |
|---|---|---|
| Signs | Pulmonary function tests | ↓ lung compliance, ↓ lung volumes: ↓ TLC, ↓ VC, ↓ RV<br>↓ FEV1 and ↓ DLCO |
| | Chest radiograph | Irregularities or linear opacities are distributed throughout lung fields in lower zones |
| | | Loss of distinct heart and diaphragm borders (shaggy appearance) |
| | | Diaphragmatic and pericardial calcification |
| | | Late in disease: cyst formation, honeycomb appearance |
| | Arterial blood gases | ↓ $PaO_2$ with exercise; late in disease ↓ $PaO_2$ at rest |
| | | $PaCO_2$ within normal limits |
| | Breath sounds | Bibasilar rales and ↓ breath sounds |
| | | Percussion dull at bases |
| | Cardiovascular | Pulmonary hypertension develops as pulmonary capillary bed destroyed: ↑ work on RV |
| | | Clubbing present; may develop cyanosis and cor pulmonale |
| Symptoms | | Dyspnea on exertion: progresses to dyspnea at rest |
| | | Recurrent infections, chronic cough with or without sputum |
| | | Weight loss, ↓ appetite, and ↓ exercise tolerance |

*DLCO, diffusing capacity of the lungs for carbon monoxide; FEV1, forced expiratory volume in 1 second; RV, residual volume; TLC, total lung capacity; VC, vital capacity.*

now been recognized that can occur in persons from 20 to 80 years of age and has a wider variety of causes. In the adult, bronchiolitis obliterans may be caused by toxic fume inhalation (nitrogen dioxide) or by viral, bacterial, or mycobacterial infectious agents, particularly *Mycoplasma pneumoniae*. It may be associated with connective tissue diseases, such as rheumatoid arthritis; related to organ transplantation and graft versus host reactions; or allied with other diseases, such as idiopathic pulmonary fibrosis. It also may be idiopathic, with no known cause.[17]

## Pathophysiology

Bronchiolitis obliterans is characterized by necrosis of the respiratory epithelium in the affected bronchioles. This necrosis allows fluid and debris to enter the bronchioles and alveoli, causing alveolar pulmonary edema and partial or complete obstruction of these small airways. With complete obstruction, the trapped air is absorbed gradually, and the alveoli then collapse, causing areas of atelectasis. When the destruction of the respiratory epithelium is severe or widespread, it may be followed by a significant inflammatory response. This causes fibrotic changes in the adjacent peribronchial space, the alveolar walls, and the air spaces. The fibrotic changes are patchy and usually occur primarily within the bronchial tree and alveoli rather than in the interstitial lung tissue, as happens in IPF. All these changes combine to increase ventilation–perfusion mismatching; decrease lung compliance; impair gas transport; and, in some patients, cause demonstrable airway obstruction.[17]

## Clinical Manifestation

The clinical manifestation of bronchiolitis obliterans can be found in Table 5-7.

## Treatment

In children, treatment is supportive, usually consisting of hydration and supplemental oxygen. If the child is unable to clear secretions, postural drainage and suctioning are employed. Mechanical ventilation is rarely needed. If respiratory syncytial virus is the causative pathogen, then the antiviral agent ribavirin may be administered via aerosol.[26] Corticosteroids, antibiotics, and bronchodilators are not recommended in the treatment of pediatric bronchiolitis obliterans. In adults, supplemental oxygen and proper fluid balance are also very important. Corticosteroids have proved very effective in treating adult bronchiolitis obliterans that is idiopathic, caused by toxic fume inhalation, or associated with connective tissue disease.

For additional therapeutic management see practice pattern 6C (Impaired Ventilation, Respiration/Gas Exchange, and Aerobic Capacity/Endurance Associated with Airway Clearance Dysfunction) or 6E (Impaired Ventilation and Respiration/Gas Exchange Associated with Ventilatory Pump Dysfunction or Failure).[11]

## Atelectasis

Atelectasis means incomplete expansion of the lung or loss of volume of part (or all) of a lung. The incomplete expansion

## Table 5-7 Clinical Manifestation of Bronchiolitis Obliterans

| | | Findings |
|---|---|---|
| Signs | Pulmonary function tests | Lung volumes normal or ↓, flow rates normal or ↓<br>↓ DLCO, ↑ RR |
| | Chest radiograph | Variable depending on cause and extent of BO<br>Pediatric BO:<br>  Hyperinflation and ↑ bronchial markings<br>  With subsegmental consolidation and collapse<br>  Some have patchy alveolar infiltrates, some with diffuse nodular or<br>    reticulonodular pattern and interstitial inflammation and scarring<br>Adults:<br>  Pulmonary edema and bilateral patchy alveolar infiltrates.<br>  Late in course<br>  Nodular pattern with fibrotic changes in bronchi and alveoli |
| | Arterial blood gases | Hypoxemia (↓ PaO$_2$)<br>PaCO$_2$ normal or ↑ |
| | Breath sounds | Rales and expiratory wheezing. Some areas of ↓ sounds |
| | Cardiovascular | Tachycardia |
| Symptoms | | Dyspnea, ↑ RR and hacking, nonproductive cough |
| | | Infants: chest wall retractions |
| | | Cyanosis in some patients, chronic infections in others |

*BO, bronchiolitis obliterans; DLCO, diffusing capacity of the lungs for carbon monoxide; RR, respiratory rate.*

can be due to a variety of causes that can prevent alveoli from fully expanding (Fig. 5-6). Primary atelectasis is the failure of the lung to expand at birth. Compression atelectasis occurs as a result of changes in transpulmonary distending pressure found in individuals with other pathologies, including pleural effusion, pneumothorax, or interstitial or pulmonary edema. Atelectasis can also occur as a result of excess secretions and the failure to get rid of secretions.

### Etiology

Atelectasis (obstructive) may result from extrabronchial compression from tumors or enlarged lymph nodes, or endobronchial diseases such as bronchial tumors, inflammatory strictures, or an intrabronchial mass (foreign body or mucous plug). Atelectasis (scar and/or postoperative) occurs in the absence of obstruction and usually as a complication of either a lobar or segmental pneumonia. The main contributing factor is the inability or unwillingness (often because of pain or mental confusion) of the patient to cough effectively and to take deep breaths throughout the day. This type of atelectasis could be prevented with good pulmonary hygiene.

Atelectasis (compression) occurs as a result of expanding volume outside of the alveoli (in pleural space, interstitial space, etc.) that presses on the alveoli and prevents complete expansion. In all these cases, the alveoli may lose their surfactant and therefore demonstrate reduced alveolar surface tension, causing the alveoli to collapse.

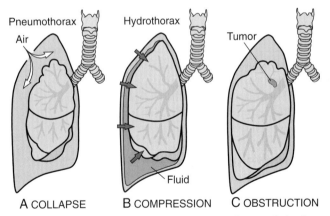

**Figure 5-6** Mechanism of atelectasis. **A,** Collapse of the lung in pneumothorax. **B,** Compression of the lung by pleural fluid. **C,** Resorption of the air from alveoli distal to an obstructed bronchus. Obstructive atelectasis is usually focal. Atelectasis of premature infants, which is caused by a deficiency of pulmonary surfactant, is not shown. (From Damjanov I. Pathology for the Health Professions, ed 3. St. Louis, 2006, Saunders.)

### Clinical Manifestation

Chest radiograph may show opacification of the atelectatic segment or lobe, or with significant lung collapse, the radiograph will show elevation of the hemidiaphragm on the affected side, shift of the mediastinum toward the affected side, and a decrease in size of the rib interspaces over the affected hemithorax. The symptoms the patient experiences with atelectasis are more likely from the cause of the atelectasis, such as postoperative pain and low-grade fever; however, if obstruction is the cause, the patient may be extremely dyspneic and demonstrate increased work of breathing.

## Treatment

Acute atelectasis, such as in postoperative or in other hospitalized patients, can respond to deep breathing or incentive spirometry exercises as well as coughing. Other airway clearance techniques may help with improving atelectasis. If simple measures do not improve the lung collapse, fiberoptic bronchoscopy can be performed to suction secretions that may be causing the atelectasis. Prevention of atelectasis should be the goal for all hospitalized patients who are unconscious or who may have poor airway clearance techniques, have postoperative pain preventing adequate inspiration and cough, or who demonstrate respiratory muscle weakness.

For additional therapeutic management, see practice pattern 6C (Impaired Ventilation and Respiration/Gas Exchange Associated with Airway Clearance Dysfunction) or 6B (Impaired Aerobic Capacity/Endurance Associated with Deconditioning).[11]

## Pneumonia

Pneumonia is an inflammatory process of the lung parenchyma. This inflammation usually begins with an infection in the lower respiratory tract that may be caused by various microbes, including bacteria, mycoplasmas, viruses, protozoa, or a psittacosis agent. There are two categories of pneumonias: community-acquired pneumonias and hospital-acquired or nosocomial pneumonias.[13,28]

## Etiology

Community-acquired pneumonias can be traced to the causative agent in approximately 50% of cases.[26] Although bacteria account for the majority of these pneumonias, viruses cause about one third of the pneumonias in this category.[26] More than 1 million cases of bacterial pneumonia occur each year in the United States. Approximately 50,000 people die of this disease, making it the fifth most common cause of death in the nation.[2] The most common agent causing bacterial pneumonia is *Streptococcus pneumoniae*, commonly called pneumococcus. Other bacterial agents that cause community-acquired pneumonias are *Legionella pneumophila*, *Haemophilus influenzae*, enteric gram-negative bacteria, *Staphylococcus aureus*, and anaerobic bacteria often found in the oropharynx. The mycoplasmal agent *M. pneumoniae*, the psittacosis agent *Chlamydia psittaci*, and the protozoan *Pneumocystis carinii* can also cause community-acquired pneumonias. The viruses that are most commonly involved in community-acquired pneumonias are adenovirus, influenza virus, herpes group viruses (including cytomegalovirus), parainfluenza virus, respiratory syncytial virus, and Hantavirus, which can lead to severe ARDS. Hantavirus was the cause of multiple deaths during an epidemic in the southwestern United States in 1993.[9]

Although there are many infectious agents in the environment, few pneumonias develop because of the efficient defense mechanisms in the lung. Those who develop community-acquired pneumonias usually have been infected with an exceedingly virulent organism or a particularly large inoculum or have impaired or damaged lung defense mechanisms.[26]

Hospital-acquired or nosocomial pneumonias are defined as infections in the lower respiratory tract with an onset of 72 hours or more after hospitalization; they are characterized by the development of a new or progressive lung infiltrate.[26] Nosocomial pneumonias account for 10% of all nosocomial infections.[8] These opportunistic infections prey on the sickest patients in the hospital. The rate of nosocomial infections in the United States is 5.7 per 100 admissions or more than 2 million per year.[8] The most commonly identified causative agent of nosocomial pneumonias is a gram-negative bacillus, *Pseudomonas aeruginosa*.[26] Other microbes also capable of causing hospital-acquired pneumonias are *S. aureus*, *Klebsiella pneumoniae*, and *P. carinii*. The patients most likely to develop a nosocomial pneumonia have one or more of the following risk factors: nasogastric tube placement; intubation; dysphagia; tracheostomy; mechanical ventilation; thoracoabdominal surgery; lung injury; diabetes; chronic cardiopulmonary disease; intraabdominal infection; uremia; shock; history of smoking; advanced age; poor nutritional status; or certain therapeutic interventions, such as the administration of broad-spectrum antibiotics, corticosteroids, antacids, or high oxygen concentrations.

## Pathophysiology

Bacteria and other microbes commonly enter the lower respiratory tract. It has been estimated that during sleep, 45% of healthy people aspirate oropharyngeal secretions into the lower respiratory tract.[8] However, microbial entrance into the lower respiratory tree usually does not lead to pneumonia because of the elaborate defense mechanisms within the pulmonary system. The mechanical defenses include cough, bronchoconstriction, angulation of the airways favoring impaction and subsequent transport upward, and action of the mucociliary escalator. The immune defenses include bronchus-associated lymphoid tissue, phagocytosis by polymorphonuclear cells and macrophages, immunoglobulins A and G, complement, surfactant, and cell-mediated immunity by T lymphocytes.[26]

The most common routes for infection leading to pneumonia are inhalation and aspiration (Table 5-8). When the causative agent is bacterial, the first response to infection is an outpouring of edema fluid. This is followed rapidly by the appearance of polymorphonuclear leukocytes that are involved in active phagocytosis of the bacteria, and then fibrin is deposited in the inflamed area. Usually by Day 5, specific antibodies are in the area fighting the bacterial infection. Clinically, bacterial pneumonia usually has an abrupt onset and is characterized by lobar consolidation, high fever, chills, dyspnea, tachypnea, productive cough, pleuritic pain, and leukocytosis.[1,25,26] When the causative

## Table 5-8 Pneumonia Transmission and Treatment

| Pneumonia Type | Transmission Route | Susceptible Populations | Preferred Drug |
|---|---|---|---|
| **Bacterial** | | | |
| *Streptococcus pneumonia* | Droplet inhalation<br>Direct contact with infected respiratory secretions<br>Indirect contact with articles soiled by infected respiratory secretions | Infants, elderly<br>Patients having congestive heart failure, COPD, splenectomy, alcoholism, multiple myeloma, or a predisposing viral infection | Penicillin G<br>Tetracyclines<br>Ampicillin |
| *Legionella pneumophila* | Inhalation of an aerosolized infected water source (drinking water, air conditioning, shower heads, lakes) | Elderly<br>Patients having diabetes, COPD, AIDS, renal transplantation, malignancy, and alcoholism<br>Smokers | Erythromycin |
| *Haemophilus influenzae* | Droplet inhalation<br>Direct contact with infected respiratory secretions<br>Indirect contact with articles soiled by infected respiratory secretions | Elderly<br>Patients having chronic bronchitis, AIDS, alcoholism, splenectomy, chronic debilitation, or a predisposing viral infection | Ampicillin<br>Cephalosporins |
| *Klebsiella pneumoniae* | Droplet inhalation<br>Direct contact with infected respiratory secretions<br>Indirect contact with articles soiled by infected respiratory secretions | Elderly in nursing homes<br>Patients having COPD, alcoholism, diabetes, malignancy, chronic renal failure, and chronic debilitation | Aminoglycosides<br>Cephalosporins |
| *Pseudomonas aeruginosa* | Droplet inhalation<br>Direct contact with infected respiratory secretions<br>Indirect contact with articles soiled by infected respiratory secretions<br>Hematogenously<br>Wound infection | Patients having cystic fibrosis, ARDS, or neutropenia<br>Patients on mechanical ventilation | Carbenicillin<br>Aztreonam<br>Aminoglycosides |
| *Staphylococcus aureus* | Droplet inhalation<br>Direct contact with infected respiratory secretions<br>Indirect contact with articles soiled by infected respiratory secretions<br>Hematogenously<br>Aspiration | Patients having cystic fibrosis, drug addictions, splenectomy, or a predisposing viral infection | Antistaphylococcal penicillin<br>Cephalosporins<br>Vancomycin<br>Clindamycin<br>Gentamicin |
| **Mycoplasmal** | | | |
| *Mycoplasma pneumoniae* | Droplet inhalation<br>Direct contact with infected respiratory secretions<br>Indirect contact with articles soiled by infected respiratory secretions | School children<br>College students<br>Patients with AIDS | Erythromycin<br>Tetracycline<br>Streptomycin |
| **Viral** | | | |
| Respiratory syncytial virus | Droplet inhalation<br>Direct contact with infected respiratory secretions<br>Indirect contact with articles soiled by infected respiratory secretions | Infants 2–5 months of age and school-aged children | Ribavirin |

## Table 5-8 Pneumonia Transmission and Treatment—cont'd

| Pneumonia Type | Transmission Route | Susceptible Populations | Preferred Drug |
|---|---|---|---|
| Adenovirus | Droplet inhalation<br>Direct contact with infected respiratory secretions or infected feces<br>Indirect contact with articles soiled by infected respiratory secretions or feces | Children 6 months to 5 years and military recruits | None |
| Cytomegalovirus | Contact with infected body fluids, including tears, saliva, blood, breast milk, urine, semen<br>Can be infected in utero and by infected transplanted organs | Fetuses<br>Patients having malignancy, AIDS, major organ transplantation, or chronic debilitation | Acyclovir analogue |
| Influenza virus | Droplet inhalation<br>Direct contact with infected respiratory secretions<br>Indirect contact with articles soiled by infected respiratory secretions | Women in the third trimester of pregnancy<br>Elderly<br>Patients having malignancy, heart disease, COPD, diabetes, chronic renal failure, neuromuscular disorders, or chronic debilitation | Amantadine |
| **Fungal** | | | |
| *Pneumocystis carinii* | Unknown, probably droplet inhalation | Premature infants<br>Patients with AIDS, or chronic debilitation | Trimethoprim-sulfamethoxazole<br>Pentamidine |
| **Chlamydial** | | | |
| *Chlamydia psittaci* | Inhalation of infected droplets, droplet nuclei, or dust from the desiccated dropping of infected birds (parrots, parakeets, turkeys, pigeons, chickens) | Persons with pet birds and workers on poultry farms and in poultry processing plants | Tetracycline<br>Chloramphenicol |

*AIDS, acquired immunodeficiency syndrome; ARDS, adult respiratory distress syndrome; COPD, chronic obstructive pulmonary disease.*
*From Cottrell GP, Surkin HB. Pharmacology for Respiratory Care Practitioners. Philadelphia, 1995, FA Davis.*

agent is viral, the virus first localizes in respiratory epithelial cells and causes destruction of the cilia and mucosal surface, leading to the loss of mucociliary function. This impairment may then predispose the patient to bacterial pneumonia. If viral infection reaches the level of the alveoli, there may be edema, hemorrhage, hyaline membrane formation, and possibly the development of adult respiratory distress syndrome. Primary viral pneumonia is a serious disease with diffuse infiltrates, extensive parenchymal injury, and severe hypoxemia. Clinically, viral pneumonia usually has an insidious onset and is characterized by patchy diffuse bronchopulmonary infiltrates, moderate fever, dyspnea, tachypnea, nonproductive cough, myalgia, and a normal white blood cell count.[26] Usually, it is impossible to identify the specific pathogen by clinical signs and symptoms or chest radiographic findings. Specific laboratory test results and other data are needed.

## Clinical Manifestation
The clinical manifestation of pneumonia can be found in Table 5-9.

## Treatment
Drug therapy is the primary focus in the treatment of pneumonia, particularly antibiotics for treating bacterial pneumonia. Antibiotic therapy should be pathogen specific if the pathogen can be determined; if not, an empiric regimen of multiple antibiotics may be needed. Oxygen and temporary mechanical ventilation or noninvasive ventilation may be necessary in patients with refractory hypoxemia ($PaO_2$ less than 60 mm Hg). Other supportive therapy includes postural drainage, percussion, vibration, and assisted coughing techniques for patients who are producing more than 30 mL per day of mucus or have an impaired cough mechanism.[26] Adequate hydration and nutrition are also

## Table 5-9 Clinical Manifestation of Pneumonia

| | | Findings |
|---|---|---|
| Signs | Pulmonary function tests | ↓ lung volumes, ↓ lung compliance, ↓ gas exchange ↑ RR, ↑ inspiratory pressure, ↑ work of breathing |
| | | ↑ ventilation–perfusion mismatching, ↓ oxygen uptake |
| | | Pulmonary capillary leakage |
| | | Resolution of pneumonia may result in fibrosis & scarring |
| | Chest radiograph | Bacterial: |
| | |   Lobar consolidation in one or more lobes |
| | | Viral |
| | |   Bilateral bronchopneumonia: diffuse scattered fluffy shadows indicating patchy alveolar infiltrates |
| | |   Necrotizing pneumonia: when cavities present |
| | Arterial blood gases | ↓ $PaO_2$, may have ↓ $PaCO_2$ as a result of breathing pattern blowing off $CO_2$ |
| | Breath sounds | May have bronchial sounds above lobar pneumonia, absent breath sounds over pneumonia and dull to mediate percussion |
| | | May also have bubbling rales, rhonchi, decreased or absent sounds, egophony, and whispering pectoriloquy |
| | Cardiovascular | Usually have ↑ HR, especially in presence of fever |
| Symptoms | | Bacterial: high fever, chills, dyspnea, tachypnea, productive cough, pleuritic pain |
| | | Viral: moderate fever, dyspnea, tachypnea, nonproductive cough, myalgias |

*HR, heart rate; $PaCO_2$, arterial partial pressure of $CO_2$; $PaO_2$, arterial partial pressure of $O_2$; RR, respiratory rate.*

important. Nosocomial pneumonias can also be prevented by rigorous environmental controls in hospitals. Such controls include strict guideline adherence for the prevention of contamination of ventilators and other respiratory equipment, careful aseptic patient care practices, and surveillance of infections and antibiotic susceptibility patterns in high-risk areas.

Pneumonia is simply an inflammatory process of some part of the lung where gas exchange occurs that progresses beyond inflammation and develops into infection. The key to treatment of pneumonia is to first identify the microbe (virus vs gram-positive or gram-negative bacteria). Specific medical treatment (specific antibiotic) is based on identification of the microbe, although broad-spectrum medications may be initiated before identification has been made.

> **Clinical Tip**
> The problem with treating pneumonia in recent years is the identification of microbes that are resistant to many forms of antibiotics. These microbes can be spread via aerosol or physical contact and can cause severe disability and even death in immunosuppressed individuals. (Some of the common ones are methicillin-resistant *Staphylococcus aureus* (MRSA) and Clostridium difficile [C-diff].)

For additional therapeutic management see practice pattern 6C (Impaired Ventilation and Respiration/Gas Exchange Associated with Airway Clearance Dysfunction) or 6B (Impaired Aerobic Capacity/Endurance Associated with Deconditioning).[11]

## Specific Pneumonias
### Bacterial Pneumonias

**Streptococcus pneumoniae.** *Streptococcus pneumoniae* (*S. pneumoniae*) is more common in the elderly, in alcoholics, and in those with asplenia, multiple myeloma, congestive heart failure, or chronic obstructive lung disease. Seventy percent of patients report a preceding viral illness.[26] This type of pneumonia occurs more frequently during the winter and early spring. Specific signs and symptoms include rusty-colored sputum, hemoptysis, bronchial breath sounds, egophony, increased tactile fremitus, pleural friction rub, severe pleuritic chest pain, pleural effusion in 25% of patients, and slight liver dysfunction.[10,26] Complications can include lung abscess, atelectasis, delayed resolution in the elderly, pericarditis, endocarditis, meningitis, jaundice, and arthritis.[25] Streptococcal pneumonia is treated with penicillin G, ampicillin or tetracyclines.[29] There is also a pneumococcal vaccine; this injection provides lifetime protection against serotypes of the pneumococcus that account for 85% of all cases of pneumococcal pneumonia.[26,29]

**Legionella Pneumophila.** *Legionella pneumophila* (*L. pneumophila*) can occur in epidemic proportions because the organism is water-borne and can emanate from air-conditioning equipment, drinking water, lakes, river banks, water faucets, and shower heads. *L. pneumophila* accounts for 7% to 15% of all community-acquired pneumonias.[26] It is found commonly in patients who are on dialysis; in persons who have a malignancy, a chronic obstructive pulmonary disease (COPD), a smoking history, or are older than 50 years; and in persons who are alcoholics or diabetics. Transplant recipients, of any organ, are at the highest risk.[10] Signs and symptoms in addition to those characteristic of bacterial pneumonias include headache, myalgias, preceding diarrhea, mental confusion, hyponatremia, bradycardia, and liver function abnormalities. Productive coughs with purulent sputum and hemoptysis can develop in 50% to 75% of patients.[10] However, most patients (90%) begin with a nonproductive cough.[10] The chest radiograph may show lobar consolidation or unilateral or bilateral bronchopneumonia; rounded densities with cavitation may also be seen. Fifteen percent of these patients have pleural effusions. The antibiotic of choice is erythromycin. Rifampin may also be used in addition to erythromycin.[26]

**Haemophilus Influenzae.** *Haemophilus influenzae* (*H. influenzae*) causes pneumonia particularly in children who have had their spleen removed, in patients with COPD, in alcoholics, in AIDS patients, in those with lung cancer, in patients with hypogammaglobulinemia, and in the elderly.[9] In addition to the expected signs and symptoms of bacterial pneumonia, *H. influenzae* often causes a sore throat. The chest radiograph may show focal lobar, lobular, multilobar, or patchy bronchopneumonia or segmental pneumonia that usually involves the lower lobes. Complications can include empyema, lung abscess, epiglottitis, otitis media, pericarditis, meningitis, and arthritis. The preferred antibiotic is ampicillin; however, 20% of patients have been shown to be resistant to ampicillin. In these cases, cephalosporins, trimethoprim–sulfamethoxazole, and chloramphenicol are used.[25,26]

**Klebsiella Pneumoniae.** *Klebsiella pneumoniae* (*K. pneumoniae*) may cause either a community-acquired pneumonia or a nosocomial pneumonia. The community-acquired Klebsiella pneumonia is seen most commonly in men over the age of 40 who are alcoholic or diabetic or who have underlying pulmonary disease. These patients may show purulent blood-streaked sputum, hemoptysis, cyanosis, and hypotension. Chest radiographic findings most frequently show right-sided involvement of the posterior segment of the upper lobe or the lower lobe segments. There may be outward bulging of a lobar fissure as a result of edema, and 25% to 50% of these patients have lung abscesses.[25] Complications include empyema, lung abscess, pneumothorax, chronic pneumonia, pericarditis, meningitis, and anemia. Treatment includes a two-drug therapy: an aminoglycoside and a cephalosporin. Oxygen is also used to maintain an oxygen saturation level of 80% to 85%. The mortality rate for this gram-negative pneumonia is 20%.[25]

Nosocomial Klebsiella pneumonia is a fulminant infection that causes severe lung damage and has a 50% mortality rate.[26] It affects debilitated patients in hospitals and nursing homes, middle-aged or older, who suffer from concomitant alcoholism, diabetes, malignancy, or chronic renal or cardiopulmonary disease. Their sputum is thick, purulent, and bloody or is thin and has a "currant jelly" texture. Tachycardia is common. The chest radiograph can show lobar consolidation, usually in the upper lobes, with lung abscesses, cavities, scarring, and fibrosis. A bronchopneumonia appearance may also occur. Complications are the same as those in community-acquired Klebsiella pneumonia. Drug therapy includes the use of aminoglycosides, cephalosporin, and antipseudomonal penicillin.[25,26]

**Pseudomonas Aeruginosa.** *Pseudomonas aeruginosa* (*P. aeruginosa*) is a gram-negative bacillus and is the most common cause of nosocomial pneumonias. It causes 15% of all hospital-acquired pneumonias and affects 40% of all mechanically ventilated patients.[26] Those at most risk for this infection are patients with cystic fibrosis, bronchiectasis, tracheostomy, or neutropenia or those who are on mechanical ventilation or corticosteroid therapy. This necrotizing pneumonia causes alveolar septal necrosis, microabscesses, and vascular thrombosis and has a mortality rate of 70% in postoperative patients.[26] Signs and symptoms include confusion, bradycardia, and hemorrhagic pleural effusion. The chest radiograph shows bilateral patchy alveolar infiltrates, usually in the lower lobes with nodular infiltrates and cavitation.[26] Treatment always involves two drugs. Aminoglycosides, carbenicillin, and aztreonam are used to overcome this bacterium.[29]

**Staphylococcus Aureus.** *Staphylococcus aureus* (*S. aureus*) causes approximately 5% of community-acquired pneumonias and can also cause nosocomial pneumonia.[26] This type of pneumonia is usually seen in infants and children under the age of 2 years, in patients with cystic fibrosis or COPD, or in patients who are recovering from influenza. The hallmark lesion seen in this pneumonia is ulcerative bronchiolitis with necrosis of the bronchiolar wall.[29] Signs and symptoms include cough with dirty salmon-pink purulent sputum, high fever, dyspnea, and pleuritic chest pain.[29] Other manifestations commonly seen in children are cyanosis, labored breathing, grunting, flaring of the nostrils, and chest wall retractions. The chest radiograph shows a diffuse bronchopneumonia, with bilateral infiltrates, cavitary lung abscesses, pneumatoceles, and pleural effusions. Complications include pneumothorax, lung abscess, endocarditis, and meningitis. Treatment is with antistaphylococcal penicillin, cephalosporin, vancomycin, clindamycin, and gentamicin.[25,26,29]

**Mycoplasma Pneumonias.** Mycoplasmas are the smallest free-living organisms that have yet been identified. This class of organisms is intermediate between bacteria and viruses. Unlike bacteria they have no rigid cell wall, and unlike viruses they do not require the intracellular machinery of a host cell to replicate.

**Mycoplasma Pneumoniae.** *Mycoplasma pneumoniae* (*M. pneumoniae*) is seen in all age groups but is more common in persons less than 20 years old. Mycoplasma pneumonias account for 20% of all community-acquired pneumonias.[26] This infection is common year round, but usually the incidence increases in the fall and winter. Mycoplasma pneumonia has also been termed walking pneumonia because the respiratory symptoms are often not severe enough for people to seek medical attention. The course of the disease is approximately 4 weeks, and it is very infectious; whole families may become ill once a child brings it into the home. The signs and symptoms often include many extrapulmonary manifestations that are not common in bacterial or viral pneumonias. Patients may have fever, shaking chills, dry cough, headache, malaise, sore throat, ear ache, arthralgias, arthritis, immune dysfunction with an autoantibody response, meningoencephalitis, meningitis, transverse myelitis, cranial nerve palsies, Guillain–Barré syndrome, myocarditis, pericarditis, gastroenteritis, pancreatitis, glomerulonephritis, hepatitis, generalized lymphadenopathy, and erythema multiforme, including Stevens–Johnson syndrome.[10] The chest radiograph shows interstitial infiltrates, usually unilateral in the lower lobe; 20% of patients have a pleural effusion. Treatment is with erythromycin, tetracycline, or streptomycin.[26,29]

### Viral Pneumonias

Cytomegalovirus, varicella zoster, and herpes simplex cause viral pneumonias most commonly in immunocompromised hosts, such as patients who have had major organ transplants or who have AIDS or malignancy. The respiratory syncytial virus and the parainfluenza virus cause viral pneumonias in children. The adenovirus is a source of viral pneumonias in children and in military recruits. Viral pneumonias in the debilitated elderly are most commonly caused by the influenza virus. Persons most at risk for a viral pneumonia are those who have an underlying cardiopulmonary disease or who are immunosuppressed or pregnant. Complications of viral pneumonias include secondary bacterial infections, bronchial hyperreactivity and possibly asthma, chronic air flow obstruction, tracheitis, bronchitis, bronchiolitis, and acellular hyaline membrane formation.

Some antiviral agents are now available. Acyclovir is used against herpes simplex and varicella-zoster. Amantadine is the drug of choice for influenza A. Ribavirin is used in children to treat the respiratory syncytial virus. Cytomegalovirus is treated with acyclovir analogue dihydroxyphenylglycol (DHPG). No drug therapy is available for all the varieties of viral agents, so treatment is often limited to supportive measures.[25,26]

### Fungal Pneumonias

**Pneumocystis carinii.** *Pneumocystis carinii* (*P. carinii*), originally described as a protozoan, is now thought to be a fungal organism.[10] *Pneumocystis carinii* pneumonia (PCP) is closely associated with AIDS because nearly 75% of AIDS patients have at least one episode of PCP during their lifetime.[10] Patients with AIDS have impairment of T-cell function as well as humoral immune dysfunction and thus are susceptible to infection from bacteria, viruses, fungi, and parasites. PCP is also seen in transplant patients, especially those on cyclosporine, and in patients with lymphoreticular hematologic malignancies.[9] The chest radiograph most commonly shows bilateral diffuse interstitial or alveolar infiltrates, more prominent in the perihilar regions, and a solitary pulmonary nodule.[9] PCP damages the parenchymal cells within the lung and alters the alveolar-capillary permeability. This type of pneumonia usually has a subacute course of fever, dyspnea, cough, chest pain, malaise, fatigue, weight loss, and night sweats, but the symptoms can progress to include tachypnea, reduced $PaO_2$, and cyanosis.[9] Treatment is with trimethoprim-sulfamethoxazole. If this drug is not tolerated, then pentamidine is prescribed.[9,13,26]

### Chlamydial Pneumonias

**Chlamydia psittaci.** *Chlamydia psittaci* (*C. psittaci*) causes approximately 12% of the community-acquired pneumonias in the student population and about 6% of the community-acquired pneumonias in the elderly.[26] The onset is usually insidious, with cough, sputum, hemoptysis, dyspnea, headache, myalgia, and hepatosplenomegaly.[9,10] Complications include laryngitis, pharyngitis, encephalitis, hemolytic anemia, bradycardia, hepatitis, renal failure, and macular rash. Treatment is with tetracycline or chloramphenicol.[9,10]

## Adult Respiratory Distress Syndrome/Acute Lung Injury

Adult respiratory distress syndrome (ARDS) is a clinical syndrome caused by acute lung injury (ALI) and characterized by severe hypoxemia (acute respiratory failure) and increased permeability of the alveolar-capillary membrane. It also has been known as noncardiogenic pulmonary edema, shock lung, ALI, increased permeability pulmonary edema, and posttraumatic pulmonary insufficiency.[2,8,26,28,30]

### Etiology

Adult respiratory distress syndrome can result from a variety of causes. Some of the primary causes of ARDS include[2,8,26,28,30]:

- Trauma: Fat emboli, lung contusion, heart–lung transplantation, head injury
- Aspiration: Drowning, gastric contents
- Drug associated: Heroin, barbiturates, narcotics, Amiodarone
- Inhaled toxins: Smoke, high oxygen concentrations
- Shock: Any cause
- Massive blood transfusion: Sepsis
- Metabolic: Acute pancreatitis, uremia
- Primary pneumonias: Viral, bacterial, *P. carinii*
- Other: Increased intracranial pressure, post–cardiopulmonary bypass, amniotic fluid embolism, ascent to high altitudes

Approximately 150,000 cases of ARDS are diagnosed annually in the United States.[26]

> **Clinical Tip**
> A diagnosis of ARDS is a serious, life-threatening diagnosis, as these patients have a high in-hospital mortality rate and poor in-hospital prognosis. Less than 50% of the patients with this diagnosis live.

## Pathophysiology

The primary pathologic change is an increase in the permeability of the microvascular pulmonary membrane (Fig. 5-7). The specific cause of this change is unknown. It seems that a variety of mechanisms can be involved, depending on the specific associated etiology. Therefore, the exact mechanisms that damage the pulmonary capillary endothelial cells and the alveolar epithelial cells are still under investigation. The current theories under investigation involve the role of the neutrophils, the complement pathway, the superoxide radicals, the proteolytic enzymes, and the coagulation system.[2] When the permeability of the microvascular membrane increases, excess fluid and plasma proteins are allowed to

move out of the vascular channel. This fluid leaks into the interstitial tissue and then crosses the usually tight alveolar epithelium to fill the alveoli. The change from an air-filled to a fluid-filled organ decreases markedly the compliance of the lung and all lung volumes and capacities; the work of breathing is increased. The alveoli lose their ability to exchange $O_2$ and $CO_2$. Pulmonary vascular resistance is increased; an intrapulmonary right-to-left shunt takes place; ventilation–perfusion mismatching is increased; and gas exchange is drastically reduced. In addition, surfactant production is decreased. The significant atelectasis due to edema in the interstitial spaces leads to increased pressure on the adjacent bronchioles and alveoli.[6,26]

Following this acute phase, ARDS may resolve completely so that the patient regains normal lung function after a period of a few months. However, some patients enter a subacute phase following ARDS. During this phase, alveolar fibrosis and capillary obliteration develop within the lung, which leads to chronic significant restrictive dysfunction. It is not

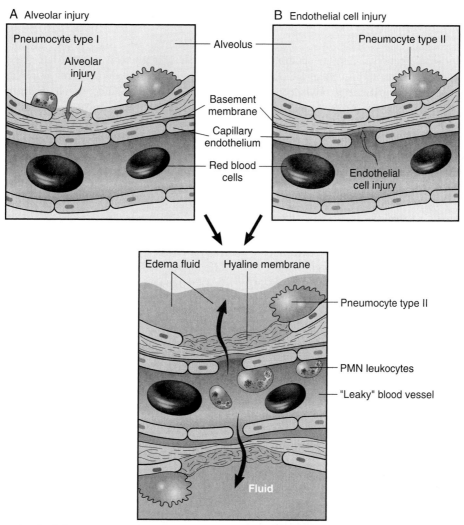

**Figure 5-7** Pathogenesis of adult respiratory distress syndrome. **A,** Alveolar cell injury. **B,** Endothelial cell injury. Regardless of the initial injury, the established lesions appear identical and comprise hyaline membranes, ruptured alveolar walls, and intraalveolar edema fluid. PMN, polymorphonuclear neutrophil. (From Damjanov I. Pathology for the Health Professions, ed 3. St. Louis, 2006, Saunders.)

## Table 5-10 Clinical Manifestation of Adult Respiratory Distress Syndrome

| | | Findings |
|---|---|---|
| Signs | Pulmonary function tests | ↓ FRC, ↓ VC, ↓ VT and ↓ lung compliance with ↑ work of breathing and ↑ RR |
| | | Flow rates normal or ↓ slightly, ↓ DLCO |
| | Chest radiograph | Symmetric bilateral diffuse fluffy infiltrates |
| | | May coalesce into diffuse haze or lung white out |
| | | May also have findings of COPD, atelectasis, or pneumonia |
| | Arterial blood gases | ↓ $PaO_2$ (<60 mm Hg),[8] ↓ $PaCO_2$ unless patient had previous $CO_2$ retention issues; then $PaCO_2$ is ↑ |
| | Breath sounds | ↓ breath sounds over fluid-filled areas of lungs, wet rales, wheezing and rhonchi may also be heard |
| | Cardiovascular | Tachycardia, may have arrhythmias due to hypoxemia |
| Symptoms | | Appear acutely ill; dyspneic at rest and with any activity |
| | | Breathing pattern fast and labored |
| | | Cyanotic |
| | | May have impaired mental status, restlessness, headache, and ↑ anxiety |

*COPD, chronic obstructive pulmonary disease; DLCO, diffusing capacity of the lungs for carbon monoxide; FRC, functional residual capacity; $PaCO_2$, arterial partial pressure of $CO_2$; $PaO_2$, arterial partial pressure of $O_2$; RR, respiratory rate; VC, vital capacity; VT, tidal volume.*

clear why ARDS in some patients resolves completely whereas in others significant permanent lung damage occurs. It is known that the longer the patient is on mechanical ventilation and high concentrations of oxygen, the poorer is the long-term prognosis.[26]

### Clinical Manifestation

The clinical manifestation of ARDS can be found in Table 5-10.

### Treatment

The treatment of ARDS can be divided into four areas, each with a distinct goal. The first area is treatment of the precipitating cause of the ARDS. Because of the wide variety of causes for ARDS, there is a wide range of treatment protocols used to address the underlying cause. The second area of treatment is aimed at supporting adequate gas exchange and tissue oxygenation until the ARDS resolves. Maintaining an adequate airway and oxygenation is usually accomplished by intubating and mechanically ventilating the patient. Most often the patient is placed on a volume-cycled ventilator with supplemental oxygen. Positive end-expiratory pressure (PEEP) of approximately 5 to 15 cm $H_2O$ is often utilized.[26] The PEEP helps inflate poorly ventilated alveoli, improves gas exchange, and permits the inspired oxygen concentration to be lowered, decreasing the risk of oxygen toxicity. Positioning the patient in the prone position is also recommended, even with the presence of mechanical ventilation, to improve the ventilation in posterior lobes/lung fields.[31] Sixty-day survival rates were improved in prone-positioned patients and $PaO_2/FIO_2$ was higher in those patients positioned prone versus supine. The third area of treatment is supportive, managing the patient's nutritional status and fluid balance. Fluid and electrolyte balance is very

important in these patients. Management may mean monitoring input and output and using diuretics. Or because ARDS can be associated with multiorgan failure, it may mean the use of highly technical interventions such as continuous arteriovenous hemofiltration (CAVH) or dialysis in patients with chronic renal insufficiency.[8] The final focus of treatment is to prevent and treat complications of the patient's condition along with intensive care measures. Complications common in patients with ARDS are nosocomial infections, pulmonary barotrauma due to the use of PEEP, and coagulation disturbances. The prognosis in ARDS is always guarded; mortality can be as high as 50% to 70%, especially if this syndrome is associated with failure in other organ systems or is complicated by serious or repeated infections.[8,26]

Predictors of poor prognosis include the elderly (>70 years of age), the immunocompromised, individuals with chronic liver disease, and those with increased dead space formation. Only 34% of individuals with and ARDS or ALI diagnosis are discharged directly from hospital to home. In addition, all patients with ARDS suffer some degree of muscle wasting and weakness, which continues past 1 year postdischarge. Corticosteroids are believed to play a role in some of this muscle wasting/weakness.[32]

For additional therapeutic management, see practice pattern 6E (Impaired Ventilation and Respiration/Gas Exchange Associated with Ventilatory Pump Dysfunction or Failure).[11]

### Bronchogenic Carcinoma

Bronchogenic carcinoma is a malignant growth of abnormal epithelial cells arising in a bronchus.[26] This growth or tumor may spread by infiltrating surrounding tissues or by metastasizing to other body organs, or both (Fig. 5-8). The

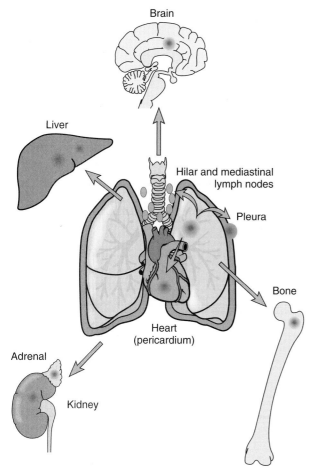

**Figure 5-8** Primary lung cancer metastasizes to pleura, lymph, bone, brain, kidney, and liver. (From Damjanov I. Pathology for the Health Professions, ed 3. St. Louis, 2006, Saunders.)

and continue smoking, after 50 years they have a 100-fold increased risk of lung cancer over that of a nonsmoker.[10] Passive smoking, that is, exposure to cigarette smoke exhaled by a smoker as well as side-stream smoke, also has been shown to increase the incidence of lung cancer by approximately 20%. Like active smoking at an early age, passive smoking during childhood and adolescence may pose a significantly increased risk.[10] It is currently estimated that there are 500 to 5000 lung cancer deaths per year in the United States due to passive smoking.[9,10]

Occupational agents have also been implicated in the development of bronchogenic carcinoma. The known carcinogens present in the workplace include radioactive material, asbestos, chromates, nickel, mustard gas, isopropyl oil, hydrocarbons, arsenic, hematite, vinyl chloride, and bischloromethyl ether.[26] Increased exposure to radon or significant air pollution also increases the incidence of lung cancer, although the relationship is very difficult to quantify. It is interesting that diets containing beta carotene (found in many green, yellow, and orange fruits and vegetables) have been shown to modestly decrease the risk for lung and other cancers.[20] In some individuals and families, a genetic predisposition for the development of lung cancer seems to be present.

Globally, it is estimated that one death occurs each minute as a result of lung cancer.[10] Currently, lung cancer accounts for 33% of all cancer deaths in men and 23% of all cancer deaths in women and is the second most common cancer. Over the past 20 years the male–female ratio of lung cancer deaths has dropped from 5.7:1 to 1.4:1 as a result of the striking increase in lung cancer among women, which began about 1965.[9] It is now the leading cause of death from cancer in both men and women (surpassing breast cancer). In 2008, approximately 159,400 Americans died of lung cancer, 88,900 men and 70,5000 women.[20] In the same year, almost 219,000 new cases of lung cancer were diagnosed.[26] Lung cancer prognosis is bleak and unchanging. About 41% of patients die within 1 year of the diagnosis. The 5-year survival rates have not changed significantly over the past 3 decades (15%). This means that of the 219,000 Americans diagnosed with lung cancer in 2008, only 30,000 will live to see the year 2013.[20] The majority of these people could have been spared this diagnosis, with its pain, health care costs, morbidity, and unrelenting fatal conclusion, if they had given up smoking.

## Pathophysiology

Each of the four major types of bronchogenic carcinoma is discussed separately (see Fig. 5-9).

Squamous cell carcinoma accounts for 15% to 25% of all lung cancer. It arises from the bronchial mucosa after repeated inflammation or irritation caused by cancer stimuli. It is therefore the type of lung cancer most closely associated with cigarette smoking. Squamous cell carcinoma often arises in the segmental or subsegmental bronchi but can also cause a hilar tumor. It is considered a centrally located tumor and occurs in the peripheral lung only about 30% of the time. Squamous cell tumors are bulky. They cause obstructive

World Health Organization (WHO) previously established a standard classification system that organizes bronchogenic carcinoma into four major types. They are squamous cell carcinoma, small cell carcinoma, adenocarcinoma, and large cell carcinoma (Fig. 5-9).[26] Currently, the International Association for the Study of Lung Cancer (IASLC) has now revised the WHO classification system and defines two main types of lung cancer: non–small cell lung cancer (includes squamous cell, adenocarcinoma, bronchioalveolar and large cell undifferentiated) which accounts for 80% of lung cancers and small cell lung cancer (which accounts for 20% of lung cancers).

## Etiology

The causes of lung cancer are many. However, it has now been well established through numerous studies that the primary causative factor is tobacco use. Approximately 80% to 90% of lung cancers are caused by tobacco.[10] The average cigarette smoker has 10 times the risk of developing lung cancer as the nonsmoker. The heavy cigarette smoker may have up to 25 times the risk of developing lung cancer as the nonsmoker.[10,26] Most disturbing is the finding that lung cancer risk is closely related to starting to smoke at an early age. When children start smoking at 15 years of age or younger

| Type | Squamous cell carcinoma | Small cell carcinoma Oat cell | Adenocarcinoma | Large cell carcinoma |
|---|---|---|---|---|
| Incidence % of all lung CA | 50% | 30% | 15% | 15% |
| Male/female ratio | 4:1 | 3:1 | 3:2 | 3:1 |
| Frequent sites of incidence | 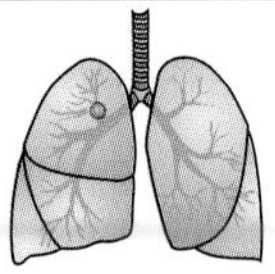 Hilium | 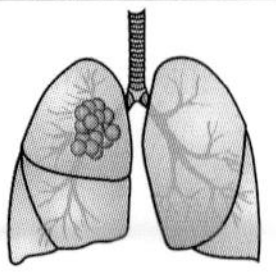 Hilum, but frequently involves lymph nodes— When detected: already metastatic | 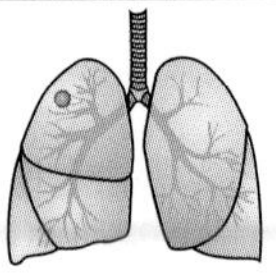 Periphery usually 4 cm or less in diameter | 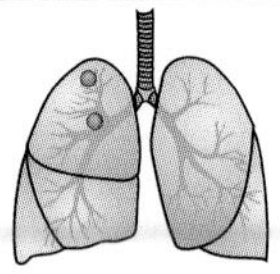 Various— either peripheral or central |
| Relationship with smoking | great | GREAT | LOW | GREAT |
| Growth rate | relatively slow | extremely rapid | moderate | rapid |
| Metastatic tendencies | slow, metastasis to hilar lymph nodes | extremely rapid... to mediastinal and distal lymph nodes | moderate | rapid |
| Operability | good | almost none | poor | poor |

**Figure 5-9** The four most common types of lung cancer are described and compared in regard to several features, including incidence, pattern of development, growth rate, and gender representation.

dysfunction because they extend into the bronchial lumen, which can prevent airflow and lead to atelectasis and pneumonia. They cause restrictive dysfunction because the tumor can compress the surrounding lung tissue; cause atelectasis and pneumonia, both of which decrease the ventilation–perfusion matching; and impair gas exchange. These tumors often cavitate but do not metastasize early. When squamous cell cancer does metastasize, it most often involves the liver, adrenal gland, central nervous system, and pancreas.[26]

Small cell carcinoma, also called oat cell carcinoma, accounts for 20% to 25% of all lung cancer.[2] It may arise in any part of the bronchial tree; however, 75% of the time it presents as a centrally located proximal lesion.[26] It often has hilar or mediastinal lymph node involvement. This tumor usually does not extend into the bronchial lumen but spreads through the submucosa and can cause obstructive and restrictive dysfunction through compression of the surrounding lung tissue. This type of lung cancer rapidly involves the vascular channels, lymph nodes, and soft tissue. It is known to metastasize widely and early and in most patients has metastasized by the time the diagnosis is made. This tumor rarely cavitates but commonly produces hormones that can lead to a wide variety of symptoms in many different body systems not involved in direct metastasis.

A number of body organs, however, are involved in direct metastasis. Seventy-five percent of small cell carcinoma metastasizes to the central nervous system, 65% to the liver, 58% to the adrenal gland, 30% to the pancreas, 28% to bone, 20% to the genitourinary system, 10% to the thyroid, and 10% to the spleen.[26] The metastases to the central nervous system and the bone often produce clinical symptoms such as hemiplegia, epilepsy, personality changes, confusion, speech deficits, headache, bone pain, and pathologic fractures. Metastases to the liver and the adrenal glands are often clinically silent.[8] Other clinical symptoms caused by tumor hormone production that are of particular interest to the physical therapist include abnormalities in the neurologic or musculoskeletal systems. These complications of small cell carcinoma can include progressive dementia, ataxia, vertigo, sensory neuropathy with numbness and loss of reflexes, motor neuropathy with progressive muscle weakness and wasting, atrophic paresis of the proximal limb girdle musculature, marked fatigability, osteoarthropathy, arthralgia, and peripheral edema.[26]

Adenocarcinoma includes acinar adenocarcinoma, papillary adenocarcinoma, and bronchoalveolar carcinoma and accounts for 40% to 50% of all lung cancer.[9] This is now the most common type of lung cancer in the United States.[10] The majority of these tumors are located in the periphery of the lung and may not be spatially related to the bronchial tree. These tumors may arise as a solitary nodule and may involve the pleura, causing a carcinogenic pleural effusion. Adenocarcinomas metastasize widely and often involve the central nervous system, which produces neurologic symptoms

**Table 5-11 Clinical Manifestation of Bronchogenic Carcinoma**

| | | | Findings |
|---|---|---|---|
| Signs | | Pulmonary function tests | No specific characteristic abnormalities: depends on location and size of cancer |
| | | Chest radiograph | Squamous: hilar or perihilar cavitary lesion with bronchial obstruction, atelectasis, or postobstructive consolidation[8,26] |
| | | | Small cell: central mass, bulky hilar and mediastinal adenopathy[8] |
| | | | Adenocarcinoma: peripheral tumor with pleural involvement and pleural effusions[26] |
| | | | Large cell: sharply defined, large, lobulated mass in periphery that may have cavitated[26] |
| | | | Diaphragms may be elevated if tumor compresses on phrenic nerve and causes paralysis |
| | | Arterial blood gases | Hypoxemia ($\downarrow$ $PaO_2$) and hypocapnia ($\downarrow$ $PaCO_2$) |
| | | Breath sounds | Wheezing and stridor heard if bronchial obstruction |
| | | | May have atelectasis (rales) or postobstructive pneumonia (consolidation) |
| | | Cardiovascular | Superior vena cava syndrome if tumor pressing superior vena cava (neck enlargement, JVD, edema in one or both arms) |
| | | | Anemia |
| | | | Recurrent or migratory thrombophlebitis |
| | | | Cardiac arrhythmias and tamponade may also complicate condition |
| Symptoms | | | Extremely variable due to: |
| | | | Location and growth of tumor and compression surrounding tumor |
| | | | Regional extension into mediastinum |
| | | | Metastases to other body organs |
| | | | Tumor-produced hormones that affect a number of systems[8] |
| | | | Most common pulmonary symptoms: |
| | | | Cough (productive or nonproductive—often blood streaked) |
| | | | Chest pain (acute or dull) |
| | | | Central lesions cause dull, vague, persistent, poorly localized type of chest pain[8] |
| | | | Peripheral lesions usually have more localized, sharp, pleuritic-type chest pain[8] |
| | | | Clubbing of digits |
| | | | Dyspnea |
| | | | Unexplained weight loss |

*JVD, jugular venous distention; $PaCO_2$, arterial partial pressure of $CO_2$; $PaO_2$, arterial partial pressure of $O_2$.*

already listed under small cell carcinoma. Approximately half of these tumors involve the hilar and mediastinal lymph nodes.[26]

Large cell carcinoma includes all tumors not categorized in the first three groups and accounts for 15% to 18% of all lung cancer.[2] These tumors are most frequently subpleural in location. Peripheral tumors are often large, lobulated, and bulky, causing compression of the normal lung tissue. They are usually sharply defined lesions, which may be necrotic or cavitate. This type of tumor spreads locally by invasion and also metastasizes widely, with more than 50% metastasizing to the brain.[26]

Prognosis for lung cancer is usually discussed in terms of 5-year survival rates according to the stage of the disease. The assigned stage number is determined by the International Cancer Staging System and is determined by the degree of lung involvement, the location of the lesion, and the metastatic spread of the disease. The 5-year survival rate for stage I is 50%, for stage II is 30%, for stage IIIa is 17%, and for stage IIIb and stage IV is less than 5%.

## Clinical Manifestation

The clinical manifestation of bronchogenic carcinoma can be found in Table 5-11.

## Treatment

The three most widely accepted forms of therapy remain surgery, radiation, and chemotherapy. Newer treatment interventions being applied to patients with lung cancer include immunotherapy (also called targeted therapy), laser, brachytherapy, and nutritional therapy. Unfortunately, none of these newer treatment options has affected the overall survival rate of lung cancer patients. Surgical removal of the tumor remains the treatment of choice for all non–small cell lung carcinoma when the location of the tumor makes resection possible.[26] The more defined and smaller the lesion, the better the surgical success rate. Radiation has been used to treat all types of lung cancer. However, small cell lung carcinoma is the most radiosensitive, followed by squamous cell carcinoma and adenocarcinoma. Large cell carcinoma is the least responsive to radiation.[26] The response to radiation therapy depends on the size of the tumor and the intrathoracic spread of the cancer. Chemotherapy does not significantly benefit non–small cell lung carcinoma. The response rates are low, and the toxicity rates for the drugs used are high. Chemotherapy is the treatment of choice for small cell lung carcinoma.[26] Because small cell carcinoma metastasizes so early, surgery has little to offer patients with this type of cancer. Chemotherapy and radiation in combination with chemotherapy are often used to treat small cell carcinoma. See Chapter 7 for the effects of chemotherapy and radiation on the cardiopulmonary system.

For additional therapeutic management, see practice pattern 6C (Impaired Ventilation and Respiration/Gas Exchange Associated with Airway Clearance Dysfunction), 6E (Impaired Ventilation and Respiration/Gas Exchange Associated with Ventilatory Pump Dysfunction or Failure), or 6B (Impaired Aerobic Capacity/Endurance Associated with Deconditioning).[11]

## Pleural Effusion

Pleural effusion is the accumulation of fluid within the pleural space (Fig. 5-10). The fluid is a transudate if it has a low protein content and accumulates owing to changes in the hydrostatic pressure within the pleural capillaries. The fluid is an exudate if it has a high protein content and accumulates because of changes in the permeability of the pleural surfaces.[27]

## Etiology

Numerous disease entities can cause pleural effusions. Transudative pleural effusions can be caused by congestive heart failure, left ventricular failure, cirrhosis, nephrotic syndrome, pericardial disease, myxedema, pulmonary emboli, peritoneal dialysis, or atelectasis.[10] Exudative pleural effusions can be caused by bacterial or viral pneumonias, parasitic or fungal infections, tuberculosis, mesotheliomas, bronchogenic carcinoma, systemic lupus erythematosus (SLE), rheumatoid arthritis (RA), acute pancreatitis, esophageal perforations, intraabdominal abscess, asbestos exposure, uremia, sarcoidosis, or drug hypersensitivity.[20,25,27]

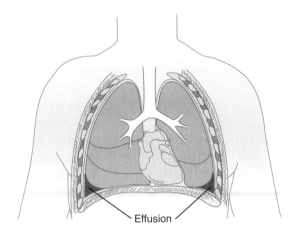

**Figure 5-10** Pleural effusion, a collection of fluid in the pleural space between the membrane encasing the lung and the membrane lining the thoracic cavity, as seen on upright x-ray examination. Pleurisy (pleuritis) is an inflammation of the visceral and parietal pleurae. When there is an abnormal increase in the lubricating fluid between these two layers, it is called pleurisy with effusion. (From Goodman CC. Pathology: Implications for the Physical Therapist, ed 3. St. Louis, 2009, Saunders.)

## Pathophysiology

The capillaries in the parietal pleura receive blood via the high-pressure systemic arterial circulation.

The capillaries in the visceral pleura receive blood via the low-pressure pulmonary circulation. Because of this pressure gradient, fluid is constantly moving from the parietal pleural capillaries into the pleural space and is then reabsorbed into the visceral pleural capillaries. Approximately 5 to 10 L of fluid pass through the pleural space each day using this route.[2] Additionally, each day up to 0.5 L of fluid and solutes can be moved out of the pleural space via the pleural lymphatics.[2,26] Normally pleural fluid formation and pleural fluid resorption are balanced, so fluid does not accumulate in the pleural space. When this balance is disrupted by any cause and a significant amount of fluid is allowed to accumulate in the pleural space, a restrictive pulmonary impairment results.[2] The excess pleural fluid within the thorax does not allow the lungs to expand fully.

> ### Clinical Tip
> The diagnosis of pleural effusion is not an indication for bronchopulmonary hygiene techniques. Instead, prevention of further pulmonary complications can be achieved with change of position, breathing exercises in different positions, and increasing activity. However, until the fluid is removed or reabsorbed, compression of the alveoli will occur, and atelectasis will be present.

Transudative pleural effusions are associated with an elevation in the hydrostatic pressure in the pleural capillaries. This is most commonly due to left-sided heart failure, right-sided heart failure, or both. Because of the increase in the hydrostatic pressure, more fluid is moved out of the pleural capillaries and less fluid is reabsorbed. There is therefore

## Table 5-12 Clinical Manifestation of Pleural Effusions

| | | Findings |
|---|---|---|
| Signs | Pulmonary function tests | Depends on the size of pleural effusion |
| | | Large: ↓ lung volumes |
| | Chest radiograph | Small effusions: blunting of costophrenic angles |
| | | Large: homogenous opacity of fluid density, pronounced at bases |
| | Arterial blood gases | Usually normal because of reflex vasoconstriction in hypoventilated areas of the lung |
| | Breath sounds | Bronchial breath sounds and egophony heard just above pleural effusion |
| | | Directly over pleural effusion, breath sounds are ↓ |
| | | Pleural friction rub may be present if pleura inflamed |
| | Cardiovascular | No specific findings |
| Symptoms | | May exhibit no symptoms |
| | | If large pleural effusion: dyspnea |
| | | If inflammation present, may have pleuritic chest pain |
| | | May have dry, nonproductive cough because of irritation |

excess fluid in the pleural space, causing a bilateral pleural effusion. Congestive heart failure is the single most common cause of transudative pleural effusions.[2]

Exudative pleural effusions are associated with an increase in the permeability of the pleural surfaces that allows protein and excess fluid to move into the pleural space. Therefore, in exudative pleural effusions, the pleurae are in some way involved in the pathologic process. Most commonly, the pleurae may be involved in an inflammatory process or with neoplastic disease. Inflammatory processes such as pneumonia, tuberculosis, or pulmonary emboli with infarction can begin in the lung but extend into the visceral pleura, causing disruption of the normal pleural permeability. Cancer can also cause disruption of the normal pleural permeability, either by direct extension of a lung tumor to the pleural surface or by hematogenous dissemination of tumor cells to the pleural surface from a distant source. Tumor cells are also spread via the lymphatic system and therefore can alter the normal lymphatic clearance of the pleural space or be brought into the pleural space by the pleural lymphatics (Fig. 5-11).[2]

### Clinical Manifestation

The clinical manifestation of pleural effusions can be found in Table 5-12.

### Treatment

The underlying cause of the pleural effusion must be identified and treated. In many cases, this treatment causes the pleural effusion to resolve secondarily.[9] Diagnostic thoracentesis, a procedure during which a needle is inserted into the chest wall to extract fluid, and tissue samples can be used to determine if the fluid is a transudate or exudate.[9] Thoracentesis can also be used therapeutically to remove excess pleural fluid via a large-bore needle. However, there is little evidence that patients benefit from this intervention, and it is being

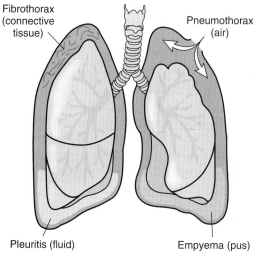

**Figure 5-11** Pleural diseases. Pleuritis is usually associated with pleural effusion. Fibrothorax is an encasement of the lungs with fibrous tissue that obliterates the pleural cavity. Pneumothorax denotes the entry of air into the pleural cavity. Empyema involves pockets of pus enclosed in fibrous adhesions. (From Damjanov I. Pathology for the Health Professions, ed 3. St. Louis, 2006, Saunders.)

used less frequently.[20] A new procedure, thoracoscopy, uses a rigid scope with a light source to explore the entire hemithorax. Thoracoscopy can be used to biopsy the pleura, biopsy the lung, obtain pleural fluid samples, remove pleural fluid, and perform a pleurodesis, and if necessary lysis of adhesions can be accomplished (Fig. 5-12).[9] Another treatment option that is used if a large infected pleural effusion (empyema) is present is the placement of a pleural space chest tube for drainage of this fluid.[20] For additional therapeutic management, see practice pattern 6B (Impaired Aerobic Capacity/Endurance Associated with Deconditioning).[11]

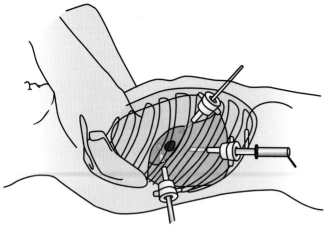

**Figure 5-12** Thoracoscopy for lung biopsy. (From Phillips N. Berry and Kohn's Operating Room Technique, ed 11. St. Louis, 2008, Mosby.)

## Sarcoidosis

Sarcoidosis is an enigmatic multisystem disease that is characterized by the presence of noncaseating epithelioid granulomas in many organs. Clinically the lung is the most involved organ (Fig. 5-13).[17,18]

### Etiology

The etiology of this disease is unknown. Infectious agents, chemicals or drugs, allergy, autoimmunity, and genetic factors have all been researched as possible causes.[10] Sarcoidosis most commonly affects young adults, with 70% of the cases diagnosed in persons 20 to 40 years of age. Sarcoidosis is more common in women than in men. The incidence is increased tenfold in black Americans when compared with whites. It is rare in Native American Indians.[27]

### Pathophysiology

This disease presents with three distinctive features within the lung: alveolitis, formation of well-defined round or oval granulomas, and pulmonary fibrosis.[17] The alveolitis usually appears earliest and is an infiltration of the alveolar walls by inflammatory cells, especially macrophages and T lymphocytes. The core of the sarcoid granuloma contains epithelioid cells and multinucleated giant cells; there is rarely any necrosis in the core. The core is surrounded by monocytes, macrophages, lymphocytes, and fibroblasts. These granulomas may resolve without scarring, but many go on to become obliterative fibrosis, which is characterized by the accumulation of fibroblasts and collagen around the granuloma. Diffuse fibrosis of the alveolar walls is not typical in this disease, although it can occur late in the disease progression. Approximately 25% of patients with pulmonary sarcoidosis experience a permanent decrease in lung function, which over time proves fatal in 5% to 10% of patients.[17] This loss of lung function is due to restrictive lung impairment primarily, but this disease also has an obstructive component. Prognosis seems to be better if the onset of pulmonary symptoms is acute. If the onset is insidious, with progressive dyspnea, then the progno-

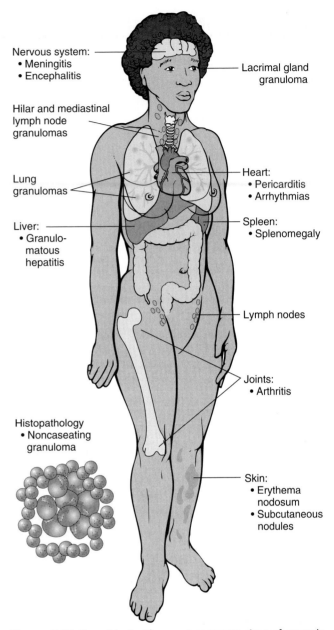

**Figure 5-13** Sarcoidosis. The most common sites of granulomas are the lungs and the thoracic lymph nodes. Other extrathoracic sites are less commonly involved. The inset shows a granuloma composed predominantly of epithelioid cells, macrophages, and lymphocytes. In contrast to tuberculosis, there is no central necrosis. (From Damjanov I. Pathology for the Health Professions, ed 3. St. Louis, 2006, Saunders.)

sis is worse (patients will have more impairments, less function, and may have higher mortality rates).

Sarcoidosis is a multisystem disease, and although the pulmonary system is the most commonly involved (90%), other systems are affected also. Seventeen percent of patients have ocular involvement, which can lead to blindness.[17] The most common ocular presentation is granulomatous uveitis, which causes redness and watering of the eyes, cloudy vision, and photophobia.[33] Five percent of patients have neurologic involvement, which can include encephalopathy,

## Table 5-13 Clinical Manifestation of Sarcoidosis

|  |  | Findings |
|---|---|---|
| Signs | Pulmonary function tests | ↓ TLC, ↓ all lung volumes, ↓ RV, ↓ lung compliance |
|  |  | ↓ DLCO due to ↑ ventilation/perfusion mismatching |
|  |  | Late in disease may find obstructive deficits with ↓ flow rates and/or 20%–30% ↓ in PFT values[20] |
|  | Chest radiograph | Bilateral hilar lymphadenopathy |
|  |  | Lung parenchyma show diffuse infiltrates with interstitial reticulonodular pattern |
|  | Arterial blood gases | Remain in normal limits until late in disease when ↓ PaO₂ |
|  | Breath sounds | Chest expansion ↓, ↑ RR |
|  |  | Auscultation: bibasilar rales and ↓ sounds in apices as a result of bullae with occasional wheezing |
|  | Cardiovascular | 15% develop pulmonary hypertension[17] |
|  |  | Dysrhythmias, CHF, and papillary muscle dysfunction |
| Symptoms |  | One third develop dyspnea during course of disease[27] |
|  |  | Cough (±sputum) |
|  |  | Complaint of vague retrosternal discomfort |
|  |  | Fever, fatigue, weight loss, erythema nodosum |

*CHF, congestive heart failure; DLCO, diffusing capacity of the lungs for carbon monoxide; PFT, pulmonary function test; RR, respiratory rate; RV, residual volume; TLC, total lung capacity.*

granulomatous meningitis, or involvement of the cranial nerves.[17] Other organ systems that can be involved are the liver (60% to 80%), the lymphatics (50% to 75%), the heart (30%), the skin (30%), the spleen (15%), the kidney, muscles, joints, and the immune system.[2,7,17,18,27,33]

The progression of this disease is extremely variable. The disease can be active and resolve spontaneously, both clinically and radiographically. The disease can be inactive and stable for long periods of time with no change in clinical symptoms. The disease also can be persistent and active, with progressive loss of lung function leading to a fatal outcome.[9,17]

### Clinical Manifestation

The clinical manifestation of sarcoidosis can be found in Table 5-13.

### Treatment

Treatment of this disease is difficult because it is known that some cases resolve spontaneously and others can go into long periods of remission. In treating the three pulmonary manifestations of this disease, corticosteroids are used early to suppress the alveolitis and granuloma formation, especially if the patient has respiratory symptoms and/or a 20% to 30% reduction in PFT values.[9,20] Established granulomas with pulmonary fibrosis are relatively fixed lesions and do not respond to therapy. Corticosteroid therapy is indicated for extrapulmonary sarcoidosis involving the eyes, heart, or nervous system.[20]

For additional therapeutic management, see practice pattern 6B (Impaired Aerobic Capacity/Endurance Associated with Deconditioning).[11]

## Cardiovascular Causes of Restrictive Lung Dysfunction

### Pulmonary Edema

Pulmonary edema is an increase in the amount of fluid within the lung. Usually the pulmonary interstitium is affected first and then the alveolar spaces.[24,26]

### Etiology

Pulmonary edema has two primary causes. One is an increase in the pulmonary capillary hydrostatic pressure secondary to left ventricular failure (see Fig. 4-8). This is called cardiogenic pulmonary edema and is discussed in this section. Pulmonary edema can also be caused by increased alveolar capillary membrane permeability secondary to various causes. This type of pulmonary edema is also named ARDS and was discussed under the section on Pulmonary Causes of RLD. Cardiogenic pulmonary edema is also known as high-pressure pulmonary edema, hydrostatic pulmonary edema, and hemodynamic pulmonary edema.[8,26]

### Pathophysiology

As the left ventricle fails, its ability to contract and pump blood into the systemic circulation efficiently is diminished. This results in an increase in left atrial pressure, which is transmitted back to the pulmonary circulation. Because of this impedance to blood flow, the pressure in the microcirculation of the lung is increased, which increases the transvascular flow of fluid into the interstitium of the lung. The interstitial space can accommodate a small amount of excess

## Table 5-14 Clinical Manifestation of Pulmonary Edema

| | | Findings |
|---|---|---|
| Signs | Pulmonary function tests | ↓ Lung volumes, ↑ RR , Flow rates normal, DLCO normal or ↓ |
| | Chest radiograph | ↑ vascular markings in hilar region |
| | | Kerly B lines present |
| | | Interstitial and alveolar infiltrates are diffuse and pleural effusions common |
| | Arterial blood gases | ↓ $PaO_2$, ↓ $PaCO_2$, ↑ pH Respiratory alkalosis |
| | | Possible ↑ $PaCO_2$ late in clinical course |
| | Breath sounds | Wet rales with ↓ breath sounds |
| | | Some patients present with bronchospasm and wheezing |
| | Cardiovascular | Most have significant cardiac dysfunction[20] |
| | | Arrhythmias common in this population |
| Symptoms | | Appear in respiratory distress, report sense of suffocation |
| | | Short of breath, cyanotic, ↑ RR, labored breathing, pallor, diaphoresis |
| | | Cough: pink frothy sputum |

*DLCO, diffusing capacity of the lungs for carbon monoxide; $PaO_2$, arterial partial pressure of $O_2$; PFT, pulmonary function test; RR, respiratory rate.*

fluid, approximately 500 mL.[26] The lymphatic drainage can be enhanced to move some excess fluid out of the thorax. However, when the left atrial pressure rises above 30 mm Hg, these protective mechanisms are overcome.[26] The interstitial edema fluid disrupts the tight alveolar epithelium, floods the alveolar spaces, and moves through the visceral pleura, causing pleural effusions. The pulmonary edema fluid in cardiogenic pulmonary edema is characterized by low-protein concentrations. This finding is in contrast to that in ARDS in which the pulmonary edema fluid has elevated protein concentrations. With fluid in the alveoli and the interstitium, lung compliance is decreased; ventilation–perfusion mismatching is increased; gas exchange is disrupted; the work of breathing is increased; and there is restrictive lung dysfunction.[8,24,26]

### Clinical Manifestation

The clinical manifestation of pulmonary edema can be found in Table 5-14.

### Treatment

Treatment is aimed at decreasing the cardiac preload and maintaining oxygenation of the tissues. To decrease cardiac preload, venous return to the heart is decreased, which decreases the left ventricular filling pressure. Venodilators, such as morphine sulfate or sodium nitroprusside, and diuretics, such as furosemide, are used to decrease the venous return. Other drugs, for example, dopamine, dobutamine, and digitalis may be given to improve cardiac contractility. To maintain oxygenation, supplemental oxygen is provided. Intubation with mechanical ventilation may also be necessary.[20]

For additional therapeutic management, see practice pattern 6D (Impaired Aerobic Capacity/Endurance Associated with Cardiovascular Pump Dysfunction or Failure).[11]

## Pulmonary Emboli

Pulmonary emboli are a complication of venous thrombosis, in which blood clots or thrombi travel from a systemic vein through the right side of the heart and into the pulmonary circulation, where they lodge in branches of the pulmonary artery (Fig. 5-14).[2,18]

### Etiology

Pulmonary embolism is the most common acute pulmonary problem among hospitalized patients in the United States. Each year 500,000 to 1 million Americans have a pulmonary embolic event.[26] Many of these events may go unnoticed because they are clinically silent. However, approximately 10% of pulmonary embolisms result in the patient's death.[26] Thus, between 50,000 and 100,000 Americans die annually because of a pulmonary embolism, making it the third most common cause of death in the United States.[26] About one third of the deaths occur within 1 hour of the acute event. And more than half of these fatalities occur in patients in whom the diagnosis was not clinically suspect.[26]

In more than 95% of the cases, the thrombi that caused the pulmonary emboli were formed in the lower extremities.[2] In the remaining 5% of the cases, the thrombi may be formed in the pelvis, the arms, or the right side of the heart. Numerous risk factors increase the likelihood of thrombus formation in the lower extremities (Box 5-4). The highest risk group for thrombophlebitis is orthopedic patients. Studies have shown that the frequency of deep-vein thrombosis perioperatively is 80% in patients after hip or knee surgery.[20]

### Pathophysiology

The pathophysiologic changes that occur following pulmonary embolism affect the pulmonary system and the cardiovascular system. The occlusion of one or more pulmonary

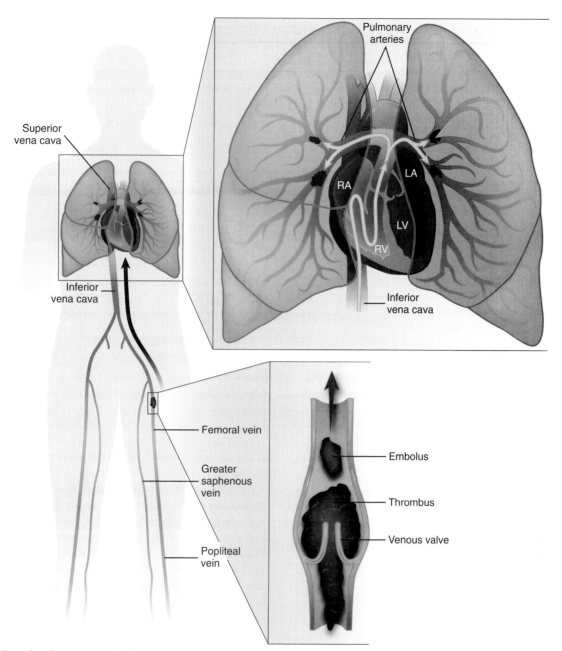

**Figure 5-14** Pathophysiology of pulmonary embolism. Pulmonary embolism usually originates in the deep veins of the legs, most commonly the calf veins. These venous thrombi originate predominantly in venous valve pockets and at other sites of presumed venous stasis (inset). If a clot propagates to the knee vein or above or if it originates above the knee, the risk of embolism increases. Thromboemboli travel through the right side of the heart to reach the lungs. LA, left atrium; LV, left ventricle; RA, right atrium; RV, right ventricle. (From Tapson VF. Acute pulmonary embolism. N Engl J Med 358(10):1037-52, 2008.)

arterial branches causes edema and hemorrhage into the surrounding lung parenchyma. This is known as congestive atelectasis. The lack of blood flow causes coagulative necrosis of the alveolar walls; the alveoli fill with erythrocytes, and there is an inflammatory response. Another change within the pulmonary system is the increase in the alveolar dead space because a portion of the lung is being ventilated but no longer perfused. Pneumoconstriction of the affected area occurs, with a marked decrease in alveolar carbon dioxide owing to the lack of gas exchange and the patient's respiratory pattern of hyperventilation. In addition, the

alveolar surfactant decreases over a period of approximately 24 hours, which results in alveolar collapse and regional atelectasis. These changes combine to cause an acute increase in ventilation–perfusion mismatching, a decrease in lung compliance, and impaired gas exchange. If the oxygen supply is completely cut off to a portion of the lung, then frank necrosis and infarction of lung tissue results. This happens in less than 10% of all pulmonary embolisms because lung tissue has three sources of oxygen: the pulmonary vascular system, the bronchial vascular system, and the alveolar gas.[26] However, infarction of lung tissue is

## Table 5-15 Clinical Manifestation of Pulmonary Emboli

| | | Findings |
|---|---|---|
| Signs | Pulmonary function tests | ↓ lung volumes, ↓ lung compliance, ↓ expiratory flow rates, ↑ RR changes will resolve with resolution of PE |
| | Chest radiograph | May appear normal. Only permanent change is scar formation secondary to lung infarction[20] |
| | | Possible changes include cone-shaped fanning out with extension to pleura or a rounded nodular lesion, one pulmonary artery may be larger, may see small pleural effusion, one diaphragm may be elevated |
| | Arterial blood gases | ↓ $PaO_2$, ↓ $PaCO_2$, ↑ pH (respiratory alkalosis)[20] |
| | Breath sounds | ↓ sounds in area of pneumoconstriction, possible wheezing |
| | | Occasional rales due to atelectasis from loss of surfactant[20] |
| | Cardiovascular | Tachycardia |
| | | ECG: minor nonspecific changes, possible arrhythmias |
| | | With massive PE: right ventricular failure and cardiac arrest may occur[20] |
| Symptoms | | Acute onset of dyspnea[26] |
| | | Severity of dyspnea is related to amount of pulmonary vasculature involved. |
| | | Rapid shallow breathing and tachycardia are present |
| | | Apprehension, cough, pleuritic chest pain and possibly syncope |
| | | Hemoptysis and low-grade fever may occur several hours after infarct |

ECG, electrocardiograph; PE, pulmonary emboli; RR, respiratory rate.

## Box 5-4

### Risk Factors for Lower Extremity Thrombus Formation

- Immobilization:
  - Bedrest
  - Long periods of travel
  - Fracture stabilization
- Injuries to leg (blow to leg, athletic injury, surgery, radiation therapy)
- Increased age
- Inherited clotting disorders
  - Factor 5V Leiden
  - Prothrombin gene mutation
- Infections and inflammatory diseases
  - Systemic lupus erythematosus
  - Rheumatoid arthritis
  - Crohn disease
  - Glomerulonephritis
- Pregnancy and individuals taking oral contraceptives
- Cancer (ovaries, pancreas, lymphatics, liver, stomach, and colon)
- Smoking
- Obesity
- Thrombocytosis
- Sickle cell anemia
- Highest risk
  - Orthopedic patients: post hip or knee surgery

From George RB, RW Light, Matthay MA, et al. Chest Medicine: Essentials of Pulmonary and Critical Care Medicine, ed 5. Baltimore, 2005, Lippincott Williams & Wilkins.

followed by contraction of the affected tissue and scar formation.

The first cardiovascular change that occurs because of a pulmonary embolism is an increase in the pulmonary arterial resistance due to a decrease in the cross-sectional area of the pulmonary arterial bed. If this cross-sectional area is decreased by more than 50%, then the pressure needed to maintain pulmonary blood flow rises and pulmonary hypertension results.[26] This also increases the work of the right ventricle and can lead to right ventricular failure. If the pulmonary embolus is massive, right ventricular failure and cardiac arrest can occur within minutes.[8,24,26]

### Clinical Manifestation

The clinical manifestation of pulmonary emboli can be found in Table 5-15.

### Treatment

Treatment begins with prevention of deep-vein thrombosis. There are two methods used in preventing or minimizing deep-vein thrombosis. The mechanical approach includes ankle pumping exercises in bed, early ambulation, use of gradient compression stockings, pneumatic calf compression, and electrical stimulation of calf muscles. The pharmacologic approach includes the use of agents that decrease the hypercoagulability of the blood, such as warfarin, dextran, low-molecular-weight heparin, heparinoids, and heparin.[20] With repeated thrombus formation and embolic events, surgical placement of a transvenous device (e.g., Greenfield filter) to prevent migration of thrombi may be utilized.

Heparin therapy is most commonly used to treat pulmonary embolism. Heparin does not lyse existing clots, but it prevents formation and propagation of further clots.[20] To maintain adequate tissue oxygenation, mechanical ventilation with supplemental oxygen may be required. In addition, if the patient is hypotensive or in shock, fluid therapy and vasopressors may be needed. Mild sedation and analgesia may be used to decrease anxiety and pain. Thromboembolic lysing agents (e.g., streptokinase) can be used to lyse the emboli, but this therapeutic intervention is no more effective than heparin therapy in terms of the patient's morbidity or mortality.[20] Pulmonary embolectomy is being performed less frequently owing to the increased mortality rate (50% to 94%) when compared with the mortality rate (24%) for conventional medical treatment.[20] However, this emergent surgical intervention may be indicated in patients who have large emboli and cannot receive heparin therapy or have overt right ventricular heart failure leading to cardiac arrest. The ultimate prognosis following pulmonary embolism is extremely variable. In patients who experience no shock and are treated medically, the mortality rate is 18%.[20] Patients who have pulmonary embolism and a simultaneous cardiac arrest have a 45% mortality rate. Patients who have a pulmonary embolism with extreme increases in right ventricular pressures have a 90% mortality rate.[26]

## Neuromuscular Causes of Restrictive Lung Dysfunction

### Spinal Cord Injury

Spinal cord injury (SCI) is damage to or interruption of the neurologic pathways contained within the spinal cord.[24,34]

### Etiology

A spinal cord injury can result from an acute traumatic event, often a motor vehicle accident or a diving accident, or from a pathologic process that invades the spinal cord and damages it or in some way interrupts the neurologic transmissions.

### Pathophysiology

For this discussion, spinal cord injuries include cervical injuries only. A spinal cord injury in the cervical region produces paralysis or paresis in the arms, legs, and trunk, therefore resulting in tetraplegia. With this type of injury, the expiratory muscles are paralyzed or very weak, leading to an inability to cough. This ineffective cough may cause an increase in the incidence of pulmonary infections. The external intercostals are inactive, and the patient may have a functional, weak, or absent diaphragm, depending on the level of the injury (Table 5-16).[8,34] Weakness in the inspiratory muscles results in alveolar hypoventilation, hypoxemia, and hypercapnia. Because the alveoli are not well ventilated, the patient is prone to atelectasis, particularly in the dependent lung regions, which could lead to recurrent pulmonary infections. With parts of the lung underventilated, the ventilation–perfusion matching is impaired and the diffusing capacity

**Table 5-16 Innervation Levels of the Respiratory Muscles**

| | Muscles | Level |
|---|---|---|
| Inspiratory | Diaphragm | C3, C4, C5 (phrenic nerve) |
| | External intercostals | TI–TI2 |
| | Sternocleidomastoids | Cranial nerve XI (spinal accessory nerve) |
| | Scalenes | C1, C2 |
| Expiratory | Internal intercostals | T1–T12 |
| | Abdominals | T7–L1 |

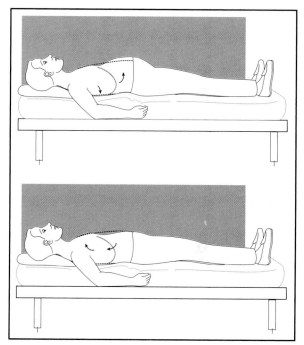

**Figure 5-15** Paradoxical breathing. Note the position of the rib cage and abdomen. *Top,* Paradoxical breathing when the diaphragm is strong, but the accessory muscles are absent. *Bottom,* Paradoxical breathing during paralysis of the diaphragm.

reduced. A cervical injury also results in the loss of the sigh reflex, which increases the incidence of atelectasis and contributes to alveolar collapse. If the patient retains use of the diaphragm, breathing dynamics are altered markedly, resulting in paradoxical breathing (Fig. 5-15). In paradoxical breathing, the diaphragm descends on inspiration, causing the abdomen to rise and the paralyzed thoracic wall to be pulled inward. The diaphragm relaxes on exhalation, causing the abdomen to fall and the chest wall to move outward. Immediately after a cervical injury, the VC and the maximum voluntary ventilation are markedly reduced.

**Table 5-17 Clinical Manifestation of Spinal Cord Injury**

| | | Findings |
|---|---|---|
| Signs | Pulmonary function tests | ↓ TLC, ↓ VC, ↓ IC, ↑ RV, ↓ flow rates, ↓ peak inspiratory and expiratory pressures, ↑ RR, VT diminished; if no active expiratory muscles, RV = FRC |
| | Chest radiograph | May be normal, or may show evidence of infiltrates and infections. Over time ribs become more horizontal |
| | Arterial blood gases | ↓ $PaO_2$, ↑ $PaCO_2$ with respiratory muscle weakness |
| | Breath sounds | Diminished breath sounds; adventitious breath sounds when presence of infiltrates and infections |
| | Cardiovascular | Above T7 have autonomic dysreflexia (hyperreflexia). This results in vasoconstriction below lesion and hypertension. CNS above lesion compensates with vasodilation and bradycardia |
| Symptoms | | Fatigue (as a result of inefficiency of breathing pattern and ↑ accessory muscle use and work); shortness of breath, inability to cough, poor voice volume, morning headaches (secondary to overnight hypoxia) |
| | | Restlessness and irritability with ↑ $PaCO_2$ |

*CNS, central nervous system; FRC, functional residual capacity; IC, inspiratory capacity; $PaCO_2$, arterial partial pressure of $CO_2$; $PaO_2$, arterial partial pressure of $O_2$; RR, respiratory rate; RV, residual volume; TLC, total lung capacity; VC, vital capacity; VT, tidal volume.*

Approximately 6 months after injury, the VC has improved significantly if the patient has an intact diaphragm. And although it may not be normal, the VC may have doubled since the acute postinjury period. Paradoxical breathing is also diminished or eliminated because of the developing spasticity in the thorax and abdomen.[8,13,34]

Over time, pulmonary compliance is decreased owing to the shallow breathing and atelectasis within the lung, and chest wall compliance is decreased as a result of paralysis of the thoracic musculature and the developing thoracic spasticity. This increases the work of breathing and can lead to diaphragmatic fatigue. All these pathophysiologic alterations lead to RLD and a chronic state of hypoxemia. The patient may therefore need mechanical ventilation part-time or full-time or an enriched $FIO_2$.[2,8,25]

## Clinical Manifestation

The clinical manifestation of SCI can be found in Table 5-17.

## Treatment

Patients with spinal cord injuries must be taught ways to strengthen and increase the endurance of any remaining ventilatory muscles via use of an inspiratory muscle trainer, resistance exercises to the diaphragm, or an incentive spirometer. Patients must learn how to perform active and passive chest wall stretching, using rolling, positioning, side leaning, and air shift maneuvers. Patients, family members, or caregivers need to know how to assist the patient in clearing excess secretions with postural drainage, percussion, assisted coughing, and possibly suctioning. Learning how to perform glossopharyngeal breathing or how to operate a portable ventilator may also be necessary for selected patients.[34]

For additional therapeutic management, see practice pattern 6E (Impaired Ventilation and Respiration/Gas Exchange Associated with Ventilatory Pump Dysfunction or Failure) or 6F (Impaired Ventilation and Respiration/Gas Exchange Associated with Respiratory Failure).[11]

## Amyotrophic Lateral Sclerosis (ALS)

Amyotrophic lateral sclerosis (ALS) is a progressive degenerative disease of the nervous system that involves both upper and lower motor neurons, causing both flaccid and spastic paralysis.[1,2]

## Etiology

The cause of the disease is unknown. It occurs worldwide, and onset is usually after the age of 40. Men are affected 1.7 times as often as women.[24]

## Pathophysiology

The anterior horn cells of the cervical, lower thoracic, and lumbosacral spinal segments usually are the most involved, which means that the respiratory muscles may be affected severely. Muscles innervated by the cranial nerves as well as the spinal nerves frequently are involved, causing problems with dysarthria and dysphagia. Muscle weakness and wasting are profound. Following the onset of neurologic symptoms, the average life expectancy is 3.6 years.[30] Death is often the result of acute respiratory failure.[25]

## Clinical Manifestation

The clinical manifestation of ALS can be found in Table 5-18.

## Treatment

There is no treatment for this disease except supportive therapy to make the patient more comfortable. Physical

## Table 5-18 Clinical Manifestation of Amyotrophic Lateral Sclerosis

| | | Findings |
|---|---|---|
| Signs | Pulmonary function tests | TLC, ↓ IC, ↓ VC, ↓ ERV, ↑ RV, FRC normal |
| | | RR with weakness of ventilatory muscles, ↓ VT |
| | | ↓ MVV, ↓ MIP and MEP |
| | Chest radiograph | May be normal or show retained secretions/infiltrates as a result of poor airway clearance |
| | Arterial blood gases | ↓ $PaO_2$, ↑ $PaCO_2$ |
| | Breath sounds | ↓breath sounds, with rales and rhonchi due to infiltrates |
| | Cardiovascular | Nothing specific |
| Symptoms | | Onset begins with weakness or wasting of muscles of hands or of legs. Atrophy follows. Progressive weakness and atrophy occur and patients fatigue easily, have poor activity endurance and complain of dyspnea with mild exertion |

*ERV, expiratory reserve volume; FRC, functional residual capacity; IC, inspiratory capacity; MEP, maximal expiratory pressure; MIP, maximal inspiratory pressure; MVV, maximum voluntary ventilation; $PaCO_2$, arterial partial pressure of $CO_2$; $PaO_2$, arterial partial pressure of $O_2$; RR, respiratory rate; RV, residual volume; TLC, total lung capacity; VC, vital capacity; VT, tidal volume.*

exertion is not recommended because it tires the patient so rapidly. However, the patient should be encouraged to get out of bed and be as mobile as possible. Patients eventually develop weakness of respiratory muscles that follows with need for mechanical ventilation to maintain adequate gas exchange.

For additional therapeutic management, see practice pattern 6E (Impaired Ventilation and Respiration/Gas Exchange Associated with Ventilatory Pump Dysfunction or Failure) or 6F (Impaired Ventilation and Respiration/Gas Exchange Associated with Respiratory Failure).[11]

## Poliomyelitis

Poliomyelitis (polio) is a viral disease that attacks the motor nerve cells of the spinal cord and brain stem and can result in muscular paralysis.[2]

## Etiology

Polio is caused by an acute viral infection, which can reach epidemic proportions in at-risk populations. It is reported most commonly in children. This infection can now be prevented by vaccine.

## Pathophysiology

The virus is neurotropic and has a predilection for the motor cells of the anterior horn and the brain stem. The lesions are patchy and asymmetric, and microscopically healthy and diseased cells can be seen side by side. This results in a patchy flaccid paralysis or paresis of the lower motor neuron type. Both the diaphragm and intercostal muscles may be affected, resulting in a respiratory muscle weakness that can progress to respiratory failure. One form of polio, bulbar polio, affects the brain stem and can result in the loss of the swallowing reflexes, thus leading to aspiration problems. There are two stages in polio. The preparalytic stage is characterized by

fever, headache, malaise, and symptoms in the gastrointestinal and upper respiratory tracts. For some patients, this stage is followed by the paralytic stage, which includes tremulousness of the limbs, tenderness in the muscles, and swollen painful joints, as well as flaccid paralysis of from one to two muscles to all four limbs and the trunk.[1,2,25]

## Clinical Manifestation

The clinical manifestation of polio with respiratory involvement can be found in Table 5-19.

## Treatment

There is no specific treatment for poliomyelitis. Prevention through the use of oral or parenteral vaccine is very effective. Supportive therapy consisting of rest during the acute phase, with proper positioning, pain relief, good nutrition, and ventilatory support, as needed, is appropriate. Later, active range-of-motion exercises, strengthening exercises, bracing, and other equipment evaluation are required for patients with paralysis.

Post-polio syndrome (PPS) is a condition that affects survivors of polio years (21 plus) after recovery from the initial illness. The clinical manifestation of PPS include new weakening of muscles that were previously affected as well as muscles that were not affected. The onset is slow and progressive muscle weakness, general fatigue, and possibly muscle atrophy and joint pain. Problems occur if respiratory muscle weakness develops and the patient develops hypoxemia and low ventilation or weakness of swallowing muscles, making them at increased risk of aspiration pneumonia. It is estimated that PPS affects 25% to 50% of the polio survivors (approximately 440,000 individuals).[35]

For additional therapeutic management, see practice pattern 6B (Impaired Aerobic Capacity/Endurance Associated with Deconditioning), 6E (Impaired Ventilation and Respiration/Gas Exchange Associated with Ventilatory Pump

### Table 5-19 Clinical Manifestation of Poliomyelitis

|  |  | Findings |
|---|---|---|
| Signs | Pulmonary function tests | ↓ lung volumes, ↑ RR, ↓ VT<br>↓ MIP, ↓ MEP, ↓ DLCO |
|  | Chest radiograph | May show presence of atelectasis or infiltrates, elevated diaphragm (if paralyzed), may develop kyphoscoliosis |
|  | Arterial blood gases | ↓ $PaO_2$, ↑ $PaCO_2$ |
|  | Breath sounds | Diminished sounds, rhonchi may be present if aspiration |
|  | Cardiovascular | May see transient rise in systolic and diastolic pressures |
| Symptoms |  | Short of breath, anxious, weak cough, and poor airway clearance |

DLCO, diffusing capacity of the lungs for carbon monoxide; MEP, maximal expiratory pressure; MIP, maximal inspiratory pressure; MVV, maximum voluntary ventilation; PaCO₂, arterial partial pressure of CO₂; PaO₂, arterial partial pressure of O₂; RR, respiratory rate; VT, tidal volume.

### Table 5-20 Clinical Manifestation of Guillain–Barré Syndrome

|  |  | Findings |
|---|---|---|
| Signs | Pulmonary function tests | All dynamic lung volumes ↓. ↓ TLC, ↓ VC, ↓IRV, ↓ERV, ↓ VT, ↑ RR<br>Peak inspiratory and expiratory pressures ↓, ↓ |
|  | Chest radiograph | Variable; may demonstrate atelectasis, infiltrates, pneumonia, or pulmonary edema |
|  | Arterial blood gases | ↓ $PaO_2$, ↑ $PaCO_2$ |
|  | Breath sounds | Diminished breath sounds, ↓ at bases; may have adventitious sounds if infiltrates present |
|  | Cardiovascular | May have dysrhythmias, hypertension, and/or postural hypotension |
| Symptoms |  | Weakness in both lower extremities, paresthesias of fingers and toes, dyspnea, anxiousness and suffocation. Poor cough and poor airway clearance, ↓ endurance and ↑ fatigue |

ERV, expiratory reserve volume; IRV, inspiratory reserve volume; PaCO₂, arterial partial pressure of CO₂; PaO₂, arterial partial pressure of O₂; RR, respiratory rate; TLC, total lung capacity; VC, vital capacity; VT, tidal volume.

Dysfunction or Failure), or 6F (Impaired Ventilation and Respiration/Gas Exchange Associated with Respiratory Failure).[11]

## Guillain–Barré Syndrome

Guillain–Barré syndrome is a demyelinating disease of the motor neurons of the peripheral nerves.[25]

## Etiology

This idiopathic polyneuritis is a disorder that seems to be linked to the immune system. The history of most patients with Guillain–Barré syndrome includes a viral illness followed by the ascending paralysis of this syndrome. However, the specific cause of the syndrome remains unknown.[2]

## Pathophysiology

Guillain–Barré syndrome is characterized by a rapid bilateral ascending (begins with distal involvement and progresses proximal) flaccid motor paralysis. The loss of muscular strength is usually fully realized within 30 days, often within 10 to 15 days, and may leave the patient so involved that mechanical ventilation is required. Approximately 10% to 20% of all patients with Guillain–Barré syndrome develop acute respiratory failure and must be placed on a ventilator.[8] The duration of mechanical ventilation is variable but is usually between 2 weeks and 2 months.[1,2,8,25]

## Clinical Manifestation

The clinical manifestation of Guillain–Barré syndrome can be found in Table 5-20.

## Treatment

Patients are supported throughout the syndrome's progression. Heat may be used to decrease muscular pain. Passive range of motion is begun immediately. Active exercises, including breathing exercises to assist the patient in weaning from the ventilator, should be begun as soon as the patient's

## Table 5-21 Clinical Manifestation of Myasthenia Gravis

|  |  | Findings |
|---|---|---|
| Signs | Pulmonary function tests | All dynamic lung volumes and capacities are ↓ |
|  |  | Peak inspiratory and expiratory pressures are ↓, ↑ RR, ↓ VT, ↓ DLCO |
|  | Chest radiograph | May show atelectasis or pneumonia |
|  | Arterial blood gases | ↓ PaO$_2$, ↑ PaCO$_2$ |
|  | Breath sounds | ↓ breath sounds, may have adventitious sounds if patient cannot clear secretions |
|  | Cardiovascular | No specific findings |
| Symptoms |  | Weakness and fatigue of voluntary muscles, SOB, weak and ineffective cough |

DLCO, diffusing capacity of the lungs for carbon monoxide; PaCO$_2$, arterial partial pressure of CO$_2$; PaO$_2$, arterial partial pressure of O$_2$; RR, respiratory rate; SOB, shortness of breath; VT, tidal volume.

condition has stabilized. Although exercise is important, patients with Guillain–Barré syndrome fatigue easily and should not be overly stressed. This polyneuropathy usually leads to complete recovery with minimal permanent sequelae. Recurrence of Guillain–Barré syndrome in the same patient is possible; in fact, patients with this syndrome are at slightly higher risk than the general public. However, even a second bout of the syndrome usually resolves.[2,24]

For additional therapeutic management, see practice pattern 6E (Impaired Ventilation and Respiration/Gas Exchange Associated with Ventilatory Pump Dysfunction or Failure) or 6F (Impaired Ventilation and Respiration/Gas Exchange Associated with Respiratory Failure).[11]

## Myasthenia Gravis

Myasthenia gravis is a chronic neuromuscular disease characterized by progressive muscular weakness on exertion.[1]

### Etiology

Myasthenia gravis is caused by an autoimmune attack on the acetylcholine receptors at the postsynaptic neuromuscular junction. What causes the production of this antibody is unknown. This disease predominantly affects women, and its onset is usually between 20 and 40 years of age.[24]

### Pathophysiology

The antibody IgG binds to the acetylcholine receptor sites, which impairs the normal transmission of impulses from the nerves to the muscles. The muscles most characteristically involved are those innervated by the cranial nerves. This causes ptosis, diplopia, dysarthria, dysphagia, and proximal limb weakness. The signs and symptoms of this disease may fluctuate over a period of hours or days. Severe generalized quadriparesis may develop. Approximately 10% of patients develop respiratory muscle involvement that can be life threatening.[24,36]

### Clinical Manifestation

The clinical manifestation of myasthenia gravis can be found in Table 5-21.

### Treatment

Treatment of the disease's symptoms is with an anticholinesterase (pyridostigmine or neostigmine) and plasmapheresis. Corticosteroids, immunosuppressive drugs, and thymectomy are used in an effort to alter the disease's progression by interfering with the autoimmune abnormality.[24,25]

## Tetanus

Tetanus is a disease of the neuromuscular system caused by the neurotoxin produced by Clostridium tetani.[1] This anaerobic bacillus is found in the soil and the excreta of humans and animals and usually enters via a contaminated wound. The neurotoxin binds to the ganglioside membranes of the nerve synapses and blocks release of the inhibitory transmitter. This action causes severe muscle spasticity with superimposed tonic convulsions. This muscle rigidity can become so severe that the chest wall is immobilized, resulting in asphyxia and death. Tetanus can produce the most severe example of decreased chest wall compliance, leading to a restrictive impairment incompatible with life. The best treatment for tetanus is prevention via immunization. Prompt and careful wound debridement is also important. Once a patient has developed the disease, the tetanus antitoxin can be used to neutralize nonfixed toxin in the system. Once fixed or bound, the toxin cannot be neutralized. Supportive therapy is primarily focused on maintaining an airway and ensuring adequate ventilation.[1,24]

## Pseudohypertrophic (Duchenne) Muscular Dystrophy

Pseudohypertrophic muscular dystrophy is a genetically determined, progressive degenerative myopathy.[24,36]

### Etiology

Pseudohypertrophic muscular dystrophy is a sex-linked (X chromosome) recessive disorder that occurs only in boys and is transmitted by female carriers. It is the most common of the muscular dystrophies, with a prevalence rate of 4 per 100,000 in the United States.[24,36]

## Pathophysiology

Pseudohypertrophic muscular dystrophy typically appears when boys who have this recessive gene are 3 to 7 years of age.[24] Muscle biopsy at this time shows both muscle fiber hypertrophy and necrosis with regeneration. There is also excessive infiltration of the muscle with fibrous tissue and fat. Muscle innervation is not normal in this disease, but the abnormality is due to loss of motor end plates when muscle fibers degenerate and not to neurogenic disease. The pelvic girdle is affected first, and then the shoulder girdle muscles become involved. Although the calf often shows pseudohypertrophy, the quadriceps usually appear atrophied. The progression of the disease is steady, and most patients are confined to wheelchairs by 10 to 12 years of age. Involvement of the diaphragm occurs late in the course of this disease. However, respiratory failure and infection are the causes of death in 75% of these patients, which occurs usually by age 20.[8,24,36]

## Clinical Manifestation

The clinical manifestation of Pseudohypertrophic muscular dystrophy can be found in Table 5-22.

## Treatment

There is no curative treatment. Supportive treatment is aimed at preserving the patient's mobility as long as possible and making the patient comfortable. Respiratory treatment involves prevention of infection with maintenance of good inspiratory effort and good airway clearance to mobilize any secretions.

For additional therapeutic management, see practice pattern 6C (Impaired Ventilation, Respiration/Gas Exchange, and Aerobic Capacity/Endurance Associated with Airway Clearance Dysfunction), 6E (Impaired Ventilation and Respiration/Gas Exchange Associated with Ventilatory Pump Dysfunction or Failure), or 6F (Impaired Ventilation and Respiration/Gas Exchange Associated with Respiratory Failure).[11]

## Other Muscular Dystrophies

### Facioscapulohumeral Muscular Dystrophy

Facioscapulohumeral muscular dystrophy is an autosomal dominant disorder characterized by weakness of the facial and shoulder girdle muscles. Respiratory involvement or failure is uncommon in this type of muscular dystrophy.[8,24]

### Limb-Girdle Muscular Dystrophy

Limb-girdle muscular dystrophy is a disorder in which adults exhibit weakness of the pelvic and shoulder girdle musculature. There can be severe involvement of the diaphragm early in the course of this disease.[8,24]

### Myotonic Muscular Dystrophy

Myotonic muscular dystrophy is an autosomal dominant disorder that combines myotonia with progressive peripheral muscle weakness. Respiratory involvement and failure are common as this disease progresses.[8,24]

## Musculoskeletal Causes of Restrictive Lung Dysfunction

### Diaphragmatic Paralysis or Paresis

Diaphragmatic paralysis or paresis is the loss or impairment of motor function of the diaphragm because of a lesion in the neurologic or muscular system. The paralysis or paresis may be temporary or permanent.[25,26]

### Etiology

Unilateral paralysis or paresis of the diaphragm is most commonly caused by invasion of the phrenic nerve by

## Table 5-22  Clinical Manifestation of Pseudohypertrophic Muscular Dystrophy

|  |  | Findings |
|---|---|---|
| Signs | Pulmonary function tests | All lung volumes ↓ except ↑RV, ↓ TLC, ↓ VC, ↑ RR, ↓ VT |
|  |  | Max inspiratory and expiratory pressures are ↓. ↓ MVV, ↓ chest wall compliance, ↓ lung compliance, ↓ gas diffusion |
|  | Chest radiograph | May show atelectasis, pulmonary infection or infiltrates |
|  | Arterial blood gases | ↓ $PaO_2$, ↑ $PaCO_2$ |
|  | Breath sounds | Diminished breath sounds; adventitious sounds when retention of secretions |
|  | Cardiovascular | Abnormalities in ECG indicating conduction block. Cardiac muscle is involved with fibrosis of myocardium |
| Symptoms |  | Waddling gait, toe walking, lordosis, frequent falls and difficulty standing up from floor and climbing stairs (related to proximal pelvic girdle muscle weakness). Dyspnea on exertion and progressive ↓ in activity. Progresses to dyspnea at rest. Weak cough, ineffective clearing of secretions |

*MVV, maximum voluntary ventilation; $PaCO_2$, arterial partial pressure of $CO_2$; $PaO_2$, arterial partial pressure of $O_2$; RR, respiratory rate; RV, residual volume; TLC, total lung capacity; VC, vital capacity; VT, tidal volume.*

bronchogenic carcinoma.[26] Another very common cause is open heart surgery. An estimated 20% of patients who undergo cardiac surgery suffer injury to the phrenic nerve owing to either cold or stretching of the nerve.[20,26] In hemiplegic patients it is not uncommon to find paralysis of the corresponding hemidiaphragm. The left hemidiaphragm is involved in left hemiplegia more frequently than the right hemidiaphragm is involved in right hemiplegia.[25] Other causes of unilateral diaphragmatic dysfunction include poliomyelitis; Huntington chorea; herpes zoster; or peripheral neuritis associated with measles, tetanus, typhoid, or diphtheria. Bilateral paralysis or paresis of the diaphragm may result from high spinal cord injury, thoracic trauma, Guillain–Barré syndrome, multiple sclerosis, muscular dystrophy, or anterior horn cell disease.[20,25,26]

## Pathophysiology

Normally as the crural portion of the diaphragm contracts, the pleural space pressure decreases; the central tendon moves caudally; the lungs inflate; and the abdominal pressure increases, which moves the abdominal wall outward (Fig. 5-16). Contraction of the costal portion of the diaphragm accomplishes these same effects and in addition causes the anterior lower ribs to expand and move in a cephalad

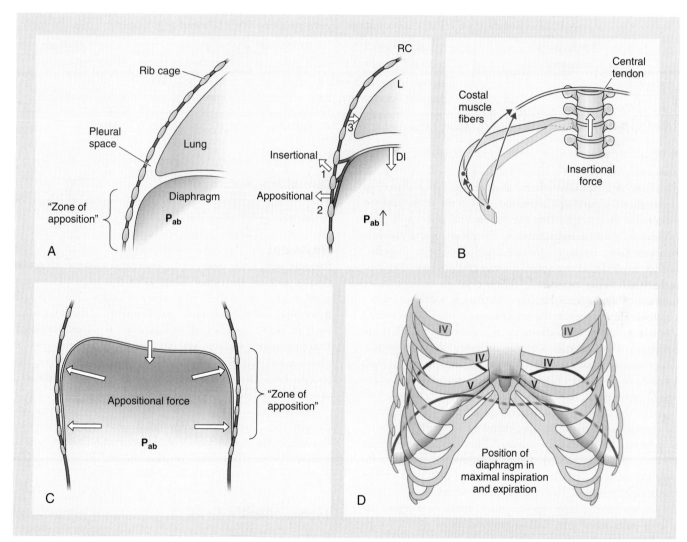

**Figure 5-16** Actions of the diaphragm. **A,** Zone of apposition and summary of diaphragm's actions. When the diaphragm contracts, a caudally oriented force is being applied on the central tendon and the dome of the diaphragm descends (DI). Furthermore, the costal diaphragmatic fibers apply a cranially oriented force to the upper margins of the lower six ribs that has the effect of lifting and rotating them outward (insertional force, *arrow 1*). The zone of apposition makes the lower rib cage part of the abdomen, and the changes in pressure in the pleural recess between the apposed diaphragm and the rib cage are almost equal to the changes in abdominal pressure. Pressure in this pleural recess rises rather than falls during inspiration because of diaphragmatic descent, and the rise in abdominal pressure is transmitted through the apposed diaphragm to expand the lower rib cage (*arrow 2*). All these effects result in expansion of the lower rib cage. On the upper rib cage, isolated contraction of the diaphragm causes a decrease in the anteroposterior diameter, and this expiratory action is primarily caused by the fall in pleural pressure (*arrow 3*). **B,** Insertional force; **C,** appositional force; **D,** shape of the diaphragm and the bony thorax at maximum inspiration and expiration. (From Albert RK, Spiro SG, Jett JR. Clinical Respiratory Medicine, ed 2. St. Louis, 2005, Mosby.)

## Table 5-23 Clinical Manifestation of Diaphragmatic Paralysis or Paresis

| | | Findings |
|---|---|---|
| Signs | Pulmonary function tests | ↓ All lung capacities and dynamic lung volumes (in proportion to degree of diaphragmatic dysfunction) |
| | | Unilateral paralysis: ↓ TLC, ↓ volume (25%) |
| | | Full diaphragmatic paralysis: ↓ VC below VT, therefore requiring mechanical ventilation |
| | | Lung volumes further decreased with change in position: VC ↓ 30% when sit → supine[25] |
| | | Flow rates ↓ in proportion to ↓ in lung volumes |
| | Chest radiograph | Elevated hemidiaphragm is classic finding. Diaphragm may be ↓, absent or paradoxical motion with inspiration. Atelectasis may be present |
| | Arterial blood gases | ↓ $PaO_2$, especially in supine position. With bilateral involvement, ↑ $PaCO_2$ |
| | Breath sounds | ↓ breath sounds on side of paralysis or paresis at base |
| | Cardiovascular | Severe hypoxemia can cause pulmonary hypertension leading to cor pulmonale[20] |
| Symptoms | | Dyspnea, worsened with supine position. Orthopnea, difficult or labored inspiration, anxiety, insomnia, daytime somnolence, and morning headaches[20] |

*$PaCO_2$, arterial partial pressure of $CO_2$; $PaO_2$, arterial partial pressure of $O_2$; TLC, total lung capacity; VC, vital capacity; VT, tidal volume*

direction.[8] In diaphragmatic paralysis or significant weakness, the negative pleural space pressure moves the diaphragm in a cephalad direction so that the diaphragm's resting position is elevated. During inspiration, as the pleural space pressure becomes more negative, the paralyzed diaphragm is pulled farther upward and the anterior lower ribs are pulled inward rather than being expanded.[26] These changes in ventilatory mechanics cause alveolar hypoventilation with secondary changes that are seen in the lung parenchyma. The decreased inspiratory capacity leads to microatelectasis, ventilation–perfusion mismatching, alveolar collapse, and hypoxemia. The atelectasis leads to a decrease in lung compliance and an increase in the work of breathing. These pathologic changes are heightened in the supine position. The rib cage is elevated in the supine position, putting the rib cage musculature at a mechanical disadvantage, thereby decreasing its ability to generate an inspiratory volume.[9] Therefore, in the supine position, diaphragmatic dysfunction produces a more significant decrease in alveolar ventilation than that produced in the upright position. The changes in the ventilatory mechanics and within the lung parenchyma combine to increase the risk of pulmonary infection or pneumonia in patients with diaphragmatic dysfunction.[8,25,26]

The degree of weakness of the diaphragm is best measured by transdiaphragmatic pressure. The normal transdiaphragmatic pressure is higher than 98 cm $H_2O$.[18,25] When the transdiaphragmatic pressure is lower than 20 cm $H_2O$, the patient exhibits significant respiratory distress.[25] The maximum transdiaphragmatic pressure is decreased 50%, and the maximum inspiratory pressure is decreased 40% with unilateral paralysis.[20,26] The reduction is even more profound with bilateral involvement.

## Clinical Manifestation

The clinical manifestation of diaphragmatic paralysis or paresis can be found in Table 5-23.

## Treatment

Patients with unilateral diaphragmatic involvement usually do not require treatment because of the large pulmonary reserve and the other respiratory muscles that are still functional. With bilateral involvement, either full-time or part-time mechanical ventilation is often required. Diaphragmatic pacing via an intact phrenic nerve is also a possibility for some of these patients; however, the success rate with this treatment intervention is estimated at only 50%.[20,25]

For additional therapeutic management, see practice pattern 6E (Impaired Ventilation and Respiration/Gas Exchange Associated with Ventilatory Pump Dysfunction or Failure) or 6F (Impaired Ventilation and Respiration/Gas Exchange Associated with Respiratory Failure).[11]

## Kyphoscoliosis

Kyphoscoliosis is a combination of excessive anteroposterior and lateral curvature of the thoracic spine (Fig. 5-17A).[2,8] This bony abnormality occurs in 3% of the population. However, lung dysfunction occurs in only 3% of the population with kyphoscoliosis (Fig. 5-17B).[20,26]

## Etiology

The cause of kyphoscoliosis is unknown or idiopathic in 85% of the cases. Idiopathic kyphoscoliosis is usually divided into three groups by age at onset: infantile, juvenile, and

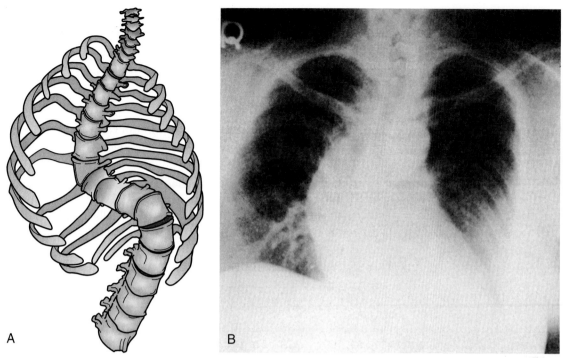

A          B

**Figure 5-17** Kyphoscoliosis. **A,** Schema showing the rotation of the spine and rib cage in kyphoscoliosis. (From Bergofsky EH, Turino GM, Fishman AP. Cardiorespiratory failure in kyphoscoliosis. Medicine (Baltimore) 38:263-317, 1959.) **B,** This chest radiograph of a patient with kyphoscoliosis reveals a markedly abnormal, reverse-S-shaped curve of the thoracic spine that is deforming the mediastinal structures and the ribs. This patient is breathing primarily with the diaphragm. (From Frownfelter D, Dean E. Cardiovascular and Pulmonary Physical Therapy: Evidence and Practice, ed 4. St. Louis, 2006, Mosby.)

adolescent (10 to 14 years of age), with most cases appearing in the adolescent group. There is a 4:1 ratio of females to males in this group. The other 15% of the cases are due to known congenital causes (e.g., hemivertebrae) or develop in response to a neuromuscular disease (e.g., poliomyelitis, syringomyelia, muscular dystrophy).[20,26]

## Pathophysiology

In addition to the excessive anteroposterior and lateral curvature, the lateral displacement causes two additional structural changes. A second lateral curve develops to counterbalance the primary curve. In addition, the spine rotates on its longitudinal axis so that the ribs on the side of the convexity are displaced posteriorly and splayed, creating a gibbous hump, whereas the ribs on the side of the concavity are compressed. Significant spinal curvature must be present before pulmonary symptoms develop. Usually angles less than 70 degrees do not produce pulmonary symptoms. Angles between 70 degrees and 120 degrees cause some respiratory dysfunction, and respiratory symptoms may increase with age as the angle increases and as the changes associated with aging affect the lung. Angles greater than 120 degrees are commonly associated with severe RLD and respiratory failure.[8] These skeletal abnormalities decrease the chest wall compliance, which may be as low as 25% of predicted.[8] Lung compliance is also decreased and dead space increased. The distribution of ventilation is disturbed, with more air going to the apices. Ventilation–perfusion matching is markedly impaired. These changes lead to a state of alveolar hypoventilation and a profound increase in the work of breathing—as high as 500% over normal.[8] The hypoventilation causes pulmonary hypertension, which over time causes structural changes in the vessels and thickening of the pulmonary arteriolar walls, leading to cor pulmonale. Although the respiratory muscles need to work harder to overcome the decreased pulmonary compliance, they are impaired because of the mechanical disadvantages from the thoracoabdominal deformity. When the VC is decreased to less than 40% of the predicted value, cardiorespiratory failure is likely to occur.[25] This usually occurs in the fourth or fifth decade of life. Sixty percent of deaths are due to respiratory failure or cor pulmonale.[25]

## Clinical Manifestation

The clinical manifestation of kyphoscoliosis can be found in Table 5-24.

## Treatment

Kyphoscoliosis is treated conservatively with orthotic devices and an exercise program. Surgical intervention includes placement of Harrington distraction strut bars. Pulmonary compromise is treated with preventive and supportive measures, including immunizations, good hydration, aggressive treatment of pulmonary infections, avoidance of sedatives, supplemental oxygen, and respiratory muscle training.[9] Serious pulmonary involvement, including recurrent episodes

**Table 5-24 Clinical Manifestation of Kyphoscoliosis**

| | | Findings |
|---|---|---|
| Signs | Pulmonary function tests | All dynamic lung volumes and capacities ↓ (in proportion to deformity). RV is normal or ↑. Flow rates ↓ in proportion to ↓ in VC. ↓ VT, ↑ RR; DLCO is normal unless angle >120° |
| | Chest radiograph | Grossly abnormal because of severe deformity of ribs and spine. Often view some compressed lung tissue with increased vascular markings, and other lung tissue distended and emphysema-like |
| | Arterial blood gases | ↓ $PaO_2$, ↑ $PaCO_2$ due to chronic alveolar hypoventilation |
| | Breath sounds | ↓ breath sounds over compressed lung |
| | Cardiovascular | Pulmonary hypertension usually present, arteriolar walls thicken, and cor pulmonale is common. Often with chronic hypoxemia, polycythemia may develop[2,20] |
| Symptoms | | Dyspnea on exertion, ↓ exercise tolerance, muscle spasms, and overuse of respiratory accessory muscles. Muscle wasting present with long-term respiratory involvement due to high caloric expenditure necessary for ventilation |

*DLCO, diffusing capacity of the lungs for carbon monoxide; $PaCO_2$, arterial partial pressure of $CO_2$; $PaO_2$, arterial partial pressure of $O_2$; RR, respiratory rate; RV, residual volume; VC, vital capacity; VT, tidal volume.*

of respiratory failure, seems to benefit from long-term nocturnal mechanical ventilation either through a chest cuirass or a positive pressure ventilator.[25,26] Studies have shown that nasal continuous positive airway pressure (CPAP) is also beneficial, and it is now the preferred therapy.[20]

## Ankylosing Spondylitis

Ankylosing spondylitis is a chronic inflammatory disease of the spine characterized by immobility of the sacroiliac and vertebral joints and by ossification of the paravertebral ligaments.[1,13]

## Etiology

Ankylosing spondylitis is an inherited arthritic condition that ultimately immobilizes the spine and results in a fixed thoracic cage.[26] It occurs predominantly in men aged 20 to 40 years.[9]

## Pathophysiology

The pulmonary impairment caused by this disease results from the markedly decreased compliance of the chest wall. With thoracic expansion so markedly decreased, ventilation becomes dependent almost entirely on diaphragmatic movement. Displacement of the abdomen during inspiration may be increased to compensate for the lack of rib expansion. Because the diaphragm is the major muscle of inspiration, the restrictive impairment involving the chest wall may result in only minimal respiratory symptoms.[8,26] However, approximately 6% of patients with ankylosing spondylitis develop specific fibrosing lesions in the upper lobes as part of this disease process.[7] Why these lesions occur in some patients is unknown, but the immune system may be involved.[27] The

pulmonary lesions may be unilateral or bilateral; they begin as small irregular opacities in the upper lobes. These lesions then increase in size, coalesce, and contract the lung parenchyma. Cavitation is frequent. The lung architecture becomes distorted, showing dense fibrosis that can lead to bronchiectasis and repeated pulmonary infections and an obstructive pulmonary deficit superimposed on the RLD.[7,27] Apical pleural thickening is invariably present.[9]

## Clinical Manifestation

The clinical manifestation of ankylosing spondylitis can be found in Table 5-25.

## Treatment

There is no curative treatment for ankylosing spondylitis. It is important to maintain good body alignment and as much thoracic mobility as possible. If there is direct lung involvement, then treatment of repeated pulmonary infections is required.

## Pectus Excavatum

Pectus excavatum (funnel chest) is a congenital abnormality characterized by sternal depression and decreased anteroposterior diameter (Fig. 5-18). The lower portion of the sternum is displaced posteriorly, and the anterior ribs are bowed markedly. Pulmonary function values are normal or near normal, and respiratory symptoms are uncommon. If the deformity is very severe, the patient may have decreased TLC, VC, and maximum voluntary ventilation and may complain of dyspnea on exertion, precordial pain, palpitation, and dizziness. Usually no treatment is indicated because the deformity is only cosmetic, with no functional deficits.[1,25,26]

## Table 5-25 Clinical Manifestation of Ankylosing Spondylitis

|  |  | Findings |
| --- | --- | --- |
| Signs | Pulmonary function tests | ↓ VC, ↓ IC, ↑ RV, ↑ FRC |
|  | Chest radiograph | May see upper-lobe fibrosis |
|  | Arterial blood gases | Usually no abnormalities |
|  | Breath sounds | Usually normal |
|  | Cardiovascular | No typical abnormalities |
| Symptoms |  | Dyspnea on exertion. Pleuritic chest pain in 60% of patients. If upper lobes involved, may have a productive cough, progressive dyspnea, fever, and possible hemoptysis. May also have low back pain, weight loss, and anorexia[9] |

*FRC, functional residual capacity; IC, inspiratory capacity; RV, residual volume; VC, vital capacity.*

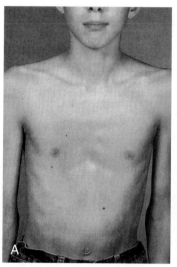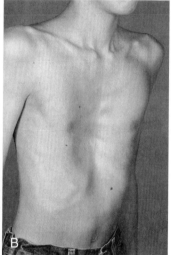

**Figure 5-18** Twelve-year-old boy with the most frequent form of pectus excavatum: the thorax is symmetric, with a depression in the inferior portion of the sternum. Pictures courtesy of Dr. Dickens St-Vil. (From Gilbert-Barness E, Kapur R, Oligny LL, et al. [eds.]. Potter's Pathology of the Fetus, Infant and Child, ed 2. St. Louis, 2007, Mosby.)

## Pectus Carinatum

Pectus carinatum (pigeon breast) is a structural abnormality characterized by the sternum protruding anteriorly (Fig. 5-19). Fifty percent of patients with atrial or ventricular septal defects have pectus carinatum. It also has been associated with severe prolonged childhood asthma. There is no pulmonary compromise associated with this structural abnormality, and no treatment is indicated.[26]

## Connective Tissue Causes of Restrictive Lung Dysfunction

### Rheumatoid Arthritis

Rheumatoid arthritis is a chronic process characterized by inflammation of the peripheral joints that results in progressive destruction of articular and periarticular structures.[1,26]

### Etiology

The etiology is unknown. There is a high prevalence of RA in the United States; 4 to 6 million adults have been diagnosed with this chronic condition.[17] One third of these patients, almost 2 million people, have some pulmonary involvement as part of their disease, although it remains unclear why one or more pulmonary lesions may develop in a given patient.[27] Lung involvement with RA usually occurs between 50 and 60 years of age and is very rare in children who have RA.[17] Another distinction is that although RA is more prevalent in women, pulmonary involvement, particularly pulmonary fibrosis, is more common in men.[27]

### Pathophysiology

Pulmonary involvement in RA was first recognized and reported by Ellman and Ball in 1948.[33] Rheumatoid arthritis can affect the lungs in seven different ways: pleural involvement, pneumonitis, interstitial fibrosis, development

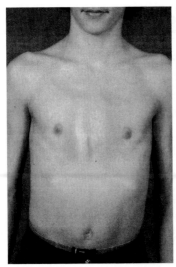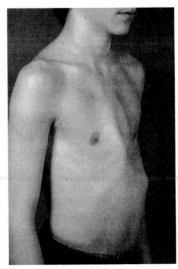

**Figure 5-19** Thirteen-year-old boy with pectus carinatum. Bilateral depressions are seen laterally to the cartilage of the costo-chondral junction, which is bilaterally hypertrophic; the sternum projects anteriorly. Pictures courtesy of Dr. Dickens St-Vil. (From Gilbert-Barness E, Kapur R, Oligny LL, et al. [eds.]. Potter's Pathology of the Fetus, Infant and and Child, ed 2. St. Louis, 2007, Mosby.)

of pulmonary nodules, pulmonary vasculitis, obliterative bronchiolitis, and an increased incidence of bronchogenic cancer.[9] These different pulmonary manifestations of RA may occur individually or in combination within the lungs.[33] Pleural involvement may include pleuritis, pleural friction rub, repeated small exudative pleural effusions, and pleural thickening and fibrosis.[17,27,28] These pulmonary abnormalities can result in pain and some RLD. Pneumonitis causes an inflammatory reaction in the lung, including patchy infiltrates, which can resolve spontaneously or can progress to fibrotic changes. The cause of interstitial fibrosis in the patient with RA is unknown but seems to correlate with increased manifestations of autoimmunity.[33] Patients with a high titer of rheumatoid factor are more likely to develop interstitial fibrosis.[17]

There seems to be a temporal relationship between joint involvement and development of fibrosing alveolitis, with the joint involvement usually coming first.[17] Interstitial fibrosis can be diffuse but predominates in the lower lobes. Rheumatoid (necrobiotic) nodules usually occur subpleurally in the upper lung fields or in the interlobular septa. They may be single, multiple, unilateral, or bilateral. Spontaneous resolution of these nodules can occur. Cavitation is common.[25,33] If a patient with RA is exposed to coal dust, pulmonary nodules known as Caplan's syndrome can develop. These multiple peripheral pulmonary nodules have a pigmented ring of coal dust surrounding the lesion. Rheumatoid nodules and Caplan's syndrome rarely produce significant RLD.[27,33]

Pulmonary vasculitis often occurs adjacent to pulmonary nodules. There is intimal fibrosis in the pulmonary arterioles.[7,33] Obliterative bronchiolitis is rare; however, the onset is usually acute and progresses within 2 years to a fatal outcome. The bronchioles become inflamed and edematous and are then replaced with granulation tissue. The bronchial lumen is severely narrowed or obliterated.[7,25] The increased

incidence of bronchogenic cancer in RA is related to coexisting interstitial fibrosis in both smokers and nonsmokers.[9]

In addition to lung involvement with RA, chest wall compliance may be decreased significantly owing to increased rigidity of the thorax because of RA, decreased inspiratory muscle power because of rheumatoid myopathy, or decreased mobility because of pain caused by pleurisy. Therefore, the RLD that can result in RA patients may be due to a decrease both in lung and in chest wall compliance.[17]

### Clinical Manifestation
The clinical manifestation of RA can be found in Table 5-26.

### Treatment
Corticosteroids and immunosuppressant drugs are commonly used to treat pulmonary involvement in RA.[25,33]

## Systemic Lupus Erythematosus

Systemic lupus erythematosus (SLE) is a chronic inflammatory connective tissue disorder.[1,24,25]

### Etiology
The etiology is unknown, although the immune system seems to be involved.[1,25] Ninety percent of cases occur in women, and SLE is more common in black women.[8] It usually occurs between the ages of 15 and 45, most frequently in the second and third decades of life.[8] It is interesting that certain drugs (procainamide hydrochloride, phenytoin, hydralazine hydrochloride, penicillamine, isoniazid) can evoke a clinical syndrome indistinguishable from spontaneous SLE.[17]

### Pathophysiology
This disorder involves the autoimmune system and is characterized by a variety of antigen–antibody reactions.[1]

## Table 5-26  Clinical Manifestation of Rheumatoid Arthritis

| | | Findings |
|---|---|---|
| Signs | Pulmonary function tests | ↓ VC, ↓ DLCO, ↓ lung compliance |
| | Chest radiograph | Pleural thickening or effusion (unilateral in 80% of cases) Rheumatoid nodules present (round, homogenous densities seen in peripheral lung fields of upper lobes). |
| | | When interstitial fibrosis develops, a dense reticular or reticulonodular pattern with honeycomb appears[9] |
| | Arterial blood gases | ↓ PaO$_2$, normal PaCO$_2$ |
| | Breath sounds | Bibasilar rales and possibly ↓ breath sounds |
| | Cardiovascular | Pulmonary hypertension develops in presence of pulmonary vasculitis |
| Symptoms | | Warm, swollen, painful joints. Progressive dyspnea with nonproductive cough. May have pleuritic pain, fever, cyanosis[17,25,28] |

*DLCO, diffusing capacity of the lungs for carbon monoxide; PaCO$_2$, arterial partial pressure of CO$_2$; PaO$_2$, arterial partial pressure of O$_2$; VC, vital capacity.*

Systemic lupus erythematosus can involve the skin, joints, kidneys, lung, nervous tissue, and heart. In 50% to 90% of the cases, it does involve the lungs or pleura; this incidence of pulmonary involvement is higher than that of any other connective tissue disorder.[10,28] The most common lung involvement is pleurisy, often with the development of small bilateral exudative pleural effusions that may be recurrent, may be associated with pericarditis, and may lead to fibrinous pleuritis.[8,28] Acute lupus pneumonitis is another manifestation of lung involvement. It usually causes hypoxemia, severe shortness of breath, cyanosis, tachypnea, and tachycardia.[8,25,28] There may be an accompanying pleuritis with or without pleural effusion. Acute lupus pneumonitis may resolve or may lead to chronic interstitial pneumonitis and fibrosis. Alveolar hemorrhage is a rare but life-threatening pulmonary manifestation of SLE. It can occur suddenly with no prior hemoptysis and can carry a mortality as high as 70%.[8] The reasons some patients develop recurrent pulmonary hemorrhages or have a massive intraalveolar hemorrhage are not known. Recurrent hemorrhages can lead to interstitial fibrosis.

It has been found that diaphragmatic weakness is relatively common in SLE patients. It is now appreciated that the "shrinkage" of the lower lobes, elevated diaphragms, and bibasilar atelectasis can be attributed largely to diaphragmatic weakness. The diaphragm may show muscle atrophy and fibrosis with minimal inflammation.[8] Other ventilatory muscles may also be weak, even with no noticeable weakness in the muscles of the extremities. This muscle involvement may cause a marked restrictive ventilatory impairment in 25% of SLE patients.[9] Nephritis occurs in more than 50% of patients and is the major cause of mortality in SLE.[8]

## Drug-Induced Systemic Lupus Erythematosus

Nearly 50 drugs have been reported to induce SLE, but only six regularly induce antinuclear antibodies and therefore symptomatic SLE. They are procainamide hydrochloride, hydralazine hydrochloride, practolol, penicillamine, isoniazid, and hydantoins. Patients who take one of these drugs for months or years may develop clinical SLE, and of these, 50% develop pleuropulmonary involvement, including interstitial lung disease. In the majority of patients, these changes are reversible by discontinuing the drug. Use of corticosteroids may accelerate the resolution.[17]

### Clinical Manifestation

The clinical manifestation of SLE can be found in Table 5-27.

### Treatment

Corticosteroids cause rapid improvement of acute lupus pneumonitis and, together with plasmapheresis, are also used to treat alveolar hemorrhage.[8,28] Fibrotic changes in the lungs are irreversible, so only supportive therapy is indicated.

## Scleroderma

Scleroderma (progressive systemic sclerosis) is a progressive fibrosing disorder that causes degenerative changes in the skin, small blood vessels, esophagus, intestinal tract, lung, heart, kidney, and articular structures.[1,25]

## Etiology

The etiology is unknown, and the pattern of involvement, progression, and severity of the disease varies widely. It is four times more common in women than in men and is rare in children. The majority of patients are diagnosed between 30 and 50 years of age.[28]

## Pathophysiology

Within the lung, scleroderma appears as progressive diffuse interstitial fibrosis, in which collagen replaces the normal connective tissue framework of the lung. There is fibrotic

## Table 5-27 Clinical Manifestation of Systemic Lupus Erythematosus

| | | Findings |
|---|---|---|
| Signs | Pulmonary function tests | ↓ lung volumes, ↓ lung compliance, ↓ DLCO |
| | Chest radiograph | Atelectatic pneumonitis with alveolar consolidation (especially at bases), elevated hemidiaphragms, reticulonodular pattern of interstitial infiltrates, pleural effusions & in presence of pericardial effusion would see cardiomegaly |
| | Arterial blood gases | ↓ PaO$_2$ and PaCO$_2$ usually within normal limits |
| | Breath sounds | Bibasilar rales may be present or pleural friction rub |
| | Cardiovascular | Often have pericarditis, may have pericardial effusions and /or pulmonary hypertension |
| Symptoms | | 90% have articular symptoms, including arthralgias and polyarthritis. Often have dyspnea, cough with or without sputum production, hemoptysis, fever, pleuritic pain. May also have fatigue, weight loss, Raynaud phenomenon, and photosensitivity |

*DLCO, diffusing capacity of the lungs for carbon monoxide; PaCO$_2$, arterial partial pressure of CO$_2$; PaO$_2$, arterial partial pressure of O$_2$.*

## Table 5-28 Clinical Manifestation of Scleroderma

| | | Findings |
|---|---|---|
| Signs | Pulmonary function tests | ↓ TLC, ↓ VC, ↓ all lung volumes, ↓ lung compliance, ↓ chest wall compliance ↓ DLCO, ↑ work of breathing |
| | Chest radiograph | Pulmonary infiltrates early in course; later in course see interstitial reticular pattern with honeycombing, especially at bases. Pleural thickening and aspiration pneumonia (as a result of ↓ esophageal motility); pericardial effusion and right-sided heart enlargement |
| | Arterial blood gases | ↓ PaO$_2$, PaCO$_2$ within normal limits |
| | Breath sounds | Bibasilar rales, breath sounds may be diminished and rhonchi present if infiltrates present |
| | Cardiovascular | Pulmonary hypertension common, can progress to cor pulmonale. May have pericarditis with pericardial effusions, arrhythmias, and conduction disturbances |
| Symptoms | | Exertional dyspnea (in 40% of cases), and more common in individuals with Raynaud phenomenon[27] |
| | | Nonproductive cough and clubbing of digits are common |

*DLCO, diffusing capacity of the lungs for carbon monoxide; PaCO$_2$, arterial partial pressure of CO$_2$; PaO$_2$, arterial partial pressure of O$_2$; TLC, total lung capacity; VC, vital capacity.*

replacement of the connective tissue within the alveolar walls. The pulmonary arterioles undergo obliterative changes; however, necrotizing vasculitis is rare.[25] These changes may be accompanied by parenchymal cystic sclerosis, thus increasing the restrictive impairment in the lung. At autopsy, 75% to 80% of scleroderma victims show evidence of interstitial pulmonary fibrosis.[27] Pleuritis and pleural effusions are unusual, unlike in the other collagen diseases that have pulmonary involvement.[27] Carcinoma of the lung also has been reported in association with scleroderma.[25]

Esophageal dysfunction is the most frequent visceral disturbance and occurs in most patients.[28] Lung dysfunction is the second most common visceral disturbance, occurring in approximately 90% of scleroderma patients.[9,10] The disease is often slowly progressive. However, if cardiac, pulmonary, or renal involvement is early, the prognosis is poor. Death is usually due to cardiac or renal failure.[27]

## Clinical Manifestation

The clinical manifestation of scleroderma can be found in Table 5-28.

## Treatment

There is no effective drug treatment for sclerodermatous pleuropulmonary disease. The interstitial fibrosis is progressive and nonreversible. There is also no drug therapy that has

## Table 5-29 Clinical Manifestation of Polymyositis

| | | Findings |
|---|---|---|
| Signs | Pulmonary function tests | ↓ lung volumes, ↓ DLCO |
| | Chest radiograph | Lower lobe interstitial fibrosis in periphery with honeycombing[10] |
| | Arterial blood gases | ↓ PaO$_2$ due to ventilatory pump weakness |
| | Breath sounds | Late inspiratory bibasilar rales[9] |
| | Cardiovascular | Nothing significant |
| Symptoms | | Progressive shortness of breath with a nonproductive cough. When neck flexors weaken, patient has difficulty supporting or lifting head. Weakness of laryngeal and pharyngeal muscles can cause dysphonia and dysphagia. With ↑ respiratory muscle weakness breathing is labored. Possible muscle pain and tenderness |

*DLCO, diffusing capacity of the lungs for carbon monoxide; PaO$_2$, arterial partial pressure of O$_2$.*

been shown to be effective in altering the course of scleroderma. A number of agents are used to treat specific symptoms in affected organs.[28] Lung transplantation may be an option, particularly if the scleroderma has not affected any other organ system.[9] Otherwise, only supportive treatment of pulmonary symptoms is available.

## Polymyositis

Polymyositis is a systemic connective tissue disease characterized by symmetric proximal muscle weakness and pain.[24,25,28]

### Etiology

The etiology is unknown but may involve an autoimmune reaction. The disease can occur throughout life but most commonly appears before age 15 or between 40 and 60 years of age. The disease is twice as common in women.[24,28]

### Pathophysiology

Approximately 5% to 20% of patients exhibit involvement of the lung parenchyma.[10] Aspiration pneumonia is the most common pulmonary abnormality and is seen in 15% to 20% of patients.[10] Other changes can include interstitial pneumonitis and fibrosis, bronchiolitis obliterans, or diffuse pulmonary infiltrates. The pleura is usually not involved. In addition to these changes, which result in a restrictive pulmonary impairment, the respiratory muscles may be weak, which increases the restrictive dysfunction. Striated muscle involvement includes inflammation, degeneration, atrophy, and necrosis. This results in profound weakness of the limb girdle muscles, the respiratory muscles, the laryngeal muscles, and the pharyngeal muscles. When the disease occurs in children, diffuse soft tissue calcification may occur also, which could decrease chest wall compliance further. Dysphagia and aspiration problems are common. Although characteristics of the disease are similar in children and adults, the onset is often more acute in children and more insidious in adults. The disease may enter long periods of remission. However, it seems to be more severe and unrelenting in patients with pulmonary or cardiac involvement.[25,27,28]

## Clinical Manifestation

The clinical manifestation of polymyositis can be found in Table 5-29.

## Treatment

Pulmonary involvement is treated with corticosteroids, with good results if started early during the inflammatory phase.[25]

## Dermatomyositis

Dermatomyositis is a systemic connective tissue disease characterized primarily by inflammatory and degenerative changes in the skin. The pulmonary involvement that occurs with this disease mirrors the involvement that occurs with polymyositis described earlier. The incidence of lung involvement in dermatomyositis patients is also 5% to 20%.[10,13,27]

# Immunologic Causes of Restrictive Lung Dysfunction

## Goodpasture's Syndrome

Goodpasture's syndrome is a disease of the immune complex that is characterized by interstitial or intraalveolar hemorrhage, glomerulonephritis, and anemia.[27]

## Etiology

This rather rare disease is most often brought on by the presence of antiglomerular basement membrane (anti-GBM) antibodies that react with the vascular basement membranes of the alveolus and the glomerulus, causing pulmonary hemorrhage and glomerulonephritis. How these antibodies come to be formed is still unknown. Prodromal viral infections or exposure to chemical substances such as hydrocarbon solvents may be involved. Why these anti-GBM antibodies cannot be demonstrated in all patients with Goodpasture's syndrome is another mystery. This syndrome is approximately four times more prevalent in men than in women. The onset of the disease occurs between the ages of 17 and 27 in 75% of the cases.[26]

## Table 5-30 Clinical Manifestation of Goodpasture's Syndrome

|  |  | **Findings** |
|---|---|---|
| Signs | Pulmonary function tests | ↓ lung volumes in proportion to amount of pulmonary fibrosis present |
|  | Chest radiograph | Shows distribution, volume, and temporal sequence of repeated pulmonary hemorrhages. Appear as diffuse, fluffy infiltrates during remission of disease. When pulmonary fibrosis develops, permanent reticulonodular infiltrates are seen.[9,20] |
|  | Arterial blood gases | ↓ $PaO_2$, may see ↓ $PaCO_2$ |
|  | Breath sounds | With active pulmonary hemorrhage breath sounds are ↓ |
|  |  | Over permanent pulmonary fibrosis, ↓ breath sounds and dry inspiratory rales |
|  | Cardiovascular | ECG normal |
| Symptoms |  | Hemoptysis is the most common symptom (and usually the first symptom). Dyspnea, cough, and substernal chest pain often occur. Patients may also experience weakness, fatigue, hematuria, pallor, and fever and 5% report arthralgias.[9,10] |

*ECG, electrocardiograph; $PaCO_2$, arterial partial pressure of $CO_2$; $PaO_2$, arterial partial pressure of $O_2$.*

## Pathophysiology

Whatever the cause of these autoantibodies, it has been shown that when they are present in the circulating blood, they cross-react with the basement membrane of the alveolar wall and deposit along the glomerular basement membrane. This results in the release of cytotoxic substances that damage the pulmonary and glomerular capillaries. Blood leaks from the damaged pulmonary capillaries into the interstitium and the alveolar spaces, which over time can lead to significant and widespread pulmonary fibrosis. The pulmonary hemorrhages are episodic and seem to be precipitated by nonimmunologic factors such as fluid overload, smoking, toxic exposure, or infection. Within the kidney, the damaged glomerular capillaries lead to a rapidly progressive, often necrotizing type of glomerulonephritis and renal failure.[8,26,27]

## Clinical Manifestation

The clinical manifestation of Goodpasture's syndrome can be found in Table 5-30.

## Treatment

Treatment usually combines plasmapheresis and immunosuppressive therapy to lower the levels of anti-GBM antibodies circulating in the blood. Cyclophosphamide with prednisone is the regimen of choice. Methylprednisolone may be used to treat pulmonary hemorrhage. Dialysis is used to counteract renal failure. The overall prognosis for Goodpasture's syndrome is poor. Until recently, approximately 50% of the patients died within 1 year of diagnosis. One half of the deaths were due to pulmonary hemorrhage and the other half to renal failure.[8,26,27] Currently, however, it has been recognized that there can be milder forms of the disease and that the disease's responsiveness to treatment can be variable. Therefore, early aggressive therapy encompassing plasmapheresis, drugs, ventilator support, acute hemodialysis, treatment of infection, and careful avoidance of cardiogenic edema has been used to increase survival rates to 70% to 80%.[9]

## Wegener's Granulomatosis

Wegener's granulomatosis is a multisystem disease characterized by granulomatous vasculitis of the upper and lower respiratory tracts, glomerulonephritis, and widespread small vessel vasculitis.[26]

## Etiology

The etiology is unknown. Some studies seem to indicate that the disease may be due to a hypersensitivity reaction to an undetermined antigen. During the active disease process, circulating immune complexes have been identified. Immune reactants and complex-like deposits have also been identified in renal biopsies of patients with Wegener's granulomatosis. Although histologically the immune system and hypersensitivity reactions seem to be involved, the disease appears clinically as an infectious process due to some unknown pathogen. This disease can occur at any age, but the average age at onset is 40 years. The disease is twice as common in males as in females.[26]

## Pathophysiology

The disease often seems to start in the upper respiratory tract with necrotizing granulomas and ulceration in the nasopharynx and paranasal areas. Inflammation with perivascular exudative infiltration and fibrin deposition in the pulmonary arteries and veins causes focal destruction. Multiple nodular cavitary infiltrates develop in one or both lungs. These lesions often consist of a necrotic core surrounded by granulation tissue. Early in the disease, the kidney shows acute focal or segmental glomerulitis with hematuria. As the disease progresses, necrotizing glomerulonephritis leading to kidney failure often occurs.[18,26]

**Table 5-31 Clinical Manifestation of Wegener's Granulomatosis**

|  |  | Findings |
|---|---|---|
| Signs | Pulmonary function tests | ↓ lung volumes, impaired gas diffusion |
|  | Chest radiograph | Pulmonary infiltrates may appear in any lobe, bilaterally or unilaterally, and may appear hazy or with sharply defined borders. Cavitation of these lesions is common.[18,26] Pleural effusions in 20% of patients[9] |
|  | Arterial blood gases | ↓ $PaO_2$ |
|  | Breath sounds | Variable |
|  |  | Depending on size and location of lesions |
|  | Cardiovascular | Variable |
|  |  | Depends on severity of disseminated small vessel vasculitis. Myocardial infarction may occur |
| Symptoms |  | Upper respiratory tract symptoms initially: rhinorrhea, paranasal sinusitis, nasal mucosal ulcerations, otitis media, and hearing loss. Dyspnea, cough, hemoptysis, vague chest pain, or pleuritic pain. Also complaints of fever, fatigue, weight loss, anorexia, and arthralgias[9] |

$PaO_2$, arterial partial pressure of $O_2$.

## Clinical Manifestation

The clinical manifestation of Wegener's granulomatosis can be found in Table 5-31.

## Treatment

The treatment of choice is with cyclophosphamide. This drug can produce marked improvement or partial remissions in 91% of patients and complete remissions in 75% of patients.[9] Without drug therapy, this disease progresses rapidly and is fatal. The mean duration between diagnosis and death is 5 months when not treated.[26] Death is most often due to renal disease progressing to kidney failure. Kidney transplantation has been used successfully in cases of renal failure.

## Pregnancy as a Cause of Restrictive Lung Dysfunction

During the third trimester of pregnancy, ventilation to the dependent regions of the lungs is impaired by the growth and position of the developing fetus. This restrictive change in ventilation is due to a decrease in chest wall compliance caused primarily by the decreased downward excursion of the diaphragm (Fig. 5-20). The decreased ventilation in the bases of the lungs results in early small airway closure and increased ventilation–perfusion mismatching. The voluntary lung volumes are decreased, particularly the ERV (8% to 40%).[9] The work of breathing is increased, and the woman may feel that she is unable to take a deep breath, particularly in the supine position. To counteract some of these changes and to keep the $PaO_2$ within the normal range, the body increases the progesterone level during this trimester. The increased level of progesterone increases the woman's ventilatory drive, which in turn increases the tidal volume and

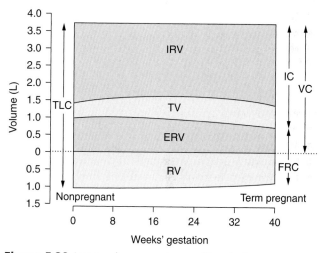

**Figure 5-20** Lung volumes and capacities during pregnancy. ERV, expiratory reserve volume; FRC, functional residual capacity; IC, inspiratory capacity; IRV, inspiratory reserve volume; RV, residual volume; TLC, total lung capacity; VT, tidal volume; VC, vital capacity. (From Chestnut DH. Obstetric Anesthesia, ed 4. St. Louis, 2009, Mosby.)

respiratory rate, thereby increasing the minute ventilation. This increase results in a decrease in $PaO_2$ and a rise in $PaO_2$, which ensures that the mother and the fetus do not become hypoxemic.[9,13]

## Nutritional and Metabolic Causes of Restrictive Lung Dysfunction

### Obesity

Obesity is defined as a condition in which the body weight is 20% or more over the ideal body weight.[24]

## Etiology

Obesity is the result of an imbalance between the calories ingested and the calories expended. This imbalance may be due to overeating, inadequate exercise, a pathologic process that alters metabolism, or a psychological need or coping mechanism.

## Pathophysiology

The increase in body weight represents a significant increase in body mass, and this extra tissue requires additional oxygen from the lungs and produces additional carbon dioxide, which must be eliminated by the lungs. The excess soft tissue on the chest wall decreases the compliance of the thorax and therefore increases the work of breathing. The excess soft tissue in the abdominal wall exerts pressure on the abdominal contents, forcing the diaphragm up to a higher resting position. This shift results in decreased lung expansion and early closure of the small airways and alveoli, especially at the bases or the dependent regions of the lung. These areas are hypoventilated relative to their perfusion, which can markedly increase the ventilation–perfusion mismatching and result in hypoxemia.[2,8] In addition, some overweight individuals have demonstrated an obesity-hypoventilation syndrome, which results when there is an imbalance between the ventilatory drive and the ventilatory load.[9]

## Clinical Manifestation

The clinical manifestation of obesity can be found in Table 5-32.

## Treatment

It is becoming better recognized that obesity is a very complex disorder. It involves virtually all the body's systems via the patient's metabolism, the psychological and mental processes within the patient, and the patient's behaviors and habits. Treatment consisting of dieting and will power is usually not effective over an extended period of time. Patients who have been markedly obese over a long period usually can demonstrate expertise in dieting and remarkably significant will power. It is not unusual for these patients to have lost three or four times their body weight over their lifetime, only to regain the lost weight and more. Current treatment strategies for the obese patient combine interventions. Weight loss programs now often include extensive medical evaluation and a variety of therapeutic interventions, including diet, increased activity, behavior modification, psychological support, nutritional counseling, and family involvement. Weight loss will decrease the work of breathing, increase the vital capacity, and increase the ventilatory drive in these patients.[9] Sleep apnea is most commonly treated with weight loss, avoidance of ethanol, position therapy, dental devices, nasal CPAP, increased $FIO_2$, and tracheostomy.[9,10]

A great deal is still to be learned and understood about the body's metabolism: how food is broken down, stored, and eliminated and how obesity can be reversed so that recurrence is not the norm. Currently two surgical procedures are being utilized for morbid obesity which are showing promising results: gastric bypass surgery and the lap band procedure. Both procedures help with weight loss: the former by bypassing the stomach and effectively decreasing the amount of food that can be absorbed and the latter by decreasing the actual size of the stomach, again decreasing the amount of food that can be absorbed. See Chapter 7 for more details on obesity.

## Diabetes Mellitus

Diabetes mellitus is a syndrome that results from abnormal carbohydrate metabolism and is characterized by inadequate insulin secretion and hyperglycemia.[24]

## Table 5-32 Clinical Manifestation of Obesity

|  |  | Findings |
| --- | --- | --- |
| Signs | Pulmonary function tests | ERV, ↓ all lung capacities and volumes slightly<br>↓ VT, ↑ RR, ↓ MVV, ↓ lung volumes in supine position (often causing problems with sleeping) |
|  | Chest radiograph | ↑ in adipose tissue overlying ribs, compression of lung tissue in dependent lung regions. Over time may show enlarged heart and small lung fields with congestion[9] |
|  | Arterial blood gases | ↓ $PaO_2$, some with ↑ $PaCO_2$ |
|  | Breath sounds | Diminished in bases |
|  | Cardiovascular | ↑ in cardiac output and circulating volume. Common to see systemic and pulmonary hypertension. May develop arrhythmias and CHF |
| Symptoms |  | Dyspnea on exertion; sleep apnea |

*CHF, congestive heart failure; ERV, expiratory reserve volume; MVV, maximum voluntary ventilation; PaCO₂, arterial partial pressure of CO₂; PaO₂, arterial partial pressure of O₂; RR, respiratory rate; VT, tidal volume.*

## Etiology

Diabetes mellitus has no distinct etiology but seems to result from a variable interaction of hereditary and environmental factors.[24]

## Pathophysiology

The most common pathologic changes seen in diabetes mellitus result from hyperglycemia, large vessel disease, microvascular disease (particularly involving the retina and kidney), and neuropathy.[24] The effects of this metabolic disorder on the lungs have been reported, and although the incidence of pulmonary involvement does not seem to be high, it can be significant in some patients. Hyperglycemic patients have an increased incidence of pulmonary infections and tuberculosis, which is manifest more frequently in the lower lobes.[25] Diffuse alveolar hemorrhage has also been reported in diabetics and may be due to inflammation and necrosis of the pulmonary capillary endothelium. This could then be followed by fibrotic changes.[17] In a study of more than 31,000 patients with diabetes mellitus, pulmonary fibrosis was found in 0.8% of the diabetic population, which is a moderately greater incidence than that reported for the general population.[25] Juvenile diabetics have shown a decrease in elastic recoil of the lungs and in lung compliance, causing a decrease in TLC.[25,33] These abnormalities in ventilatory mechanics are thought to be due to changes in the elastin and collagen within the lung. Another mechanism that can cause a restrictive impairment in the lung is diabetic ketoacidosis, which can produce a noncardiogenic pulmonary edema. The physiologic cause for this change is unclear but may be an alteration in the pulmonary capillary permeability.[25] See Chapter 7 for more details on diabetes.

## Traumatic Causes of Restrictive Lung Dysfunction

### Crush Injuries

Crush injuries to the thorax are usually caused by blunt trauma that results in pathologic damage, particularly rib fractures, flail chest, or lung contusion.[1]

## Etiology

The leading cause of blunt trauma to the thorax is motor vehicle accidents. The second most common cause of thoracic crush injuries is falls, which usually occur in the home.[26]

## Pathophysiology

### Rib Fractures

Rib fractures most commonly involve the fifth through the ninth ribs because they are anchored anteriorly and posteriorly and are less protected than ribs 1 through 4 from the kinetic energy of a traumatic blow.[26] Even nondisplaced rib fractures can be very painful, and it is the pain on any movement of the chest wall that causes the restrictive impairment. Patients with rib fractures breathe very shallowly in an effort to keep the thoracic wall still. The muscular splinting around the fracture site also decreases chest wall excursion and lung expansion. In addition, fractured ribs may be accompanied by a hemothorax (blood in the pleural cavity), which can progress to a large sanguinous effusion and empyema. This fluid in the pleural space compresses the underlying lung parenchyma and can cause fibrosis and scarring of the pleura, leading to permanent restrictive dysfunction.[8] More frequently, the pain of the rib fractures decreases significantly during the first 2 weeks after the injury, atelectasis improves, and normal lung function is restored, although coughing may cause pain for up to 6 months. Patients who have multiple rib fractures, are older than 50 years, or have underlying pulmonary or cardiovascular disease are at greater risk of developing a pneumonia following rib fracture.[4,26]

### Flail Chest

Flail chest refers to a free-floating segment of ribs due to multiple rib fractures both anteriorly and posteriorly that leave this part of the thoracic wall disconnected to the rest of the thoracic cage (Fig. 5-21).[26] This segment can usually be identified by its paradoxical movement during the respiratory cycle. It moves inward during inspiration, drawn by the increase in the negative pleural space pressure. It moves outward during expiration, as the pleural space pressure approaches atmospheric pressure. Both the pain and the paradoxical movement of a part of the thoracic cage during the

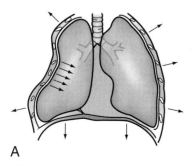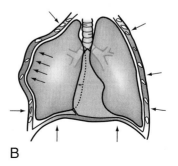

**Figure 5-21** Forces producing disordered chest wall motion in flail chest. **A,** During inspiration, the lowering of pleural pressure produces inward motion of the flail segment. **B,** During expiration, the increase in pleural pressure produces an outward displacement of the flail segment. (From Mason RJ, Broaddus VC, Murray JF, et al. Murray & Nadel's Textbook of Respiratory Medicine, ed 4. St. Louis, 2005, Saunders.)

respiratory cycle contribute to the restrictive dysfunction. Lung volumes are decreased, and the distribution of ventilation is altered, causing an increase in ventilation–perfusion mismatching. The force of the blunt trauma that causes a flail chest is usually greater than that causing a simple rib fracture. Because the force is greater, flail chest is often associated with lung contusion.[4,20,26] Long-term pulmonary disability following flail chest is common; 60% of these patients have chest wall pain, chest wall deformity, dyspnea on exertion, and mild restrictive pulmonary dysfunction for months to years following the injury.[20]

### Lung Contusion

Lung contusion occurs when the lung strikes directly against the chest wall. The local pulmonary microvasculature is damaged, causing red blood cells and plasma to move into the alveoli.[26] This immediately decreases the compliance of the lung, changes the distribution of inspired gases, and increases ventilation–perfusion mismatching. Although the injury due to the lung contusion may resolve in approximately 3 days, patients are at high risk for serious pulmonary complications. Approximately 50% to 70% develop a pneumonia in the contused segment, 35% develop an empyema, and some patients develop ARDS, with complete "white out" of the injured lung on chest radiograph.[4,20,26]

## Clinical Manifestation

The clinical manifestation of lung contusion, fracture, and flail chest can be found in Table 5-33.

## Treatment

### Rib Fractures

Pain control is the primary treatment and can be accomplished by oral analgesics, intercostal nerve block, or epidural anesthesia depending on the extent of the injury.[26] The goal is to allow the patient to reestablish a normal breathing pattern. In patients at high risk for developing pneumonia, hospital admission may be indicated for close observation and for aggressive pulmonary hygiene in addition to pain relief.[20]

### Flail Chest

Flail chest may have to be managed by mechanical ventilation when the patient's respiratory rate exceeds 40 breaths per minute, the VC progressively decreases to less than 10 to 15 mL/kg of body weight, the arterial oxygenation falls to less than 60 mm Hg with an FIO2 of 40% and hypercapnia develops with the PaCO2 higher than 50 mm Hg, or other injuries sustained in the trauma necessitate its use.[26] Mechanical ventilatory support may be needed for 2 to 4 weeks. With severe chest wall injuries or marked displacement of the fracture fragments, surgical stabilization may be required. Surgery usually shortens the time the patient needs to be on mechanical ventilation, decreases the pain, and increases anatomic alignment during the healing process.[26] When the injuries are less severe injuries, it might be possible to treat the flail chest with excellent pain control and aggressive breathing exercises, use of an incentive spirometer, positioning, and coughing.

### Lung Contusion

Treatment is supportive and preventive. Mechanical ventilation and supplemental oxygen may be required. Fluid monitoring to ensure against volume overload, which could lead to pulmonary edema, is important. Although corticosteroids have been used, there are no current data that show corticosteroids improve the morbidity or mortality rates in these patients.[20] Deep breathing exercises, positioning, and coughing are also used to assist in clearing infiltrates and to decrease the incidence of pneumonia.[26]

## Table 5-33 Clinical Manifestation of Lung Contusion/Fracture/Flail Chest

|  |  | Findings |
|---|---|---|
| Signs | Pulmonary function tests | ↑ RR, ↓ VT, ↓ FRC, ↓ VC, ↓ TLC |
|  | Chest radiograph | May appear normal if rib fractures are not displaced. If displaced, best seen on posteroanterior view of chest film. Lung contusion shows as focal infiltrates in nonsegmental and nonlobar distribution. If infiltrates remain for >3 days, patient may be developing pneumonia or ARDS |
|  | Arterial blood gases | ↓ $PaO_2$, ↑ ventilation–perfusion mismatching[20] |
|  | Breath sounds | Diminished breath sounds and possible fluid in pleural space. Rales with atelectasis |
|  | Cardiovascular | Variable |
| Symptoms |  | Chest wall pain and tenderness to palpation. Pain exacerbated with movement of chest wall, especially coughing and sneezing. Patients splint chest wall, RR ↑, and with large injuries appear in respiratory distress |

*ARDS, acute respiratory distress syndrome; FRC, functional residual capacity; $PaO_2$, arterial partial pressure of $O_2$; RR, respiratory rate; TLC, total lung capacity; VC, vital capacity; VT, tidal volume.*

## Penetrating Wounds

Penetrating wounds to the thorax are usually caused by shooting or stabbing and result in pathologic damage, particularly pneumothorax, hemothorax, pulmonary laceration, tracheal or bronchial disruption, diaphragmatic injury, esophageal perforation, or cardiac laceration. Only the first three are discussed within the scope of this chapter.[1,4]

## Etiology

The leading cause of penetrating wounds to the thorax is gunshot wounds and stab wounds. Penetrating wounds to the chest are usually more specific and defined and are less likely to have the multisystem involvement more commonly seen with thoracic crush injuries.[4,26]

## Pathophysiology

### Pneumothorax

Traumatic pneumothorax is defined as the entry of free air into the pleural space (see Fig. 1-9). This often occurs after a penetrating wound to the thorax. A traumatic pneumothorax can be further classified as an open pneumothorax or a tension pneumothorax.[1]

An open pneumothorax means the air in the pleural space communicates freely with the outside environment. When air can move freely through the chest wall, into and out of the pleural space, the patient is unable to maintain a negative pleural space pressure. Because an effective negative pleural space pressure cannot be maintained in both the affected and unaffected hemithorax, the patient's ability to move air into the lungs is severely diminished. Lung volumes are decreased, lung compliance is decreased, ventilation–perfusion mismatching is increased, and gas exchange is impaired.[1]

A tension pneumothorax means air can enter the pleural space but cannot escape into the external environment. This is an acute life-threatening situation.[27] As air continues to enter and become trapped in the pleural space, the intrapleural pressure rapidly increases. This causes the lung on the involved side to collapse. The mediastinal structures are pushed away from the affected side. The increased thoracic pressure causes a decrease in venous return, cardiac output falls, and systemic hypotension and shock are the result. Lung volumes are significantly reduced, lung compliance is decreased, and the alveolar-capillary surface area available for gas exchange is cut by more than 50%.[1,4,26]

### Hemothorax

Hemothorax is the presence of blood in the pleural space. It can occur with both penetrating wounds and crush injuries to the thorax. Approximately 70% of patients with chest trauma develop a hemothorax.[20] Collection of blood in the pleural space causes compression of the underlying lung tissue and prevents lung expansion. This process usually affects the lower lobes because the blood in the pleural space is pulled by gravity to the most dependent area. Compression of the lung tissue causes an increase in ventilation–perfusion mismatching, decreases lung compliance, and promotes

atelectasis. Occasionally, trauma to the thorax results in a massive hemothorax, which almost always means that the heart or great vessels were injured directly.

Hemothorax can have serious sequelae if all the blood is not evacuated from the pleural space. The residual blood becomes organized into nonelastic fibrous tissue, which can form a restrictive pleural rind. This condition is known as fibrothorax and can limit lung expansion markedly, causing a restrictive lung dysfunction and predisposing the patient to atelectasis and pneumonic complications.[20] In addition, approximately 5% of patients with hemothorax develop an infection within the pleural space called an empyema, which can lead to further scarring of the pleural surfaces.[1,4,26]

## Pulmonary Laceration

A laceration directly into the lung parenchyma is usually caused by a penetrating wound. It results in air and blood escaping from the lung into the pleural space and often into the environment. Therefore, a pulmonary laceration most commonly appears in combination with a pneumothorax and hemothorax. The hemothorax is usually not massive because the lung is perfused at low pressures, so the bleeding is not profuse. The restrictive impairments caused by pneumothorax and hemothorax described earlier are present, and in addition the damaged lung tissue is not participating in gas exchange.[26]

## Clinical Manifestation

The clinical manifestation of pneumo- or hemothorax can be found in Table 5-34.

## Treatment

### Pneumothorax

The definitive treatment of an open pneumothorax is the application of an airtight, sterile dressing over the sucking chest wound and the placement of a chest tube into the pleural space of the affected hemithorax. The chest tube is connected to suction so that the air and any fluid or blood within the pleural space can be evacuated. These measures will reexpand the collapsed lung. Mechanical ventilation and supplemental oxygen may be required until the patient can maintain tissue oxygenation independently.[20,26]

A tension pneumothorax is treated as an emergency by inserting a needle into the pleural space to allow air to escape. This is immediately followed by placement of a chest tube connected to suction so that air can be continuously evacuated from the pleural space along with any blood or fluid.[4,20,26]

### Hemothorax

The definitive treatment for hemothorax is to evacuate the blood from the pleural space by placement of a dependent chest tube. This chest tube is connected to suction. Autotransfusion devices are becoming more common so that the patient's own blood can be returned to the cardiovascular system to replace lost blood volume.[20] If the wound involves

**Table 5-34  Clinical Manifestation of Pneumo- or Hemothorax**

|  |  | Findings |
|---|---|---|
| Signs | Pulmonary function tests | $\uparrow$ RR, $\downarrow$ lung volumes |
|  | Chest radiograph | Pneumothorax: lung collapse seen. Tension pneumothorax: diaphragm may be flattened, mediastinal structures shifted, trachea deviated, and neck veins distended. Hemothorax difficult to visualize on radiograph; best seen on upright and decubitus films[4,26] |
|  | Arterial blood gases | $\downarrow$ PaO$_2$ (degree of hypoxemia depends on extent of injury); may have $\uparrow$ PaCO$_2$ |
|  | Breath sounds | Pneumothorax: marked $\downarrow$ or absent breath sounds; $\downarrow$ breath sounds in hemothorax, fibrothorax, and empyema |
|  | Cardiovascular | Tachycardia is common; $\downarrow$ cardiac output and systemic hypotension in tension pneumothorax |
| Symptoms |  | SOB; if in respiratory distress: $\uparrow$ RR, intercostal retractions, cyanosis, anxiety, and agitation. Pain at site of chest wound expected. May also be pale, cyanotic, systemic hypotension, hypoxemic, and shock-like. |

*PaCO$_2$, arterial partial pressure of CO$_2$; PaO$_2$, arterial partial pressure of O$_2$; RR, respiratory rate; SOB, shortness of breath.*

the lung parenchyma, the bleeding in most patients stops because of clotting and internal repair mechanisms. Only 4% of these patients require thoracotomy and surgical intervention to control the bleeding.[26] If the wound involves the heart or great vessels, then emergency surgery may be required to stop massive bleeding; this surgery takes precedence over all other treatment other than respiratory and cardiac resuscitation. Following placement of the chest tube, the patient should be monitored carefully by chest radiograph to be sure all the blood is evacuated from the pleural space. An additional chest tube may be required to accomplish this goal. If a fibrothorax does develop and impairs lung expansion, a surgical procedure known as a decortication may be required. A decortication removes the restrictive pleural rind, which is usually done through a minithoracotomy.[26,27] An empyema may also develop if the hemothorax is not completely resolved. The empyema would be treated with placement of a chest tube and antibiotics.[26]

## Thermal Trauma

Thermal trauma involving the pulmonary system is usually due to inhalation injuries, direct burn injuries to the thorax, or a combination of both.[13]

## Etiology

Thermal trauma is usually caused by exposure to fire and smoke, particularly in an enclosed space. The effects of this exposure are dependent on what is burning, the intensity of or the temperatures generated by the fire, the length of the exposure, and the amount of body surface involved.[37]

## Pathophysiology

Smoke inhalation causes pulmonary dysfunction in three different ways. First is a direct injury from inhaling hot, dry air containing heated particulate matter. This injury is localized in the upper airway because most of the heat is dissipated in the nasopharynx. Nasal hairs may be scorched. There is usually edema of the laryngeal and tracheal mucosa, with laryngospasm and bronchospasm almost always present. Mucus production is increased, and commonly there is damage to the mucociliary clearance mechanism. This can lead to bronchopneumonia.[13,37]

The second cause of pulmonary dysfunction is the inhalation of carbon monoxide, a gas present in smoke. Carbon monoxide is a colorless, odorless, tasteless, nonirritating gas. Exposure to carbon monoxide can be life threatening: Many suicides are committed by overexposure to carbon monoxide. This gas has more than 200 times the affinity for hemoglobin when compared with oxygen.[13] This means that when carbon monoxide is taken into the lungs it diffuses quickly into the pulmonary capillaries, enters the red blood cells, and binds with hemoglobin to form carboxyhemoglobin. This abnormal process decreases the available hemoglobin-binding sites for oxygen and significantly decreases the oxygen-carrying capacity of the blood.[9]

The third cause of pulmonary dysfunction is the inhalation of noxious and toxic gases, the effects from which are dependent on the materials being burned. The specific pulmonary abnormalities depend on the specific gas inhaled and the length of time exposed to the gas. However, exposure to noxious gases often results in surfactant inactivation and chemical pneumonitis.[13,30,37] Later in the clinical course, the lungs may develop an obliterative bronchiolitis. Although this complication is uncommon, when it occurs it causes significant RLD.[9]

Direct burn injuries to the thorax cause pulmonary dysfunction in five ways.

- The pain of the burn decreases chest wall mobility.
- If the depth of the burn is third degree, involving chest wall musculature, then the effectiveness of the respiratory pump is diminished.

**Table 5-35 Clinical Manifestation of Thermal Injuries**

|  |  | Findings |
|---|---|---|
| Signs | Pulmonary function tests | ↓ flow rates, ↓ lung volumes, ↓ lung compliance (surfactant is inactivated), ↓ chest wall compliance, ↓ gas diffusion, ↑ RR |
|  | Chest radiograph | Diffuse interstitial and intraalveolar infiltrates. May have bronchopneumonia or atelectasis |
|  | Arterial blood gases | ↓ $PaO_2$, if exposed to carbon monoxide for extended time, ↓↓↓ $PaO_2$ and incompatible with life |
|  | Breath sounds | ↓ breath sounds, wet rales, and rhonchi may be present |
|  | Cardiovascular | Tachycardia, may have arrhythmias, hypertension, hypotension or may develop myocardial infarction[37] |
| Symptoms |  | Dyspnea, repetitive hacking, productive cough. Sputum usually carbonaceous[37] |
|  |  | Stridor and wheezing may be present. May be anxious and cyanotic |

$PaO_2$, arterial partial pressure of $O_2$; RR, respiratory rate.

- Major burns involving 25% of the body surface area or more result in a massive shift of fluid from the intravascular to the interstitial spaces, causing pulmonary edema and possibly acute pulmonary insufficiency.
- With circumferential burns of the thorax, eschar formation may severely restrict chest wall expansion.
- Because these patients may have to be on bed rest for protracted periods of time, the pulmonary system is at risk for atelectasis and bronchopneumonia.[13,37]

## Clinical Manifestation

The clinical manifestation of thermal injuries can be found in Table 5-35.

## Treatment

Treatment of the seriously burned patient is usually divided into emergency, acute, and rehabilitative care and involves monitoring and providing support and care for every body system. Treatment of the pulmonary system includes humidification, supplemental oxygen, bronchodilators, appropriate positioning, and pulmonary hygiene techniques.[37] Bronchoscopy, intubation, ventilatory support using high-frequency ventilation (HFV) and PEEP, suctioning, and perhaps hyperbaric oxygen may be necessary in some patients.[9]

# Therapeutic Causes of Restrictive Lung Dysfunction

## Surgical Therapy

*Surgery* can be defined as a planned entry into the human body by a trained practitioner under well-controlled conditions.[1]

## Etiology

The pulmonary dysfunction that results from surgical therapy is due to three primary factors: (1) the anesthetic agent, (2) the surgical incision or procedure itself, and (3) the pain caused by the incision or procedure.[1,26]

## Pathophysiology

The anesthetic agent causes a decrease in the pulmonary arterial vasoconstrictive response to hypoxia. This increases ventilation–perfusion mismatching and decreases pulmonary gas exchange. Anesthesia also depresses the respiratory control centers so that ventilatory response to hypercapnia and hypoxia is decreased.[20] Placement of an endotracheal tube increases airway resistance.[26] Placing the patient in a supine position reduces the functional residual capacity by 20%.[20] During surgery, the shape and configuration of the thorax change. The anteroposterior diameter decreases, and the lateral diameter increases. The vertical diameter of the thorax also decreases, with the diaphragm moving in a cephalad direction owing to the effect of general anesthesia on central nevous system innervation of diaphragmatic tone.[20] These changes in configuration result in a further decrease in thoracic volumes; the FRC is decreased an additional 15%.[20]

If the site of surgery is in the upper abdomen or the thorax, the surgical incision causes a significant, although temporary, restrictive impairment. Following upper abdominal surgery, the VC is decreased by 55% and the FRC by 30%.[26] These decreases in lung volumes reach their greatest values 24 to 48 hours following surgery. Lung volumes then return to relatively normal values in 5 days, although full recovery may take 2 weeks.[26] Postoperative lung volume changes after upper abdominal surgery resemble changes seen in patients with unilateral diaphragmatic paralysis. In fact, diaphragmatic dysfunction has been demonstrated in some abdominal surgery patients. Diaphragmatic dysfunction also can occur following thoracic surgery, particularly if the phrenic nerve experiences hypothermic damage because of external cardiac cooling. Some studies have shown that a transverse abdominal incision results in better postoperative lung volumes and fewer postoperative pulmonary complications than the vertical midline abdominal incision. This is not a universal finding.[26] However, it is well accepted that the median sternotomy incision is better tolerated and results in fewer pulmonary complications than the posterolateral thoracotomy.[26]

The surgical procedure itself can result in a permanent restrictive impairment when lung tissue is excised. Because pulmonary reserves are significant, a pneumonectomy or possibly a lobectomy has to be performed before any measurable restrictive dysfunction results. Thoracoplasty is another surgical procedure that results in restrictive dysfunction. This procedure removes portions of several ribs so that the soft tissue of the chest wall can be used to collapse underlying lung parenchyma. Thoracoplasty was used to treat tuberculosis and was designed to close cavities caused by tuberculosis in the upper lobes. Currently this procedure is rarely performed, although it has been used to treat bronchopulmonary fistulas.[1] Another surgical procedure that can result in significant restrictive lung dysfunction is lung transplantation. This therapeutic cause of RLD is discussed later in this section.

Surgical incisions invariably cause pain, particularly abdominal incisions and posterolateral thoracotomies. Because of the pain, the tone in the muscles of the thorax and the abdominal wall increases, thereby decreasing the chest wall compliance. This change contributes to decreased lung volumes and increased work of breathing during the postoperative period. The phenomenon of increased muscle tone in and around the incision is known as muscular splinting of the incision (Fig. 5-22).

## Clinical Manifestation

The clinical manifestation of surgery on the lungs can be found in Table 5-36.

## Treatment

The pulmonary status of surgical patients should be evaluated before surgery. Many patients require preoperative treatment, including deep breathing and coughing exercises and practice with an incentive spirometer. In addition, patients should abstain from smoking for a minimum of 6 weeks before surgery. To prevent aspiration pneumonia, patients usually fast for 12 hours or longer before surgery. Drugs such as cimetidine or ranitidine can be used preoperatively to increase gastric pH and decrease gastric volume.[38] Postoperatively,

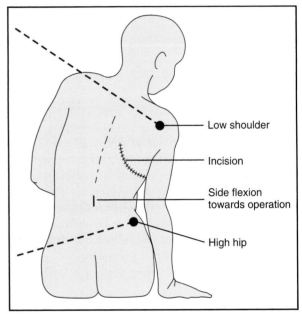

**Figure 5-22** Increased muscle tone in and around the incision is known as muscular splinting of the incision.

## Table 5-36 Clinical Manifestation of Effect of Surgeries on Lungs

| | | Findings |
|---|---|---|
| Signs | Pulmonary function tests | ↓ all lung volumes, ↓ VC by 55%, and ↓ FRC by 30% following upper abdominal surgery. Flow rates normal |
| | | ↓ gas exchange temporarily due to V/Q mismatching |
| | Chest radiograph | Atelectasis (in approximately 95% of patients following abdominal and thoracic surgery).[20] May also show pneumonia, especially of lower lobes, or even pulmonary embolism |
| | Arterial blood gases | ↓ $PaO_2$; $SpO_2$ <90% found in 35% of postoperative patients |
| | Breath sounds | ↓ breath sounds; may have rhonchi or rales |
| | Cardiovascular | May have myocardial infarction, arrhythmias, and possible cardiac arrest. If significant portion of lung removed, patients develop pulmonary hypertension.[8] |
| Symptoms | | Altered breathing patterns, ↓ VT, and ↑ RR. Cough reflex suppressed due to anesthesia. Cough productive of blood-streaked sputum if patient was intubated. |

*FRC, functional residual capacity; $PaO_2$, arterial partial pressure of $O_2$; RR, respiratory rate; $SpO_2$, saturation of peripheral oxygen; VC, vital capacity; V/Q, ventilation–perfusion; VT, tidal volume.*

hypoxia can be treated with inflation-hold breathing techniques, PEEP, CPAP, and occasionally with increased oxygen concentrations. Common techniques used to treat postoperative atelectasis include deep breathing exercises, early mobilization of the patient out of bed, incentive spirometry, and CPAP.[20] Nosocomial pneumonias following surgery are not uncommon following upper abdominal surgery, and 12% to 20% of patients experience this complication.[20] Nosocomial pneumonias are treated with an appropriate antibiotic and possibly with postural drainage, percussion, and vibration if the patient's secretion clearance mechanisms are impaired. Postoperative pulmonary embolism is usually treated with low-dose heparin. Prevention of venous thromboembolism may include simple leg exercises (ankle dorsi and plantar flexion), low-dose subcutaneous or adjusted-dose heparin, external pneumatic compression devices, and gradient compression stockings.[20]

## Lung Transplantation

Lung transplantation can be defined as the replacement of poorly functioning lung tissue in the recipient with better-functioning lung tissue (the lung tissue is never normal, there is always some preservation injury) from the donor.[39] The many aspects of this surgical therapeutic intervention are discussed in Chapter 12. Only the possible development of obliterative bronchiolitis after lung transplantation will be discussed in this section.

## Etiology

Obliterative bronchiolitis (OB) is primarily a restrictive lung impairment and the major long-term complication of lung transplantation. Recent evidence suggests that chronic pulmonary rejection may be the major determinant in the cause of OB.[23] A variety of other processes may also be involved in the development of OB, including viral and bacterial pneumonias, toxic inhalants, bronchial obstruction, chronic aspiration, and cytomegalovirus mismatch (seronegative recipient vs seropositive donor).[23]

## Pathophysiology

Obliterative bronchiolitis clinically shows both restrictive and obstructive pulmonary function deficits and histologically shows obliteration of the terminal bronchioles.[20] This late complication of lung transplantation is seen in 20% to 40% of single-lung-transplant recipients.[20] It occurs most commonly between 8 and 12 months after transplant and is often preceded by an upper respiratory infection.[20] A transbronchial biopsy (TBB) is used to confirm the diagnosis (sensitivity ranging from 5% to 99%).[20,23] In OB there is fibrotic narrowing of the bronchiolar lumen that may be irregular, regular, or totally obliterative. The smooth muscle is often destroyed and there is extension of the fibrosis into the interstitium. Early in OB there is mononuclear cell infiltration, epithelial damage, and ulceration. Later, as this complication develops and becomes more chronic, the fibrosis is more acellular, and the terminal bronchioles are completely obliterated.[39] This decreases the surface area for gas exchange. Although the patchy fibrosis seen in OB may not involve the entire transplanted lung, it does decrease lung compliance, decrease lung volumes, and increase ventilation–perfusion mismatching, all hallmarks of a restrictive lung impairment. Obliterative bronchiolitis is often accompanied by bronchiectasis, and recurrent respiratory infections. Death is usually due to pneumonia from gram-negative bacteria or Aspergillus.[39] Infection and OB are currently the most frequent causes of post–lung transplantation death.[9]

## Clinical Manifestation

The clinical manifestation of bronchiolitis obliterans can be found in Table 5-37.

## Treatment

Optimal maintenance of the immunosuppressive drug regimen, prompt diagnosis and treatment of infections and episodes of acute rejection, and careful cytomegalovirus matching may all contribute to the prevention of OB.[23] Once diagnosed, OB is usually treated with high-dose

## Table 5-37 Clinical Manifestation of Bronchiolitis Obliterans

|  |  | Findings |
|---|---|---|
| Signs | Pulmonary function tests | ↓ IRV, ↓ ERV, ↓ RV, ↓ flow rates, ↓ FEV1 >20%, ↓ gas exchange[23] |
|  | Chest radiograph | May be unchanged or may show central bronchietasis[20,39] |
|  | Arterial blood gases | ↓ $PaO_2$, $PaCO_2$ within normal limits |
|  | Breath sounds | Often have decreased breath sounds with rhonchi and rales |
|  | Cardiovascular | Pulmonary hypertension due to destruction of pulmonary capillary beds. Pulmonary arterioles and veins in transplanted lung also often experience chronic vascular rejection.[39] |
| Symptoms |  | Dyspnea, decreased exercise tolerance and eventually dyspnea at rest. Often have cough with sputum production[39] |

*ERV, expiratory reserve volume; FEV1, forced expiratory volume in 1 second; IRV, inspiratory reserve volume; $PaCO_2$, arterial partial pressure of $CO_2$; $PaO_2$, arterial partial pressure of $O_2$; RV, residual volume.*

methylprednisolone followed by a tapering course of oral corticosteroids. If there is no clinical response to this regimen, then azathioprine and lympholytic agents such as antilymphocyte globulin (ALG) or muromonab-CD3 (Ortho-clone OKT3) may be used. Drug therapy may stabilize the pulmonary function test results but rarely is there any improvement in lung function. Relapses of OB occur in 50% of these patients. Often infections complicate the intensive immunosuppression used to treat OB and frequently result in death. Because most cases of OB can only be stabilized when treated, early diagnosis and treatment are paramount in preserving lung function.[20] In the most severe cases, single-lung retransplantation has been used with limited success.[23]

## Pharmaceutical Causes of Restrictive Lung Dysfunction

More than 100 drugs are capable of causing RLD. Approximately 80 of these drugs adversely affect the lung parenchyma directly, causing drug-induced interstitial lung disease.[17] Other drugs affect the ventilatory pump, ventilatory drive, or chest wall compliance.[1] Most drug-induced interstitial lung disease is reversible if it is recognized early and the drug is discontinued. Drug-induced RLD contributes to the morbidity of an estimated several hundred thousand patients in the United States annually. Approximately 50% of patients treated with chemotherapeutic drugs develop some degree of interstitial pneumonitis.[17] Some patients who take chemotherapeutic drugs demonstrate pathologic alterations with no radiologic, symptomatic, or physiologic abnormalities. Therefore, probably less than 5% of all adverse drug-induced interstitial lung disease is reported or recognized.[17]

It is very difficult to predict which drugs may affect a particular person's lung adversely. The basic reason for this difficulty is insufficient knowledge. First, knowledge of the metabolites of different drugs and their effects on the lung is lacking. Second, some patients seem to have a genetic predisposition to react adversely to certain drugs, but this is not well understood. Third, many patients are on multiple drugs, and the interaction of the various metabolites has not been well studied.[17]

Drug-induced interstitial lung disease probably results from a combination of mechanisms including:
- Toxic effects of the drug or its metabolites
- Interference with the oxidant-antioxidant system[10]
- An indirect inflammatory reaction
- Altered immunologic processes[17]

Drugs capable of causing drug-induced interstitial lung disease are discussed here by drug category and found in Box 5-5.

### Oxygen

High concentrations of oxygen for more than 24 hours can produce interstitial lung disease. The lung damage occurs in

---

**Box 5-5**

### Drugs Capable of inducing Interstitial Lung Disease
- Oxygen
- Antibiotics
- Nitrofurantoin
- Sulfasalazine
- Antiinflammatory drugs
- Cardiovascular drugs
- Chemotherapeutic drugs
- Poisons
- Anesthetics
- Muscle relaxants
- Illicit drugs

---

two phases. First is the exudative phase, which begins after using high oxygen concentrations for 24 to 72 hours. During this phase, perivascular, interstitial, and alveolar edema and alveolar hemorrhage and atelectasis occur. The second or proliferative phase is marked by hyperplasia of the type II pneumocytes and deposition of collagen and elastin in the interstitium, and is irreversible. Oxygen toxicity can result in significant RLD. Treatment is primarily preventive. Oxygen toxicity can be minimized by keeping the $FIO_2$ less than 40% and the $PaO_2$ less than 120 mm Hg.[17]

### Antibiotics

Some antibiotics used to fight infections can be neurotoxic. Drugs such as polymyxin, gentamicin, and kanamycin, when given intravenously, can cause neuromuscular blockade. This neuromuscular blockade can result in respiratory muscle paralysis, failure of the ventilatory pump, and such significant restrictive lung impairment that assisted ventilatory support may be necessary. The significance of the respiratory impairment is even greater when these drugs are used with anesthetic agents or muscle relaxants.[38]

### Nitrofurantoin

This drug is an antiseptic agent used to fight specific urinary tract infections. It can cause acute or chronic interstitial pneumonitis and is responsible for more reported cases of drug-induced pulmonary disease than any other drug.[10] There seems to be no relation between the acute and chronic reactions. The acute pneumonitis is characterized by fever, dyspnea, cough, and rales; approximately 35% of patients experience pleuritic pain. The acute pneumonitis (90% of reported cases) is completely reversible if the drug is discontinued.[10] Chronic pneumonitis (10% of reported cases) mimics IPF and usually begins 6 to 12 months after initiation of the drug. Patients complain of dyspnea and a mild, nonproductive cough. There can be diffuse fibrosis with lower zone predominance. Treatment includes discontinuation of the drug, lung biopsy, and possibly corticosteroids. Therapeutic results are inconsistent and the mortality rate is 10%.[10,17,38]

## Sulfasalazine

This drug is used to treat inflammatory bowel disease (chronic ulcerative colitis) and more recently to treat rheumatologic disorders.[10] Patients who develop lung complications complain of dyspnea and cough approximately 1 to 8 months after the initiation of the drug. Approximately half the patients also complain of fever. This can develop into interstitial pulmonary fibrosis. Treatment is to discontinue the drug. Pulmonary involvement and symptoms are reversible in most patients. Corticosteroids hasten improvement in some patients.[10] Three fatalities have been recorded as caused by sulfasalazine-induced diffuse pulmonary fibrosis.[10,17]

## Antiinflammatory Drugs

### Gold

Gold is used in the treatment of rheumatoid arthritis, and is also being used to treat osteoarthritis and asthma, but in some patients it causes diffuse interstitial pneumonitis and fibrosis.[10] These patients develop dyspnea and a nonproductive cough approximately 6 weeks to many months after initiation of gold therapy. Treatment is the discontinuation of the drug, which allows the reaction to regress spontaneously. Some patients with respiratory distress are given corticosteroids to speed up this process.[7,17]

### Penicillamine

This drug is used to treat Wilson disease, cystinuria, primary biliary cirrhosis, scleroderma, and severe rheumatoid arthritis in patients who have failed to respond to conventional therapy.[10] However, it can cause bronchiolitis obliterans, which contributes to both obstructive and restrictive lung dysfunction; Goodpasture's syndrome; or penicillamine-induced SLE. The drug is discontinued in patients who develop any of these pulmonary complications. Patients who have developed Goodpasture's syndrome are also treated with hemodialysis, immunosuppression, and plasmapheresis. Patients who have penicillamine-induced SLE may also receive corticosteroids to accelerate the resolution of this pulmonary complication.[17,38]

## Cardiovascular Drugs

### Amiodarone

This antiarrhythmic drug is given for ventricular dysrhythmias that are refractory to other antiarrhythmic drugs. The pulmonary complications seem to be dose related and rarely occur if the dose is under 400 mg per day. The incidence of pulmonary complications is approximately 6%, and the pulmonary complications may be fatal in 10% to 20% of patients.[10] Patients with pulmonary involvement experience an insidious onset of dyspnea and a nonproductive cough with occasional fever and chills. Rales are heard on auscultation, and the chest radiograph shows asymmetric lesions in the lung, which appear mostly in the upper lung fields. Treatment is to discontinue the drug; the value of corticosteroids is uncertain.[10,17]

## Chemotherapeutic Drugs

These cytotoxic drugs used in cancer chemotherapy are a major cause of morbidity and mortality in the immunocompromised individual. It has been reported that the majority of these drugs can cause pulmonary fibrosis.[7] They are also responsible for causing pulmonary infiltrates, secondary neoplasms, and non-Hodgkin lymphoma, all of which compromise lung function. The precise mechanism that incites the inflammatory and fibrotic response in the lung is unknown.

Dyspnea appears gradually, usually within a few weeks of the drug therapy, followed by fever and a nonproductive cough. With some drugs, symptoms may be delayed for months or years (e.g., cyclophosphamide). Early chest radiographs show asymmetric parenchymal changes in one lobe or lung; eventually, these changes progress and become diffuse and uniform in distribution. Pulmonary function tests show a classic restrictive impairment. The DLCO usually falls before the patient experiences the onset of any overt symptoms (except with methotrexate). Rales are heard on auscultation. Treatment consists of the discontinuation of the drug and in some cases the use of corticosteroids.[17]

### Bleomycin

Bleomycin is an antibiotic used as an antineoplastic agent against squamous cell carcinomas, seminomas, and lymphomas. Ten percent of patients on this drug develop parenchymal lung disease, which proves to be fatal in 1% of the patients. The risk of lung involvement increases with higher dosages of bleomycin, if it is used with previous or concomitant thoracic radiation, if it is prescribed with current or subsequent use of high oxygen concentrations, if it is used in combination with cyclophosphamide, or if it is used in patients more than 70 years old.[10,17,38]

### Mitomycin C

Mitomycin C is an antibiotic used in conjunction with other chemotherapeutic drugs, particularly for adenocarcinoma of the esophagus, stomach, pancreas, or colon.[10] It is also used to treat breast and lung malignancies.[10] Approximately 3% to 12% of patients on this drug develop pulmonary complications. Frequency of lung involvement increases if this drug is used with radiation or with other drugs, particularly fluorouracil or the Vinca alkaloids.[17,38]

### Busulfan

Busulfan is an alkylating agent used to treat myeloid leukemia. Pulmonary toxicity occurs in 4% to 6% of patients. Pulmonary complications commence an average of 41 months after initiation of therapy.[10] Clinical symptoms appear insidiously; however, prognosis is poor, with an estimated mortality rate of 84%.[10]

### Cyclophosphamide

Cyclophosphamide is an alkylating agent used in the treatment of malignant lymphomas, multiple myeloma, and leukemias. Diffuse interstitial fibrosis can occur a few months to a few years after use of this drug; however, pulmonary toxicity is uncommon (less than 1%).[10] There seems to be no age or dose correlation with the development of pulmonary complications. The drug-induced pulmonary disease can range from one with a very long-term course to one with a rapid downhill course resulting in death.[17,38]

## Chlorambucil

Chlorambucil is an alkylating agent used to treat chronic lymphatic malignancies. If pulmonary complications develop, it is usually 1 to 12 months before symptoms appear.[17]

## Melphalan

Melphalan is an alkylating agent used in the treatment of multiple myeloma. Significant RLD has been reported in only a few patients, but more than half of these patients died of respiratory failure despite termination of drug therapy.[10,17]

## Azathioprine

Azathioprine is an antimetabolite used for treating neoplastic disease, regional enteritis, ulcerative colitis, chronic active hepatitis, rheumatoid arthritis, systemic lupus erythematosus, Wegener's granulomatosis, and rejection episodes in organ transplant patients.[10] This drug rarely causes interstitial lung disease; however, six cases have been reported in the literature.[17]

## Cytarabine

Cytarabine is an antimetabolite used primarily to induce a remission in acute leukemia. Unlike the other drugs under discussion, cytarabine causes minimal parenchymal abnormalities. However, it can cause a noncardiac pulmonary edema, which results in RLD and has a fatality rate of 69%.[10]

## Methotrexate

Methotrexate is an antimetabolite taken for acute lymphatic leukemia and osteogenic sarcoma in children. More recently, it is being used as an anti-inflammatory agent to treat rheumatoid arthritis, psoriasis, and asthma.[10] The complication of interstitial lung disease is not dose or age related. Symptoms begin a few days to a few weeks after drug initiation, and approximately one third of patients who develop interstitial pneumonitis have poorly formed granulomas. Treatment is the discontinuation of the drug; in almost all patients the lung involvement is spontaneously resolved. Corticosteroids are sometimes used.[17]

## Nitrosoureas

Nitrosourea drugs (bis-chloronitrosourea [BCNU; carmustine], 1-(2-chloroethyl)-3-cyclohexyl-1-nitrosourea [CCNU; lomustine], methyl-CCNU [semustine]) are used against a variety of neoplasms, particularly intracranial neoplasm.[10] Anywhere from 1% to 50% of patients on these drugs develop interstitial lung disease. Patients have a higher risk of developing pulmonary complications when higher dosages are prescribed or when these drugs are prescribed along with other agents, particularly cyclophosphamide.[17] A history of

cigarette smoking or preexisting lung disease increases the risk of nitrosourea-induced lung disease.[10]

## Poisons

### Paraquat

Paraquat is used as a weed killer. If it is ingested, it causes acute pulmonary fibrosis. There are usually no symptoms for 24 hours after ingestion, and then the person experiences progressive respiratory distress leading to death in 1 to 38 days.[7]

Other drugs can cause RLD via a variety of pathophysiologic mechanisms other than that of producing alveolar pneumonitis and fibrosis. A few of these drug categories or specific drugs are discussed.

## Anesthetics

Anesthetic agents such as halothane (Fluothane), methoxyflurane (Penthrane), or thiopental sodium (Pentothal) are used to provide anesthesia during surgical procedures. These agents also inhibit the respiratory centers in the medulla and therefore depress ventilation so that lung volumes are significantly reduced. Assisted mechanical ventilation is usually required with the use of these drugs. The effects of these drugs and the effects of the assisted mechanical ventilation usually result in significant but brief RLD.[1,38]

## Muscle Relaxants

Muscle relaxants such as pancuronium bromide (Pavulon), dantrolene sodium (Dantrium), diazepam (Valium), and cyclobenzaprine hydrochloride (Flexeril) are used to enhance surgical relaxation, overcome muscle spasm, and control shivering (with systemic hypothermia). However, because these drugs act on skeletal muscle, they also decrease thoracic expansion, decrease chest wall compliance, and decrease pulmonary ventilation. As soon as the drug effects have worn off, the transient RLD also disappears.[1,38]

## Illicit Drugs

### Cocaine

It is estimated that there are more than 5 million regular cocaine users in the United States.[10] Cocaine became affordable and very popular in the 1980s with the introduction of the alkaloidal form of cocaine hydrochloride, known as "freebase" or "crack." Crack is smoked, is usually 30% to 90% pure, and produces a rapid and intense euphoria that is extremely addictive. Lung disease is much more common among crack smokers than other cocaine users.[10] Pulmonary pathologic conditions caused by crack use include acute pulmonary hemorrhage (58%), interstitial pneumonia with or without fibrosis (38%), vascular congestion (88%), and intraalveolar edema (77%).[10] The major symptoms of lung involvement are dyspnea (63%), cough (58%), cough with blood-stained or black sputum (34%), and chest pain (25%).[10]

Fever, bronchospasm, perihilar infiltrates, hypoxemia, and respiratory failure also occur. In fact, the term *crack lung* is used to describe acute pulmonary eosinophilia or acute respiratory failure, both of which can occur after smoking free-base cocaine. These different pulmonary disorders cause acute or chronic restrictive lung dysfunction with decreased lung compliance, increased ventilation–perfusion mismatching, decreased DLCO, hypoxemia, and hypercapnia.

Treatment of acute pulmonary diseases with corticosteroids (prednisone) can result in rapid improvement. When lung tissue is repeatedly involved in hemorrhage, edema, and pneumonia, then fibrosis may result. Chronic fibrosis of the lung does not seem to respond to corticosteroids. A number of deaths have been attributed to pulmonary involvement following crack cocaine use.[10]

## Heroin

An overdose of methadone hydrochloride, propoxyphene hydrochloride, or heroin can lead to a noncardiac pulmonary edema with interstitial pneumonitis. This reaction can begin within minutes of an intravenous injection or within an hour of oral ingestion. Respiration is depressed, lung compliance is decreased, and hypoxemia and hypercapnia result. Treatment includes mechanically assisted ventilation and usually antibiotics to deal with the invariable aspiration pneumonia.[17] It is estimated that there are 800,000 heroin users in the United States.[10]

## Talc

Talc (magnesium silicate) is used as a filler in oral medications such as amphetamines, tripelennamine hydrochloride, methadone hydrochloride, meperidine, and propoxyphene hydrochloride (Darvon). When addicts inject these drugs intravenously, talc granulomatosis results. Talc granulomatosis is characterized by granulomas in the arterioles and the pulmonary interstitium. The clinical picture includes dyspnea, pulmonary hypertension, and restrictive lung impairment with a decreased DLCO. Treatment is abstinence from further intravenous talc exposure. Use of corticosteroids has afforded variable results.[17]

# Radiologic Causes of Restrictive Lung Dysfunction

## Radiation Pneumonitis and Fibrosis

Radiation pneumonitis or fibrosis is a primary complication of irradiation to the thorax. It usually occurs 2 to 6 months after this treatment intervention.[10,26]

## Etiology

Irradiation of the thorax is a treatment option for lymphoma (Hodgkin disease), breast cancer, lung cancer, and esophageal cancer. Not all patients who receive irradiation to the thorax develop radiation pneumonitis or fibrosis. This serious pulmonary complication of irradiation seems to depend on the rate of delivery of the irradiation, the volume of lung being irradiated, the total dose, the quality of the radiation, and the concomitant chemotherapy.[2,8,17] Time–dose relationships are extremely important in predicting the occurrence of radiation pneumonitis or fibrosis. The number of fractions into which a dose is divided seems to be the most important factor.[8] Also important is the total dose and the span of time over which the radiation is delivered. Approximately 50% of patients undergoing irradiation of the thorax show radiologic abnormalities in the lung.[10] Only 5% to 15% of patients who receive radiation to the thorax actually develop signs and symptoms of radiation pneumonitis.[2,10]

Currently one group of patients seems to be at higher risk for developing radiation pneumonitis or fibrosis. Bone marrow transplant patients receive whole lung irradiation. They are also on cytotoxic chemotherapeutic agents that can intensify the pneumonitis, and these patients often have a graft versus host reaction that can add to radiation damage.[8]

## Pathophysiology

The pathogenesis of radiation pneumonitis or fibrosis is uncertain.[10] It is known that irradiation causes breaks in the DNA strands. When these breaks are double stranded, the cell cannot correctly repair the damage, and so the integrity of the chromosome is disrupted.[10] Chromosomal aberrations do not affect the survival or function of the cell until it tries to replicate itself. Cell death usually occurs with cell mitosis during the first or subsequent mitotic divisions. Radiation responses are seen first in cells with rapid rates of cell replication. In the lung, this would include the capillary endothelial cells, the type I alveolar epithelial cells, and the type II pneumocytes. In addition to cellular death caused by molecular changes, irradiation causes an inflammatory syndrome. This inflammation may be initiated by the release of free radicals.[10]

Pulmonary injury following radiation of the thorax is usually divided into two clinical syndromes: acute radiation pneumonitis and chronic radiation fibrosis.[9] The onset of acute radiation pneumonitis is insidious, beginning 2 to 3 months after radiation. It is characterized by swelling of endothelial cells, capillary engorgement and disruption, intimal proliferation, subintimal accumulation of macrophages, and capillary occlusion and thrombosis.[9] Endothelial injury may lead to increased vascular permeability, which may have a profound effect on gas exchange and ventilation–perfusion matching.

Chronic radiation fibrosis occurs 6 to 9 months after radiation and is characterized by basement membrane damage, fibroblastic proliferation, collagen deposition, capillary endothelium hyalinization and sclerosis, obliteration of alveoli, dense fibrosis, and contraction of lung volume.[8,9,17] There is evidence that the pneumonitis and fibrosis are two separate phases and that radiation fibrosis may not always be preceded by radiation pneumonitis.[10] It seems that the earlier the onset, the more serious and protracted the complications.[9,27] Usually one third to one half of the volume of one lung must be irradiated for pneumonitis to develop and show any clinical symptoms.[8] Some patients have a complete resolution of

**Table 5-38 Clinical Manifestation of Radiation Pneumonitis and Fibrosis**

| | | Findings |
|---|---|---|
| Signs | Pulmonary function tests | ↓ lung volumes, ↓ flow rates. Maximum impairment occurs 4–6 months after irradiation.[2,3,26] Regional irradiation: ↓ VC, ↓ ERV. As more lung is irradiated, ↓ all lung volumes, ↓ TLC, ↓ VC, ↓ IC, ↓ RV, ↓ DLCO, ↓ capillary-alveolar surface area. ↑ RR, ↓ VT, ↓ lung compliance[9] |
| | Chest radiograph | Alveolar and/or interstitial parenchymal infiltrates limited to the radiation port.[26] Lungs may have ground-glass or soft appearance and lung markings may appear hazy or indistinct. Progresses to a reticulonodular pattern (found in location of lung irradiated). Irradiated regions may look bronchiectatic, cystic or honeycomb-like.[25] Patients may develop additional changes outside field of irradiation and even contralateral lung tissue.[25] |
| | Arterial blood gases | ↓ $PaCO_2$ (as a result of ↑ RR); ↓ $PaO_2$ |
| | Breath sounds | Rales and rhonchi or wheezes may be present. Breath sounds diminished over involved area. Pleural rubs may be present |
| | Cardiovascular | Pulmonary hypertension develops, leading to cor pulmonale. Thrombolytic occurrences are common. Tachycardia often present |
| Symptoms | | SOB on exertion progressing to dyspnea with minimal effort. Cough is repetitive and irritating to patient. HR ↑ and exercise tolerance ↓. Patients may develop a low-grade fever or even temperature spikes. Some complain of pleuritic pain or even sharp chest wall pain and can develop fractured ribs from coughing.[17,25] |

*DLCO, diffusing capacity of the lungs for carbon monoxide; ERV, expiratory reserve volume; HR, heart rate; IC, inspiratory capacity; $PaCO_2$, arterial partial pressure of $CO_2$; $PaO_2$, arterial partial pressure of $O_2$; RV, residual volume; SOB, shortness of breath; TLC, total lung capacity; VC, vital capacity.*

the pneumonitis, but many go on to develop permanent fibrosis. Occasionally pleural effusion, spontaneous pneumothorax, bronchial obstruction, rib fractures, pericardial effusion, or tracheoesophageal fistula may further complicate the clinical picture.[9] With whole-lung irradiation, the involved fibrotic lung may contract to a remarkable degree, even causing shifts in the mediastinal structures, overexpansion of the other lung, and death. It has been reported that a late complication of radiation fibrosis may be the rapid development of adenocarcinoma of the lung. Bilateral adenocarcinoma of the lung has been described 2 years following radiation therapy for Hodgkin disease (patient had also received chemotherapy). Malignant fibrous histiocytoma may also complicate radiation fibrosis.[10]

## Clinical Manifestation

The clinical manifestation of radiation pneumonitis and fibrosis can be found in Table 5-38.

## Treatment

Asymptomatic patients with radiologic abnormalities do not require treatment.[9] Corticosteroids are used to treat acute radiation pneumonitis and may produce dramatic results. However, there are reports of a lack of response to corticosteroids, even during the acute radiation pneumonitis phase.[9] Corticosteroids offer no help in treating chronic radiation fibrosis and should not be used prophylactically because terminating corticosteroid therapy may actually precipitate

radiation pneumonitis. Pneumonectomy has been reported to treat severe unilateral radiation fibrosis. Otherwise treatment is supportive and consists of oxygen therapy, cough suppression medications, analgesics, and antibiotics to treat any superimposed infection.[2,8,9,25] Prophylactic antibiotics should not be used because they could predispose patients to aggressive antibiotic-resistant organisms.[9]

Prevention is the ultimate treatment, and the occurrence of radiation injury to the lung is decreasing with the refinement of radiotherapy techniques, particularly the careful tailoring of radiation fields.[7,8]

## Summary

- Restrictive lung dysfunction (RLD) is not a disease: It is an abnormal reduction in pulmonary ventilation.
- Restrictive lung dysfunction can be caused by a variety of disease processes occurring in different body systems, trauma, or therapeutic measures.
- In RLD, one or more of the following is abnormal: lung compliance, chest wall compliance, lung volumes, or the work of breathing.
- The classic signs of RLD include tachypnea, hypoxemia, decreased breath sounds, dry inspiratory rales, decreased lung volumes, decreased diffusing capacity, and cor pulmonale.
- The hallmark symptoms of RLD include shortness of breath; cough; and a wasted, emaciated appearance.

- Treatment interventions for RLD vary and are dependent on the cause of the restrictive impairment. Sometimes corrective measures are possible. However, once the lung has undergone fibrotic changes, the pathologic alterations are irreversible and only supportive interventions are used.
- Idiopathic pulmonary fibrosis is the pulmonary disease entity most commonly associated with RLD.
- Pneumonia is an inflammatory process within the lung that can be caused by bacteria, mycoplasmas, viruses, fungi, or chlamydial agents.
- There are four major types of lung cancer: squamous cell carcinoma, small cell carcinoma, adenocarcinoma, and large cell carcinoma. All types can cause a restrictive impairment within the lung. This restrictive impairment may be due to direct pressure from the tumor, may result from susceptibility to other disease processes in the weakened cancer patient, may be related to changes that occur as the tumor metastasizes to other body systems, or may be produced by hormones arising from the tumor, which can cause a variety of symptoms in different body systems.
- Cigarette smoking has been linked to a variety of pathologic conditions, including bronchogenic carcinoma, cancer of the mouth and larynx, esophageal cancer, kidney and urinary bladder cancer, pancreatic cancer, chronic bronchitis, emphysema, increased incidence of respiratory infection, increased frequency and severity of asthmatic attacks, coronary artery disease, myocardial infarction, peripheral vascular disease, hypertension, stroke, low birth weights in infants, increased incidence of stillbirths, impotence, burn injuries, and reduced exercise capacity.
- Neuromuscular causes of RLD include spinal cord injury, ALS, polio, Guillain–Barré syndrome, muscular dystrophy, and myasthenia gravis, and any of these disease entities can cause such a significant decrease in alveolar ventilation that a mechanical ventilator is required to maintain life.
- Crush injuries and penetrating wounds to the thorax can cause significant RLD but are almost always reversible with corrective interventions.
- More than 100 drugs have the side effect of causing restrictive lung impairment, including oxygen and the majority of drugs used in the treatment of cancer.
- Radiation fibrosis of the lung is a complication of radiation therapy and is dependent on the number of fractions into which the radiation dose is divided, the total dose of radiation, the volume of lung being irradiated, and the quality of the radiation.

## References

1. Hercules PR, Lekwart FJ, Fenton MV. Pulmonary Restriction and Obstruction. Chicago, 1979, Year Book Medical Publishers.
2. Weinberger SE, Cockrill BA, Mandel J. Principles of Pulmonary Medicine. Philadelphia, 2008, Saunders.
3. Whipp BJ, Wasserman K. Exercise Pulmonary Physiology and Pathophysiology. New York, 1991, Marcel Dekker.
4. Divertie MB. Respiratory System. The CIBA Collection of Medical Illustrations, ed 2. Summit, NJ, 1980, CIBA Pharmaceutical Company.
5. Basmajian JV. Therapeutic Exercise, ed 3. Baltimore, 1978, Williams & Wilkins.
6. Hamilton H. Respiratory Disorders (Nurse's Clinical Library). Springhouse, PA, 1984, Springhouse.
7. Dunhill MS. Pulmonary Pathology, ed 2. New York, 1987, Churchill Livingstone.
8. Fishman AP. Pulmonary Diseases and Disorders, ed 2. New York, 1988, McGraw-Hill.
9. Bordow RA, Ries AL, Morris TA. Manual of Clinical Problems in Pulmonary Medicine, ed 2. Boston, 2005, Little, Brown.
10. Hasleton PS. Spencer's Pathology of the Lung, ed 5. New York, 1996, McGraw-Hill.
11. American Physical Therapy Association. Guide to Physical Therapist Practice, ed 2. Phys Ther 81:9–744, 2001.
12. Fishman AP. Update: Pulmonary Diseases and Disorders. New York, 1982, McGraw-Hill.
13. Scully RM, Barnes MR. Physical Therapy. Philadelphia, 1989, JB Lippincott.
14. Castillo-Garzón MJ, Ruiz JR, Ortega FB, et al. Anti-aging therapy through fitness enhancement. Clin Interv Aging 1(3):213–20, 2006.
15. Drewnowski A, Evans WJ. Nutrition, physical activity, and quality of life in older adults. J Gerontol A Biol Sci Med Sci 56(2):89–94, 2001.
16. DiPietro L. Physical activity in aging: changes in patterns and their relationship to health and function. J Gerontol A Biol Sci Med Sci 56(2):13–22, 2001.
17. Schwarz MI, King TE Jr. Interstitial Lung Disease. Philadelphia, 1993, BC Decker.
18. Glauser FL. Signs and Symptoms in Pulmonary Medicine. Philadelphia, 1983, JB Lippincott.
19. Phan SH, Thrall RS. Pulmonary Fibrosis. New York, 1995, Marcel Dekker.
20. George RB, Light RW, Matthay MA, et al. Chest Medicine: Essentials of Pulmonary and Critical Care Medicine, ed 5. Baltimore, 2005, Williams & Wilkins.
21. Agarwal R, Jindal SK. Acute exacerbation of idiopathic pulmonary fibrosis: a systematic review. Eur J Intern Med 19(4):227–35, 2008.
22. Taskar VS, Coultas DB. Is idiopathic pulmonary fibrosis an environmental disease? Proc Am Thorac Soc 3(4):293–298, 2006.
23. Derenne JP, Whitelaw WA, Similowski T. Acute Respiratory Failure in Chronic Obstructive Pulmonary Disease. New York, 1996, Marcel Dekker.
24. Beers MH, Fletcher AJ. The Merck Manual of Diagnosis and Therapy, ed 2. Rahway, NJ, 2003, Merck Sharp and Dohme Research Laboratories.
25. Baum GL, Wolinsky E. Textbook of Pulmonary Diseases, ed 3. Boston, 1983, Little, Brown.
26. George RB, Light RW, Matthay MA, et al. Chest Medicine: Essentials of Pulmonary and Critical Care Medicine, ed 2. Baltimore, 1990, Williams & Wilkins.
27. Hinshaw HC, Murray JF. Diseases of the Chest, ed 4. Philadelphia, 1980, WB Saunders.
28. Mitchell RS. Synopsis of Clinical Pulmonary Disease, ed 2. St. Louis, 1978, CV Mosby.
29. Cottrell GP, Surkin HB. Pharmacology for Respiratory Care Practitioners. Philadelphia, 1995, FA Davis.

30. Boyda EK. Respiratory Problems. Oradell, NJ, 1985, Medical Economics Company.

31. Fernandez R, Trenchs X, Klamburg J, et al. Prone positioning in acute respiratory distress syndrome: a multicenter randomized clinical trial. Intensive Care Med 34(8):1487–91, 2008.

32. Rubenfeld GD, Caldwell E, Peabody E, et al. Incidence and outcomes of acute lung injury. N Engl J Med 353(16):1685–1693, 2005.

33. Cannon GW, Zimmerman GA. The Lung in Rheumatic Diseases. New York, 1990, Marcel Dekker.

34. Peat M. Current Physical Therapy. Philadelphia, 1988, BC Decker.

35. Willén C, Thorén-Jönsson AL, Grimby G, et al. Disability in a 4-year follow-up study of people with post-polio syndrome. J Rehabil Med 39(2):175–80, 2007.

36. Adams JH, Corsellis JAN, Duchen LW. Greenfield's Neuropathology, ed 4. New York, 1984, John Wiley & Sons.

37. McDonald K, Wisniewski JM. Basic Burn Seminar Notebook (unpublished). Ann Arbor, Physical Therapy Division, 1988, University of Michigan Medical Center.

38. Physicians' Desk Reference, ed 62. Oradell, NJ, 2008, Medical Economics Company.

39. Sheppard M. Practical Pulmonary Pathology. London, 1995, Edward Arnold.

# CHAPTER 6

# Chronic Obstructive Pulmonary Diseases

*Susan Garritan*

## Chapter Outline

The symptoms of many obstructive pulmonary diseases have been described in the medical literature of centuries past by physicians considered to be "the fathers" of modern medicine. However, an incomplete understanding of the disease process limited their clinical ability to help alleviate patients' symptoms. Today we are more fortunate because the etiology and pathophysiology of obstructive pulmonary disease is becoming increasingly understood. With our increased understanding of mechanisms leading to various pulmonary diseases, more effective medical and physical therapy interventions are available to improve the quality of life for affected individuals. Our enhanced understanding of obstructive pulmonary diseases has resulted in recommendations for preventive strategies, which are expected to reduce incidences of this disease in future generations. In the future, our knowledge and understanding of a variety of medical conditions will result in necessary changes to current treatment approaches. Therefore, it is critical that physical therapists treating patients with cardiovascular and pulmonary disorders keep current with medical research, review meta-analysis articles, and practice evidence-based physical therapy to provide the best possible care to clients with obstructive pulmonary disease.

Table 6-1 outlines the American Physical Therapy Association (APTA) preferred practice patterns that categorize the obstructive pulmonary disorders physical therapists encounter in their practice.[1] Primary practice patterns for each pulmonary disorder are listed first. Other practice patterns also may become applicable if disease severity progresses over time.

Chronic obstructive pulmonary diseases (COPDs) are diseases of the airways, which produce obstruction to expiratory airflow. Airflow obstruction can be related to any or all of the following problems:

- Retained secretions
- Inflammation of the mucosal lining of airway walls
- Bronchial constriction related to increased tone or spasm of bronchial smooth muscle
- Weakening of the support structure of airway walls

All of these conditions have the potential to decrease the size of the bronchial lumen and increase the resistance to expiratory airflow. Therefore, regardless of the mechanism, obstructive lung diseases generally result in incomplete emptying of the lung, which produces the classic signs of lung hyperinflation seen in chest radiographs (CXRs).

The CXRs shown in Figure 6-1 illustrate the most common signs of lung hyperinflation associated with obstructive lung diseases. These signs include the following:

- Elevation of the shoulder girdle
- Horizontal ribs
- Barrel-shaped thorax (increased anterior–posterior diameter)
- Low, flattened diaphragms

> ### Clinical Tip
> CXR findings such as those shown in Figure 6-1 are present only in severe obstructive lung disease; therefore, a CXR is of limited value in diagnosing obstructive lung disease. Results of spirometry testing are more important in identifying the presence of most obstructive lung diseases. One type of obstructive pulmonary disease, bronchiectasis, is best diagnosed by computed tomography (CT). More information about bronchiectasis can be found later in this chapter.

## Lung Function in Obstructive Lung Diseases

Lung hyperinflation affects both the mechanical function of the respiratory muscles and the gas exchange capabilities of the lung. Abnormalities in gas exchange are seen by examining the arterial blood gas (ABG) values. Oxygenation levels

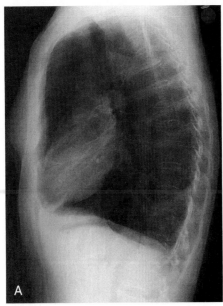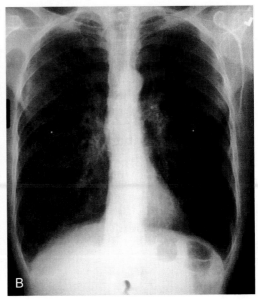

**Figure 6-1** Radiographic signs of lung hyperinflation. (From Hess D, MacIntyre NR, Mishoe SC, et al. Respiratory Care Principles and Practice. St. Louis, 2002, Saunders.)

### Table 6-1 Preferred Practice Patterns Associated with Chronic Obstructive Lung Diseases

| | ICD-9-CM Code | Primary Practice Patterns | Secondary Practice Patterns |
|---|---|---|---|
| Cystic fibrosis | 277.0 | 6C | 6E, 6F |
| Chronic bronchitis | 491 | 6C, 6B | 6F |
| Emphysema | 492 | 6B, 6C | 6E, 6F |
| Asthma | 493 | 6C, 6B | 6E, 6F |
| Bronchiectasis | 494 | 6C, 6B | 6F |
| COPD (not elsewhere classified [NEC]) | 496 | 6B, 6C | 6F |

*6B: impaired aerobic capacity/endurance associated with deconditioning; 6C: impaired ventilation, respiration/gas exchange and aerobic capacity/endurance associated with airway clearance dysfunction; 6E: impaired ventilation and respiration/gas exchange associated with ventilatory pump dysfunction or failure; 6F: impaired ventilation and respiration/gas exchange associated with respiratory failure.*
*Data from American Physical Therapy Association. Preferred physical therapist practice patterns: cardiovascular/pulmonary. In Guide to Physical Therapist Practice, ed 2. Alexandria, VA, 2003, American Physical Therapy Association.*

($PaO_2$) become decreased as disease severity progresses and $CO_2$ levels vary according to either the type or stage of disease. $CO_2$ levels can be decreased (in emphysema), normal in early obstructive pulmonary disease, or elevated (in chronic bronchitis or impending respiratory failure). Disease-specific abnormalities in lung function will be discussed in detail in the section for each of the obstructive diseases.

## Symptoms Associated with Obstructive Lung Diseases

In general, individuals with obstructive lung diseases frequently complain of dyspnea on exertion (DOE), especially during functional activities such as stair climbing or long-distance or fast walking. The sensation of DOE can be so uncomfortable and occasionally frightening for individuals with obstructive lung disease that the onset can lead to an increased anxiety level. In some obstructive diseases, secretion production and cough are prominent features. Disease-specific symptoms will be discussed in the relevant sections for each disease.

## Quantification of Impairment in Obstructive Lung Diseases

### Pulmonary Function Testing

Spirometry tracings measure time–volume relationships in the lung (see Chapter 10). Typically obstructive diseases are characterized by delayed and incomplete emptying of the lung during exhalation. To assess the progression of COPD, two forced spirometry measures that can be followed over time are the forced expiratory volume in 1 second ($FEV_1$; Fig. 6-2) and the forced vital capacity (FVC; see Chapter 10 for further information). Another way of expressing airflow limitation is to measure the amount of air that can be exhaled in 1 second as a percentage of the total amount of air that can be forcefully exhaled, or the $FEV_1$/FVC ratio $\times$ 100%. A normal $FEV_1$/FVC ratio is considered to be >75%,[2] and the ratio's value reflects the increased time it takes to expel air as an obstructive disease becomes more severe. The $FEV_1$/FVC ratio decreases as the severity of lung obstruction increases.

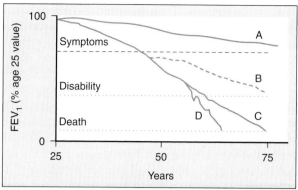

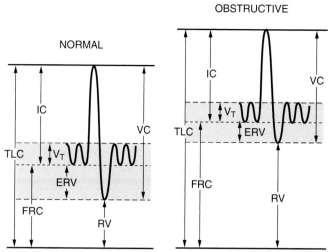

**Figure 6-2** The progression of COPD over time. Natural history of COPD as measured by FEV1 as a percentage of the baseline value at age 25. Normal nonsmoking individuals (A) have a progressive loss of $FEV_1$ but never become symptomatic with airway obstruction. Patients with COPD who quit smoking (B) experience an $FEV_1$ decline that parallels a nonsmoking, age-matched person. Patients with progressive COPD (C) can develop a loss of $FEV_1$, which may eventually produce symptoms, disability, and death. Some COPD patients (D) have steep declines in lung function during discreet clinical episodes. (From Heffner JE: Chronic obstructive pulmonary disease on an exponential curve of progress. Respir Care 47:586, 2002.)

**Figure 6-3** Lung volumes in chronic obstructive pulmonary disease compared with normal values. In the presence of obstructive lung disease, the vital capacity (VC) is normal to decreased, the residual volume (RV) and functional residual capacity (FRC) are increased, the TLC (total lung capacity) is normal to increased, and the RV/TLC ratio is increased. ERV, expiratory reserve volume; IC, inspiratory capacity; VT, tidal volume. (From Hines & Marshall: Stoelting's Anesthesia and Co-Existing Disease, ed 5. Philadelphia, 2008, Churchill Livingstone.)

Forced flow rates measured during exhalation are used to
- quantify the degree of airway obstruction present,
- document improvements in lung function following the administration of medications, and
- follow the progression, or worsening, of an obstructive lung disease.

> **Clinical Tip**
> Individuals with obstructive pulmonary disease require increased time to expel air from their lungs. As the severity of lung obstruction increases, less and less air can be exhaled in 1 second.

## Lung Volumes

Pulmonary function tests (PFTs) provide information regarding the volume of air the lung contains, after different levels of inhalation or exhalation, and information regarding the lung capacities (the sums of different lung volumes). In general, individuals with COPD show larger than normal total lung capacities (TLCs) and larger residual volumes (RVs) when compared to individuals of the same age, height, gender, and race (Fig. 6-3).[3] See Chapter 10 for more detailed information on PFTs.

> **Clinical Tip**
> Individuals with obstructive lung disease demonstrate an increased total lung capacity and an increased RV as a result of air trapping and lung hyperinflation.

## Disease-Specific Obstructive Lung Conditions

In the sections that follow, the obstructive lung diseases will be considered separately to highlight the unique features, such as etiology, pathophysiology, and variations in clinical presentation, medical management, and prognosis. Knowledge of disease-specific differences is important to help determine appropriate physical therapy interventions and the best sequence of intervention application to help individuals attain their maximal functional potential and reduce their symptoms of shortness of breath.

## Cystic Fibrosis

"The infant that tastes of salt will surely die. This observation from ancient European folklore is probably the first recognition of cystic fibrosis (CF), a disease that is characterized by abnormal salt transport, and in early times, death in infancy."[4]

Today, CF is recognized as a multisystem disorder affecting both children, and increasingly young adults.[5] In 2007, 45% of the individuals in the CF Patient Registry were adults (18 years and older).[6] Cystic fibrosis affects every organ system that has epithelial surfaces,[7] with the most prominent symptoms in clinical presentation relating to pulmonary and pancreatic involvement. The pulmonary system is affected by chronic airway obstruction and inflammation, thick tenacious mucus, and recurrent bacterial infections. In addition, the pancreas develops exocrine pancreatic insufficiency, which affects both gastrointestinal function (fat maldigestion) and the growth and development of individuals with CF.[8] Other organs affected include the upper airway (sinus infections), male reproductive tract (obstructive azoospermia), and sweat glands (elevated sweat chloride levels).[8,9]

## Epidemiology

Cystic fibrosis is the most common life-threatening genetic trait in the Caucasian population.[10] It is estimated that 30,000 people in the United States have CF.[6] In the United States, the incidence of CF is as follows[11]:

- Caucasians: 1 in 3200 live births
- African Americans: 1 in 15,000 live births
- Asian Americans: 1 in 31,000 live births

Mutations of the CF gene are most prevalent in individuals of northern and central European ancestry, and the incidence of CF is considered rare in American Indians, Asian populations, and in black natives of Africa.[8] Cystic fibrosis transmission follows the pattern for transmission of autosomal recessive traits. When parents are both carriers of CF trait mutations, 25% of their offspring will have CF, 50% will be carriers, and 25% will neither have CF nor be carriers.

Numerous mutations and many combinations of mutations of a single gene locus are responsible for the CF syndrome and for variations in its severity.[8] The affected gene is located on the long arm of chromosome.[7,10] The gene encodes a membrane protein called the cystic fibrosis transmembrane conductance regulator (CFTR).[8] CFTR functions mainly as a chloride channel, but it also regulates the activity of other ion channels in some tissues.[8] The first described CFTR mutation is a deletion that eliminates phenylalanine at position 508, the ΔF 508 mutation.[8,12] The ΔF 508 deletion has been detected in 66% of 20,000 CF patient chromosomes analyzed worldwide.[10] At this time, more than 1500 other mutations of the CF gene have been reported, but the functional importance of only a small number are known.[13] The large number of possible CF mutations makes DNA testing for carriers more difficult.[13]

## Pathology

Mucus stasis has been described at a number of different sites throughout the body: including the conducting airways of the lung, nasal sinuses, sweat glands, small intestine, pancreas, and biliary system (Fig. 6-4). Disease in the conducting airways in CF is acquired postnatally, as infants who have died within the first few days of life display only subtle abnormalities.[8] Either increased production of secretions or failure to clear secretions at an early age accounts for the mucus accumulation seen in bronchial regions and in bronchioles. Failure to clear secretions from airway lumens can often

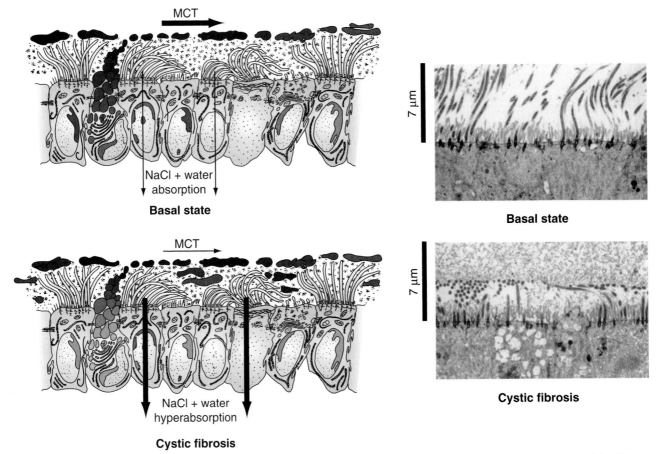

**Figure 6-4** Mucociliary transport in normal and cystic fibrosis airway epithelia. (From Mason RJ, Murray JF, Broaddus VC, et al. Murray & Nadel's Textbook of Respiratory Medicine, ed 4. Philadelphia, 2005, Saunders.)

initiate infection.[8] As the lung disease progresses, submucosal glands hypertrophy, goblet cells become more numerous, and small airways often become completely obstructed by secretions.[14] Bronchiolectasis and finally bronchiectasis are the outcome of repeated obstructive-infection cycles.[8]

In the pancreas, obstruction of the ducts by inspissated secretions occurs early, followed by dilation of secretory ducts and flattening of the epithelium. Acinar cells are destroyed and replaced by fibrous tissue and fat.[8] The pancreas is abnormal in almost all patients with CF and is virtually destroyed in approximately 90% of CF patients studied at autopsy.[8]

## Pathophysiology

The CFTR protein appears to have multiple functions. It serves as a chloride channel[15] and modulates the activity of other plasma membrane channels, such as sodium channels.[16] Abnormal function of CFTR results in abnormal salt and water transport.[8] Cystic fibrosis affects the epithelial lining of various organs in the body, but because epithelial function can vary from one organ to another, the physiologic consequences of mutant CFTR can also vary widely.[8] Several hypotheses attempt to explain how CFTR dysfunction leads to the disease presentations seen in CF. It is possible that elements of all the hypotheses may contribute to the pathogenesis of CF.[13]

- The low-volume hypothesis postulates that CFTR dysfunction causes loss of inhibition of sodium channels so that excessive sodium and water are reabsorbed, which results in dehydration of the airway surface. In addition, loss of chloride efflux prevents correction of low surface water volume, which results in a reduction of the lubricating layer between the epithelium and mucus and compression of the cilia by mucus, which inhibits ciliary and cough clearance of mucus.[8]
- The high-salt hypothesis argues that in the absence of CFTR, excess sodium and chloride are retained in airway surface liquid, and the increased concentration of chloride disrupts the function of innate antibiotic molecules, which allows bacteria to persist in the airways of the lung.[17]

Two additional hypotheses include dysregulation of the host inflammatory response and primary predisposition to infection.[13]

Failure of the airways to clear mucus normally is likely the primary pathophysiologic event in CF.[8] The resulting mucus stasis, adhesion and obstruction are likely responsible for severe and unrelenting chronic bacterial infections that are prominent clinical features of CF.[8] The most common bacterial pathogens include *Pseudomonas aeruginosa* and *Staphylococcus aureus*.[6,8,12] Less common pathogens include *Haemophilus influenzae*, methicillin-resistant *S. aureus* (MRSA), and *Burkholderia cepacia*.[6] Once established, infection of the lung in CF is rarely eradicated, despite prolonged administration of antibiotic, bacteria frequently persist, especially Pseudomonas.[6,12] By adulthood, 70% to 80% of those with CF are colonized with Pseudomonas.[6] Infection with *B. cepacia* complex carries the worst prognosis for survival, with some patients experiencing a sepsis-like syndrome with necrotizing pneumonia (cepacia syndrome) and rapid deterioration, leading to death.[4]

## Clinical Presentation

Usual clinical presentations in CF include early onset of respiratory tract symptoms, such as persistent cough and recurrent lung infiltrates. Usual gastrointestinal presentations include meconium ileus (intestinal obstruction caused by viscous meconium stool) at birth in approximately 15% of patients and failure to thrive with steatorrhea (excessive fat in the feces).[8]

### Pulmonary System: Lower and Upper Respiratory Tract Disease

The earliest manifestation of CF is cough, initially associated with episodes of acute lower respiratory tract infection but over time, the cough becomes chronic.[8] With progression of lung disease, the cough becomes productive of tenacious, purulent, green sputum (reflecting *P. aeruginosa* infection) and paroxysmal, often associated with gagging and emesis.[8] In the upper respiratory tract both nasal polyps and sinusitis are common in individuals with CF.[8]

### Gastrointestinal System: Pancreas, Gallbladder, and Intestinal Tract Disease

In addition to the presence of meconium ileus at birth in 15% of infants with CF, abnormalities in intestinal mucins beyond the newborn period contribute to malabsorption of nutrients in the intestinal tract and a decrease in intestinal transit time. This results in maldigestion and fecal impaction in the terminal ileum or distal intestinal obstruction syndrome (meconium ileus equivalent). Intussusception (infolding of one segment of the intestine into an adjacent part) and rectal prolapse are other possible intestinal complications.[8,12]

Ninety percent of individuals with CF have pancreatic insufficiency.[12] Pancreatic insufficiency in infants results in failure to thrive, and in older children enzyme deficiency results in fat and protein maldigestion, producing a distended abdomen and frequent bulky, greasy, foul-smelling stools.[8] In the pancreas of individuals with CF, thick, viscous secretions from the exocrine portion of the pancreas progressively obstruct the pancreatic ducts. This results in pancreatic autodestruction by the pancreatic enzymes. Endocrine function of the pancreas is usually preserved in children, but in adults pancreatic fibrosis may obliterate the islets of Langerhans and cause diabetes mellitus.[12] Approximately 50% of adults with CF are diabetic by the age of 30 years.[12]

In the gallbladder, obstruction of the biliary tract by viscid secretions may produce biliary cirrhosis. Some newborns develop inspissated bile syndrome, characterized by prolonged obstructive jaundice, which often clears without medical therapy. In adults with CF, the risk for development of cholelithiasis (gallbladder stones) or cholecystitis (inflammation of the gallbladder) is increased compared to age-matched controls.[12]

## Table 6-2  Results of Sweat Test Values

| | Normal | Borderline | Cystic Fibrosis | |
|---|---|---|---|---|
| Sweat Chloride Concentrations | <40 mEq/L | 40–60 mEq/L | ≥60 mEq/L | |
| | | | Nonclassic | 60–90 mEq/L |
| | | | Classic | 90–110 mEq/L |

*Adapted from Knowles MR, Durie PR. What is cystic fibrosis? N Engl J Med 347:439–442, 2002.*

### Reproductive System: Genitourinary
Almost all male patients with CF have congenital absence of the vas deferens and obstructive azoospermia.[18] Fertility is generally not affected in women with CF and they can successfully complete the term of pregnancy provided they have adequate nutritional and pulmonary reserve.[19]

## Symptoms
Cystic fibrosis should be considered as a possible diagnosis in any child with recurrent or chronic cough, recurrent pneumonia, or recurrent wheezing when other causes such as asthma, bronchitis, and bronchiolitis have been ruled out.[18]

## Physical Examination
Lung sounds are often unremarkable, except for diminution in the intensity of the breath sounds, which correlates with the degree of hyperinflation present.[8] Adventitious breath sounds are usually heard first over the upper lobes, and increased respiratory rate and retraction of the chest during inspiration may be observed during new bacterial infections. Digital clubbing occurs in virtually all patients with CF and its severity generally correlates with the severity of lung disease.[18]

### Diagnostic Tests
Newborn screening for CF is becoming more prevalent in the United States and is done through blood spot analysis from infant heel sticks, followed by a limited CFTR mutation screen if immunoreactive trypsin levels in the blood sample are elevated. Final diagnosis requires a sweat test or DNA mutation analysis.[4] Early diagnosis of CF has been beneficial in instituting early intervention. The gold standard for diagnosing CF is based on demonstrating elevated sweat chloride levels (≥60 mEq/L) in individuals with a medical history consistent with CF, specifically the presence of meconium ileus, chronic pulmonary disease, and pancreatic insufficiency. A family history of CF, particularly in a sibling, supports the diagnosis and two positive sweat tests using the quantitative pilocarpine iontophoresis method establishes the diagnosis with certainty.[12] In children, chloride concentration levels are usually less than 40 mEq/L, with average chloride concentrations of 20 mEq/L in normal cases and 95 mEq/L for those with CF (Table 6-2).[12] Other conditions that may cause elevated chloride levels must be ruled out, such as malnutrition and adrenal insufficiency.[12]

Genetic analysis may also be used to confirm the diagnosis of CF, especially in those with minimal symptoms. The presence of two CF-associated alleles is considered sufficient to diagnose classic CF with certainty.[12] A milder form of CF, or non-classic CF, may be seen in individuals with only one copy of a mutant gene who have some CFTR function preserved. These individuals have no overt signs of maldigestion because some pancreatic function is preserved. The sweat chloride levels for those with non-classic CF are usually in the 60 to 90 mEq/L range, whereas those with classic CF have chloride levels of approximately 90 to 110 mEq/L.[9]

### Radiographic Tests
Early in the course of CF, mild hyperinflation and minimal peribronchial thickening is seen, usually first in the upper lobes of the lung. As the disease progresses, peribronchial thickening extends to involve all lobes. In advanced disease, ring shadows, cystic lesions, nodular densities, bronchiectasis, and atelectasis are evident.[12] Subpleural blebs may be evident in the second decade of life and are most prominent along the mediastinal border.[8] High-resolution computed tomographic (HRCT) scans are more sensitive than plain CXRs and they may detect early bronchiectasis or mucoid impaction (retained secretions) before the x-ray becomes abnormal.[12]

### Pulmonary Function Tests
Prior to age 6, ABG analysis is used to as a measure of overall lung function in CF.[12] Children older than 6 years are able to perform PFTs reliably, with spirometry testing in CF showing an obstructive pattern, initially in the small airways, with increases in RV, functional residual capacity (FRC), and TLC.[12] In general, patients progress from initial reductions in maximum midexpiratory flow rates to reductions in $FEV_1$/FVC and then to diminished vital capacity and total lung volumes.[8] This progression from peripheral airway obstruction to more generalized obstruction and finally the addition of a restrictive component is illustrated in Table 6-3.

### Arterial Blood Gases
By the time the diagnosis of CF is made, many children with CF show mild decreases in arterial $PO_2$, with oxygenation declining slowly throughout life.[8] Elevation of arterial $PCO_2$ generally occurs with $FEV_1$ volumes of <30% of predicted and constitutes an end-stage event for most patients.[8]

## Medical Management
Guidelines for CF Care (CFF Annual Report 2007) for both children and Adults with CF include

**Table 6-3 Representative Pulmonary Function Test Results from Three Young Adult Males with Mild, Moderate, and Severe Lung Disease**

| Test | Mild | Moderate | Severe |
|---|---|---|---|
| FVC | 98 | 72 | 48 |
| $FEV_1$ | 92 | 46 | 34 |
| $FEV_1/FVC$ | (0.81) | (0.70) | (0.64) |
| MMEF | 83 | 15 | 6 |
| $Vmax_{50}$ | 91 | 19 | 11 |
| $Vmax_{25}$ | 52 | 10 | 5 |
| FRC | 162 | 112 | 75 |
| RV | 189 | 200 | 120 |
| TLC | 131 | 105 | 62 |
| RV/TLC | (0.29) | (0.45) | (0.50) |
| $PaO_2$ (room air) | [87] | [74] | [48] |
| Patient Function | Coughs several times a day | Coughs frequently | Chronic right heart failure |
| | Cough is occasionally productive | Expectorates moderately large amounts of mucus | Able to work daily as a hair stylist |
| | No restriction of activity | Able to jog 3 miles daily | |
| | | Is a full-time student in a professional school | |

*Note: Values are percentage predicted, except those in parentheses, which are simple ratios, and those in square brackets, which are mmHg. FRC, functional residual capacity; MMEF, maximal mid-expiratory flow; RV, residual volume; TLC, total lung capacity.*
*Adapted from Mason RJ, Murray JF, Broaddus VC, et al. Murray & Nadel's Textbook of Respiratory Medicine, ed 4. Philadelphia, 2005, Saunders.*

- Clinic visits: four or more per year
- PFTs: two or more per year
- Respiratory cultures: at least one per year
- Glucose monitoring: every year if age ≥14
- Liver enzymes monitoring: every year
- Influenza vaccine: every year if ≥6 months of age 6 years

The goals of medical management of CF include controlling lung infection, promoting mucus clearance, and improving nutritional status.[20] Other interventions may also include treating additional medical complications that may develop in adolescence and young adulthood, such as CF-related diabetes, bone disease (osteopenia), or depression.[6]

To reduce the chance of pulmonary infections, the Cystic Fibrosis Foundation recommends the following[6]:

- Using airway clearance techniques to keep the lungs as free of mucus as possible
- Taking all recommended medications, including the flu shot
- Participating in a regular exercise program to maintain muscle strength
- Minimizing germ contact by using good hand hygiene and properly cleaning and disinfecting equipment
- Avoiding secondhand smoke exposure

*Pulmonary Infection*

When signs and symptoms of a pulmonary infection are present, treatment is initiated (Box 6-1).

**Box 6-1**

**Signs and Symptoms of an Acute Pulmonary Exacerbation**

- Increased cough
- Increased sputum production
- Increased temperature: low-grade rise in body temperature
- Increased respiratory rate
- Increased white blood cell count
- New findings on auscultation or on CXR
- Decrease in $FEV_1$
- Decrease in appetite
- Decrease in weight
- Decrease in activity level

Treatment of acute pulmonary infection includes administration of antibiotics (oral, inhaled, or intravenous), increasing the frequency of secretion clearance techniques, and improved nutrition.[13] The choice of antibiotics is guided by sputum culture, with antibiotic selection directed at staphylococcal and pseudomonas organisms; however, antibiotic resistance frequently develops after a few courses of treatment. In resistant cases, a combination antibiotic treatment with agents that have different modes of action is preferred to single antibiotic treatment. In these resistant cases, antibiotics are given intravenously for a 2-week time frame to avoid relapse.[12,21] In-hospital combination antibiotic treatment for *P. aeruginosa* usually includes a β-lactam (which interferes with cell wall biosynthesis) and an aminoglycoside (which inhibits protein production).[21] Use of combined oral and inhaled antibiotics without hospital admission may be sufficient for milder exacerbations. In individuals with persistent Pseudomonas infections, the inhaled antibiotic tobramycin (TOBI) is recommended twice daily on a 28-day on–off cycle for patients with moderate to severe CF.[22] The Cystic Fibrosis Foundation recommends the use of oral azithromycin (Zithromax) for the treatment of persistent *P. aeruginosa*–positive patients.[6]

Sputum viscosity is decreased in CF patients by the use of mucolytic medications such as rhDNase (Pulmozyme), a DNA-cleaving mucolytic. Inhaled hypertonic saline solution is also being used to decrease sputum viscosity in CF. The hypertonic saline draws water into the airways, rehydrating the periciliary layer, and this sustained hydration promotes increased mucociliary clearance.[23] The use of oral ibuprofen is recommended by the Cystic Fibrosis Foundation to control inflammation.[6]

Although pulmonary function may be restored to baseline after treatment for infection, the cumulative effect of these repeated infections usually leads to the development of bronchiectasis, atelectasis, and an irreversible decrease in pulmonary function over time.[12]

### Pancreatic Status and Nutritional Supplementation

Management of pancreatic insufficiency in CF is partially accomplished by ingestion of pancreatic enzyme replacements, which should be taken with food containing protein, fat, or complex carbohydrates. The enzyme dosage is adjusted to attempt maintain an ideal weight while decreasing the likelihood of developing abdominal cramping or flatulence. Enzyme replacement therapy does not totally correct pancreatic insufficiency, so individuals with CF also require increased caloric intake to maintain optimal growth. This may be accomplished through the use of nutritional supplements taken orally or via a gastrostomy tube. Fat-soluble vitamin supplementation is essential in all individuals with pancreatic insufficiency.[13] Because of the strong correlation between nutritional status and pulmonary function, attention to nutritional well-being should be regarded as one of the cornerstones of good lung health in CF.[13]

Management of the other possible complications in CF includes restoring electrolyte balance when electrolyte imbalance is caused by hot weather. Fecal impaction can occur as a result of decreased water and chloride content in the feces, and it may result in partial or complete small bowel obstruction. Pulmonary complications include pneumothorax from ruptured bronchiectatic cysts or subpleural blebs. Pneumothorax can cause an abrupt decline in pulmonary function and requires placement of a chest tube for lung reexpansion with the possible need for surgery if the pneumothorax recurs. Hemoptysis (coughing up blood) can occur in CF, usually related to infection, but massive hemoptysis is uncommon in CF.

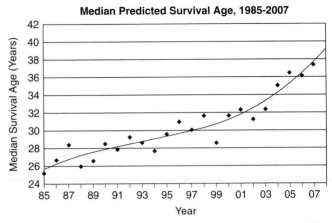

**Figure 6-5** Cystic fibrosis median predicted survival age 1985–2007. (From Consumer Fact Sheet. It's All About Suzy: Quality Improvement in CF Care. Bethesda, MD, 2010, Cystic Fibrosis Foundation.)

### Prognosis

Comprehensive, multidisciplinary evidence-based CF treatment programs have led to a dramatic increase in the median age of survival, which is reported to be 37.4 years in 2007.[6] The graph shown in Figure 6-5 illustrates the increase in median survival age since 1985.

Aggressive nutritional support in CF has become a major component of this increase in survival,[24] along with centralization of care at CF centers and aggressive management of symptoms.[13] However, despite the increases in years of survival, CF is characterized by a gradual decline in pulmonary function over the life span with abrupt deterioration in pulmonary function when infection is present. Cystic fibrosis is invariably fatal, with more than 90% of individuals dying from pulmonary complications.[12] Disease progression includes hypercapnic and hypoxemic respiratory failure due to progressive airway obstruction with alveolar hypoventilation and ventilation–perfusion mismatching.[8] Cor pulmonale is a late complication of severe airway obstruction. Ventilatory assistance is effective in CF patients with acute respiratory failure due to reversible and treatable conditions or patients awaiting lung transplantation.[8]

For selected individuals with CF and end-stage lung disease, lung transplantation (see Chapter 12) has become an option, with 178 lung transplants performed in 2007 on CFF Registry patients, 174 of which were bilateral lung transplants.[6]

### Prevention

The role of genetic counseling is very important in families who have had a child, or first cousin, diagnosed with CF. Ideally screening for CF carrier status of potential parents should be done prior to conception. A screening panel is done for 25 mutations that have both a known association with CF and an allele frequency in the affected U.S. population of ≥0.1% based on data from the Cystic Fibrosis Foundation and others researchers.[25] However, screening for CF carrier status is complicated by the large number of different mutations (>1500) that can contribute to CF. For example, genetic testing for the presence of the Δ F 508 mutation identifies only 50% to 60% of couples at risk of having a child with CF.[26]

## Implications for Physical Therapy Treatment

The following elements of physical therapy treatment should be included in the care of individuals with CF:

- Secretion clearance techniques
  - Postural drainage with percussion, shaking and vibration
  - Acapella
  - Positive expiratory pressure (PEP)
  - High-frequency chest wall oscillation (the Vest)
  - Autogenic drainage
  - Active cycle breathing technique
  - Forced expiratory technique
- Controlled breathing techniques (during episodes of shortness of breath)
- Exercise and strength training
- Inspiratory muscle training
- Thoracic stretching exercises
- Postural reeducation to avoid round-shouldered postures

## Asthma

The word *asthma* is derived from the ancient Greek word for "panting." The currently understood basis of asthma is summarized in the National Heart, Lung, and Blood Institute's definition in the 1995 "Global Initiative for Asthma"

Asthma is a chronic inflammatory disorder of the airways in which many cells and cellular elements play a role, in particular, mast cells, eosinophils, T lymphocytes, macrophages, neutrophils, and epithelial cells. In susceptible individuals, this inflammation causes recurrent episodes of wheezing, breathlessness, chest tightness, and coughing, particularly at night or in the early morning. These episodes are usually associated with widespread but variable airflow obstruction that is often reversible either spontaneously or with treatment. The inflammation also causes an associated increase in the existing bronchial hyperresponsiveness to a variety of stimuli.[27]

Asthma is considered an "episodic" obstructive lung condition, with periods of relatively normal lung function occurring in many asthmatics between episodes of wheezing, breathlessness, chest tightness, and coughing.

### Epidemiology

Although asthma has long been recognized as a distinct disease, it has only emerged as a major health problem in the last 35 years.[28] Research has indicated worldwide increases in the prevalence of asthma since 1960.[29] In the United States, data from the National Health Interview Survey show that the overall prevalence of asthma increased from 3.1% in 1980 to 5.5% in 1996.[30] There is also evidence that increases in the prevalence of asthma is related to a general increase in the prevalence of allergic disease.[28]

Asthma may have a genetic component as an increased prevalence of asthma is noted in first-degree relatives compared to the prevalence of asthma in the general population.[31] In addition to a family history of atopic disease, other risk factors for developing asthma include low or high birth weight, prematurity, maternal smoking during pregnancy, parental smoking, high intake of salt, pet ownership, and obesity.[32] Additional factors related to the development of asthma come from comparisons of varying rates of allergies and asthma in different countries worldwide. The International Study of Asthma and Allergies in Childhood (ISAAC) involved 155 centers in 55 countries.[33] The ISAAC survey, a one-page questionnaire and a video demonstrating signs and symptoms of asthma, was used to survey nearly half a million children 13 to 14 years of age. Results of the ISAAC survey showed wide variation in the prevalence of asthma, allergic rhinoconjunctivitis, and atopic eczema among the centers surveyed. Prevalence of asthma was highest in the United Kingdom, Ireland, Australia, and New Zealand and lowest in China, Russia, Greece, and Indonesia (Fig. 6-6).[33]

The results of the ISAAC study indicate that the factors responsible for allergies and asthma are more common in Westernized countries.[28] Allergic asthma is associated with sensitivities to indoor allergens such as house dust mites, cats, dogs, and molds, which are more common in Western styles of housing. In early studies, increased exposure to indoor allergens during infancy and early childhood had been considered a primary cause of the rise in asthma.[34,35] However, in later studies, the effect of exposure to cats and dogs during the first year of life was reported to actually reduce the risk of allergies and asthma later in life.[36,37]

Another feature of Westernized societies is the shift in population from agricultural to industrial settings. Several studies have shown that children living on farms have a lower prevalence of hay fever and asthma than peers not living in an agricultural environment. This finding suggests the presence of protective factors in the rural environment, such as increased exposure to bacterial compounds in stables or exposure to livestock.[28]

Another possible explanation is that the increase in asthma and allergies in children is an unintended consequence of the success of domestic hygiene in reducing the rate of infections in early childhood.[28] The "hygiene hypothesis" suggests that early-life infections may protect against allergic asthma. However, in a more hygienic environment, there are fewer early-life respiratory infections. According to this hypothesis, the reduction in early-life infections increases the likelihood of developing asthma.

Another area being investigated to explain the increase in asthma in Westernized societies is diet. Studies have indicated an association between obesity and newly diagnosed asthma in school-age children, adolescents, and adult women (Fig. 6-7).[38-40]

### Pathology

Chronic, stable asthma is characterized by inflammation of the airway wall, with abnormal accumulation of eosinophils,

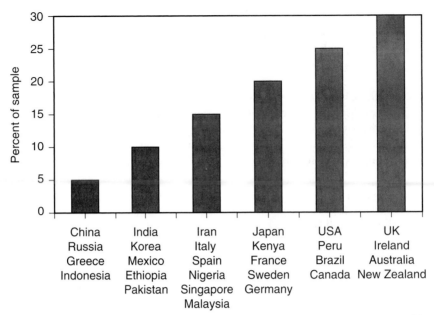

Figure 6-6 Prevalence of wheeze in the last 12 months among 12- to 14-year-old children as measured in the International Study of Asthma and Allergies in Childhood (ISAAC) studies. Only subsections of the 56 participating countries are shown. (Redrawn from Peat JK, Li J. Reversing the trend: reducing the prevalence of asthma. J Allergy Clin Immunol 103(1 Pt 1):1–10, 1999.)

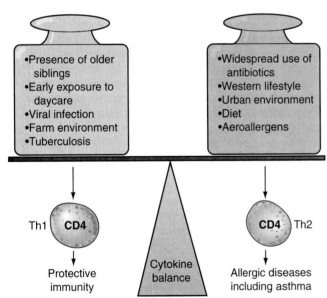

Figure 6-7 Determinants of the direction of differentiation of precursor T cells in neonatal life. The concept is that environmental factors in early life can have key influences on the direction of differentiation of precursor T cells. Several factors favor development of a Th1 phenotype, leading to the absence of allergy and asthma. (From Mason RJ, Murray JF, Broaddus VC, et al. Murray & Nadel's Textbook of Respiratory Medicine. 4th ed. Philadelphia, 2005, Saunders.)

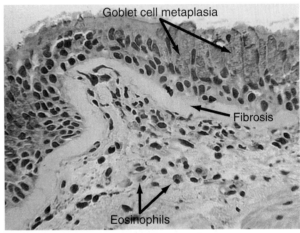

Figure 6-8 Airway pathology in asthma is detected in this photomicrograph of a section from an endobronchial biopsy taken during bronchoscopy from a subject with mild chronic asthma. Goblet cell metaplasia, subepithelial fibrosis, and eosinophilic infiltration of the submucosa are shown. (Hematoxylin and eosin stain; ×1200.) (From Mason RJ, Murray JF, Broaddus VC, et al. Murray & Nadel's Textbook of Respiratory Medicine. ed 4. Philadelphia, 2005, Saunders.)

## Pathophysiology

Asthma is a complex disease with airway inflammation being a key component.[28] Episodes of acute inflammation resulting from viral or allergen exposures may result in further cycles of inflammation that contribute over time to airway remodeling.[28] The term *airway remodeling* describes structural changes that take place in the airway in asthma. The overall result is thickening of the airway walls in both large (cartilaginous) and small (membranous) airways.[28] Thickening of the airway wall can profoundly affect airway narrowing caused by smooth

lymphocytes, mast cells, macrophages, dendritic cells, and myofibroblasts. The inflammatory mediators and proteins secreted by these cells contribute to the changes seen in airway structure and function.[28] Structural changes include abnormal deposition of collagen in the subepithelium and hypertrophy of goblet cells, submucosal glands, smooth muscle cells, and blood vessels (Fig. 6-8).[28]

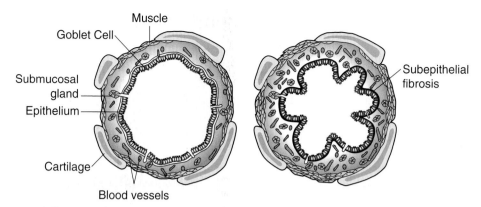

**Figure 6-9** Airway remodeling in asthma is depicted through representations of the airway wall in health (*left*) and in asthma (*right*). In asthma there is goblet cell hyperplasia/hypertrophy, subepithelial fibrosis, increased vascularity, and smooth muscle hypertrophy and hyperplasia. Not shown is the increased collagen deposition throughout the airway wall, smooth muscle proliferation throughout the airway wall, degenerative changes in cartilage, and pericartilaginous fibrosis. (From Mason RJ, Murray JF, Broaddus VC, et al. Murray & Nadel's Textbook of Respiratory Medicine. ed 4. Philadelphia, 2005, Saunders.)

muscle[41] and may explain persistent and incompletely reversible airway narrowing seen in some asthmatics (Fig. 6-9).[42]

The physiologic consequences of airway remodeling are clearly seen during severe asthma attacks, with diffuse narrowing of airways at all levels of the tracheobronchial tree, and increased airway resistance to airflow. Maximal expiratory flow is reduced at all lung volumes; maximal inspiratory flow is also reduced but less affected than expiratory flow.[28] Narrowing of peripheral airways results in their premature closure, causes a marked increase in RV,[43] which results in a tendency to breathe at higher lung volumes. The advantage of breathing at higher lung volumes is that airways are held open and there is an increase in the elastic recoil of the lungs, which increases the driving pressure for exhalation.[28] However, at high thoracic volumes, the diaphragm and intercostal muscles must function over a suboptimal range of their length-tension curve which increases the work of breathing and fatigue. The inappropriateness of the length-tension relationship of respiratory muscles is perceived by the patient as dyspnea.[28]

Airway narrowing in asthma also impairs gas exchange. Some airways are completely occluded; some are narrowed, while others remain unobstructed. This results in ventilation–perfusion mismatching and widens the alveolar–arterial $O_2$ difference [$(A - a) PO_2$], which results in hypoxia in acute severe asthma. Hypocapnia (low $CO_2$ level) is also typically found during an asthma attack because of an increased respiratory drive. Hypercapnia (high $CO_2$ level) occurs in an asthma attack of extreme severity and requires aggressive treatment with bronchodilators and preparation for possible intubation and mechanical ventilation.[28]

## Clinical Presentation

### Symptoms

The most prominent symptoms of asthma are
- wheezing,
- chest tightness, and
- shortness of breath.

These symptoms are often precipitated by exercise, inhalation of cold air, and exposure to allergens or viral respiratory infections.[28] Variability in symptoms from day to day is almost universal, but many patients note variations within a day, with symptoms worsening at night.[44] Examples of terms used by asthmatics to describe the sensation of bronchoconstriction are *throat tightness*, *choking*, *stuffed chest*, and *chest congestion*.[45]

## Physical Examination

### Diagnostic Tests

In taking the history of patients with asthma, specific questions should be asked regarding aspirin or sulfite sensitivities (present in dried fruit, restaurant salads, and some wines and beers), because ingestion of aspirin or sulfites can provoke life-threatening asthma attacks.[46,47] In addition, information should be obtained regarding exposure in the home or workplace to substances known to worsen asthma, such as pets, cockroaches, house dust mites, and environmental tobacco smoke.[28]

Auscultation of the lungs during an asthma attack commonly reveals polyphonic expiratory wheezing, but as airway narrowing increases, wheezing may disappear altogether or be faint in patients making little effort to move air. Overinflation of the thoracic cage may be present during an asthma attack because of air trapping.[28]

Pulmonary function tests (PFTs; see Chapter 10) performed between attacks usually show reductions in maximal expiratory flow. The volume of air expired in the first second of a forced expiratory maneuver from total lung capacity ($FEV_1$) is the best standardized, most widely used test for airflow obstruction.[28] An improvement in $FEV_1$ of >12% and an increase in $FEV_1$ of more than 200 mL after bronchodilator administration are considered reversibility of airway obstruction.

This reversibility of airway obstruction is the hallmark of asthma.[48] Reversibility helps to distinguish asthma from other obstructive lung diseases, such as emphysema and chronic bronchitis.[28] In asthma, the reduction in $FEV_1$ usually exceeds the reduction in FVC, so typically the $FEV_1$/FVC ratio is low.[28] The maximum midexpiratory flows (between 25% and 75% of the FVC) is usually also reduced in asthma, indicating obstruction in the small airways.[49] Reversibility of airway obstruction helps to distinguish asthma from other obstructive pulmonary diseases.[28]

> **Clinical Tip**
> The reversibility of airway obstruction following the use of bronchodilator medications is the hallmark of asthma.

Airway responsiveness is another characteristic of asthma. Airway responsiveness occurs when the airways demonstrate excessive bronchoconstriction in response to inhalation of an irritating substance. Tests of airway responsiveness are conducted by delivering progressively increasing doses of a provocative stimulus, usually methacholine, until the airway diameter changes by a fixed amount. Methacholine is delivered as a nebulized aerosol in doubling concentrations at 10-minute intervals until the $FEV_1$ falls by >20%. This concentration is called the PC20 (provocative concentration causing 20% fall in $FEV_1$). The degree of bronchial responsiveness correlates roughly with the severity of asthma. Greater levels of airway responsiveness indicate increased severity of asthma.[50]

Asthma can also be categorized in terms of severity as mild intermittent, mild persistent, moderate persistent, or severe persistent based on the results of PFTs and in both the severity and frequency of symptoms (Table 6-4).

### Special Types of Asthma

The term *seasonal asthma* is used to describe asthma symptoms that develop only in the presence of high levels of certain allergens, such as grass or birch pollen, which occur during specific seasons of the year.[28] *Exercise-induced bronchospasm* is a term used to describe airway narrowing provoked by exercise, with asthma symptoms appearing during or immediately after exercise. Drug-induced asthma is used to describe asthma triggered by drugs such as aspirin, nonsteroidal anti-inflammatory drugs, β-blockers, and angiotensin-converting enzyme inhibitors. Another type of asthma, cough-variant asthma, is characterized by the absence of wheezing and chest

### Table 6-4 Classification of Asthma Severity

| Classification | Symptoms[b] | Nighttime Symptoms | Lung Function |
|---|---|---|---|
| | **CLINICAL FEATURES BEFORE TREATMENT[A]** | | |
| Step 4: Severe persistent | Continual symptoms<br>Limited physical activity<br>Frequent exacerbations | Frequent | $FEV_1$ or PEF ≤60% predicted<br>PEF variability >30% |
| Step 3: Moderate persistent | Daily symptoms<br>Daily use of inhaled short-acting $β_2$-agonist<br>Exacerbations affect activity<br>Exacerbations ≥2 times a week; may last days | >1 time a week | $FEV_1$ or PEF >60%–<80% predicted<br>PEF variability >30% |
| Step 2: Mild persistent | Symptoms >2 times a week but <1 time a day<br>Exacerbations may affect activity | >2 times a month | $FEV_1$ or PEF ≥80% predicted<br>PEF variability 20%–30% |
| Step 1: Mild intermittent | Symptoms ≤2 times a week<br>Asymptomatic and normal PEF between exacerbations<br>Exacerbations brief (from a few hours to a few days):<br>Intensity may vary | ≤2 times a month | $FEV_1$ or PEF ≥80% predicted<br>PEF variability <20% |

PEF, peak expiratory flow
[a]The presence of one of the features of severity is sufficient to place a patient in that category. An individual should be assigned to the most severe grade in which any feature occurs. The characteristics noted are general and may overlap because asthma is highly variable. Furthermore, an individual's classification may change over time.
[b]Patients at any level of severity can have mild, moderate, or severe exacerbations. Some patients with intermittent asthma experience severe and life-threatening exacerbations separated by long periods of normal lung function and no symptoms.
From National Asthma Education and Prevention Program (NAEPP). Clinical Practice Guidelines. Expert Panel Report 2: Guidelines for the Diagnosis and Management of Asthma (NIH Publication No. 91-4051). Bethesda, MD, 1997, National Institutes of Health, National Heart Lung and Blood Institutes.

tightness, because cough is the sole presenting symptom. Cough-variant asthma is more common in children, with up to 75% of these children developing wheezing within 5 to 7 years.[51] The cough associated with asthma is typically nonproductive, nocturnal, and chronic, sometimes persisting for years.[28] Finally, the term *asthmatic bronchitis* is used to describe individuals with prominent features of both asthma and bronchitis.[28]

## Medical Management

Guidelines for the medical management of asthma emphasize the importance of long-term control as a goal of therapy, as opposed to simply treating symptomatic episodes.[28]

Treatments are organized around four basic recommendations:

1. The use of objective measures of pulmonary function to assess severity and to monitor the effectiveness of therapy;
2. Identification and elimination of factors that worsen symptoms, precipitate exacerbations, or promote ongoing airway inflammation;
3. Comprehensive pharmacologic therapy to reverse bronchoconstriction and to reverse and prevent airway inflammation; and
4. Creation of a therapeutic partnership between the patient and care provider.[52]

Pharmacologic therapy can be divided into two classes of medications:

- Short-term "relievers" or "rescue "medications (inhaled medications that reverse acute bronchospasm)
- Long-term "controllers" (antiinflammatory, long acting bronchodilators that improve overall asthma control when taken regularly).[53]

The most effective short-term "reliever" medications are the short-acting β-adrenergic agonists, such as albuterol (Proventil, Ventolin) or levalbuterol (Xopenex), or anticholinergics, such as ipratropium bromide (Atrovent) or tiotropium (Spiriva). They increase airway diameter by relaxing airway smooth muscle.[28]

The most effective long-term controllers are the inhaled corticosteroids, which are believed to produce benefits through their antiinflammatory action. These medications are not fast-acting, so they must be taken on a daily basis to obtain the full benefit. Examples of inhaled corticosteroids include beclomethasone (Qvar), budesonide (Pulmicort), flunisolide (AeroBid), Fluticasone (Flovent), Mometasone (Asmanex), and triamcinolone (Azmacort). Taking corticosteroids by inhalation minimizes the risk of adverse systemic effects but does not entirely eliminate them.[28]

It should be noted that new medications are constantly being introduced. To obtain a relatively current list of available medications from an Internet search, type "asthma medications" and a choice of several websites from large medical centers are available to help physical therapists become familiar with the names of commonly used medications for treating asthma.

Nonpharmacologic therapy includes reduction of allergen exposure in the home and, in the United States, allergen immunotherapy (allergy shots). Prevention and prompt treatment of viral infections are very important as they can precipitate an asthma attack (Table 6-5).[28]

## Prognosis

Although some individuals who have asthma as children appear to outgrow their asthma, approximately 50% of adults who recall having asthma as a child continue to have

## Table 6-5 Major Components of Asthma Management

| | |
|---|---|
| Periodic assessment and monitoring | Monitor signs and symptoms of asthma |
| | Monitor pulmonary function (spirometry, peak flow) |
| | Monitor quality of life and functional status |
| | Monitor history of asthma exacerbations |
| | Monitor pharmacotherapy (adverse effects, inhaler technique, frequency of quick reliever use) |
| | Monitor patient–provider communication and patient satisfaction |
| Avoidance of contributing factors | Skin testing to identify allergens |
| | Control of household and workplace allergens and irritants |
| | Prevention and treatment of viral infections |
| | Prevention and treatment of gastroesophageal reflux |
| Pharmacotherapy | Explain and reinforce role of medications (quick relief, long-term agents) |
| | Stepwise therapy recommended with provision for step-up and step-down in therapy |
| Patient education | Provide basic asthma education |
| | Teach and reinforce inhaler and peak flow technique |
| | Develop action plans |
| | Encourage self-management |

*From Mason RJ, Murray JF, Broaddus VC, et al. Murray & Nadel's Textbook of Respiratory Medicine, ed 4. Philadelphia, 2005, Saunders.*

symptoms in adulthood.[54] In a longitudinal study conducted in New Zealand, more than 1000 children born over a 12-month period in 1972 to 1973 were evaluated annually from birth to age 26.[55] The percentage of children reporting wheezing at more than one evaluation was 51%, confirming the high incidence of asthma in New Zealand. Among subjects who reported wheezing, the wheezing persisted until adulthood in 15%, whereas wheezing appeared and then remitted in 27% of subjects. However, the remission was not sustained in approximately half of those in whom it had remitted, and wheezing recurred by age 26.[55] Factors associated with the persistence of asthma into adulthood were sensitization to house dust mites, low $FEV_1$, airway hyperresponsiveness, being female, and a positive smoking history.[55]

In individuals who appear to have a "spontaneous remission" of their asthma symptoms and have been without medication for more than 12 months, bronchial biopsies reveal increases in eosinophils, T cells, and mast cells as well as thickening of the basement membrane.[56] These findings indicate that although symptoms are in remission, markers for asthma are still present.

### Prevention

Prevention of episodes of bronchospasm in asthma depends on adhering to the medical and pharmacological recommendations for asthma management made by the physician (internist or pulmonary specialist) and avoidance of personal asthma-triggering substances, both in the workplace and at home. Use of a peak-flow meter is recommended to assist in monitoring reductions in airway flow rates, indicating airway narrowing (Fig. 6-10). Asthmatic individuals are given guidelines based on the degree of narrowing recorded by the peak-flow meter. These results can indicate the need for increasing medications, or going directly to the physician's office or a hospital emergency room for more aggressive management of an asthmatic episode. Clues that an asthma attack is life-threatening include confusion, upright posture due to breathing difficulty, diaphoresis, speech difficulties due to shortness of breath, cyanosis, and fatigue.[28]

### Implications for Physical Therapy Treatment

The most important treatment for asthma management involves the use of appropriate medications to reduce inflammation, stabilize airways, and relieve bronchospasm. Physical therapy interventions should not begin unless an appropriate regime of medication has been initiated. Individuals with exercise-induced asthma may require the use of bronchodilator medication 30 minutes prior to exercise. Following medical therapy, the following physical therapy interventions may be helpful:

- Secretion clearance techniques (Active cycle of breathing and gentle manual techniques, shaking and vibration work well with this population)
- Controlled breathing techniques
- Exercise and strength training
- Thoracic stretching exercises
- Postural reeducation to avoid round-shouldered postures

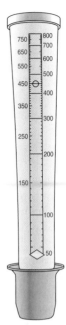

**Figure 6-10** Peak flow meter. (From Hess D, MacIntyre NR, Mishoe SC, et al. Respiratory Care Principles and Practice. St. Louis, 2002, Saunders.)

## Adult Obstructive Lung Conditions

### Chronic Obstructive Pulmonary Disease

Chronic Obstructive Pulmonary Disease (COPD) is currently the fourth-leading cause of death in the world. It continues to increase in the adult population, and additional increases in prevalence and mortality are predicted in the coming decades.[57]

"Chronic Obstructive Pulmonary Disease (COPD) is a preventable and treatable disease with some significant extrapulmonary effects that may contribute to the severity in individual patients. Its pulmonary component is characterized by airflow limitation that is not fully reversible. The airflow limitation is usually progressive and associated with an abnormal inflammatory response of the lung to noxious particles and gases."[58]

The chronic airflow limitation that characterizes COPD is caused by a mixture of parenchymal alveolar disease (emphysema) and small-airway disease (obstructive bronchiolitis). Most commonly, these conditions occur in combination, with proportions varying from individual to individual.[58] However, in some cases, either emphysema or chronic bronchitis is clearly dominant. These two disorders are discussed separately below.

### Emphysema

"In emphysema of the lungs, the size of the vesicles (alveoli) is much increased, and is less uniform. The greater number equal or exceed the size of a millet seed, while some attain the magnitude of hemp-seed or cherry-stones, or even french beans (haricot vert). These latter are probably produced by the reunion of several of the air cells through rupture of the intermediate partitions; sometimes, however they appear

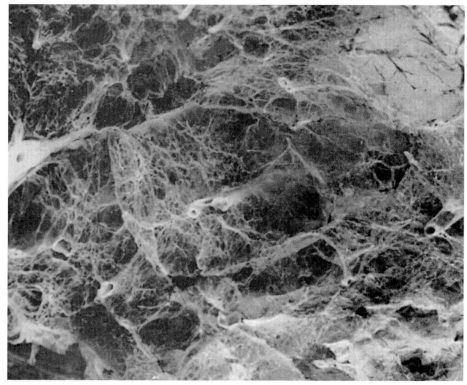

**Figure 6-11** Panlobular emphysema is shown. Close-up view of the cut surface of an inflation-fixed lung of a patient with severe generalized panlobular emphysema. Note the extensive enlargement, distortion, and coalescence of the respiratory air spaces. (From Snider GL. Clinical Pulmonary Medicine. Boston, 1981, Little, Brown.)

to arise from the simple enlargement of a single vesicle." R. T. H. Laennec (1821)[59]

Today emphysema is defined similarly. In anatomic terms, emphysema is defined as a condition of the lung characterized by destruction of alveolar walls and enlargement of the air spaces distal to the terminal bronchioles, including the respiratory bronchioles, alveolar ducts and alveoli.[60] The key role inflammatory cells play in activating potentially destructive mechanisms within the lung has been clearly recognized (see pathophysiology of COPD). The concept that the lung has some ability to repair itself has recently emerged, with emphysema representing an imbalance between destruction and repair.[60] This is especially true in $\alpha_1$-antitrypsin deficiency, a genetic condition which predisposes affected individuals to the early development of emphysema.

There are three subtypes of emphysema: centrilobular, panlobular, and distal acinal (or subpleural):

- Centrilobular emphysema describes proximal dilation of the respiratory bronchioles, with alveolar ducts and sacs remaining normal. It is most common in the upper lobes and posterior portions of the lung.
- Panlobular emphysema describes dilation of all the respiratory airspaces in the acinus and occurs most frequently in the lung bases. Panlobular emphysema is seen in emphysema associated with $\alpha_1$-antitrypsin deficiency (Fig. 6-11).
- Distal acinar (subpleural) emphysema describes dilation of airspaces underneath the apical pleura, associated with apical bullae (large air collection contained within a thin outer wall), which can lead to spontaneous pneumothorax.

*Pathology*

Cigarette smoking, which is a major cause of emphysema, leads to inflammatory cell recruitment, proteolytic injury (the hydrolysis of proteins by enzymes) to the extracellular matrix, and cell death. In addition, airway walls become perforated, and in the absence of repair, the walls become obliterated and small distinct airspaces appear, changing into larger abnormal airspaces.[60]

Three types of emphysema are named for the location of airspace enlargement within the acinus. The acinus includes all the lung tissue distal to the terminal bronchiole and is composed of respiratory bronchioles, alveolar ducts, and alveolar sacs, all of which participate in gas exchange (Fig. 6-12).[60]

*Centrilobular and Panlobular Emphysema*

- Centrilobular emphysema describes proximal dilation of the respiratory bronchioles, with alveolar ducts and sacs remaining normal. It is most common in the upper lobes and posterior portions of the lung.
- Panlobular emphysema describes dilation of all the respiratory airspaces in the acinus and occurs most frequently in the lung bases. Panlobular emphysema is seen in emphysema associated with $\alpha_1$-antitrypsin deficiency (see Fig. 6-11).
- Distal acinar (subpleural) emphysema describes dilation of airspaces underneath the apical pleura, associated with apical bullae (large air collection contained within a thin outer wall), which can lead to spontaneous pneumothorax.

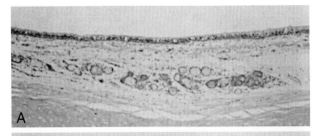

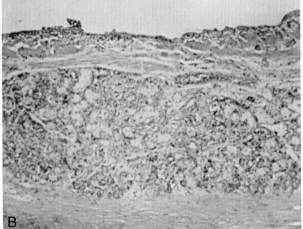

**Figure 6-12** Photomicrographs showing the left main bronchus from a patient without respiratory symptoms (**A**) and from a patient with many years of productive cough and airflow obstruction (**B**). Serous acini (*dark staining*) and mucous acini (*light staining*) constitute the submucosal gland in **A**. The average gland thickness represents about one third the distance between the epithelial basement membrane and the perichondrium. The submucosal gland in **B** is markedly thickened, is made up mostly of mucous acini, and constitutes most of the wall thickness between the epithelial basement membrane and the perichondrium; note also that the epithelium has desquamated. (From Snider GL. Clinical Pulmonary Medicine. Boston, 1981, Little, Brown.)

## Chronic Bronchitis

### Bronchitis

"Pulmonary catarrh is inflammation of the mucous membranes of the bronchia. … This inflammation is attended, from the commencement, with a secretion of mucus more abundant than natural … it obstructs, more or less completely, the bronchial tubes, especially those of small calibre … and the impeded transmission of air … produces the sound usually denominated the rattles." R. T. H. Laennec (1821).[59]

Today chronic bronchitis is defined in clinical terms, as the presence of a chronic productive cough for 3 months in each of two successive years, provided that other causes of chronic mucus production (CF, bronchiectasis and tuberculosis) have been ruled out.[61] Hypersecretion of mucus begins in the large airways and is not associated with airway obstruction (simple bronchitis). Later hypersecretion progresses to smaller airways, where airway obstruction begins as chronic bronchitis. Obstruction of the small airways in COPD is associated with thickening of the airway wall. This remodeling, which involves tissue repair and malfunction of the mucociliary clearance system, results in the accumulation of inflammatory mucous exudates in the airway lumen.[62] The

progression of COPD is strongly associated with this increase in the volume of tissue in the walls of small airways and the accumulation of inflammatory mucous exudates.[62]

### Pathology

In chronic bronchitis, there is hypertrophy of the submucosal glands and the gland-to-bronchial wall thickness ratio, or Reid index, is used as an indicator of mucous gland hypertrophy. In individuals with chronic bronchitis, this ratio may be as high as 8 to 10, whereas it normally is <3 to 10.[63] Surface epithelial secretory cells are increased and patchy areas of squamous metaplasia may replace normally ciliated epithelium. The degree of small-airway involvement (bronchioles) determines the degree of disability (Fig. 6-13).[63]

## Chronic Obstructive Pulmonary Disease: The Combination Disease

### Etiology

Cigarette smoking is the most common risk factor worldwide contributing to the development of COPD, although in many countries air pollution from the burning of wood and other biomass fuels has also been identified as a risk factor for COPD.[58] COPD is a term that describes obstructive airway disease caused by a combination of emphysema and chronic bronchitis (including small airways disease). Clinical presentation and symptoms can vary from individual to individual (Fig. 6-14).

> **Clinical Tip**
> Spirometry is considered the "gold standard" for diagnosing COPD and monitoring its progression. Decreases in expiratory flow rates result in decreased $FEV_1$ and $FEV_1/FVC$ values. Spirometry is the best standardized, reproducible, and objective measure of airflow limitation available.[58]

Smokers lose lung function in a dose-dependent manner, with heaviest smokers sustaining greater loss of lung function. However, many other factors, both genetic and environmental, affect individual susceptibility to develop COPD.[60] The onset of COPD usually begins in midlife.[58] When the onset of COPD occurs at a young age (<45 years) in Caucasian individuals or those who have a strong family history of COPD, screening for the genetic condition $\alpha_1$-antitrypsin deficiency is warranted.[58]

### Pathophysiology

The inhalation of cigarette smoke or noxious particles results in inflammation of the lung, a normal response that seems amplified in those who develop COPD.[58] A characteristic pattern of inflammation is seen in individuals with COPD, with increased numbers of inflammatory cells, such as neutrophils, macrophages, T and B lymphocytes, and eosinophils, present in various parts of the lung.[58]

Chronic inflammation results in structural changes and narrowing of the small airways. Chronic inflammation also results in destruction of lung parenchyma, the respiratory bronchioles, and alveoli, leading to the loss of alveolar

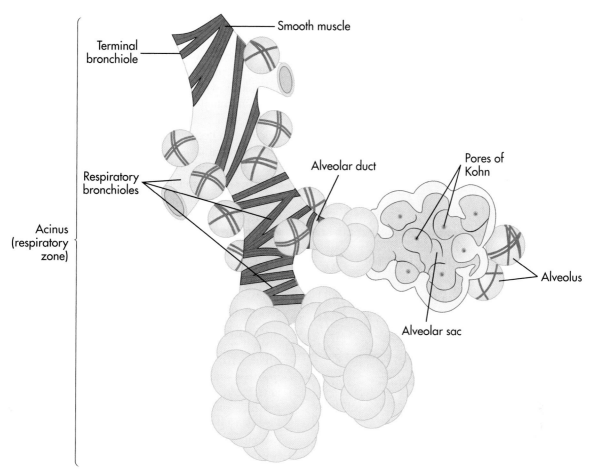

**Figure 6-13** Chronic bronchitis may lead to the formation of misshapen or large alveolar sacs with reduced space for oxygen and carbon dioxide exchange. The client may develop cyanosis and pulmonary edema. (From Goodman CC, Snyder TE. Differential Diagnosis for Physical Therapists: Screening for Referral, ed 4. St. Louis, 2006, Saunders.)

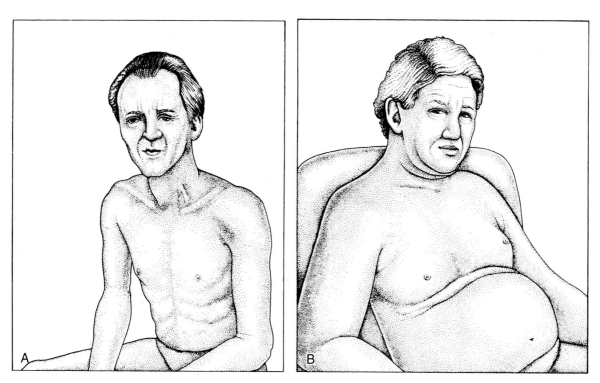

**Figure 6-14** Comparison of appearance of individuals with emphysema-dominant (*left*) and chronic bronchitis–dominant (*right*) chronic obstructive pulmonary disease. (From Goodman CC, Snyder TEK. Differential Diagnosis in Physical Therapy. Philadelphia, 1990, Saunders.)

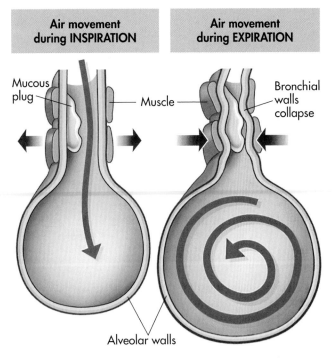

**Figure 6-15** Mechanisms of air trapping in chronic obstructive pulmonary disease (COPD). Mucous plugs and narrowed airways cause air trapping and hyperinflation on expiration. During inspiration the airways are pulled open, allowing gas to flow past the obstruction. During expiration decreased elastic recoil of the bronchial walls results in collapse of the airways and prevents normal expiratory airflow. (From McCance KL. Pathophysiology: The Biologic Basis for Disease in Adults and Children, ed 6. St. Louis, 2010, Mosby.)

attachments (tethers that hold the airways open), and this decreases lung recoil. Both of these inflammation-related changes reduce the ability of the airways to remain open during expiration, which leads to air trapping, hyperinflation, and progressive airflow limitation (Fig. 6-15).[58]

Lung inflammation is further amplified by oxidative stress and an excess of proteases (enzymes capable of cell destruction) in the lung, with evidence for an imbalance between proteases that break down connective tissue components and antiproteases that protect against this.[58]

### Clinical Presentation

**Symptoms.** Although coughing is the most frequent symptom reported by individuals with COPD, they usually seek medical attention when they begin to experience dyspnea.[60] Dyspnea is described by patients as an "increased effort to breathe," "heaviness," "air hunger," or "gasping," and this breathlessness is typically persistent and progressive.[58] Usually dyspnea is first noticed during strenuous exercise, when attempting to climb stairs or inclines, or when hurrying on level surfaces. Dyspnea may limit the distance walked and make individuals with COPD walk at a slower pace than other people of the same age.[64] As the disease progresses, shortness of breath is more easily triggered by walking or functional activities that involve bilateral overhead arm activities, such as dressing, grooming and/or bathing. Many

patients try to avoid dyspnea by avoiding exertion and as a result become more and more sedentary.[60] Eventually, many individuals with COPD become confined to their homes, with a minimum of outside activities.[58]

Coughing initially may be intermittent but as the disease progresses it becomes present daily and often throughout the day.[58] Sputum production is usually described as "scanty," or less than several tablespoons of mucoid, thin, watery secretions per day. Purulence secretions, containing pus, are seen during episodes of infection.[60] The most common pathogens cultured from the sputum are *Streptococcus pneumoniae* and *H. influenzae*.[60] As COPD progresses, it is characterized by acute exacerbations, including increased cough, increased dyspnea, purulent sputum, and on occasion, the presence of wheezing.[60]

### Physical examination

DIAGNOSTIC TESTS. Auscultation of the lungs of individuals with COPD reveals a prolonged expiratory phase. Normal exhalation time is considered to be 4 seconds; exhalation beyond 4 seconds is indicative of significant obstruction, which can be quantified more precisely by spirometry testing.[60] Breath sounds in COPD are diminished in intensity in all lung fields, often noted as "distant breath sounds." In the presence of secretion retention, rhonchi and occasionally localized wheezing may also be heard over affected areas. Mediate percussion of the thorax is often hyperresonant because of lung hyperinflation. As COPD becomes more severe, the chest becomes more barrel shaped, with widening of the xiphosternal angle because of lung hyperinflation. Flattening of the hemidiaphragms may be associated with paradoxical in-drawing of the lower rib cage with inspiration.[58]

Individuals with COPD may assume a forward-leaning posture resting on their elbows or supporting their upper body on extended arms, a position known as "tripoding." Tripoding stabilizes the shoulder girdle and allows accessory muscles of respiration to help maximize lung volume.[60] Use of the accessory muscles (scalene and sternocleidomastoid muscles) to augment breathing as well as pursed-lip expiration may be present even at rest in patients with severe COPD. Inspection of mucosal membranes and lips may reveal central cyanosis (bluish tint), which indicates the need to further assess the oxygenation status through arterial blood gas analysis ($PaO_2$) or pulse oximetry ($SpO_2$). In advanced COPD, inspection of the neck may reveal jugular vein distension as well as ankle or lower leg swelling when cor pulmonale (right heart failure) is present.

As previously noted, CXR changes are noted late in the disease progression. Evidence of lung hyperinflation consists of flattening of the diaphragms, an increased anterior–posterior diameter, and an increase in the width of the retrosternal air space.[2] HRCT can help detect early changes in the lung associated with focal emphysema or regional air trapping associated with small airways disease (obliterative bronchiolitis).[2] Air trapping of the type seen in obliterative bronchiolitis is best identified by comparing full inspiratory with full expiratory scans.[2] CT scans can also help to detect the presence of bullae (bubble-like, air-filled lung) which, if ruptured, can lead to pneumothorax.

## Table 6-6 Classification of COPD Severity

| Stage | LUNG FUNCTION[A] | | General Pattern of Symptoms |
|---|---|---|---|
| | FEV$_1$ (% Predicted) | FEV$_1$/FVC | |
| I (mild) | >80 | <0.7 | Chronic cough, ± sputum production |
| II (moderate) | 50–80 | <0.7 | Chronic cough, ± sputum, and dyspnea |
| III (severe) | 30–50 | <0.7 | Chronic cough, ± sputum, and ↑ dyspnea |
| IV (very severe) | <30[b] | <0.7 | Chronic cough, ± sputum, and ↑↑ dyspnea Respiratory or right heart failure, weight loss |

COPD, chronic obstructive pulmonary disease
[a]Based on post-bronchodilator function
[b]A postbronchodilator FEV$_1$ <30% predicted or FEV$_1$<50% with respiratory failure
Adapted from Global Initiative for Chronic Obstructive Lung Disease (GOLD Report 2008).

PULMONARY FUNCTION TESTS. Spirometry tracings measure time–volume relationships and are useful in exploring severity in obstructive lung diseases, such as COPD where delayed and incomplete emptying of the lung during exhalation and lung hyperinflation are present. To determine the presence and severity of COPD, two forced spirometry measures are routinely used: the FEV$_1$ and the FVC (see Chapter 10 for information on PFTs). The decrease in FEV$_1$ seen in COPD primarily results from inflammation.[58] The presence of a post-bronchodilator FEV$_1$ <80% of predicted along with a calculated FEV$_1$/FVC <0.7 confirms the presence of an airflow limitation that is not fully reversible. Criteria for determining the impairment level in COPD, as outlined in the Global Initiative for Chronic Obstructive Lung Disease, are shown in Table 6-6.[58]

In some individuals with COPD, there is a strong asthmatic component (reversibility of airflow limitation) in addition to components of chronic bronchitis. Individuals with these characteristics are usually described as having "asthmatic bronchitis."

Lung volumes may be determined by body plethysmography (see Chapter 10). In general, total lung capacity is increased in emphysema because the loss of lung recoil allows the lungs to stretch to an increased maximal volume.[60] The RV and FRC of the lungs are also increased.[60]

Decreased O$_2$ levels (PaO$_2$), as determined by arterial blood gas measurements, characterize disease progression in individuals with COPD. The CO$_2$ (PaCO$_2$) level may initially be normal in mild COPD or even decreased in individuals with a strong emphysematous component. In individuals with a strong bronchitis component, PaCO$_2$ levels will gradually increase as the disease progresses. Blood gas abnormalities usually worsen during acute exacerbations and may also worsen during sleep[65] or exercise.[66] It should be noted that information regarding CO$_2$ levels is needed to diagnosis the risk of impending respiratory failure. Respiratory failure is defined as a PaO$_2$ of <60 mmHg with or without PaCO$_2$ levels >50 mmHg in arterial blood gases measured while breathing air at sea level.[58] Polycythemia, or an hematocrit of >55% can develop in the presence of arterial hypoxemia, in an attempt to increase O$_2$-carrying capacity.[58] Modified exercise testing, such as hallway walking or bicycling, may be used to help determine if a need for O$_2$ supplementation exists. More formal exercise testing is usually done in conjunction with pulmonary rehabilitation and used as a pre- and posttest measure to determine if gains in exercise capacity were achieved (see Chapter 19).

Comorbidities are common in COPD; some are related to the aging process, such as arthritis, diabetes, reflux esophagitis, whereas others are more likely to occur when COPD is present, such as bronchial carcinoma, osteoporosis, and ischemic heart disease.[58] An association between reduced lung function and atherosclerotic heart disease has also been noted. Conditions resulting in reduced lung function are often associated with low-grade systemic inflammation. Furthermore, a reduced FEV$_1$ has been found to be a marker for cardiovascular mortality independent of age, gender, and smoking history.[67]

There is growing evidence that COPD is a multiorgan-system disease, with skeletal muscle dysfunction contributing to exercise intolerance.[68] The mechanisms accounting for muscle weakness and muscle wasting, as well as for weight loss in COPD, have not yet been fully explained.[60] Psychologically, the impact of COPD on the individual's life may often result in feelings of depression and/or anxiety.[58]

### Medical Management

The goals of medical treatment are to relieve symptoms, prevent disease progression, improve exercise tolerance, enhance health status, prevent and treat complications, and reduce mortality.[58]

Smoking cessation is essential to the medical management of COPD and can slow the rate of deterioration of lung function.[68] Health education is considered to have an important role in smoking cessation and in improving the ability to cope with illness and improve health status.[58]

Pharmacotherapy for COPD is used to decrease symptoms, reduce the frequency of exacerbations, and improve health status and exercise tolerance.[58] None of the existing medications used in treating COPD have been shown to modify the long-term decline in lung function that characterizes

---

**Box 6-2**

**Classes of Medications Used in Chronic Obstructive Pulmonary Disease**

- Bronchodilator medications alter smooth muscle tone. Short acting and long acting include: $\beta_2$-agonists and anticholinergics.
- Antiinflammatory medications to reduce inflammation. Inhaled glucocorticosteroids are used for stage III and IV COPD, and those with repeated exacerbations (see Asthma treatment for specific names of medications). In some cases, the use of IV steroids (prednisone) or oral steroids may be necessary to reduce inflammation.
- Combination medications (combine an inhaled steroid with a bronchodilator) such as fluticasone and salmeterol (Advair) or budesonide and formoterol (Symbicort)
- Antibiotics to treat lung infections

---

COPD.[58] Classes of medications used in COPD can be found in Box 6-2.

The use of medications to reduce airflow limitations, including bronchodilators and antiinflammatory agents, may help many patients manage their symptoms, but reduction in airflow obstruction is usually modest.[68] To obtain an updated list of COPD medications by an Internet search, type "COPD medications" and a choice of several websites from large medical centers are available to help physical therapists become familiar with the names of commonly used medications for treating COPD.

The influenza vaccine is recommended yearly, as well as the pneumococcal vaccine (one-time vaccine) to help prevent respiratory infections. Respiratory infections may trigger exacerbations of the inflammatory response and worsening of patient's symptoms.

Treatment of sleep disorders such as sleep apnea, in individuals with COPD, is important because nocturnal hypoxemia tends to be more severe than in the general population because of their baseline hypoxemia.[60] The use of supplemental $O_2$ usually begins with nighttime use. Long-term $O_2$ therapy (>15 hours per day) is used for individuals with stage IV COPD who have a resting $PaO_2$ ≤55 mmHg or an $SpO_2$ ≤88%.[58] $O_2$ administration may also be used in less-severe COPD to improve exercise tolerance or to relieve episodes of acute dyspnea.[58]

Pulmonary rehabilitation and exercise training has been shown to improve exercise tolerance and reduce symptoms of dyspnea and fatigue (see Chapter 19).[58]

Surgical excision of bullae may be necessary to reduce dyspnea and improve lung function. For carefully selected patients with upper lobe emphysema, lung volume reduction surgery (LVRS) may help to improve lung mechanics and the function of respiratory muscles by reducing lung hyperinflation. However, LVRS is a costly palliative procedure and should be recommended only in carefully selected patients.[58]

*Prognosis*
COPD is a progressive disease and lung function can be expected to worsen over time, even in individuals who receive the best available medical care.[58] Following exacerbations, those with COPD rarely return fully to their baseline functional status; this results in a gradual progressive downhill course. A composite score based on body mass index (B), Obstruction (O), Dyspnea (D), and Exercise (E), or the BODE index, has been found to be better than the $FEV_1$ value alone in predicting death from any cause and from respiratory causes in COPD.[69] This composite BODE score includes the respiratory and systemic effects of COPD on the individual, as well as considering the physiological variable of $FEV_1$. Points for degree of obstruction ($FEV_1$), degree of dyspnea rated on the modified Medical Research Council dyspnea scale, and distance walked during 6 minutes range from 0 to 3, while body mass index is rated either 0 or 1.[69] Adding the points in each BODE category results in scores ranging from 0 to 10, with 0 representing less-severe disease and 10 representing more severe COPD. The highest BODE scores (7 to 10) were associated with a mortality rate of 80% in 52 months.[69]

End-stage COPD results in cor pulmonale, or right heart failure.[60] The response to alveolar hypoxia is vasoconstriction, which in turn causes increased pulmonary vascular resistance, pulmonary hypertension, and ultimately right heart failure.[60]

*Prevention*
Smoking cessation is the single most effective intervention in most people to reduce the risk of developing COPD and to stop its progression. Reduction of personal exposure to tobacco smoke, occupational dusts and chemicals, and avoidance of exposure to smoke from home cooking and heating fuels can prevent the onset and progression of COPD.[58] Adequate ventilation should be encouraged when solid fuels are used for cooking and heating, and protective respiratory equipment should be used in the workplace to minimize exposure to toxic gases or particles.[58]

*Implications for Physical Therapy Treatment*
- Secretion clearance techniques, when indicated (postural drainage, Acapella instruction, and active cycle of breathing)
- Controlled breathing techniques (pursed lips and paced breathing) at rest
- Controlled breathing techniques coordinated with position changes, ambulation, and stair climbing
- Ambulation with use of a rolling walker
- Instruction in the use of recovery from shortness of breath positions
- Endurance exercise training
- Strength and weight training
- Thoracic stretching exercises
- Postural reeducation to avoid round-shouldered postures

## Obstructive–Restrictive Lung Conditions

### Bronchiectasis
*Dilatation of the Bronchia*
"This affection of the bronchia is always produced by chronic catarrh (inflammation of the mucous membranes of the

bronchia), or by some other disease attended by long, violent, and often repeated fits of coughing." R. T. H. Laennec (1821)[59]

Bronchiectasis, once thought to be decreasing in prevalence, is now resurging in the developed world and continues to be a common respiratory disease in areas of the world where people have limited access to health care.[70] Bronchiectasis is characterized by irreversible dilation of one or more bronchi with chronic inflammation and infection.[71] Bronchiectasis is also associated with distortion of the conducting airways, thickening, herniation, or dilation, with some airways being dilated up to 6 times their normal size.[72] Thus, bronchiectasis describes an anatomic abnormality rather than a single disease.[73]

### Epidemiology

Establishing the cause of bronchiectasis in some cases may be difficult. Even with extensive clinical, laboratory, and pathologic testing, many cases of bronchiectasis are currently still considered idiopathic (unknown cause). When a cause can be determined, bronchiectasis is found to occur as a complication of a prior lung infection or injury to the bronchial wall, or it may be related to an underlying anatomic or systemic disease.[70]

Bronchiectasis can be localized or diffuse depending on the cause of the bronchial dilation. Distinguishing localized from diffuse bronchiectasis is an important part of the diagnostic workup. Localized bronchiectasis is due to either an intraluminal obstructive process, such as an inhaled foreign body (e.g., peanut, chicken bone, or tooth), or an airway tumor. It could also be caused by extrinsic compression from a lung tumor or lymph adenopathy, which would prevent clearance of mucus distal to the obstruction. Infection and inflammation would then follow.[71] Middle lobe syndrome describes airway obstruction to either the right middle lobe or lingula, with recurrent atelectasis and/or opacification, which may eventually lead to the development of bronchiectasis.[71] Localized bronchiectasis may require bronchoscopy to exclude endobronchial obstruction. Diffuse bronchiectasis requires further testing to attempt to identify an underlying systemic cause.[74]

### Pathology

Several mechanisms can lead to development of the permanent, pathologic dilation and damage of the airways, seen in bronchiectasis. Three common mechanisms include

1. bronchial wall injury/structural weakness of bronchial walls,
2. traction from adjacent lung fibrosis, and
3. bronchial lumen obstruction.[75]

**Bronchiectasis associated with bronchial wall injury.** Injury to the bronchial wall can occur following infection or inhalation accidents. Injury to the bronchial wall can also occur when genetic conditions causing structural defects of the airway or abnormal mucociliary clearance predispose individuals to recurring and chronic lung infections. The destructive effect of chronic airway infections was described by Cole in 1986, as the "vicious cycle theory." Cole's theory proposed that when a short-lived inflammatory

response fails to eliminate infection, chronic bacterial colonization can occur. Inflammation is further amplified in an attempt to eliminate the organisms, and this uncontrolled inflammation can result in damage to surrounding normal, "bystander" lung tissue which can lead to more progressive disease.[76]

In the past, childhood respiratory infections (pneumonia, pertussis, complicated measles, and tuberculosis) were considered the primary cause of bronchiectasis.[77] Lung damage post infection is now less likely due to widespread use of antibiotics in childhood. Currently increasing emphasis has been placed on investigation of intrinsic defects or primary immunodeficiency that predisposes an individual to bronchial inflammation/infection and result in the development of bronchiectasis.[77] See Table 6-7 for a summary of conditions associated with bronchiectasis due to airway wall injury.

**Bronchiectasis associated with traction from lung fibrosis.** In the normal lung, airways are held open by a combination of negative intrapleural pressure, which maintains the lungs in an inflated state, and the cartilaginous rings of the trachea and large and medium airways.[78] If the lung undergoes fibrotic changes as a result of a restrictive lung disease (sarcoidosis or interstitial fibrosis) or infections like tuberculosis, the airway is pulled outward by local retractile forces resulting in fixed dilation of the airways or traction bronchiectasis (Box 6-3).

**Bronchiectasis associated with bronchial lumen obstruction.** Airway obstruction is related to slow-growing tumors in the airway or fibrotic strictures related to prior infection, such as histoplasmosis, or TB.[75] Atelectasis or postobstructive pneumonia can develop behind these airway obstructions.

Bronchiectasis tends to occur in different locations within the lung depending on its cause. Table 6-8 outlines some common presentations of lung involvement.

### Clinical Presentation

**Symptoms.** The most common symptoms of bronchiectasis care are cough with chronic sputum production that can vary from small to large quantities of mucopurulent (containing both mucus and pus) secretions; these secretions form three layers: a white frothy top layer, a mucoid inner layer, and a purulent

---

**Box 6-3**

**Conditions Associated with Bronchiectasis due to Traction**

- Restrictive pulmonary diseases
- Sarcoidosis
- Usual interstitial pneumonitis (idiopathic pulmonary fibrosis)
- Infections
- Tuberculosis
- Radiation fibrosis

Adapted from Javidan-Nejad C, Bhalla, S. Bronchiectasis. Rad Clin N Am 47:289–306, 2009.

## Table 6-7 Conditions Associated with Bronchiectasis due to Airway Wall Injury/Weakness

| | |
|---|---|
| Postinfectious conditions | Atypical Mycobacterium (*Mycobacterium avium* intracellulare complex [MAC]) |
| | Necrotizing pneumonia |
| | Pertussis (whooping cough) |
| | Tuberculosis |
| Injury or inhalation accidents | Chronic gastroesophageal reflux and aspiration |
| | Foreign body aspiration |
| | Smoke and gaseous toxin inhalation |
| Congenital structural defect (anatomic disease) | Mounier–Kuhn syndrome (Tracheobronchomegaly, enlargement of the trachea and bronchi in the first to fourth generations) |
| | Williams–Campbell syndrome (defective cartilage in the fourth-, fifth-, and sixth-generation bronchi) |
| Congenital abnormal mucociliary clearance (systemic disease) | Cystic fibrosis |
| | Primary ciliary dyskinesia (immotile cilia syndrome) |
| Decreased systemic immunity disorders | Primary: Hypogammaglobulinemia |
| | Secondary: Immune modulation following lung or bone marrow transplantation |
| Exaggerated immune response disorders | Allergic bronchopulmonary aspergillosis (ABPA) |
| | Inflammatory bowel disease |
| | Rheumatoid arthritis |

*Adapted from Javidan-Nejad C, Bhalla, S. Bronchiectasis. Rad Clin N Am 47:289–306, 2009.*

## Table 6-8 Bronchiectasis Distribution by Disease

| | Location | Disease |
|---|---|---|
| Focal | | Foreign body |
| | | Endobronchial tumor |
| Diffuse | Upper lung | Cystic fibrosis |
| | | Sarcoidosis |
| | | Radiation fibrosis |
| | Right middle lobe and lingual | Atypical mycobacterial infection |
| | | Immotile cilia syndrome (also lower lobes) |
| | Lower lobes | Chronic aspiration |
| | | Usual interstitial pneumonitis (IPF) |
| | | Hypogammaglobulinemia |
| | | Lung and bone transplantation |

*Adapted from Javidan-Nejad C, Bhalla, S. Bronchiectasis. Rad Clin N Am 47:289–306, 2009.*

(containing pus) bottom layer, composed of thick yellow-green plugs.[79] Sputum production is often greatest in the morning, because of mucus accumulation during sleep in the recumbent position. During episodes of infection, sputum increases in both volume and purulence. Rarely, sputum production is not present, and this is referred to as "dry bronchiectasis."

Individuals with bronchiectasis usually have a history of recurrent, chronic, or recurring lung infections.[77,78] Blood-streaked sputum or larger amounts of hemoptysis (coughing up blood) can occur in bronchiectasis. These symptoms are usually related to erosive airway damage caused by an acute infection.[79] When blood-streaked sputum is present, it is common practice to withhold percussion of the chest wall during physical therapy treatment to avoid further bleeding episodes and to urge the individual to call his or her physician for proper treatment of the new infection. If bleeding is moderate, patients will require hospital treatment. Elevation of the head of the bed and placing the individual in the lateral decubitus position with the area of suspected bleeding side down are recommended, with the airway protected by intubation.[71] If life-threatening bleeding occurs surgery may be necessary to control the bleeding.

Other symptoms associated with bronchiectasis include breathlessness and tiredness.[77] Sinusitis is frequently associated with bronchiectasis, especially in CF and immotile cilia syndromes.

### Physical Examination
#### Results of diagnostic tests

CT SCANS. Bronchiectasis is diagnosed by HRCT, and the criterion for the presence of bronchiectasis is "when the internal luminal diameter of one or more bronchi exceeds the diameter of the adjacent pulmonary artery."[75] This finding is called the signet ring sign (Fig. 6-16), where the artery simulates a jewel attached to the thick-walled, dilated bronchus (the ring). The tram-track sign is another common finding on HRCT in bronchiectasis, with tram-tracks describing the

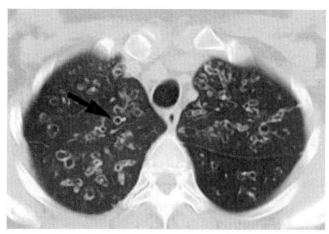

**Figure 6-16** CT findings of diffuse bronchiectasis in a 27-year-old woman with cystic fibrosis. Transaxial images show the dilated bronchus and adjacent arteriole, seen along their short axis, creating the signet ring sign (*arrow*). (From Javidan-Nejad C, Bhalla S. Bronchiectasis. Radiol Clin North Am 47(2):289–306.)

parallel thickened walls of a dilated bronchus.[75] Nodules may also be present, which indicates mucus inspissation (dried, impacted mucus) in the airways.[72]

Bronchiectasis is classified into three types based on the appearance of the bronchial walls on HRCT: cylindrical, varicose (or varicoid), and saccular.

- Cylindrical bronchiectasis is characterized by smooth, parallel bronchial walls that fail to taper progressive in their distal course[78] and often end squarely and abruptly (Fig. 6-17A).[73]
- Varicose or varicoid bronchiectasis is characterized by bronchi that are distorted and bulging, in a similar manner to varicose veins (Fig. 6-17B).[73]
- Saccular bronchiectasis is characterized by bronchial dilation that increases progressively toward the lung periphery, almost to the pleura, where the bronchus has a ballooned outline.[73] Saccular or cystic bronchiectasis may be isolated or may form a "honeycomb" pattern (Fig. 6-17C).[78] Saccular bronchiectasis is considered the most severe form of bronchiectasis.[73]

Computed tomography of the nasal sinuses is also frequently done as many people with bronchiectasis also have chronic rhinosinusitis, which must be treated as well.[78]

Pulmonary function test results depend on the extent of disease present and the coexistence of other lung diseases, such as COPD or asthma. Spirometry testing should also include postbronchodilator studies to check for the presence of asthma. Individuals with mild or localized bronchiectasis may have relatively normal pulmonary function. However, in diffuse bronchiectasis, patterns of airway obstruction are usually seen, with reductions in FVC, $FEV_1$, and FEF 25% to 75% and an increased RV. In individuals with associated atelectasis or fibrosis, or more advanced disease, a mixed obstructive–restrictive is usually present.[74]

BLOOD WORK. Arterial blood gases become abnormal with extensive bronchiectasis as a result of ventilation–perfusion mismatching. This can result in hypoxemia, but $CO_2$ retention is rare in bronchiectasis unless chronic bronchitis is also present. Laboratory tests to assess immunoglobulin (Ig) levels are also important, as immune deficiency may promote the development of bronchiectasis.[78]

SPUTUM TESTING. Sputum microbiology reveals the predominant organisms in the sputum of individuals with bronchiectasis to be *H. influenzae* and *P. aeruginosa*.[77,79] If *S. aureus* is cultured from the sputum of individuals with bronchiectasis, clinicians should consider testing for the possibility of CF.[77] Mycobacterial sputum cultures may reveal the presence of environmental mycobacteria such as *M. avium* complex, *M. chelonae*, and *M. abscessus*, which appear to be increasingly common in individuals with bronchiectasis.[78] Fungal sputum cultures, especially in individuals with an asthmatic component to their bronchiectasis, may also reveal the presence of Aspergillus.[78]

EVALUATION FOR GASTROESOPHAGEAL REFLUX DISEASE. The use of pH probe tests are frequently ordered for individuals suspected of having gastroesophageal reflux disease, which may contribute to lung congestion and the development of bronchiectasis.[78]

### Physical examination signs

AUSCULTATION FINDINGS. Auscultation of the lungs of individuals with bronchiectasis usually reveals crackles over the involved lobes. Rhonchi are present during periods of mucus retention, with dullness to percussion and decreased or absent breath sounds when mucus plugging occurs. Wheezing is present in a smaller percentage of patients and bronchovesicular or bronchial breath sounds may be heard during episodes of pneumonia. It is common for individuals with bronchiectasis to breathe very shallowly when their lungs are being auscultated, to avoid triggering coughing episodes. As a result of shallow breathing, diminished breath sounds are detected in all lung fields.

### *Medical Management*

The goals of bronchiectasis management are to reduce the number of exacerbations and improve quality of life.[70]

The first step is medical management of the underlying condition, after it has been identified. For example, giving Ig replacement therapy for documented cases of immunodeficiency and giving steroid therapy for the treatment of allergic bronchopulmonary aspergillosis both involve management of the underlying condition.[70] The second step in the medical management of acute exacerbations involves chronic maintenance therapy.[71] Antibiotic therapy should be considered when an acute exacerbation occurs, noted by any of the following: a change in sputum production (consistency, color, quantity, or hemoptysis); increased cough, dyspnea, or wheezing; fever >38° C; fatigue; decreased $FEV_1$ values; or new x-ray or auscultation findings. To assist in the selection of the most effective antibiotic therapy, the sputum should be cultured to identify the bacterial organism.[70,71]

Long-term maintenance therapy includes the use of nebulized medication, bronchodilators if indicated; increased hydration; and secretion clearance techniques to promote

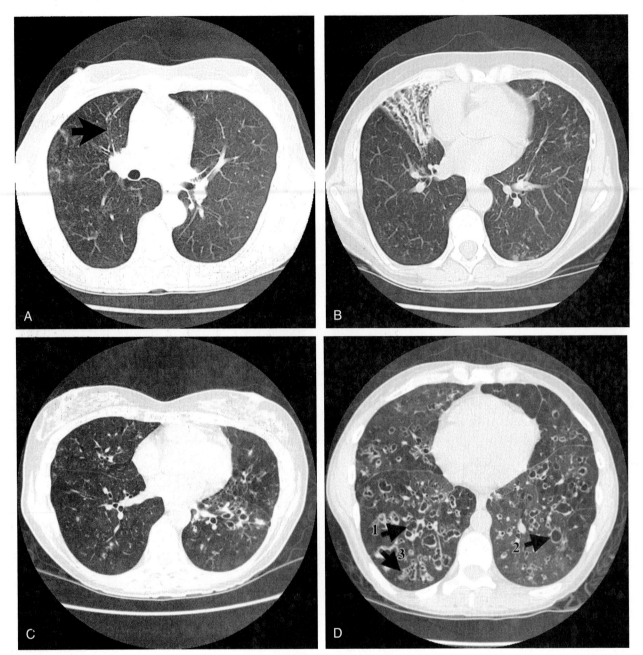

**Figure 6-17** Three types of bronchiectasis. **A,** Cylindrical bronchiectasis (BXSIS). **B,** Varicoid bronchiectasis. **C,** Saccular bronchiectasis. **D,** Saccular, cylindrical, and varicoid bronchiectasis. (From Mason RJ, Murray JF, Broaddus VC, et al. Murray & Nadel's Textbook of Respiratory Medicine. ed 4. Philadelphia, 2005, Saunders.)

good pulmonary hygiene and prevent stasis of secretions (see implications for physical therapy).

Surgery for individuals with bronchiectasis may be necessary to control massive hemoptysis; otherwise surgery is not generally recommended, except in some cases of localized bronchiectasis when symptoms cannot be managed by medical therapy.

### Prognosis

The prognosis for individuals with bronchiectasis depends on the underlying disease or condition contributing to the anatomical abnormality in the bronchi. Those with CF and bronchiectasis will have the poorest prognosis. Few studies

have been published regarding outcomes in individuals with non-CF bronchiectasis. With aggressive medical management and diligent secretion clearance routines, many individuals with bronchiectasis have been documented living into their seventies and eighties.

### Prevention

At this time, our understanding of the conditions that can predispose individuals to the development of bronchiectasis is continuing to evolve. Genetic conditions associated with bronchiectasis or associated with disorders of immunity, which set the stage for development of bronchiectasis, may potentially be screened for in future generations. At this time, this is the only measure that can be taken to prevent bronchiectasis in future generations.

### Implications for Physical Therapy Treatment
Management of bronchiectasis can include all of the following physical therapy interventions:

- Secretion clearance techniques
- Controlled breathing techniques coordinated with activity
- Strength training
- Endurance exercise

---

## CASE STUDY 6-1

MA is a 31-year-old man who was diagnosed with asthma at age 7.

### Past Medical History
Intermittent wheezing over the past 24 years, symptoms of shortness of breath precipitated by exercise, change in temperature, and exposure to smoke, perfume, and animals. A history of allergies related to dogs, cats, and dust. Hospitalization in June 1997 for an episode of severe bronchospasm. Pneumonia recurring four times in 1998, with a left lower lobe collapse in August 1998.
- Past surgical history: none
- Smoking history: none
- Medications: Ventolin inhaler three times a day, Intal inhaler three times a day

### Results of Pulmonary Function Tests

| Spirometry | PREBRONCHODILATOR TREATMENT Actual (Predicted) | % Pred | POSTBRONCHODILATOR TREATMENT Actual (Predicted) | % Pred |
|---|---|---|---|---|
| $FEV_1$ (L) | 3.33 (4.37) | 76 | 3.77 (4.37) | 86 |
| FEF 25%–75% (L/second) | 2.07 (4.50) | 46 | 2.50 (4.50) | 56 |

### Interpretation of Medical Data
Improvement is seen in both the $FEV_1$ and FEF 25% to 75% following administration of a bronchodilator medication. This illustrates the importance of medications in managing the bronchoconstriction seen in individuals with asthma. This case also provides an opportunity for physical therapists to reinforce several important educational points regarding living with asthma. There is evidence that mucus retention may be an issue (history of lobar collapse and recurrent pneumonia) and physical therapy can be helpful in resolving secretion retention, as well as encouraging participation in regular physical activity without triggering asthma symptoms by using medications prior to exercise.

### Physical Therapy Evaluation
- Auscultation: Expiratory wheezes in bilateral upper lobes, otherwise lungs are clear with good aeration throughout.
- Assessment with peak flow meter: Able to achieve a flow rate of 820 mL peak flow, but reports that he does not use the peak flow meter at home.
- HR = 68 bpm, BP = 120/80 mmHg, $O_2$ saturation = 99% on room air
- Postural assessment: Slightly rounded shoulders
- Activity level: Reports being able to jog 2 miles continuously in all seasons, except winter. Therefore, he never exercises in the winter. Always uses Ventolin inhaler prior to exercise.

- Interview: MA reports missing work occasionally because of respiratory symptoms and coughing spasms. Reports that his pulmonologist has added an inhaled steroid to his medication regimen 3 weeks ago, but he has not started to use it.

### Physical Therapy Treatment Goals
By the end of his physical therapy treatment, MA will understand the importance of
1. Taking medications as prescribed to manage asthma
2. Avoiding all asthma triggers
3. Detecting changes in airway caliber using the peak flow meter as a guide
4. Performing secretion clearance techniques when needed
5. Performing regular aerobic exercise
6. Early entry into the medical system when respiratory symptoms are worsening

### Physical Therapy Program
1. Reinforce the importance of using prescribed medications prior to any secretion clearance or exercise intervention. Pharmacologic support is essential to avoid triggering increased bronchospasm in asthmatic individuals.
2. Reinforce the importance of avoiding animals, smoke, perfumes, and dust.
3. Encourage daily use of the peak flow meter to gain understanding of MA's range of normal flow rates, which will make it easier to detect significant decreases in airway caliber. Instruct MA to be aware of the need to treat episodes of wheezing with appropriate use of medications followed by secretion clearance techniques if his cough sounds congested.
4. Instruct MA in the active cycle of breathing secretion clearance technique to clear lung congestion. Secretion clearance may be accomplished by either expectoration or by swallowing. MA's cough should sound clear if this has been accomplished.
5. Instruct MA in postural exercises and pectoral stretching to improve his round-shouldered posture.
6. Explore an alternate form of exercise for the winter months, such as an exercise bicycle, indoor swimming, stair climbing, or use of a health club so exercise can be continued all year round.
7. Reinforce the importance of going early to an emergency room or calling 911 if respiratory symptoms are unable to be controlled. Assure MA that it is better to allow his doctor to decide how serious an asthma attack is, rather than attempting to make that judgment on his own. This will also reduce anxiety on MA's part.

## CASE STUDY 6-1—cont'd

*Program Measures and Ongoing Evaluation in the Home Setting*
1. Monitor and record daily peak flows achieved with the peak flow meter
2. Keep a daily exercise log
3. Monitor absences from work

*Expected Program Outcomes*
MA will feel confident in his ability to participate in all activities of daily living while managing his asthma effectively, with assistance as needed, from his physician.

## References

1. American Physical Therapy Association. Preferred physical therapist practice patterns: cardiovascular/pulmonary. In Guide to Physical Therapist Practice, ed 2. Alexandria, VA, 2003, American Physical Therapy Association.
2. Rondinelli R. The pulmonary system. In Rondinelli R. Guides to the Evaluation of Permanent Impairment, ed 6. Chicago, 2008, American Medical Association.
3. Pellegrino R, Viegi G, Brusasco V, et al. Interpretative strategies for lung function tests. Eur Respir J 26(5):948–68, 2005.
4. Strausbaugh SD, Davis PB. Cystic fibrosis: a review of epidemiology and pathobiology. Clin Chest Med 28(2):279–88, 2007.
5. Davis PB, Drumm M, Konstan MW. Cystic fibrosis. Am J Respir Crit Care Med 154(5):1229–56, 1996.
6. Cystic Fibrosis Foundation (CFF) Patient Registry. Annual Data Report 2007. Bethesda, MD, 2008, Cystic Fibrosis Foundation.
7. Orenstein DM, Noyes BE. Cystic fibrosis. In Casaburi R, Petty T. Principles and Practice of Pulmonary Rehabilitation. Philadelphia, 1993, Saunders.
8. Boucher RC, Knowles MR, Yankaskas JR. Cystic fibrosis. In Mason RJ, Murray JF, Broaddus VC, et al. Murray & Nadel's Textbook of Respiratory Medicine, ed 4. Philadelphia, 2005, Saunders.
9. Knowles MR, Durie PR. What is cystic fibrosis? N Engl J Med 347(6):439–42, 2002.
10. Zielenski J, Tsui LC. Cystic fibrosis: genotypic and phenotypic variations. Annu Rev Genet 29:777–807, 1995.
11. Orenstein D, Rosenstein B, Stern R. Diagnosis of cystic fibrosis. In Orenstein D, Rosenstein B, Stern R. Cystic Fibrosis Medical Care. Philadelphia, 2000, Lippincott, Williams & Wilkins.
12. Bellini LM, Grippi MA. Cystic fibrosis. In Fishman AP. Fishman's Manual of Pulmonary Diseases and Disorders, ed 3. New York, 2002, McGraw-Hill.
13. O'Sullivan BP, Freedman SD. Cystic fibrosis. Lancet 393:1891–904, 2009.
14. Baker D, Kupke KG, Ingram P, et al. Microprobe analysis in human pathology. Scan Electron Microsc 2:659–80, 1985.
15. Anderson MP, Gregory RJ, Thompson S, et al. Demonstration that CFTR is a chloride channel by alteration of its anion selectivity. Science 253:202–5, 1991.
16. Stutts, MJ, Canessa CM, Olsen JC, et al. CFTR as a cAMP-dependent regulator of sodium channels. Science 269:847–50, 1995.
17. Goldman MJ, Anderson GM, Stolzenberg ED, et al. Human beta-defensin-1 is a salt-sensitive antibiotic in lung that is inactivated in cystic fibrosis. Cell 88:553–60, 1997.
18. Quittell L. Cystic fibrosis. In Burg FD, Inglefinger JR, Polin RA, et al. (eds.): Gellis & Kagan's Current Pediatric Therapy, ed 17. Philadelphia, 2002, Saunders.
19. McMullen AH, Pasta DJ, Frederick PD, et al. Impact of pregnancy on women with cystic fibrosis. Chest 129:706–11, 2006.
20. Yankaskas JR, Marshall BC, Sufian B, et al. Cystic fibrosis adult care: consensus conference report. Chest 125:S1–39, 2004.
21. Doring G, Conway S, Heijerman H, et al. Antibiotic therapy against Pseudomonas aeruginosa in cystic fibrosis: a European consensus. Eur Respir J 16:749–67, 2000.
22. Flume PA, O'Sullivan BP, Robinson KA, et al. Cystic fibrosis pulmonary guidelines: chronic medications for maintenance of lung health. Am J Respir Crit Care Med 176:957–69, 2007.
23. Donaldson SH, Bennett WD, Zehman K, et al. Mucus clearance and lung function in cystic fibrosis with hypertonic saline. N Engl J Med 354:241–50, 2006.
24. Corey M, McLaughlin FJ, Williams M, et al. A comparison of survival, growth and pulmonary function in patients with cystic fibrosis in Boston and Toronto. J Clin Epidemiol 41:583–91, 1988.
25. Grody WW, Cutting GR, Watson MS. The cystic fibrosis mutation "arms race": when less is more. Genet Med 9(11):739–44, 2007.
26. Wilfond BS, Fost N. The cystic fibrosis gene: medical and social implications for heterozyote detection. JAMA 263:2777–83, 1990.
27. National Heart, Lung, and Blood Institute, World Health Organization. Global Initiative for Asthma. National Institutes of Health pub no. 95-3659. Bethesda, MD, 1995.
28. Boushey HA, Corry DB, Fahy JV, et al. Asthma. In Mason RJ, Murray JF, Broaddus VC, et al. Murray & Nadel's Textbook of Respiratory Medicine, ed 4. Philadelphia, 2005, Saunders.
29. Grant EN, Wagner R, Weiss KB. Observations on emerging patterns of asthma in our society. J Allergy Clin Immunol 104:S1–9, 1999.
30. Mannino DM, Homa DM, Akinbami LJ, et al. Surveillance for asthma—United States, 1980–1999. MMWR Surveill Summ 51(1):1–13, 2002.
31. Sanford A, Weir T, Pare P. The state of the art: the genetics of asthma. Am J Respir Crit Care Med 153:1749–65, 1996.
32. Ariff AA, Delclos GL, Lee ES, et al. Prevalence and risk factors of asthma and wheezing among US adults: an analysis of the NHANES III data. Eur Respir J 21:827–33, 2003.
33. The International Study of Asthma and Allergies in Childhood (ISAAC) Steering Committee. Worldwide variation in prevalence of symptoms of asthma, allergic rhinoconjunctivitis, and atopic eczema. Lancet 351:1225–32, 1998.
34. Peat JK, Tovey E, Toelle BG, et al. House dust mite allergens: a major risk factor for childhood asthma in Australia. Am J Respir Crit Care Med 153:141–6, 1996.
35. Custovic A, Smith AC, Woodcock A. Indoor allergens are a primary cause of asthma: asthma and the environment. Eur Respir Rev 53:155–8, 1998.
36. Celedon JC, Litonjua AA, Ryan L, et al. Exposure to cat allergen, maternal history of asthma, and wheezing in the first 5 years of life. Lancet 360:781–2, 2002.

37. Perzanowski MS, Ronmark E, Platts-Mills TA, et al. Effect of cat and dog ownership on sensitization and development of asthma among preteenage children. Am J Respir Crit Care Med 166:696–702, 2002.

38. Camargo CA, Weiss ST, Zhang S, et al. Prospective study of body mass index and risk of adult-onset asthma. Am J Respir Crit Care Med 157(Suppl):A47, 1998.

39. Guerra S, Sherrill DL, Bobadilla A, et al. The relation of body mass index to asthma, chronic bronchitis, and emphysema. Chest 122:1256–63, 2002.

40. Gilliland FD, Berhane K, Islam T, et al. Obesity and the risk of newly diagnosed asthma in school-age children. Am J Epidemiol 158:406–15, 2003.

41. Wiggs BR, Bosken C, Pare PD, et al. A model of airway narrowing in asthma and chronic obstructive pulmonary disease. Am Rev Respir Dis 145:1251–8, 1992.

42. Brown PJ, Greville HW, Finucane KE. Asthma and irreversible airflow obstruction. Thorax 39:131–6, 1984.

43. McFadden ER. Pulmonary structure, physiology, and clinical correlates in asthma. In Middleton E, Reed C, Elliser E, et al. Allergy: Principles and Practice. St. Louis, 1993, Mosby.

44. Turner-Warwick M. Epidemiology of nocturnal asthma. Am J Med 85(Suppl 1B):6–8, 1988.

45. Hardie GE, Janson S, Gold WM, et al. Ethnic differences: word descriptors used by African-American and white asthma patients during induced bronchoconstriction. Chest 117:935–43, 2000.

46. Baker GJ, Collette P, Allen DH. Bronchospasm induced by metabisulfite-containing foods and drugs. Med J Aust 2:614, 1981.

47. Stevenson DD, Mathison DA. Aspirin sensitivity in asthmatics: when may this drug be safe? Postgrad Med 78:111–17, 1985.

48. American Thoracic Society. Lung function testing: selection of reference values and interpretative strategies. Am Rev Respir Dis 144:1202–16, 1991.

49. McFadden ER, Linden DA. A reduction in maximum mid-expiratory flow rate: a spirographic manifestation of small airways disease. Am J Med 52:725–37, 1972.

50. Cockcroft DW, Killian DN, Mellon JJ, Hargreave FE. Bronchial reactivity to inhaled histamine: a method and clinical survey. Clin Allergy 7:235–43, 1977.

51. Johnson D, Osborn LM. Cough variant asthma: a review of the clinical literature. J Asthma 28:85–90, 1991.

52. National Asthma Education and Prevention Program Expert Panel. Highlights of the Expert Panel Report 2: Guidelines for the Diagnosis and Management of Asthma. Bethesda, MD, 1997, National Heart, Lung, and Blood Institute, National Institutes of Health.

53. National Asthma Education and Prevention Program. Executive Summary of the NAEPP Expert Panel Report: Guidelines for the Diagnosis and Management of Asthma: Update on Selected Topics. Bethesda, MD, 2002, National Heart, Lung, and Blood Institute, National Institutes of Health.

54. Barbee RA, Murphy S. The natural history of asthma. J Allergy Clin Immunol 102:S65–72, 1998.

55. Sears MR, Greene JM, Willian AR, et al. A longitudinal, population based, cohort study of childhood asthma followed to adulthood. N Engl J Med 349:1414–22, 2003.

56. Van den Toorn LM, Overbeek SE, de Jongste JC, et al. Airway inflammation is present during clinical remission of atopic asthma. Am J Respir Crit Care Med 164:2107–13, 2001.

57. Lopez AD, Shibuya K, Rao C, et al. Chronic obstructive pulmonary disease: current burden and future projections. Eur Respir J 27(2):397–412, 2006.

58. Global Initiative for Chronic Obstructive Lung Disease (GOLD Report 2008).

59. Laennec RTH. A treatise on the disease of the chest. Forbes J (trans.). New York, 1962, Hafner Publishing.

60. Shapiro SD, Snider GL, Rennard SI. Chronic bronchitis and emphysema. In Mason RJ, Murray JF, Broaddus VC, et al. Murray & Nadel's Textbook of Respiratory Medicine, ed 4. Philadelphia, 2005, Saunders.

61. American Thoracic Society. Standards for the diagnosis and care of patients with chronic obstructive pulmonary disease. Am J Respir Crit Care Med. 152:S77–121, 1995.

62. Hogg JC, Chu F, Utokaparch S, et al. The nature of small-airway obstruction in chronic obstructive pulmonary disease. N Engl J Med 350(26):2645–53, 2004.

63. Reid LM. Chronic obstructive pulmonary diseases. In Fishman AP. Pulmonary Diseases and Disorders, ed 2. New York, 1988, McGraw-Hill.

64. Bestall JC, Paul EA, Garrod R, et al. Usefulness of the Medical Research Council (MRC) dyspnea scale as a measure of disability in patients with chronic obstructive pulmonary disease. Thorax 54(7):581–6, 1999.

65. Mulloy E, McNicholas WT. Ventilation and gas exchange during sleep and exercise in severe COPD. Chest 109:387–94, 1996.

66. Belman MJ. Exercise in patients with chronic obstructive pulmonary disease. Thorax 48:936–46, 1993.

67. Sin DD, LieLing W, Paul Man SF. The relationship between reduced lung function and cardiovascular mortality. Chest 127(6):1952–9, 2005.

68. American Thoracic Society. Skeletal muscle dysfunction in chronic obstructive pulmonary disease. A statement of the American Thoracic Society and European Respiratory Society. Am J Respir Crit Care Med 159:S1–40, 1999.

69. Celli, BR, Cote CG, Marin JM, et al. The body-mass index, airflow obstruction, dyspnea, and exercise capacity index in chronic obstructive pulmonary disease. N Engl J Med, 350:1005–12, 2004.

70. O'Donnell AE. Bronchiectasis. Chest 134:815–23, 2008.

71. Lazarus A, Myers J, Fuhrer G. Bronchiectasis in adults: a review. Postgrad Med 120(3):113–21, 2008.

72. Morrisey BM. Pathogenesis of bronchiectasis. Clin Chest Med 28:289–96, 2007.

73. Reid LM. Reduction in bronchial subdivision in bronchiectasis. Thorax 5:233–47, 1950.

74. Prasad M, Tino G. Nontuberculous mycobacteria are an increasingly common cause—Bronchiectasis, part 1: presentation and diagnosis. J Respir Dis 28(12):545–54, 2007.

75. Javidan-Nejad C, Bhalla S. Bronchiectasis. Rad Clin N Am 47:289–306, 2009.

76. Cole PJ. Inflammation: a two-edged sword—the model of bronchiectasis. Eur J Respir Dis 147(Suppl):6–15, 1986.

77. Pasteur, MC, Helliwell SM, Houghton SJ, et al. An investigation into causative factors in patients with bronchiectasis. Am J Respir Crit Care Med 162:1277–84, 2000.

78. Iseman MD. Bronchiectasis. In Mason RJ, Murray JF, Broaddus VC, et al. (eds.): Murray & Nadel's Textbook of Respiratory Medicine. 4th ed. Philadelphia, Saunders, 2005.

79. Barker AF. Bronchiectasis. N Engl J Med 346(18):1383–93, 2002.

# CHAPTER 7

# Cardiopulmonary Implications of Specific Diseases

*Joanne Watchie*

## Chapter Outline

Many diseases of body systems other than the heart and lungs also affect cardiopulmonary function. Some, like diabetes or neuromuscular diseases, have well-known associations with cardiopulmonary dysfunction; others, such as rheumatoid arthritis and the other connective tissue diseases, are not routinely recognized as having cardiovascular (CV) and pulmonary manifestations. This chapter will present the cardiopulmonary complications of a number of specific diseases and medical problems as well as their clinical implications for physical therapy intervention. The medical information presented is merely a synopsis of current knowledge and therefore is meant only as an introduction to each topic. The goal of this chapter is to emphasize the potential for cardiovascular and pulmonary limitations in patients with the described diagnoses and to suggest appropriate interventions and treatment modifications. Further reading may be beneficial for the physical therapist who is treating patients with any of these medical problems.

## Obesity

Obesity is defined as an excessive accumulation of adipose tissue such that body mass index (BMI) is 30 kg/m² or more (Box 7-1). Overweight is characterized by BMIs of 25.0 to 29.9 kg/m²; however, some overweight individuals may not be overfat, if their excess weight is due to increased lean body mass.

Obesity is a chronic disorder that is caused by a complex interplay between environmental and genetic factors, which leads to a positive energy balance resulting from an excess of energy intake compared with energy expenditure. Even small but chronic differences between caloric intake and energy expenditure can lead to large increases in body fat; for example, the ingestion of just 8 kcal/day more than expended for 30 years can theoretically produce the 10-kg weight gain typically seen in Americans between the ages of 25 and 55 years.[1] In fact, experts believe that in 90% of adults, this weight gain is attributable to a positive energy balance of 100 kcal/day or less.[2]

See Table 7-1 for components of total daily energy expenditure. Between 1980 and 2006, the prevalence of obesity more than doubled, whereas the percentage of adults with BMIs of 25.0 to 29.9 kg/m² (i.e., overweight) has remained stable.[3–5] According to the data from the National Health and Nutrition Examination Survey (NHANES), it is estimated that 32.7% of adults 20 years or older are overweight, 34.3% are obese, and 5.9% are extremely obese.[3,4] The increments in obesity affect males and females of all ethnic groups, all ages, and all educational and socioeconomic levels.[5,2]

**Table 7-1 Components of Total Daily Energy Expenditure (TDEE)**

| Component | Description | % of TDEE | Effect of Obesity |
|---|---|---|---|
| Resting energy expenditure (REE) | Energy required for basic physiologic functions | 60%–75% | Usually increased due to increased fat and lean body mass |
| Diet-induced thermogenesis (DIT) | Increase in metabolic rate associated with processing of ingested food | 10% | Appears to be decreased, though much conflicting data |
| Physical activity | Energy expended on volitional and nonvolitional activities | 15%–30% | Tends to be decreased, although the energy cost of performing weight-bearing activities is increased. |

---

**Box 7-1**

**Calculation of Body Mass Index**

Weight (kg)/Height ($m^2$) = BMI
[Weight (lbs)/Height ($in^2$)] × 701 = BMI

---

Obesity increases with age and is higher in minority groups, particularly African Americans and Hispanics, when compared with Caucasians in the United States.[5,6] In addition, the prevalence of obesity in children has more than tripled from 5.5% to 17%.[4,7] Obesity is also a widespread global epidemic with a prevalence of overweight of 35.2% and obesity of 20.3% in developed countries as of 2005 versus 19.6% and 6%, respectively, in developing countries.[8,9]

## Factors Related to the Development of Obesity

The major factors involved in the marked increase in the prevalence of obesity since the 1980s are environmental (Table 7-2). Dietary factors that promote obesity include increases in the energy density of foods (high fat, high sugar), portion size, availability, and variety of highly palatable sweets, snacks, entrees, and caloric beverages, as well as lower cost. Changes in activity level are also important and consist of more time spent on sedentary activities, particularly television watching, video games, and computer use; expansion of labor-saving devices to assist with activities of daily living and mobility; and reductions in occupational and recreational physical activities.

Genetics also play an important role in the pathogenesis of obesity, most often through multiple and interacting phenotypes, which provide input that influences such factors as energy expenditure, appetite control, and eating behavior.[10] Thus, it appears that there are subpopulations of individuals who have a genetic susceptibility to obesity, achieving higher BMIs in similar environments of excess energy intake compared to energy expenditure than individuals with a normal genetic background. In addition, gene–gene interactions and alterations in gene expression induced by environmental factors, such as type of ingested nutrients and level of physical activity, may have an effect on energy balance, and these effects might be influenced by ethnicity, age, and gender. Furthermore, hormonal and metabolic factors, as well as other medical conditions (e.g., hypothyroidism, Cushing syndrome, and growth hormone deficiency) and some medications (e.g., antidepressants, antipsychotics, steroid hormones, and antidiabetic drugs) may contribute to the problem.

Other factors also affect energy balance. Several hormones produced by the central nervous system (CNS), gastrointestinal (GI) tract, and adipose tissue ultimately act via the hypothalamus to regulate energy balance (Table 7-3).[2,11-13] Some of the hormones that signal hunger include ghrelin, a gastric hormone that appears to be involved in long-term regulation of body weight, and neuropeptide Y and orexin, which are produced in the hypothalamus; these hormones stimulate food intake and may suppress energy expenditure. Some of the hormones that signal satiety include cholecystokinin, peptide YY, and glucagon-like peptide-1 (GLP-1), which are produced in the gut, and leptin, which is mostly secreted by adipocytes (see description in next section); these hormones tend to reduce energy intake and induce weight loss. Insulin also plays a role in long-term regulation of appetite by acting with leptin to provide negative feedback signals to central receptors regarding food intake in relation to body energy stores. Of note, these hormones are affected by a number of other signaling molecules, enzymes, and factors and can be overridden by psychosocial and environmental influences. Of particular importance is the influence of highly palatable foods, especially sweet foods and soft drinks, which activate the reward system and can cause uncontrolled stimulation of appetite, "food addiction," and cravings.

Another important factor is calcium and dairy food intake, which has been noted to have an inverse relationship with body fat levels via its influence on many components of energy and fat balance. A recent review of calcium-related research suggests that calcium and dairy product intake has the potential to increase fat oxidation, decrease fat absorption, promote adipocyte apoptosis, and increase satiety and decrease food intake, thus favoring a healthier metabolic profile, a stable or negative energy balance, and ultimately a decrease or maintenance of fat mass over time.[14] Importantly, the ingestion of dairy products may have greater effects than

## Table 7-2 Factors That Contribute to Obesity

| Contributory Factors | Comments |
| --- | --- |
| Environmental | Affected by visual, olfactory, social, and emotional stimuli |
|   Increased caloric intake | Increased energy density of food, portion size, availability, and variety of highly tasty foods and caloric beverages that override satiety signals, along with the low cost of fast food contribute to the consumption of excess calories. |
|   Decreased physical activity | Increased time spent on sedentary activities (TV, video games, computer), increased availability of automated devices for ADLs and mobility, and decreased activity related to occupation and often recreation result in reduced energy expenditure |
| Genetic | It is estimated that genetic factors play a role in the development of 40% to 70% of obesity.[68] |
|   Monogenic mutations | Mutations in single genes (e.g., for leptin production and the leptin receptor) have been associated with rare types of obesity. |
|   Polygenic abnormalities | Input of multiple genes that influence food intake and energy expenditure appear to confer susceptibility in an obesogenic environment. |
| Hormonal | Many hormones and peptides produced by the hypothalamus, gastrointestinal tract, and adipocytes are involved in the regulation of food intake and energy expenditure (see Table 7-3). |
| Metabolic | |
|   Medical conditions | Hypothyroidism, Cushing syndrome, and growth hormone deficiency are associated with obesity. |
| Other | |
|   Medications | Certain antidepressants, antipsychotics, steroid hormones, and antidiabetic drugs are associated with weight gain. |
|   Low calcium/dairy intake | Calcium and dairy food intake are inversely related to body fat levels. |
|   Sleep deprivation | Short sleep duration is associated with a dose-dependent increase in BMI. |
|   Novel possibilities | Additional environmental factors may play a role in the development of obesity, including prenatal and early postnatal environmental factors, viral infection, and environmental toxin. |

calcium supplementation alone, implying that other nutrients, such as milk peptides and proteins, may also be involved. In addition, higher amounts of dairy intake have been associated with lower risk of abnormal glucose homeostasis, hypertension (HTN), and dyslipidemia in young overweight individuals and may protect them from the development of obesity and the metabolic syndrome.[15]

Sleep deprivation appears to affect both sides of the energy balance equation, increasing appetite and decreasing energy expenditure. A number of cross-sectional analyses and a few prospective studies have revealed that there is a U-shaped curvilinear relationship between hours of sleep and BMI such that sleeping less or more than 7 to 8 hours per night is associated with a dose-dependent increase in BMI.[16–18] It appears that short sleep duration results in metabolic changes, including decreased leptin and increased ghrelin (both of which increase appetite, among other actions), that may contribute to the development of obesity, insulin resistance, type 2 diabetes mellitus (DM), and cardiovascular disease (CVD).[19] Sleeping only 5 hours per night compared to 8 hours is associated with an average 4% to 5% increase in body weight.[17,18]

Last, additional factors that may be related to the development of obesity include a number of prenatal and early postnatal environmental factors: maternal smoking during pregnancy, low birth weight relative to gestational age, and higher maternal BMI at the onset of pregnancy are associated with increased risk, whereas breastfeeding appears to reduce risk (the recent Endocrine Society clinical practice guideline for prevention and treatment of pediatric obesity[20] recommends breastfeeding for at least 6 months). Furthermore, viral infection (e.g., adenovirus-36, AD-36) and environmental toxins, such as endocrine-disrupting chemicals (EDCs, such as bisphenol A [BPA] in polycarbonate plastic, organotins, and phytoestrogens) may be contributory factors.

## Health Hazards of Obesity

Obesity represents a major health problem because of its association with higher prevalences of HTN, coronary artery disease (CAD), stroke, insulin resistance, glucose intolerance, type 2 DM, dyslipidemia, gallbladder disease, osteoarthritis and other orthopedic problems, sleep-related breathing

## Table 7-3 Hormones and Peptides That Affect Energy Balance

| Signal | Hormone/Peptide | Produced By | Action(s) |
|---|---|---|---|
| Hunger | Ghrelin | Stomach | Stimulates the seeking and collection of food |
| | | | Diverts energy to adipose tissue and restricts energy flow to skeletal muscle |
| | Neuropeptide Y Orexin | Hypothalamus | Stimulate food intake |
| | | | May suppress energy expenditure |
| Satiety | Cholecystokinin | Gastrointestinal tract | Short-term regulation of feeding via signals regarding fullness of stomach and composition of diet |
| | Peptide YY | | |
| | Glucagon-like peptide-1 (GLP-1) | | |
| | Amylin | | |
| | Enterostatin | | |
| | Leptin | Adipocytes | Decreases expression of hunger peptides, increases secretion of satiety peptides |
| | | | Inhibits food intake and increases energy consumption through action on receptors in hypothalamus |
| | | | Influences the production of other adipokines involved in metabolic regulation |
| | Insulin | Pancreas | Inhibits food intake when acting through central receptors |

problems, gynecologic problems, obesity hypoventilation syndrome, pulmonary HTN, and certain forms of cancer, as listed in Table 7-4.[1,21,22] Yet, it is not only obesity that increases risk of disease, but weight gain of 5 kg or more since age 18 to 20 years increases the risk of developing DM, HTN, and CAD, and the risk increases with the amount of weight gained.[1] Also of importance, obesity is associated with increased mortality rates, usually as a result of atherosclerotic heart disease, stroke, DM, digestive diseases, or cancer.[23-26]

Increasing BMI is directly related to greater disease risk, as depicted in Table 7-5. The National Heart, Lung, and Blood Institute (NHLBI) and the World Health Organization (WHO) have identified subcategories of obesity: BMI 30 to 34.9 kg/m$^2$ is considered Class I obesity, 35.0 to 39.9 kg/m$^2$ denotes Class II obesity, and 40 kg/m$^2$ or more is deemed Class III (extreme or morbid) obesity; and these subcategories are related to degree of disease risk.[27] Of note, because changes in the spine with aging result in loss of height, BMI based on height measured earlier in life is less likely to overestimate BMI in older individuals.

Even more important than the amount of body fat is the location of excess fat. Substantial evidence indicates that abdominal (or central) obesity, particularly intraabdominal or visceral adiposity, is a better predictor of CVD and type 2 DM than BMI.[8,23,25,28-30] It is known that visceral adipose tissue (VAT) is associated with increased release of free fatty acids (FFAs) by adipocytes through lipolysis, which enter the circulation and may become deposited as ectopic

fat in the skeletal muscle, liver, heart, and pancreas and ultimately induce insulin resistance (reduced ability of cells, especially muscle, hepatic, and fat cells, to respond to the effects of insulin, which are described in the section on DM).[23,29] Conversely, the accumulation of fat in the gluteofemoral areas in not associated with increased CVD risk and may even be metabolically protective by acting as a "sink" for excess circulating FFAs and thus prevent ectopic fat storage.[23,29,30]

Therefore, the use of waist circumference (WC) or waist–hip circumference ratio (WHR), which takes into account the distribution of body fat, is recommended when defining disease risk. The NHLBI recommends using WC cutoff points of 40 in. (102 cm) for men and 35 in. (88 cm) for women, measured along the horizontal plane at the level of the iliac crest, to define central obesity,[27] although these are arbitrary cutoff values on the continuous relationship between WC and disease risk. The effect of WC on disease risk relative to BMI is shown in Table 7-5, which reveals a graded relationship with CVD and DM at all levels of BMI, including in so-called lean individuals.[8] This is particularly true in the elderly and in Asian ethnic groups, who generally have more visceral fat at smaller WCs than do younger Caucasian populations, and thus may require lower cutoff points to more accurately define risk.[23] A meta-regression analysis of prospective studies of CVD has revealed that a 1-cm increase in WC is associated with a 2% increase in risk of future CVD and a 0.01 increase in WHR is associated with a 5% increase

## Table 7-4 Health Complications Associated with Obesity

| Health Complication | Possible Contributory Factors |
| --- | --- |
| Hypertension (HTN) | Increased cardiac output |
| | Endothelial dysfunction |
| | Renal function abnormalities |
| | Genetic predisposition |
| | Increased leptin, proinflammatory cytokines, FFAs, aldosterone, angiotensinogen and angiotensin II, and insulin levels + decreased adiponectin leading to overactivity of SNS and RAAS |
| | Insulin resistance, decreased adiponectin as independent risk factors, chronic kidney disease, and obstructive sleep apnea |
| Dyslipidemia (increased triglycerides, decreased HDL cholesterol, increased fraction of small, dense LDL particles) | Insulin resistance, hyperinsulinemia, decreased adiponectin, increased levels of circulating FFAs, and inadequate adipocyte fatty acid oxidation |
| Insulin resistance | Increased release of FFAs, glycerol, leptin, TNF-$\alpha$, IL-6, resistin, and proinflammatory cytokines + decreased adiponectin from VAT |
| | Accumulation of FFAs in nonadipose tissue |
| Diabetes mellitus (DM), type 2 | Insulin resistance, decreased adiponectin |
| | Genetic predisposition |
| Atherosclerotic cardiovascular disease (CVD) Coronary artery disease (CAD) Stroke Chronic kidney disease | HTN, dyslipidemia, insulin resistance (which leads to impaired thrombolysis, inflammation, and endothelial dysfunction), DM, and decreased adiponectin (which normally acts to reduce inflammation and protect the vasculature from endothelial dysfunction as well as modulates the production of other adipokines involved in the regulation of inflammation, insulin resistance, and atherosclerosis) |
| | Increased leptin levels (which may stimulate vascular remodeling and endothelial dysfunction, enhance platelet aggregation, and initiate macrophage recruitment to the vessel wall as well as affect the secretion of other adipokines involved in inflammation and metabolic regulation) |
| Left ventricular dysfunction, heart failure | HTN, CAD, DM, obstructive sleep apnea |
| Obesity cardiomyopathy | Diastolic and later systolic dysfunction due to increased blood volume and cardiac output, obesity-related metabolic disturbances (e.g., insulin resistance, increased SNS and RAAS activity, and lipotoxicity), endothelial dysfunction, leptin resistance, decreased adiponectin, and proinflammatory mediators |
| | Fat deposition in the myocardium |
| Pulmonary function test abnormalities Restrictive lung dysfunction Increased airway resistance and airway responsiveness Impaired gas exchange | Increased pulmonary compliance as a result of restriction of thoracic expansion by excessive abdominal and chest wall adipose tissue and increased pulmonary blood flow; impaired respiratory muscle function |
| | Reduced airway caliber, early airway closure, and ventilatory–perfusion mismatching due to excessive weight impeding chest expansion |
| | Proinflammatory effects of some adipokines |
| Obstructive sleep apnea–hypopnea syndrome (OSAHS) | Excessive fat accumulation in the neck, causing pharyngeal lumen narrowing |
| | Hypoventilation and impaired response to hypercapnia induced by leptin resistance. |

## Table 7-4 Health Complications Associated with Obesity—cont'd

| Health Complication | Possible Contributory Factors |
|---|---|
| Obesity hypoventilation syndrome (OHS) | OSAHS, abnormal ventilatory drive. |
| Orthopedic problems (osteoarthritis, plantar fasciitis) | Mechanical stress induced by excess body weight |
| Gastrointestinal disease (GERD, gallstones, nonalcoholic fatty liver, and steatohepatitis) | Unknown. Possible factors include excessive abdominal adiposity and resultant cytokines as well as insulin resistance and hyperinsulinemia. |
| Increased incidence of breast, prostate, colon, endometrial, and other cancers | Unknown. Obesity-related cytokines that cause insulin resistance (e.g., increased leptin, IL-6, TNF-α, insulin-like growth factor-1 [IGF-1], and FFAs and decreased adiponectin) are involved in the promotion of cellular proliferation and in the inhibition of apoptosis, which could lead to cancer. Other factors that may be important include increased levels of estrogen and vascular endothelial growth factor. |

*CAD, coronary artery disease; DM, diabetes mellitus; FFAs, free fatty acids; HDL, high-density lipoprotein; HTN, hypertension; IL-6, interleukin-6; LDL, low-density lipoprotein; RAAS, renin–angiotensin–aldosterone system; SNS, sympathetic nervous system; TNF-α, tumor necrosis factor-α; VAT, visceral adipose tissue*

## Table 7-5 Classification of Overweight and Obesity by BMI and Associated Disease Risk Relative to BMI and Waist Circumference

| | BMI (kg/m²) | Disease Risk Relative to Normal Weight and Waist Circumference | |
|---|---|---|---|
| | | M ≤40 in (102 cm) F ≤35 in (88 cm) | M >40 in (102 cm) F >35 in (88 cm) |
| Underweight | <18.5 | — | — |
| Normal weight | 18.5–24.9 | — | — |
| Overweight | 25.0–29.9 | Increased | High |
| Obesity | | | |
| Class I | 30.0–34.9 | High | Very high |
| Class II | 35.0–39.9 | Very high | Very high |
| Class III (extreme obesity) | ≥40 | Extremely high | Extremely high |

*BMI, body mass index; F, female; M, male.*
*Data from North American Association for the Study of Obesity (NAASO), National Heart, Lung, and Blood Institute (NHLBI): Practical Guide on the Identification, Evaluation, and Treatment of Overweight and Obesity in Adults. NIH Publication No. 00-4084. Bethesda, MD, 2000, National Institutes of Health.*

in risk.[28] Commonly accepted cutoff points for WHR are 0.8 for women and 0.9 for men.[6]

Abnormal blood glucose (BG) regulation is a common complication of abdominal obesity, with most individuals progressing from insulin resistance in skeletal muscle, liver, and adipose tissue to prediabetes with impaired glucose tolerance (IGT; 2-hour oral glucose tolerance test, OGTT, values >120 mg/dL but <200 mg/dL after ingestion of 75 g glucose) and/or impaired fasting glucose (IFG; fasting blood glucose [FBG] level of 100 to 125 mg/dL).[31,32] In the majority of individuals, functional β-cells are able to increase insulin

secretion to compensate for insulin resistance so normal glucose tolerance (NGT) is maintained.[33] Eventually though, usually in those with a genetic predisposition, progressive β-cell failure often develops, and relative or absolute deficiency in insulin secretion causes hyperglycemia, and some patients develop type 2 DM.[34,35]

The development of cardiometabolic complications in obese patients appears to be related to changes in adipocyte function induced by hyperplasia and hypertrophy of fat cells, particularly those in VAT. Rather than simply serving as the body's major energy storage depot, adipose tissue is now recognized as the largest endocrine organ in the body, which secretes numerous proteins, including hormones, cytokines, complement factors, enzymes, and other proteins, that are essential for energy homeostasis, glucose and lipid metabolism, cell viability, control of feeding, thermogenesis, neuroendocrine function, reproduction, immune system function, and cardiovascular function.[25,36] VAT is an important source of several adipokines, including adiponectin, leptin, resistin, visfatin, angiotensinogen and angiotensin II, and FFAs, and macrophages that infiltrate VAT produce interleukin-6 (IL-6), tumor necrosis factor-alpha (TNF-α), and plasminogen activator inhibitor-1 (PAI-1), which may exert effects on many body systems, as listed in Table 7-6.[30,37–49] Research elucidating the role of these cytokines is very active, and the effects of many of them in humans is still unclear; however, it is clear that they exert a number of effects on each other and their actions.

## Cardiovascular and Pulmonary Complications of Obesity

The CV problems associated with overweight and obesity include HTN, CAD, stroke, heart failure (HF), and sudden death. Typically, the major complications are related to atherosclerotic CVD, the risk of which is directly related to BMI, WC, and WHR, as discussed in the previous section. Causative factors include obesity's association with a number of traditional risk CVD factors, including HTN, dyslipidemia, and insulin resistance, as well as with nontraditional risk factors, such as C-reactive protein (CRP) and interleukin-6, that promote inflammation and a procoagulatory state.[39–41,50] As discussed previously, reduced adiponectin and elevated levels of leptin and several other adipokines likely play important roles in the development of these risk factors, as shown in Figure 7-1 and listed in Table 7-6, and also contribute to endothelial dysfunction.[1,25,36,51,52] All of these abnormalities can promote CV events, and there is an increased incidence of myocardial infarction (MI) and stroke with obesity, which tend to occur at younger ages in obese individuals and are associated with worse outcomes.[50]

The prevalence of HTN in obese individuals is three times greater than in those of normal weight, and the incidence is five to six times higher.[40,53] There is a direct linear relationship between magnitude of weight gain and increases in BP, and even a moderate gain of weight is associated with an increased risk of developing HTN, which is particularly evident in studies involving children and adolescence with obesity.[39] In as much as many obese individuals do not develop HTN, it appears that genetic susceptibility must also play a role.

Obesity can provoke a number of alterations in cardiac structure and function, even in the absence of comorbidities. Obesity is associated with an increased incidence of left ventricular (LV) dysfunction and HF and is now recognized as a risk factor for HF in the American College of Cardiology (ACC)/American Heart Association (AHA) heart failure guidelines.[54,55] Moreover, there is a distinct obesity

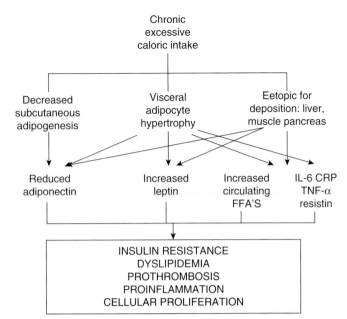

**Figure 7-1** The pathophysiology of adiposity. (From Schelbert KB. Comorbidities of obesity. Prim Care Clin Office Pract 2009; 36(2):271–85.)

cardiomyopathy, which is characterized by myocardial disease ranging from asymptomatic LV dysfunction to overt dilated cardiomyopathy that cannot be explained by DM, HTN, CAD, or other etiologies.[56,57] Circulating blood volume and cardiac output are increased with obesity because of the circulatory and metabolic requirements of the expanded adipose tissue and the additional lean body mass needed for movement, which leads to elevated end-diastolic volumes and filling pressures, especially during exertion. In addition, various obesity-related metabolic alterations, such as insulin resistance (which decreases myocardial glucose uptake and oxidation, increases fatty acid oxidation, and alters myocyte gene expression), augmented renin–angiotensin–aldosterone system (RAAS) and sympathetic nervous system (SNS) activity (which promotes myocardial cell proliferation, hypertrophy, apoptosis, and/or fibrosis), and lipotoxicity (due to FFA and lipid accumulation within cardiomyocytes), as well as other abnormalities associated with obesity, such as endothelial dysfunction, leptin resistance, reduced adiponectin levels, and proinflammatory mediation, may mediate the development of this cardiomyopathy. All of these factors can contribute to biventricular hypertrophy, dilation, and remodeling, which occur in proportion to the degree and duration of obesity, especially VAT, and are associated with diastolic and often systolic dysfunction.[53,55,58] If HTN is also present, left ventricular hypertrophy (LVH) will be more marked and congestive heart failure (CHF) may develop.

Pulmonary problems that are associated with obesity include altered respiratory physiologic parameters, obstructive sleep apnea–hypopnea syndrome (OSAHS), the obesity hypoventilation syndrome (OHS), and pulmonary venous and arterial HTN at rest or during exercise.[58,59] Again, the location of body fat is usually related to the severity of

**Table 7-6 Major Adipokines and Other Substances Secreted by Adipocytes or Adipose Tissue Macrophages and Their Functions**

| Adipokine | Site of Action | Functions |
|---|---|---|
| Adiponectin | Cardiovascular system | Protects arteries against atherogenesis through effects on endothelial cell function |
| | | Protects myocardium from ischemia-reperfusion injury |
| | Immune system | Suppresses release of proinflammatory adipokines that affect endothelial cells |
| | Liver | Inhibits gluconeogenesis and increases fatty acid oxidation |
| | Skeletal muscle | Stimulates glucose uptake and fatty acid oxidation |
| Leptin | Hypothalamus | Suppresses appetite and increases energy consumption (see Table 7-3) |
| | Cardiovascular system | Promotes atherosclerotic plaque formation and arterial thrombosis; stimulates vascular smooth muscle proliferation and hypertrophy |
| | | Promotes production of proinflammatory adipokines |
| | | Promotes the development of HTN via activation of the renin-angiotensin system |
| | Immune system | Upregulates immune function |
| | Endocrine system | Regulates puberty and reproduction |
| | Liver, skeletal muscle | Improves insulin sensitivity by reducing intracellular lipid levels |
| Resistin | Cardiovascular system | May promote atherosclerosis via proinflammatory mediation and induction of endothelial dysfunction |
| | Immune system | Promotes the expression of several proinflammatory cytokines |
| | Liver, skeletal muscle | May contribute to insulin resistance |
| Visfatin | Cardiovascular system | May promote atherosclerotic plaque destabilization and endothelial dysfunction |
| | Immune system | Induces production of several proinflammatory cytokines |
| | Skeletal muscle | May bind to and activate insulin receptors and thus mimic insulin |
| Angiotensinogen and angiotensin II | Cardiovascular system | Promotes the development of HTN |
| | | Contributes to obesity-induced cardiac remodeling and ischemia/reperfusion injury |
| | Adipose tissue | Exerts proinflammatory effects; may stimulate visceral adipose tissue growth and differentiation |
| Retinol-binding protein 4 (RBP4) | Blood | Transports vitamin A |
| | Cardiovascular system | May promote atherosclerosis via proinflammatory mediation and induction of endothelial dysfunction |
| | Liver, skeletal muscle | May promote insulin resistance |
| FFAs | Cardiovascular system | Promote prothrombotic state; stimulate aldosterone production to increase blood pressure |
| | Liver, skeletal muscle | May promote insulin resistance |
| Interleukin 6 (IL-6) | Cardiovascular system | May promote atherosclerosis via proinflammatory mediation |
| | Immune system | Mediates the acute phase response to injury and infection |
| | Skeletal muscle | May improve insulin resistance |
| Tumor necrosis factor alpha (TNF-α) | Cardiovascular system | May promote atherosclerosis via proinflammatory mediation |
| | Immune system | Stimulates the acute phase response to injury and infection |
| | Liver, skeletal muscle | May promote insulin resistance |
| Plasminogen activator inhibitor-1 (PAI-1) | Cardiovascular system | Inhibits fibrinolysis and thus promotes atherothrombosis |
| | Liver, skeletal muscle | May contribute to insulin resistance |

*FFAs, free fatty acids; HTN, hypertension.*

pulmonary problems, with upper body or central fat distribution having a greater effect on pulmonary function and sleep-disordered breathing, as does increasing age.

In obesity, standard pulmonary function tests (PFTs) typically reveal only minimal changes unless obesity is severe; however, reduced pulmonary compliance, respiratory muscle inefficiency, exaggerated demand for ventilation, and increased work of breathing may be evident at lesser degrees of obesity.[60-62] Total pulmonary compliance is decreased by 25% in simple obesity and by as much as 67% in individuals with OHS reductions in both thoracic compliance and lung compliance. Thoracic expansion is restricted by excessive abdominal fat that elevates the diaphragm and limits its descent and excessive chest wall fat that impedes chest expansion, leading to lower lung volumes, whereas lung compliance may be reduced by augmented pulmonary blood volume and early closure of distal airways; these changes are more pronounced in recumbency. The same mechanical factors that reduce thoracic expansion may also impair respiratory muscle function; the diaphragm is most often affected, because of its elevated position, with evidence of reduced strength and endurance, which increases the risk of inspiratory muscle fatigue, especially during exercise. The extra effort required to overcome the abnormal pulmonary compliance and respiratory muscle inefficiency, as well as increased airway resistance (discussed later), results in higher minute ventilation and an increase in the energy cost of breathing by four- to sevenfold. In addition, obese individuals tend to have a rapid, shallow breathing pattern, which further increases the work of breathing. The disproportionately high amount of energy required for breathing impairs exercise tolerance and may place obese persons at greater risk for respiratory failure when conditions provoking increased ventilatory demands develop (e.g., acute infection or diabetic ketoacidosis).

Other pulmonary abnormalities that may be observed in obese individuals include increases in airway resistance and airway responsiveness and impaired gas exchange.[60-62] Airway resistance rises with increasing obesity, likely as a result of relatively reduced airway caliber caused by mechanically induced lower lung volumes. The same mechanism may be responsible for an increase in airway responsiveness that may occur in obesity, in as much as the airway smooth muscle is at a shorter length throughout the respiratory cycle when breathing at lower lung volumes, which may increase its contractility. It is also possible that alterations in levels of adipokines (e.g., high leptin and low adiponectin) may promote airway hyperreactivity.[61] There is also evidence that the incidence of asthma, possibly with unique characteristics, increases with the degree of adiposity in a dose-dependent fashion, which may be related to enhanced airway responsiveness as well as to the proinflammatory effects of certain adipokines.[63] Finally, gas exchange can become impaired because of increasing ventilation–perfusion mismatching induced by airway closure and atelectasis of underventilated alveoli. Hypoxemia may be mild in simple obesity but is more pronounced in severe obesity, particularly in those with OHS.

The rapid, shallow breathing pattern that is commonly used by patients with OHS contributes to hypercapnia, as discussed later.

Thus, the most common alterations seen on PFTs are decreased expiratory reserve volume (ERV) and functional residual capacity (FRC), which can occur even in modest obesity, and diminished total lung capacity (TLC) in morbid obesity. Abdominal obesity of any degree is also associated with reductions in vital capacity (VC) and forced expiratory volume in 1 second (FEV$_1$), which are accelerated by increasing weight gain.[61] The FEV$_1$/FVC ratio is usually normal, but occasionally an obstructive ventilatory impairment is observed. In patients with the OHS, more severe restrictive lung dysfunction is observed with more marked reductions in TLC and VC, as well as in maximum voluntary ventilation (MVV) and peak inspiratory flow rate, which are most likely related to respiratory muscle inefficiency. Fortunately, most parameters of pulmonary function improve with weight loss.

Obesity is the strongest risk factor for obstructive sleep apnea–hypopnea syndrome (OSAHS); a 10% increase in body weight in 4 years is associated with a sixfold greater risk in developing sleep apnea (complete absence of airflow) or hypopnea (i.e., temporary reduction of respiratory flow of at least 50% compared to baseline amplitude, or decrease in air flow of less than 50% associated with either arousal or oxygen desaturation of at least 3%).[59] The most likely cause is excess fat accumulation in the neck, which causes pharyngeal lumen narrowing; however, hypoventilation and impaired response to hypercapnia provoked by leptin resistance may also play a role. OSAHS is characterized by five or more episodes per hour of sleep-disordered breathing lasting at least 10 s in adults, with apnea (complete obstruction) versus loud snoring or choking (partial obstruction), accompanied by hypersomnolence during the day and often morning headaches. The severity of OSAHS is determined by the symptoms, frequency of apnea-hypopnea episodes, and degree of oxygen desaturation.

OSAHS produces both acute and chronic cardiovascular responses. During the apneic periods, marked impairment of gas exchange may occur, leading to hypoxemia and hypercapnia, as well as increased SNS activity. These changes may provoke cardiac arrhythmias, including sinus arrest, asystole up to 6 seconds, atrioventricular block, and ventricular tachycardia, and significant variations in cardiac output, systemic and pulmonary arterial pressures, and cerebral perfusion pressure. In addition, the greater respiratory effort required to maintain air flow in totally or partially obstructed airways may result in greater negative intrathoracic pressures, which increases LV preload and afterload. The major consequence of chronic OSAHS is arterial HTN, and there is an increased risk of MI, HF, stroke, and pulmonary HTN.[59]

Patients with obesity hypoventilation syndrome (OHS) are by definition obese and have sleep-disordered breathing and chronic daytime alveolar hypoventilation (defined as PaCO$_2$ ≥45 mm Hg and PaO$_2$ <70 mm Hg) not resulting from other known causes; there is growing evidence that abnormal ventilatory drive is involved.[60] Patients with OHS almost always have OSAHS, although some patients have sustained periods of hypoventilation, particularly during rapid eye movement sleep (i.e., sleep hypoventilation syndrome), instead, or a combination of the two problems.[64,65] Clinically, OHS includes hypoventilation, cyanosis, and daytime somnolence, with chronic hypoxemia, hypercapnia, respiratory acidosis, and polycythemia. Chronic hypoxemia and hypercapnia stimulate pulmonary vasoconstriction, leading to worsening of pulmonary HTN and biventricular hypertrophy with pulmonary and systemic congestion. Sleep-disordered breathing along with hypoxemia and hypercapnia also affects central respiratory drive, reducing the ventilatory responses to apneic and hypoventilatory episodes, and thus may create a viscous cycle of OHS and attenuation of central ventilatory drive.

## Treatment of Obesity

The most successful strategy for the treatment of obesity is a stepped-care approach, in which the level of intervention is based on the severity of obesity. Mild to moderate obesity is traditionally treated using caloric restriction and other diet modifications, increased physical activity, and behavioral modifications that can be maintained for life, such as self-monitoring of eating and shopping behaviors (e.g., avoiding distractions during meals, eating slowly and purposefully, limiting portion sizes, not shopping while hungry or without a list, and not buying tempting foods), stress management to cope with emotional eating, cognitive restructuring, and relapse prevention training. For individuals with more severe obesity, medications aimed at normalizing the regulatory and metabolic disturbances that are involved in the pathogenesis of obesity may be added to lifestyle modifications. For patients with extreme obesity, bariatric surgery is the most effective treatment, inducing impressive long-term weight loss.

The goals of obesity treatment are not only to produce and maintain loss of adipose tissue, while preserving fat-free (lean body) mass (FFM) and resting metabolic rate (RMR), and to improve appearance and physical function, but even more important in terms of decreasing morbidity and mortality is to reduce cardiovascular risk and improve cardiorespiratory fitness. It is important to emphasize that clients need not achieve optimal weight to obtain significant health benefits. Modest but sustained weight loss of 5% to 10% of baseline weight is associated with clinically significant effects on several hormonal, metabolic, and cardiovascular risk factors and results in reduced blood pressure and improved insulin sensitivity and lipid profile.[66] Thus, the goal of weight loss therapy is typically set at 10% from baselines. However, as will be discussed, this goal is hard to achieve and even more difficult to maintain. Factors that are positively related to weight loss maintenance include a physically active lifestyle, regular meal rhythm including breakfast, internal motivation to lose weight, self-monitoring of behaviors, reaching a self-determined goal weight, social support, and better coping

strategies.[66] When attempts at weight reduction are not successful, prevention of further weight gain becomes an important goal.

> **Clinical Tip**
> Modest sustained weight loss (5% to 10% of baseline weight) reduces many of the medical risk factors and complications associated with obesity.

Diet modification is the most common intervention used to reduce weight and consists of altering total caloric intake and/or dietary composition to create a negative energy balance. Energy-restricted diets commonly reduce energy intake by 500 to 1000 cal/day, which effects the loss of 1 to 2 lb of fat per week (a caloric deficit of 3500 cal is required to lose 1 lb of adipose tissue).[67] Such modest calorie restricted diets are generally successful in producing <5 kg of short-term weight loss, which is typically followed by weight regain of almost 50%. Very low-calorie diets (total energy intake of 400 to 800 cal/day) produce greater short-term weight loss but show no advantage in the long run; in addition, they are associated with higher risks of micronutrient deficiencies, blood chemistry abnormalities, and cardiac arrhythmias, and when used repeatedly, creating cycles of starvation and feeding, may actually result in additional weight gain once caloric restriction ends (see note on yo-yo dieting).[66,68,69]

The most important factor related to success is consistent and long-term compliance with diet modifications, which has been found to be higher with high-protein diets and lower with low-fat diets,[70,71] although evidence supporting the advantages of one particular type of diet over another for long-term weight loss is lacking, with all diets producing modest weight loss of less than 5 kg after 2 to 5 years.[69,72,73] Therefore, individualized diets tailored to client needs and preferences is likely the best approach.

## Yo-Yo Dieting

The pattern of losing and regaining weight is known as yo-yo dieting, so named because the body weight goes up and down, like a yo-yo. Because very-low-calorie diets often result in a reduction of the resting metabolic rate and an increase in the efficiency of absorption, dieting may become less effective. Not only does weight loss become more difficult, but weight regain may occur more easily following each weight loss attempt, and a subset of those who engage in yo-yo dieting actually end up weighing more than their baseline due to adjustment of the set point for each individual's weight to a higher level once caloric restriction ends.

Many forms of exercise, when used in combination with dietary modification, have been shown to produce weight loss and improve cardiorespiratory fitness, including continuous and intermittent aerobic exercise, resistance training, and increasing lifestyle activities.[74] Weight loss associated with physical activity occurs in a dose–response relationship, such that weight loss increases with increasing energy expenditure (i.e., higher intensity, duration, and/or frequency). Unfortunately, studies evaluating the efficacy of exercise, either as a single modality or combined with dietary restriction, are very disappointing because of the modest amounts of short- and long-term weight loss achieved (<5 kg) and the high dropout rates (typically 20% to 60%).[75-77] Meta-analyses of randomized clinical trials assessing the effectiveness of exercise plus diet versus diet only have revealed that combination treatment results in significantly greater short- and long-term weight loss than diet interventions alone among obese and overweight adults.[78,79] Unfortunately, weight regain of almost 50% occurs over the long term after both interventions. Furthermore, although observational studies show that physical activity is associated with prevention of weight regain after weight loss, these analyses did not support this finding. Yet, a number of studies indicate that the addition of aerobic or resistance exercise to diet restriction preserves FFM, but only resistance exercise showed a tendency to maintain RMR.[80]

In more severe obesity (i.e., BMI ≥30 kg/m$^2$ or BMI of 27.0 to 29.9 kg/m$^2$ with one or more obesity-related medical complications), pharmacotherapy may be added to a comprehensive program of diet, exercise, and behavior modification. Drugs used to promote weight loss work through suppression of appetite, enhancement of energy expenditure (by stimulating activity or thermogenesis), or inhibition of lipid digestion and absorption, as described in Table 7-7. Currently, very few drugs have been approved by the Food and Drug Administration (FDA) for the treatment of obesity, and all produce extra weight loss of less than 5 kg at 1 year and have high rates of attrition (30% to 40%) because of side effects and poor efficacy.[81-83] Because discontinuation of these drugs usually results in weight regain, long-term if not lifelong treatment is required, but FDA guidelines allow the long-term use of only two agents. However, long-term safety and efficacy data are still lacking, so patients must be made aware of the potential risks associated with their use, as with earlier medications that had to be removed from the market because of safety concerns.

Bariatric surgery, most commonly in the form of Roux-en-Y gastric bypass (RYGB) and laparoscopic adjustable gastric banding (LAGB), is an effective treatment for individuals with morbid obesity.[1,84,85] RYGB involves stapling the stomach into a small (15- to 30-mL) proximal gastric pouch that empties into a segment of jejunum; it is performed either laparoscopically or via abdominal incision. On average, patients lose approximately 60% of their excess body weight (~30% of actual body weight), which is achieved through gastric restriction, mild malabsorption induced by bypassing the upper small intestine, and neuroendocrine changes. Complications include various surgical complications (e.g., GI leak, staple line disruption, internal or incisional hernias, and stomal stenosis), pulmonary embolism, wound infection, dumping syndrome (i.e., rapid gastric emptying), and nutritional deficiencies, particularly in iron, calcium, folic acid, and vitamins D and B$_{12}$. LAGB involves laparoscopic placement of an adjustable silicone gastric band around the uppermost part of the stomach to create a small pouch. The band circumference is adjusted via a balloon within the band that is connected to a subcutaneous port, which allows percutaneous inflation or deflation with saline. Band adjustment is based on the rate of weight loss and GI symptoms and may continue for several years. Mean weight loss after LAGB is about 50% of excess body weight (~25% of actual body weight) at 2 years and eventually similar to RYGB. Complications are less frequent and severe than other bariatric surgical procedures and consist of esophageal dilation, gastric erosion, band slippage or prolapse, band or port infection, or band or system leaks that lead to inadequate weight loss.

Weight loss produced by bariatric surgery is associated with significant improvements and often complete resolution of HTN, dyslipidemias, metabolic syndrome, type 2 DM, OSAHS, and OHS.[85,86] Remarkably, the improvement and sometimes remission of DM occurs within days of surgery, resulting from changes in the production of gut-derived hormones triggered by the rerouting of nutrients.[87] In addition, bariatric surgery appears to slow the progression of atherosclerotic CVD, resulting in reduced incidences of coronary events and numbers of percutaneous and surgical revascularization procedures, improves the functional and physiologic indices of HF, and reduces overall mortality as a result of decreased CV and cancer deaths.[57,86]

## Exercise and Obesity

The physiologic responses to exercise are affected by obesity, and the common association of obesity with cardiovascular and metabolic comorbidities may further affect the exercise responses.[60,61] Because obesity increases the physiologic stress of activity as a result of greater body mass, the heart rate (HR), respiratory rate, minute ventilation (VE), and absolute oxygen consumption (VO$_2$) are usually higher at any given workload than in nonobese individuals (as they are at rest). However, when VO$_2$ is standardized to body weight (i.e., expressed as mL O$_2$/kg), values are lower than normal. Importantly, cardiovascular and ventilatory reserves are frequently limited in their ability to meet the increasing demand for VO$_2$ during exercise, because the heart and lungs do not increase in size in proportion to the increase in body mass. Therefore, obese individuals commonly experience dyspnea on exertion and their exercise capacity is reduced. These impediments are rarely caused by ventilatory limitation in uncomplicated obesity; rather the major limiting factor is probably a reduced capacity to increase blood flow and oxygen delivery to the exercising muscles.[88] In fact, deep breathing during exercise expands atelectatic lung units and normalizes ventilation–perfusion relations in uncomplicated obesity, so that arterial oxygenation improves.

Although the literature cites disappointing results for exercise as a sole means of reducing obesity (without any dietary intervention), it is important to note that exercise training offers health benefits even if no weight is lost, including improvements in serum lipid profile, BP, insulin sensitivity, and psychological well-being.[80,89-91] As with other populations, exercise training also increases cardiorespiratory fitness, protects against the loss of lean body mass, and

## Table 7-7 Medications Used for Weight Loss

| Drug | Mechanism of Action | Adverse Side Effects |
| --- | --- | --- |
| Orlistat[a,b] (Xenical, Alli) | Lipase inhibitor: decreased absorption of fat. | GI symptoms: fatty/oily stools, flatulence, fecal urgency, loose stools<br><br>Reduced absorption of fat-soluble vitamins (A, D, E, K, and β-carotene) and lipophilic medications (e.g., amiodarone and cyclosporine) |
| Sibutramine[a,b] (Meridia) | Appetite suppressant: norepinephrine, serotonin, and dopamine uptake inhibitor. Possible increase in resting energy expenditure | Dry mouth, constipation, drowsiness, insomnia, headache, dizziness, and nausea<br><br>Possible increased HR and BP |
| Benzphetamine[a] (Didrex) | Appetite suppressant: sympathomimetic amine | CNS effects (restlessness, dizziness, insomnia, tremor, sweating, headache), CV effects (palpitations, increased HR and BP), dry mouth, unpleasant taste, and GI symptoms |
| Diethylpropion[a] (Tenuate) | Appetite suppressant: sympathomimetic amine | CNS effects (insomnia, restlessness, dizziness, headache), mild CV effects, mild GI symptoms, and rash |
| Phendimetrazine[a] (Bontril, Plegine, Prelu-2, X-Trozine, and others) | Appetite suppressant: sympathomimetic amine | CNS effects (restlessness, insomnia, agitation, flushing, tremor, sweating, dizziness, headache, blurring of vision), CV effects, dry mouth, GI symptoms, and urinary frequency. |
| Phentermine[a] (Adipex-P, Fastin Ionamin, and others) | Appetite suppressant: sympathomimetic amine | Dizziness, dry mouth, insomnia, irritability, CV effects, and GI effects |
| Bupropion (Wellbutrin, Zyban) | Appetite suppressant: dopamine and norepinephrine reuptake inhibitor | Dry mouth, insomnia, diarrhea, and constipation |
| Fluoxetine (Prozac) | Appetite suppressant: selective serotonin reuptake inhibitor | CNS effects (agitation, nervousness, sweating, tremors, somnolence, and insomnia), fatigue, weakness, and GI symptoms |
| Sertraline (Zoloft) | Appetite suppressant: selective serotonin reuptake inhibitor | Agitation, nervousness, and GI upset |
| Topiramate (Topamax) | Unknown; carbonic anhydrase inhibitor—inhibition of lipogenesis? | Paresthesia, dry mouth, headache, taste disturbance, cognitive problems, dizziness, somnolence, fatigue, and GI upset |
| Zonisamide (Zonegran) | Unknown; carbonic anhydrase inhibitor—inhibition of lipogenesis? | Dizziness, confusion, difficulty concentrating, somnolence, and nausea |

*BP, blood pressure; CNS, central nervous system; CV, cardiovascular; GI, gastrointestinal; HR, heart rate.*
[a]*Approved by the U.S. Food and Drug Administration for weight loss.*
[b]*Approved for long-term use for weight loss.*

increases muscular efficiency, so daily activities can be performed more easily. This improvement is particularly important for obese individuals, who tend to use more energy with exaggerated cardiovascular and respiratory stress to perform any form of physical work. Notably, exercise without weight loss has been shown to reduce VAT and prevent further weight gain.[92] Furthermore, overweight and obese adults with the highest levels of fitness have a lower risk of CVD than those with an optimal BMI but low level of fitness. There is also evidence that higher levels of physical fitness level reduce mortality risk in older adults (≥60 years), irrespective of overall obesity and fat distribution.[93]

## Clinical Implications for Physical Therapy

Because of the prevalence of obesity-related complications, careful evaluation and treatment modifications are often required when obese individuals are referred to PT. Consideration should be given to the presence of any cardiovascular risk factors and medical comorbidities, the medications and supplements the individual is taking, the presence of orthopedic complications that might affect treatment, and past exercise experience and attitudes.

A number of specific considerations, when prescribing exercise for obese individuals, will maximize both safety and effectiveness. Because of the increased prevalence of HTN and atherosclerotic heart disease in obese individuals, monitoring of the physiologic responses to exercise is indicated during PT evaluation and initial treatments. Obese individuals may exhibit a hypertensive response to exercise even when resting BP is normal, whereas those with impaired ventricular function may show a drop in BP with exercise because of reduced cardiac output. Also, a tendency toward exercise-induced syncope due to fluid imbalance resulting from calorie-restricted diets and exacerbated by exercise-induced fluid loss further emphasizes the need for BP monitoring. Furthermore, obese adults are at higher risk for myocardial ischemia during exercise. Last, because of the many comorbidities associated with obesity, patients are often taking a variety of medications, many of which may have adverse effects on exercise responses and tolerance.

An endurance training program should be prescribed for all obese patients in order to increase energy expenditure, lower cardiovascular risk factors, and improve respiratory muscle and functional efficiency. Moderate-intensity exercise is usually recommended (40% to 60% of heart rate reserve [HRR] or maximal oxygen consumption [$VO_2max$]), which is usually lower than the anaerobic threshold, in order to utilize predominantly FFAs as fuel. However, the inclusion of some sessions with more vigorous exercise (≥60% HRR or $VO_2max$) may be more effective for maintaining weight loss.[94] Exercise duration should be emphasized over intensity, allowing for gradual increases to targeted levels before advancing to more vigorous activities. To achieve and maintain long-term weight loss, at least 45 to 60 minutes/day of at least moderate exercise totaling at least 250 to 300 minutes/week may be required. Intermittent exercise (several 10- to 15-min bouts per day) that achieves these targets appear to be just as effective as continuous exercise and may enhance exercise adherence.[95,96] Non–weight-bearing exercise programs, such as cycling, swimming, or water aerobics, will decrease the stress on joints, which often suffer from osteoarthritis. Resistance exercise also improves endurance as well as muscle strength and thus enhances the performance of functional tasks and weight loss.

Because injuries are one of the primary reasons for discontinuing exercise in obese individuals, injury prevention is extremely important during treatment planning and exercise interventions. Special considerations include obtaining a detailed history of previous injuries and joint problems; prescribing adequate warm-up, cool-down, and stretching; and encouraging a gradual progression of duration and intensity.

Another concern when working with people who are obese is impaired thermoregulation due to excess body fat, so exercise is best performed during the cooler times of day or in a controlled environment with neutral temperature and humidity. In addition, individuals should be encouraged to wear loose-fitting clothing and drink plenty of water.

---

**Clinical Tip**

Physical therapists who are familiar with the use of brain natriuretic peptide (BNP) and N-terminal pro–brain natriuretic peptide (NT-proBNP) levels as a screening tool for LV dysfunction should be aware that these levels are inversely proportional to BMI, regardless of the presence or severity of HF.[56] Thus, BNP levels are decreased in obese individuals even when LV end-diastolic pressure is elevated, and their levels are less likely to be useful for diagnosis and monitoring of LV dysfunction.

---

## Metabolic Syndrome

The metabolic syndrome (MetS) refers to a cluster of inter-related risk factors that is found in one third of American adults and a growing number of children and is associated with increased risk of CVD events and death, type 2 DM, and chronic kidney disease (CKD).[53,97-99] Among the most commonly recognized metabolic risk factors are central or visceral obesity, atherogenic dyslipidemia (i.e., elevated serum triglyceride, apolipoprotein B, and small low-density lipoprotein particles and reduced high-density lipoprotein cholesterol), HTN, insulin resistance, and IGT. In addition, persons with these abnormalities usually manifest hypercoagulable and proinflammatory states (Table 7-8).

The prevalence of the MetS continues to increase along with that of obesity and rises with the severity of adiposity. Of major concern is its expansion in the pediatric population, in which nearly 50% of severely obese youngsters have the syndrome.[100] These individuals have an extremely high risk of developing future obesity, nonalcoholic fatty liver disease, type 2 DM, and early morbidity and mortality due to CVD. Once CVD is present, the number of components of the MetS contributes to disease progression and greater risk of CV events.

As discussed in the preceding section on obesity, increased visceral adiposity is associated with insulin resistance and elevated plasma FFA levels, which appear to be related to changes in adipocyte function leading to abnormal secretion of various adipokines (decreased adiponectin and increased leptin, IL-6, TNF-α, resistin, and other proinflammatory cytokines). In addition, increased lipolysis of stored triglycerides from the large adipocytes that characterize VAT generates more circulating FFAs; these FFAs interfere with insulin receptor signaling and impairs glucose uptake, reducing

## Table 7-8 Criteria for Clinical Diagnosis of the Metabolic Syndrome[a]

| Measure | Categorical Cutoff Points |
|---|---|
| Increased waist circumference[b] | Population- and country- specific definitions |
| Elevated triglycerides (or drug treatment for it[c]) | ≥150 mg/dL (1.7 mmol/L) |
| Reduced HDL-C (or drug treatment for it[c]) | Males: <40 mg/dL (1.0 mmol/L) |
| | Females: <50 mg/dL (1.3 mmol/L) |
| Elevated blood pressure (or antihypertensive drug treatment in patient with history of HTN) | Systolic BP ≥130 mm Hg and/or |
| | Diastolic BP ≥85 mm Hg |
| Elevated fasting glucose[d] (or drug treatment for it) | ≥100 mg/dL |

Modified from Alberti KGMM, Eckel RH, Grundy SM, et al. Harmonizing the metabolic syndrome. A joint interim statement of the International Diabetes Federation Task Force on Epidemiology an Prevention; National Heart, Lung, and Blood Institute; American Heart Association; World Heart Federation; International Atherosclerosis Society; and International Association for the Study of Obesity. Circulation 120:1640–1645, 2009.

HDL-C, high-density lipoprotein cholesterol; HTN, hypertension

[a]Must meet three of the five criteria for clinical diagnosis of the metabolic syndrome

[b]It is recommended that the IDF cutoff points be used for non-Europeans and either the IDF or AHA/NHLBI cutoff points used for people of European origin until more data are available.

[c]The most commonly used drugs for elevated triglycerides and reduced HDL-C are fibrates and nicotinic acid. A patient taking one of these drugs can be presumed to meet these two criteria. High-dose ω-3 fatty acids presumes high triglycerides.

[d]Most patients with type 2 diabetes mellitus will meet this criterion.

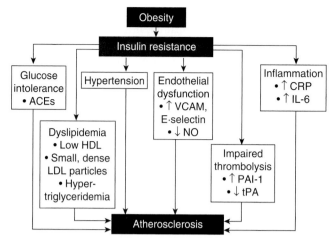

**Figure 7-2** Association of obesity and insulin resistance with cardiovascular risk factors and atherosclerosis. AGEs, advanced glycation end-products; CRP, C-reactive protein; HDL, high-density lipoprotein; IL-6, interleukin-6; LDL, low-density lipoprotein; NO, nitric oxide; PAI-1, plasminogen activator inhibitor-1; tPA, tissue plasminogen activator; VCAM, vascular adhesion molecule; ↑, increased; ↓, decreased. (Adapted from McFarlane SI, Banerji M, Sowers JR. Insulin resistance and cardiovascular disease. J Clin Endocrinol Metab 86(2):713–8, 2001 in Rader DJ. Effect of insulin resistance, dyslipidemia, and intra-abdominal adiposity on the development of cardiovascular disease and diabetes mellitus. Am J Med 120(3 Suppl 1):S12–8, 2007.)

energy production for cellular function (often referred to as lipotoxicity). The ultimate result is insulin resistance, which causes cells, particularly in muscle, liver, and adipose tissue, to be less responsive to the effects of insulin (see section on DM).[30,101,102] In the liver, glycogen synthesis and suppression of glucose production are impaired, resulting in excessive increases in BG levels, which then stimulate the pancreas to produce more insulin (hyperinsulinemia) to compensate for the rising blood sugar.

Thus, most affected individuals progress from insulin resistance in skeletal muscle, liver, and adipose tissue to prediabetes, which consists of IGT (defined as BG >120 mg/dL but <200 mg/dL after ingestion of 75 g glucose during a 2-hour oral glucose tolerance test, OGTT) and/or impaired fasting glucose (IFG, defined as fasting blood glucose [FBG] of 100 to 125 mg/dL).[31,32] In the majority of these individuals, functional β-cells are able to increase insulin secretion to compensate for insulin resistance so normal glucose levels are maintained.[33,34] Eventually though, progressive β-cell failure often develops, usually in those with a genetic predisposition,

and relative or absolute deficiency in insulin secretion causes hyperglycemia. The cause is either inadequate insulin secretion from each β-cell or loss of adequate β-cell mass, likely resulting from glucotoxicity (whereby chronic hyperglycemia provokes slow and progressive irreversible damage to β-cells) or lipotoxicity (whereby accumulated fatty acids and their metabolic products deleteriously affect β-cells).[34,35] Thus, over 10 to 20 years of follow-up, approximately 35% to 50% of individuals with prediabetes go on to develop type 2 DM (FBG levels exceeding 125 mg/dL or a BG level of at least 200 mg/dL on casual blood sample [along with symptoms of DM] or at 2 hours of an OGTT).

Visceral obesity is also strongly associated with the development of insulin resistance and both of these are major factors in the development of the other features of the MetS and thus play a central role in the pathogenesis of CVD, as illustrated in Figure 7-2.[103,104] The link between VAT and the adipokines that induce endothelial dysfunction and hypercoagulable and proinflammatory states has been described under obesity. Furthermore, the VAT-induced increment in FFAs also stimulates the liver to produce more LDL cholesterol, particularly the small, dense particles that are more easily embedded in atherosclerotic plaques, while producing less HDL cholesterol that normally removes cholesterol from these plaques. Moreover, glucose intolerance and hyperglycemia facilitate the formation of advanced glycation end products (AGEs), which alter the function of endothelial, macrophage, and arterial smooth muscle cells, whereas insulin resistance is associated with the development of HTN, dyslipidemia, blunted production of nitric oxide and thus endothelial dysfunction, impaired thrombolysis, and a proinflammatory state. All of these factors also contribute to the pathogenesis of atherosclerotic CVD and explain why the risk for CVD increases with the progression from insulin resistance to IGT to IFG to DM.

Several definitions of the MetS have been proposed over the past decade, and recently several major organizations came to an agreement on common criteria for its clinical diagnosis, three of five of which must be present: central obesity, elevated triglycerides, low high-density lipoprotein cholesterol, HTN, and elevated FBG (see Table 7-8 for specific criteria for abnormal values).[105] This definition recognizes that the cardiometabolic risk associated with abdominal obesity varies in different ethnic groups and that defining thresholds for WC is complicated by these differences and their relationship to other metabolic risk factors, as well as by the practical considerations of the public health and economic implications of a particular cutoff point. The current recommended thresholds for weight circumference range from 85 to 90 cm for Asian men and up to 102 cm for Caucasian men and from 80 cm up to 88 cm for most Asian and Caucasian women, respectively.[105] According to these criteria, most patients with type 2 DM have the MetS; however, there is debate as to whether these are two different entities, at least in regards to CV risk, or a continuum of a primary metabolic disorder.

Because even minimal elevations in these risk factors significantly increase morbidity and mortality, aggressive lifestyle modification and pharmacologic therapy are recommended for those with the MetS to reduce CV risk and delay or prevent the development of type 2 DM and CKD.[53,106–111] Fortunately, these interventions are often successful in reducing disease risk. Studies have shown that combined lifestyles interventions that include weight loss and physical activity can improve BG levels or return them to normal and reduce the risk of developing DM by up to 58%, or even 71% among adults aged 60 years or older.[107,112–114] However, there is concern about the reality of achieving similar success in routine clinical practice, given the inability to provide the considerable multidisciplinary support offered in clinical trials and the challenges of long-term adherence to lifestyle modifications. Regardless, exercise training to improve cardiorespiratory fitness is beneficial, as higher levels of fitness attenuate much of the all-cause and CVD mortality risk associated with the MetS, at least in men.[115]

## Diabetes Mellitus

Diabetes mellitus is a group of chronic metabolic diseases characterized by hyperglycemia, which results from defects in insulin production, insulin action, or both. The major functions of insulin serve to control the rise in blood sugar following meals, as described in the next section. A deficiency of insulin or resistance to its action results in elevated BG levels, which eventually causes damage to the blood vessels, heart, kidneys, eyes, and peripheral nerves, as well as increased susceptibility to periodontal disease and other infections, particularly pneumonia, influenza, and skin infections.[31]

There are at least four types of DM. Type 1 DM (formerly insulin-dependent diabetes) and type 2 DM (formerly non–insulin-dependent diabetes) are the most common types, which differ in etiology, clinical presentation, and pathophysiology. Gestational diabetes mellitus is a form of glucose intolerance that develops in some women during pregnancy and almost always resolves after parturition; however, women with gestational diabetes mellitus have a 40% to 60% risk of developing DM in the next 5 to 10 years.[112] In rare cases, DM results from secondary causes, such as genetic defects (e.g., cystic fibrosis, hemochromatosis), drug or chemical toxicity (e.g., Dilantin, glucocorticoids, estrogens, many antihypertensive agents), pancreatic disease, infections, hormonal syndromes (e.g., acromegaly, Cushing syndrome, pheochromocytoma), and other immune-mediated and genetic syndromes associated with DM.

Type 1 DM is caused by autoimmune destruction of the β-cells in the pancreas resulting in complete lack of insulin secretion, usually by the age of 10 to 25, although it can occur at any age. Approximately 85% to 90% of patients have antibodies to islet cells or glutamic acid decarboxylase (GAD) or other autoantibodies.[116] These individuals develop extreme hyperglycemia, ketosis (the presence of ketone bodies in the blood), and the associated symptomatology (polyuria, polydipsia, weight loss, and sometimes polyphagia), making their survival dependent on insulin therapy. Diabetic ketoacidosis (DKA) is the most serious acute complication of uncontrolled type 1 DM, and it is manifested by marked hyperglycemia, nausea and vomiting, polydipsia, polyuria, abdominal pain, fruity-scented (ketotic) breath, dry skin and mouth, weakness or fatigue, and rapid, deep (Kussmaul) breathing.

Type 2 DM, which accounts for 90% to 95% of all cases of DM, is a genetically heterogenous disease that is characterized by insulin resistance, relative insulin deficiency, and progressive decline in β-cell function over time.[117] Hyperglycemia results from an increased rate of hepatic glucose production as a consequence of hepatic insulin resistance as well as β-cell dysfunction and eventual failure. There is also evidence of α-cell dysfunction with excessive glucagon release occurring concomitantly with reductions in insulin secretion.[118] Before fulfilling the criteria for the diagnosis of type 2 DM, most individuals experience a period of prediabetes with IGT or IFG or both, as described for the metabolic syndrome. The chief risk factors for developing type 2 DM are obesity (85% to 90% of patients are overweight or obese), particularly abdominal obesity, age, sedentary lifestyle, and genetic predisposition.

The symptoms of type 2 DM are often insidious and mild, consisting of fatigue, weakness, dizziness, blurred vision, and other nonspecific complaints. Individuals with type 2 DM, particularly obese adolescents, may exhibit overt signs of insulin resistance, such as acanthosis nigricans, which is a velvety, dark hyperpigmentation of the skin occurring in the folds of the neck, axilla, and other areas, or skin tags.[119] DKA is rare in patients with type 2 DM, except when stressed by a severe intercurrent illness (e.g., acute MI or septicemia), because they retain some endogenous insulin secretion. Instead uncontrolled hyperglycemia leads to dehydration and a hyperosmolar hyperglycemic nonketotic syndrome, which is manifested as postural hypotension and focal neurologic deficits and hallucinations and is often fatal. Previously, type 2 DM was typically diagnosed after the age of 40, but with the recent surge in obesity, it is now found in some children and adolescents.

Recently, a type 1 variant of DM, sometimes termed latent diabetes of adults (LADA) or sometimes type 1.5 DM, has been recognized, which has clinical, metabolic, and phenotypic features that fall somewhere between those of type 1 and type 2 DM.[116,119,120] LADA typically develops in adults aged 30 to 50 years and is caused by autoimmune destruction of β-cells, as indicated by anti-GAD or other islet cell autoantibodies, which progresses more slowly and more selectively than in classic type 1 DM, so patients do not require insulin therapy for at least 6 months and often for many years after diagnosis. Because the onset of hyperglycemia is insidious without an acute ketoacidotic crisis, patients with LADA are frequently misdiagnosed as having type 2 DM.[119] However, these patients typically have a BMI <25 and lack signs of insulin resistance and a significant family history of diabetes; however, they often have a personal or family history of autoimmune disease.

According to 2007 data from the NHANES, the prevalence of diagnosed and undiagnosed diabetes among U.S. adults aged 20 years or older was 10.7% (23.1% of adults aged 60 years or older).[112] In addition, in 1988 to 1994, NHANES found that among adults aged 40 to 74 years in the United States, 33.8% had IFG, 15.4% had IGT, and 40.1% had prediabetes; unfortunately, more recent data are not available for IGT, but in 2003 to 2006, data indicate that 25.9% of U.S. adults aged 20 years or older had IFG (35.4% of adults aged 60 years or older), so a large proportion of the population is at risk for developing DM. Fortunately, the Diabetes Prevention Program has shown that lifestyle intervention to lose weight and increase physical activity can reduce the risk of developing DM by 58% during a 3-year period and by 71% among adults aged 60 years or older.

The measurement of glycosylated hemoglobin (HbA1c, or simply A1c) is considered the gold standard as an indicator of the degree of glycemic control achieved by an individual over the preceding 2- to 3-month period. The test does not rely on the patient's ability to monitor or accurately record blood glucose levels, and it is not influenced by acute changes in blood glucose or by the interval since the last meal. During hyperglycemia, some hemoglobin molecules become glycosylated (bound with glucose), which is a relatively irreversible process. Therefore, the level of HbA1c within the red blood cells reflects the average level of glucose that the cell has been exposed to during its life cycle (about 120 days). In normal healthy individuals, HbA1c levels are 2.5% to 6%, and with intensive glycemic control in DM, the goal is to achieve levels of <7% in order to reduce the risk of diabetic complications.

## Insulin and Glucose Physiology

The major actions of insulin are the suppression of glucose production by the liver and the promotion of glucose transport across the cell membrane and its subsequent metabolism within the cell. Insulin also plays a role in the synthesis of glycogen, fat, and protein. In DM, insulin deficiency results in an inability to utilize glucose as fuel, impaired protein metabolism, and increased fat mobilization with increased levels of FFAs in the blood. When the FFAs are metabolized in the liver, ketone bodies are formed. Uncontrolled DM (usually type 1) can lead to diabetic ketoacidosis, an acute, life-threatening metabolic complication caused by the production of ketones from the catabolism of triglycerides for cellular fuel when insulin deficiency prevents cellular uptake of glucose; it can develop quickly and without treatment can progress to coma and death within a few hours. When insulin resistance is present, as in type 2 DM, cells in muscle, liver, and adipose tissue are less responsive to insulin, so not only is glucose utilization impaired but hepatic glucose production continues despite rising blood glucose levels, which provokes the pancreatic β-cells into producing even more insulin (hyperinsulinemia); when β-cell mass and function are not able to produce enough insulin to compensate for the insulin resistance, hyperglycemia develops.[33]

Two major incretin hormones that are secreted by the gut, glucose-dependent insulinotropic polypeptide and GLP-1, play a major role in maintaining glucose homeostasis after food is ingested.[120] Both hormones enhance glucose-stimulated insulin secretion. In addition, GLP-1 stimulates β-cell proliferation and is a potent inhibitor of glucagon secretion.

A number of counterregulatory hormones also participate in the regulation of glucose metabolism to prevent hypoglycemia and maintain adequate cellular fuel sources for energy production: glucagon, growth hormone, cortisol, and catecholamines. Of these, glucagon plays the most important role in terms of DM, in which its levels are increased. Glucagon release is stimulated by hypoglycemia (as in periods of fasting and overnight), amino acids, neural influences, and stress. In the liver, it promotes the breakdown of glycogen to glucose (glycogenolysis), the formation of glucose or glycogen from proteins and fats (gluconeogenesis), and the production of ketone bodies (ketogenesis).

Of note, not all tissues utilize glucose as the preferred substrate for energy production, or at least not under all conditions. Although the brain and red blood cells rely on glucose at all times, at rest, particularly in the postabsorptive state, skeletal muscle and other tissues favor FFAs, which are derived from adipose tissue. During low- to moderate-intensity exercise, FFAs continue to serve as the predominant fuel source, but as exercise intensity rises, increasing SNS-stimulated catecholamine levels (about two to four times baseline) causes a shift to greater proportions of BG (derived from carbohydrate intake during exercise, hepatic glycogenolysis, and hepatic gluconeogenesis) and muscle glycogen.[121–124] These changes are accomplished by adjustments in the levels of circulating insulin and the counter-regulatory hormones (primarily glucagon and catecholamines), which usually correspond to the intensity of exercise, as described later in the section on exercise. During high-intensity exercise inducing anaerobic metabolism, further SNS stimulation provokes a dramatic increase in circulating catecholamines (up to 14 to 18 times baseline), which promotes augmented release of hepatic glucose, FFAs, and ketone bodies and impairs glucose utilization by skeletal muscle, resulting in a rise in BG level both during and immediately after exercise. Following exercise, muscle and hepatic glycogen stores are replenished, which occurs more quickly after intense exercise because of increased insulin release but can take as long as 24 hours after prolonged low- to moderate-intensity exercise.

## Cardiovascular and Pulmonary Complications of Diabetes

Cardiovascular disorders are the most common cause of morbidity and mortality in people with both types of DM. Vascular disease develops as the result of insulin resistance and endothelial dysfunction, which are caused, at least in part, by hyperglycemia-induced glucotoxicity.[125] Proinflammatory states also play an important role. The vast majority of patients with DM will develop CVD[112] as a result of atherosclerosis (macroangiopathies) that commonly manifests as CAD, stroke, and peripheral arterial disease (PAD),[112] which tend to occur at an earlier age and with greater severity than in nondiabetics. Moreover, abnormalities of the small blood vessels (microangiopathies caused by thickening or damage to the capillary basement membrane) often induce damage to the eyes, kidneys, and nerves. Other CV abnormalities that are more prevalent in diabetic patients include HTN, cerebrovascular disease, sinus node dysfunction and AV conduction abnormalities, CHF, PAD, and autonomic neuropathy.

Microvascular disease is much more prevalent than macrovascular disease and occurs earlier in type 1 DM but is often present at the time of diagnosis with type 2 DM[126]; the frequency and degree of damage increase with greater duration of DM. Diabetic retinopathy in the form of microaneurysms, hemorrhages, proliferative retinopathy, and other abnormalities is the most common microvascular complication of diabetes and is the leading cause of new blindness among adults aged 20 to 74 years; its prevalence is estimated to be approximately 40% of adults age 40 years or older known to have DM.[112,127] DM is also the leading cause of chronic renal failure, accounting for 44% of new cases in 2005.[112] Diabetic nephropathy, which develops in approximately half of patients with DM (African Americans, Hispanics, and Native Americans appear to be at particularly high risk) is characterized by progressively increasing proteinuria, which is first manifested as microalbinuria.[128] Last, about 60% to 70% of patients with DM have diabetic neuropathy due to structural damage to nerve fibers induced by metabolic and vascular factors; it is manifested as impaired sensation or pain in the feet or hands, slowed digestion of food in the stomach, carpal tunnel syndrome, erectile dysfunction, autonomic dysfunction, or other nerve problems.[112,129] The combination of peripheral neuropathy and arterial insufficiency gives rise to the common complication of chronic, nonhealing foot ulcers, which affect about 15% of diabetics and may lead to lower extremity amputation.[126] Fortunately, strict glycemic control reduces the risks of developing microvascular disease and its progression: Each percentage point reduction in HbA1c level can decrease the risk of microvascular disease by 40%.[112]

Hyperglycemia and insulin resistance accelerate the development of atherosclerosis, so macrovascular disease, mostly in the form of CAD and stroke, accounts for about two thirds of all deaths in people with DM.[112,130] CAD, which probably results from both macro- and microangiopathy, is often diffuse and may present as angina pectoris, MI, sudden death, and occasionally as unexplained left ventricular failure. Importantly, symptoms associated with myocardial ischemia and infarction are frequently atypical in DM: Both may present "silently," that is, with little or no discomfort, or ischemia may appear as fatigue or dyspnea in the absence of pulmonary disease, which comes on with exertion and resolves within minutes with rest (i.e., angina equivalents). Up to 80% of asymptomatic patients with type 2 DM have been found to have CAD on noninvasive coronary angiography and at autopsy, and more than 50% have multivessel disease.[131,132] Thus, DM is considered a coronary risk equivalent to established CAD. PAD is also common in diabetics, and the risk of PAD complications is increased in patients with a combination of abnormal lipid levels and impaired fibrinolytic activity.[129]

The mortality rate associated with acute MI is approximately two to four times that of adults without diabetes, with the highest risk occurring in women.[112] The majority of deaths result from pump failure or arrhythmias and conduction disturbances and frequently occur up to 1 to 2 months after acute MI. Diabetics appear to have twice the risk of ventricular fibrillation, which often occurs after transfer from the cardiac care unit and is nearly always fatal. Furthermore, diabetic patients with no history of previous CVD have the same long-term morbidity and mortality as nondiabetic individuals with established CVD after hospitalization for unstable CAD or acute MI.[133]

Hypertension is 1.5 to 3 times more prevalent in diabetics as in nondiabetics, and 75% of adults with DM have BP of above the goal of <130/80 mm Hg or take antihypertensive medications.[112,134] This finding is particularly significant because HTN accelerates both the microvascular and macrovascular complications of DM and causes irreversible myocardial damage. Aggressive treatment of even borderline HTN is indicated in diabetics and can reduce the risk of diabetes-related macrovascular disease by 33% to 50% and microvascular disease by approximately 33%.[112,135] In general, for every 10 mm Hg reduction in SBP, the risk for diabetic complications is reduced by 12%.[112]

Diabetes is an independent risk factor for CHF, particularly in women. Both CHF and DM are believed to share the same pathophysiologic processes, including neurohumoral activation, endothelial dysfunction, and increased oxidative stress.[136] DM predisposes patients to the development of CHF, and CHF predisposes patients to the development of DM. CHF is also related to CAD, HTN, obesity, left ventricular hypertrophy, and autonomic dysfunction. There is also a specific diabetic cardiomyopathy that occurs in the absence of CAD and HTN, which appears to result from hyperglycemia-induced myocardial fibrosis and collagen deposition and is characterized by diastolic dysfunction due to impaired myocardial relaxation and subtle systolic dysfunction.[137] Although these changes appear to be reversible with tight glycemic control in the early stages, they become irreversible as the disease process becomes more established. Diabetic patients who develop CHF have a worse prognosis than those without DM, with increased mortality and hospitalizations.

Autonomic neuropathy results from damage to vagal and sympathetic neurons as well as their supporting glia. Diabetic autonomic neuropathy results in reduced awareness of the signs and symptoms of hypoglycemia (which greatly increases the risk of exercise-induced hypoglycemia), impaired thermoregulation as a result of abnormal sweating and cutaneous blood flow regulation, diminished thirst and increased risk of dehydration, impaired night vision due to delayed pupillary reaction, gastroparesis with unpredictable food delivery, and genitourinary dysfunction.[138,139] Cardiovascular autonomic neuropathy (CAN) is common in DM (affecting about one fourth of type 1 and one third of type 2 diabetics), appears early, and its presence is significantly associated with age, duration of DM, microangiopathy, peripheral neuropathy, and with obesity in type 2 DM.[138,139] It should be suspected in all individuals with type 2 DM and in those with type 1 DM for more than 5 years. Once established, CAN is associated with increased morbidity and mortality and a significant deterioration in quality of life.[140,141] Clinical manifestations of CAN include impaired exercise tolerance, orthostatic hypotension, and painless myocardial ischemia and infarction (due to cardiac denervation).[138] Parasympathetic-mediated HR control is affected earlier than sympathetically mediated vasomotor control, giving rise to higher resting HRs and reduced HR variability. When sympathetic dysfunction is added, HRs become slower and the response to exercise is further blunted, and with advanced CAN, the HR becomes fixed and does not change with stress, exercise, or postural changes.[142] CAN is also associated with LV diastolic and sometimes systolic dysfunction in the absence of cardiac disease and an increased risk of sudden death, which may be caused by silent myocardial ischemia, a prolonged QT interval, or other mechanisms.[122,141] Techniques for assessing autonomic function are presented later in this chapter.

The lungs are also affected by DM, with thickening of alveolar endothelial and capillary basal laminae as a result of pulmonary microangiopathy.[143,144] PFTs often shows mild abnormalities in lung elastic recoil, lung volumes, diffusion capacity, and pulmonary capillary blood volume, which are directly related to the duration of DM. In addition, patients with type 1 DM may exhibit reduced respiratory muscle strength and endurance. Individuals with DM are more prone to pulmonary infections, particularly bacterial and viral infections and tuberculosis, and some infections may be associated with increased morbidity and mortality.[143] Diabetics, especially those with autonomic neuropathy, have a higher incidence of sleep-related breathing disorders and central hypoventilation. Diabetic ketoacidosis is related to a number of pulmonary problems, including hyperventilation, pneumomediastinum, mucous plugging of the major airways, and pleuritic chest pain.

## Diabetes and Exercise

Normally, sustained physical activity induces a reduction in insulin secretion and enhanced secretion of the glucagon and the other counterregulatory hormones, which result in stimulation of hepatic glucose production and enhanced mobilization of muscle glycogen and FFAs, so there is adequate fuel to energize the exercising muscles. Reduced insulin secretion is compensated for by a heightened sensitivity and responsiveness of the peripheral tissues to insulin to allow rapid uptake of glucose. Hepatic glucose production intensifies according to glucose requirements such that blood glucose levels remain nearly constant despite large increases in glucose uptake. An exception is continuous high-intensity exercise (>80% of $VO_2$max), which invokes anaerobic metabolism and greater SNS stimulation. The markedly increased catecholamine levels induce increased hepatic glucose production that can exceed peripheral uptake, so BG levels frequently rise during exercise, especially in trained athletes, reaching a peak during the immediate postexercise period.[145-147] In addition, high-intensity exercise is associated with a lesser degree, if any, of reduction in insulin secretion compared to moderate-intensity exercise. It has been hypothesized that the hyperglycemia and relative hyperinsulinemia that occurs with high-intensity exercise may be important in promoting rapid replenishment of depleted muscle glycogen stores. The rising BG levels after cessation of exercise provoke increased insulin secretion, which, combined with the rapid decline in circulating catecholamines, slowly lowers BG to baseline levels during the first hour of recovery. In DM, glucoregulatory defects lead to marked disturbances in glucose homeostasis during exercise, which vary with the type of diabetes and the type, intensity, and duration of activity as well as the levels of circulating insulin and glucose counterregulatory hormones.

In type 1 DM, exercise may have beneficial effects on metabolic control, aerobic capacity, body composition, BP, blood lipids, sense of well-being, quality of life, and ability to cope with stress; in addition, participation in sports promotes social interaction and peer group assimilation, which are important for children and adolescents.[148,149] However, the management of physical activity is complicated in these individuals by the abnormal glucoregulatory responses that require close attention to BG levels and frequent modification of insulin doses and food intake in order to avoid major complications, the most common being hypoglycemia. The metabolic responses to activity are determined by the levels of circulating insulin and the counterregulatory hormones, as indicated by the BG level, both at the onset of exercise (which are determined by the type and dose of insulin administered before exercise and the timing of previous insulin injection and carbohydrate intake relative to the onset of exercise) and during exercise (which are affected by the injection site and the intensity, type, and duration of exercise).

Individuals with type 1 DM are unable to reduce plasma insulin concentration during exercise and are dependent on the level of previously injected insulin. Commonly, there is an excess of circulating insulin in relation to need at the onset of physical activity (Fig. 7-3), which prevents the large increase in peripheral glucose uptake induced by exercise to be matched by augmented hepatic glucose production and impedes the mobilization of FFAs for gluconeogenesis, leading to exercise-induced hypoglycemia.[146,149,150] After exercise, persistent increased insulin sensitivity and mandatory repletion of muscle and liver glycogen stores can lead to late-onset hypoglycemia. Thus, hypoglycemia can occur during, immediately after, or up to at least 24 hours afterwards. Risk factors include intensive insulin therapy and tight glycemic control (so smaller safety margin), inadequate food intake preceding exercise (e.g., when a meal is delayed or skipped), rapid absorption of depot insulin from an injection site near exercising muscle, exercising at the time of peak insulin effect, and prolonged moderate-intensity exercise. Furthermore, in individuals with autonomic neuropathy, the secretion of glucagon and other counterregulatory hormones during exercise may be permanently reduced, and these patients are at even greater risk.

On the other hand, when there is an insulin deficiency with marked hyperglycemia at the onset of exercise (as occurs right after a meal or with poorly controlled DM), glucose uptake by the exercising muscle is hindered, and the release of counterregulatory hormones that is stimulated by exercise provokes additional glucose production by the liver. Thus, hyperglycemia is further aggravated, which can last for several hours after intense exercise.[146,149,150] In addition, the excessive mobilization of FFAs can lead to accelerated ketogenesis and DKA. Therefore, exercise may be contraindicated if resting BG level is above 250 mg/dL, as described in the section on Implications for PT. Furthermore, even well-controlled diabetics may develop hyperglycemia during high-intensity exercise as the result of SNS-activated hepatic glucose production that exceeds the rate of peripheral glucose utilization, and in extremely intense exercise, rising catecholamine levels also promote excessive FFA and ketone body production, which can lead to DKA. Under most circumstances, this is a transient response that resolves within 1 hour.[121]

To allow safe participation in physical activity and high-level athletic performance, persons with type 1 DM must carefully match insulin administration, food intake, and exercise in order to avoid either hypo- or hyperglycemia.[149,151–153] Dietary considerations include carbohydrate control of meals and supplemental carbohydrates (CHO) for exercise. The BG response to a meal varies with its composition. Whereas fats and proteins consumed in healthful amounts have little effect on BG levels, CHO ingestion produces significant postprandial BG excursions and thus increases insulin requirements.[154]

Likewise, adjustments of the dosages of the pre-meal and sometimes the following short-acting insulin boluses may be required to prevent exercise-induced hypoglycemia or, less commonly, hyperglycemia. Insulin dose reductions (typically 30% to 50%) are usually required for the premeal insulin bolus that is administered 1 to 3 hours before low- to moderate-intensity exercise that will be performed for more than 30 minutes during the postmeal period when insulin levels are relatively high; reduction of the insulin dose following exercise may also be needed, especially with prolonged (>60 to 90 minutes) or higher-intensity aerobic exercise. Of note, reductions in insulin dose to prevent hypoglycemia may cause a rebound effect during the recovery period after exercise, resulting in hyperglycemia.

In patients with type 2 DM, exercise plays a central role in the management of their disease because of its beneficial effects on glycemic control and weight loss. Most individuals with type 2 DM have some endogenous insulin secretion, which vary according to need, and contraction-mediated glucose uptake is normal in skeletal muscle (only insulin-mediated glucose uptake is impaired).[155] Therefore, their glucoregulatory responses to exercise differ somewhat from those of type 1 diabetics, although they, too, depend on the type, intensity, and duration of exercise, disease severity and hypoglycemic medications being taken, the timing of exercise onset relative to medication(s) and food intake, and the insulin and BG levels at the onset of exercise. When there is mild to moderate hyperglycemia at the onset of exercise, low- to moderate-intensity exercise increases glucose uptake by the exercising muscle via increased insulin sensitivity, as well as muscle contraction-mediated mechanisms,[145,153] and thus reduces hyperglycemia, especially when performed after eating a meal.[155] Because most medications used for type 2 DM have little or no effect on the counterregulatory responses to impending hypoglycemia, the risk of hypoglycemia is low. Only the insulin secretagogues (sulfonylureas and glinides) are associated with a higher risk of hypoglycemia and may require dose reduction on days of exercise. However, the risk is increased when patients are taking a combination of antihyperglycemic medications that include a sulfonylurea or insulin.[156] Furthermore, the frequency of hypoglycemic reactions increases progressively as serious β-cell dysfunction develops, and most episodes of hypoglycemia that occur in patients referred to physical therapists, including severe episodes, are likely to occur in individuals with type 2 DM. There are limited data describing the responses of individuals

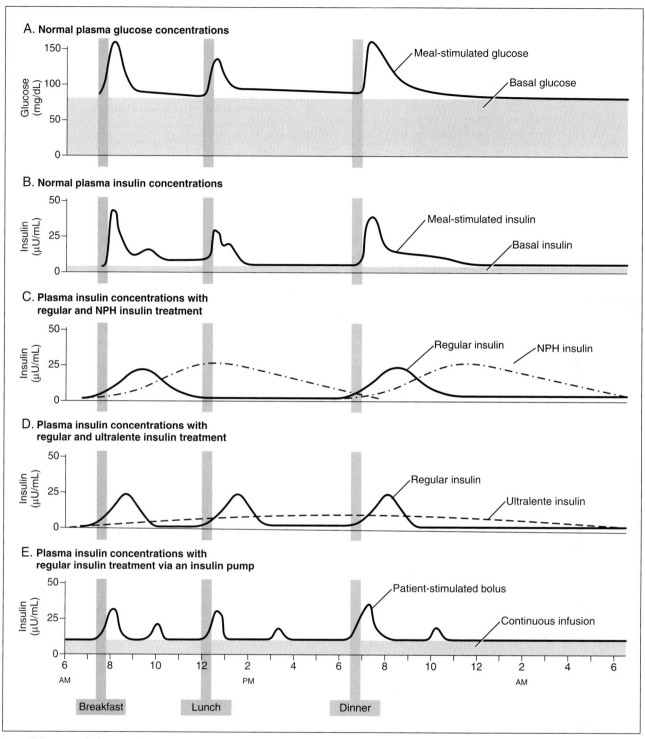

**Figure 7-3** Normal plasma glucose concentrations, endogenous insulin secretion, and exogenous insulin levels produced by various treatment regimens as a function of time and food intake. **A,** Normal plasma glucose concentrations consist of the basal level and meal-stimulated increases. **B,** In healthy individuals, insulin is secreted as the postprandial glucose concentration rises, which acts to increase glucose utilization and return the blood glucose concentration to its basal level. **C-E,** In patients with diabetes mellitus, insulin treatment seeks to mimic the natural secretion of insulin as closely as possible, with different treatment regimens producing different curves, as shown. **C,** Insulin levels resulting from two daily injections of regular insulin and neutral protamine Hagedorn (NPH) insulin, which are given before breakfast and the evening meal. **D,** Insulin levels produced by treatment based on three daily injections of regular insulin, administered before each meal, and one injection of ultralente insulin given at bedtime. **E,** Insulin levels resulting from treatment via an insulin pump, which delivers a constant infusion to fulfill basal insulin requirement as well as patient-activated small bolus injections before meals, snacks, and bedtime. (From Brenner GM. Pharmacology, ed 2. Philadelphia, 2006, Saunders.)

with type 2 DM to high-intensity or intermittent high-intensity exercise.

Resistance exercise is also recommended for all individuals with DM.[157] With appropriate exercise prescription and instruction, resistance training offers many benefits for diabetics, including improved muscle strength and endurance, enhanced flexibility, improved insulin sensitivity and glucose tolerance, enhanced body composition, and reduced CVD risk factors.[158-161] In patients with type 2 DM, the increase in insulin sensitivity induced by resistance training results from enhanced insulin action as well as altered translocation and synthesis of glucose transporters, and beneficial adaptations in muscle fiber area and capillary density were also noted.[158,161,162] Most often, patients participate in moderate-intensity, high-volume training or circuit-type resistance training, although some data indicate that high-intensity training may produce better results.[157,163] A combination of aerobic and resistance exercise provides the greatest benefits.[164,165]

Beyond the complex problems associated with abnormal BG regulation during exercise, individuals with DM often exhibit abnormal CV responses to exercise, especially if they have autonomic neuropathy. In individuals with type 2 DM, exercise capacity is reduced by about 20% compared to nondiabetic controls matched for age, weight, and physical activity level, which appears to be related to diastolic dysfunction.[166,167]

In summary, exercise creates both benefits and risks in patients with DM, as listed in Box 7-2. With proper monitoring of cardiovascular and metabolic responses to exercise and appropriate adjustments in antidiabetic medications and carbohydrate intake, regular physical exercise is safe and extremely beneficial for individuals with DM. In addition to providing the typical cardiovascular and musculoskeletal benefits that are well known, regular physical exercise results in tissue-specific effects that may impede diabetic pathology. In animal models, aerobic training has been shown to increase the level of renal antioxidants, reverse LV contractile abnormalities, and improve myocardial glucose oxidation and glycolytic rate, and thus ameliorate conditions that lead to microvascular complications, especially when initiated early in the disease process.[129]

Studies indicate that higher-intensity aerobic exercise (65% to 80% of VO$_2$max) may have a greater effect on glycemic control and improve aerobic fitness compared with moderate exercise.[147,163,168]

## Treatment of Diabetes

The major goal of treatment for DM is to control hyperglycemia, dyslipidemia, and HTN and thus minimize the resultant long-term damage, dysfunction, and failure of various organs, especially the eyes, kidneys, nerves, heart, and blood vessels. Treatment is individualized and varies according to the type of DM and metabolic status; it may include education, diet modification (high monounsaturated fatty acid [MUFA] and high-fiber diets are particularly beneficial

---

**Box 7-2**

**Benefits and Risks of Regular Exercise in Diabetes**

| Benefits | Risks |
|---|---|
| Possible improved glycemic control, as evidenced by lower HbA1c | Hypoglycemia |
| Increased insulin sensitivity | Worsening hyperglycemia, possible ketoacidosis if poor BG control prior to exercise, especially with high-intensity exercise |
| Reduced risk of CVD, HTN, obesity, osteoporosis, and colon cancer | Abnormal exercise responses (hypertensive BP response during exercise, postexercise orthostatic hypotension) |
| Increased exercise tolerance, muscle strength and endurance, and flexibility | Cardiovascular events (myocardial ischemia or infarction, arrhythmia, sudden death) |
| Enhanced sense of well-being, stress reduction | Possible aggravation of underlying retinopathy or nephropathy |
| Increased overall life expectancy | Musculoskeletal injury, especially if neuropathy is present |
| Reduced risk of developing microvascular disease (retinopathy, nephropathy, and neuropathy) and of its progression | |

BG, blood glucose; CVD, cardiovascular disease; HbA1c, glycosylated hemoglobin; HTN, hypertension.

---

because of improved glycemic control and improved lipoprotein profile),[101] exercise, and insulin therapy and/or oral hypoglycemic agents.

For patients with type I DM, insulin therapy is required for survival and can be provided in a variety of forms. The most common insulin therapy consists of daily injections of insulin preparations, which are listed in Table 7-9. Usually some combination of short-, intermediate-, or long-acting insulin is used in an attempt to mimic a normal physiologic insulin profile, with sharp peaks at mealtimes and maintenance of basal levels between meals and at night (see Fig. 7-3).[152,169-172] The most common regimen for individuals who are reticent to perform frequent BG monitoring consists of twice-daily injections of short-acting and intermediate-acting insulin, with the best results produced using this regimen with a rigid meal schedule.[169] The most effective regimens involve intensive insulin therapy. When compared to the normal insulin profile, it can be seen that patients using insulin injections often oscillate between states of insulin excess and insulin deficiency. Intensive insulin therapy, which allows for the adjustment of insulin doses throughout the day based on the results of frequent blood glucose monitoring (at least three times a day) and other factors, achieves the most normal physiologic levels but requires maximal patient participation and cooperation.

Hypoglycemia is the major problem associated with insulin therapy, because the level of available insulin can exceed the

**Table 7-9 Common Insulin Preparations and Their Properties**

| Type | Agents | Action[a] | | |
|---|---|---|---|---|
| | | Onset | Peak Effect | Duration |
| Rapid-acting insulin analogs | Aspart (NovoLog) | 5–15 min | 30–90 min | 3–5 hr |
| | Glulisine (Apidra) | 5–15 min | 30–90 min | 3–5 hr |
| | Lispro (Humalog) | 5–15 min | 30–90 min | 3–5 hr |
| Short-acting insulin | Regular (Humulin R, Novalin R) | 30–60 min | 2–3 hr | 3–8 hr |
| Intermediate-acting insulin | NPH (Humulin N, Novolin N) | 1.5–4 hr | 4–6 hr | 10–18 hr |
| Long-acting insulin analogs | Glargine (Lantus) | 2–4 hr | None | 20–24 hr |
| | Detemir (Levemir) | 1–4 hr | Mild peak at 6–9 hr | 12–24 hr |
| Premixed insulin preparations | Humulin 70% NPH/30% regular | 30–60 min | 2–3 hr + 4–10 hr | 10–16 hr |
| | Novolin 70% NPH/30% regular | 30–60 min | 2–3 hr + 4–10 hr | 10–16 hr |
| | Humulin 50% NPH/50% regular | 30–60 min | 2–3 hr + 4–10 hr | 10–16 hr |
| | Humalog Mix 75% NPL/25% lispro | 5–15 min | 30–90 min + 4–10 hr | 10–16 hr |
| | NovoLog Mix 70% NPA/30% aspart | 5–15 min | 1–3 hr + 4–10 hr | 10–16 hr |
| | Humalog Mix 50% NPL/50% lispro | 5–15 min | 30–90 min + 4–10 hr | 10–16 hr |

*NPA, neutral protamine aspart (insulin aspart protamine); NPH, neutral protamine Hagedorn; NPL, neutral protamine lispro (insulin lispro protamine)*
[a]*These are approximate figures for human insulins and insulin analogs. There is considerable variation from patient to patient and from time to time in a given patient.*

individual's need at times, especially during the hour or so immediately prior to mealtime or overnight, as shown in Figure 7-3. The risk of hypoglycemia, which is usually mild but can be severe and life-threatening, increases when a meal is delayed or skipped or less food than expected is eaten following insulin injection, an inappropriately large dose of insulin is injected, or glucose uptake is increased (e.g., exercise performed during peak insulin effect, fever, or hypothyroidism). The risk of hypoglycemia is also increased with intensive insulin therapy, which induces severe hypoglycemia (blood glucose <50 mg/dL) more often than standard insulin treatment, and also with autonomic neuropathy, as discussed later.

Newer treatments for type 1 DM that eliminate the need for insulin therapy include pancreas and islet cell transplantation. Because of the need for long-term immunosuppression, with its increased risk of infection, malignancy such as lymphoma, and specific drug toxicity, pancreas transplantation is offered mainly to patients who also require immunosuppression for kidney transplantation.[173]

The treatment of type 2 DM consists of diet, exercise, oral hypoglycemic agents, and sometimes injectables (amylin agonists and insulin). The cornerstones of treatment are diet and exercise, especially for the control of obesity. Antidiabetic agents are prescribed for patients who fail to control their hyperglycemia through diet and exercise. These medications act by increasing insulin sensitivity and improving peripheral glucose uptake (biguanides and thiazolidinediones [also referred to as glitazones]), increasing insulin secretion (insulin secretagogues [sulfonylureas and non-sulfonylurea

secretagogues, or glinides]), inhibiting glucose absorption in the GI tract (α-glucosidase inhibitors; incretin potentiators, i.e., glucagon-like peptide-1 [GLP-1] receptor agonists and dipeptidyl-peptidase-4 [DPP-4] inhibitors; and amylase agonists), reducing hepatic glucose release (biguanides, incretin potentiators, DPP-4 inhibitors, amylin agonists, and insulin), and replacing endogenous insulin secretion (insulin), as listed in Table 7-10).[120,152,169,174–177]

During the early stages of type 2 DM, therapies to improve β-cell function using an oral antihyperglycemic agent, along with diet and exercise interventions, are usually effective in controlling blood glucose levels. However, as the disease progresses, combinations of agents are often required. Because glucoregulatory control changes continuously throughout the course of type 2 DM, constant monitoring and adjustments of the therapy are crucial to maintain glycemic control, which typically worsens within 5 years of initiating antihyperglycemic therapy.

For patients with extreme obesity, bariatric surgery produces marked weight loss as well as amelioration of many of the metabolic abnormalities in type 2 DM. Most patients are able to reduce their dosage of antidiabetic medications or go into complete remission within 1 year after surgery. Interestingly, there is a dramatic improvement in metabolic status within just a few days of surgery, even before any meaningful weight loss has occurred, which are due to changes in the release of gut-derived hormones induced by rerouting of nutrients.[85,87] In addition, bariatric surgery appears to slow the progression of macroangiopathies, resulting in reduced incidences of coronary events and numbers of revascularization

**Table 7-10 Antihyperglycemic Medications for Type 2 Diabetes Mellitus**

| | Type and Drugs | Mechanism of Action | Adverse Effects |
|---|---|---|---|
| Insulin sensitizers | Biguanides<br><br>Metformin (Glucophage) | Decreased hepatic gluconeogenesis,<br>Decreased intestinal absorption of glucose,<br>Increased peripheral insulin sensitivity | GI symptoms (anorexia, nausea, abdominal discomfort, diarrhea), especially during initiation of treatment<br>Rare lactic acidosis, mainly if renal insufficiency<br>Hypoglycemia only if combination therapy |
| | Thiazolidinediones or glitazones<br><br>Rosiglitazone (Avandia)<br>Pioglitazone (Actos) | Decreased peripheral and hepatic insulin resistance so increased insulin-dependent glucose uptake and decreased gluconeogenesis | Generally well tolerated<br>New or worsening peripheral edema, possible increased HF risk<br>Occasional hepatotoxicity<br>Possible hypoglycemia several weeks after adding a TZD to a sulfonylurea |
| Insulin secretagogues | Sulfonylureas<br><br>Acetohexamide (Dymelor)<br>Chlorpropamide (Diabinese)<br>Tolazamide (Tolinase)<br>Tolbutamide (Orinase, Oramide)<br>Glipizide (Glucotrol)<br>Glyburide (Micronase, DiaBeta)<br>Glimepiride (Amaryl) | Stimulate pancreatic β-cells to an increase in insulin production (independent of BG level)<br>May also increase peripheral insulin sensitivity<br>Glipizide, Glyburide, and Glimepiride are second-generation, more potent sulfonylureas, and act as above | Hypoglycemia, usually subclinical or minor but occasionally life-threatening, with increased risk in patients with irregular eating habits and excessive alcohol intake<br>Uncommon sensitivity reactions<br>Weight gain (~1–4 lb) |
| | Glinides[a]<br><br>Repaglinide (Prandin)<br>Nateglinide (Starlix) | Stimulate rapid but short-lived release of insulin following ingestion of food | Hypoglycemia (lower incidence than sulfonylureas)<br>Sensitivity reactions (usually transient)<br>Possible small weight gain |

| | | | |
|---|---|---|---|
| Glucose absorption inhibitors | α-Glucosidase inhibitors | Acarbose (Precose, Glucobay) Miglitol (Glyset) | Delay absorption of carbohydrates in small intestine, so decreased rise in postprandial BG | GI symptoms (flatulence, abdominal cramps, sometimes diarrhea), which subside over time; hypoglycemia only if therapy combined with sulfonylurea or insulin |
| | Incretin potentiators | GLP-1 receptor agonists Exenatide (Byetta) | Increased insulin secretion with glucose ingestion, decreased postprandial glucagon secretion, delay gastric emptying | Nausea, which usually improves over time, but rare instances of unremitting nausea, mainly in patients with gastroparesis |
| | | DPP-4 inhibitors Sitagliptin (Januvia) | Increased insulin release and decreased glucagon secretion in glucose-dependent manner | Generally well tolerated Stuffy or runny nose, sore throat, URI, headache, diarrhea, joint pain, UTI |
| | Amylin agonists | Pramlintide (Symlin) | Slow gastric emptying, decreased glucagon secretion, suppress appetite | Nausea, which usually improves over time Hypoglycemia, especially during first month of treatment |
| Combination drugs | | Glyburide/metformin (Glucovance) Glipizide/metformin (Metaglip) Metformin/rosiglitazone (Avandamet) Rosiglitazone/glimepiride (Avandaryl) Pioglitazone/metformin (Actoplus Met) | Per individual drugs | See individual drugs |

*DPP-4, dipeptidyl-peptidase-4; GI, gastrointestinal; GLP-1, glucagon-like peptide-1; HF, heart failure; TZDs, thiazolidinediones; URI, upper respiratory tract infection; UTI, urinary tract infection.*
[a]*Also referred to as non-sulfonylurea or rapid-acting secretagogues.*

procedures, improves the functional and physiologic indices of HF, and reduces overall mortality, including CV and cancer deaths.[57,86]

Lastly, the reduction of other CV risk factors, such as HTN, dyslipidemias, and smoking, is crucial in patients with DM for limiting morbidity and mortality.

## Clinical Implications for Physical Therapy

Given the abnormal glucoregulatory responses of diabetics to exercise and the prevalence of cardiovascular complications, caution is required when providing physical therapy (PT) to patients with DM. Therefore, patients should be questioned to determine if they have DM and if so, further information should be obtained including the type and duration of DM, presence of any diabetes complications and CV risk factors, and how their disease is managed, including frequency of self-monitoring of BG levels and most recent HbA1c level. Based on each patient's specifics, several factors need to be considered, including the necessity of pretreatment medical screening; the importance of HR, BP, and blood glucose monitoring; the potential for exercise-induced hypoglycemia; attention to the timing of exercise; and the intensity, mode, and duration of exercise.

Because of the increased incidence of CVD, including asymptomatic myocardial ischemia and infarction, higher-risk patients (age >40 years, age >30 years with known CVD risk factors, any age if known or suspected CVD, autonomic neuropathy, or advanced nephropathy) should have a thorough medical evaluation, including exercise testing whenever possible, prior to starting exercise training at intensities greater than brisk walking. Ideally, adequate metabolic control should also be established before an exercise program is initiated. In the acute care setting, these precautions are frequently ignored, especially when the admitting diagnosis is not cardiac in nature. In any event, in as much as so many patients with DM exhibit abnormal hemodynamic responses to activity, HR and BP monitoring should be included in all PT evaluations and at least during the initial treatment sessions as well. Exercise is contraindicated if resting SBP is >200 mm Hg or DBP is >100 mm Hg. Diabetics who do not have autonomic dysfunction frequently have hypertensive responses to exercise, as well as postexercise hypotension. As described in the section on exercise and DM, patients with autonomic dysfunction exhibit impaired exercise tolerance with abnormal HR and BP responses and hypoglycemia unawareness.

Autonomic dysfunction, including cardiovascular autonomic neuropathy, is fairly common in diabetics and is associated with increased risk for silent ischemia and impaired exercise tolerance, so assessment of HR control and vascular dynamics as indicators of autonomic function is recommended as part of the PT evaluation for individuals with type 1 DM for more than 5 years and all patients with type 2 DM (Table 7-11).

A simple method of assessing SNS function is to measure the BP response to standing from the supine position, which normally produces a fall in SBP of less than 10 mm Hg in 30 seconds and a rise in diastolic BP of more than 16 mm Hg.[139] A drop in SBP of more than 30 mm Hg within 2 minutes of standing or in DBP of more than 10 mm Hg may be indicative of SNS dysfunction.[141]

A more reliable technique involves the measurement of the DBP response to sustained isometric contraction using a handgrip dynamometer; after determining maximum force, the individual squeezes the grip at 30% max for 5 min, toward the end of which a BP is obtained on the opposite arm. The normal response is a rise in diastolic BP of more than 16 mm Hg and a drop in DBP of more than 10 mm Hg is indicative of abnormal SNS function.[139,141]

Monitoring of BG levels is recommended before, after, and several hours after new patterns of exercise are undertaken, at least until the glycemic response can be predicted, given a stable exercise schedule relative to insulin dose and timing as well as food intake. BG monitoring is essential for determining appropriate strategies to prevent hypo- and hyperglycemia. By taking measurements 60 and 30 minutes before exercise, the trend of BG changes can be identified and it will be clear whether the patient is likely to require adjustments in carbohydrate intake or insulin dosage to avoid hypoglycemia or is likely to develop hyperglycemia.[147,150] Postexercise BG monitoring should be performed every 2 hours to avoid late-onset hypoglycemia.[147] Clearly, both patients and clinicians will benefit from the availability of continuous glucose monitors, but current technology produces a significant time delay and often fails to provide accurate BG values.[146]

When BG levels are elevated before PT, adjustments in treatment may be indicated. If BG values are 250 to 300 mg/dL and the patient is using insulin, she or he should check for ketosis (via urine stick or BG meter that measures ketones). If no ketones are detected and the BG is stable or falling, or if the patient is taking oral medications, and she or he feels good and is well hydrated, the individual can proceed with low- to moderate-intensity exercise for 10 to 15 minutes and then should recheck the BG level.[150] If BG has risen, exercise should be terminated, but if it has dropped, exercise can be continued with repeat BG monitoring every 15 minutes and adequate hydration. Of note, the risk of aggravated hyperglycemia is increased during sports competitions, beginning with anticipation of performance, because of stress-induced augmented catecholamine release. If ketones are detected or if BG exceeds 300 mg/dL, no exercise should be performed, at least until more insulin is administered and hyperglycemia and ketoacidosis resolve.[147,150]

If BG levels are low (70 to 100 mg/dL) and levels are falling before PT, the individual should eat a carbohydrate snack and wait until the hypoglycemia has been corrected before initiating exercise (typically 20 to 30 minutes). If marked hypoglycemia is present (<70 mg/dL), exercise is contraindicated and a snack should be ingested.

Because PT activities may cause either hypoglycemia or hyperglycemia in diabetics, therapists must be cognizant of the signs and symptoms of these abnormal states, as described

**Table 7-11 Simple Tests of Cardiovascular Autonomic Neuropathy**

| Test | PNS vs SNS | Methods and Diagnostic Parameters |
|---|---|---|
| Resting HR | PNS–SNS balance | >100 bpm is abnormal |
| HR variability with deep breathing | PNS | With the patient resting in supine position, she or he performs paced deep breathing at 6/min while HR is measured by ECG or other device to determine HR variability<br>Normal response:<br>  15–20 bpm[a]<br>Abnormal response:<br>  <10 bpm or R-R expiration/R-R inspiration >1.17[b] |
| HR response to standing | PNS | ECG is recorded continuously with the patient at rest and supine and with rising to stand to compare the R-R intervals measured at beats 15 and 30 after standing<br>Normal response:<br>  Tachycardia followed by reflex bradycardia, producing a 30:15 ratio >1.03<br>Abnormal response:<br>  Ratio of ≤1.0 |
| BP response to standing | SNS | BP is measured with the patient supine and again 2 min after rising to stand<br>Normal response:<br>  Decrease in SBP of <10 mm Hg and increase in DBP of >16 mm Hg<br>Abnormal response:<br>  Decrease in SBP of >30 mm Hg or decrease in DBP of >10 mm Hg |
| DBP response to sustained isometric exercise | SNS | After establishing maximum force by performing a maximal contraction on a handgrip dynamometer, the grip is squeezed at 30% maximum for 5 min and toward the end a BP is obtained in the other arm<br>Normal response:<br>Increase in DBP of >16 mm Hg<br>Abnormal response:<br>Decrease in DBP of >10 mm Hg |

*BP, blood pressure; bpm, beats per minute; DBP, diastolic blood pressure; ECG, electrocardiogram; HR, heart rate; PNS, parasympathetic nervous system; SBP, systolic blood pressure; SNS, sympathetic nervous system.*
*[a]All indexes of HR variability are age-dependent.*
*[b]Lowest normal value of R-R expiration/inspiration ratio is 1.17 for ages 25–29 years, 1.15 for ages 30–34, 1.13 for ages 35–39, 1.10 for ages 40–44, 1.08 for ages 45–49, 1.07 for ages 50–54, 1.06 for ages 55–59, 1.04 for ages 60–64, 1.03 for ages 65–69, and 1.02 for ages 70–74.*

in Tables 7-12 and 7-13. Notably, some of the same symptoms occur with both hypo- and hyperglycemia. In addition, individuals with poor glycemic control often have an impaired ability to sense even major changes in BG levels. The bottom line is that any change in a patient's symptoms or behavior should be an indication to check BG level. No universal guidelines can be applied to daily diabetes management; however, general recommendations based on exercise intensity and duration have been published (Table 7-14).[149,150,178]

To reduce risk of hypoglycemia related to the injection site, diabetics should avoid injecting insulin into tissue near the exercising muscles particularly if patient will be exercising within 40 minutes after regular insulin or within 90 minutes after intermediate insulin. Injection in the abdomen or arm is preferable to the leg, and rotation within the same site is recommended over using different sites.[149]

Interestingly, exercise does not appear to affect the absorption rate of the long-acting insulin analogue glargine.[147]

In individuals with type 2 DM who take oral antihyperglycemic agents, the risk of hypoglycemia is generally very low. Only the insulin secretagogues (sulfonylureas and glinides) are associated with a higher risk of hypoglycemia, and typically a 50% dose reduction is recommended on the days of exercise (unless patient exercises on a daily basis and dosages have already been adjusted accordingly).[123] Patients with type 2 DM should avoid exercise if BG is more than 400 mg/dL, which is usually related to overeating.

Dietary adjustments are important for diabetics to prevent hypo- and hyperglycemic reactions as well as to meet their increased caloric and fluid requirements. To maximize endogenous energy stores, a meal containing 200 to 350 g of CHO along with fats and protein should be ingested about 3 to 6 hours before a sports competition. In addition, in the

## Table 7-12 Signs and Symptoms of Hypoglycemia

| Hypoglycemic reactions | Adrenergic[a] | Neuroglycopenic[b] |
|---|---|---|
| Mild<br>(BG ≤60–70 mg/dL) | Tremor or shakiness<br>Anxiety and nervousness<br>Tachycardia<br>Palpitations<br>Increased sweating<br>Excessive hunger | |
| Moderate<br>(BG ~40–50 mg/dL) | Irritability and abrupt mood changes<br>Weakness<br>Dizziness<br>Numbness or tingling of lips and tongue<br>Nausea or vomiting (rare) | Headache<br>Lethargy, drowsiness<br>Impaired concentration and attentiveness<br>Blurred vision<br>Mental confusion<br>Nightmares<br>Nighttime restlessness or inability to go back to sleep<br>Night sweats |
| Severe[c] | | Loss of consciousness<br>Seizures<br>Coma<br>Death |

[a]*Caused by increased activity of the autonomic nervous system*
[b]*Caused by decreased activity of the central nervous system*
[c]*Definitions of severe hypoglycemia vary and include hypoglycemia, resulting in a seizure or a coma, reactions that require the intervention of another person, or a reaction that requires the administration of intravenous glucose, intramuscular glucagon, or hospitalization.*

## Table 7-13 Signs and Symptoms of Hyperglycemia and Ketoacidosis

| | Adrenergic[a] | Neuroglycopenic[b] |
|---|---|---|
| Mild to moderate hyperglycemia[c] | Frequent urination<br>Dry mouth, increased thirst | Weakness or fatigue |
| More marked hyperglycemia | Increased hunger<br>Flu-like achiness | Headache<br>Blurred vision |
| Serious ketoacidosis | Facial flushing<br>Dry skin<br>Nausea or vomiting<br>Abdominal pain<br>Deep, rapid breathing<br>Fruity-smelling breath | Coma<br>Death |

[a]*Caused by increased activity of the autonomic nervous system*
[b]*Caused by decreased activity of the central nervous system*
[c]*Perceptions of hyperglycemia vary among individuals: Some persons notice symptoms only when blood glucose is very high, whereas others notice symptoms with more mild degrees of hyperglycemia.*

absence of hyperglycemia, excessive heat and humidity, or competition stress, the performance of moderate-to-high intensity exercise is enhanced by a CHO beverage containing 6% to 8% simple sugar, which optimizes absorption, or a low-fat CHO snack (e.g., crackers, fruit, yogurt) that provides 1 g CHO/kg body weight ingested approximately 1 hour before exercise; alternatively, for exercise lasting less than 45 minutes, a pre-exercise CHO snack of about 15 to 30 g consumed 15 to 30 minutes before exercise is usually adequate.[123,147,179]

## Table 7-14 General Strategies for Limiting Blood Glucose Excursions Associated with Exercise

| | |
|---|---|
| Before exercise | Determine the timing, mode, duration, and intensity of exercise |
| | Eat a carbohydrate meal (CHO = 60% of total calories) 1–3 hr before exercise |
| | Assess BG control 60 and 30 min before planned exercise to determine the trend in BG control: |
| |     If BG is <70 mg/dL, supplemental CHO should be consumed (generally 15–30 g) and BG should be reassessed after 15–30 min. If BG is still low, repeat process until hypoglycemia resolves |
| |     If BG is 70–90 mg/dL and levels are falling, supplemental CHO may be needed. |
| |     If BG is 90–250 mg/dL, supplemental CHO may not be needed, depending on the duration and intensity of exercise and individual response to exercise. |
| |     If BG is >250 mg/dL and ketones are present, additional insulin is required (inject into site away from exercising muscle), and delay exercise until BG level is normalized. |
| | If anticipated exercise is aerobic, estimate energy expenditure and determine if adjustment in insulin dose and/or additional CHO will be needed based on peak insulin activity. |
| | If aerobic exercise is to be performed for at least 30 min, the premeal insulin dose given 1–3 hr before exercise should be reduced according to the exercise intensity and duration: 25% dose reduction for mild exercise (~25%–40% VO$_2$max) lasting 30 min, 50% dose reduction for mild exercise lasting 60 min or moderate exercise (~40%–60% VO$_2$max) lasting 30 min, and 75% dose reduction for moderate exercise lasting 60 min or higher-intensity exercise (~60%–70% VO2max) lasting 30 min.[a] |
| | If CSII is provided using a pump and anticipated exercise is higher-intensity and longer-duration, consider reducing basal insulin dose by up to 50%, depending on exercise intensity, at least 90 min before the onset of exercise. |
| | If supplemental CHO is to be ingested, the goal is to match utilization of glucose by the exercising muscle, generally estimated at 1 g/kg body weight/hr of moderate- to high-intensity aerobic exercise performed during peak insulin activity and less CHO as the time since insulin injection increases. The total dose of CHO should be divided equally and consumed at 20- to 30-min intervals. The amount of CHO can be adjusted on subsequent exercise days based on the measured individual response. |
| | If anticipated exercise is anaerobic (≈15 min at >65%–80% VO$_2$max) or will occur during heat or accompanied by competition stress, no reduction in insulin dose or supplemental CHO should be used. If anaerobic exercise is prolonged, additional insulin may be required. If using CSII via a pump, consider administering a correction insulin bolus using the sensitivity index for the immediate postexercise BG at least 90 min before exercise; if such correction boluses are needed on a consistent basis, the basal insulin dose can be increased beginning 90 min before such exercise. |
| | Consider fluid intake to maintain hydration (~250 mL 20 min before exercise) |
| During exercise | Monitor BG every 30 min |
| | If required, consume CHO at 20- to 30-min intervals |
| | Alternatively, consider inserting short bouts of intense anaerobic exercise periodically throughout aerobic exercise to blunt exercise-induced hypoglycemia |
| | If using SCII via a pump, continue reduced basal insulin dose, adjusting according to measured individual response |
| | Continue fluid intake (250 mL every 20–30 min) |
| After exercise | Monitor BG, including overnight, if amount of exercise is not habitual |
| | Consider reducing insulin dose to decrease immediate and delayed insulin action |
| | If using SCII via a pump, continue reduced basal insulin dose, adjusting according to measured individual response, for at least 90 min after exercise |
| | Consider consuming additional slow-acting CHO to protect against postexercise late-onset hypoglycemia |
| | If anaerobic or competitive exercise or exercise performed in warm and humid conditions is known to produce prolonged or pronounced hyperglycemia, consider administering additional insulin immediately after exercise |

BG = blood glucose concentration; CHO = carbohydrate.
[a]Adjustment of insulin dose varies according to individual responses to exercise and dose adjustment. It is a trial-and-error process that requires experience, such that dosages are adjusted on subsequent exercise days based on the measured response.

Resistance training is most effective at improving glycemic control when high-intensity exercise targeting all major muscle groups is performed in 3 sets of 8 to 10 repetitions at a weight that induces near fatigue after 8 to 10 reps three times a week.[157,180] Greater CVD risk reduction is achieved with at least 4 hours/week of moderate to vigorous aerobic, resistance, or combined exercise,[163] but larger volumes of exercise (7 hours/week) are more successful in achieving and maintaining major weight loss.[97]

A few other factors should be emphasized in the care of diabetics. First, diabetics should practice good foot care by wearing proper shoes and cotton socks, inspecting feet after exercise, and maintaining good hygiene. Patients with severe peripheral neuropathy should engage in non–weight-bearing exercise to reduce the risk of skin breakdown, infection, and the development of Charcot joint destruction. Second, diabetics should never exercise alone and should always carry medical identification and supplemental CHO. Lastly, patients should be alerted to the possibility of delayed exercise-induced hypoglycemia, which may occur up to 24 or more hours after exercise.

In patients with type 2 DM, medications used to treat comorbidities can affect exercise responses. Diuretics can decrease or increase potassium levels, leading to various arrhythmias. Diuretics and β-blockers may impair thermoregulation during exercise, particularly when it is hot and humid. β-Blockers attenuate the HR response to exercise and may reduce exercise capacity and exercise performance. Aspirin and angiotensin-converting enzyme (ACE) inhibitors may increase the patient's susceptibility to hypoglycemia.

## Chronic Kidney Disease and Failure

The kidneys are complex organs whose major functions include the control of extracellular fluid volume, the regulation of serum osmolality, electrolyte and acid–base balances, and the secretion of hormones such as renin and erythropoietin. Thus, when renal function becomes impaired, the resultant metabolic disturbances affect virtually every other body system. Impairment of glomerular filtration results in renal insufficiency or failure, which can be staged according to severity (Table 7-15). Chronic kidney disease (CKD) is usually an insidious process that is generally asymptomatic initially (Stages 1 and 2), being manifested only as microalbuminuria and increasing glomerular filtration rate (GFR), and later presents with symptoms of only vague general malaise and ill health (Stages 3 and 4) until late in its progression. Only when renal failure becomes marked (Stage 5), with the accumulation of water, crystalloid solutes and waste products, are the symptoms of uremia manifested: altered electrolyte homeostasis and acid–base imbalance, GI distress, severe anemia, and multiple other abnormalities involving the skin, respiratory, cardiovascular, neurological, musculoskeletal, endocrine, genitourinary, and immune systems.

Risk factors for CKD include DM, HTN, CVD, and obesity.[181] Other less common but important etiologies include primary glomerulonephritis, lupus, and polycystic kidney disease. On rare occasions, CKD can develop as a complication of overuse of some common drugs, such as aspirin, ibuprofen, acetaminophen, and cocaine. The major sequelae of CKD include development and progression of CVD (the most common cause of morbidity and mortality), anemia, bone disease, and continued progression of the disease toward CRF.

Renal failure sometimes results from acute kidney injury (AKI), such as poor renal blood flow while on cardiopulmonary bypass or drug overdose, and is characterized by rapidly progressive loss of renal function, which is potentially reversible with proper treatment, including dialysis until the kidneys recover sufficient function. More commonly, it results from a progressive and irreversible chronic disease that affects the kidneys, such as DM (~40% of cases), HTN (~25% of cases), and CHF (~50% of cases).[182–185] On occasion, AKI can occur on top of CKD, which is referred to as acute-on-chronic renal failure (AoCRF).

## Table 7-15 Stages of Chronic Kidney Disease and Corresponding CV Risk

| Stage | Description | GFR (mL/min per 1.73 m$^2$) | CV Risk[a] (Odds Ratio, Univariate) |
|-------|-------------|------------------------------|--------------------------------------|
| 1[b] | Kidney damage with normal or increased GFR | ≥90 | Depends on degree of proteinuria |
| 2 | Kidney damage with mildly decreased GFR | 60–89 | 1.5 |
| 3 | Moderately decreased GFR | 30–59 | 2–4 |
| 4 | Severely decreased GFR | 15–29 | 4–10 |
| 5 | Kidney failure | <15 or dialysis | 10–50–1000 if ESRD |

Data from Schiffrin EL, Lipman ML, Mann JFE. Chronic kidney disease: Effects on the cardiovascular system. Circulation 116:85–97, 2007.
CKD, chronic kidney disease; CV, cardiovascular; ESRD, end-stage renal disease (indicating the need for renal replacement therapy); GFR, glomerular filtration rate
[a]The increase in CV risk in comparison with people free of CKD depends on the age of the population studied: the younger the person, the higher the relative risk. Microalbuminemia increases the CV risk two- to fourfold.
[b]Stage 1 CKD is mostly recognized by either albuminuria or structural renal abnormality (usually identified using ultrasound).

Chronic renal failure (CRF) is associated with a number of major health problems: HTN, pericarditis with pericardial effusion and sometimes cardiac tamponade, accelerated atherosclerosis, anemia, bleeding disorders, renal osteodystrophy (bone changes resembling osteomalacia and rickets occurring in patients with chronic renal failure), proximal myopathy (wasting and weakness of the proximal skeletal muscles), peripheral neuropathy, peptic ulceration, and immunosuppression leading to intercurrent infections.[186] Although most of these complications are reversible with frequent dialysis, patients maintained on dialysis can develop other problems, as will be described later.

## Cardiovascular and Pulmonary Complications of Chronic Kidney Disease

Chronic kidney disease and renal failure are associated with a number of cardiovascular and pulmonary complications.

### Cardiovascular Complications

Chronic kidney disease increases the risk of major CV events, which appears even with relatively minor renal abnormalities, such as slightly reduced GFR or microalbuminuria occurring within the normal range, and intensifies in proportion to the severity of the disease, as shown in Table 7-15. Decreasing renal function results in a number of abnormalities involving changes in coagulation, fibrinolysis, endothelial dysfunction, anemia, calcium–phosphorous balance, renin–angiotensin–aldosterone system, lipid abnormalities, and arrhythmia.[182,183,187] By the time patients require dialysis, 40% have evidence of CAD and 85% of these patients have abnormal LV structure and mass.[183] The annual mortality rate for patients with end-stage renal disease (ESRD) is above 20%, and approximately 50% of deaths are related to CVD, particularly MI, CHF, and stroke.[182,183,187] In fact, death due to CVD complications is more common in patients with CKD than progression to CRF.

Hypertension is almost invariably present as it is both a cause and a consequence of renal disease and greatly aggravates renal dysfunction in CKD, particularly in African Americans. About 50% to 75% of individuals with Stage 3 or greater CKD have HTN and left ventricular hypertrophy (LVH), which accelerates CV morbidity and mortality due to CAD, stroke, and PAD.[188] Additionally, LVH increases the incidence of myocardial ischemia, leading to further impairment of LV function. LVH is also aggravated by anemia, and there is some evidence that treatment of anemia with erythropoietin ameliorates LVH and improves survival.[189] Treatment is usually initiated for BP ≥130/≥80 mm Hg and almost always consists of ACE inhibitors or ARBs, which are known to delay progression of CKD and reduce CV mortality; most patients require multiple antihypertensive medications, often three to four, to achieve adequate BP control. Also, HTN commonly develops in kidney transplant recipients, often as a complication of the antirejection medication cyclosporine and contributes to graft loss and premature death; newer immunosuppressive regimens are associated with lower rates of HTN.

Accelerated atherosclerosis is related to numerous CV risk factors commonly seen in patients with CKD: DM and insulin resistance, HTN, dyslipidemia, and obesity. Endothelial dysfunction, low-grade inflammation, enhanced coagulability, and hyperhomocysteinuria observed in CKD contribute to higher prevalences of CAD, cerebrovascular accident (CVA) and TIA, and PAD.[182,183] Morbidity and mortality rates are elevated following acute MI and coronary revascularization procedures and are directly related to the degree of renal dysfunction.[183,187]

Heart failure is also prevalent in CKD, occurring in about 40% of those more than 65 years of age, and 65% to 70% of patients with ESRD have CHF.[184] Not only is it likely that CKD itself is a major contributor to severe cardiac damage, but it also appears that CHF is a major cause of progressive CKD, as about half of patients with CHF have some degree of CKD. The codependence between the kidneys and heart also leads to the cardiorenal syndrome, which includes the presence of renal insufficiency, diuretic resistance, anemia, tendency to hyperkalemia, and low SBP and is related to anemia, microalbuminuria, and calcium–phosphorous imbalance.[190] Treatment with ACE inhibitors and ARBs reduces mortality rates for both CHF and CKD. Other causes of CHF in individuals with CKD include HTN, CAD, DM and increased insulin resistance, anemia, and hypervolemia between renal replacement treatments.

Other CV abnormalities that occur as complications of CKD and CRF include coronary microvascular dysfunction (producing myocardial ischemia), cardiac autonomic neuropathy (~75% of patients show reduced HR variability),[178] and uremia-induced pericarditis and pericardial effusion (which occasionally leads to cardiac tamponade).

### Pulmonary Complications

Acute or chronic renal failure is also associated with a number of pulmonary complications. Pulmonary edema is the most serious problem and may be due to fluid overload hypoalbuminemia, and possibly increased pulmonary microvascular permeability (in addition to CHF). Fibrinous pleuritis is found in 20% to 40% of patients who die of CRF and is manifested as pleuritic chest pain with pleural rubs, pleural effusion, or fibrothorax.[191] Other pulmonary complications that occur in patients with CRF include pulmonary calcification that may be induced by secondary hyperparathyroidism, pleural effusion due to uremia, and an increased risk of respiratory tract infection, especially tuberculosis and pneumonia, probably caused by pathological changes in the respiratory tract and impaired immune function. There is evidence of respiratory muscle weakness, contributing to restrictive lung dysfunction, in patients with ESRD, which improves following renal transplantation.

The treatment of ESRD is often associated with pulmonary complications. The majority of patients treated with hemodialysis show a decrease in arterial oxygen concentration ($PaO_2$) during treatment, which results from hypoventilation induced by loss of $CO_2$ or metabolic alkalosis, depending on the type of dialysate used.[192]

Other forms of treatment are also associated with pulmonary abnormalities. Peritoneal dialysis is commonly associated with pleural effusions and an elevated diaphragm. Renal transplantation is complicated by pulmonary problems in an estimated 18% to 24% of patients, which include opportunistic pulmonary infections (pneumonia and tuberculosis) due to immunosuppression, pulmonary edema, pulmonary thromboembolism, and pulmonary calcification.[193,194] In addition, immunosuppression with sirolimus following transplantation is sometimes complicated by pleural effusion and interstitial pneumonitis.

## Treatment of Chronic Renal Failure

The primary goals of treatment for CKD are to retard the rate of progressive deterioration in renal function and to minimize the complications of CRF. Preventive measures to limit disease progression include ACE inhibitors or angiotensin–receptor blockers to thwart the renin–angiotensin–aldosterone system and control BP, statins for dyslipidemia, early treatment of anemia to achieve hemoglobin levels of 11 to 12 g/dL, intensive hyperglycemia management, and smoking cessation.[127,182,188] Primary and secondary prevention strategies to reduce the risk of CVD and associated mortality are also essential, and patients are usually prescribed a number of medications: β-blockers, calcium channel blockers, and ACE inhibitors or angiotensin-receptor blockers to control BP and HF and to provide secondary prevention following MI, and statins to improve lipid abnormalities and inhibit inflammatory processes involved in plaque formation.

When the symptoms or complications of CKD become unacceptable, renal replacement therapy (RRT) is indicated and is most commonly accomplished using hemodialysis or peritoneal dialysis. Dialysis is a process that replaces the excretory functions of the kidney through the use of a semipermeable membrane and a rinsing solution (dialysate) to filter out toxic waste substances from the blood. Dialysis also allows for control of fluid and electrolyte balances. However, RRT fails to adequately provide the regulatory and endocrine functions normally afforded by the kidneys and is associated with renal osteodystrophy, anemia, vascular access infections and thromboses, pericarditis, and ascites.

In standard hemodialysis, patients go to an outpatient dialysis center, typically three days/week to be connected to a dialysis machine (dialyzer) through an arteriovenous fistula or venous graft; the treatment typically takes 3 to 4 hours, but can take longer in very large individuals. The same treatment is used for inpatients when they are hospitalized for some reason. Many patients undergo peritoneal dialysis, whereby a dialysis fluid is introduced into the peritoneal cavity via a permanent catheter placed in the abdominal wall and remains for several hours while waste products and extra fluid are filtered out from the vascular system through the peritoneal membrane into the dialysate solution. In continuous ambulatory peritoneal dialysis (CAPD), the used fluid from the previous treatment is drained from the abdomen after a few hours of "dwell time" and new fluid is introduced;

this is a manual procedure that requires no machine and the fluid exchanges are performed four times/day.

Although many patients do well for more than 10 years on dialysis, success is limited by the impaired clearance of waste products and other substances and the marked impairment of the regulatory and endocrine functions normally provided by the kidneys. Therefore, the treatment of choice for ESRD, particularly in younger patients, is kidney transplantation. It offers the best opportunity for normalization of renal function and lifestyle, but its application is dependent on organ availability. Furthermore, transplantation can be complicated by a number of early and late immunologic, surgical, and medical events, as well as problematic side effects of the immunosuppressive medications that are required.

## Exercise and Chronic Kidney Disease and Failure

Patients with CKD exhibit impaired exercise tolerance and reduced muscle strength and endurance, which become more limiting as kidney disease progresses. Contributory factors include anemia, CVD, chronic physical inactivity, skeletal muscle dysfunction, and metabolic acidosis. In most patients with ESRD, exercise capacity is reduced to approximately 50% to 60% of normal.[178,195,196] However, it is important to keep in mind that these values were determined from studies that included only the highest functioning patients, with exclusion of patients with DM and/or CVD comorbidities; therefore, they are not representative of the larger percentage of patients who are more physically limited.[196] In addition, many dialysis patients suffer from mild to severe neuropathy, which is compounded by diabetic neuropathy in a large percentage of patients and is a major cause of disability.[197] Lastly, patients are frequently limited by reduced flexibility and impaired coordination.[198] Thus, many activities of daily living (ADLs) and lower levels of employment are challenging for the majority of individuals, especially those with DM.

Typically, the limiting symptom is skeletal muscle fatigue, and patients with CKD have notable skeletal muscle atrophy and weakness. Biopsy studies indicate that skeletal muscles frequently have abnormal structure and function, referred to as uremic myopathy. Contributory factors include malnutrition because of inadequate protein and/or energy intake and increased protein catabolism (protein-restricted diets are recommended for patients with CKD, as they have been shown to delay the progression of the disease and alleviate uremic symptoms), impaired protein synthesis and amino acid metabolism, chronic deconditioning, and side effects of excess parathyroid hormone and other uremic toxins, among others.[199-202] This skeletal muscle wasting results in multiple functional, metabolic, and psychologic deficits, as illustrated in Figure 7-4.

For patients with ESRD, compliance is highest when exercise sessions are performed during dialysis, which is well tolerated when performed within the first 1 to 2 hours of a dialysis session. However, because the intensity is lower with intradialytic exercise, the effects are less pronounced.[195,203,204]

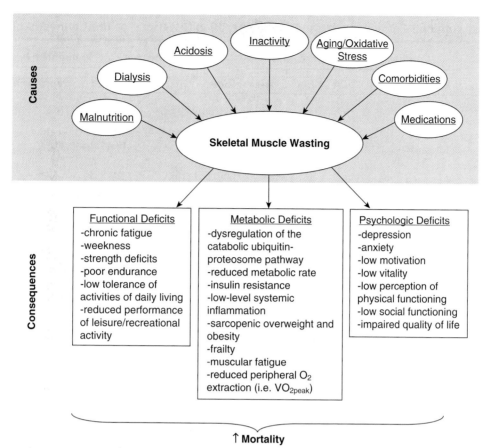

**Figure 7-4** Causes and consequences of muscle wasting in end-stage renal disease. (From Cheema BSB. Review article: Tackling the survival issue in end-stage renal disease: Time to get physical on haemodialysis. Nephrology 13(7):560–9, 2008.)

In patients with chronic renal insufficiency, resistance training has been reported to improve muscle strength and mass, functional performance (6-minute walk test, normal and maximal gait speed, sit-to-stand test), peak exercise capacity, and possibly GFR; it also reduces inflammation, maintains body weight, and increases protein utilization and nitrogen retention to counteract the catabolic effects of protein restriction, low energy intake, and uremia.[200,205] In dialysis patients, resistance exercise produces additional benefits, as well, including enhanced cardiac vagal tone at rest, leading to lower resting HR and reduction in the incidence of cardiac arrhythmias, increased body weight, and improved quality of life.[190,199,206–208] Combined aerobic exercise and resistance training appear to provide augmented benefits, increasing VO$_2$max by 41% to 48% (more accurately referred to as VO$_2$peak because most patients cannot exercise intensely enough to reach their true maximum), augmenting HR variability, and reducing risk of arrhythmia.[209,210] More randomized clinical trials are needed to identify optimal training regimens according to patient characteristics and the effects on specific outcomes in patients with CKD.

## Clinical Implications for Physical Therapy

As discussed, patients with CRF are often debilitated and have poor tolerance for activity. A major contributing factor appears to be physical inactivity. Approximately 60% of patients with ESRD participate in no physical activity beyond basic ADLs and their sedentary behavior may contribute to a number of adverse effects, as illustrated in Figure 7-4. Sedentary patients show a 62% greater risk of mortality over 1 year compared with nonsedentary patients, given adjustments for other variables associated with survival.[208,211] Fortunately, there is evidence that dialysis patients will increase their physical activity if given specific information and encouragement to do so, generating the improvements in physical functioning and exercise capacity already described.[208]

Laboratory values should be reviewed prior to each treatment, especially in dialysis patients. Particular attention should be directed to hemoglobin, hematocrit, glucose, potassium, calcium, creatinine and BUN, WBC, and platelets (see Chapter 9), and appropriate treatment modifications should be made if values are abnormal. Treatment of anemia with erythropoietin improves exercise tolerance and quality of life and possibly survival.[182] Fluid status should also be assessed, as hypervolemia may reduce exercise tolerance.

In patients with CKD, maximal exercise capacity and muscle strength decrease as renal disease progresses, long before they develop ESRD. Exercise training, using both aerobic and resistance exercise, is beneficial for the prevention of physical deterioration as the disease progresses.[198,212] As with the general population, exercise prescription incorporates four parameters: mode, intensity, duration, and frequency. Yet, in dialysis patients, a fifth exercise parameter

**Table 7-16 Most common Cardiovascular and Pulmonary Manifestations of the Connective Tissue Diseases**

| | Cardiovascular Manifestations | | | | | | | Pulmonary Manifestations | | | | | |
|---|---|---|---|---|---|---|---|---|---|---|---|---|---|
| | P | M | E/V | CA | ECG | Art | Other | Pl. | I | F | Pn. | Vasc. | Mm. |
| Rheumatoid Arthritis | ++ | + | + | + | + | +/− | Rare intrapulm. nodules | ++ | + | + | + | +/− | − |
| Systemic Lupus Erythematosus | ++ | +/− | ++ | + | +/− | + | HTN, CHF | ++ | + | +/− | + | +/− | + |
| Systemic Sclerosis | + | ++ | + | ++ | + | ++ | HTN, CHF, pulm HTN | ++ | ++ | ++ | + | ++ | − |
| Ankylosing Spondylitis | − | +/− | ++ | − | + | + | Ankylosis of thorax | − | + | − | + | − | − |
| Polymyositis | − | ++ | − | + | +/− | − | CHF | + | ++ | − | + | − | ++ |
| Dermatomyositis | − | ++ | − | + | +/− | − | CHF | + | ++ | − | + | − | ++ |
| Marfan's Syndrome | − | − | ++ | + | − | ++ | Aortic dissection | − | − | − | − | − | − |
| Osteogenesis Imperfecta | − | − | ++ | − | + | − | AI, MVP, MR | − | − | − | − | − | − |

P, pericardial; M, myocardial; E/V, endocardial/valvular; CA, coronary arteries; ECG, ECG changes, arrhythmias and conduction disturbances; Art, abnormalities affecting the arterial system; Pl., pleural; I, interstitial; F, fibrosis; Pn., pneumonitis; Vasc., vascular; Mm., respiratory muscle weakness; HTN, hypertension; CHF, congestive heart failure; AI, aortic incompetence; MVP, mitral valve prolapse; MR, mitral regurgitation; pulm., pulmonary
+, convincing association; ++, very common; +/−, possible association; −, no association reported for specific disease/disorder.

should also be considered: the timing of exercise relative to the patient's dialysis treatment. Patients who perform exercise during dialysis benefit from improved dialysis efficacy (by 10% to 15%), with greater removal of waste products produced by augmented flux between the blood and the dialyzer because of increased cardiac output as well as expanded capillary blood flow as a result of exercise-induced vasodilation in the exercise muscle bed.[203]

Because of the prevalence of DM in patients with CKD, the clinical implications previously discussed for diabetics should be noted when appropriate. Furthermore, in as much as patients with CKD often have CVD and DM, they are often taking multiple medications that may have adverse effects on exercise responses and tolerance, which are also described at the end of the section on diabetes.

## Other Specific Diseases and Disorders

A wide variety of other specific diseases may be associated with cardiopulmonary complications. The presence of CV or pulmonary complications may affect patient tolerance for physical activity and many PT interventions. Tables 7-16 to 7-20 summarize the CV and pulmonary manifestations of a number of specific diseases and disorders that are commonly encountered by physical therapists, as well as those associated with various cancer treatments.

## Connective Tissue Diseases

The connective tissue diseases (CTDs) are a diverse group of disease in which CT cells or extracellular matrix proteins,

particularly collagens, proteoglycans, and elastins, are damaged by various genetic mutations, inflammatory mechanisms, or degenerative processes. Because of the wide distribution of connective tissues throughout the body, CTDs often have diffuse systemic effects, and all have the potential for CV and pulmonary involvement. Cardiopulmonary effects are often subclinical or found only at autopsy, although this may be due, at least in part, to limitations imposed by the musculoskeletal features that mask their presence.

## Autoimmune Rheumatic Diseases

The autoimmune rheumatic diseases are systemic diseases that are characterized by immune-mediated inflammatory abnormalities that affect the joints, muscles, and connective tissues. The autoimmune rheumatic diseases can affect all pulmonary structures (the respiratory muscles, the pleura, the small airways, the interstitium, and the pulmonary vessels), either separately or in combination, and all cardiac structures (endocardium, myocardium, conduction system, pericardium, and coronary arteries), as shown in Table 7-16, and this involvement is often responsible for increased morbidity and mortality.[213-215] Not infrequently, pulmonary involvement precedes the musculoskeletal manifestations by several months to several years and appears as pleuritis, infection, pneumonitis, interstitial disease, and pulmonary vascular disease. Pulmonary disease can also develop from a toxic reaction to drugs used to treat autoimmune rheumatic diseases (e.g., D-penicillamine, methotrexate, gold, cyclophosphamide, sulfasalazine, nonsteroidal antiinflammatory drugs). Pericarditis is the most common cardiac manifestation, appearing as pericardial effusion or pericardial thickening. In addition, involvement of the endocardium can induce arrhythmias and valvular dysfunction, myocardial involvement can lead to cardiomyopathy, and involvement of the coronary arteries can result in myocardial ischemia and on rare occasions infarction. Of note, as improved therapies and preventive measures have reduced the incidence and severity of cardiopulmonary complications of these diseases and extended the longevity of these patients, atherosclerotic CVD has become an even greater cause of death and disability.[216] Inflammatory mechanisms along with physical inactivity are important contributory factors, along with acceleration of atherosclerosis by corticosteroid treatment.[217]

## Rheumatoid Arthritis

The chronic inflammation of rheumatoid arthritis (RA) frequently affects other organ systems, including the CV and respiratory systems, particularly when the disease is severe and long-standing. The most prevalent pulmonary manifestations are pleural effusions (40% to 70% of patients), which are usually small but occasionally can be massive, causing shortness of breath and/or pleural chest pain; interstitial lung disease (80% of cases by lung biopsy), which is typically mild but sometimes evolves into progressive pulmonary fibrosis; bronchiectasis (20% to 35% of cases); and rheumatoid lung nodules (20% to 30% of patients).[213] Although evidence of CV involvement is commonly seen during echocardiography and at autopsy, it is seldom clinically evident. Pericarditis can be detected in 30% to 50% of patients, valvular disease is found in 30% to 80% of patients, and cardiomyopathy is noted in 3% to 30% of RA patients on postmortem studies.[218] Dyspnea is the most common symptom followed by cough, and digital clubbing is found in many patients. Increased CV mortality results from CHF and ischemic heart disease and associated arrhythmias.

## Systemic Lupus Erythematosus

Systemic lupus erythematosus (SLE) results in diffuse and widespread inflammation involving the skin, joints, brain, kidney, heart, and virtually all serous membranes. CVD is the most common cause of death in patients with SLE.[219] Pericarditis can be found in 62% of patients, becoming symptomatic with chest pain and sometimes a rub mainly at the onset of SLE or during flares; constriction or tamponade is rare. More than 50% of patients have valvular disease (usually regurgitation or rarely stenosis), which is clinically apparent in about 20% of patients.[214] Another common problem is premature atherosclerotic CAD, which sometimes produces myocardial ischemia or infarction. More uncommon cardiac manifestations include myocarditis, which can lead to dilated cardiomyopathy, and endocarditis (both infective and pseudoinfective), which can result in valvular disease. Cardioembolism from valvular vegetations or left heart thrombi causes ischemic stroke in 10% to 20% of patients. Pleurisy is the most prevalent pulmonary complication, occurring in at least 45% to 60% of patients at some time during the disease[213]; it is often asymptomatic but sometimes causes recurrent or intractable pleuritic chest pain, pleural rub, and effusion. Inflammation of the lung parenchyma sometimes causes diffuse lung disease, with cough, hemoptysis, and pulmonary infiltrates. Restrictive lung dysfunction due to "shrinking lung syndrome" is a well-recognized complication of SLE that is thought to result from limited thoracic compliance. Uncommon but potentially lethal complications of SLE include pulmonary HTN due to either vasoconstriction or recurrent thromboembolism, diffuse alveolar hemorrhage, and chronic lupus pneumonitis.

## Scleroderma

Systemic sclerosis (SSc, or scleroderma) produces slowly progressive fibrosis and vascular obliteration of the skin, subcutaneous tissues, and often the visceral organs. It is known most for its pulmonary complications, which are the leading cause of morbidity and mortality, but CV involvement also occurs. Accumulation of CT matrix cells and proteins in the lungs leads to interstitial lung disease with progressive fibrosis, affecting 75% of patients at autopsy, and subsequent pulmonary HTN in up to 50% of cases.[213] The incidence of lung cancer is increased 4- to 16-fold in patients with SSc and pulmonary fibrosis. Overt heart disease occurs in less than 25% of patients but is found in up to 80% at autopsy and results from either primary involvement of the heart or secondary involvement by SSc affecting the kidneys or lungs.[214] Myocardial fibrosis (resulting from vasospasm and small vessel disease producing ischemia/reperfusion damage, as well as occlusive arterial disease) leads to cardiomyopathy.[220] Other cardiac manifestations of SSc include myocarditis, pericarditis, and occasionally conduction disturbances and arrhythmias and valvular abnormalities. Dyspnea is the most frequent symptom, occurring in more than 60% of patients, particularly those with vascular disease. However, a sedentary lifestyle due to skin and joint restrictions often masks the symptoms of dyspnea on exertion until late in the disease process. Exercise testing frequently reveals subclinical pulmonary abnormalities not detected during routine PFTs.[221]

## Ankylosing Spondylitis

Ankylosing spondylitis mainly affects the spine and sacroiliac joints and is only occasionally associated with significant pulmonary or cardiac manifestations. Thoracic restriction due to severe rib cage immobility and kyphosis leads to restrictive lung dysfunction, which is usually surprisingly mild; symptoms of shortness of breath or chest wall pain are uncommon. On rare occasions, patients develop upper lobe fibrobullous lung disease or nonapical interstitial lung disease[222]; progressive dyspnea and cough are the usual symptoms, though cyst formation and subsequent infection may cause hemoptysis. Lastly, ankylosing hyperostosis of the cervical spine can cause dysphagia, foreign-body sensation, and aspiration. Cardiac involvement typically takes the form of sclerosing inflammatory lesions involving the aortic cusps, proximal aortic root, and adjacent atrioventricular nodal tissue, which can be identified in up to 100% of patients and induces aortic regurgitation in 10% of cases and varying degrees of atrioventricular conduction disturbances in about 5% of patients.[214] Left ventricular dilatation and diastolic dysfunction are very common. Mitral regurgitation may also develop.

## Mixed Connective Tissue Disease

Mixed connective tissue disease is an overlap syndrome with clinical features of SLE, SSc, and myositis. Pulmonary involvement occurs in 20% to 85% of patients, according to the most dominant clinical pattern, and most often consists of interstitial lung disease and pulmonary fibrosis, pleural effusion, and pulmonary HTN, which is a major cause of morbidity and mortality.[213] The most common cardiac manifestations are pericarditis and mitral valve prolapse.

## Inflammatory Myopathies

The inflammatory myopathies are often included in the CTDs. Two types, polymyositis and dermatomyositis, are particularly likely to be associated with cardiopulmonary complications. Pulmonary involvement, which bears a poor prognosis, includes respiratory muscle dysfunction, interstitial lung disease (one form of which evolves quickly into acute respiratory failure while others lead to progressive fibrosis), aspiration pneumonia (due to pharyngolaryngeal muscle weakness), and lung cancer. Death due to respiratory insufficiency occurs in 30% to 66% of patients.[213] The muscle inflammation that is characteristic of the myositis also affects the heart, resulting in myocarditis and cardiomyopathy. The most common clinical manifestations seen in polymyositis and dermatomyositis are those of CHF and CAD (because of vasculitis, small vessel disease, and vasospasm, as well as atherosclerosis), which are major causes of mortality.[223]

## Inherited Connective Tissue Diseases

The inherited CT diseases are characterized by abnormalities of the connective tissues that affect the great arteries, cardiac valves, skeletal system, and skin. The most common of these include Marfan syndrome, Ehlers–Doanlos syndrome, and osteogenesis imperfecta. These diseases may cause minimal CV dysfunction, such as mitral valve prolapse or mild aortic root dilatation, or severe problems, such as severe aortic or mitral insufficiency or aortic aneurysm and dissection, depending on the degree of CT abnormalities and their response to prolonged hemodynamic stress. Some patients develop serious ventricular or supraventricular arrhythmias. Pulmonary problems may also develop as a result of bullous emphysema, chest wall deformities, kyphoscoliosis, and obstructive sleep apnea due to increased upper airway collapsibility.

## Infiltrative Diseases

Some diseases affect the heart and/or lungs through the infiltration or deposition of various substances within these organs (as well as other organs of the body). Amyloidosis, sarcoidosis, and hemochromatosis are the most recognized of these diseases, and their effects on the CV and pulmonary system are presented in Table 7-17.

## Amyloidosis

Amyloidosis results from the overproduction of certain proteins leading to the deposition of amyloid fibrils in various organs. It can occur as a primary process and also as a complication of some inflammatory processes, as in rheumatoid arthritis, inflammatory bowel disease, and bronchiectasis. Pulmonary amyloidosis can occur along with systemic disease

## Table 7-17 Pulmonary and Cardiac Complications of the Common Infiltrative Diseases

| Disease | Pathology | Pulmonary Manifestations | Cardiac Manifestations |
|---|---|---|---|
| Amyloidosis | Deposition of amyloid fibrils | Progressive diffuse parenchymal infiltrates<br>Localized tracheobronchial plaques<br>Diaphragm weakness, respiratory failure | Diastolic and sometimes systolic dysfunction, restrictive or dilated CM<br>Myocardial infarction, sudden death<br>Arrhythmias—atrial fibrillation, brady- and tachyarrhythmias |
| Sarcoidosis | Noncaseating granulomas leading to inflammation or scarring | Parenchymal granulomas<br>Bronchostenosis | Cardiomyopathy with impaired LV function, CHF<br>Arrhythmias—ventricular tachycardia |
| Hemochromatosis | Deposition of iron | | Myocardial fibrosis, restrictive or dilated CM<br>Conduction disturbances or arrhythmias |

*CHF, congestive heart failure; CM, cardiomyopathy.*

or as a localized entity, resulting in progressive diffuse parenchymal infiltrates, RLD, and impaired gas exchange versus localized tracheobronchial plaques or diffuse parenchymal nodules; and possible pulmonary HTN, obstructive sleep apnea caused by massive infiltration of the tongue, and respiratory failure induced by infiltration of the diaphragm. Cardiac involvement is commonly manifested as diastolic dysfunction due to infiltration of rigid amyloid fibrils and sometimes systolic dysfunction. Cardiomyopathy may occur as a result of restrictive dysfunction or dilation. Other CV problems include atrial arrhythmias, particularly atrial fibrillation, which has a high risk of thromboembolism; syncope caused by orthostatic hypotension or brady- or tachyarrhythmias; and myocardial infarction and sudden death provoked by involvement of the coronary arteries.

## Sarcoidosis

Sarcoidosis is a chronic inflammatory disease characterized by the presence of noncaseating granulomas in multiple organ systems with resultant combinations of inflammation and scarring, which can vary from mild and asymptomatic with spontaneous resolution to severe progressive disease leading to organ failure and death. Pulmonary manifestations consist of granulomas within the lung parenchyma (more often in the upper rather than the lower lobes) and within the bronchi, which can lead to bronchostenosis. Typical symptoms are dyspnea and nonproductive cough. Cardiac involvement is noted in up to 50% of patients at autopsy, but clinical manifestations are found in <10% of patients and include ventricular tachyarrhythmias and cardiomyopathy appearing as impaired LV function or CHF.

## Hemochromatosis

Hemochromatosis is a common inherited disorder of iron metabolism that leads to iron deposition in various organs, including the liver, heart, pancreas, joints, skin, and endocrine organs. Excess deposition of iron in the liver can be fatal but can be prevented by regular therapeutic phlebotomy to reduce circulating iron levels. Involvement of the heart can lead to secondary myocardial fibrosis, cardiomyopathy (either restrictive or dilated), and conduction disturbances or arrhythmias.

## Neuromuscular Diseases and Neurologic Disorders

A number of diseases and disorders affecting the neurologic or neuromuscular systems are associated with cardiovascular and pulmonary dysfunction (Table 7-18). Among the most notable are spinal cord injury (SCI), stroke, Parkinson disease (PD), amyotrophic lateral sclerosis (ALS), Guillain–Barré syndrome (GBS), myasthenia gravis, the muscular dystrophies, and Friedreich ataxia. The incidence and severity of dysfunction in all the disorders vary widely.

Pulmonary compromise is a common complication of many neuromuscular and neurologic disorders and is the major cause of morbidity and mortality.[224-227] Respiratory muscle weakness or paralysis, or abnormal tone, restricts chest

expansion and ventilation and reduces cough force and effectiveness, leading to retained secretions, atelectasis, and high risk of pneumonia. Abnormally low pulmonary compliance, which may result from chronically impaired chest wall mobility and low lung volumes, makes the chest wall stiffer and adds to the difficulty in expanding the lungs. Hypoventilation, which is particularly common at night, and microatelectasis give rise to $CO_2$ retention and hypoxemia, which may be exacerbated by different positions (e.g., laying flat in high cervical SCI, sitting in lower cervical SCI). Bulbar muscle weakness with dysfunction of the pharyngeal and laryngeal muscles, which is common in such diseases as ALS, myasthenia gravis, and MS, increases the risk of recurrent aspiration and resultant pneumonia and interferes with cough effectiveness (due to poor glottic closure). Sleep-disordered breathing, including central apneas and hypopneas and obstructive sleep apnea, is seen in many patients, including those with quadriplegia, postpolio syndrome, ALS, and the muscular dystrophies. Nocturnal hypoventilation is often an indication of chronic respiratory muscle fatigue and increased risk of ventilatory failure, which can be ameliorated with the use of nocturnal ventilatory assistance, usually via nocturnal noninvasive positive pressure ventilation in most cases. Pulmonary embolism is a constant threat to patients with SCI, stroke, and other neurological and neuromuscular diseases because of reduced peripheral blood flow and limited activity level.

---

> **Clinical Tip**
> It is important to realize that respiratory symptoms often do not correlate well with the degree of respiratory dysfunction in slowly progressive disorders.

---

Measures of maximal inspiratory and expiratory pressures can be used to detect and monitor respiratory muscle weakness and are more sensitive than spirometric measures of lung volume. Patients with neuromuscular and myopathic disorders involving the respiratory muscles are particularly prone to hypoventilation and oxygen desaturation during sleep. Therefore, clinicians should be attentive to the development of symptoms such as sleep disturbances, morning headache, excessive daytime somnolence, impaired concentration, and loss of appetite and alert the patient's physician if they are noted.

Cardiovascular dysfunction also occurs in many patients with neuromuscular and neurologic disorders, although the typical symptoms of dyspnea and reduced exercise tolerance are difficult to appreciate in nonambulatory patients. Instead, these patients may exhibit increased fatigue, difficulty sleeping, impaired concentration, and more subtle variants of poor performance.[228] Cardiac abnormalities found in this population include cardiomyopathy associated with neuromuscular diseases, arrhythmias, and conduction disturbances. Disruption of autonomic nerve fibers in SCI with lesions above T1 or nerve involvement by other neurologic pathologies, such as multiple sclerosis, ALS, PD, and GBS, can result in

**Table 7-18 Cardiac and Pulmonary Manifestations of Some Neurological and Neuromuscular Diseases**

| Disease/Disorder | Cardiac Manifestations | | | Pulmonary Manifestations | | | |
|---|---|---|---|---|---|---|---|
| | Myocardial | Cond | Other | Mm | Bulb | RLD | Sleep |
| Spinal cord injury | – | – | According to level of lesion<br>Autonomic dysfunction above T7 | ++ | – | ++ | ++ |
| Hemiplegia | + | ++ | HTN, CAD if vascular pathology | + | +/– | + | +/– |
| Parkinson's disease | – | – | Dyskinetic respiration<br>Upper airway obstruction | ++ | +/– | + | + |
| Amyotrophic lateral sclerosis | – | – | Progressive ventilatory failure | ++ | ++ | ++ | ++ |
| Guillain–Barré syndrome | – | – | Ventilatory failure (temporary) | ++ | + | ++ | ++ |
| Multiple sclerosis | – | – | Correlates with severity of disease | ++ | ++ | + | + |
| Myasthenia gravis | + | ++ | Arrhythmias, rare CHF<br>Ventilatory failure | + | ++ | ++ | + |
| Progressive muscular dystrophy | ++ | ++ | Arrhythmias, dilated cardiomyopathy<br>Pulmonary infections | ++ | ++ | ++ | ++ |
| Becker muscular dystrophy | ++ | ++ | Arrhythmias, heart blocks<br>Dilated cardiomyopathy, CHF | ++ | – | + | ++ |
| Myotonic dystrophy | – | ++ | Arrhythmias, sudden cardiac death<br>Occasional CHF<br>Dyskinetic breathing, possible respiratory failure | ++ | – | + | + |
| Fascioscapulohumeral dystrophy, scapuloperoneal myopathies | + | ++ | Sinus arrest, atrial paralysis<br>AV blocks | +/– | – | +/– | + |
| Limb-girdle syndromes | + | + | ECG abnormalities | +/– | – | +/– | + |
| Postpolio syndrome | – | – | Same muscles as original infection | + | + | + | ++ |
| Friedreich ataxia | ++ | ++ | Arrhythmias, CHF<br>Scoliosis, chest deformity<br>Respiratory failure | + | – | + | ++ |

*AV, atrioventricular; Bulb, bulbar muscle involvement; CA, coronary arteries; CHF, chronic heart failure; Cond, conduction system; ECG, electrocardiogram; Mm, respiratory muscle weakness or paralysis; RLD, restrictive lung dysfunction; Sleep, sleep-disordered breathing.*
*+, convincing association, ++, very common, +/–, possible association, –, no association reported for specific disease/disorder.*

orthostatic hypotension and impaired thermoregulation. In older individuals, the presence of HTN and CAD often adds to CV dysfunction. In addition, abnormal movement patterns due to muscle weakness or abnormal neural input increase the energy cost of mobility and daily activities; and impaired mobility induces a more sedentary lifestyle, which leads to cardiovascular and muscular deconditioning and diminished efficiency. Both of these factors contribute to exaggerated physiologic demands of mobility and ADLs and increase the risk of activity intolerance, as well as that of

CVD morbidity and mortality. Appropriate exercise training provides many benefits for these patients.[229–236]

Hemiplegia can result from a number of events, including CVA due to thrombosis, embolism, or hemorrhage, surgical excision of a brain tumor, and trauma. Regardless of cause, weakness or spastic paralysis of the affected side of the body can include the diaphragm and intercostal muscles, leading to altered respiratory mechanics and reduced respiratory muscle efficiency. Left diaphragmatic dysfunction is more common than right. PFTs reveal decreased volumes and flows to about 60% to 70% predicted normal values[224–227,237]; these abnormalities take on additional clinical significance in the presence of preexisting pulmonary disease. Respiratory failure can develop in patients whose vital capacity decreases to 25% or less of predicted normal values, and mechanical ventilation will be required. The major pulmonary complications associated with stroke occur when the facial and pharyngeal muscles are affected, causing impairments in secretion management, proper swallowing, airway protection, and cough effectiveness. The vast majority of patients with ischemic stroke also have CVD, particularly HTN and CAD, although most patients are asymptomatic and not diagnosed; CVD is responsible for the majority of deaths following transient ischemic attacks, stroke, and carotid endarterectomy.[238–241] There is also some evidence that both hemorrhagic and ischemic strokes are associated with nonischemic cardiac damage, most likely related to stress-induced release of catecholamines and possibly corticosteroids.[242,243] The usual lack of clinical symptoms in hemiplegic patients is probably due to their low level of physical exertion; however, strenuous exertion or PT activities may elicit dyspnea and other signs of exercise intolerance, especially when lying flat.

Spinal cord injury is associated with significant pulmonary dysfunction, according to the severity and level of injury.[224,227,244] SCI at or above C3 to C5 interferes with phrenic nerve function, causing partial or complete bilateral hemidiaphragmatic paralysis, and diminishes intercostal muscle forces, leading to marked reductions in ventilation and cough force; ventilatory assistance is almost always required for lesions above C4. Abnormal respiratory mechanics result in a paradoxical breathing pattern characterized by inward movement of the abdomen as the upper chest rises on inspiration. Lesions below C5 will have corresponding intercostal muscle involvement and therefore some restrictive lung dysfunction (VC may be reduced to 60% of predicted normal in high thoracic lesions and to 78% of predicted normal in low thoracic lesions),[227] but because diaphragmatic and accessory muscle function is preserved, hypoventilation usually does not occur. In this case, strong contraction of the diaphragm produces a paradoxical breathing pattern marked by inward movement of the upper chest on inspiration. The work done by the diaphragm is up to nine times normal in lower cervical and high thoracic injuries, which is due in large part to the work required to displace the abdominal viscera, and dyspnea on exertion is common.[224,227] The major problems with weakness of the expiratory muscles (internal intercostals and abdominals) are poor cough and impaired clearance of airway secretions.

Cardiovascular abnormalities, mostly related to interruption of autonomic nervous system signals, also occur in patients with SCI. Acute injury to the cervical spine is frequently accompanied by cardiac arrhythmias and occasionally by sudden death. Patients with SCI at or above the T6 level often experience serious disturbances of BP. Orthostatic hypotension is common in the early phase of recovery but usually resolves over time. Autonomic dysreflexia (hyperreflexia) can produce marked elevation of BP when noxious visceral or cutaneous stimuli, such as a full bladder, are sensed below the level of the lesion. Furthermore, autonomic denervation interferes with temperature regulation so that body temperature tends to fluctuate according to the ambient temperature, especially in higher lesions; therefore, hypo- and hyperthermia can develop. In addition, SCI above the T1 level is associated with reductions in both preload and afterload, which leads to atrophy of the LV and reduced systolic efficiency.[233] Moreover, limited physical activity promoting a sedentary lifestyle and exercise intolerance increases the risk of CV morbidity and mortality.

## Parkinson Disease

Parkinson disease (PD) is a common dyskinetic disorder of the extrapyramidal system, which is characterized by resting muscle tremors, rigidity, slowness and poverty of motion, gait impairment, and postural instability. Secondary Parkinsonism may develop following some cases of encephalitis and as a result of drug abuse and repeated brain trauma. Although rarely recognized clinically, impaired ventilatory function occurs in 50% to 87% of patients and tends to be proportional to the severity of the skeletal muscle disease and improves with effective treatment.[245–248] Erratic, or chaotic, breathing due to the rigidity and weakness of the respiratory muscles, as well as abnormal control of ventilation, is common and results in restrictive lung dysfunction, decreased maximal inspiratory and expiratory forces and peak expiratory flow rate, and reduced maximum voluntary ventilation on PFTs. Upper airway obstruction is found in 5% to 62% of patients, most likely due to involvement of the upper airway musculature.[246,249] In addition, an obstructive pulmonary disease may be associated with PD. Furthermore, medications used to treat PD are also associated with pulmonary dysfunction: Overtreatment with levodopa causes dyskinetic breathing and abnormal central control of ventilation, and the ergot-derivatives can cause pleuropulmonary fibrosis.[245,248] Lastly, pneumonia resulting from pulmonary complications is a significant cause of morbidity and mortality in PD.[248] There are no specific cardiac complications associated with Parkinson disease; however, patients often have the same cardiovascular problems (HTN, ASHD, etc.) that commonly occur in their same-aged peers. Exercise testing has shown that individuals with mild to moderate PD who regularly exercise can maintain normal exercise tolerance; more involved patients exhibit significantly lower exercise capacity.[250] Moreover, it is possible to improve exercise capacity in patients with mild to moderate PD with exercise training.

## Amyotrophic Lateral Sclerosis

Amyotrophic lateral sclerosis (ALS, or Lou Gehrig disease) is the most common motor neuron disease in the United States and is characterized by progressive neurologic deterioration without remission due to loss and degeneration of both upper and lower motor neurons. Patients experience a combination of spasticity and hyperreflexia and muscle wasting, weakness, and fasciculations. Irreversible hypoventilation results from weakness of the intercostal muscles and diaphragm, but the insidious onset of gradually developing dyspnea may delay the diagnosis.[226,227] Nocturnal hypoventilation can occur despite only mild respiratory muscle dysfunction and normal gas exchange. With bulbar involvement, which occurs eventually in 80% of patients, swallowing becomes impaired, leading to aspiration pneumonia. Mechanical ventilator dependence and fatal respiratory failure is common in the later stages of the disease, producing an average life expectancy of 4 years after diagnosis.[251]

## Guillain–Barré Syndrome

Guillain–Barré syndrome, or acute inflammatory polyneuropathy, is an autoimmune demyelinating disease of motor neurons that is usually triggered by an infectious process and is the most common cause of acute neuromuscular paralysis. Clinical manifestations include progressive symmetric ascending weakness and dyspnea, difficulty in coughing, and, later on, dysphagia and difficulty with speech. However, many patients do not notice respiratory dysfunction even in the presence of significant respiratory insufficiency because of the gradual onset and slow progression of the respiratory muscle weakness. Respiratory complications develop in approximately half of patients as a result of hypoventilation, impaired coughing, airway secretion retention, and atelectasis, and 30% of all patients progress to ventilatory failure and require mechanical ventilatory support during the course of their disease.[227,252,253] There is a poor correlation between peripheral muscle strength and the presence or absence of respiratory muscle weakness. In addition, bulbar dysfunction causes upper airway obstruction and aspiration and increases the risk of ventilatory failure.

## Multiple Sclerosis

Multiple sclerosis (MS) is an autoimmune disease that causes demyelination of the CNS and is characterized clinically by periods of remissions and relapses of symptoms, although on occasion its course can be chronic and progressive. MS is the most common neurologic disease affecting young adults. Its classic clinical symptoms include paresthesias, motor weakness, blurred and double vision, dysarthria, bladder incontinence, and ataxia. Because MS can cause focal lesions anywhere in the CNS, different patterns of respiratory impairment can occur but are relatively rare. The three most common pulmonary manifestations are respiratory muscle weakness, bulbar dysfunction, and abnormalities of respiratory control.[227,254-256] Pulmonary dysfunction correlates with the severity of the disease, so that quadriplegic patients with bulbar involvement are at highest risk for developing respiratory failure. Even with severe disability and impaired respiratory muscle strength, patients with MS seldom complain of dyspnea, most likely due to their low activity level and greater expiratory than inspiratory muscle dysfunction. Clinical signs that may be helpful in predicting respiratory muscle impairment are weak cough and inability to clear secretions, limited ability to count to 10 on a single breath, and upper extremity involvement. There are no specific cardiovascular abnormalities associated with MS.

## Myasthenia Gravis

Myasthenia gravis is an acquired autoimmune disorder with specific autoantibodies that attack the nicotinic acetylcholine receptors in the neuromuscular junction, producing muscle weakness that is aggravated by repetitive muscle contractions. The disease may affect only the ocular or bulbar muscles, but the limb and respiratory muscles are often involved. Respiratory muscle weakness occurs in about 10% of patients, and ventilatory failure may necessitate prolonged ventilatory assistance.[224] The risk of ventilatory insufficiency is increased by surgery, acute infection, and the administration of corticosteroids or antimicrobial drugs. Of note, patients may have severe respiratory muscle involvement even with mild peripheral muscle weakness; however, most patients with moderate, generalized myasthenia gravis exhibit mild to moderate reductions in forced vital capacity and maximal inspiratory and expiratory forces.[224,227] Cardiac involvement occurs in 10% to 40% of patients, especially those with thymoma, and appears to be caused by heart-reactive autoantibodies.[257,258] Focal inflammation and necrosis are found on autopsy. Clinical symptoms include tachycardia and other arrhythmias and dyspnea. Notably, drugs used to treat cardiovascular problems, such as quinidine, procainamide, lidocaine, and morphine, may adversely affect myasthenia gravis. Treatment with acetylcholine esterase inhibitors (e.g., neostigmine and pyridostigmine) results in improvements in cardiac function and respiratory muscle strength and pulmonary function, but may have relatively little effect on respiratory muscle endurance. Plasmapheresis to remove the IgG antibody is sometimes used.

## Duchenne Muscular Dystrophy

Progressive (Duchenne) muscular dystrophy (DMD) is the most common inherited progressive myopathy and is caused by a lack of dystrophin. It is characterized by delayed motor development or early onset of progressive, generalized muscle weakness and pseudohypertrophy of certain muscle groups, especially the calves, resulting in increasing orthopedic, pulmonary, and cardiac complications and the inability to ambulate by the age of 10 or 11. Respiratory impairment becomes clinically manifest as chronic alveolar ventilation and poor cough caused by respiratory muscle weakness in the advanced stages of the disease, usually in the late teens.[226,227,259] Sleep-disordered breathing occurs in up to two thirds of patients during the early teenage years and is associated with transient hypoxemic dips. Progressive kyphoscoliosis resulting from severe muscle weakness contributes to the respiratory decline. Finally, loss of the diaphragm late in the disease leads to hypercapnia and rapid deterioration. The most common cause of death is respiratory failure, which is usually precipitated by respiratory infection and occurs by the age of 20 unless ventilatory support is provided. Virtually all patients with DMD develop a dilated cardiomyopathy by age 10, but clinical recognition may be masked by severe skeletal muscle weakness.[228,260-263] Dystrophic myocardial changes occur most prominently in the posterobasal and adjacent lateral left ventricle and consist of vacuolar degeneration and fibrous replacement of the muscle fibers, as well as fatty infiltration of the heart muscle and peripheral circulatory system. Arrhythmias and conduction disturbances are common findings. Involvement of the posteromedial papillary muscle sometimes causes mitral valve prolapse and mitral regurgitation. CHF usually develops in the preterminal stage of the disease.

Becker's muscular dystrophy is a milder variant of DMD with more variable clinical manifestations. It presents later in life and is slower in progression, so that 50% of patients survive to age 40 and some have a near-normal life expectancy. Cardiac involvement, which is also more variable and unrelated to the extent of the musculoskeletal disease, is often more severe than in DMD.[228,260,263] Dilated cardiomyopathy, bundle branch block, complete heart block, or tachyarrhythmias may develop.[263,264] About 30% of patients develop dilated cardiomyopathy and CHF, and some patients have received heart transplants.[264,265] Respiratory impairment develops similar to DMD, although its onset is later and its course is more slowly progressive.

## Myotonic Dystrophy

Myotonic dystrophy (Steinert disease), an autosomal dominant multisystem disease, is the most common adult form of muscular dystrophy. Symptoms usually present during adolescence or early adulthood, with premature death usually resulting from cardiopulmonary complications. Respiratory muscle weakness is common in patients with myotonic dystrophy and can be severe, despite mild limb weakness. Myotonia of the respiratory muscles produces a chaotic breathing pattern, increased work of breathing, and often hypercapnia.[226–228,259,266] Bulbar dysfunction and sleep-related breathing disturbances also occur. These patients are particularly susceptible to respiratory failure with general anesthesia and sedatives. Respiratory failure can also result from chronic respiratory muscle weakness, altered central control of breathing, and pneumonia. Myotonic dystrophy is associated with cardiac involvement, especially ECG abnormalities and arrhythmias, in at least two thirds of patients; high-grade heart block or ventricular tachycardia may cause sudden death.[264,267,268] Occasionally, there is acute left ventricular failure or CHF.

## Additional Types of Muscular Dystrophy

Other types of muscular dystrophy are also associated with cardiopulmonary dysfunction.[226,227,259,264] Cardiomyopathy may occur in fascioscapulohumeral (FSH) dystrophy and the limb-girdle syndromes, but they are usually less prominent and CHF is unusual. There may be cardiac gallop sounds, cardiac enlargement, and ECG abnormalities. Atrial abnormalities are present in all patients with X-linked scapuloperoneal myopathy (Emery–Dreifuss dystrophy) and result in sinus arrest, atrial arrhythmias, varying atrioventricular block, and permanent atrial paralysis with junctional bradycardia. Because sudden death is common in young adults, permanent pacing is recommended for ventricular rates below 50, regardless of atrial activity. FSH dystrophy and the scapuloperoneal syndromes have also been associated with atrial paralysis. Pulmonary function has not been studied in much detail in most of the other muscular dystrophies. FSH dystrophy affects the pelvic girdle and trunk muscles in approximately 20% of patients, and this involvement may be associated with impairment of pulmonary function, which tends to be mild and complicated by an increased incidence of obstructive sleep apneas related to upper airway muscle weakness. Facial muscle weakness makes spirometric measures unreliable. Limb girdle dystrophy may be accompanied by chronic hypoventilation but rarely requires assisted ventilation. Finally, oculopharyngeal muscular dystrophy is associated with swallowing dysfunction, complicated by repeated aspiration, which may improve after cricopharyngeal myotomy.

## Postpolio Syndrome

Postpolio syndrome (PPS) is a late sequela of poliomyelitis, which afflicts from 15% to 80% of polio survivors and develops 30 to 40 years after the acute enterovirus infection.[269,270] Factors known to precipitate PPS include overuse syndromes, recent weight gain, acute illnesses, trauma, exposure to toxic agents, and hormonal changes. The most common symptoms reported by PPS patients include fatigue and weakness, joint and muscle pain, respiratory difficulties, cold intolerance, and dysphagia. In general, PPS affects the same muscle groups that were originally involved with the disease; however, because patients with mild to moderate respiratory muscle involvement often went undetected, there is a higher incidence of late onset respiratory symptoms, which occur in up to 40% of PPS patients[271] and range from mildly reduced pulmonary function, dyspnea, morning headaches, and daytime hypersomnolence to frank respiratory failure requiring ventilatory assistance. Individuals who required ventilatory assistance in the acute phase or had an onset of polio after 10 years of age and those with chest deformities are at highest risk of respiratory impairment, which often occurs without shortness of breath.[269,272] Sleep-disordered breathing, including obstructive sleep apnea and nocturnal hypoventilation, is common. Weakening of bulbar muscles leads to dysphagia in at least 15% of patients. Patients with PPS benefit from supervised muscular training that avoids muscular overuse, as well as recognition of respiratory impairment, use of respiratory muscle training, and early introduction of noninvasive ventilatory aids.[269] No specific CV complications are associated with PPS.

## Friedreich Ataxia

Friedreich ataxia is a hereditary disease characterized by progressive spinocerebellar degeneration beginning during adolescence. Progressive weakness and ataxia of the upper and lower extremities gradually develop, resulting in difficulty walking, unsteadiness of the arms and hands, and problems with writing and using eating utensils. Cardiac involvement occurs in 50% to 100% of patients and is characterized by cardiomyopathy with decreased ventricular compliance and varying degrees of hypertrophy and occasionally obstruction to ventricular outflow.[260,261,273,274] Cardiac problems often present as the initial manifestation of the disease, although most patients are asymptomatic, except for dyspnea, which could be explained on the basis of their neurologic disability. When other symptoms are noted, they usually consist of palpitations and angina. Arrhythmias are common, especially premature atrial contractions, atrial flutter/fibrillation, and premature ventricular contractions. Progression of the neuromuscular disease usually results in the development of ventilatory failure. Death is usually caused by CHF or intercurrent infections and usually occurs within 20 to 30 years after onset of symptoms.[227,260]

## Hematologic Disorders

Many hematologic disorders are associated with CV and pulmonary dysfunction because of reduced oxygen-carrying capacity, reduced immune function, or coagulopathy or other forms of vascular obstruction.

## Anemia

Anemia is defined as a reduced circulating red blood cell (RBC) mass relative to an individual's gender and age and can result from impaired RBC production, excessive destruction of RBCs (hemolysis), loss by hemorrhage, or a combination of these factors. Causes include dietary deficiency, acute or chronic blood loss, genetic defects of hemoglobin, exposure to toxins or certain drugs, diseases of the bone marrow, and a variety of chronic inflammatory, infectious, or neoplastic diseases.

## Sickle Cell Disease

Sickle cell disease (SCD) is a genetic disease found most commonly in individuals of Equatorial African ancestry, which is characterized by structurally abnormal hemoglobin that causes the RBCs to become less pliable and some become crescent or sickle shaped with deoxygenation.[275-278] Hemolytic anemia develops because of shortened circulatory survival of damaged RBCs (10 to 12 days rather than 120 days), which are destroyed intravascularly by macrophages and extravascularly in the spleen. Acute painful episodes resulting from occlusion of small capillaries and venules by the adherence of sickled RBCs to the vascular endothelium, termed *vasoocclusive crises*, are the most common complication of SCD, which typically occur one to six times a year and last for a few days up to several weeks. These episodes may be precipitated by cold, dehydration, infection, stress, menses, or alcohol consumption, although the cause is frequently unknown. They result in tissue ischemia–reperfusion injury and infarction that affect nearly all organs, particularly the spleen, kidneys, CNS, bones, liver, lungs, and heart, leading to progressive systemic vasculopathy and chronic organ failure. Most patients are anemic but asymptomatic except during painful episodes.

Cardiopulmonary dysfunction is common in sickle cell disease, as shown in Table 7-19. As with anemia, cardiac output and tissue oxygen extraction increase, but in SCD the reduction in oxygen content of the RBCs induces further sickling and compounds the cardiopulmonary complications. The leading cause of death in SCD is the acute chest syndrome, which occurs in approximately 30% of patients and is induced by vasoocclusion, infection, and pulmonary fat embolism from infarcted bone marrow. It typically presents with dyspnea, chest pain, fever, tachypnea, hypoxemia, leukocytosis, pulmonary infiltrates on chest radiography, and airflow limitation on PFTs, but sometimes it is insidious, with nonspecific signs and symptoms.[279-281] It progresses to acute respiratory failure in 13% of patients and has a mortality rate of 4.3% to 23%.

The heart is also affected by SCD. Biventricular hypertrophy and dilatation are induced by chronic anemia and the compensatory volume overload that increases cardiac output.[282,283] Clinical manifestations include diminished exercise tolerance, dyspnea on exertion, and progressive loss of cardiac reserve. Diastolic dysfunction, most likely due to relative systemic HTN, has been noted in 18% of patients and increases the mortality risk, especially when combined with pulmonary HTN.[284] CHF is a late occurrence. Systolic cardiac murmurs are common. Venoocclusion can cause myocardial infarction. Arrhythmias and second-degree AV block may occur during painful episodes and increase the risk of sudden death. Exercise capacity is reduced most likely because of ongoing lung injury and diminished oxygen-carrying capacity of the blood and may be associated with an exercise-induced drop in cardiac output or myocardial ischemia.[284,285]

## Human Immunodeficiency Virus and Acquired Immune Deficiency Syndrome

Patients with human immunodeficiency virus (HIV) are living much longer and suffering less disability than in the 1990s as a result of highly active antiretroviral therapy (HAART), which aims to preserve immune function and minimize viral replication in order to delay the progression to acquired immune deficiency syndrome (AIDS). Thus, HIV has become a chronic illness with episodes of exacerbations and remissions, which often affects the neurologic, cardiopulmonary, integumentary, and musculoskeletal systems.

Although the success of HAART has sharply reduced the incidence of opportunistic infections, pulmonary complications continue to be a major cause of morbidity and mortality in individuals with HIV/AIDS.[286] Noninfectious pulmonary complications are common in HIV and include malignancies (lung, Kaposi sarcoma, and non-Hodgkin lymphoma), pulmonary HTN (possibly through increased production of inflammatory cytokines and chemokines by infected lymphocytes and alveolar macrophages, as well as due to endothelial dysfunction), and lymphoproliferative disorders (lymphocytic interstitial pneumonitis and alveolitis).[287] HIV also increases the risk of developing active tuberculosis (TB) and TB recurrence, which are associated with accelerated progression and mortality of HIV, partially due to a number

**Table 7-19 Cardiac and Pulmonary Manifestations of Some Other Specific Diseases**

| Disease | Cardiac Manifestations | | | | Pulmonary Manifestations | | | |
|---|---|---|---|---|---|---|---|---|
| | P | M | CA | Other | Pl. | I | Pn. | Vasc. |
| Anemia | − | − | +/− | Dyspnea on exertion<br>Increased angina if CAD, rare CHF | − | − | − | − |
| Sickle cell disease | − | ++ | + | Cardiomegaly, late CHF<br>Decreased exercise capacity | − | − | ++ | + |
| HIV and AIDS | + | + | + | Metastasis of Kaposi sarcoma to heart and lungs, vascular thrombosis and embolism, non–Hodgkin's lymphoma, opportunistic infections | − | + | + | − |
| Hepatic disease | − | + | − | Alcoholic cardiomyopathy<br>HTN, arrhythmias, chest pain<br>Mild–moderate hypoxemia<br>Pulmonary shunting and HTN<br>Pleural effusion, ascites leads to RLD | + | − | + | − |
| Anorexia nervosa | − | ++ | − | Arrhythmias, sudden death | − | − | − | − |
| Bulimia nervosa | − | +/− | − | Arrhythmias, sudden death<br>Aspiration pneumonia<br>Ipecac-induced cardiomyopathy | − | − | + | − |

*CA, coronary arteries; E/V, endocardial/valvular; H, hypertension; I, interstitial; M, myocardial; P, pericardial; Pl., pleural; Pn., pneumonitis; Vasc., vascular*

*+, convincing association; ++, very common; +/−, possible association; −, no association reported for specific disease/disorder.*

of drug–drug interactions between the various medications used to treat the two diseases.[286] Fungal (e.g., *Pneumocystis pneumonia* [PCP]) and bacterial infection (e.g., *Streptococcus pneumoniae, Haemophilus influenzae, Staphylococcus aureus,* Pseudomonas, and *Mycobacterium avium*) also occur more frequently and are a major problem where HAART is not available. In addition, reactivation of cytomegalovirus (CMV) may occur in conjunction with PCP and is a marker of poor prognosis.

Cardiovascular complications also occur in many patients with HIV and are fatal in some patients.[288] The most common CV problem seen in HIV, particularly in children with AIDS, is pericardial effusion, which may be induced by opportunistic infection or malignancy, but more often no definitive cause can be identified.

## Hepatic Diseases

Several diseases of the liver, including cirrhosis and hepatitis, produce or are associated with multiple cardiac and pulmonary abnormalities, as shown in Table 7-19. Patients with cirrhosis have a hyperdynamic systemic circulation, particularly in the supine position, which is characterized by increased HR and cardiac output, expanded plasma volume, and reduced systemic vascular resistance and low-normal BP. These alterations contribute to cardiopulmonary dysfunction.

As many as 70% of patients with chronic liver diseases suffer from pulmonary problems.[289] Certain liver diseases have known associations with specific pulmonary pathologies: primary biliary cirrhosis is associated with fibrosing alveolitis, diffuse interstitial pneumonitis, airflow limitation and emphysema, and bronchiectasis; chronic active hepatitis and possibly chronic hepatitis C are associated with fibrosing alveolitis; sclerosing cholangitis is associated with bronchiectasis and fibrosing alveolitis; and $\alpha_1$-proteinase deficiency is associated with chronic airflow limitation and emphysema.[290] Patients with cirrhosis, the most prevalent type of chronic liver disease in the United States, may experience the pulmonary effects of pleural effusions and ascites as well as two unique disorders, the hepatopulmonary syndrome and portopulmonary HTN.[192,289] Between 5% and 10% of patients with cirrhosis develop pleural effusions, most commonly on the right side, which are usually mild to moderate in size and asymptomatic, but occasionally they can be massive and provoke shortness of breath. The hepatopulmonary syndrome (HPS) consists of the clinical triad of advanced chronic liver disease, intrapulmonary vascular dilation (in the absence of intrinsic cardiopulmonary disease), and hypoxemia, which occurs in 8% to 29% of patients with cirrhosis, and it may also be found in some patients with noncirrhotic portal HTN and occasionally in acute hepatic conditions, such as viral hepatitis and ischemic hepatitis. The symptoms of HPS are not specific, consisting of insidious onset of dyspnea on exertion and often on standing (platypnea), which may progress to dyspnea at rest in more severely affected patients. Arterial hypoxemia, which is found in 30% to 70% of patients with cirrhosis, is usually mild to moderate but oxygen desaturation may occur during exercise. Digital clubbing and cyanosis are seen in many patients. The presence of ascites further compromises pulmonary function due to diaphragmatic elevation and reduced lung volumes, resulting in tachypnea and dyspnea. Additionally, 2% to 10% of patients with cirrhosis may develop portopulmonary HTN (POPH, the coexistence of pulmonary HTN and portal HTN), which is characterized by pulmonary HTN induced by increased pulmonary blood flow, which results from splanchnic vasodilatation and a hyperdynamic high-flow circulatory state that are provoked by portal HTN. Both HPS and POPH can become fatal as hepatic damage progresses.

Chronic alcohol consumption is associated with pulmonary and cardiac abnormalities. It increases the risk of developing pulmonary tuberculosis, chronic bronchitis, aspiration pneumonitis, lung abscess, and the pulmonary complications of alcoholic cirrhosis and alcoholic cardiomyopathy.[291] ARDS also occurs more frequently in patients with a history of alcohol abuse. Furthermore, chronic alcohol consumption is associated with higher prevalences of HTN, cerebrovascular accident, cardiac arrhythmias, sudden death, and CHF. The major cardiac abnormality specific to hepatic disease is alcoholic cardiomyopathy (or alcoholic heart muscle disease), which is the leading cause of dilated cardiomyopathy in the United States, accounting for approximately one third of cases.[292] In addition, up to 50% of asymptomatic alcoholics demonstrate subclinical systolic and diastolic dysfunction, with LV hypertrophy and dilation and impaired contractility.[293] Autonomic dysfunction is also common. Abstaining from alcohol consumption early in the course of alcoholic CM may halt the progression of or even reverse LV systolic dysfunction.

A distinct cirrhotic cardiomyopathy that differs from alcoholic cardiomyopathy has also been identified in patients with nonalcoholic cirrhosis, which is associated with hyperdynamic circulatory function, patchy myocardial fibrosis, subclinical diastolic and systolic dysfunction, an impaired myocardial response to an erect posture, and eventually high cardiac output failure.[294] These individuals also exhibit autonomic dysfunction with enhanced SNS tone and vagal dysfunction, which is directly related to the severity of cirrhosis.

Patients with both alcoholic and nonalcoholic cirrhosis exhibit significantly impaired cardiovascular responses to exercise, marked by blunted HR response, reduced myocardial contractility, subnormal increases in LV ejection fraction and cardiac output, and abnormally elevated cardiac pres-

sures.[294,295] Furthermore, profound wasting of skeletal muscle impairs oxygen extraction and utilization.

## Eating Disorders

The two most common eating disorders are anorexia nervosa and bulimia. Both disorders occur predominantly in young, previously healthy females and have specific behavioral and psychological features as well as physiologic abnormalities, including those involving the heart and lungs, as summarized in Table 7-19. The medical complications caused by eating disorders occur as a result of starvation, purging behaviors, and binge eating and involve almost all organ systems. Cardiac complications occur in 80% of patients with an eating disorder and include bradycardia and other cardiac arrhythmias, hypotension, decreased cardiac mass, and mitral valve prolapse. Arrhythmias are the leading cause of death.[296]

### Anorexia Nervosa

Anorexia nervosa is characterized behaviorally by severe self-induced weight loss (at least 15% below ideal body weight) through extreme restriction of food intake and sometimes ritualized exercise and purging. The major psychological manifestations are a distorted body image and an unreasonable concern about being "too fat," as well as denial of hunger, fatigue, and emaciation. A number of medical problems besides the characteristic amenorrhea have been reported in anorexia nervosa: salivary gland enlargement, pancreatitis, pancreatic insufficiency, liver dysfunction, thiamine deficiency, coagulopathies, electrolyte imbalance, decreased gastric emptying and intestinal mobility, hypophosphatemia, bilateral peroneal nerve palsies, hypoglycemia, osteoporosis, hypothalamic dysfunction, and cardiac abnormalities.[297] Furthermore, anorexia nervosa has a significant mortality rate, which is approximately 6% over a 5-year period and 15% to 20% at 15 years, and these deaths are often sudden due to cardiac arrhythmias.[298] Cardiac complications account for most of these deaths. Nutritional depletion due to starvation can result in wasted cardiac muscle and reduced LV mass, diminished glycogen stores, and evidence of myofibrillar atrophy and destruction.[296,299] Both systolic and diastolic ventricular dysfunction may occur.[296,300-302] Mitral valve prolapse is found in one-third of patients, resulting from wasted cardiac muscle disproportionate to mitral valve size. Clinically, bradycardia, hypotension, and impaired exercise tolerance (approximately 50% of predicted normal) with blunted HR and BP responses are common.[297,302,303]

### Bulimia Nervosa

Bulimia nervosa is a much more common disorder, which is characterized behaviorally by binge eating counterposed with purging by self-induced vomiting, laxative abuse, or diuretic abuse. In addition, many patients participate in fasting and extreme exercise. Psychologically, there is an awareness that the eating pattern is abnormal, a fear that eating cannot be controlled, and feelings of depression following binge eating. Because severe weight loss is not a problem for the majority of patients, many of the physiologic abnormalities seen in anorexia nervosa do not occur in most bulimic patients. However, there are major complications associated with bulimia, including electrolyte disorders resulting from the abuse of diuretics and laxatives, tooth decay, aspiration pneumonia, esophageal or gastric rupture, pneumomediastinum, pancreatitis, and neurologic abnormalities. Hypokalemia occurs in approximately 14% of patients with bulimia and sometimes leads to arrhythmias, which can be fatal, and the degeneration of cardiac and skeletal muscle.[296] In addition, the chronic use of ipecac to induce vomiting can cause cardiomyopathy, arrhythmias, and death.[304]

## Cardiopulmonary Toxicity of Cancer Treatment

The development of more aggressive treatments for a number of malignancies using chemotherapy, irradiation, and biologic agents, as well as hematopoietic stem cell or bone marrow transplantation and other medications to support patients during cancer treatments has yielded higher survival rates and longer survival periods but has also increased the incidence of cardiac and pulmonary toxicity causing acute and late complications. There is hope that the development of cardioprotective agents, such as the free-radical scavenger dexrazoxane currently under investigation, and medications that can reduce the incidence of radiation pneumonitis will reduce treatment-related toxicity that affect the lungs and heart.

A number of chemotherapeutic agents are associated with cardiac and pulmonary toxicity, which can occur acutely or may become apparent months to years following the completion of treatment. As with other situations involving cardiopulmonary complications, damage is found on autopsy much more frequently than is clinically apparent. The most notable complications are presented here.

Chemotherapy is often complicated by pulmonary toxicity, as indicated in Table 7-20.[305-310] Despite a variety of mechanism by which chemotherapeutic agents can injure the lungs, the clinical presentations are often similar, with dyspnea, nonproductive cough, and frequently fever, which develop weeks to years after treatment. Bleomycin has the highest incidence of pulmonary toxicity (up to 20% of patients), which is sometimes severe and can be fatal.[308] Acute bleomycin-induced hypersensitivity pneumonitis occurs in a small number of patients even with very low doses. More commonly pneumonitis develops that mainly appears as chronic pulmonary fibrosis; risk factors include higher cumulative dose (especially if >450 to 500 mg), patient age, smoking, renal dysfunction, prior or concomitant thoracic irradiation, and administration of oxygen. Bleomycin can also produce a number of other patterns of interstitial lung

disease. Other chemotherapeutic agents that can induce interstitial pneumonitis include
- Busulfan
- Chlorambucil
- Cyclophosphamide
- Methotrexate
- Mitomycin C
- The nitrosoureas (particularly carmustine and lomustine)
- Sometimes fludarabine, irinotecan (Camptosar), paclitaxel (Taxol), and procarbazine (Matulane, Natulan).

A number of other agents are also associated with other types of lung injury: Busulfan (Myleran) can cause pulmonary fibrosis and sometimes an alveolar-interstitial process with alveolar proteinosis, which is often fatal. Noncardiac pulmonary edema develops in 13% to 28% of patients during the administration of cytosine arabinoside (Cytarabine) and in a few patients months after treatment with mitomycin C. Pneumothorax occurs in some patients treated with the nitrosoureas. Acute hypersensitivity reactions have occurred with docetaxel (Taxotere) and procarbazine. Gemcitabine (Gemzar) causes dyspnea, which can be severe, in up to 10% of patients, and there have been reports of acute hypersensitivity reaction with bronchospasm, diffuse alveolar damage, and ARDS, and a rare severe idiosyncratic reaction with pulmonary infiltrates and marked dyspnea that may progress to life-threatening respiratory insufficiency. Procarbazine and vincristine (and theoretically cytarabine and chlorambucil) can cause neuropathies that may affect the respiratory muscles, inducing weakness. Zinostatin can produce a unique drug reaction involving hypertrophy of the pulmonary vasculature. In addition, sometimes pulmonary toxicity develops when specific chemotherapeutic agents are used in combination (e.g., vinblastine [Velban, Velsar] combined with mitomycin C induces bronchospasm, interstitial pneumonitis, and noncardiac pulmonary edema).

A number of chemotherapeutic agents are also known to cause cardiovascular dysfunction, as listed in Table 7-21.[306,311,312] The most well-recognized agents linked with cardiotoxicity are the anthracycline antibiotics:
- Doxorubicin (Adriamycin)
- Daunorubicin (Cerubidine)
- Epirubicin (Ellence, Pharmorubicin)
- Idarubicin (Idamycin)
- Mitoxantrone (Novantrone)

Radiation therapy (XRT) to the chest, as for the treatment of Hodgkin disease (HD), lymphoma, lung, breast, esophageal, and head and neck cancers, necessarily exposes the heart and lungs to varying degrees and dosages of radiation, depending on the extent of disease. Fortunately, modern treatment techniques instituted in 1985, particularly for HD, have drastically reduced cardiac and pulmonary complications. Radiation-induced pulmonary toxicity is usually related to the volume of lung tissue radiated, total dose of radiation, and the dose per treatment fraction (see Table 7-20).[310,313] The advent of three-dimensional treatment planning has

## Table 7-20 Pulmonary Toxicity Associated With Cancer Treatments

| | Cancer Treatment | Notable Pulmonary Side Effects | Incidence |
|---|---|---|---|
| Chemotherapeutic Agents | Bleomycin | Acute hypersensitivity pneumonitis, chronic pulmonary fibrosis. | Up to 20%, dose dependent |
| | Busulfan (Myleran) | Interstitial pneumonitis, alveolar-interstitial process with proteinosis | ~4% |
| | Chlorambucil (Leukeran) | Interstitial pneumonitis, pulmonary fibrosis | Rare |
| | Cyclophosphamide, CTX (Cytoxan) | Subacute pneumonitis, late-onset pulmonary fibrosis, ARDS | <5% |
| | Cytosine arabinoside (Cytarabine) | Subacute noncardiogenic pulmonary edema ± pleural effusion | 13–28% |
| | Docetaxel (Taxotere) | Acute hypersensitivity reaction, diffuse alveolar damage | 1–20% (less if premedication), dose related |
| | Fludarabine (Fludara) | Increased risk of opportunistic infections, diffuse pneumonitis, ARDS | Rare-18% |
| | Gemcitabine (Gemzar) | Acute hypersensitivity reaction with bronchospasm, nonspecific interstitial pneumonitis, diffuse alveolar damage/ARDS | <1– up to 10% |
| | Melphalan (Alkeran) | Diffuse pneumonitis 1–48 mo. after therapy | Rare |
| | Methotrexate, MTX | Hypersensitivity pneumonitis, respiratory failure | 2–8% |
| | Mitomycin (Mutamycin) | Acute and subacute pneumonitis, chronic pneumonitis; late noncardiac pulmonary edema, ARDS occur with hemolytic uremic syndrome | 3–14%, esp with higher doses |
| | Nitrosureas (carmustine [BCNU], lomustine [CCNU]) | Acute alveolitis/pneumonitis, chronic pulmonary fibrosis, pneumothorax | up to 20–30% if preexisting lung disease |
| | Paclitaxel (Taxol) | Anaphylactoid hypersensitivity at or near time of infusion (caused by suspension vehicle not the drug); hypersensitivity pneumonitis days to weeks after treatment; enhanced XRT-related lung damage? | 3–10+% (less if premedication), dose related |
| | Procarbazine (Metulane) | Acute hypersensitivity pneumonitis, pleural effusion, respiratory muscle weakness | 1–5% |
| | Vinca alkaloids: vinblastine (Velban, Velsar), vincristine (Oncovin, Vincasar, Vincrex) and vindesine (Eldisine, Fildesin), vinorelbine (Navelbine) | Acute interstitial pneumonitis, pulmonary fibrosis; respiratory muscle weakness (vincristine) | up to 5%, esp if combined treatment with mitomycin or single agent vinorelbine |

## Table 7-20 Pulmonary Toxicity Associated With Cancer Treatments—cont'd

| | Cancer Treatment | Notable Pulmonary Side Effects | Incidence |
|---|---|---|---|
| Biologic Agents | Interferon-α | Hypotension, ischemia, LV dysfn | |
| | Interleukin–2 (IL-2) | Acute noncardiac pulmonary edema, pleural effusion | ~20% |
| | Monoclonal antibodies | | |
| | Alemtuzumab (Campath) | Dyspnea, neutropenia-associated pneumonia | up to 15–28% |
| | Bevacizumab (Avastin) | Hemoptysis in lung cancer patients | 20% |
| | Cetuximab (Erbitux) | Acute dyspnea, which may be severe; delayed dyspnea | 5–13% |
| | Gemtuzumab (Mylotarg) | Acute hypersensitivity pneumonitis, pleural effusion, noncardiac pulmonary edema, ARDS, neutropenia-associated pneumonia | up to 10% |
| | Ibritumomab (Zevalin) | Acute hypersensitivity pneumonitis | 1–5% |
| | Rituximab (Rituxan, Mabthera) | Interstitial pneumonitis, COP, alveolar hemorrhage | Rare |
| | Tosituzumab (Bexxar) | Subacute hypersensitivity pneumonitis, bronchospasm, neutropenia-associated pneumonia | up to 29% |
| | Trastuzumab (Herceptin) | Bronchospasm, ARDS, pneumonitis, pleural effusion occurring during or after infusion | Rare |
| Miscellaneous | Etoposide (VP-16) | Alveolar hemorrhage | Rare |
| | Thalidomide (Thalomid) | Dyspnea, thromboembolic disease, interstitial pneumonitis, pleural effusion | 4–54% |
| Radiation Therapy to Chest | | Acute radiation pneumonitis developing 4–6 wks after treatment, late radiation fibrosis, cryptogenic organizing pneumonia (COP) | Lung: 5–15%, HD: 3–11%, Breast: >1% |
| Hematopoietic Stem Cell Transplantation | | Pulmonary edema due to fluid overload with infusion, chemotherapy-induced pulmonary toxicity (see above), increased risk of infection, diffuse alveolar hemorrhage, radiation pneumonitis with total body radiation, idiopathic pneumonia syndrome, bronchiolitis obliterans, delayed pulmonary toxicity syndrome, COP, respiratory muscle weakness. | Up to 65% |

permitted higher radiation doses to be delivered to the tumor while sparing surrounding normal tissue and is associated with a marked reduction in pulmonary toxicity. Acute radiation pneumonitis, which usually develops 4 to 6 weeks after XRT and is manifested clinically as a nonproductive cough, dyspnea (often at rest), and fever, occurs in 5% to 15% of patients who receive high-dose external beam radiation for lung cancer, 3% of those treated for HD with radiation alone and 11% of those who received combined modality treatment with XRT and chemotherapy, and less than 1% of women treated for breast cancer using breast XRT as part of a breast conserving approach.[306,313] Most patients with acute radiation

**Table 7-21 Cardiotoxicity Associated With Cancer Treatments**

| | Cancer Treatment | Notable Cardiovascular Side Effects | Incidence |
|---|---|---|---|
| Chemotherapeutic agents | Anthracyclines (doxorubicin [Adriamycin, Rubex], daunorubicin [Cerubidine], epirubicin [Ellence, Pharmorubicin], idarubicin [Idamycin, Zavedos], mitoxantrone [Novantrone]) | Acute myocarditis ± pericarditis causing CHF, delayed-onset (up to 20+ years after treatment) cardiomyopathy with chronic CHF. Early detection of falling ejection fraction can prevent dysfunction. | 6%–57%, dose dependent.<5% with mitoxantrone |
| | Busulfan (Myleran) | Endocardial fibrosis, cardiac tamponade | 1%–2% |
| | Capecitabine (Xeloda) | Ischemia, arrhythmias, especially in those with cardiac history | 3%–6% |
| | Cisplatinum (Platinol) | Ischemia, hypertension, CHF | 5%–15% |
| | Cyclophosphamide, CTX (Cytoxan) | Acute myocarditis, acute/subacute CHF; usually transient and reversible | 5%–10% |
| | Cytarabine, Aca-C (Cytosar) | Pericarditis, CHF | Rare |
| | Fluorouracil, 5-FU (Adrucil) | Ischemia, arrhythmias, MI, cardiogenic shock | 1%–8%, increased if cardiac history |
| | Iphosphamide (Ifex) | Myocarditis, CHF, arrhythmias; generally transient and reversible | 1%–5% |
| | Mitomycin (Mutamycin) | LV dysfunction, CHF | 1%–5% |
| | Paclitaxel (Taxol) | Acute or subacute arrhythmias, hypotension, ischemia, hypertension | <1%–5% |
| | Vinca alkaloids: vinblastine (Velban, Velsar), vincristine (Oncovin, Vincasar, Vincrex) and vindesine (Eldisine, Fildesin) | Ischemia, MI, autonomic cardioneuropathy | 5%–25% |
| Biologic agents | Interferons | Hypotension, arrhythmias, LV dysfunction, ischemia | 5%–10% |
| | Interleukins (IL-2, denileukin deftitox [Ontak]) | Capillary leak syndrome, hypotension, arrhythmias | 1%–15% |
| | Monoclonal antibodies | | |
| | Alemtuzumab (Campath) | Hypotension, CHF | 6%–17% |
| | Bevacizumab (Avastin) | Hypertension (may be severe), CHF, DVT | 7%–10% |
| | Cetuximab (Erbitux) | Hypotension | Rare |
| | Gemtuzumab (Mylotarg) | Hypertension, hypotension | 8%–9% each |
| | Ibritumomab (Zevalin) | Hypotension, chest pain, arrhythmias | 1%–5% |
| | Rituximab (Rituxan) | Hypotension, angioedema, arrhythmias, hypertension | 1%–5% |
| | Trastuzumab (Herceptin) | LV dysfunction, CHF | 3%–5% |
| Miscellaneous | All-trans-retinoic acid, ATRA (Tretinoin) | Hypotension, CHF | 1%–5% |
| | Arsenic trioxide (Trisenox) | QT prolongation, tachycardia | 8%–55% |
| | Etoposide (VP-16) | Hypotension, esp. with rapid infusion | 1%–4% |
| | Imatinib (Gleevec) | Pericardial effusion, CHF, edema | 6%–10% |
| | Pentostatin (Nipent) | CHF | 1%–5% |
| | Thalidomide (Thalomid) | Edema, hypotension, bradycardia, DVT | 1%–5% |

**Table 7-21 Cardiotoxicity Associated With Cancer Treatments—cont'd**

| Cancer Treatment | Notable Cardiovascular Side Effects | Incidence |
| --- | --- | --- |
| Radiation therapy to chest | Pericarditis with effusion, which is usually delayed, possible pericardial tamponade or constriction; premature CAD and MI; valve disease, myocardial disease, arrhythmias and conduction disturbances | 2%–12%, volume and dose dependent |
| Hematopoietic stem cell transplantation | Acute arrhythmias, conduction disturbances, pericardial effusion; late-onset cardiomyopathies; usually related to prior chemotherapy or drugs used to prepare for HSCT | Up to 57% |

*CAD, coronary artery disease; CHF, congestive heart failure; DVT, deep vein thrombosis; HSCT, hematopoietic stem cell transplantation; LV, left ventricular; MI, myocardial infarction.*

pneumonitis require no treatment and show complete resolution within 6 to 8 weeks, but a few patients develop severe pneumonitis requiring hospitalization and aggressive supportive care.

Radiation therapy to the chest can damage all structures of the heart (see Table 7-21), with the highest risk occurring in survivors of pediatric HD.[306,311] Late sequelae, which may not become clinically apparent for up to 25 or more years following treatment, often involve more than one cardiac structure in affected individuals, so that a number of conditions occur together. An estimate of the aggregate incidence of radiation-induced cardiac dysfunction is between 10% and 30% by 5 to 10 years post-treatment, although asymptomatic abnormalities of the heart muscle, valves, pericardium, conduction system, and the vascular system are detected in up to 88% of patients.[306] Factors that increase the risk of cardiac sequelae after mediastinal irradiation include cotreatment with anthracycline chemotherapy, location of tumor close to the heart border, age less than 18 years at the time of treatment, presence of CV risk factors or preexisting cardiac disease, treatment occurring more than 10 years earlier, and a number of radiation factors (use of orthovoltage radiation [mostly prior to 1970s], increased volume of irradiated heart, total dose to heart >30 Gy or daily dose fraction >2 Gy/day, or absence of subcarinal blocking). Cardiotoxicity typically manifests as pericarditis with pericardial effusion in 2% to 5% of patients receiving modern XRT for HD, which usually has a delayed onset (4 months to years after treatment). Approximately 10% to 20 % of patients with pericardial effusion develop tamponade and require pericardiocentesis.[311] Interferons (IFNs: -α, -β, -γ) are used in a wide variety of malignant, idiopathic, infectious, and inflammatory conditions, and their administration is associated with a variety of pulmonary reactions: severe exacerbation of bronchospasm in patients with preexisting asthma and a granulomatous reaction similar to sarcoidosis occur with IFN-α therapy;

interstitial lung disease, possibly cryptogenic organizing pneumonia, develops weeks to months after initiation of IFN therapy; and severe radiation pneumonitis can develop with multimodality therapy when IFN-γ is used.[305,307,308] Adverse cardiovascular effects are sometimes noted with IFNs: acute toxicity may be manifested as hypotension with compensatory tachycardia or, more rarely, as HTN, and in severe cases, as angina and MI, and there are rare reports of cardiomyopathy.[311,312]

Cardiotoxicity following hematopoietic stem cell transplantation and bone marrow transplantation is usually related to previous chemotherapy or that used as part of the conditioning regimen.[314,315] Acute toxicity is usually manifested by ECG abnormalities, such as arrhythmias and conduction disturbances, and pericardial effusion, which are usually asymptomatic but occasionally cause more serious problems. Some patients develop chemotherapy-induced cardiomyopathies, which may not become clinically apparent for many years to decades following treatment. A study involving the longitudinal evaluation of cardiopulmonary performance during exercise after bone marrow transplantation in children has revealed a number of functional defects, including significantly reduced maximal cardiac index, oxygen consumption, work performed, and ventilatory threshold, compared to age-matched, healthy control subjects.[314] Whereas the percentage of predicted VO$_2$max, maximum work performed, and ventilatory threshold increased over time for most patients, maximal cardiac index did not, providing evidence of subclinical myocardial dysfunction.

Finally, some treatments used to support cancer patients during treatment also have the possibility of inducing pulmonary complications. The hematopoietic growth factors, granulocyte and granulocyte-macrophage colony stimulating factors (G/GM-CSF; e.g., Filgrastim), used to facilitate neutropenia recovery and prevent infection following high-dose

---

**Box 7-3**

**Guidelines for Physical Therapy Intervention and Endurance Training**

### Guidelines for Physical Therapy Intervention

HR, BP, and signs and symptoms of exercise intolerance should be monitored during every PT evaluation.

If the patient's responses are normal, it is safe to proceed with typical treatment planning (including endurance training).

If the responses are abnormal, caution is indicated. They may be so abnormal that physician consultation is warranted, or they may signal that the patient's tolerance is compromised and that he or she will require treatment modifications, such as frequent rests during more strenuous activities and careful attention to maintain coordinated breathing during exertion.

Patients with moderate to severe cardiopulmonary dysfunction will usually display symptoms of dyspnea, fatigue, or weakness, and possibly lightheadedness or dizziness during activity, which should be associated with the physiologic responses detected during monitoring and then used during future treatment sessions as indicators of patient tolerance.

A few patients will require continued monitoring of HR, BP, and/or $O_2$ saturation during further treatment sessions, until their responses normalize or their symptoms become predictable indicators of physiologic status.

Some patients may benefit more from two shorter treatment sessions per day rather than one intense or prolonged session.

### Guidelines for Endurance Training

Regarding endurance training, the following guidelines are suggested:

Patients should start with low-intensity exercise and increase their activity gradually.

The mode can consist of any form of aerobic exercise, including walking, jogging, cycling, swimming, cross-country skiing, and aerobics classes, and can vary during the week.

Intensity may be most easily monitored by using a rating of perceived exertion (RPE) scale. A good starting place is "somewhat hard" (13 on the Borg scale of 6 to 20)[323] or "moderate" (3 to 4 on the Borg 0–10 scale).[324] (See Chapter 16.)

Duration starts with the length of time a patient can exercise until fatigue begins to occur and increases about 1 or 2 min per day.

Short rest periods (1 to 2 min) can be alternated with the exercise intervals if a patient has very limited endurance.

Patients will benefit most from twice-daily exercise periods until the duration increases to at least 20 min of continuous peak activity.

Once a patient can perform the peak aerobic portion of the program for at least 30 min continuously, the frequency can be reduced to 3 to 5 or more d per wk, depending on the intensity and the goals of the patient (for control of HTN or reduction of body weight, lower-intensity, longer-duration exercise programs are more successful).

Any amount of activity is better than no activity. If a patient has a hectic day and cannot fit the entire workout in, a partial workout or multiple short bouts are preferable to skipping the workout.

Exercise time or distance can be recorded on a calendar in order to keep track of progress and provide motivation. Include totals for each week and month.

Finally, exercise should be fun! Identify activities patients enjoy or create a social aspect to their exercise program so it will not seem like a chore.

BP, blood pressure; HR, heart rate; PT, physical therapy.

---

chemotherapy and stem cell transplantation are associated with an increased risk of respiratory deterioration as a result of acute lung injury or ARDS (when used in patients with pulmonary infiltrates), as well as arterial thrombosis and the vascular leak syndrome. Platelet and blood transfusions sometimes cause pulmonary edema.

## Clinical Implications for Physical Therapy

The most obvious implication of all the information presented in this chapter is that many patients with many different primary diagnoses may exhibit cardiopulmonary dysfunction. Yet, the symptoms of dysfunction are often nonspecific, such as shortness of breath, lightheadedness, and fatigue, or there may not be any symptoms at all, as in HTN. Furthermore, many patients will not complain of symptoms despite significant exercise intolerance, because they have gradually limited their physical activity in order to avoid discomfort.

Worthy of particular mention based on prevalence are the benefits of exercise for patients with cancer. Increased levels of physical activity during and after cancer treatment has been shown to reduce fatigue, enhance physical performance and improve quality of life.[316–318] Exercise therapy may also mitigate the adverse effects of treatment for cancer on the CV system.[319] Resistance training likely helps to improve muscle function, lean tissue mass, and bone mineral density. Furthermore, there is evidence that regular physical activity improves survival in patients with breast and colorectal cancers.[320–322]

To summarize and reduce to the basics for practical application, recommendations are offered in Box 7-3.

## CASE STUDY 7-1

JF is a 76-year-old woman admitted 2 days ago because of confusion, incoherent speech, and lethargy. CT scan revealed a large parietal lobe infarct on the left. Her past medical history is significant for HTN for 30 years, treated with hydrochlorothiazide 75 mg once a day and captopril 50 mg once a day. She has had type 2 diabetes for 15 years, treated with glyburide 5 mg every morning. Positive smoking history: 90 pack-years. The PT assessment reveals a lethargic-appearing 76-year-old woman with obvious right facial paresis, severe dysarthria, flaccid right upper extremity, decreasing tone right lower extremity through positive clonus of right ankle. She requires moderate assistance to roll supine, right side, maximal assistance to roll to left, and maximal assistance of one to come to sitting at edge of bed. Sitting balance is poor, with trunk lean to right.

### Discussion

Admitting diagnosis of CVA indicates carotid or cerebrovascular disease. Comorbidities: diabetes (treated with an oral insulin secretagogue), HTN (treated with a diuretic and ACE inhibitor). Other risk factors for CAD and CVA: Smoking history (90 pack-years, may also have underlying COPD).

Current medical problem of CVA with hemiparesis and functional limitations implies increased work required to perform activities and possible ventilatory limitation due to restrictive lung dysfunction, which increases the risk of atelectasis and pneumonia. The risk of atelectasis and pneumonia is compounded by the patient's marked limitation of physical activity. Probable speech and swallowing dysfunction increases the risk for aspiration pneumonia and may impair cough effectiveness.

This patient, who presents with CVA and also has multiple risk factors for CAD should be monitored closely for signs and symptoms of CAD and cardiac pump dysfunction, as well as abnormal responses to exercise. She may also benefit from diabetic education. Patients with long-standing smoking history may have underlying COPD and may need to have oxygen saturation monitored, arterial blood gases, and CXR.

## Summary

A great number of medical problems are associated with cardiovascular and pulmonary complications, many of which are not recognized by either the individual or his primary medical provider. The symptoms of cardiopulmonary dysfunction are often nonspecific, such as shortness of breath, fatigue and weakness, and lightheadedness, and many patients are unaware of symptoms of activity intolerance despite significant dysfunction because they are unwittingly avoiding activities that cause discomfort. Yet, it is important for physical therapists to recognize the presence of cardiopulmonary dysfunction when prescribing physical therapy (PT) interventions in order to optimize safety and effectiveness. A summary of the most important points provided in this chapter includes the following:

- Several factors are known to affect energy balance and contribute to the development of overweight and obesity, the most important of which are environmental factors, particularly excessive caloric intake and reduced physical activity, and genetic, hormonal, and metabolic factors also play a role. In addition, calcium intake, particularly in dairy products, is inversely related to body fat levels, and sleep deprivation is associated with higher body fat levels.
- Overweight and obesity represent major health problems in this country because of their association with increased prevalences of hypertension (HTN), coronary artery disease (CAD), stroke, osteoarthritis, and other orthopedic problems, gastrointestinal (GI) problems, glucose intolerance, insulin resistance, type 2 diabetes mellitus (DM), dyslipidemia, gallbladder disease, sleep-related breathing disorders, gynecologic problems, pulmonary dysfunction, and certain forms of cancer.
- Increased body fat, particularly intraabdominal or visceral adiposity, is directly related to cardiovascular disease (CVD) risk and type 2 DM. The measurement of waist circumference (WC) provides a simple index of disease risk, with commonly accepted cutoff points of 40 in. (102 cm) for men and 35 in. (88 cm) for women to define central obesity. Risk of future CVD increases by 2% per 1 cm increase in WC.
- Treatments for obesity include caloric restriction and other diet modifications, increased physical activity, behavioral modification, pharmacotherapy, and bariatric surgery, depending on the degree of obesity. With the exception of bariatric surgery, the goal is usually set at a 10% reduction in body weight, which is associated with significant health benefits; however, this goal is hard to achieve and even more difficult to maintain.
- Obesity is associated with both pulmonary and cardiovascular dysfunction, and obese individuals usually exhibit abnormal physiological responses to exercise and reduced exercise tolerance. Thus, obese individuals require clinical monitoring and often treatment modifications when referred to PT.
- Aerobic and resistance exercise are important interventions for all individuals who are obese as means of increasing energy expenditure, improving cardiorespiratory fitness, ameliorating CV risk factors, protecting against loss of lean body mass during caloric restriction, and increasing muscular efficiency, even if no weight loss is achieved.
- To achieve and maintain long-term weight loss, at least 45 to 60 minutes/day of at least moderate-intensity exercise may be required, such that a total of 250 to 300 minutes of exercise is performed each week.

- The metabolic syndrome refers to a cluster of interrelated risk factors, including abdominal obesity, atherogenic dyslipidemia, HTN, insulin resistance, and impaired glucose tolerance, that is associated with increased risk of CVD events and death, type 2 DM, and chronic kidney disease. Lifestyle interventions to lose weight and increase physical activity can markedly reduce the risk of developing DM.

- Diabetes mellitus is a chronic metabolic disorder characterized by hyperglycemia and caused by inadequate insulin production or ineffective insulin action. Abnormalities in the metabolism of carbohydrates, fats, and proteins result. In addition, chronically elevated blood glucose (BG) levels and other associated abnormalities result in damage to the arteries, heart, kidneys, eyes, and peripheral and autonomic nerves.

- Cardiovascular disorders are the most common cause of morbidity and mortality in people with both type 1 and type 2 DM. Microvascular disease results in retinopathy, renal damage, and neuropathy, and macrovascular disease due to accelerated atherosclerosis causes CAD, stroke, and peripheral arterial disease (PAD). Strict glycemic control can reduce the risk of developing vascular complications related to DM.

- Glycosylated hemoglobin (HbA1c, or simply A1c) provides a reliable indication of the degree of glycemic control achieved by an individual over the preceding 2- to 3-month period. For individuals with DM, the goal is to achieve levels of <7% (normal levels are 2.5% to 6%) through intensive glycemic control in order to reduce the risk of diabetic complications.

- Type 1 DM requires insulin therapy, whereas other antihyperglycemic medications are used for the treatment of type 2 DM, at least until there is significant β-cell dysfunction, when insulin will also be needed.

- The major problem associated with insulin therapy is hypoglycemia, which occurs when the level of circulating insulin exceeds need, such as during the hour or so immediately before mealtime or when there is persistent increased insulin sensitivity and mandatory repletion of muscle and liver glycogen stores following exercise. Risk factors for exercise-related hypoglycemia include intensive insulin therapy and tight glycemic control (so smaller safety margin), inadequate food intake preceding exercise (e.g., when a meal is delayed or skipped), rapid absorption of depot insulin from an injection site near exercising muscle, exercising at the time of peak insulin effect, and prolonged moderate-intensity exercise.

- The glucoregulatory responses to exercise are abnormal in DM. A number of important variables affect these responses in individuals with type 1 diabetes: the preexercise levels of circulating insulin and the counterregulatory hormones, as indicated by the BG level, both at the onset of exercise (which are determined by the type and dose of insulin administered before exercise and the timing of previous insulin injection and carbohydrate intake relative to the onset of exercise) and during exercise (which

is affected by the injection site and the intensity, type, and duration of exercise).

- To allow safe participation in physical activity and high-level athletic performance, persons with type 1 DM must carefully match insulin dose, carbohydrate intake, and exercise in order to avoid either hypo- or hyperglycemia. Thus, it is important to monitor BG level 60 and 30 min before exercise in order to identify the individual's glucoregulatory status. If BG levels are low, supplemental carbohydrates may be required to prevent exercise-induced hypoglycemia. If BG levels are high, there is a risk of further aggravation of hyperglycemia during exercise, particularly with higher-intensity or longer-duration exercise. Both situations require BG monitoring during exercise to clarify the individual's glucoregulatory responses and need for treatment modifications. If BG levels are excessively low (<70 mg/dL) or high (>300 mg/dL) or if ketones are present, exercise is contraindicated, at least until corrective measures have taken effect.

- Adjustments in insulin dose before and sometimes after exercise may be required to prevent exercise-associated hypoglycemia, or less commonly hyperglycemia.

- The concerns for patients with type 2 DM differ from those for type 1 DM. They should avoid exercise if BG is more than 400 mg/dL because of the risk of hyperosmolar hyperglycemic nonketonic syndrome. In addition, only the insulin secretagogues (sulfonylureas and glinides) are associated with a higher risk of hypoglycemia and may require dose reduction on the day of exercise.

- Cardiac autonomic neuropathy (CAN) should be suspected in all individuals with type 2 DM and in those with type 1 DM for more than 5 years. Clinical manifestations include higher resting HR and reduced HR variability, orthostatic hypotension, impaired exercise tolerance, and painless myocardial ischemia and infarction (due to cardiac denervation). Simple tests are available to determine the presence of CAN and should be included in the PT evaluation of susceptible individuals.

- The kidneys are complex organs whose major functions include the control of extracellular fluid volume; the regulation of serum osmolality, electrolyte, and acid–base balances; and the secretion of hormones, such as renin and erythropoietin. Thus, when renal function becomes impaired, the resultant metabolic disturbances affect virtually every other body system.

- Chronic renal failure (CRF) is associated with a number of major complications: HTN, pericarditis with pericardial effusion and sometimes cardiac tamponade, accelerated atherosclerosis, anemia, bleeding disorders, renal osteodystrophy, proximal myopathy, peripheral neuropathy, peptic ulceration, and immunosuppression leading to intercurrent infections. Pulmonary edema can also occur as a result of fluid overload as well as increased capillary permeability.

- Although many patients do well for more than 10 years on dialysis, success is limited by the impaired clearance of waste products and other substances and the marked impairment of the regulatory and endocrine functions normally provided by the kidneys.

- Most patients with CRF have very limited exercise tolerance and many have difficulty doing more than self-care activities. Contributory factors include anemia, CVD, chronic physical inactivity, skeletal muscle dysfunction, and metabolic acidosis. The limiting symptom is usually skeletal muscle fatigue, and patients have notable skeletal muscle atrophy and weakness.

- Connective tissue diseases affects all pulmonary and CV structures, either separately or in combination. Not infrequently, pulmonary involvement precedes the musculoskeletal manifestations by several months to several years. Cardiovascular abnormalities most often involve the pericardium, arterial vasculature, and cardiac valves and usually causes minimal cardiovascular dysfunction (e.g., asymptomatic mitral valve prolapse or mild aortic root dilatation) but occasionally results in significant problems (e.g., cardiomyopathy producing CHF, myocardial infarction, severe aortic or mitral insufficiency, or dissecting aortic aneurysm).

- Many neurological and neuromuscular diseases and disorders are associated with pulmonary and cardiac complications, and symptoms often do not correlate well with the degree of dysfunction in slowly progressive disorders. Sleep-disordered breathing is often an indication of chronic respiratory muscle fatigue and increased risk of ventilatory failure, which can be ameliorated with the use of nocturnal ventilatory assistance. Therefore, PTs should be attentive to relevant symptoms, such as sleep disturbances, morning headache, excessive daytime somnolence, impaired concentration, and loss of appetite, and alert the patient's physician if they are noted.

- The clinical manifestations of anemia depend upon the cause of anemia, its extent, the rapidity of onset, and the presence of any other medical problems that compromise the individual's health. Most cases of chronic anemia are asymptomatic other than vague fatigue until the hemoglobin concentration falls below 50% of normal, whereupon more notable symptoms appear, including fatigue and weakness, exertional dyspnea and diminished exercise tolerance, palpitations, pallor, and sometimes tachycardia. Patients with CAD may develop myocardial ischemia with mild anemia.

- Sickle cell disease is characterized by hemolytic anemia and periodic acute painful crises resulting from occlusion of small capillaries and venules, which result in progressive systemic vasculopathy and chronic organ failure.

- Pulmonary complications are the leading cause of morbidity and mortality in patients with HIV and AIDS; cardiovascular complications also occur in many patients and are sometimes fatal.

- The vast majority of patients with chronic liver disease exhibit pulmonary abnormalities, particularly arterial hypoxemia, which is usually mild, although oxygen desaturation may occur during exercise. Pleural effusions and ascites will compound pulmonary dysfunction as a result of restriction of ventilation, resulting in tachypnea and dyspnea. Chronic alcohol consumption is associated with numerous pulmonary and CV complications, some of which cause serious dysfunction and death; alcoholic cardiomyopathy (or alcoholic heart muscle disease) is the leading cause of dilated cardiomyopathy in the Western world.

- Eating disorders are associated with numerous medical complications. Cardiac complications are responsible for most of the deaths, which may be sudden due to arrhythmias induced by electrolyte imbalances. In addition, the chronic use of ipecac to induce vomiting can cause cardiomyopathy, arrhythmias, and death.

- Nearly all therapies used to treat cancer are associated with cardiac and pulmonary toxicity, which can cause acute or late complications that may be serious and/or fatal. There is often a synergistic effect of radiation therapy and some chemotherapeutic agents, and also of some of the drugs when used in combination, which can increase the extent of cardiac or pulmonary injury. Regular exercise provides a number of benefits for individuals during and after cancer treatment, possibly including increased survival.

- The only way to determine if a patient is responding to exercise appropriately is to assess his or her physiologic responses. This is achieved by monitoring HR, BP, and other signs and symptoms of exercise intolerance during every PT evaluation. Abnormal responses indicate the need for treatment modifications.

- Endurance and resistance training should be included as components of the PT program for every patient who is not already performing regular aerobic exercise, except those who have cardiopulmonary instability or debilitating neuromuscular diseases that are adversely affected by exercise.

## References

1. Klein S, Romijn JA. Obesity. In Kronenberg HM, Melmed S, Polonsky KS, Larsen PR (eds.): Williams Textbook of Endocrinology. 11th ed. Philadelphia, Saunders, 2008.

2. Catenacci VA, Hill Jo, Wyatt HR. The obesity epidemic. Clin Chest Med 30:415–44, 2009.

3. National Center for Health Statistics Health E-Stat. Prevalence of overweight, obesity and extreme obesity among adults: United States, trends 1976–1980 through 2005–2006.

4. Ogden CL, Carroll MD, Curtin LR, et al. Prevalence of overweight and obesity in the United States, 1999–2004. JAMA 295:1549–55, 2006.

5. Wang Y, Beydoun MA. The obesity epidemic in the United States—gender, age, socioeconomic, racial/ethnic, and geographic characteristics: a systematic review and meta-regression analysis. Epidemiol Rev 29:6–28, 2007.

6. Boardley D, Pobocik RS. Obesity on the rise. Prim Care Clin Office Pract 36:243–55, 2009.

7. Bradford NF. Overweight and obesity in children and adolescents. Prim Care Clin Office Pract 36:319–39, 2009.

8. Balkau B, Deanfield JE, Després J-P, et al. International Day for the evaluation of abdominal obesity (IDEA). A study of

waist circumference, cardiovascular disease, and diabetes mellitus in 168,000 primary care patients in 63 countries. Circulation 116:1942–51, 2007.

9. Kelly T, Yang W, Chen CS, et al. Global burden of obesity in 2005 and projections to 2030. Int J Obes (Lond) 32:1431–7, 2008.

10. Maes HH, Neale MC, Eaves LJ. Genetic and environmental factors in relative body weight and human adiposity. Behav Genet 27:325–51, 1997.

11. Erlanson-Albertsson C. Appetite regulation and energy balance. Acta Paediatr 94(Suppl 448):40–1, 2005.

12. King PJ. The hypothalamus and obesity. Curr Drug Targets 6:225–40, 2005.

13. Spiegelman BM, Flier JS. Obesity and the regulation of energy balance. Cell 104:531–43, 2001.

14. Major GC, Chaput J-P, Ledoux M, et al. Recent developments in calcium-related obesity research. Obesity Rev 9:428–45, 2008.

15. Pereira MA, Jacobs DR, Van Horn L, et al. Dairy consumption, obesity, and the insulin resistance syndrome in young adults. JAMA 287:2081–9, 2002.

16. Gangwisch JE, Malaspina D, Boden-Alala B, et al. Inadequate sleep as a risk factor for obesity: analyses of the NHANES I. Sleep 28:1289–96, 2005.

17. Knutson KL, Spiegel K, Penev P, et al. The metabolic consequences of sleep deprivation. Sleep Med Rev 11:163–78, 2007.

18. Taheri S, Lin L, Austin D, et al. Short sleep duration is associated with reduced leptin, elevated ghrelin, and increased body mass index. PLoS Med 1:e62 (210–17), 2004.

19. Taheri S. The link between short sleep duration and obesity: we should recommend more sleep to prevent obesity. Arch Dis Child 91:881–4, 2006.

20. August GP, Caprio S, Fennoy I, et al. Prevention and treatment of pediatric obesity: an endocrine society clinical practice guideline based on expert opinion. J Clin Endocrinol Metab 93:4576–99, 2008.

21. Bessesen DH. Update on obesity. J Clin Endocrinol Metab 93:2027–34, 2008.

22. Jensen MD. Obesity. In Goldman L, Auseillo D (eds.). Cecil Textbook of Medicine. 23rd ed. Philadelphia, Saunders Elsevier, 2008.

23. Canoy D, Boekholdt SM, Wareham N, et al. Body fat distribution and risk of coronary heart disease in men and women in the European Prospective Investigation into Cancer and Nutrition in Norfolk cohort. A population-based prospective study. Circulation 116:2933–43, 2007.

24. Kannel WB, D'Agostino RB, Cobb JL. Effect of weight on cardiovascular disease. Am J Clin Nutr 63:419S–22S, 1996.

25. Schelbert KB. Comorbidities of obesity. Prim Care Clin Office Pract 36:271–85, 2009.

26. Van Itallie TB. Health implications of overweight and obesity in the United States. Ann Intern Med 103:983–8, 1985.

27. North American Association for the Study of Obesity (NAASO), National Heart, Lung, and Blood Institute (NHLBI). Practical Guide on the Identification, Evaluation, and Treatment of Overweight and Obesity in Adults. NIH Publication No 00-4084. Bethesda, MD: National Institutes of Health; 2000. http://www.nhlbi.nih.gov/guidelines/obesity/prctgd_c.pdf.

28. de Koning L, Merchang AT, Pogue J, et al. Waist circumference and waist-to-hip ration as predictors of cardiovascular events: multi-regression analysis of prospective studies. Eur Heart J 28:850–6, 2007.

29. Snijder MB, van Dam RM, Seidell JC. What aspects of body fat are particularly hazardous and how do we measure them? Int J Epidemiol 35:83–92, 2006.

30. Westphal SA. Obesity, abdominal obesity, and insulin resistance. Clin Cornerstone 9:23–31, 2008.

31. American Diabetes Association. Diagnosis and classification of diabetes mellitus. Position statement. Diabetes Care 30(Suppl 1):S42–7, 2007.

32. Nathan DM, Davidson MB, DeFronzo A, et al. Impaired fasting glucose and impaired glucose tolerance: implications for care. Diabetes Care 30:753–9, 2007.

33. Abdul-Ghani MA, DeFronzo RA. Plasma glucose concentration and prediction of future risk of type 2 diabetes. Diabetes Care 32(Suppl 2):S194–8, 2009.

34. Fonseca VA. Defining and characterizing the progression of type 2 diabetes. Diabetes Care 32(Suppl 2):S151–6, 2009.

35. Poitout V, Robertson RP. Minireveiws: secondary beta-cell failure in type 2 diabetes–a convergence of glucotoxicity and lipotoxicity. Endocrinology 143:339–42, 2002.

36. Gualillo O, González-Juanatey JR, Lago F. The emerging role of adipokines as mediators of cardiovascular function: physiologic and clinical perspectives. Trends Cardiovasc Med 17:275–83, 2007.

37. Antuna-Puente B, Feve B, Fellahi S, et al. Adipokines: the missing link between insulin resistance and obesity. Diabetes Metab 34:2–11, 2008.

38. Boden G. Obesity and free fatty acids. Endocrinol Metab Clin N Am 37:635–46, 2008.

39. Bogaert YE, Linas S. The role of obesity in the pathogenesis of hypertension. Nat Clin Pract Nephrol 5:101–11, 2009.

40. Cannon CP. Obesity-related cardiometabolic complications. Clin Cornerstone 9:11–22, 2008.

41. Franssen R, Monajemi H, Stroes ESG, et al. Obesity and dyslipidemia. Endocrinol Metab Clin North Am 37:623–33, 2008.

42. Goldstein BJ, Scalia RG, Ma XL. Protective vascular and myocardial effects of adiponectin. Nat Clin Pract Cardiovasc Med 6:27–35, 2009.

43. Kurukulasuriya LR, Stas S, Lastra G, et al. Hypertension in obesity. Endocrinol Metab Clin North Am 37:647–62, 2008.

44. Moschen AR, Kaser A, Enrich B, et al. Visfatin, an adipocytokine with proinflammatory and immunomodulating properties. J Immunol 178:1748–58, 2007.

45. Omoigui S. The interleukin-6 inflammatory pathway from cholesterol to aging—Role of statins, bisphosphonates and plant polyphenols in aging and age-related diseases. Immunity & Aging 4:1–22, 2007.

46. Rabe K, Lehrke M, Parhofer KG, et al. Adipokines and insulin resistance. Mol Med 14:741–51, 2008.

47. Romero-Corral A, Sierra-Johnson J, Lopez-Jiminez F, et al. Relationship between leptin and C-reactive protein with cardiovascular disease in the adult general population. Nat Clin Pract Cardiovasc Med 5:418–25, 2008.

48. Skurk T, Hauner H. Obesity and impaired fibrinolysis: role of adipose production of plasminogen activator inhibitor-1. Int J Obes 28:1357–64, 2004.

49. Stehno-Bittel L. Intricacies of fat. Phys Ther 88:1265–78, 2008.

50. Zalesin KC, Franklin BA, Miller WM, et al. Impact of obesity on cardiovascular disease. Endocrinol Metab Clin North Am 37:663–84, 2008.

51. Hoene M, Weigert C. The role of interleukin-6 in insulin resistance, body fat distribution, and energy balance. Obes Rev 9:20–9, 2008.

52. Rocha VZ, Libby P. Obesity, inflammation, and atherosclerosis. Nat Rev Cardiol 6:399–409, 2009.

53. Gallagher EJ, LeRoith D, Karnieli E. The metabolic syndrome—from insulin resistance to obesity and diabetes. Endocrinol Metab Clin North Am 37:559–79, 2008.

54. Dela Cruz CS, Matthay RA. Role of obesity in cardiomyopathy and pulmonary hypertension. Clin Chest Med 30:509–23, 2009.

55. Hunt SA, Baker DW, Chin MH, et al. ACC/AHA guidelines for the evaluation and management of chronic heart failure in the adult: executive summary. A report of the American College of Cardiology/American Heart Association Task Force on Practice Guidelines. Circulation 104:2996–3007, 2001.

56. Wong C, Marwick TH. Obesity cardiomyopathy: pathogenesis and pathophysiology. Nat Clin Pract Cardiovasc Med 4:436–43, 2007.

57. Wong C, Marwick TH. Obesity cardiomyopathy: diagnosis and therapeutic interventions. Nat Clin Pract Cardiovasc Med 4:480–90, 2007.

58. Haque AK, Gadre S, Taylor J, et al. Pulmonary and cardiovascular complications of obesity. An autopsy study of 76 obese subjects. Arch Pathol Lab Med 132:1397–404, 2008.

59. de Sousa AGP, Cercato C, Mancini MC, et al. Obesity and obstructive sleep apnea-hypopnea syndrome. Obesity Rev 9:340–54, 2008.

60. Parameswaran K, Todd DC, Soth M. Altered respiratory physiology in obesity. Can Respir J 13:203–10, 2006.

61. Sood A. Altered resting and exercise respiratory physiology in obesity. Clin Chest Med 30:445–54, 2009.

62. Tzelepis GE, McCool FD. The lungs and chest wall disease. In Mason RJ, Murray JF, Broaddus VC, et al (eds.): Mason: Murray & Nadel's Textbook of Respiratory Medicine. 4th ed. Philadelphia, Elsevier Saunders, 2004.

63. Beuther DA. Obesity and asthma. Clin Chest Med 30:479–88, 2009.

64. Littleton SW, Mokhlesi B. The Pickwickian syndrome—obesity hypoventilation syndrome. Clin Chest Med 30:467–78, 2009.

65. Olson AL, Zwillich C. The obesity hypoventilation syndrome. Am J Med 118:948–56, 2005.

66. Rössner S, Hammarstrand M, Hemmingsson E, et al. Long-term weight loss and weight-loss maintenance strategies. Obes Rev 9:624–30, 2008.

67. Expert Panel on the Identification, Evaluation, and Treatment of Overweight and Obesity in Adults. Executive summary of the clinical guidelines on the identification, evaluation, and treatment of overweight and obesity in adults. Arch Intern Med 158:1855–67, 1998.

68. Hainer V, Toplak H, Mitrakou A. Treatment modalities of obesity. What fits whom? Diabetes Care 31(Suppl 2):S269–77, 2008.

69. Shewmake RA, Huntington MK. Nutritional treatment of obesity. Prim Care Clin Office Pract 36:357–77, 2009.

70. Hession M, Rolland C, Kulkarni U, et al. Systematic review of randomized controlled trials of low carbohydrate vs. low-fat/low-calorie diets in the management of obesity and its comorbidities. Obes Rev 10:36–50, 2009.

71. Westerterp-Plantenga MS, Nieuwenhuizen A, Tomé D, et al. dietary protein, weight loss, and weight maintenance. Annu Rev Nutr 29:21–41, 2009.

72. Brehm BJ, D'Alessio DA. Weight loss and metabolic benefits with diets of varying fat and carbohydrate content: separating the wheat from the chaff. Nat Clin Pract Endocrinol Metab 4:140–6, 2008.

73. Douketis JD, Macie C, Thabane L, et al. Systematic review of long-term weight loss studies in obese adults: clinical significance and applicability to clinical practice. Int J Obes 29:1153–67, 2005.

74. Donnelly JE, Blair SN, Jakicic JM, et al. Appropriate physical activity intervention strategies for weight loss and prevention of weight regain for adults. Med Sci Sports Exerc 41:459–71, 2009.

75. Garrow JS, Summerbell CD. Meta-analysis: effect of exercise, with or without dieting, on the body composition of overweight subjects. Eur J Clin Nutr 49:1–10, 1995.

76. Miller WC, Koceja DM, Hamilton EJ. A meta-analysis of the past 25 years of weight loss research using diet, exercise, or diet plus exercise intervention. Int J Obes Relat Metab Disord 21:941–7, 1997.

77. Wing RR. Physical activity in the treatment of the adulthood overweight and obesity: current evidence and research issues. Med Sci Sports Exerc 31:S547–52, 1999.

78. Curioni CC, Lourenco PM. Long-term weight loss after diet and exercise: a systematic review. Int J Obes (Lond) 29:1168–74, 2005.

79. Wu T, Gao X, Chen M, et al. Long-term effectiveness of diet-plus-exercise interventions vs. diet-only interventions for weight loss: a meta-analysis. Obes Rev 10:313–23, 2009.

80. Stiegler P, Cunliffe A. The role of diet and exercise for the maintenance of fat-free mass and resting metabolic rate during weight loss. Sports Med 36:239–62, 2006.

81. Dickerson LM, Carek PJ. Pharmacotherapy for the obese patient. Prim Care Clin Office Pract 36:407–15, 2009.

82. Idelevich E, Kirch W, Schindler C. Current pharmacotherapeutic concepts for the treatment of obesity in adults. Ther Adv Cardiovasc Dis 3:75–90, 2009.

83. Li Z, Maglione M, Tu W, et al. Meta-analysis: pharmacologic treatment of obesity. Ann Intern Med 142:532–46, 2005.

84. Fabrini E, Klein S. Fundamentals of cardiometabolic risk factor reduction: achieving and maintaining weight loss with pharmacotherapy or bariatric surgery. Clin Cornerstone 9:41–51, 2008.

85. Maggard MA, Shugarmann LR, Suttorp M, et al. Meta-analysis: surgical treatment of obesity. Ann Intern Med 142:547–59, 2005.

86. Mathier MA, Ramanathan RC. Impact of obesity and bariatric surgery on cardiovascular disease. Med Clin North Am 91:415–31, 2007.

87. Knop FK. Resolution of type 2 diabetes following gastric bypass surgery: involvement of gut-derived glucagon and glucagonotropic signaling? Diabetologia 52:2270–6, 2009.

88. Salvadori A, Fanari P, Palmulli P, et al. Cardiovascular and adrenergic response to exercise in obese subjects. J Clin Basic Cardiol 2:229–36, 1999.

89. Donnelly JE, Jacobsen DJ, Heelan KS, et al. The effects of 18 months of intermittent vs continuous exercise on aerobic capacity, body weight and composition, an metabolic fitness

in previously sedentary, moderately obese females. Int J Obes 24:566–72, 2000.

90. Pedersen BK, Saltin B. Evidence for prescribing exercise as therapy in chronic disease [Review]. Scand J Med Sci Sports 16(Suppl 1):3–63, 2006.

91. Wadden TA, Vogt RA, Andersen RE, et al. Exercise in the treatment of obesity: effects of four interventions on body composition, resting energy expenditure, appetite, and mood. J Consult Clin Psychol 65:269–77, 1997.

92. Okay DM, Jackson PV, Marcinkiewicz M, et al. Exercise and obesity. Prim Care Clin Office Pract 36:379–93, 2009.

93. Sui X, LaMonte MJ, Laditka JN, et al. Cardiorespiratory fitness and adiposity as mortality predictors in older adults. JAMA 298:2507–16, 2007.

94. Klem ML, Wing RR, McGuire MT, et al. A descriptive study of individuals successful at long-term maintenance of substantial weight loss. Am J Clin Nutr 66:239–46, 1997.

95. Jakicic JM, Winters C, Lang W, et al. Effects of intermittent exercise and use of home exercise equipment on adherence, weight loss, and fitness in overweight women: a randomized trial. JAMA 282:1554–60, 1999.

96. Jakicic JM, Otto AD. Treatment and prevention of obesity: what is the role of exercise? Nutr Rev 64:S57–61, 2006.

97. Gami AS, Witt BJ, Howard DE, et al. Metabolic syndrome risk and incident cardiovascular events and death. A systematic review and meta-analysis of longitudinal studies. J Am Coll Cardiol 49:403–14, 2007.

98. Kurella M, Lo JC, Chertow GM. Metabolic syndrome and the risk for chronic kidney disease among nondiabetic adults. J Am Soc Nephrol 16:2134–40, 2005.

99. Rashidi A, Ghanbarian A, Azizi F. Are patients who have metabolic syndrome without diabetes at risk for developing chronic kidney disease? Evidence based on data from a large cohort screening population. Clin J Am Soc Nephrol 2:976–83, 2007.

100. Weiss R, Kaufman FR. Metabolic complications of childhood obesity. Diabetes Care 31(Suppl 2):S310–16, 2008.

101. Henry RR, Mudaliar S. Obesity and type 2 diabetes mellitus. In Eckel RH (ed.): Obesity—Mechanisms and Clinical Management. Philadelphia, Lippincott, Williams & Wilkins, 2003:229–72.

102. Ye J, Kraegen T. Insulin resistance: central and peripheral mechanisms. The 2007 Stock Conference Report. Obes Rev 9:30–4, 2008.

103. Bansilal S, Farkouh ME, Fuster V. Role of insulin resistance and hyperglycemia in the development of atherosclerosis. Am J Cardiol 99(4A):6B–14B, 2007.

104. Rader DJ. Effect of insulin resistance, dyslipidemia, and intra-abdominal adiposity on the development of cardiovascular disease and diabetes mellitus. Am J Med 120:S12–8, 2007.

105. Alberti KGMM, Eckel RH, Grundy SM, et al. Harmonizing the metabolic syndrome. A joint interim statement of the International Diabetes Federation Task Force on Epidemiology an Prevention; National Heart, Lung, and Blood Institute; American Heart Association; World Heart Federation; International Atherosclerosis Society; and International Association for the Study of Obesity. Circulation 120:1640–5, 2009.

106. Bassuk SS, Manson JE. Epidemiological evidence for the role of physical activity in reducing risk of type 2 diabetes and cardiovascular disease. J Appl Physiol 99:1193–204, 2005.

107. Garber AJ. Combined pharmacologic/nonpharmacologic intervention in individuals at high risk of developing type 2 diabetes. Diabetes Care 32(Suppl 2):S184–8, 2009.

108. Hafidh S, Senkottaiyan N, Villarreal D, et al. Management of the metabolic syndrome. Am J Med Sci 330:343–51, 2005.

109. Jandeleit-Dahm KAM, Tikellis C, Reid CM, et al. Why blockade of the rennin-angiotensin system reduces the incidence of new-onset diabetes. J Hypertens 23:463–73, 2005.

110. LaMonte MJ, Blair SN, Church TS. Physical activity and diabetes prevention. J Appl Physiol 99:1205–13, 2005.

111. Pi-Sunyer FX. Use of lifestyle changes treatment plus drug therapy in controlling cardiovascular and metabolic risk factors. Obesity 14(Suppl):135S–42S, 2006.

112. Centers for Disease Control and Prevention. National diabetes fact sheet: General information and national estimates on diabetes in the United States, 2007. Atlanta, GA: U.S. Department of Health and Human Services, Centers for Disease Control and Prevention, 2008. http://www.cdc.gov/diabetes/pubs/pdf/ndfs_2007.pdf.

113. Deedwania PC, Fonseca VA. Diabetes, prediabetes, and cardiovascular risk: shifting the paradigm [Review]. Am J Med 118:939–47, 2005.

114. Tuomilehto J. Nonpharmacologic therapy and exercise in the prevention of type 2 diabetes. Diabetes Care 32(Suppl 2):S189–93, 2009.

115. Katzmarzyk PT, Church TS, Blair SN. Cardiorespiratory fitness attenuates the effects of the metabolic syndrome on all-cause and cardiovascular disease mortality in men. Arch Intern Med 164:1092–7, 2004.

116. Kirk JK. Diabetes: rethinking risk and the Dx that fits. J Fam Pract 58:248–56, 2009.

117. DeFronzo RA. Pathogenesis of type 2 diabetes mellitus. Med Clin North Am 88:787–835, 2004.

118. Del Prato S, Marchetti P. Beta- and alpha-cell dysfunction in type 2 diabetes. Horm Metab Res 36:775–81, 2004.

119. Appel SJ, Wadas TM, Rosenthal RS, et al. Latent autoimmune diabetes of adulthood (LADA): an often misdiagnosed type of diabetes mellitus. J Am Acad Nurs Pract 21:156–9, 2009.

120. Green DE. New therapies for diabetes. Clin Cornerstone 8:58–65, 2007.

121. Chansky ME, Corbett JG, Cohen E. Hyperglycemic emergencies in athletes. Clin Sports Med 28:469–78, 2009.

122. Chipkin SR, Klugh SA, Chasan-Taber L. Exercise and diabetes. Cardiol Clin 19:489–505, 2001.

123. MacKnight JM, Mistry DJ, Pastors JG, et al. The daily management of athletes with diabetes. Clin Sports Med 28:479–95, 2009.

124. Riddell MC, Iscoe KE. Physical activity, sport, and pediatric diabetes. Pediatr Diabetes 7:60–70, 2006.

125. Kim J, Montagnani M, Koh KK, et al. Reciprocal relationships between insulin resistance and endothelial dysfunction. Molecular and pathophysiological mechanisms. Circulation 113:1888–904, 2006.

126. Deshpande AD, Harris-Hayes M, Schootman M. Epidemiology of diabetes and diabetes-related complications. Phys Ther 88:1254–64, 2008.

127. The Eye Diseases Research Prevalence Research Group. The prevalence of diabetic retinopathy among adults in the United States. Arch Opthal 122:552–63, 2004.

128. McCullough PA, Bakris GL, Owen WF Jr, et al. Slowing the progression of diabetic nephropathy and its cardiovascular consequences. Am Heart J 148:243–51, 2004.

129. Loganathan R, Searls YM, Smirnova IV, et al. Exercise-induced benefits in individuals with type 1 diabetes. Phys Ther Rev 11:77–89, 2006.

130. Buse JB, Ginsberg HN, Bakris GL, et al. Primary prevention of cardiovascular disease in people with diabetes mellitus. A scientific statement from the American Heart Association and the American Diabetes Association. Circulation 115:114–26, 2007.

131. Goraya TY, Leibson CL, Palumbo PJ, et al. Coronary atherosclerosis in diabetes mellitus. A population-based autopsy study. J Am Coll Cardiol 40:946–53, 2002.

132. Scholte AJHA, Schuijf JD, Kharagjitsingh AV, et al. Prevalence of coronary artery disease and plaque morphology assessed by multi-slice computed tomography coronary angiography and calcium scoring in asymptomatic patients with type 2 diabetes. Heart 94:290–5, 2008.

133. Malmberg K, Yusuf S, Gerstein HC, et al. Impact of diabetes on long-term prognosis in patients with unstable angina and non-Q-wave myocardial infarction. Results of the OASIS (Organization to Assess Strategies for Ischemic Syndromes) Registry. Circulation 102:1014–19, 2000.

134. Mancia G. The association of hypertension and diabetes: prevalence, cardiovascular risk, and protection by blood pressure reduction. Acta Diabetol 42:S17–25, 2005.

135. Arauz-Pacheco C, Parrott MA, Raskin P. The treatment of hypertension in adult patients with diabetes. Diabetes Care 25:134–47, 2002.

136. Fonarow GC. An approach to heart failure and diabetes mellitus. Am J Cardiol 96(Suppl):47E–52E, 2005.

137. Aneja A, Wilson Tang WH, Bansilal S, et al. Diabetic cardiomyopathy: insights into pathogenesis, diagnostic challenges, and therapeutic options. Am J Med 121:748–57, 2008.

138. Vinik AI, Freeman R, Erbas T. Diabetic autonomic neuropathies. Diabetes Care 26:1553–79, 2003.

139. Vinik AI, Erbas T. Neuropathy. In Ruderman N, Devlin JT, Schneider SH, et al. (eds.): Handbook of Exercise in Diabetes. 2nd ed. Alexandria, VA, American Diabetes Association, 2002.

140. Valensi P, Pariès J, Attali JR, et al. Cardiac autonomic neuropathy in diabetic patients: influence of diabetes duration, obesity, and microangiopathic complications—the French Multicenter Study. Metabol 52:815–20, 2003.

141. Vinik AI, Ziegler D. Diabetic cardiovascular autonomic neuropathy. Circulation 115:387–97, 2007.

142. Maser RE, Lenhard MJ. Review: cardiovascular autonomic neuropathy due to diabetes mellitus: clinical manifestations, consequences, and treatment. J Clin Endocrinol Metab 90:5896–903, 2005.

143. Prakash UBS, King TE Jr. Endocrine and metabolic disorders. In Crapo JD, Glassroth J, Karlinsky JB, et al. (eds.): Baum's Textbook of Pulmonary Disease. 7th ed. Philadelphia, Lippincott Williams & Wilkins, 2004.

144. Zimmerman L. Pulmonary complications of endocrine disease. In Mason RJ, Murray JF, Broaddus VC, et al. (eds.): Murray & Nadel's Textbook of Respiratory Medicine. 4th ed. Philadelphia, Elsevier Saunders, 2004.

145. Marliss EB, Vranic M. Intense exercise has unique effects on both insulin release and its role in glucoregulation: implications for diabetes. Diabetes 51(Suppl 1):S271–83, 2002.

146. Riddell MC, Perkins BA. Exercise and glucose metabolism in persons with diabetes mellitus: perspectives on the role of continuous glucose monitoring. J Diabetes Sci Tech 3:914–23, 2009.

147. Riddell MC, Perkins BA. Type 1 diabetes and vigorous exercise: applications of exercise physiology to patient management. Can J Diabetes 30:63–71, 2006.

148. Guelfi KJ, Jones TW, Fournier PA. New insights into managing the risk of hypoglycemia associated with intermittent high-intensity exercise in individuals with type 1 diabetes mellitus. Sports Med 37:937–46, 2007.

149. Toni S, Reali MF, Barni F, et al. Managing insulin therapy during exercise in Type 1 diabetes mellitus. Acta Biomed 77(Suppl 1):34–40, 2006.

150. Giannini C, de Giorgis T, Mohn A, et al. Role of physical exercise in children and adolescents with diabetes mellitus. J Pediatr Endocrinol Metab 20:173–84, 2007.

151. DeWitt DE, Hirsch IB. Outpatient insulin therapy in type 1 and type 2 diabetes mellitus. Scientific review. JAMA 289:2254–64, 2003.

152. Diaz-Collins M. Managing the diabetic patient. Today in PT 26:32–8, 2009.

153. Gulve EA. Exercise and glycemic control in diabetes: benefits, challenges, and adjustments to pharmacotherapy. Phys Ther 88:1297–321, 2008.

154. Gillespie SJ, Kulani KD, Daly AE. Using carbohydrate counting in diabetes clinical practice. J Am Diet Assoc 98:897–905, 1998.

155. Galbo H, Tobin L, van Loon LJC. Responses to acute exercise in type 2 diabetes, with an emphasis on metabolism and interaction with oral hypoglycemic agents and food intake. Appl Physiol Nutr Metab 32:567–75, 2007.

156. Cryer PE. Insulin therapy and hypoglycemia in type 2 diabetes mellitus. Insulin 2:127–33, 2007.

157. Campaigne BN. Exercise and diabetes mellitus. In American College of Sports Medicine (ed.): ASCM's Resource Manual for Guidelines for Exercise Testing and Prescription. 4th ed. Philadelphia, Lippincott Williams & Wilkins, 2001.

158. Colberg SR, Grieco CR. Exercise in the treatment and prevention of diabetes. Curr Sports Med Rep 8:169–75, 2009.

159. Gordon BA, Benson AC, Bird SR, et al. Resistance training improves metabolic health in type 2 diabetes: a systematic review. Diabetes Res Clin Pract 83:157–75, 2009.

160. Sigal RJ, Kenny GP, Wasserman DH, et al. Physical activity/exercise and type 2 diabetes: a consensus statement from the American Diabetes Association. Diabetes Care 29:1433–8, 2006.

161. Tresierras MA, Balady GJ. Resistance training in the treatment of diabetes and obesity. J Cardiopulm Rehabil Prev 29:67–75, 2009.

162. Wang Y, Simar D, Fiatarone Singh MA. Adaptations to exercise training within skeletal muscle in adults with type 2 diabetes or impaired glucose tolerance: a systematic review. Diabetes Metab Res Rev 25:13–40, 2009.

163. Sigal RJ, Kenny GP, Wasserman DH, et al. Physical activity/exercise and type 2 diabetes. Diabetes Care 27:2518–39, 2004.

164. Lambers S, Van Laethem C, Van Acker K, et al. Influence of combined exercise training on indices of obesity, diabetes, and cardiovascular risk in type 2 diabetes patients. Clin Rehabil 22:483–92, 2008.

165. Sigal RJ, Kenny GP, Boule NG, et al. Effects of aerobic exercise training, resistance exercise, or both on glycemic control in type 2 diabetes: a randomized trial. Ann Intern Med 147:357–69, 2007.

166. Baldi JC, Aoina JL, Whalley GA, et al. The effect of type 2 diabetes on diastolic function. Med Sci Sports Exerc 28:1384–8, 2006.

167. Kjær M, Hollenbeck B, Frey-Hewitt B, et al. Glucoregulation and hormonal responses to maximal exercise in non-insulin-dependent diabetes. J Appl Physiol 68:2067–74, 1990.

168. Boulé NG, Kenny GP, Haddad E, et al. Meta-analysis of the effect of structured exercise training on cardiorespiratory fitness in type 2 diabetes mellitus. Diabetologia 46:1071–81, 2003.

169. Crasto W, Jarvis J, Khunti K, et al. New insulins and new insulin regimens: a review of their role in improving control in patients with diabetes. Postgrad Med J 85:257–67, 2009.

170. Hirsch IB. Insulin analogues. N Engl J Med 352:174–83, 2005.

171. Oiknine R, Bernbaum M, Mooradian AD. A critical appraisal of the role of insulin analogues in the management of diabetes mellitus. Drugs 65:325–40, 2005.

172. Physician's Desk Reference 2009. 63rd ed. Montvale, NJ, Thomson PDR, 2009.

173. White SA, Shaw JA, Sutherland DER. Pancreas transplantation. Lancet 373:1808–17, 2009.

174. Cefalu WT. Pharmacotherapy for the treatment of patients with type 2 diabetes mellitus: rationale and specific agents. Clin Pharm Ther 81:636–49, 2007.

175. Deeg MA. Basic approach to managing hyperglycemia for the nonendocrinologist. Am J Cardiol 96(Suppl):37E–40E, 2005.

176. Nathan DM, Buse JB, Davidson MB, et al. Medical management of hyperglycaemia in type 2 diabetes mellitus: a consensus algorithm for the initiation and adjustment of therapy. Diabetologia 52:17–30, 2009.

177. Nauck MA, Vilsbøll T, Gallwitz B, et al. Incretin-based therapies. Diabetes Care 32(Suppl 2):S223–31, 2009.

178. Deligiannis A. Cardiac adaptations following exercise training in hemodialysis patients. Clin Nephrol 61(Suppl 1):S39–45, 2004.

179. Iscoe KE, Perkins BA, Riddell M. Type 1 diabetes and aerobic exercise: strategies for optimal glycemic control. 2007. http://www.sseh.uwa.edu.au/_data/page/151951/.

180. Boulé NG, Haddad E, Kenny GP, et al. Effects of exercise on glycemic control and body mass in type 2 diabetes mellitus. JAMA 286:1218–27, 2001.

181. Weiner DE. Causes and consequences of chronic kidney disease: implications for managed health care. J Manag Care Pharm 13(Suppl 3):S1–9, 2007.

182. Best PJM, Reddan DN, Berger PB, et al. Cardiovascular disease and chronic kidney disease: insights and updates. Am Heart J 148:230–42, 2004.

183. Schiffrin EL, Lipman ML, Mann JFE. Chronic kidney disease. Effects on the cardiovascular system. Circulation 116:85–97, 2007.

184. Silverberg D, Wexler D, Blum M, et al. The association between congestive heart failure and chronic renal disease. Curr Opin Nephrol Hypertens 13:163–70, 2004.

185. US Renal Data System. USRDS 2009 Annual Data Report: Atlas of End-Stage Renal Disease in the United States. Bethesda, MD: National Institutes of Health, National Institute of Diabetes and Digestive and Kidney Diseases, 2009.

186. Luke RG. Chronic renal failure. In Goldman L, Ausiello D (eds.): Cecil Textbook of Medicine. 22nd ed. Philadelphia, Saunders, 2004:708–16.

187. Go AS, Chertow GM, Fan D, et al. Chronic kidney disease and the risks of death, cardiovascular events, and hospitalization. N Engl J Med 351:1296–305, 2004.

188. Chanda R, Fenves AZ. Hypertension in patients with chronic kidney disease. Curr Hypertens Rep 11:329–36, 2009.

189. Pendse S, Singh AK. Complications of chronic kidney disease: anemia, mineral metabolism, and cardiovascular disease. Med Clin North Am 89:549–61, 2005.

190. Obialo CI. Cardiorenal consideration as a risk factor for heart failure. Am J Cardiol 99(Suppl):21D–4D, 2007.

191. Rodriguez-Roisin R, Barberá JA. Pulmonary complications of abdominal disease. In Mason RJ, Murray JF, Broaddus VC, et al. (eds.): Murray & Nadel's Textbook of Respiratory Medicine. 4th ed. Philadelphia, Elsevier Saunders, 2004.

192. Bouffard Y, Viale JP, Annat G, et al. Pulmonary gas exchange during hemodialysis. Kidney Int 30:920–3, 1986.

193. Ettinger NA, Trulock EP. Pulmonary considerations of organ transplantation (part I). Am Rev Respir Dis 144:1386–413, 1991.

194. Kotloff RM, Ahya VN, Crawford SW. Pulmonary complications of solid organ and hematopoietic stem cell transplantation. Am J Respir Crit Care Med 170:22–48, 2004.

195. Konstantinidou E, Koukouvou G, Kouidi E, et al. Exercise training in patients with end-stage renal disease on hemodialysis: comparison of three rehabilitation programs. J Rehabil Med 34:40–5, 2002.

196. Painter P. Physical functioning in end-stage renal disease patients: update 2005. Hemodial Int 9:218–35, 2005.

197. Tawney KW, Tawney PJ, Kovach J. Disablement and rehabilitation in end-stage renal disease. Semin Dial 16:447–52, 2003.

198. Fuhrman I, Krause R. Principles of exercising in patients with chronic kidney disease, on dialysis, and for kidney transplant recipients. Clin Nephrol 61(Suppl 1):S14–25, 2004.

199. Adams GR, Vaziri ND. Skeletal muscle dysfunction in chronic renal failure: effects of exercise. Am J Physiol Renal Physiol 290:F753–61, 2006.

200. Castenada C, Gordon PL, Uhlin KL, et al. Resistance training to counteract the catabolism of a low-protein diet in patients with chronic renal insufficiency. A randomized controlled trial. Ann Intern Med 135:965–76, 2001.

201. Deligiannis A. Exercise rehabilitation and skeletal muscle benefits in hemodialysis patients. Clin Nephrol 61(Suppl 1):S46–50, 2004.

202. Leikis MJ, McKenna MJ, Peterson AC, et al. Exercise performance falls over time in patients with chronic kidney disease despite maintenance of hemoglobin concentration. Clin J Am Soc Nephrol 1:488–95, 2006.

203. Parsons TL, King-VanVlack CE. Exercise and end-stage kidney disease: functional exercise capacity and cardiovascular outcomes. Adv Chronic Kidney Dis 16:459–81, 2009.

204. Daul AE, Schäfers RF, Daul K, et al. Exercise during hemodialysis. Clin Nephrol 61(Suppl 1):S26–30, 2004.

205. Moinuddin I, Leehey DJ. A comparison of aerobic exercise and resistance training in patients with and without chronic kidney disease. Adv Chronic Kidney Dis 15:83–96, 2008.

206. Cheema B, Abas H, Smith B, et al. Progressive Exercise for Anabolism in Kidney disease (PEAK): a randomized, controlled trial of resistance training during hemodialysis. J Am Soc Nephrol 18:1594–601, 2007.

207. Kouidi E. Health-related quality of life in end-stage renal disease patients: the effects of renal rehabilitation. Clin Nephrol 61(Suppl 1):S60–71, 2004.

208. Painter P, Carlson L, Carey S, et al. Physical functioning and health-related quality of life changes with exercise training in hemodialysis patients. Am J Kidney Dis 35:482–92, 2000.

209. Cheema BSB, Fiatarone Singh M. Exercise training in patients receiving maintenance hemodialysis: a systematic review of clinical trials. Am J Nephrol 25:352–64, 2005.

210. Johansen KL. Exercise and chronic kidney disease. Current recommendations. Sports Med 35:485–99, 2005.

211. O'Hare AM, Tawney K, Bachetti P, et al. Decreased survival among sedentary patients undergoing dialysis: Results from the dialysis morbidity and mortality study wave 2. Am J Kidney Dis 41:447–54, 2003.

212. Clyne N. The importance of exercise training in predialysis patients with chronic kidney disease. Clin Nephrol 61(Suppl 1):S10–3, 2004.

213. Crestani B. The respiratory system in connective tissue disorders. Allergy 60:715–34, 2005.

214. Goodson NJ, Solomon DH. The cardiovascular manifestations of rheumatic diseases. Curr Opin Rheumatol 18:135–40, 2006.

215. Rayner CFJ, Grubnic S. Pulmonary manifestations of systemic autoimmune disease. Best Pract Res Clin Rheumatol 18:381–410, 2004.

216. Shoenfeld Y, Gerli R, Doria A, et al. Accelerated atherosclerosis in autoimmune rheumatic diseases. Circulation 112:3337–47, 2005.

217. Turesson C, Matteson EL. Cardiovascular risk factors, fitness, and physical activity in rheumatic diseases. Curr Opin Rheumatol 19:190–6, 2007.

218. Voskuyl AE. The heart and cardiovascular manifestations in rheumatoid arthritis. Rheumatology 45:iv4–7, 2006.

219. Tincani A, Rebaioli CB, Taglietti M, et al. Heart involvement in systemic lupus erythematosus, anti-phospholipid syndrome, and neonatal lupus. Rheumatology 45:iv8–13, 2006.

220. Kahan A, Allanore Y. Primary myocardial involvement in systemic sclerosis. Rheumatology 45:iv14–17, 2006.

221. Schwaiblmair M, Behr J, Fruhmann G. Cardiorespiratory responses to incremental exercise in patients with systemic sclerosis. Chest 110:1520–5, 1996.

222. Tanoue LT. Pulmonary involvement in collagen vascular disease: a review of the pulmonary manifestations of the Marfan syndrome, ankylosing spondylitis, Sjogren's syndrome, and relapsing polychondritis. J Thorac Imaging 7:62–77, 1992.

223. Lundberg LE. The heart in dermatomyositis and polymyositis. Rheumatology 45:iv18–21, 2006.

224. Aldrich TK, Tso R. The lungs and neuromuscular diseases. In Mason RJ, Murray JF, Broaddus VC, et al. (eds.): Murray & Nadel's Textbook of Respiratory Medicine. 4th ed. Philadelphia, Elsevier Saunders, 2005.

225. O'Donnell DM. Pulmonary complications in neuromuscular disease. Adolesc Med 11:633–45, 2000.

226. Perrin C, Unterborn JN, D'Ambrosio C, et al. Pulmonary complications of chronic neuromuscular diseases and their management. Muscle Nerve 29:5–27, 2004.

227. Prakash UBS, King TE Jr. Neurologic diseases. In Crapo JD, Glassroth J, Karlinsky JB, et al. (eds.): Baum's Textbook of Pulmonary Disease. 7th ed. Philadelphia, Lippincott Williams & Wilkins, 2004.

228. Dellefave LM, McNally EM. Cardiomyopathy in neuromuscular disorders. Prog Pediatr Cardiol 24:35–46, 2007.

229. Crizzle AM, Newhouse IJ. Is physical exercise beneficial for persons with Parkinson's disease? Clin J Sports Med 16:422–5, 2006.

230. Cup EH, Peiterse AJ, ten Broek-Pastoor JM, et al. Exercise therapy and other types of physical therapy for patients with neuromuscular diseases: a systematic review. Arch Phys Med Rehabil 88:1452–64, 2007.

231. Eldar R, Marincek C. Physical activity for elderly persons with neurological impairment: a review. Scand J Rehab Med 32:99–103, 2000.

232. Hirsch MA, Toole T, Maitland CG, et al. The effects of balance training and high-intensity resistance training on persons with idiopathic Parkinson's disease. Arch Phys Med Rehabil 84:1109–17, 2003.

233. Jacobs PL, Nash MS. Exercise recommendations for individuals with spinal cord injury. Sports Med 34:727–51, 2004.

234. MacKay-Lyons MJ, Howlett J. Exercise capacity and cardiovascular adaptations to aerobic training early after stroke. Top Stroke Rehabil 12:31–44, 2005.

235. Rampello A, Franceschini M, Piepoli M, et al. Effect of aerobic training on walking capacity and maximal exercise tolerance in patients with multiple sclerosis: a randomized crossover controlled study. Phys Ther 87:545–55, 2007.

236. Rimmer JH, Wang E. Aerobic exercise training in stroke survivors. Top Stroke Rehabil 12:17–30, 2005.

237. Oppenheimer S, Hachinski V. Complications of acute stroke. Lancet 339:721–4, 1992.

238. Chimowitz MI, Mancini GB. Asymptomatic coronary artery disease in patients with stroke. Prevalence, prognosis, diagnosis, and treatment. Stroke 23:433–6, 1992.

239. Di Pasquale G, Andreoli A, Pinelli G, et al. Cerebral ischemia and asymptomatic coronary artery disease: a prospective study of 83 patients. Stroke 17:1098–101, 1986.

240. Hertser NR, Young JR, Beven EG, et al. Coronary angiography in 506 patients with extracranial cerebrovascular disease. Arch Intern Med 145:849–52, 1985.

241. Love BB, Grover-McKay M, Biller J, et al. Coronary artery disease and cardiac events with asymptomatic and symptomatic cerebrovascular disease. Stroke 23:939–45, 1992.

242. Leary MC, Caplan LR. Cerebrovascular disease and neurologic manifestations of heart disease. In Fuster V, Alexander RW, O'Rourke RA (eds.): Hurst's the Heart. 11th ed. New York, McGraw-Hill, 2004.

243. Oppenheimer SM, Hachinski VC. The cardiac consequences of stroke. Neurol Clin 10:167–76, 1992.

244. Massery M. Multisystem consequences of impaired breathing mechanics and/or postural control. In Frownfelter D, Dean E (eds.): Cardiovascular and Pulmonary Physical Therapy. Evidence and Practice. 4th ed. St. Louis, MO, Mosby Elsevier, 2006.

245. Brown LK. Respiratory dysfunction in Parkinson's disease. Clin Chest Med 15:715–27, 1994.

246. Sabate M, Gonzalez I, Ruperez F, et al. Obstructive and restrictive pulmonary dysfunctions in Parkinson's disease. J Neurol Sci 138:114–9, 1996.

247. Sathyaprabha TN, Kapavarapu PK, Thennarasu K, et al. Pulmonary function in Parkinson's disease. Indian J Chest Dis Allied Sci 47:251–7, 2005.

248. Shill H, Stacy M. Respiratory complications of Parkinson's disease. Semin Respir Crit Care Med 23:261–5, 2002.

249. Izquierdo-Alonso JL, Jimenez-Jimenez FJ, Cabrera-Valdivia F, et al. Airway dysfunction in patients with Parkinson's disease. Lung 172:47–55, 1994.

250. Canning CG, Alison JA, Allen NE, et al. Parkinson's disease: an investigation of exercise capacity, respiratory function, and gait. Arch Phys Med Rehabil 78:199–207, 1997.

251. Gay PC, Westbrook PR, Daube JR, et al. Effects of alterations in pulmonary function and sleep variables on survival in patients with amyotrophic lateral sclerosis. Mayo Clin Proc 6:686–94, 1991.

252. Ng KK, Howard RS, Fish DR, et al. Management and outcome of severe Guillain-Barré syndrome. QJM 88:243–50, 1995.

253. Sharshar T, Chevret S, Bourdain F, et al. Early predictors of mechanical ventilation in Guillain-Barré syndrome. Crit Care Med 31:278–83, 2003.

254. Buyse B, Demedts M, Meekers J, et al. Respiratory dysfunction in multiple sclerosis: a prospective analysis of 60 patients. Eur Respir J 10:139–45, 1997.

255. Carter JL, Noseworthy JH. Ventilatory dysfunction in multiple sclerosis. Clin Chest Med 15:693–703, 1994.

256. Foglio K, Clini E, Facchetti D, et al. Respiratory muscle function and exercise capacity in multiple sclerosis. Eur Respir J 7:23–8, 1994.

257. Hofstad H, Ohm OJ, Mork SJ, et al. Heart disease in myasthenia gravis. Acta Neurol Scand 70:176–84, 1984.

258. Owe JF, Gilhus NE. Myasthenia gravis and the heart. ACNR 8:9–10, 2008.

259. Lynn DJ, Woda RP, Mendell JR. Respiratory dysfunction in muscular dystrophy and other myopathies. Clin Chest Med 15:661–74, 1994.

260. Groh WJ, Zipes DP. Neurological disorders and cardiovascular disease. In Zipes DP, Libby P, Bonow PO, et al. (eds.). Braunwald's Heart Disease. 7th ed. Philadelphia, Elsevier Saunders, 2005.

261. Perloff JK, de Leon ACJ, O'Doherty D. The cardiomyopathy of progressive muscular dystrophy. Circulation 33:625–48, 1966.

262. Perloff JK, Henze E, Schelbert HR. Alterations in regional myocardial metabolism, perfusion, and wall motion in Duchenne muscular dystrophy studied by radionuclide imaging. Circulation 69:33–42, 1984.

263. Towbin JA, Roberts R, et al. Cardiovascular diseases due to genetic abnormalities. In Alexander RW, Schlant RC (eds.): Hurst's the Heart, Arteries and Veins. 9th ed. New York, McGraw-Hill, 1998:1877–923.

264. Steare SE, Dubowitz V, Benatar A. Subclinical cardiomyopathy in Becker muscular dystrophy. Br Heart J 68:304–8, 1992.

265. Quinlivan RM, Dubowitz V. Cardiac transplantation in Becker muscular dystrophy. Neuromuscul Disord 2:165–7, 1992.

266. Begin P, Mathieu J, Almirall J, et al. Relationship between chronic hypercapnia and inspiratory-muscle weakness in myotonic dystrophy. Am J Respir Crit Care Med 156:133–9, 1997.

267. Moorman JR, Coleman RE, Packer DL, et al. Cardiac involvement in myotonic muscular dystrophy. Medicine (Baltimore) 64:371–87, 1985.

268. Perloff JK, Stevenson WG, Roberts NK, et al. Cardiac involvement in myotonic muscular dystrophy (Steinert's disease): a prospective study of 25 patients. Am J Cardiol 54:1074–81, 1984.

269. Farbu E, Gilhus NE, Barnes MP, et al. EFNS guideline on diagnosis and management of post-polio syndrome. Report of an EFNS task force. Eur J Neurol 13:795–801, 2006.

270. LeCompte CM. Post polio syndrome: an update for the primary health care provider. Nurs Practitioner 22:133–54, 1997.

271. Halstead LS, Rossi CD. New problems in old polio patients: Results of a survey of 539 polio survivors. Orthopedics 8:845–50, 1985.

272. Dean E, Ross J, Road JD, et al. Pulmonary function in individuals with a history of poliomyelitis. Chest 100:118–23, 1991.

273. Alboliras ET, Shub C, Gomez MR, et al. Spectrum of cardiac involvement in Friedreich's ataxia: clinical, electrocardiographic and echocardiographic observations. Am J Cardiol 58:518–24, 1986.

274. Harding AE, Hewer RL. The heart disease of Friedreich's ataxia: a clinical and electrocardiographic study of 115 patients, with an analysis of serial electrocardiographic changes in 30 cases. Q J Med 52:489–502, 1983.

275. Zuckerman KS. Approach to anemias. In Goldman L, Auseillo D (eds.): Cecil Textbook of Medicine. 23rd ed. Philadelphia, Saunders Elsevier, 2008.

276. Lubin BH. Sickle cell anemia. In Humes HD, DuPont HL, Gardner LB, et al. (eds.): Kelley's Textbook of Internal Medicine. 4th ed. Philadelphia, Lippincott Williams & Wilkins, 2000.

277. Serjeant GR. Sickle-cell disease. Lancet 350:725–30, 1997.

278. Stuart MJ, Nagel RL. Sickle-cell disease. Lancet 364:1343–60, 2004.

279. Bernard AW, Yasin Z, Venkat A. Acute chest syndrome of sickle cell disease. Hosp Physician 43:15–23, 44, 2007.

280. Graham LM. The effect of sickle cell disease on the lung. Clin Pulm Med 11:369–78, 2004.

281. Vichinsky EP, Neumayr LD, Earles AN, et al. Causes and outcomes of the acute chest syndrome in sickle cell disease. N Engl J Med 342:1855–65, 2000.

282. Wenger NK, Abelmann WH, Roberts WC. Cardiomyopathy and specific heart muscle disease. In Hurst JW, Alexander RW, Schlant RC (eds.): Hurst's the Heart, Arteries and Veins. 9th ed. New York, McGraw-Hill Information Services, 1998:1278–347.

283. Sachdev V, Machado RF, Shizukuda Y, et al. Diastolic dysfunction is an independent risk factor for death in patients with sickle cell disease. J Am Coll Cardiol 49:472–9, 2007.

284. Covitz W, Eubig C, Balfour IC, et al. Exercise-induced cardiac dysfunction in sickle cell anemia. A radionuclide study. Am J Cardiol 51:570–5, 1983.

285. Pianosi P, D'Souza SJ, Charge TD, et al. Cardiac output and oxygen delivery during exercise in sickle cell anemia. Am Rev Respir Dis 143:231–5, 1991.

286. Boyton RJ. Infectious lung complications in patients with HIV/AIDS. Curr Opin Pulm Med 11:203–7, 2005.

287. Kanmogne GD. Noninfectious pulmonary complications of HIV/AIDS. Curr Opin Pulm Med 11:208–12, 2005.

288. Restrepo CS, Diethelm L, Lemos JA, et al. Cardiovascular complications of human immunodeficiency virus infection. RadioGraph 26:213–31, 2006.

289. Yeshua H, Blendis LM, Oren R. Pulmonary manifestations of liver diseases. Semin Cardiothorac Vasc Anesth 13:60–9, 2009.

290. Muers MF. Gastrointestinal, hepatic and pancreatic diseases. In Gibson GJ, Geddes DM, Costabel U, et al. (eds.): Respiratory Medicine. 3rd ed. Edinburgh, Saunders, 2003.

291. Prakash UBS, King TE Jr. Gastrointestinal diseases. In Crapo JD, Glassroth J, Karlinsky JB, et al. (eds.): Baum's Textbook of Pulmonary Disease. 7th ed. Philadelphia, Lippincott Williams & Wilkins, 2004.

292. Wynne J, Braunwald E. The cardiomyopathies. In Zipes DP, Libby P, Bonow PO, et al. (eds.): Braunwald's Heart Disease, 7th ed. Philadelphia, Elsevier Saunders, 2005.

293. Mathews ECJ, Gardin JM, Henry WL, et al. Echocardiographic abnormalities in chronic alcoholics with and without overt congestive heart failure. Am J Cardiol 47:570–8, 1981.

294. Møller S, JH Henriksen. Cirrhotic cardiomyopathy: a pathophysiological review of circulatory dysfunction in liver disease. Heart 87:9–15, 2002.

295. Grose RD, Nolan J, Dillon JF, et al. Exercise-induced left ventricular dysfunction in alcoholic and non-alcoholic cirrhosis. J Hepatol 22:326–32, 1995.

296. Casiero D, Frishman WH. Cardiovascular complications of eating disorders. Cardiol Rev 14:227–31, 2006.

297. Casper RC. The pathophysiology of anorexia nervosa and bulimia nervosa. Annu Rev Nutr 6:299–316, 1986.

298. Schwartz DM, Thompson MG. Do anorectics get well? Current research and future needs. Am J Psychiatry 138:319–23, 1981.

299. Moodie DS. Anorexia and the heart. Results of studies to assess effects. Postgrad Med 81:46–55, 1987.

300. Cooke RA, Chambers JB. Anorexia nervosa and the heart. Br J Hosp Med 1995; 54:313–7.

301. de Simone G, Scalfi L, Galderisi L, et al. Cardiac abnormalities in young women with anorexia nervosa. Br Heart J 1994; 71:287–92.

302. Schocken DD, Holloway JD, Powers PS. Weight loss and the heart. Effects of anorexia nervosa and starvation. Arch Intern Med 149:877–81, 1989.

303. Nudel DB, Gootman N, Nussbaum MP, et al. Altered exercise performance and abnormal sympathetic responses to exercise in patients with anorexia nervosa. J Pediatr 105:34–7, 1984.

304. Silber TJ. Ipecac syrup abuse, morbidity, and mortality: isn't it time to repeal its over-the-counter status? J Adolesc Health 37:256–60, 2005.

305. Camus P, Fanton A, Bonniaud P, et al. Interstitial lung disease induced by drugs and radiation. Respir 71:301–26, 2004.

306. Carver JR, Shapiro CL, Ng A, et al. American Society of Clinical Oncology clinical review on the ongoing care of adult cancer survivors: cardiac and pulmonary late effects. J Clin Oncol 25:3391–4008, 2007.

307. Dimopoulou I, Bamias A, Lyberopoulos P, et al. Pulmonary toxicity from novel antineoplastic agents. Ann Oncol 17:372–9, 2006.

308. Limper AH. Chemotherapy-induced lung disease. Clin Chest Med 25:53–64, 2004.

309. Roig J, Domingo C, Gea E. Pulmonary toxicity caused by cytotoxic drugs. Clin Pulm Med 13:53–62, 2006.

310. Stover DE, Kaner RJ. Pulmonary toxicity. In DeVita VT, Hellman S, Rosenberg SA (eds.): Cancer: Principles & Practice of Oncology. 7th ed. Philadelphia, Lippincott Williams & Wilkins, 2005.

311. Yahalom J, Portlock CS. Cardiac toxicity. In DeVita VT, Hellman S, Rosenberg SA (eds.): Cancer: Principles & Practice of Oncology. 7th ed. Philadelphia, Lippincott Williams & Wilkins, 2005.

312. Yeh ETH, Tong AT, Lenihan DJ, et al. Cardiovascular complications of cancer treatment. Diagnosis, pathogenesis, and management. Circulation 109:3122–31, 2004.

313. Abratt RP, Morgan GW, Silvestr G, et al. Pulmonary complications of radiation therapy. Clin Chest Med 25:167–77, 2004.

314. Hogarty AN, Leahey A, Zhao H, et al. Longitudinal evaluation of cardiopulmonary performance during exercise after bone marrow transplantation in children. J Pediatr 136:311–7, 2000.

315. Shusterman S, Meadows AT. Long-term survivors of childhood leukemia. Curr Opin Hematol 7:217–22, 2000.

316. Galv o DA, Newton RU. Review of exercise intervention studies in cancer patients. J Clin Oncol 23:899–909, 2005.

317. McTiernan A. Physical activity after cancer: physiologic outcomes. Cancer Invest 22:68–81, 2004.

318. Watson T, Mock V. Exercise and cancer-related fatigue: a review of current literature. Rehabil Oncol 21:23–30, 2003.

319. Jones LW, Haykowsky MJ, Swarz JJ, et al. Early breast cancer therapy and cardiovascular injury. J Am Coll Cardiol 50:1435–41, 2007.

320. Courneya KS, Jones LW, Fairey AS, et al. Physical activity in cancer survivors: implications for recurrence and mortality. Cancer Ther 2:1–12, 2004.

321. Holmes MD, Chen WY, Feskanich D, et al. Physical activity and survival after breast cancer diagnosis. JAMA 293:2479–86, 2005.

322. Meyerhardt JA, Giovannucci EL, Holmes MD, et al. Physical activity and survival after colorectal cancer diagnosis. J Clin Oncol 24:3527–34, 2006.

323. Borg G. Borg's RPE Scale, Copyright Gunnar Borg 1994.

324. Borg G. Borg CR10 Scale. Copyright Gunnar Borg 1982, 1998, 2003.

## CHAPTER 8

# Cardiovascular Diagnostic Tests and Procedures

*Ellen Hillegass*

## Chapter Outline

Objective information on the patient's cardiovascular system is derived from data obtained from laboratory studies and from diagnostic tests and procedures. Physical therapists must be able to identify and interpret the results of these medical tests and procedures in order to assess the status of their patients' cardiovascular systems. This chapter provides the basis for an understanding of the importance and impact of medical tests that may be ordered to determine key disease states and impairments. In addition, these tests facilitate the achievement of a correct diagnosis, aid in the prevention of complications, develop information to determine a prognosis, identify subclinical disease states, and assist in the monitoring of the progress of treatments.

The tests and procedures that are discussed in this chapter include clinical laboratory studies (e.g., for cardiac enzymes and markers, cholesterol and triglycerides, and complete

## Table 8-1 Cardiovascular Diagnostic Tests and Procedures and Their Indications

| Tests | Indications |
| --- | --- |
| Rhythm abnormalities | Holter monitor |
| | 12-Lead ECG |
| | Exercise ECG |
| | Electrophysiologic studies (EPS mapping) |
| Ischemia | Resting ECG (if ischemia or complaints of angina are occurring at time of ECG being taken) |
| | Exercise ECG (with or without dye or stress echo) |
| | Pharmacologic stress testing |
| | Single-photon emission computed tomography (SPECT) |
| | Positron emission tomography (PET) |
| | Ergonovine challenges |
| | Contrast echocardiography |
| | Cardiac catheterization |
| | Cardiac magnetic resonance imaging (MRI) |
| | Digital subtraction angiography |
| Valve integrity | Echocardiography |
| | Contrast echocardiography |
| | Cardiac catheterization |
| Ventricular size and ejection fraction | Chest x-ray |
| | Multigated acquisition or angiogram (MUGA) imaging |
| | Echocardiography |
| Cardiac muscle pump functioning | MUGA |
| | Echocardiography |
| | Ventriculography |
| | Digital subtraction angiography |
| Acute myocardial infarction | Cardiac enzymes and markers |
| | Resting ECG |
| Vascular diagnostic testing | Ankle brachial index |
| | Segmental limb pressures |
| | Pulse volume recordings |
| | Arterial duplex ultrasonography |
| | Exercise studies |

blood cell count), Holter monitoring, echocardiography, contrast echocardiography, positron emission tomography (PET), computed tomography (CT), single-photon emission computed tomography (SPECT), electron beam computed tomography (EBCT), multigated acquisition or angiogram (MUGA) imaging, magnetic resonance imaging (MRI), perfusion imaging, exercise testing, coronary angiography and ventriculography, digital subtraction angiography (DSA), ergonovine stimulation, heart rate variability, and endocardial biopsy. Table 8-1 provides an overview of all tests and their indications found in this chapter. Electrocardiography is a separate diagnostic evaluation that is covered in Chapter 9.

## Diagnostic Test Interpretation and Probability of Disease

As all diagnostic tests are not 100% accurate, a brief description of terminology used to define accuracy of testing is included. Usually the literature will report on the sensitivity/specificity of the test or the predictive value of the test.

## Sensitivity/Specificity of Testing

Sensitivity is defined as the proportion of those individuals with the disease who have a true positive test. For example, a high sensitivity means the test will have low false-negative rates. Specificity is defined as the proportion of those individuals without the disease with a true negative test. A test with a high specificity will have a low false-positive rate.

Predictive Values are used as they are more clinically informative than sensitivity and specificity, and translates into the likelihood individuals have the disease. These values are highly dependent on the prevalence of the disease.

- A Positive Predictive Value is defined as the proportion of individuals who had a positive test and actually have the disease.
- A Negative Predictive Value is defined as the proportion of individuals who had a negative test and truly do not have the disease.

## Clinical Laboratory Studies

Laboratory studies provide important information regarding the clinical status of the patient. The laboratory tests that are specific to the patient with cardiac dysfunction measure the serum enzymes/cardiac biomarkers, blood lipids (triglycerides and cholesterol), complete blood cell count, coagulation profile (prothrombin time), electrolyte levels, blood urea nitrogen (BUN), creatinine levels, blood natriuretic peptide (BNP) testing, and serum glucose levels. Table 8-2 provides the laboratory studies and the normative values.

### Serum Enzymes and Cardiac Biomarkers

Evaluation of specific serum enzyme levels and cardiac protein markers contributes to a definitive diagnosis of myocardial necrosis and in some cases to an assessment of the degree of myocardial damage or the effectiveness of reperfusion. When damage has occurred to the myocardial tissue, cellular integrity is lost and intracellular cardiac enzymes are released into the circulation. These enzymes are released at a variable rate and are cleared by the kidney and other organs. Their presence can be measured by serum blood tests. However, owing to their variable release and clearing rate, their absence does not rule out the possibility of injury.

The markers that are diagnostic of cardiac injury include
- Creatine phosphokinase (CPK-MB isoenzyme)
- Troponin
- Myoglobin
- Carbonic anhydrase III
- Cardiac myosin light chains
- Lactic dehydrogenase (LDH isoenzyme 1)
- Aspartate aminotransferase (AST)

More specifically, isoenzymes, which are different chemical forms of the same enzyme, have been found to be most conclusive of specific muscle cell necrosis. Creatine phosphokinase (CPK; also CK) has three isoenzymes (MB, MM, BB), which are differentiated by their tissue distribution. The CPK-MB fraction is most conclusive of all three isoenzymes for myocardial injury. MM is most conclusive for skeletal muscle damage and BB for brain tissue injury. CPK-MB is

considered abnormal if its serum level is greater than 3%; MB is found in healthy skeletal muscle up to 3%. CPK-MB has been used as a cardiac marker for more than 35 years; however, it has been shown to be elevated after cardiac surgery and cardiopulmonary resuscitation (especially if the person was defibrillated) and has been shown to be abnormally elevated in patients undergoing thrombolysis with streptokinase or tissue plasminogen activator.[1] Chapter 14 discusses specific cardiac medications. False-elevated CPK-MB index >6% without myocardial infarction (MI) was evidenced in 43.3% of elective hip surgery patients.[2] Troponin I levels were elevated >3.1 ng/mL only in the patients who suffered MI postoperatively. All the patients who suffered MI had both CPK-MB index and troponin I levels elevated. Also, there was a high correlation between maximum CPK-MB levels and size of implants, which means that reaming and its heating effect may be responsible for false-elevated CPK-MB levels, except the direct muscle damage caused by the surgical incision.[2]

More recently, blood levels of the troponins have been assessed to determine myocardial damage and are now considered the gold standard. Elevated levels of troponin occur earlier[3] and may last for up to 5 to 7 days in plasma (normal range = 0 to 3.0 mg/mL).[4] The troponins are a group of structurally related proteins found in striated muscle cells and are bound to the actin filament. The troponins include the TnC, which binds calcium; TnI, which inhibits the interaction between actin and myosin; and TnT, which links the troponin complex to tropomyosin. With cell necrosis, there is a release of the troponins into the circulation. The cardiac isoforms of cTnI and cTnT are expressed only in cardiac muscle and therefore are the two troponins tested during severe ischemia and infarction.

The cTnI and cTnT are the most sensitive and specific biochemical markers of myocardial cell damage and have replaced creatine kinase MB as the preferred marker for diagnosis of myocardial injury.[5,6] Troponin, a three-protein complex consisting of troponins I, T, and C, is found in cardiac and skeletal muscle. Most of these proteins stored in myofibrils (the area actually bound to the myofibril) are key for calcium-regulated cardiac and skeletal contraction.[7] Some troponin is also found in the cytosol (unbound). Troponins I (cTnI) and T (cTnT) are cardiac tissue–specific, but troponin C (cTnC) is not.[8] Injured cardiac muscle releases troponin into the bloodstream. Thus, increased levels of cardiac troponin may suggest myocardial injury.[7] Troponin released after cardiac injury usually remains elevated (its half-life is about 2 hours), leading to better identification of cardiac injury.[7] Monoclonal antibodies can now detect cardiac troponins, resulting in immunoassays for blood measurement.

Although acute coronary syndrome (ACS) can cause elevated troponin levels, so can other conditions. Cardiac surgery can cause myocardial damage from procedures such as cross-clamping to using the cardiopulmonary bypass. Therefore, elevations in troponin are not specific to the cause of the injury; however, the more elevated the level is

## Table 8-2 Clinical Laboratory Studies with Normative Values

| | Measurement | Normative values |
| --- | --- | --- |
| Serum enzymes and cardiac biomarkers | Creatine phosphokinase (CPK) | 5–75 mU/mL |
| | CPK-MB isoenzyme | 0%–3% |
| | Lactic dehydrogenase (LDH) | 100–225 mU/mL |
| | Aspartate aminotransferase (AST) | 10–40 mU/dL |
| | Troponin | <0.2 µg/mL |
| | | troponin I: 0–0.1 ng/mL (onset: 4–6 hours, peak) |
| | | troponin T: 0–0.2 ng/mL (onset: 3–4 hours) |
| | Myoglobin | <100 ng/mL onset 1–3 hours |
| | | Male: 10–95 ng/mL |
| | | Female: 10–65 ng/mL |
| | Blood natriuretic peptide (BNP) | <100 pg/mL Normal |
| | | <500 Goal at hospital discharge |
| | | ≥700 Decompensated congested heart failure |
| | | ≈3000 During nesiritide infusion |
| | Carbonic anhydrase III | Myo/CAIII <3.2* |
| Blood lipids | Total cholesterol | <200 mg/dL |
| | High-density lipoproteins (HDL) | Male: ≥40 mg/dL |
| | | Female: ≥50 mg/dL |
| | Low-density lipoproteins (LDL) | <100 mg/dL |
| | Triglycerides | <140 mg/dL |
| Other risk factors for coronary artery disease (CAD) | Homocysteine | ≤13.0 µmol/L |
| | C-reactive protein hs-(CRP) | Low risk <1.0 mg/L |
| | | Avg risk 1.0–3.0 mg/L |
| | | High risk >3.0 mg/L |
| | | If >10.0 mg/L eval for other problems |
| | Glucose | 70–110 mg/dL |
| | HbA1C | ≤6.0% |
| Complete blood cell count | Red blood cells | Males: $4.6–6.2 \times 10^6$/µL |
| | | Females: $4.2–5.4 \times 10^4$/µL |
| | Hemoglobin | Male: 13.5–18 g/dL |
| | | Female: 12–16 g/dL |
| | Hematocrit | Male: 40%–54% |
| | | Female: 38%–47% |
| | White blood cells | 4500–11,000/µL of whole blood |
| | Platelets | 300,000/µL |
| Coagulation profile | Prothrombin time | 11.6–13.0 s |
| | Partial thromboplastin time | 21.5–34.1 s |
| | International Normalized Ratio (INR) | Prevention /treatment of venous thrombosis or PE 2.0–3.0 |
| | | Prosthetic heart valves 2.5–3.5 |
| | | Prevention of recurrent MI 2.5–3.5 |
| Electrolytes, Others | $Na^+$ | 136–143 mEq/L |
| | $K^+$ | 3.8–5.0 mEq/L |
| | Blood urea nitrogen | 8–18 mg/dL |
| | Creatinine | 0.6–1.2 mg/dL |
| | Albumin | >2.5 g |

*Myo/CAIII = myoglobin value/carbonic anhydrase III.

postoperatively, the greater the damage and the more grave the prognosis.[7] Because troponin levels are being tested more frequently, cardiac injury has been identified more often, but the causative factors are not always known. Direct damage to the heart, such as from blunt cardiac trauma, is another cause of elevated troponin levels. Also, therapies such as electrical cardioversion or defibrillation may injure the heart. Elective cardioversion usually does not raise troponin levels, but levels are more likely to be elevated after defibrillation or prolonged resuscitation.

Elevated cardiac troponin has been found in critically ill patients without a cardiac diagnosis.[9] Critically ill patients with sepsis often have increased troponin levels, although the reason is unclear. The elevated troponin could be related to underlying coronary artery disease (CAD), or the release of toxins in sepsis (such as tumor necrosis factor) that can injure the heart and cause increased troponin levels.[10] Other patient groups that show elevated troponin include patients with renal failure. The elevation may be due to musculoskeletal injury, but these patients are at high risk for cardiovascular disease as well, so a baseline troponin value that can be used as a comparison in future acute cardiac events should be obtained.[7]

Patients with heart failure also have increased levels of cardiac troponins, both in acute and chronic phases with and without coronary artery disease (CAD). In patients with ventricular hypertrophy (left or right), the ventricular wall stress or oxygen imbalances could cause troponin elevations.[7] Similarly, right ventricular strain and increased pulmonary vascular resistance may explain increased troponin levels in patients with acute pulmonary embolism (PE). The troponin elevation in PE resolves in 40 hours or less.[7]

The amount of cardiac troponin in the blood initially rises in about 4 to 6 hours. Peak concentrations appear at 18 to 24 hours after symptoms begin.[7] Usually troponin is collected on admission and then testing is repeated 6 to 9 hours later. Troponin can remain elevated for 10 days after the injury.[8] Prolonged elevation makes diagnosing cardiac injury in a patient who does not seek treatment for more than 24 hours easier, because other cardiac biomarkers, such as CPK-MB, may be normal in these patients.

Elevated troponin levels have also been found to be prognostic in the ACS patient. The risk of short-term mortality is increased in patients with ST-segment elevation MI (STEMI), although the risk of death and repeat MI is higher in patients with non-ST-segment elevation MI (NSTEMI) when troponin levels are elevated, compared with those patients without elevations. Troponin elevations have also helped clinicians detect reinfarctions and estimate infarct size.[7] Levels of troponin are not elevated in unstable angina.[9,11]

The assay used to measure cTnT levels has cardiac specificity equivalent to that of assays for cTnI. That is, troponin I: 0 to 0.1 ng/mL (onset: 4 to 6 hours, peak: 12 to 24 hours, return to normal: 4 to 7 days); troponin T: 0 to 0.2 ng/mL (onset: 3 to 4 hours, peak: 10 to 24 hours, return to normal: 10 to 14 days).[11]

Current research has demonstrated an increase in the cardiac troponins with heart failure and renal insufficiency; therefore, the troponins alone may not indicate specificity of MI.[12] Several studies have shown an increased short-term mortality rate (30 to 40 days) in individuals with elevations in cTnI and cTnT.[13–17]

Myoglobin is a heme protein found in all muscle tissue and has recently come under study as a potentially powerful diagnostic tool for acute MI. Myoglobin can be detected as early as 2 hours after injury and peaks approximately 3 to 15 hours after injury.[18] The presence of myoglobin requires ruling out possible skeletal muscle injury versus cardiac muscle injury.

Carbonic anhydrase III is a cytoplasmic protein that is present in skeletal muscle but not in cardiac muscle. In situations of skeletal muscle injury, both the myoglobin and the carbonic anhydrase III are elevated, but the ratio is constant, whereas in acute MI the ratio is not constant and changes within 2 to 15 hours after injury. This finding, although only recent, may prove to be more beneficial to emergency room monitoring of patients in the future than CPK and the troponins.

Skeletal and cardiac muscle contain two heavy chains and two light chains in the myosin molecule. Cardiac myosin light chains (CMLCs) have been shown to be released after MI[19] and may have a role in identification of cardiac injury in unstable angina pectoris.[20,21] Cardiac myosin light chains are currently difficult to separate from skeletal muscle chains and difficult to detect because of the lack of a reliable immunoassay; however, once a means of detection becomes available, this diagnostic test might prove to be the most sensitive and specific for cardiac injury.

Lactic dehydrogenase has five isoenzymes, of which LDH-1 is the most conclusive for myocardial injury. Normally LDH-2 activity exceeds that of LDH-1, but after MI, LDH-1 activity exceeds that of LDH-2.[22] More specifically, a ratio of LDH-1 to LDH-2 greater than 1.0 is strongly suggestive of MI. The other LDH isoenzymes are increased in the presence of heart failure, renal failure, and the like.

Enzyme and isoenzyme levels increase within the first 36 hours after myocardial injury, reaching their individual peaks at different rates (Table 8-3).[23] Marked elevation in CPK enzyme levels occurs whenever thrombolytic medications (streptokinase and tPA) are used to lyse clots. Clinically, an early or secondary peak in CPK levels followed by a more rapid decline in the CPK-MB levels is strongly suggestive of reperfusion after thrombolytic therapy.[24]

---

**Clinical Tip**

Troponin assessment is considered to be the gold standard for cardiac injury. In the absence of troponin information, the therapist should depend on CPK-MB information, electrocardiographic (ECG) changes, and symptoms. In any case where the CPK-MB is elevated, especially after hip surgery, confirmation of lack of troponin rise should be made prior to increasing the patient's activity.

## Table 8-3 Cardiac Enzymes

| | Normal Serum Level Values (IU)[a] | Onset of Rise (hours) | Time of Peak Rise (hours) | Return To Normal (days) |
|---|---|---|---|---|
| CPK | 55–71[b] | 3–4 | 33 | 3 |
| LDH | 127[c] | 12–24 | 72 | 5–14 |
| SGOT | 24 | 12 | 24 | 4 |
| Troponin I | <0.1 ng/ml | 4–6 | 12–24 | 4–7 |
| Troponin T | <0.2 ng/ml | 3–4 | 10–24 | 10–14 |

*From Smith AM, Theirer JA, Huang SH. Serum enzymes in myocardial infarction. Am J Nurs 73(2):277, 1973. Used with permission. All rights reserved. Copyright © 1973 The American Journal of Nursing Company.*
*[a]1 IU is the amount of enzyme that will catalyze the formation of 1 μmol of substrate per minute under the conditions of the test.*
*[b]CPK-MB, 0%–3%*
*[c]LDH-1, 14%–26%*
*CPK, creatine phosphokinase; LDH, lactic dehydrogenase; SGOT, serum glutamic oxaloacetic transaminase.*

## Table 8-4 Normal Lipid Values

| Lipids | Low Risk (0–1 RF) | Moderate Risk (2 RF) | High Risk |
|---|---|---|---|
| Total cholesterol | <200 mg/dL | <200 | <200 |
| LDL | <160 mg/dL | <130 | <100 (optimal <70) |
| HDL | ≥40 mg/dL Male | | |
| | ≥50 mg/dL Female | | |
| VLDL | 5–40 mg/dL | | |
| Triglycerides | <150 mg/dL | | |

*From NCEP Expert Panel. Detection, Evaluation and treatment of high cholesterol in adults.*
*Adult Treatment Panel III. NIH publication#01-3670 May 2001.*
*LDL, low-density lipoprotein; HDL, high-density lipoprotein; VLDL, very-low-density lipoprotein.*

## Blood Lipids

Elevation in blood lipid levels (hyperlipidemia) is considered a major risk factor contributing to CAD.[25] The concentrations of serum cholesterol and triglycerides are the blood lipids of concern. The American Heart Association defines elevated blood cholesterol levels as being higher than 200 mg/100 mL; however, the more stringent recommendations suggested by Castelli define 180 mg/100 mL as the upper end of normal (Table 8-4).[26] Elevated cholesterol levels are associated with ingestion of excess amounts of saturated fat and cholesterol as well as with hereditary influences. Elevated triglyceride levels are defined as being higher than 150 mg/100 mL. Elevated triglyceride levels are associated with increased carbohydrate ingestion and often preclude diabetes mellitus. Caution should be taken if measurements of cholesterol and triglyceride levels are taken at the time of acute injury, as research has shown these values to be inaccurate.[27] Such measurements are most accurate when obtained before a myocardial injury or a minimum of 6 weeks after an acute injury.[27]

The usefulness of clinical laboratory reports is improved by giving a breakdown of the component parts of the total cholesterol. Current information now lists the high-density lipoprotein (HDL) and low-density lipoprotein (LDL) levels as well as the ratio of total cholesterol to HDL cholesterol. High plasma levels of high-density lipoprotein cholesterol (HDL-C) are inversely related to the risk of CAD High-density lipoprotein has been further subdivided into apolipoproteins and apo A-I (A-1), which is the main protein constituent of the HDL particle and has identical results in relation to risk for coronary disease. As a result, medications to raise apo A-1 are currently in clinical trials for the primary purpose of decreasing the risk of CAD.

Research has shown that the absolute values of total cholesterol or HDL cholesterol are of less importance than the ratio of total cholesterol to HDL cholesterol in establishing an individual's relative risk for developing CAD (Table 8-5). An increased ratio of total cholesterol to HDL cholesterol identifies a person at an increased risk for development of CAD.[28] High levels of LDL (higher than 130 mg/100 mL) also increase a person's relative risk for developing CAD. Lowering total cholesterol and especially LDL cholesterol has shown to result in a 25% to 35% reduction in cardiovascular events.[29]

Recently, several new markers have been identified that are considered to be probable new risk factors, including lipoprotein a (Lpa), LDL subclasses, oxidized LDL,

## Table 8-5 Total Cholesterol to High-Density Lipoprotein (HDL) Ratio as a Predictor of Heart Disease

|  | Total Cholesterol/ HDL Ratio | Risk of Heart Disease |
|---|---|---|
| Men | 3.43 | 1/2 average |
|  | 4.97 | Average |
|  | 9.55 | 2× average |
|  | 23.39 | 3× average |
| Women | 3.27 | 1/2 average |
|  | 4.44 | Average |
|  | 7.05 | 2× average |
|  | 11.04 | 3× average |

*From Gordon T, Castelli WP, Hjortland MC, et al. Diabetes, blood lipids, and the role of obesity in coronary heart disease risk for women. Ann Intern Med 87:393, 1977.*

homocysteine, hematologic factors (primarily fibrinogen, factor VII, and tPA), inflammatory markers such as C-reactive protein (CRP), and infective agents such as *Chlamydia pneumoniae* (CPN).[30] Elevated serum levels of a lipid particle called Lpa have been strongly associated with atherosclerosis and also identified as an independent risk factor for CAD.[29] Lpa appears to have an atherogenic and prothrombic effect that interferes with plasminogen and tPA binding to fibrin. Lpa levels are thought to be genetic in origin and were found in 50% of the offspring of patients with CAD in the Framingham study.[29] Increased Lpa levels are associated with a threefold increase in the risk of a primary CAD event.[29] Response to standard treatment for lowering LDL in individuals with elevated Lpa were not successful except with LDL apheresis.[29]

In addition to Lpa, the presence of an elevated amount of small dense LDL particle subtype (phenotype B) is also associated with an elevated risk for CAD (threefold increased risk).[29,30] Small dense LDL is also associated with elevated triglyceride levels. Apparently small LDL particles can be moved into the vessel wall 50% faster than the large LDL particles. Treatment for presence of elevated small dense LDL particle subtype consists of low-fat diet, exercise, pharmacologic therapy with resins, niacin, and hormone replacement in women.[29]

Individuals with diabetes often have abnormal lipid levels. The most common pattern of lipid abnormalities in type 2 diabetes patients is elevated triglycerides and decreased LDL levels.[31] However, type 2 diabetes patients have a preponderance of smaller denser LDL particles, although their LDL cholesterol concentration is usually not significantly different than that of individuals without diabetes. Therefore, elevated triglyceride levels may be a better predictor of coronary heart disease in type 2 diabetes patients than elevated LDL levels because of the correlation with insulin resistance and small dense LDL.

## Other Potential Clinical Laboratory Risk Factors for CAD

Homocysteine, which is a type of amino acid found in the blood, has been linked to increased risk of development of cardiovascular diseases when the levels in the blood are elevated (Anderson article) Elevated levels of homocysteine have been reported to be >13 μmol/L). In addition, elevated plasma homocysteine has been associated with increased risk of death in individuals with many cardiovascular diseases, including CAD,[32] congestive heart failure,[33] first major cardiovascular event,[34,35] recurrent stroke,[36] and also persistent atrial fibrillation.[37]

Low levels of folate and vitamin B6 are related to elevated circulating homocysteine blood levels, and therefore sufficient folate intake may be an important factor in the prevention of coronary heart disease.[38,39] The odds ratio for CAD of a 5-μmol/L homocysteine increase was discovered to be 1.6 for males and 1.9 for females.[39]

Hematologic factors, such as fibrinogen, and elevated WBC counts have been associated with increased risk of CAD. Individuals with elevated fibrinogen levels in the highest quartile demonstrated a double risk of CAD, whereas the Multiple Risk Factor Intervention Trial found that an elevated WBC count is associated with increased risk.[30,40]

Inflammatory markers and infection markers have shown some relationship to CAD. Inflammatory markers such as CRP, an acute-phase reactant to inflammation, have recently been related to increased risk for CAD. CRP is one of the acute-phase proteins that increase during systemic inflammation. Testing CRP levels in the blood may be an additional way to assess cardiovascular disease risk. A more sensitive CRP test, called a highly sensitive C-reactive protein (hs-CRP) assay, is available to determine heart disease risk.

Higher hs-CRP levels also are associated with lower survival rates in these patients with CAD, and therefore may be a useful risk predictor.[41] Elevated levels of hs-CRP may increase the risk that an artery will reclose after it has been opened by balloon angioplasty. In addition, elevated levels of hs-CRP in the blood also seem to predict prognosis and recurrent events in patients with stroke or peripheral arterial disease. One study looked at CRP levels in individuals who took aspirin regularly versus those who did not take aspirin and found that CRP levels were predictive of MI in those who did *not* take aspirin.[41]

Normative values for hs-CRP are <1.0 mg/L, indicating a person has a low risk of developing cardiovascular disease. If hs-CRP is between 1.0 and 3.0 mg/L, a person has an average risk, and if hs-CRP is higher than 3.0 mg/L, a person is at high risk of developing cardiovascular disease.[32] If, after repeated testing, patients have persistently unexplained, markedly elevated hs-CRP (>10.0 mg/L), they should be evaluated to exclude noncardiovascular causes. Patients with autoimmune diseases or cancer, as well as other infectious diseases, often have elevated CRP levels.

Males with CRP levels in the highest quartile may have a fivefold increase in risk of developing an MI.[30] Infection markers, including *C. pneumoniae*, have shown a twofold increase in risk of CAD. Systemic infection may act directly on the arterial wall, or may work by local or systemic inflammation.[30]

Because these are new risk factors with insufficient evidence to support regular screening for them, they should be measured only in families with unexplained CAD or premature CAD. Future studies documenting their efficacy in identifying CAD will be necessary prior to routine screening.

In recent years B-type natriuretic peptide (BNP), a protein produced by the ventricles of the heart, has become an important tool to diagnose heart failure and may have indications with CAD. One of four known natriuretic peptides (atrial NP [ANP], BNP, C-type NP [CNP], and DNP), BNP is released from the cardiac ventricles, especially the left ventricle, during pressure or volume overload. BNP functions to dilate arteries and veins and acts as a neurohormonal modulator in decreasing vasoconstricting and sodium-retaining neurohormones. BNP also functions with ANP to promote diuresis.

B-type natriuretic peptide (BNP) and N-terminal (NT) pro-BNP are peptide fragments derived from a common precursor molecule, proBNP. Recently, BNP and NT-proBNP concentrations have been shown to be strongly predictive of short- and long-term survival in patients with ACSs.[42] BNP has now been associated with increased risk of heart failure, whereas NT-proBNP appears to be associated with increased risk of cardiovascular mortality, heart failure, and stroke. By C-statistic calculations, BNP and NT-proBNP significantly improved the predictive accuracy of the best available model for incident heart failure, and NT-proBNP also improved the model for cardiovascular death.[42]

## Complete Blood Cell Count

The physical therapist should evaluate the complete blood cell count for three components: hemoglobin, hematocrit values, and WBC count. Hemoglobin plays a major role in the transport of oxygen throughout the body, and the hematocrit (the amount of the blood that is cells) is a significant indicator of the viscosity of the blood. Hemoglobin values are reported as a concentration in the blood (in grams per 100 mL of blood). The normal range of hemoglobin for females is 12 to 16 g/100 mL, and for males it is 14 to 18 g/100 mL.[22]

Low levels of hemoglobin or a diagnosis of anemia will increase the work on the myocardium because of a lack of oxygen-carrying capacity and subsequently low levels of oxygen available to the tissues. In order to transport adequate oxygen to the tissues (even when the body is at rest) the heart rate is elevated and subsequently the cardiac output increases, thereby increasing the work on the myocardium. In addition, the mean corpuscular volume (MCV) test measures red blood cells (RBCs) in terms of individual volume. This test is used to classify anemias as microcytic (RBC size smaller than normal), normocytic, or macrocytic (larger than normal). Microcytic anemias are found in iron deficiency, chronic infections, chronic renal disease, and malignancies. Normocytic anemia (hypochromic) is found in

chronic infections, lead poisoning, chronic renal disease, and malignancies, whereas normochromic anemia is found in hemorrhage, hemolytic anemia, bone marrow hypoplasia, and splenomegaly. Macrocytic anemia is found in pernicious anemia, folic acid deficiency, hypothyroidism, and hepatocellular disease. Defining the MCV therefore assists in treatment of the cause of the anemia.[43-45]

> ### Clinical Tip
> Many facilities use a cutoff value for Hb of <8 g/100 mL as a red flag for out-of-bed activities. A Hb value <8 g/100 mL would require the individual to have an extremely low oxygen-carrying capacity and therefore be performing a lot of work even with bed and activities of daily living (ADLs). Heart rates are elevated with low Hb and the patient would also be performing a lot of work with breathing.

The lower-limit value for hematocrit is 37 g/100 mL for females and 42 g/100 mL for males.[22] Decreased levels of hemoglobin and hematocrit are often found in post–coronary artery bypass graft surgery patients. Elevated hematocrit levels suggest that the flow of blood to the tissues may be impeded because of an increase in the viscosity of the blood. Elevated hematocrit levels are often seen in individuals with chronic obstructive pulmonary disease (a response to chronic low $PO_2$).

> ### Clinical Tip
> After surgery, particularly after coronary artery bypass graft surgery, patients will demonstrate decreased hematocrit and hemoglobin values (and usually normocytic and normochromic MCV) and may be more symptomatic with activity because of low oxygen-carrying capacity.

White blood cells are monitored for the body's response to infectious diseases. Elevated levels of WBCs (leukocytosis) are found in response to leukemia, bacterial infection, or polycythemia (secondary to bone marrow stimulation). Some studies have identified a possible association between elevated WBC counts and increased risk of CAD.[40] Decreased WBC count (leukopenia) is found with bone marrow depression, acute viral infection, alcohol ingestion, and agranulocytosis. Disease processes may result in a change within individual leukocyte groups by altering morphology, function, or total numbers. Therefore, the differential WBC count is important to assess in order to determine possible causes of the abnormal WBC count.

## Coagulation Profiles

Coagulation profiles have become an important component of the patient's medical record because of the use of thrombolytic agents to dissolve clots in the early stages of MI.

Prothrombin time and partial thromboplastin time measure the coagulation of the blood. Streptokinase or tissue plasminogen activator (tPA) infusion is a means of dissolving critical clots that are blocking a coronary artery and creating a potential infarction and subsequent necrosis. These thrombolytic agents are most commonly administered intravenously but can also be injected directly into the coronary arteries. After the initial infusion of thrombolytics is begun, an intravenous infusion of heparin is started. As a result, prothrombin time and partial thromboplastin time must be monitored closely to determine the therapeutic ranges of anticoagulation.[22] partial thromboplastin time will often be elevated following any thrombolytic or heparin infusion. An elevated partial thromboplastin time indicates an increased time to form a clot, therefore, the chance of bleeding when bruised or cut is increased and caution should be taken.

Another oral anticoagulant commonly used to treat and prevent venous thrombosis and pulmonary embolism is warfarin (Coumadin). Warfarin interferes with the vitamin K–dependent activation of clotting factors II, VII, IX, and X. When the amount of anticoagulation is within narrow limits, warfarin therapy is both safe and effective; however, too little anticoagulation can lead to treatment failure or recurrence of thrombosis and too much anticoagulation can lead to serious or fatal bleeding. The amount of anticoagulation cannot be accurately predicted from the dose of warfarin because patient response is affected by several factors, so prothrombin time is the most accurate way to monitor warfarin therapy. Laboratory monitoring is critical to maintain warfarin anticoagulation within a therapeutic range; however prothrombin time values do not agree well between laboratories, making prothrombin time unsuitable for defining therapeutic ranges for warfarin therapy.

The International Normalized Ratio, or INR, was developed to standardize prothrombin time values, so that test results from different thromboplastins and coagulation analyzers become equivalent. Under the INR system, a thromboplastin is assigned an International Sensitivity Index (ISI) value (Hirsh article). Post-MI and mechanical valve patients have a target INR of 3 (2.5 to 3.5) and all other clotting problems have a target INR of 2.5 (2.0 to 3.0) (see Table 8-2).

Nonvalvular atrial fibrillation (AF) increases the risk of ischemic stroke by as much as a factor of 5, and the intensity of anticoagulation therapy reduces not only the frequency of ischemic stroke but also its severity and risk of death from stroke. Although warfarin is highly effective in preventing stroke in patients with AF by minimizing the formation of atrial thrombi, an INR of 2.0 or above decreases the risk of ischemic stroke to a higher degree than just the treatment with warfarin, emphasizing the need to follow a patient's INR regularly.[46] However, any anticoagulant therapy has the risk of hemorrhage associated with it, yet research has shown that if the INR is less than 2.0 because of the fear of bleeding, the patient is at an increased risk of having a more severe stroke and of having higher mortality poststroke.[46]

> **Clinical Tip**
> If a patient has been on thrombolytics or heparin (including low-dose heparin), the therapist should take extreme precautions against bumping extremities with all movement as the individual will be at a greater risk of bruising and bleeding.

## Electrolytes

All electrolyte levels should be observed when evaluating the laboratory results because disturbances in the electrolytes may affect the patient's performance. The electrolytes involved in maintaining cell membrane potential—$Na^+$, $K^+$, and $CO_2$—are the most important electrolytes to monitor. Hydration state, medications, and disease can affect these values. Patients receiving diuretics (e.g., for hypertension or heart failure) should have their sodium and potassium levels monitored carefully, because some diuretics act on the kidney. The action of these medications on the kidney is on the renal tubules and collecting ducts, where these electrolytes are allowed to diffuse out or are reabsorbed from the bloodstream. Dangerously low levels of potassium (lower than 3.5 mEq/L) can cause serious, life-threatening arrhythmias. Dangerously high levels of potassium (greater than 5.0 mEq/L) can affect the contractility of the myocardium. Low levels of $CO_2$ can cause an alkalotic state, muscle weakness, and dizziness.[22]

## Blood Urea Nitrogen and Creatinine

The BUN and creatinine values can be found on the same laboratory form as that reporting the electrolytes and cholesterol. The normal range for the BUN is 8 to 23 mg/dL; an elevated BUN can be an indication of heart failure or renal failure. Elevated BUN values also indicate uremia or a retention of urea in the blood. Decreased BUN values may indicate starvation, dehydration, or even other organ dysfunction such as liver disease.

> **Clinical Tip**
> Abnormal laboratory values found in heart failure include increased BUN, increased LDH, increased BNP, normal CPK-MB, and possible increased creatinine levels due to renal dysfunction.

The BUN value is unsuitable as a single measure of renal function, and therefore the creatinine value should also be noted. Normal serum creatinine levels are lower than 1.5 mg/dL. Endogenous creatinine is fully filtered in the glomerulus and is not reabsorbed in the tubules in the presence of normal renal function. Therefore, the clearance of creatinine is a measure of renal efficiency. As the glomerular filtration rate declines, the creatinine level rises and the renal function is assessed as inefficient. Severely elevated creatinine levels greater than 4.0 mg/dL indicate severe renal insufficiency or failure. The interpretation of the BUN and creatinine concentrations is an indication of the severity of the uremia.

## Serum Glucose

Serum glucose level is measured when a typical laboratory sample of blood is collected. The normal value for serum glucose is 80 to 110 mg/100 mL of blood, measured in the fasting state. The concentration is maintained within a reasonably narrow range. An elevated blood glucose level (mild hyperglycemia is 120 to 130 mg/100 mL) indicates a surplus of glucose in the blood. An elevated serum glucose value is suggestive of a prediabetic state and warrants testing for diabetes, such as administration of a glucose tolerance test (performed in the fasting individual following the ingestion of 100 g of glucose). Severe hyperglycemia (above 300 mg/100 mL) denotes a crisis situation that requires immediate insulin because cells lack the energy source to function, resulting in severe fatigue and subsequently inadequate metabolic activity. Patients should not be exercised when blood glucose measures in the severe range.

An elevated serum glucose value may also be found in a patient with diabetes who is not well controlled on oral or injectable insulin. Testing the hemoglobin A1C (HbA1C is normally 4.8% to 6.0%) measures a diabetic's insulin control during the past 90 days, which is the life of the RBCs that carry the hemoglobin.[22] See Chapter 7 for more information on diabetes.

## Other Laboratory Values

Other laboratory values may be abnormal but not usually indicative of cardiac dysfunction and instead may be related to other comorbidities. Abnormal laboratory values should be investigated to assess for comorbidity and any effect on the cardiac system. For example, albumin, a small blood protein, is the first protein detected in the urine when there is renal damage (burns, shock, low cardiac output). Elevations in albumin are rare, but low levels of albumin may be found in chronic liver disease, protein malnutrition, chronic infection, and acute stress. Elevated bilirubin may be present when there is hemorrhage or hepatic dysfunction, whereas elevations in lipase indicate pancreatic dysfunction or pancreatitis.

## Other Noninvasive Diagnostic Tests

### Holter Monitoring

Holter monitoring consists of continuous 24-hour electrocardiographic monitoring of a patient's heart rhythm, providing information that is essential to the diagnosis and management of episodes of cardiac arrhythmias and corresponding symptoms. Holter monitoring tracings must be reliable to capture, recognize, and reproduce any abnormality in heart rhythm, particularly those that threaten life or cardiac hemodynamics.

Indications for use of the Holter monitor include identifying symptoms possibly caused by arrhythmias (e.g., dizziness, syncope, shortness of breath at rest as well as with activity),

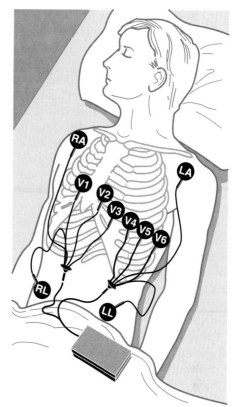

**Figure 8-1** Holter monitoring is transcutaneous, with multiple leads to record heart rhythm for 24 hours.

describing the arrhythmias noted with activity (frequency and severity), and evaluating antiarrhythmia therapy and pacemaker functioning. A common practice is to perform Holter monitoring routinely before discharging any patient who has had an MI, because arrhythmias are commonly associated with coronary disease, ischemia, and injury.

The patient's heart rhythm is monitored by means of a transcutaneous recorder applied to the patient's chest wall via multiple leads and electrodes and then recorded onto digital flash memory devices (Fig. 8-1). The patient wears the Holter monitor for 24 hours (there are 30-day monitors available as well) while performing normal activities (except bathing). All the patient's activities as well as any symptoms that may be felt during the 24 hours are documented by the patient. Once the recorder is removed from the patient, the flash memory device is processed by reproducing the recording on computer or paper for visual inspection. The physician then interprets the results and plans the treatment accordingly. Repeat Holter monitoring may be necessary once treatment has been initiated to evaluate the effectiveness of the treatment.

It is the responsibility of the physical therapist working with a patient who is wearing or has worn a Holter monitor to obtain the interpretation of the results of the Holter monitor to determine if modifications are needed in the patient's activities. For example, patients with life-threatening arrhythmias recorded by the Holter monitor should not begin physical therapy activity until treatment for the arrhythmia is initiated or modified. Increasing frequency of arrhythmias or more serious (life-threatening) arrhythmias developing with activity also require further evaluation by the physician.[47]

Patients with abnormal Holter monitor results may be referred for treadmill exercise testing to assess arrhythmias during an assessment of increased work on the heart or may be referred for echocardiography to assess valve functioning.

Patients demonstrating life-threatening arrhythmias on the Holter monitor may be referred to electrophysiologic mapping studies (EPS), particularly if they demonstrated sustained or nonsustained ventricular tachycardia. These individuals have a high risk of sudden death. EPS is performed to identify the specific area that may be initiating the arrhythmia by inducing the arrhythmia and subsequently attempting to restore normal rhythm with one or more antiarrhythmic medications. If the arrhythmia is induced and unable to be treated successfully by the antiarrhythmic medication, the patient may be referred for an ablation procedure (cauterization of the area inducing the arrhythmia) or pacing techniques, or the patient may be provided an implantable cardiac defibrillator (ICD) for rhythm control. According to the American Heart Association (AHA) guidelines, indications for ICD therapy include individuals who have ischemic cardiomyopathy and LVEF <30% or individuals with ischemic or nonischemic heart failure and NYHA (New York Heart Association) Classes II to III and LVEF <35%.[48,49]

Clinical trials have confirmed that ICDs save lives over current antiarrhythmic treatment in certain populations.[50,51] In the MUSTT trial, arrhythmic deaths or cardiac arrests were highest in inducible (able to induce sustained ventricular tachycardia under EPS study) patients randomized to no antiarrhythmic therapy; next were inducible patients receiving an ICD; and lowest were in patients who were noninducible.[52] Individuals with recurrent uncontrolled AF may be referred for similar procedures, including an implantable atrial defibrillator, or an ablation procedure.

## Echocardiography

Echocardiography is a noninvasive procedure that uses pulses of reflected ultrasound to evaluate the functioning heart. A transducer that houses a special crystal emits high-frequency sound waves and receives their echoes when placed on the chest wall of the patient. The returning echoes, reflected from a variety of intracardiac surfaces, are displayed on the ultrasonography equipment.

Echocardiography has an advantage over other cardiac diagnostic tests because the technique is completely noninvasive and gives real-time images of the beating heart. The transducer is placed on the chest wall in the third to fifth intercostal space near the left sternal border. The transducer is then tilted at various angles so that the sound waves can scan the segments of the heart. M-mode echo and two-dimensional echo (Fig. 8-2) are common techniques of echocardiography, whereas Doppler echocardiography is a newer

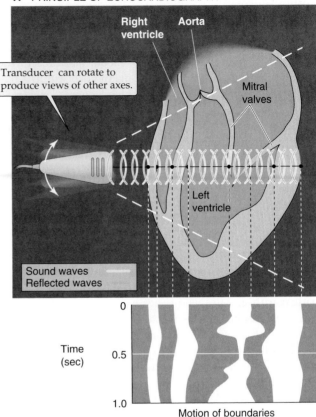

**A    PRINCIPLE OF ECHOCARDIOGRAPHY**

**Figure 8-2** M-mode and two-dimensional echocardiography. The tracing on the bottom shows the result of an M-mode echocardiogram (i.e., transducer in single position) during one cardiac cycle. The waves represent motion ("M") of heart boundaries transected by stationary ultrasonic beam. In two-dimensional echocardiography (upper panel), the probe rapidly rotates between the two extremes (broken lines), producing an image of a slice through the heart at one instant in time. (From Boron WF: Medical Physiology, Updated Edition. Philadelphia, Saunders, 2005.)

procedure. Doppler echocardiography gives information about the blood flow velocities of the heart.

Important information can be obtained from the echocardiogram, including the size of the ventricular cavity, the thickness and integrity of the interatrial and intraventricular septa, the functioning of the valves, and the motions of individual segments of the ventricular wall. Assessment of the performance of the heart muscle itself, especially the regional functioning of the left ventricle, is a valuable application of echocardiography. The degree of normal thickening of a portion of the myocardium can be assessed and is an indirect assessment of ischemia, because ischemic cardiac muscle does not thicken. Echocardiography can quantify volumes of the left ventricle, estimate stroke volume and therefore ejection fraction, and analyze motion of the valves and the heart muscle. There are numerous specific problems that can be evaluated with the echocardiogram:

- Pericardial effusion
- Cardiac tamponade

- Idiopathic congestive cardiomyopathy
- Hypertrophic cardiomyopathy
- Mitral valve regurgitation
- Mitral valve prolapse
- Aortic regurgitation
- Aortic stenosis
- Vegetation on the valves
- Intracardiac masses
- Ischemic heart muscle
- Left ventricular aneurysm
- Ventricular thrombi
- Proximal coronary disease
- Congenital heart disease
- Interventricular thickness
- Pericarditis
- Aortic dissection
- Patency of internal mammary coronary artery bypass graft (determined with Doppler technique)

Problems exist with the image quality of standard echocardiograms owing to such confounding factors as pulmonary disease, obesity, and chest deformities. Transesophageal echocardiography (TEE) has solved these problems and allows an improved view of the heart and mediastinum (Fig. 8-3). The patient begins to swallow the tube and the procedure begins. The use of anesthesia and the sedative minimizes discomfort and there is usually no pain. The tube goes down the esophagus the same way as swallowed food. Therefore, it is important that the patient swallow the tube rather than gag on it.

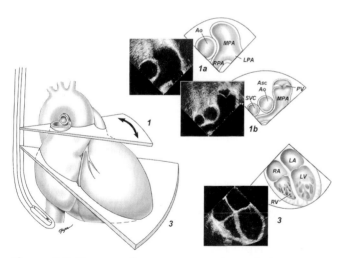

**Figure 8-3** Diagram of common scan planes during a transesophageal echocardiogram (TEE) with a two-dimensional view. Transverse plane: cross-sectional view at Level 1a depicts the proximal ascending aorta (Ao), main pulmonary artery (MPA), and left and right pulmonary arteries (LPA and RPA, respectively). A rightward tilt of the transducer shows the RPA as it passes behind the superior vena cava (SVC) and ascending aorta (Asc Ao). To obtain a four-chamber view (Level 3), the transducer is advanced in the esophagus with slight retroflexion of the scope. (From Geva T. Echocardiography and Doppler ultrasound. In Garson, A, Bricker JT, Fisher DJ, Neish SR (eds.): The Science and Practice of Pediatric Cardiology. Baltimore, MD: Williams & Wilkins, 1997:789, with permission.)

The transducer at the end of the tube is positioned in the esophagus, directly behind the heart. By rotating and moving the tip of the transducer, the physician can examine the heart from several different angles. The heart rate, blood pressure, and breathing are monitored during the procedure. Oxygen is given as a preventive measure and suction is used, as needed.

Further, TEE allows for improved visualization of cardiac structures and function and is valuable in the intraoperative and perioperative monitoring of left ventricular performance as well as the evaluation of surgical results.[53–56] In addition, TEE has become established as the imaging modality of choice for the evaluation of known or suspected cardioembolic stroke.[57] TEE may also be useful in detection of those at risk for an embolic stroke because of its ability to detect blood clots, masses, and tumors that are located inside the heart and those individuals with nonvalvular AF.[58] A TEE can also gauge the severity of certain valve problems and help detect infection of heart valves, certain congenital heart diseases such as atrial septal defect (ASD; or a hole between the atria), and a tear (dissection) of the aorta.[58]

Two-dimensional echocardiographic studies during exercise, immediately after exercise, or at both times (also known as stress echocardiography) are currently used to evaluate ischemia-induced wall motion abnormalities noninvasively. In addition to treadmill or bicycle exercise, atrial pacing or the use of pharmacologic agents provides an "artificial exercise" situation from which two-dimensional echocardiographic studies can identify the presence and location of ischemia-induced abnormalities in the ventricular wall.[59] Stress echocardiography is especially useful for the evaluation of atypical symptoms such as dyspnea and fatigue[60] as well as for the evaluation of patients with nondiagnostic ECGs with exercise or who have atypical chest pain syndromes.[61]

The development and use of three-dimensional echocardiography, the newest form of echocardiography, provides enhanced images displaying intracardiac anatomy.[62] Three-dimensional echocardiography provides accurate quantified data previously assessed by computer analysis.[62,63]

## Contrast Echocardiography

Using an intravenously injected contrast agent with the echocardiogram has improved the diagnostic accuracy of echocardiography in assessing myocardial perfusion and ventricular chambers.[64] The contrast agent used consists of a suspension of air-filled microspheres that act as an ultrasound tracer. Contrast echocardiography enhances the visualization of intracardiac and intrapulmonary shunts, endocardial wall motion, and ventricular wall thickness and improves the calculation of ejection fraction. In addition, contrast echocardiography appears to have potential for quantifying coronary flow and assessing myocardial viability.[65] It is a method for noninvasively assessing areas of the myocardium at risk for damage, presence or absence of coronary collateral flow, and revascularization of occluded arteries after coronary angioplasty. The use of contrast material also improves the visualization of endocardial borders, allowing to discrimination between the myocardial tissue and the blood pool.[66–68] The Food and Drug Administration currently has approved octafluoropropane (Optison) as a contrast agent for echo imaging as it increases the endocardial border identification.

Contrast echocardiography has also been used with transesophageal or epicardial echocardiography (only in the operating room or in the cardiac catheterization laboratory) to assess the distribution of cardioplegia and the degree of valvular regurgitation, as well as the vascular supply of bypass grafts and bypass graft patency.[65] The future of contrast agents with echocardiography may be in the performance of clot lysis and for targeted gene therapy.[69]

Studies comparing contrast echocardiography with thallium-201 SPECT imaging have demonstrated similar conclusions regarding presence and amount of jeopardized myocardium, yet it may involve one half the cost of the SPECT and therefore be more cost-effective than the SPECT imaging.[64,70]

## Other Imaging Modalities

In addition to contrast perfusion echocardiography, other imaging techniques are used in the diagnosis of cardiac dysfunction that may or may not utilize radioactive isotopes. PET, CT, SPECT, EBCT, MUGA, and MRI are all imaging techniques used for evaluation of CAD and cardiac dysfunction. Some of these modalities use high-speed scintillation cameras that can follow the transit of isotopes injected into the peripheral vein through the right side of the heart, much as the dye flow that occurs with cardiac catheterization. Other methods use a camera that times the acquisition of images according to the cardiac cycle. All these tests play an important role in the diagnostic evaluation of coronary artery status, each with their advantages and disadvantages, which will be discussed in the following paragraphs.

### Positron Emission Tomography

Positron emission tomography is a nuclear technique that provides visualization and direct measurement of metabolic functioning, including glucose metabolism and fatty acid metabolism, as well as blood flow of the heart. PET is considered to be the gold standard for blood flow measurement and metabolic assessment of the heart, but it requires specialized technologic equipment and highly trained personnel and therefore is extremely expensive and not available at many hospitals.[71] PET has the highest resolution gain, yet given the high cost associated with PET imaging, it is unlikely it will become used routinely for cardiac imaging because there are comparable tests that are more widely available and cost less than PET imaging.[72]

Positron emission tomography is a test that uses a special type of camera and a tracer (radioactive chemical) to look at organs in the body. PET imaging requires administration of dipyridamole to cause vasodilation of the coronary arteries while the patient is at rest, and often FD6 (18F-fluorodeoxyglucose a tracer liquid) is administered to allow for myocardial metabolism and blood flow to be assessed in three dimensions.[73] The tracer moves through the body, where much of it collects in the specific organ or tissue. The tracer gives off tiny positively charged particles (positrons). The camera records the positrons and turns the recording into pictures on a computer.

Further, FD6 PET imaging allows for quantification and qualification of regional myocardial tracer distribution. PET imaging demonstrates tissue viability using the metabolic tracers to detect CAD and is especially helpful in identifying the individual with severe left ventricular dysfunction who would be a candidate for revascularization or transplant.[73]

Therefore, PET imaging has advantages over thallium imaging with exercise because it can detect jeopardized but viable myocardium[74,75] without requiring the individual to perform an active exercise test. Patients can safely undergo PET imaging from 2 to 10 days after infarction, or when any question of impedance of flow is involved. Since the invention of thrombolytic medications to decrease infarct size, this technique has demonstrated great advantages in evaluating the effectiveness of the thrombolytic technique because the procedure can be performed so early after infarction.[76] Because of the inaccessibility and cost of the procedure, other procedures have been studied and compared with the results of PET to determine equally effective diagnostic tests for myocardial blood flow. Williams determined that the viable myocardium results obtained from dobutamine echocardiography were similar to the results obtained from PET imaging, and it could therefore be performed when PET imaging was not an option.[77]

In addition, PET imaging has also been used as a diagnostic tool to assess brain metabolism and ischemia/injury in cerebrovascular accident and acute trauma patients.[78]

### Computed Tomography

Computed tomography (CT) is used predominantly to identify masses in the cardiovascular system or to detect aortic aneurysms or pericardial thickening associated with pericarditis. Images are taken of anatomic structures; in this case, cardiac structures are viewed in slices and analyzed, and the slices are approximately 1 to 3 mm apart. Recently, CT scanning has been used to assess graft patency in coronary artery bypass graft surgery patients. Because nothing is injected into the patient, this procedure is completely noninvasive and harmless, although it may not be indicated in individuals with claustrophobia. One recent study looked at evaluating low-risk patients admitted to the emergency department with chest pain to see if cardiac CT scans could rule out coronary ischemia and reduce the length of stay and hospital charges.[79] Individuals who were admitted with chest pain who were identified as low risk and who had negative cardiac CT scans were discharged earlier and with reduced hospital charges, indicating that CT scans might prove beneficial for some patients admitted with chest pain.[79]

## Single-Photon Emission Computed Tomography

Single-photon emission computed tomography is a noninvasive method to detect and quantify myocardial perfusion defects and contractility defects and is used in conjunction with radioactive isotopes.[80] SPECT uses newer gated tomographic techniques and can be performed with the use of sestamibi (a radioactive perfusion agent) to improve the view of a myocardial perfusion study. Images are acquired with either a gamma camera or a camera that times or "gates" the acquisition according to the cardiac cycle (via ECG). SPECT can determine contractility defects at rest by assessing both left and right ventricular ejection fraction, regional function, and ventricular volumes.[80]

In addition, SPECT imaging, although less accurate than PET imaging, is more often the diagnostic tool of choice because of the availability of these gated imaging machines and the ease of performance. Further information on SPECT is detailed in perfusion imaging with sestamibi later in this chapter.

## Electron Beam Computed Tomography

Electron beam computed tomography (EBCT) is used to detect calcium in the coronary arteries and is a noninvasive method to detect and quantify coronary atherosclerosis.[81–84] Calcium in the coronary arteries may be an early sign of CAD. Rumberger used EBCT on older populations; however, recently O'Malley used the procedure for screening for CAD in asymptomatic active-duty U.S. Army personnel.[81,85]

A typical EBCT scanning protocol involves a 10-minute scan involving 40 slices through the heart every 3 to 6 mm.[86] Intravenous contrast medium is not used, so radiation exposure is minimal (approximately one half the radiation exposure to the average person living in the United States in 1 year).[81] EBCT detects the presence of calcium in the coronary arteries as well as the location, extent, and density of the deposits and provides a calcium-scoring system. Results are given in the form of a composite score for the entire epicardial coronary system.

Further, EBCT has been studied in individuals undergoing cardiac catheterization and has shown a sensitivity of 81% to 94% for any angiographic evidence of coronary disease and a specificity of 72% to 86%.[84,87] EBCT currently appears to have moderate discriminating power in young, symptomatic patients with a high prevalence of obstructive disease, but its reliability with asymptomatic subjects is yet to be determined. Several studies have shown the association of future cardiovascular events with an elevated amount of coronary calcifications and reported that coronary calcium predicts cardiovascular events more accurately than does risk stratification using conventional risk factors.[88–91]

The determination of coronary calcifications allows the identification of patients with a high risk for future MI and CAD within an asymptomatic population. Becker looked at the ability of EBCT to predict MI compared to ATP III risk score and found that there was higher diagnostic accuracy with the EBCT.[92] In addition, future MI or CAD during the observation period was excluded in patients without coronary calcifications independent of concomitant cardiovascular risk factors.[92–94] As accuracy of predicting CAD is still not proven with the EBCT, further studies are needed in this area.

> **Clinical Tip**
> The use of EBCT to identify individuals at risk for future MI or stroke is still very controversial and the evidence is not conclusive regarding the sensitivity of this test for identifying CAD in any population. Individuals undergoing this procedure need to know that this is not 100% reliable for all populations (those at risk versus those not at risk for CAD).

## Multigated Acquisition Imaging

Multigated acquisition imaging or gated pool imaging is a noninvasive technique to calculate left ventricular ejection fraction. The information gathered in this study is obtained from the electrical activity of the heart using an electrocardiograph. Multigated acquisition imaging obtains multiple individual ejection fractions knowing the heart rate and R-R intervals on the electrocardiogram and then measures the emptying curves of the heart via computer. This technique has advantages over others in that it is noninvasive and can therefore be used on critically ill cardiac patients (e.g., those with acute cardiac failure) when other more invasive tests such as catheterization would be dangerous.[95–98]

## Magnetic Resonance Imaging

Magnetic resonance imaging MRI is used to evaluate morphology, cardiac blood flow, and myocardial contractility.[99] However, use of cardiovascular MRI has been limited because of the existence of echocardiography and nuclear scintigraphy and the familiarity with these two techniques over MRI.

Further, MRI has similar diagnostic accuracy as PET imaging, is similarly used as a noninvasive test to assess regional blood flow problems, but is more widely available and often less expensive.[73] Nuclear magnetic resonance can produce high-resolution tomographic pictures of the heart without using any radiation. Originally MRI was used for assessing cardiac anatomy and congenital malformations and to identify masses and thrombi. Currently MRI is being used for assessment of valvular disease, cardiac shunts, quantification of cardiac flow, and coronary artery anatomy.[100] Fayed demonstrated that the human coronary vessel wall could be noninvasively imaged in vivo with MRI, thereby providing a technique to show atherosclerotic plaque without the use of coronary angiography.[101] Future work with MRI indicates it may be the choice for detection of vulnerable plaque prior to an acute clinical event.[101,102]

Yang et al. assessed the new cardiac MRI system, comparing it to echocardiography.[103] The new cardiac MRI (CMRI) system allows for continuous real-time dynamic acquisition and display. The CMRI was completed in less than 15 minutes and showed improved visualization of wall segments and left ventricular function as compared to the echocardiography results.[103,104] MRI is also being used in conjunction with pharmacologic stress testing to determine significant coronary atherosclerotic plaques.[105]

### Magnetic Resonance Angiogram

A magnetic resonance angiogram (MRA) uses magnetic and radio wave energy to take pictures of blood vessels inside your body. An MRA is a type of MRI.

An MRA can find the location of a blocked blood vessel and show how severe the blockage is; however, if an individual has a pacemaker, artificial joint, stent, surgical clips, heart valve, or any other metallic device, he or she might not be a candidate for an MRA.

## Exercise Testing

Exercise testing continues to be the single most important noninvasive procedure used in the diagnosis and management of patients with CAD, although exercise testing alone is less sensitive and specific for women versus men.

Originally exercise testing was used to measure functional capacity or to evaluate abnormalities of coronary circulation. Currently exercise testing is used for a variety of patient management problems that are listed in Box 8-1.

Exercise testing involves systematically and progressively increasing the oxygen demand and evaluating the responses to the increased demand. The technique varies with different modes of exercise chosen and different protocols used by the examiner. Formal exercise testing involves the following modes of exercise:

- Walking up and down steps
- Exercising on a stationary bicycle
- Using arm or wheelchair ergometry
- Walking or jogging on a treadmill at variable speeds and inclines
- Walking a specified distance as in the 6-minute walk test

Informal testing is performed to screen for exercise programs, sometimes on a group basis, and includes such tests as

the 12-minute walk, Cooper's 12-minute run, the pulse recovery test, or the 1.5-mile run (Table 8-6).[106–108]

### Maximal Versus Submaximal Stress Testing

The protocols that are used are described as either maximal or submaximal; the distinction between them is the termination point of the test. Submaximal tests are terminated on achievement of a predetermined end point (unless symptoms otherwise limit completion of the test). The predetermined end point may be either the achievement of a certain percentage of the patient's predicted maximal heart rate (PMHR; e.g., 75% of PMHR) or the attainment of a certain workload (e.g., 2.5 mph, 12% grade). A special subset of submaximal testing is low-level testing, performed on patients during the recuperative phase after myocardial injury or coronary bypass surgery.

Maximal stress tests usually use the end point of the PMHR or terminate when a patient is limited by symptoms. Maximal stress testing is used to measure functional capacity as well as to diagnose CAD. The protocol for testing involves performing a progressive workload until the patient perceives an inability to continue because of some limiting symptom such as shortness of breath, leg fatigue, or chest discomfort.

Exercise tests also may be described as intermittent or continuous. Intermittent testing intersperses progressive workloads with short rest periods to give the subject time to recover and decrease the effect of peripheral fatigue. Continuous tests utilize incrementally progressive workloads until the test is terminated because of patient symptoms or a defined end point.

### Low-Level Exercise Testing

Low-level exercise testing is usually performed when patients have experienced an MI recently or have undergone coronary artery bypass graft surgery. Such tests have been performed as early as 5 days after MI or surgery[109] but are more likely to be performed just before or immediately after discharge from the hospital following an acute event. Some physicians prefer to wait up to 2 weeks after the cardiac event before administering the low-level exercise test.

Low-level exercise testing may be useful in predicting the subsequent course of an MI or bypass surgery as well as for identifying the high-risk patient. High-risk patients exhibit an increased risk of complications or death as a result of myocardial ischemia or poor ventricular function. High-risk patients need more immediate intervention and should not be treated as typical patients in a cardiac rehabilitation program. After a high-risk patient is identified, the decision on optimal medical management or surgical intervention is more easily made.

Many factors have been studied from the results of the low-level exercise test to determine the most outstanding variable for identifying high-risk patients. Exercise-induced ST-segment depression of 2.0 mm or greater on low-level exercise tests has been identified as the single most valuable

---

**Box 8-1**

### Indications for Exercise Stress Testing

- Evaluation of chest pain suggestive of coronary disease
- Evaluation of atypical chest pain
- Determination of prognosis and severity of coronary artery disease
- Evaluation of the effects of medical or surgical therapy or intervention
- Evaluation of arrhythmias
- Evaluation of hypertension with activity
- Assessment of functional capacity
- Screening to provide an exercise prescription
- Providing motivation for a lifestyle change to reduce the risk of developing coronary artery disease

**Table 8-6 The 12-Minute Walk/Run Test, Which Identifies Fitness Category for the Distance Covered in 12 Minutes**

| Fitness Category | | AGE (YEARS) | | | | | |
|---|---|---|---|---|---|---|---|
| | | 13–19 | 20–29 | 30–39 | 40–49 | 50–59 | ≥60 |
| I. Very poor | M | <1.30 | <1.22 | <1.18 | <1.14 | <1.03 | <0.87 |
| | F | <1.00 | <0.96 | <0.94 | <0.88 | <0.84 | <0.78 |
| II. Poor | M | 1.30–1.37 | 1.22–1.31 | 1.18–1.30 | 1.14–1.24 | 1.03–1.16 | 0.87–1.02 |
| | F | 1.00–1.18 | 0.96–1.11 | 0.95–1.05 | 0.88–0.98 | 0.84–0.93 | 0.78–0.86 |
| III. Fair | M | 1.38–1.56 | 1.32–1.49 | 1.31–1.45 | 1.25–1.39 | 1.17–1.30 | 1.03–1.20 |
| | F | 1.19–1.29 | 1.12–1.22 | 1.03–1.18 | 0.99–1.11 | 0.94–1.05 | 0.87–0.98 |
| IV. Good | M | 1.57–1.72 | 1.50–1.64 | 1.46–1.56 | 1.40–1.53 | 1.31–1.44 | 1.21–1.32 |
| | F | 1.30–1.43 | 1.23–1.34 | 1.19–1.29 | 1.12–1.24 | 1.06–1.18 | 0.99–1.09 |
| V. Excellent | M | 1.73–1.86 | 1.65–1.76 | 1.57–1.69 | 1.54–1.65 | 1.45–1.58 | 1.33–1.55 |
| | F | 1.44–1.51 | 1.35–1.45 | 1.30–1.39 | 1.25–1.34 | 1.19–1.30 | 1.10–1.18 |
| VI. Superior | M | >1.87 | >1.77 | >1.70 | >1.66 | >1.59 | >1.56 |
| | F | >1.52 | >1.46 | >1.40 | >1.35 | >1.31 | >1.19 |

*M = Male; F = Female.*
*From Cooper K. The Aerobic Ways. New York, Bantam Books, 1981.*

indicator of prognosis after MI according to the regression analysis by Davidson and DeBusk.[110] In addition, early onset of ST-segment depression is related to increased incidence of coronary events. Starling and co-workers[111] demonstrated a significantly increased risk of death after MI when both ST-segment depression and angina were produced during low-level exercise testing in the early period after an MI. Exercise-induced angina alone was associated with subsequent coronary artery bypass surgery.[112,113] Other variables of minor prognostic significance after MI include inappropriate blood pressure response, maximum heart rate achieved, and maximum systolic blood pressure achieved.[114,115]

Low-level exercise testing can also provide information useful for optimal medical management after myocardial injury or surgery, including treatment for angina, arrhythmias, or hypertension. Exercise-induced arrhythmias on a low-level exercise test may be an indication for therapeutic management before hospital discharge. The incidence of sudden death has been reported to be 2.5 times higher in patients manifesting ventricular arrhythmias during low-level exercise testing.[116] Poor performance, such as limited exercise duration, has been highly correlated with increased incidence of heart failure and is associated with an increased mortality.[117]

Because of its great prognostic and therapeutic value, low-level testing is often used for screening patients who wish to participate in cardiac rehabilitation programs.[118] Activity levels for patients during rehabilitation in the home or hospital setting can be prescribed on the basis of the results of the low-level exercise test.

However, not all patients are appropriate candidates for low-level exercise testing. Safety of exercise testing early after

---

**Box 8-2**

**Contraindications to Low-Level Testing**

- Unstable angina or angina pectoris at rest
- Severe heart failure (overt left ventricular failure on examination with pulmonary rales and S3 heart sound)
- Serious arrhythmias at rest
- Second- or third-degree heart block
- Disabling musculoskeletal abnormalities
- Valvular heart disease
- Blood pressure >180/105 mm Hg
- Patient refuses to sign consent form

From Starling MR, Crawford MH, et al. Predictive value of early post-myocardial infarction modified treadmill exercise testing in multivessel coronary artery disease detection. Am Heart J 102(2):169, 1981.

MI has been a topic of debate because of the traditional medical belief that a recently damaged myocardium is prone to further injury, including rupture, aneurysm, extension of infarction, or susceptibility to serious arrhythmias.[119] However, the safety of properly conducted exercise testing was documented as early as 1973.[120] Knowledge of and adherence to contraindications for testing optimize the safety of exercise testing (Box 8-2).[121] See Box 8-3 for indications/contraindications for exercise testing in the emergency department.[79]

Institutions vary in the choice of an exercise testing protocol for low-level testing. However, a progressively increasing workload from 2 to approximately 6 METs (Metabolic Equivalent Tables, a multiple of the resting metabolic rate) is often used. Among the protocols for low-level exercise

**Box 8-3**

**Indications and Contraindications for Exercise ECG in the Emergency Department Setting**

**Requirements Before Exercise ECG Testing in the ED**

Two sets of cardiac enzymes at 4-hour intervals should be normal

ECG at the time of presentation, and preexercise 12-lead ECG shows no significant change

Absence of rest ECG abnormalities that would preclude accurate assessment of the exercise ECG

From admission to the time results are available from the second set of cardiac enzymes: patient asymptomatic, lessening chest pain symptoms, or persistent atypical symptoms

Absence of ischemic chest pain at the time of exercise testing

**Contraindications**

New or evolving ECG abnormalities on the rest tracing

Abnormal cardiac enzymes

Inability to perform exercise

Worsening or persistent ischemic chest pain symptoms from admission to the time of exercise testing

Clinical risk profiling indicating imminent coronary angiography is likely

### Table 8-7  Modified Naughton Treadmill Protocol

|  | TIME (MIN) | | | | | | | |
|---|---|---|---|---|---|---|---|---|
|  | 0 | 3 | 6 | 9 | 12 | 15 | 18 | 21 |
| Speed (mph) | 2 | 2 | 2 | 2 | 2 | 3 | 3 | 3 |
| Grade (%) | 3.5 | 7 | 10.5 | 14 | 17.5 | 12.5 | 15 | 17.5 |
| MET | 3 | 4 | 5 | 6 | 7 | 8 | 9 | 10 |

*MET, resting metabolic rate.*

testing, the modified Naughton (Table 8-7) and modified Sheffield-Bruce (Table 8-8) protocols appear to be most widely chosen.

Low-level exercise testing soon after MI is a safe, noninvasive method for evaluating the functional capacity for physical activity; for detecting arrhythmias, angina, and hypertensive responses with exercise; for determining optimal medical management; and for predicting the risk of subsequent cardiac events.

### Safety in Exercise Testing

The physical therapist must have a clear understanding of the rationale for terminating any exercise test. The specific criteria for termination vary from one institution to another, but the general criteria for termination of a maximal stress or low-level stress test are found in Box 8-4.

Both the patient and the discharging physician benefit when a predischarge exercise test is conducted.[118] The test can facilitate the distinction between chest wall and angina pain. In addition, improvement in exercise performance following an MI has been related to improvement in the patient's self-confidence following a successful, uneventful predischarge exercise test.

### Table 8-8  Modified Sheffield-Bruce Submaximal Protocol

| Stage | Speed (mph) | Grade (%) | Time (min) |
|---|---|---|---|
| 1 | 1.7 | 0 | 3 |
| 2 | 1.7 | 5 | 3 |
| 3 | 1.7 | 10 | 3 |
| 4 | 2.5 | 12 | 3 |

Maximal exercise testing and testing of high-risk patients or post–myocardial injury patients should be done in a setting in which emergencies can be managed expertly and efficiently. Appropriate equipment, which includes emergency medications and intravenous, intubation, and suctioning materials, should be present and updated when necessary. A direct current defibrillator should be available and functioning properly. Persons performing the testing should be certified in Advanced Cardiac Life Support, taught by the American Heart Association, and well trained in emergency cardiac response techniques such as defibrillation. Written protocols describing emergency procedures to be followed

## Box 8-4

### Criteria for Termination of Maximal and Low-Level/Submaximal Testing

#### Criteria for Termination of Maximal Testing

Increasing frequency or pairing of premature ventricular complexes

Development of ventricular tachycardia

Rapid atrial arrhythmias, including atrial fibrillation or atrial flutter, with uncontrolled ventricular response rates

Development of second- or third-degree heart block

Increased angina pain (Level 2 on a scale of 4)

Hypotensive blood pressure response (20 mm Hg or greater decrease)

Extreme shortness of breath

Dizziness, mental confusion, or lack of coordination

Severe ST-segment depression. The American College of Sports Medicine recommends termination when the ST segment is depressed 2.0 mm or more, although some testing personnel may proceed when changes of greater magnitude are demonstrated as long as there is no evidence of other abnormal responses.[100]

Observation of the patient reveals pale and clammy skin (pallor and diaphoresis)

Extremely elevated systolic or diastolic blood pressure, or both, which may or may not be associated with symptoms.

On achievement of predicted maximal heart rate; it is usually safe to proceed with the test beyond the predicted maximal heart rate if the patient is able and willing to continue and if other indications to terminate the test are absent.[106]

Presence of leg fatigue or leg cramps or claudication pain

Patient request for termination of test

#### Criteria for Termination of Low Level/Submaximal Testing

An oxygen consumption level of 17.5 mL of oxygen per kg (6 METs) achieved

70% to 75% of age-predicted maximal heart rate achieved

Fatigue or dyspnea

Maximal heart rate of 120 to 130 beats per minute

Frequent (nine or more per minute) unifocal or multifocal premature ventricular contractions, paired premature ventricular contractions, or ventricular tachycardia

ST-segment depression of 1.0 to 2.0 mm

Claudication pain

Dizziness

Decrease in systolic blood pressure of 10 to 15 mm Hg below peak value

Hypertensive blood pressure (systolic >200 mm Hg, diastolic >110 mm Hg)

Level 1 (out of 4) angina

---

should be available to all testing personnel. These can be adopted from the American Heart Association's guidelines for advanced cardiac life support.[122]

Safety is a major consideration in exercise testing, and among the most important determinants of safety are the knowledge and experience of the examiner conducting the test. The American College of Sports Medicine has published guidelines that document the knowledge and skills required for exercise testing, including a description of situations in which the involvement or presence of a physician during testing may be necessary.[123] Ellestad and Stuart published a survey of more than 500,000 exercise tests, which suggested an overall mortality rate of 0.5 per 10,000 tests and a morbidity rate of 9 per 10,000.[124]

Exercise testing by nonphysician health care professionals has been performed for more than 30 years, although the American Heart Association Committee on Stress Testing did not endorse the idea of "experienced paramedical personnel" as able to perform the tests until 1979.[125] In 1987, Cahalin published a report on the safety of testing as performed by physical therapists with advanced clinical competence.[126] In 10,577 tests performed, the mortality rate was 0.9 per 10,000 and the morbidity rate was 3.8 per 10,000. In addition, Squires reported on the safety of exercise testing of 289 cardiac outpatients with left ventricular dysfunction

(ejection fraction over 35%) by paramedical personnel with physician available on call.[127] Only one serious event occurred in 289 tests, and the outcome was a successful resuscitation. In addition, Olivotto demonstrated that exercise testing was safe in a community-based population of patients with hypertrophic cardiomyopathy and provides useful information on functional capacity, blood pressure responses to exercise, and presence or absence of inducible ischemia.[128] In 2000 the American College of Cardiology/American Heart Association and American College of physicians published a joint statement on the clinical competence required for stress testing including skills required for paramedical professionals to perform graded exercise testing that is found in Box 8-5.[129]

Factors that enhance the safety of exercise testing include the use of an informed consent to be signed by the patient, the knowledge of when to exclude a patient from proceeding with an exercise test, the knowledge of when to terminate an exercise test, the knowledge and skills to react to an abnormal response or situation, and the availability of appropriate equipment and supplies to manage an emergency (e.g., defibrillator, emergency medications, intubation, suctioning equipment).

Physical therapists wishing to conduct exercise tests on individuals older than 40 years or on persons who are at

---

**Box 8-5**

### Graded Exercise Testing Skills for Paramedical Professionals

- Knowledge of absolute and relative contraindications for exercise testing
- Ability to communicate properly with the client to complete a medical history and informed consent
- Ability to explain to the client the purpose of completing the graded exercise test (GXT), procedures of the test, and the responsibilities of the client during the test
- Competence in cardiopulmonary resuscitation certified by American Heart Association basic cardiac life support and preferably advanced cardiac life support
- Knowledge of specificity, sensitivity, and predictive value of a positive and negative test and diagnostic accuracy of exercise testing in different patient populations
- Understanding of causes that produce false-positive and false-negative test results
- Knowledge of most appropriate activity and exercise protocol (e.g., Bruce, Naughton, Blake-Ware) for each individual, based on his or her medical history
- Knowledge of normal and abnormal hemodynamic responses to graded exercise (blood pressure and heart rate response) in different age groups and with various cardiovascular conditions
- Knowledge of metabolic data collected during a GXT and knowledge of how to interpret the data (e.g., maximal oxygen uptake, metabolic equivalent) for different medical conditions
- Knowledge of 12-lead electrocardiography and changes in the electrocardiogram that may result from exercise, especially ischemia, arrhythmias, and conduction abnormalities
- Knowledge of proper lead placement and skin preparation for a 12-lead electrocardiogram
- Knowledge and skills for accurately taking blood pressure under resting and exercise conditions
- Knowledge of how to run and troubleshoot the medical equipment used for graded exercise testing (treadmill, electrocardiogram, bicycle ergometer, metabolic cart)
- Ability to communicate with the client to assess signs and symptoms of cardiovascular disease before, during, and after the GXT
- Knowledge of how to assess signs and symptoms by using appropriate scales (e.g., chest pain, shortness of breath, rating of perceived exertion)
- Knowledge of how the appropriate time to end the GXT and absolute and relative indications for test termination
- Knowledge of knowing when to ask for physician support when the physician is not directly involved in the GXT
- Ability to communicate results of the GXT to the supervising physician

Data from Rodgers GP, Ayanian JZ, Balady G, et al. American College of Cardiology/American Heart Association clinical competence statement on stress testing. A report of the American College of Cardiology/American Heart Association/American College of Physicians-American Society of Internal Medicine Task Force on Clinical Competence. Circulation 102(14):1726–1738, 2000, in Ehrman JK, Gordon P, Visich PS, et al.: Clinical Exercise Physiology. 2nd ed. Champaign, IL, Human Kinetics, 2009.

---

**Box 8-6**

### Interpretation of Exercise Testing

- Exercise time completed (and protocol used)
- Limiting factors (reason for termination)
- Presence or absence of chest pain at peak exercise: usually defined as positive, negative, or atypical for angina or extreme shortness of breath
- Maximal heart rate achieved
- Blood pressure response
- Arrhythmias: description of which type developed and when they occurred
- ST-segment changes: usually described as positive, negative, equivocal, or indeterminate for ischemia
- Positive: 1.0 mm or greater horizontal or down-sloping ST-segment depression (Fig. 8-11)
- Equivocal: more than 0.5 but less than 1.0 mm horizontal or down-sloping ST-segment depression or more than 1.5 mm up-sloping depression
- Negative: less than 0.5 mm horizontal or down-sloping ST-segment depression[106]
- Indeterminate: unable to measure the ST segment accurately because of the presence of any of the following: bundle branch block, medication (if patient is taking digoxin [Lanoxin]), resting ST-segment changes on the ECG, or cardiac hypertrophy
- Heart sounds: notation of pretest and posttest sounds and description of any change
- Functional aerobic impairment: can be determined from a nomogram if the Bruce treadmill protocol is used. This value is compared with normal values to determine impairment in functional capacity (physical work capacity).
- R wave changes: amplitude changes are considered to give additional diagnostic information in interpreting exercise test results. The normal response to exercise is a decrease in R wave amplitude. If no change or an increase in R wave amplitude occurs with exercise, the patient with CAD is considered to be at an increased risk for developing a cardiac problem in the future (Fig. 8-12).[120]
- Maximal oxygen consumption ($VO_2max$) can be calculated using formulas if not directly measured during the test; however, this method is not very accurate.

---

moderate to high risk of developing CAD should expect to obtain the required knowledge and skills in advanced training or in clinically supervised postprofessional education. However, all physical therapists should understand the procedures involved in exercise testing and interpretation of the test results because one of the major purposes of these tests is the development of exercise prescriptions. Exercise prescriptions are based on the results of the exercise test and other pertinent information (Box 8-6).

## Contraindications to Testing

Essential to safe testing is knowing who should not be tested. Thoroughly evaluating the patient before testing reveals any

## Box 8-7

### Absolute and Relative Contraindications to Exercise Testing

#### Absolute Contraindications

Recent myocardial infarction (MI; less than 4 to 6 weeks after the MI for a maximal, symptom-limited test) in most clinical settings

Acute pericarditis or myocarditis

Resting or unstable angina

Serious ventricular or rapid atrial arrhythmias (e.g., ventricular tachycardia, couplets, atrial fibrillation, or atrial flutter)

Untreated second- or third-degree heart block

Overt congestive heart failure (pulmonary rales, third heart sound, or both)

Any acute illness

#### Relative Contraindications

Aortic stenosis

Known left main coronary artery disease (CAD; or its equivalent)

Severe hypertension (defined as systolic blood pressure >165 mm Hg at rest, diastolic blood pressure >110 mm Hg at rest, or both)

Idiopathic hypertrophic subaortic stenosis

Severe depression of the ST segment on the resting electrocardiograph

Compensated heart failure

---

contraindications to testing. See Box 8-7 for absolute contraindications to maximal stress testing.

In addition to absolute contraindications, the general clinical status of the patient must be considered before determining whether the stress test is contraindicated. See Box 8-4 for contraindications to testing and low-level testing.

### Exercise Testing Equipment

Clinical monitoring tools used during exercise testing traditionally include continuous ECG monitoring and periodic measurement of blood pressure and heart rate (this can be extracted from the ECG recording; see Chapter 9), patient reported or demonstrated symptoms, and heart and lung sounds. In some testing laboratories, expired gas analysis permits the assessment of oxygen uptake during the test (Fig. 8-4). Multiple-lead ECG monitoring is used to depict the electrical activity of the heart. Detection of both arrhythmias and ischemia can be made from the ECG. A detailed discussion of the interpretation of ECG data and a description of arrhythmias are presented in Chapter 9.

### Protocols for Exercise Testing

Most institutions adopt a standard protocol to facilitate comparisons of the test subject's responses from test to test session as well as for comparisons among other subjects. Standard testing procedures require a 12-lead ECG to be obtained before any test to rule out any acute ischemia or injury before testing. The patient's ECG is continuously monitored during the test. Standard procedure is to monitor a minimum of three leads during the test. Other pretest procedures include assessment of the patient's risk factor history for CAD (see Chapter 3); assessment of the patient's symptom history; and assessment of the patient's resting blood pressure, heart rate, and heart and lung auscultation.

When exercise is initiated, the workload is increased in accordance with a specific protocol. The patient's heart rate

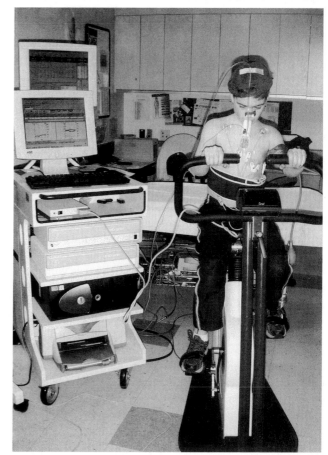

**Figure 8-4** A pediatric patient undergoing a bicycle ergometry stress test. (From Keane JF, Lock JE, Fyler DC: Nadas' Pediatric Cardiology. 2nd ed. Philadelphia, 2006, Saunders.)

and blood pressure (and in some tests, the expired gases) are periodically monitored throughout the test and during the recovery period. Most tests are symptom limited and, as such, are terminated at the request of the patient or on the identification of an abnormality in one or more of the parameters

BICYCLE TESTING PROTOCOL

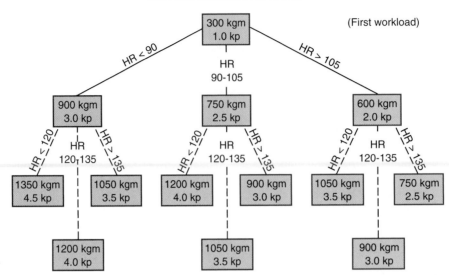

**Figure 8-5** A branching bicycle testing protocol. HR, Heart rate. (Adapted from Golding LA, Myers CR, Slinning WE [eds]. The Y's Way to Physical Fitness. Rev. ed. Chicago, The YMCA of the USA, 1982:535, with permission of the YMCA of the USA, 101 N. Wacker Dr., Chicago IL, 60606.)

being measured. The patient is monitored continuously during the recovery period until the pretest values are achieved. A written report documenting and interpreting the results is prepared following the test.

The most commonly used protocols in testing involve the use of either the stationary bicycle or the treadmill. Blood pressure is easier to auscultate on the stationary bicycle than on the treadmill. The bicycle also takes up less room, requires less coordination to operate, and is less expensive than the treadmill. The greatest disadvantage of the stationary bicycle, however, is that bicycling is not a daily functional activity for most persons. Therefore, patients develop muscular fatigue faster because they are using muscle groups that are not as "trained" as the muscles used for walking. Such patients do not achieve their best results, because the maximal heart rate may be well below what is considered diagnostic (85% of PMHR).[121] A widely used bicycle testing protocol is displayed in Figure 8-5.[130] This protocol may be used intermittently (meaning that rests are incorporated between each work stage) rather than continuously because of the peripheral fatigue that develops. Also, the workloads may be reduced by half for females or severely deconditioned individuals.

The treadmill is relatively large, requires a patient to have balance and coordination, and is extremely noisy, making the auscultation of blood pressure very difficult. However, because walking is a functional activity, the muscles do not fatigue as rapidly as they do with cycling, and therefore the treadmill is considered to have greater diagnostic benefits. The two most common treadmill protocols are the Bruce exercise test protocol and the Balke exercise protocol. The Bruce protocol (Table 8-9) is probably most widely used in the clinical setting of hospitals because it provides normative data in the form of a nomogram to

### Table 8-9  Bruce Treadmill Protocol

| Stage | Time (min) | Speed (mph) | Grade | Met[a] |
|---|---|---|---|---|
| I | 3 | 1.7 | 10% | 4–5 |
| II | 3 | 2.5 | 12% | 6–7 |
| III | 3 | 3.4 | 14% | 8–10 |
| IV | 3 | 4.2 | 16% | 11–13 |
| V | 3 | 5.0 | 18% | 14–16 |
| VI | 3 | 6.0 | 20% | 17–19 |

[a]1 MET, resting metabolic rate = 3.5 mL of oxygen per kg of body weight per minute.
From Ellestad MH. Stress Testing Principles and Practice. 4th ed. New York, Oxford University Press, 1996.

calculate functional aerobic impairment (Fig. 8-6). Previous studies have reported limitations in the ability of the functional aerobic impairment nomogram to predict functional capacity. The preferred method of predicting functional capacity is via the maximal workload performed on the treadmill test. According to Froelicher, a true test of aerobic capacity is best limited to a total exercise time of 10 minutes because of the endurance factor, which becomes significant after 10 minutes of exercise.[131]

The starting speed of the Bruce protocol is 1.7 miles per hour, which is a fairly comfortable speed for all. However, because of the rapid increases in speed and the fact the subject starts on a 10% grade, the average time a nontrained subject actually exercises during the test is between 6 and 12 minutes. In comparison, the Balke protocol (Fig. 8-7) starts

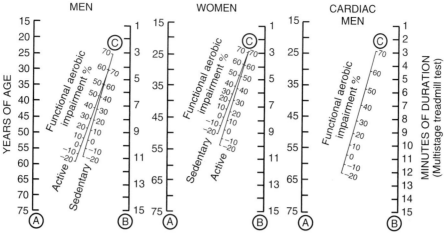

**Figure 8-6** Nomograms for evaluating functional aerobic impairment (FAI) of men, women, and men with cardiac diagnosis, according to age and by duration of exercise on the Bruce protocol for sedentary and active groups. To find the FAI, identify age (in years) in the left column and identify duration of time on the Bruce treadmill protocol in the right column. With a straight edge, line up the two points and read where the straight edge intercepts the FAI nomogram for either active or sedentary. (From Bruce RL, Kusumi F, Hosmer D. Maximal oxygen intake and nomographic assessment of functional aerobic impairment in cardiovascular disease. Am Heart J 85:545–562, 1973.)

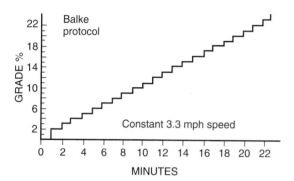

**Figure 8-7** The Balke treadmill protocol.

at a speed of 3.3 miles per hour, which is often too fast for a deconditioned patient or an older individual, but the subject starts on a level surface and only gradually is an incline added during the protocol. The gradual workload increments allow closer attainment of a steady state at each stage and facilitate the measurement of true maximal oxygen consumption. However, the Balke protocol requires a longer time to perform owing to the gradual addition of the incline. The Balke protocol is used more widely with athletes, especially with runners, because runners typically do not train on steep inclines and because this protocol allows the athlete to attain a steady state in a shorter period of time. Another exercise testing protocol often used in conjunction with functional capacity evaluations on workers is the Harbor Ramp protocol.

## Terminating the Testing Session

The person administering the exercise test must observe the patient and the ECG monitor during the test continuously to decide when the test should be terminated. See Box 8-4

for criteria for termination and for termination criteria for low-level exercise testing.

## Interpretation of Results

Once the test is concluded, the results are written on a worksheet to provide data for the interpretation (Fig. 8-8). Box 8-6 provides the parameters that are necessary for a thorough interpretation.

The final summary of the exercise test should define whether the outcome of the test is normal or abnormal; if the outcome is abnormal, the summary should provide the reasons. Although the physical therapist may not actually perform the stress test, obtaining the interpretation of the results provides valuable data for developing an exercise prescription. The interpretation also provides valuable information regarding safety during exercise for the patient.

## Prognostic Value of Maximal Exercise Testing

Maximal exercise testing is used as a noninvasive screening method for the detection of coronary disease. Its diagnostic accuracy in determining coronary disease is limited by the fact that it is a noninvasive test and therefore only reflects gross metabolic and electrical changes in the heart. Nonetheless, studies evaluating the specificity and sensitivity of stress testing have suggested that in appropriately chosen populations, it can be very helpful in identifying coronary disease and defining its severity.[121] Sensitivity is the measure of the reliability of stress testing in identifying the presence of disease. Specificity is the measure of the reliability of stress testing in identifying the population without disease. In general, testing demonstrates greater sensitivity and specificity in males over the age of 40 than in females. Females generally demonstrate a greater percentage of false-negative results,

Name _____John Doe_____ Date _____

Age __45___ Sex __M__ Height __5'10"__ Weight __190 lb.__

Diagnosis _____ Reason for test ___chest pains___

Protocol __Bruce__

Time of test __8 AM__ Time last cigarette _____ Time last meal ___12___

Medications __None__ Time last dose _____

Physician _____

RESULTS

12-Lead ECG interpretation ___Normal___

Minutes completed __7.06__ Limiting factor(s) ___Leg fatigue___

Rest HR __84__ Rest BP __140/98__ Heart sounds __Normal__

Maximum HR __170__ Maximum BP __190/102__

BP Response __Diastolic hypertension throughout__

Chest pain __None__

Summary of ST segment changes __Negative for ischemia__

Summary of arrhythmias __Rare PAC throughout__

Physical work capacity __Poor, 30% below predicted functional aerobic impairment__

Remarks/recommendations __Patient needs an exercise program to decrease blood pressure and improve__ functional aerobic impairment.

Interpreted by _____ Date _____

**Figure 8-8** Worksheet for interpretation of exercise test results. (From Scully R, Barnes ML. Physical Therapy. Philadelphia, JB Lippincott, 1989.)

but it is beyond the scope of this chapter to describe the predictive values for every potential population. However, to aid clinical judgment in predicting the risk of developing CAD, one can use Bayes theorem to assist in predicting sensitivity and specificity of testing.[132]

The value of diagnostic stress testing is tempered by the amount of variability among examiners conducting the test. Problems with testing include amount of encouragement given to the patient, a lack of strict adherence to protocols, use of handrail support, and interpretation of ST-segment deviation and symptoms.[131]

Despite its acknowledged potential limitations, several studies have attempted to identify specific single parameters or combinations of variables that might identify a group of patients with more severe disease.[121] Ischemia, reflected by ST-segment depression, that occurs during the early stages of an exercise test has been correlated with more severe disease than ischemia that occurs at peak exercise. Goldschlager and coworkers reported an increased incidence of subsequent MI in a group of patients who exhibited ST-segment depression at light workloads.[133] The severity of coronary disease has also been correlated with the length of recovery time (postexercise rest) for ST segment to return to normal.

Other subsets of patients have been identified who demonstrate certain signs and symptoms that suggest a greater risk for the subsequent development of a cardiac event. The signs and symptoms that have increased prognostic value include ST-segment depression, bradycardic heart rate responses, presence of angina, and maximal systolic blood pressure attained. Ellestad identified a population with more serious prognosis of disease when the magnitude of ST-segment depression was considered.[121] In addition, a subset of persons at high risk for progression of angina, MI, or death was identified by Ellestad. Persons with normal ST segments at peak effort who achieved maximal heart rates considerably below their predicted pulses (bradycardic heart rate response or chronotropic incompetence) demonstrated high risk of progression of angina, MI, or death. The tendency was to describe the test results as normal because the patients in Ellestad's study did not demonstrate ischemic ST-segment changes.

The presence of angina pain gives added significance when the patient demonstrates ST-segment depression during exercise. Ellestad described a subset of patients at double the risk of a subsequent coronary event when angina and ST-segment depression occurred together, as compared with patients without angina but with ST-segment depression (silent ischemia).[121]

The incidence of sudden death is increased in the following subset of patients:

- Those unable to exceed a maximal systolic blood pressure of 130 mm Hg

- Those with increased frequency and severity of arrhythmias during testing[134]

Calculating a probability score from the combination and weighing of clinical variables from the exercise test identifies the subsets of individuals at greater risk for coronary events. Many institutions are in the process of developing multiple variable analyses to increase the predictive value of exercise testing.[135] However, the use of thallium injection at peak performance also increases the information gained from the test, as well as increasing the sensitivity of the test.

An exercise time of more than 6 minutes, a maximum heart rate of more than 150 beats/min, and an ST recovery time of less than 1 minute were the variables that best identified women at low risk for developing CAD.[136]

## Exercise Testing with Ventilatory Gas Analysis

Although exercise testing alone is diagnostic for coronary disease, exercise testing with ventilatory gas analysis using a metabolic cart can provide greater information regarding oxygen exchange, breathlessness, etc. (see Fig. 8-4). A computer is used in conjunction with a system that automatically samples expired air continuously, a system for measuring the volume of expired air, a system with oxygen provided electronically, and $CO_2$ analyzers that measure the concentration of gases that are expired. The computer is programmed to compute the oxygen consumption, caloric expenditure, and $CO_2$ production during rest and during any activity. The computer can provide a printout of the gas exchange and other variables every second of activity and provide information for exercise prescription as well as for diagnosis of limitation of activity. One disadvantage of using the automatic computer-generated information is that the output data are accurate only if the electronic equipment and analyzers are accurate and calibrated against previously established standards.

Cardiopulmonary exercise testing with ventilatory gas analysis provides information on cardiac performance, functional limitation, and exercise limitations, particularly when the symptom limiting the individual is breathlessness or dyspnea. In assessing dyspnea, the ventilatory reserve and the dyspnea index are the most important variables. Normally 60% of an individual's maximal ventilatory reserve is utilized during activity; measurement of maximal voluntary ventilation (MVV) provides the information. Dyspnea occurs when the minute ventilation VE divided by the MVV is greater than 50% (otherwise known as the dyspnea index). When the VE/MVV is greater than 70%, respiratory muscle fatigue will occur within minutes. When the ratio is greater than 90% an individual cannot continue exercising more than a few seconds.[137]

Dyspnea that occurs in the presence of pulmonary disease will demonstrate early rapid and shallow breathing, with a reduction in peak ventilation and a reduction in tidal volume (VT). Both VO$_2$max and maximal volume of $CO_2$ production are reduced, and the peak exercise dyspnea index is 1.0.[137]

Dyspnea that occurs in the presence of heart failure produces a different outcome with exercise testing. Individuals with heart failure achieve their anaerobic threshold much earlier than healthy individuals of similar age, with a lower than normal maximal ventilation and maximal $CO_2$ production. The dyspnea index, however, is normal.[137]

Many advantages exist in using ventilatory gas analysis with exercise testing; however, several disadvantages exist, including the fact that the equipment (a metabolic cart) is not widely available in the clinical setting. This equipment may be in hospital settings for use with resting nutritional studies, and may be loaned for exercise testing. Another disadvantage is that many patients feel claustrophobic with the mouthpiece or headpiece and may actually hyperventilate with the mouthpiece.

## Exercise Testing with Imaging Modalities

Individuals may perform an exercise test to assess the myocardial oxygen supply and demand relationship (to determine if ischemia occurs during physiologic stress) and undergo additional noninvasive imaging immediately following the performance of the exercise. The use of imaging techniques such as thallium-201 or sestamibi scanning and SPECT allows for greater diagnostic accuracy and sensitivity, particularly in individuals with atypical chest pain syndromes, or in females who demonstrate low sensitivity to exercise testing alone.[138-140] Two-dimensional echocardiography is often used immediately after exercise testing as well. (See earlier sections on imaging and echocardiography for information.)

## Radioactive Nuclide Perfusion Imaging

As advances in cardiac medicine have evolved, assessment of coronary perfusion has been improved with the use of perfusion imaging using radioactively labeled agents. The commonly used agents include thallium-201 and technetium-99m (labeled sestamibi). These agents are taken up by the myocardium based on coronary blood flow. These agents can be injected following exercise or if the individual is not able to perform exercise following a pharmacologic stress test (described later in this chapter).

### Thallium-201 Perfusion Imaging

Thallium-201 is an excellent perfusion tracer that is injected intravenously and used to assess acute cardiac ischemia as a result of induced physiologic stress from an exercise treadmill test, a pharmacologic induced exercise test, or when ischemia occurs spontaneously. Thallium imaging assesses blood flow and cell membrane integrity as a result of the thallium being taken up by the myocardium in proportion to the coronary blood flow in the region.[141] Cells must be both perfused and metabolically intact in order to accumulate thallium-201. Nonperfused or dead myocardium appears as "cold spots" on the scan. When exercise thallium imaging is performed, a patient is exercised to maximal exercise potential and injected

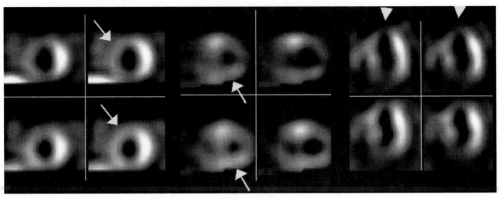

**Figure 8-9** Stress-redistribution thallium scintigram. The patient was studied several days after acute ST-segment elevation MI and medical stabilization. Besides the fixed defect representing the MI in the anterior wall and apex (*arrowheads*), there is extensive inducible ischemia both within and remote from the infarct territory (septum and inferior walls, *arrows*), involving 25% of the ventricle. Gated single-photon emission computed tomography EF was 38%. On the basis of the data in A, there is an approximately 25% risk of post-MI adverse event. SA, short axis; VLA, vertical long axis; HLA, horizontal long axis. (From Libby P, Bonow RO, Mann DL, et al. Braunwald's Heart Disease: A Textbook of Cardiovascular Medicine, ed 8. Philadelphia, 2008, Saunders.)

with the thallium-201 1 minute prior to the end of the exercise. Immediately after the exercise test, the patient is scanned using a gamma camera to assess thallium-201 uptake and scanned again 4 hours later after the thallium has been redistributed. An area without thallium uptake (cold spot) immediately after exercise as well as 4 hours afterward is considered irreversibly damaged (scarred). An area "cold" following exercise, but reperfused 4 hours later is considered "ischemic" or "reversible" and intervention usually is indicated in such cases (Fig. 8-9).

Thallium scanning is used to predict the risk of recurrent acute MI or death after the first acute MI.[142–144] The use of thallium can also identify viable myocardium that could functionally improve with revascularization.[145]

As cost-effectiveness of diagnostic tests is scrutinized in the current health care environment, the sensitivity and specificity of the use of thallium has been studied. Van der Wieken reported a high sensitivity (97%) and relatively high specificity (77%) for determining future events when used in individuals with acute chest pain and nondiagnostic ECGs.[146] The cost of thallium scanning increases the costs of evaluation of these patients by $500 to $800.[18] In addition, imaging equipment is available in most institutions.

The disadvantages of the use of thallium are related to the fact that it is not an ideal isotope; its low-energy photons are easily scattered and have a half-life of 73 hours. Because of the radiation exposure, the dose injected must be a low dose (approximately 2 to 4 mCi).[18] In addition, image scanning must commence within 15 to 20 minutes of the actual thallium injection, and experts in nuclear medicine must be available to perform the test and interpret the results.[18]

## Sestamibi

Technetium-99m or sestamibi (99mTc-sestamibi), sometimes abbreviated as MIBI, has become an alternative perfusion agent to thallium-201.[142,143,147,148] Like thallium-201,

sestamibi is used to assess acute cardiac ischemia or infarction, and like thallium, it is taken up by the myocardium in proportion to regional blood flow.[18] The tracer can then be imaged under the gamma camera.

Whereas thallium washes out of the myocardium in proportion to blood flow, 99mTc-sestamibi remains stable, and therefore images of blood flow can be scanned immediately after administration or up to several hours later.[143] Sestamibi accumulates in irreversibly damaged myocardial cells and might not demonstrate uptake in an infarction that is only a few hours old. Sestamibi is a marker of cell membrane and mitochondrial integrity as it requires active processes to occur at the level of the sarcolemma and mitochondrial membrane.[149,150] Therefore, sestamibi is not retained in acute or chronic MIs.

Sestamibi has demonstrated to be a more practical radioactive isotope because of its stability and has shown sensitivity and specificity for predicting any event to be 94% and 83%, respectively.[138] For predicting an acute MI, the sensitivity and specificity are 100% and 83%, respectively.[138]

One of the problems with sestamibi is that its accuracy is dependent on the skill of the operator and the knowledge and experience of the interpreter. The use of the isotope is slightly more expensive than the use of thallium-201, but it has demonstrated cost-effectiveness in use with patients with nondiagnostic ECGs presenting to the emergency room.[139,140]

Pharmacologic vasodilation with intravenous dipyridamole has been used in conjunction with sestamibi for diagnostic purposes.[80] This procedure can be done either while the patient is resting or in conjunction with exercise.

Sestamibi is often used in nonacute cardiac ischemic patients to assess myocardial contractility by assessing both left and right ventricular ejection fraction, regional function, and ventricular volumes.[80] SPECT, using newer gated tomographic techniques, can be performed with sestamibi to improve the perfusion study.

**Box 8-8**

### Absolute and Relative Contraindications to Pharmacologic Stress Testing

**Absolute**

Patients with active bronchospasm or patients being treated for reactive airway disease should not be administered adenosine because this can lead to prolonged bronchospasm, which can be difficult to treat or can remain refractory.

Patients with more than first-degree heart block (without a ventricular-demand pacemaker) should not undergo adenosine infusion because this may lead to worsening of the heart block. Although this is usually transient, because of the extremely short half-life of adenosine (approximately 6 seconds), cases of prolonged heart block (and asystole) have been reported.

Patients with an SBP <90 mm Hg should not undergo adenosine stress testing because of the potential for further lowering of the blood pressure.

Patients using dipyridamole or methylxanthines (e.g., caffeine and aminophylline) should not undergo an adenosine stress test because these substances act as competitive inhibitors of adenosine at the receptor level, potentially decreasing or completely attenuating the vasodilatory effect of adenosine. In general, patients should refrain from ingesting caffeine for at least 24 hours prior to adenosine administration. Patients should avoid decaffeinated products, which typically contain some caffeine, as opposed to caffeine-free products, which do not.

**Relative**

Patients with a remote history of reactive airway disease (COPD/asthma) that has been quiescent for a long time (approximately 1 year) may be candidates for adenosine. However, if a question exists concerning the status of the patients' airway disease, a dobutamine stress test may be the safer choice.

Patients with a history of sick sinus syndrome (without a ventricular-demand pacemaker) should undergo adenosine stress testing with caution. These patients are prone to significant bradycardia with adenosine; therefore, use caution if they are to undergo adenosine stress. Similarly, those patients with severe bradycardia (heart rate of 40 bpm) should undergo adenosine stress with caution.

## Pharmacologic Stress Testing

When an individual is unable to perform upright exercise on a treadmill or stationary bicycle owing to debilitating conditions such as severity of disease or heart failure, a neuromuscular insult (such as following a cerebrovascular accident), a musculoskeletal disability (e.g., following recent hip or knee surgery, back pain), being of increased age with decreased functional capacity or anyone who is unable to achieve at least 85% of their PMHR on an exercise test (as might occur in individuals taking β-blockers or other negative chronotropic agents that would inhibit the ability to achieve an adequate heart rate response), physiologic stress can be induced while the patient remains in a resting position by injection of a pharmacologic agent. Some centers prefer to use pharmacologic stress testing in conjunction with echocardiogram, MRI, or CT scanning because it avoids repositioning the patient, which may be necessary during nuclear imaging. Repositioning the patient may give a false-positive pharmacologic stress test result because of different degrees of attenuation of myocardial tissue imaging with changes in the breast positions as seen in women.

The most common agents that are used in pharmacologic stress testing are adenosine, dipyridamole (Persantine), dobutamine, and most recently regadenoson (Lexiscan).[80] Both dipyridamole and adenosine induce coronary vasodilation, a physiologic phenomenon that is difficult to occur in diseased coronary arteries, thereby affecting the perfusion image. With adenosine testing, approximately 80% of patients experience minor adverse effects from the adenosine infusion. However, absence of these effects does not imply a lack of efficacy of the adenosine with respect to coronary vasodilation. The chest pain experienced during adenosine infusion is very nonspecific and does not indicate the presence of CAD. However, approximately a third of patients with ischemia after perfusion imaging have ST-segment depression during the infusion of adenosine. Adverse effects with adenosine (and similarly dipyridamole) include dizziness, headache, symptomatic hypotension, dyspnea, and cardiac effects (chest pain or ST changes).[80]

Dobutamine acts as a stimulant (adrenergic), similar to exercise, and results in an increase in myocardial oxygen demand with the purpose of assessing myocardial oxygen supply. A dose-related increase in both heart rate and systolic blood pressure occurs with dobutamine. However, diastolic pressure falls as the dose of dobutamine increases. These hemodynamic changes are similar to those of exercise stress. Adverse effects occur in approximately 75% of patients undergoing dobutamine stress testing. Effects include ST changes (50%), chest pain (31%), palpitations (29%), and significant supraventricular or ventricular arrhythmias (8% to 10%). Typically, adverse effects requiring early termination subside within 5 to 10 minutes of discontinuation of the infusion (the half-life of dobutamine is 2 minutes). The effect of dobutamine can be reversed with β-blockers; typically, an intravenous agent with an ultrashort half-life, such as esmolol, is used. Because most patients who undergo dobutamine stress testing have bronchospastic lung disease, β-blockers should be used with caution. See Box 8-8 for absolute and relative contraindications to pharmacologic stress testing.[151]

Regadenoson (Lexiscan) is a new pharmacologic stress agent approved by the FDA in 2008 as an additional agent for use in stress testing for patients unable to perform the standard exercise stress test.[151] Regadenoson produces maximal hyperemia quickly and maintains it for an optimal duration that is practical for radionuclide myocardial perfusion imaging. Regadenoson requires a simple rapid bolus administration and has a short duration of hyperemic effect which is advantageous for a pharmacologic test.

## Adenosine or Dipyridamole-Walk Protocol

For patients who are able, combined low-level treadmill exercise during adenosine infusion has been demonstrated in several reports to be associated with a significant decrease in the frequency of adverse effects (e.g., flushing, nausea, headache). In addition, less-symptomatic hypotension and bradycardia occur. An additional advantage is that simultaneous low-level exercise allows for immediate imaging, as would be performed with exercise stress testing. This is due to the peripheral vasodilation and splanchnic vasoconstriction induced by exercise.

Safety of stress testing with pharmacologic agents is equivalent to the safety found in exercise testing. Safety in testing has been demonstrated in all populations including diabetics, as long as similar pretest and monitoring procedures are followed as in exercise testing.[152] In addition, pharmacologic stress testing has been shown to be safe in patients who have undergone thrombolysis following acute MI as soon as 2 to 5 days after initiation of thrombolysis.[151,153] The sensitivity of dipyridamole SPECT imaging, 89% (95% CI = 84% to 93%), was higher than that of dipyridamole echocardiography, but the specificity of dipyridamole SPECT imaging, 65% (95% CI = 54% to 74%), was lower than that of dipyridamole echocardiography. Dipyridamole and adenosine tests had similar sensitivities and specificities. The sensitivity of dobutamine echocardiography, 80% (95% CI = 77% to 83%), was similar to that of dobutamine SPECT imaging, but dobutamine echocardiography had a higher specificity, 84% (95% CI = 80% to 86%), than dobutamine SPECT imaging did.[151]

## Ergonovine Stimulation

Coronary artery spasm has been demonstrated to play a role in the manifestation of ischemic heart disease. To document coronary artery spasm, one must demonstrate significant or total narrowing of a segment in an artery that may or may not have partial arteriosclerotic narrowing. If increased narrowing of the artery occurs and the narrowing is relieved with the administration of a vasodilator, then coronary artery spasm has been documented. Spasm is rarely documented with coronary angiography (3%).[154] Therefore, because angiography does not frequently induce the spasm, ergonovine stimulation has become an important diagnostic test for coronary spasm.

Ergonovine stimulation is used when coronary spasm is suspected, particularly in a patient with documented ECG changes during symptoms or with documented ischemic episodes and a normal coronary angiographic study. The test has a high degree of sensitivity and specificity for coronary vasospasm.[155,156]

Ergonovine stimulation is performed in the cardiac catheterization laboratory or in the coronary care unit (if previous angiographic studies have demonstrated normal coronary arteries). Either incremental doses of ergonovine are given by intravenous injections or a single bolus of ergometrine is given while a patient is monitored continuously for ECG or hemodynamic changes (particularly ST-segment elevation or major heart rate and blood pressure changes) (Fig. 8-10). The patient is monitored throughout the injections until a maximal dosage is given or until the patient experiences symptoms.

When ergonovine stimulation is performed in the cardiac catheterization laboratory, repeat angiography is performed when symptoms or changes on the ECG develop; treatment with vasodilators is initiated after spasm is documented. In the coronary care unit, the patient is treated with vasodilators when the ECG changes or when the patient complains of symptoms. When a positive response occurs to ergonovine stimulation, the patient is managed with medications that reduce or prevent the occurrence of spasm (see discussion of calcium-channel blockers in Chapter 14).

The most sensitive test for coronary artery spasm is coronary stimulation by ergonovine, which has a greater than 90% sensitivity and specificity for the diagnosis of Prinzmetal's variant angina (PVA). This test is recommended when recurrent episodes of ischemic chest pain occur at rest without the classic ECG manifestations of PVA (i.e., ST-segment elevation) and normal or minimally abnormal coronary angiograms.

## Heart Rate Variability

Heart rate variability (HRV) is an accepted measurement of cardiac autonomic modulation.[157–159] This simple, noninvasive measurement of the interbeat variation of RR interval can provide important information regarding autonomic modulation of the SA node. De Jong provides a nice description of HRV methodologies to assess autonomic dysfunction.[160] Studies have indicated that both the sympathetic and parasympathetic branches of the autonomic nervous system affect the frequency of sudden death and cardiovascular death after MI.[161,162] Methods in the past have used heart rate variability as measured by 24-hour Holter monitoring, looking at variability over a time period from 2 to 15 minutes.

Deep breathing has been utilized to assess variations in heart rate due to the altered vagal-cardiac activity during this activity.[163] Impairments in the vagal input can depress the variability of the heart rate during deep breathing.[164] Katz found that heart rate variability below 10 beats per minute during 6 deep respirations in 1 minute was a significant predictor of death with an odds ratio of 1.38.[163] Therefore, there

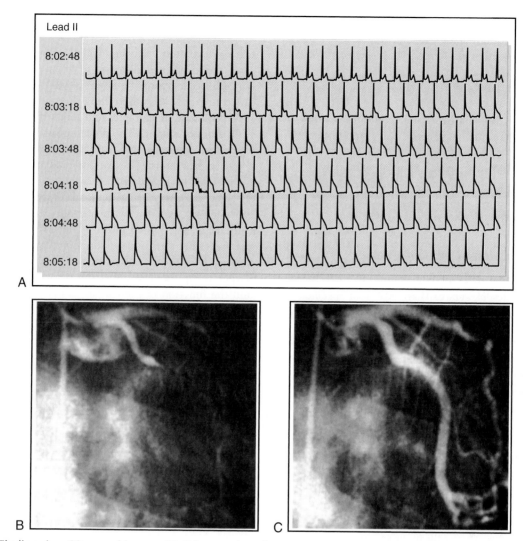

**Figure 8-10** Findings in a 39-year-old man with Prinzmetal angina. **A,** During an episode of angina, transient ST-segment elevation (in lead II) was noted on continuous telemetry. **B,** Hyperventilation-induced total occlusion of the proximal left circumflex artery (visible on angiography from the right anterior oblique caudal view). **C,** Spasm that resolved with the administration of intracoronary nitroglycerine and diltiazem. The patient's symptoms were controlled with oral nitrates and calcium channel blockade during a follow-up of 2 years. (From Chen HSV, Pinto DS: Prinzmetal angina. N Engl J Med 349:e1, 2003.)

may be some indication to follow heart rate variability in the asymptomatic at-risk population as well as the post-MI population in the future. However, reduced HR variability may also indicate reduced activity and worsening health. Therefore the prognostic capabilities of HR variability have not been proven.[165–167]

## Cardiac Catheterization: Coronary Angiography and Ventriculography

Cardiac catheterization is an invasive procedure that provides extremely valuable information for the diagnosis and management of patients with cardiac disease. The general goal of cardiac catheterization is to obtain objective information that can

- establish or confirm a diagnosis of cardiac dysfunction or heart disease,

- demonstrate the severity of CAD or valvular dysfunction, and
- determine guidelines for optimal management of the patient, including medical and surgical management as well as a program of exercise.

The data obtained from the cardiac catheterization are as follows:
- Cardiac output
- Shunt detection
- Angiography: coronary and ventriculography
- Left and right heart pressures (hemodynamics)
- Right atrial (normal = 0 to 4 mm Hg)
- Right ventricle (normal = 30/2 mm Hg)
- Pulmonary artery (normal = 30/10 mm Hg)
- Pulmonary artery wedge (normal = 8 to 12 mm Hg)
- Left ventricular end-diastolic (normal = 8 to 12 mm Hg)
- Ventricular ejection fraction (estimated) (normal = 65% ± 8%)

Specific determinations that can be made as a result of cardiac catheterization include the following:

- The presence of and severity of CAD (degree of stenosis)
- The presence of left ventricular dysfunction or aneurysm or both
- The presence of valvular heart disease and the severity of the dysfunction, including aortic valve stenosis or regurgitation, mitral valve stenosis or regurgitation or prolapse, tricuspid valve dysfunction, or pulmonary valve dysfunction (amount of backward flow across valve)
- The presence of pericardial disease

## Indications for Cardiac Catheterization

Because several noninvasive tests are now available that achieve sensitivities of greater than 90% and specificities above 70% for detection of ischemia and poor perfusion, cardiac catheterization is not indicated simply to diagnose angina. However, absolute indications for catheterization include the following[80]:

- Cardiac arrest or primary (not infarction-related) ventricular fibrillation
- Pulmonary edema, potentially of ischemic etiology
- Intolerance of or noncompliance with medical therapy for angina
- Job description mandate (such as commercial pilots or heavy-machine operators)
  In the absence of specific angina symptoms, the following are indications for catheterization:
- Significant decrease (more than 35%) in exercise duration when compared with previous exercise treadmill test or associated with significant ST-segment depression
- Progressive decline in systolic blood pressure to less than 100 mm Hg during exercise
- Evidence of symptomatic hypoperfusion during exercise such as intense diaphoresis, pallor, mental confusion, associated with decrease in blood pressure, and ST-segment depression
- Left ventricular ejection fraction below 35% with clinical evidence of ischemia
- Ventricular tachycardia emerging with exercise, especially if associated with ST-segment depression and increasing workload
  Other indications for cardiac catheterization in the presence of symptoms include the following:
- A 25% decrease in exercise duration as compared to a previous exercise test
- Prolonged chest pain not responsive to three nitroglycerine tablets and associated with ECG changes in an individual with known CAD
- A change in angina pattern occurring with less effort, or at rest, and requiring nitroglycerine for relief
- Increasing symptoms of angina despite adjustment in medications

## Procedure for Cardiac Catheterization

Cardiac catheterization involves the insertion of a catheter into the cardiovascular system to measure pressures or perform angiography (anatomic evaluation). The specific procedure includes catheterizing the right or left sides of the heart, contrast angiography, and sometimes revascularization with drugs or pacing. The procedure is invasive and is performed in a special room in the radiology department or in a special laboratory. The patient undergoing the procedure is awake but under sedation. A catheter is inserted into either the brachial artery or the femoral artery, depending on the cardiologist's expertise with an individual technique. The catheter is then passed into the great vessels and then into the great chambers under fluoroscopic control. Pressures are measured in the chambers across the valves, and cardiac output is measured to assess the competency of the valves and the function of the cardiac muscle. Finally, radiopaque contrast medium is injected into the chambers and then into the orifices of the coronary arteries (and in some cases into the aorta itself). The passage of the contrast medium is followed and filmed for closer evaluation of the integrity of the arteries and the myocardium when the procedure is completed (Fig. 8-11).

## Interpreting the Test Results

On completion of the cardiac catheterization, the cardiologist reviews the films to assess the ventricular function and the severity of coronary artery stenosis. The degree of stenosis in each arterial segment is graded during the review of the

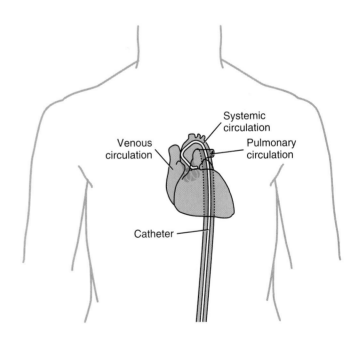

**Figure 8-11** The cardiac catheterization procedure involves the passage of a catheter through the great vessels so that radiopaque contrast medium can be injected into the orifices of the coronary arteries.

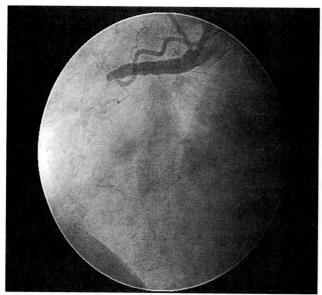

**Figure 8-12** Coronary arteriogram of an acute proximal total occlusion of the right coronary artery (RCA). The patient had sudden onset of chest pain at home and was emergently admitted to the cardiac catheterization laboratory. (From Urden LD: Critical Care Nursing: Diagnosis and Management. 6th ed. St. Louis, MO, Mosby, 2010.)

---

**Box 8-9**

**Clinical Example**

The following are findings from a cardiac catheterization, and an interpretation follows:

- Left anterior descending (LAD) artery shows 90% stenosis proximally
- First diagonal (off of LAD) shows 97% stenosis just after the origin
- Circumflex appears to be small with a 60% lesion midvessel and 50% distally
- Right coronary artery shows 70% stenosis
- LV: normal in size, antero-apical hypokinesis
- Ejection Fraction (EF): 40%
- End-Diastolic Pressure (EDP): 14
- End-Diastolic Volume (EDV): 100

**Interpretation**: Evidence of severe disease with anterior infarction from first diagonal with spontaneous reperfusion. These results indicate patient should undergo surgical revascularization to ensure adequate cardiac perfusion. In addition, EF is decreased and borderline for cardiac muscle dysfunction, and EDP and EDV are elevated. Antero-apical hypokinesis means the antero-apical region is moving sluggishly ... indicating the area that is severely ischemic or possible injury.

---

film, with total occlusion graded as 100% (Fig. 8-12). One of the problems with interpreting the cardiac catheterization film is the fact that angiography is only two-dimensional and atheromatous plaque tends to cause expansion of the internal elastic lamina, causing the degree of plaque burden to be greatly underestimated by angiography.[168,169] Angiography only reveals the edge of the atheroma that protrudes into the lumen.

Another problem concerns reliability: the film interpretation relies either on a person's subjective judgment or on a computer to measure the degree of stenosis. However, cardiac catheterization has greater sensitivity in detecting disease than other noninvasive procedures previously presented (Box 8-9).

Controversy exists over the indication for performing cardiac catheterization. Some critics in the medical field believe that the catheterization technique is overused and that less-invasive procedures should be used before catheterization.[74,170] Others note, however, that coronary angiography is the only test that provides information about the actual site, extent, and severity of obstruction in CAD. Cardiac catheterization has greater predictive accuracy in assessment of CAD than exercise testing. It also may be used to confirm diagnoses from other noninvasive tests. Cardiac catheterization must be performed before any surgical intervention. Common practice demonstrates that coronary angiography and ventriculography are being performed on the majority of patients following acute MI to assess severity of disease and amount of ventricular dysfunction resulting from the infarction. Cardiac catheterization results are very important

in determining the entire clinical picture of the patient. In addition, researchers are looking to identify prognosis based on catheterization findings. One such prognostic scoring system identifies risk for future events in individuals with previous coronary artery bypass grafting (CABG) who have undergone diagnostic catheterization and is described in the study by Liao.[171]

## Digital Subtraction Angiography

Digital subtraction angiography is a technique involving the introduction of small concentrations of iodinated contrast material into a vascular bed and then analyzed by a computer to produce an angiogram without direct injection of contrast material into an artery or cardiac chamber. This procedure has shown excellent reliability with carotid circulation and bypass grafts. It can also improve the quality of coronary angiograms obtained from coronary catheterization.[172] Three-dimensional digital angiography has become more accurate as compared to regular DSA and has been shown to give more detailed information of neurovascular lesions (cerebrovascular aneurysms). Its use in coronary angiography appears more limited at this time.

## Intravascular Ultrasonography

Intravascular ultrasonography (IVUS) involves the use of a specially designed catheter with a miniaturized ultrasound

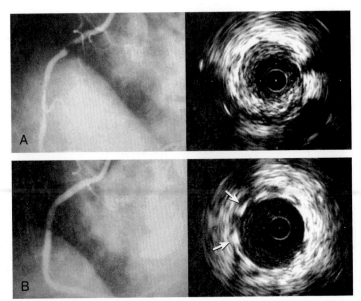

**Figure 8-13** Intravascular ultrasonographic (IVUS) images shown on the right correlated with angiography images on the left. Arrows in **B** show the echogenicity of the stent struts during IVUS. (From Frank, ED: Merrill's Atlas of Radiographic Positioning and Procedures. 11th ed. St. Louis, MO, Mosby, 2008.)

probe attached to the distal end of the catheter. The proximal end of the catheter is attached to computerized ultrasound equipment. It allows the application of ultrasound technology to see from inside blood vessels out through the surrounding blood column, visualizing the endothelium (inner wall) of blood vessels (Fig. 8-13).[173]

In addition, IVUS is of use to determine both plaque volume within the wall of the artery and/or the degree of stenosis of the artery lumen. It can be especially useful in situations in which angiographic imaging is considered unreliable; such as for the lumen of ostial lesions or where angiographic images do not visualize lumen segments adequately, such as regions with multiple overlapping arterial segments. The most valuable use of IVUS is to visualize plaque, which cannot be seen by angiography. Based on the angiographic view and long-popular medical beliefs, it had been assumed that areas of high-grade stenosis of the lumen within the coronary arteries, visible by angiography, were the likely points at which most MIs would occur.[174]

Further, IVUS enables accurately visualizing not only the lumen of the coronary arteries but also the atheroma (membrane/cholesterol-loaded white blood cells) "hidden" within the wall. Unlike angiography, IVUS generates detailed tomographic images that permit accurate size, composition, and topographic evaluation of the arterial wall and atherosclerotic plaque.[174-176] Longitudinal reconstruction and three-dimensional analysis allow further quantification of plaque and lumen area and plaque volume.[177-179]

One study looked at left main CAD detected by angiography and then by IVUS. In all subjects, the left main (LM) disease was angiographically silent yet disease detected by IVUS was an independent predictor of cardiac events and determined to be a marker for future events.[180] Obstructive disease of the left main coronary artery, angiographically defined as ≥50% diameter stenosis, is associated with a poor long-term prognosis.[180] The clinical significance of angiographically mild disease appears to have a more favorable prognosis. In addition, the gold standard for in vivo assessment of coronary artery narrowing—contrast angiography—provides only silhouette images of the artery and is therefore an imperfect tool.[180] It is especially limited when disease severity is mild[180] and when the left main coronary artery is involved.[180]

Although conventional IVUS imaging can provide real-time cross-sectional gray-scale images of coronary endovascular structures including plaque distribution, it is difficult to accurately identify coronary plaque subtypes such as fatty or fibrous plaques using IVUS gray-scale images.[175,172] IVUS radio-frequency (RF) signal analysis is useful to discriminate between fibrous and degenerated tissue in vivo with >90% sensitivity and specificity.[177] In addition, several ex vivo analyses have demonstrated that IVUS-RF parameters are useful to discriminate histologic components in a human coronary plaque.[177-179]

## Diagnostic Tests for Women

Diagnosis and assessment of CAD is especially difficult in women. The history of chest discomfort and various non-invasive tests each have particular problems, which indicate the need to consider more accurate tests such as cardiac MRI and PET. MRI of cardiac function at rest and during dobutamine stress has good accuracy and has improved predictive accuracy of heart attack and mortality for women, whereas MR myocardial perfusion imaging with gadolinium diethylenetriamine penta-acetic acid (DTPA) looks promising. MRI and SPECT revealing a low-magnetic-resonance global perfusion status was associated with a sevenfold increase in risk of death or heart attack in women.[180,181] The most exciting MR method is cineangiography (MRA), which images blood flow through the coronary arterial lumen as an intense signal. In an initial clinical trial this method showed excellent sensitivity and fair specificity in patients in whom adequate images could be obtained. Magnetic resonance spectroscopy (MRS) has imaged changes in high-energy phosphates in patients with severe coronary stenoses during handgrip exercise, but is still experimental. PET MPI corrects the images for attenuation problems that limit the use of other radionuclide imaging procedures in women more than in men. Many studies show excellent sensitivity and specificity to diagnose CAD by PET MPI. In view of its clinical validation and the safety of dipyridamole relative to dobutamine, PET MPI appears to be the best test for assessing CAD in women. The greater accuracy of PET (or perhaps of fully developed MRI/MRA systems) will produce better clinical outcomes and cost-effectiveness for most patients than will less-accurate modalities, despite their higher initial cost.[181,136]

## Endocardial Biopsy

Samples of the right or left ventricular endomyocardium may be obtained at the time of catheterization to determine myocardial rejection in patients with cardiac transplant. In addition, a myocardial biopsy may be taken to diagnose hypertrophic and congenital cardiomyopathy.[172]

## Vascular Diagnostic Testing for Aortic, Peripheral, and Carotid Disease

Adequate perfusion of muscles and organs is imperative for optimal functioning and requires optimal flow through the body's vascular system. Therefore, when disease or dysfunction is suspected in any of these vessels, evaluation of the specific vascular components is performed, including physical assessment, laboratory evaluation, and diagnostic assessment.

### Aortic Disease and Dysfunction and Diagnosis

The most common dysfunctions identified in the aorta include aneurysms, atherosclerotic disease, aortic valve dysfunction, and arteritis. The most common diagnostic tests for aortic dysfunction include ECG, angiography, CT scan, and chest x-ray. Table 8-10 presents information on clinical, physical, and laboratory features for assessment of aortic aneurysms, one of the most common dysfunction secondary to atherosclerotic disease in the aorta and aortic valve dysfunction. Because abdominal aneurysms seldom produce symptoms, they are usually detected accidentally as the result of an x-ray or a routine physical examination. Several tests can confirm a suspected abdominal aneurysm. Serial ultrasound (sonography) can accurately determine the aneurysm's

size, shape, and location. Anteroposterior and lateral x-rays of the abdomen can detect aortic calcification, which outlines the mass, at least 75% of the time. Aortography shows the condition of vessels proximal and distal to the aneurysm and the aneurysm's extent but may underestimate aneurysm diameter because it visualizes only the flow channel and not the surrounding clot. Computed tomography scan is used to diagnose and size the aneurysm. MRI can be used as an alternative to aortography. Lastly, aortic angiography may be used, which involves the use of a special dye (contrast material) and x-rays to see how blood flows through the aorta.

## Peripheral Arterial Disease and Dysfunction and Diagnosis

The presence of peripheral arterial disease (PAD) increases with age and is most often found in the form of arteriosclerosis obliterans (or atherosclerotic narrowing) of large- and medium-sized arteries supplying blood to the lower extremities, or thromboangiitis obliterans (Buerger disease; an inflammatory process causing vessel blockage) of peripheral arteries and veins.[182,183] Arteriovenous fistulas (abnormal communications between arteries and veins without connecting capillaries), Raynaud phenomena (bilateral paroxysmal ischemia of fingers and toes), arterial emboli, and trauma are other peripheral arterial dysfunction that occur in the population.

The current methods to determine presence of PAD include history of symptoms, history of risk factors for atherosclerotic disease, physical examination of pulses, and use of noninvasive vascular tests. Table 8-11 provides general clinical, physical, and laboratory features for PADs.

Noninvasive vascular tests include the ankle brachial index (ABI), segmental limb pressures, pulse volume recordings, and native vessel arterial duplex ultrasonography. If invasive tests are required, arteriography with contrast or with MRI may be used.

### Ankle Brachial Index

Ankle brachial index (ABI) is a noninvasive test that compares the blood pressure obtained with a Doppler probe in the dorsalis pedis (or posterior tibial artery) to the blood pressure in the higher of the two brachial pressures (Fig. 8-14). An ABI above 0.9 is considered normal. An ABI below 0.5 is suggestive of severe arterial occlusive disease (Table 8-12).

Research has shown that the ABI may be a marker of diffuse atherosclerosis, cardiovascular risk, and overall survival.[184] Males who had an ABI less than 0.9 demonstrated a higher relative risk of death from all causes and from cardiovascular causes. In addition, in a study of men and women older than 65, the lower the ABI, the greater the incidence of cardiovascular risk factors and clinical cardiovascular disease.[185]

## Table 8-10 Aortic Aneurysms

| Aneurysm Type | Etiology | Location | Clinical Features | Physical Findings | Laboratory Findings | Treatment |
|---|---|---|---|---|---|---|
| Arterosclerotic | Atherosclerosis | Usually abdominal (between renal arteries and aortic bifurcation) | • Older males<br>• Often asymptomatic until rupture<br>• Abdominal fullness or pulsations; back or epigastric pain, worse prior to rupture | • Palpable, pulsatile abdominal mass<br>• Peripheral emboli<br>• Abdominal bruit<br>• Associated peripheral vascular disease | • Size measured by abdominal ultrasound<br>• Angiography less accurate at estimating size but necessary to define surgical anatomy | Rupture of >6 cm diameter: surgery <4 cm diameter |
| Dissecting | Hypertension | Type I: proximal ascending aorta to descending aorta | • Severe, sudden, tearing chest pain radiating to abdomen and back (occasional patient will have no pain) | • Hypertension | • ECG may show myocardial infarction | Surgical indications |
| | Marfan's syndrome | Type II: confined to ascending aorta | • Aortic branch occlusions causing myocardial infarction, stroke, spinal infarction with paraplegia, renal impairment | • Asymmetric pulses | • Wide mediastinum on chest x-ray (not always present)<br>• Echo may be indicated | Ascending aortic involvement |
| | Cystic medial necrosis | Type III: begins in descending aorta and aorta and extends distally | • Aortic root involvement causing acute aortic insufficiency, rupture into pericardium with pericardial friction rub or tamponade | • Signs of aortic insufficiency, neurologic involvement, or tamponade if present | • CT scan usually diagnostic | Impairment of vital organs |
| | Aortic coarctation | | | | • Angiography necessary to define surgical anatomy | Etiology not hpertensive |
| | Trauma | | | | | Hemodynamic impairment Medical therapy may be tried in older patient with distal hypertension and lessen force of contraction nitroprusside + beta blocker) |

*From Andreoli TE, Carpenter CC, Plum F, Smith LH: Cecil Essentials of Medicine, ed 2. Philadelphia, 1990, Saunders.*

## Table 8-11 General Clinical, Physical, and Laboratory Features of Peripheral Arterial Disease

| Disease | Pathology | Clinical Features | Physical Features | Laboratory/ Diagnostic |
|---|---|---|---|---|
| Arteriosclerosis obliterans | Atherosclerotic narrowing of large- and medium-sized arteries of lower extremities | Males more than females Common in diabetes patients Exertional leg pain relieved with rest Cold, numb legs | Decreased or absent lower extremity pulses Aortic, iliac, or femoral Limb ischemia, cool pale, cyanotic, shiny dry skin | Doppler and arteriography |
| Thromboangiitis obliterans | Intima inflammation and infiltrates, thrombi, in small- to medium-sized vessels | Males more than females Occurs before age 30 Cool extremities | Cool extremities Ulcers of digits | Biopsy of artery |
| Arterial embolism | Emboli lodge at bifurcations, with thrombus formation | Sudden onset, painful extremity | Cold, pale extremities Absent pulses distal to embolus | Doppler |
| Raynaud phenomenon | Vasospasm of digital vessels aggravated by cold, relieved by heat | | White, cyanotic digits exposed to cold, hyperemic upon recirculation | None; diagnosis based on physical symptoms |

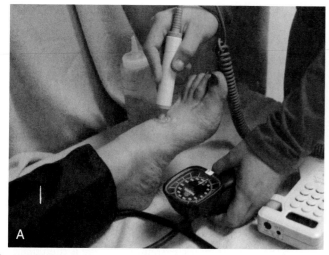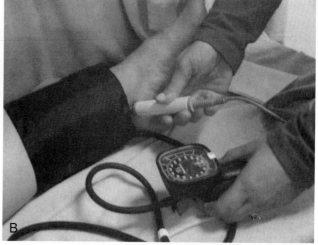

**Figure 8-14** Measurement of blood pressure at the ankle using Doppler ultrasound. **A,** At the dorsalis pedis; **B,** at the posterior tibial artery. (From Cameron MH, Monroe LG: Physical Rehabilitation: Evidence-Based Examination, Evaluation, and Intervention. St. Louis, MO, Saunders, 2008.)

## Segmental Limb Pressures

Segmental limb pressures can aid in localizing stenoses or occlusions with the placement of pressure cuffs on the thigh, calf, ankle, and transmetatarsal region of the foot and digit. The pressure is sequentially inflated in each cuff to approximately 20 to 30 mm Hg above the systolic pressure. The pressure is measured using a Doppler at each segment as the pressure in the cuff is gradually released (Fig. 8-14).

## Pulse Volume Recordings

The changes in the volume of blood flowing through a limb can be detected by plethysmographic tracings. Pressure cuffs are placed on the thigh and ankle and inflated separately to approximately 65 mm Hg while a plethysmographic tracing is recorded. The normal pulse volume recording consists of a rapid systolic upstroke and rapid downstroke with a dicrotic notch. Individuals with severe arterial disease will

**Table 8-12 Ankle Brachial Interpretation**

| ABI measurement | Possible symptoms | Clinical Presentation |
|---|---|---|
| >1.10 | None | Normal |
| 0.5–1.0 | Claudication | Pain in calf with ambulation |
| 0.2–0.5 | Critical limb ischemia | Atrophic changes |
| | | Rest pain |
| | | Wounds |
| <0.2 | Severe ischemia | Gangrene/severe necrosis |

demonstrate a more attenuated waveform with a wide downslope. Individuals with near-complete blockage will demonstrate absent waveforms.[186]

## Arterial Duplex Ultrasonography

Arterial duplex ultrasonography is a more precise diagnostic test for defining arterial stenoses and occlusions. A 5.0- to 7.5-MHz transducer is used to image the supra- and infrainguinal arteries in the sagittal plane at a 60-degree Doppler angle. The five categories, ranging from normal to occluded, are determined based on the alterations in the Doppler waveform. Duplex ultrasonography is utilized to guide the interventionist when performing endovascular therapy. One limitation cited in the literature is the potential to overestimate residual stenoses following balloon angioplasty.[187]

## Graft Surveillance

Graft surveillance is utilized in patients who have undergone surgical bypass graft revascularization. Stenoses have been reported in 21% to 33% of bypass cases.[188] However, once the stenosis is detected and repaired prior to thrombosis, more than 80% of the grafts have been salvaged.[188] The procedure for graft surveillance is similar to arterial duplex ultrasonography. Initially the inflow artery to the bypass is imaged, followed by the proximal anastomosis; proximal, middle, and distal graft; distal anastomosis; and then the outflow artery. The peak systolic and end-diastolic velocities are determined at each segment and compared to the segment of graft proximal to the area being studied. If the peak systolic velocity to normal segment proximal to graft is greater than 2, a 50% to 75% diameter reduction is assumed. If the end-diastolic velocity is less than 100 cm/second, then a greater than 75% stenosis is assumed to exist. Arteriography should be performed if either of these values are determined with graft surveillance.

Vein bypass grafts should be studied within 7 days of surgery, 1 month after surgery, and then every 3 months for the first year, and every 6 months after the first year.

## Exercise Studies

Exercise testing provides objective documentation of functional limitation from PAD as well as determining the physiologic improvement following arterial stenosis intervention (angioplasty or bypass graft surgery). However, claudication often limits activity before any cardiac symptoms are evoked, and therefore a graded exercise test may not be an effective method of evaluating cardiac disease if patients have PAD.[189] A cycle ergometer may be the choice of mode for exercise testing to reduce the effort placed on the calf muscles.[190] In the absence of a complete graded exercise test, the minimum that should be performed is an assessment of claudication during a walk on the treadmill until exercise must be ceased (sometimes referred to as the claudication time test). Ankle pressures should be assessed prior to the treadmill walk and immediately after exercise. A postexercise drop in ankle systolic pressure confirms the diagnosis of arterial disease.[189] Ankle pressures should be measured at 1-minute intervals until a return to the pre-exercise pressure. Other findings from exercise testing has shown that a hypertensive BP response during exercise testing in patients with known or suspected PAD is an important independent risk factor for all-cause long-term mortality.[191]

## Other Clinical Tests
### Rubor Dependency Test

This test assesses lower extremity arterial circulation using skin color changes and positional changes. The patient begins the test supine with legs elevated 35 to 45 degrees. The legs are assessed in this position for color (pale versus normal pink), then placed in a dependent position. Normal response is to see a rapid pink flush in the feet. Arterial insufficiency will demonstrate a deep, red color (rubor) after 30 seconds in this position.

### Venous Filling Time Test

This test measures the efficiency of arterial blood flow through the capillaries and into the veins. The patient is placed in the supine position and the leg or legs are elevated to drain the blood from the extremity. The leg is then placed in a dependent position and time for veins to refill is recorded. In the presence of arterial insufficiency, the time for veins to refill is greater than 15 seconds.

### Peripheral Venous Disease and Diagnosis

The most common disorder involving peripheral veins is thrombosis and subsequent thrombophlebitis (inflammation of the vein secondary to thrombosis, but can occur with trauma or infection). Initial diagnosis is often made with clinical signs of red color, warmth, and swelling, but diagnostic evaluation should be performed using Doppler studies and impedance plethysmography. Occasionally, venograms are performed (injected dye into the venous system rather than arterial system as in arteriography).

The second most common disorder involving peripheral veins is varicose veins, which can result from thrombophlebitis, but often occur congenitally or in conditions of increased venous pressure (such as pregnancy, prolonged standing, obesity, or ascites). Venography is recommended to assess for severity of insufficiency and prior to any surgical or chemical treatment.

## Other Clinical Venous Insufficiency Tests

### Trendelenburg Test

To assess valvular competence, the patient lies supine with the leg elevated 90 degrees to empty any blood currently in the venous system. A tourniquet is placed around the thigh to occlude venous flow, and the patient assumes a standing position while the filling of the veins is assessed. Normal venous fill should occur within 30 seconds. If superficial veins fill while the tourniquet is still in place, the communicating veins are deemed incompetent. If, when the tourniquet is removed, sudden additional filling occurs, the saphenous vein valves are determined to be incompetent.

### Homan Sign

To assess for deep-vein thrombophlebitis, the patient's gastrocnemius muscle belly is squeezed while the foot is dorsiflexed with force. If the patient indicates tenderness or pain in the gastrocnemius the test is determined to be positive for thrombophlebitis, and further diagnostic testing should be performed to determine the severity of the thrombophlebitis and initiate treatment.

## Carotid Artery Disease and Diagnosis

Significant internal carotid artery disease increases the risk for transient and permanent ischemic attacks to the neurologic system and represents an increased risk for coronary atherosclerosis and infarction.[192,193] Often, eye examinations may detect ischemia; however, carotid Doppler evaluations are most widely used, especially when bruits are auscultated during the physical examination. Recently, direct visualization with duplex ultrasonography has been used and demonstrated to have excellent accuracy (duplex ultrasonography is discussed earlier).[182] Carotid duplex examination can identify plaque, stenoses, and occlusions in the internal, common, and external carotid arteries as well as the flow direction in the vertebral arteries. Research has demonstrated that the

sensitivity of carotid duplex ultrasonography is 85% and the specificity is 90%.[194,195]

Various methods have been used to quantify atherosclerosis, beginning in the mid-1980s with ultrasound measurement of carotid intima-media thickness (IMT), and going on to coronary calcification assessed by electron-beam CT, measurement of carotid plaque by ultrasound, and measurement of carotid wall thickness by MRI. In recent years, it has become clear that carotid IMT, coronary calcification, and carotid plaque reflect biologically and genetically different aspects of the atherosclerotic process and will respond differentially to therapy. IMT represents mainly hypertensive medial hypertrophy; this measure is more predictive of stroke than of MI and is only weakly associated with traditional coronary risk factors. Carotid plaque area, on the other hand, is more strongly associated with traditional risk factors, and is more predictive of MI than of stroke. A quantitative trait, called "unexplained atherosclerosis," expresses the extent to which an individual has excess carotid plaque not explained by traditional risk factors, or the extent to which an individual is protected from traditional risk factors. Unexplained progression of plaque is an even more powerful tool for genetic research, because age, which accounts for the greatest proportion of baseline plaque, has much less influence on the rate of progression. Compared with IMT, measurement of carotid plaque volume by three-dimensional ultrasound is, therefore, an important tool for patient management, genetic research, and evaluation of new therapies for stroke prevention.

Baseline plaque area is more than 3.4 times more powerful than a Framingham risk equation, in the sense that after adjustment in multiple regression for more variables than in Framingham, patients with plaque scores in the top quartile had 3.4 times the risk of stroke, death, or MI than those in the lowest quartile.[196,197] In a prospective study, the research group found that a risk score based on age, blood pressure, smoking, and cholesterol predicted only 32% of patients with vascular events during a 5-year period, whereas 77% of events occurred among patients in the top quartile of plaque area.[196]

Two other diagnostic tests have been showing increased sensitivity and specificity to neurovascular diagnosis. Three-dimensional digital angiography has been found to be great for more detailed information of neurovascular lesions (particularly cerebrovascular aneurysms) as compared to DSA. In addition, MR angiography using time of flight or contrast enhancement helps diagnose stenotic and occlusive internal carotid arteries.[198]

## CASE STUDY 8-1

MH is a 48-year-old woman who experienced frequent symptoms of chest pain during her aerobic workouts that were not always relieved with rest. Sometimes the symptoms would develop with emotional upset. Her past medical history included elevated cholesterol, which was to be treated with diet, and a positive family history (father with MI, CHF, and pacemaker and mother with hypertension and elevated cholesterol). MH had undergone a stress exercise test 2 months prior, experienced chest pain on the test, but there was no evidence of ischemic changes or abnormal heart rate, blood pressure, or ECG changes, so it was recommended that MH follow up with her family physician if similar symptoms persisted. Because MH continued to experience chest pain that limited her activities, she was then referred for thallium-201 stress exercise test, during which she developed chest pain after 5 minutes. The results of the thallium stress test demonstrated significant inferior perfusion defects at peak exercise that were resolved on the 3-hour postexercise scan. MH subsequently underwent single-vessel (right) percutaneous transluminal coronary angioplasty (PTCA). On the day after PTCA, MH underwent a repeat thallium stress exercise test, which she performed symptom-free for 8 minutes and without any perfusion defects. MH was discharged to home and returned to her normal activities within 2 weeks.

### Discussion

This case study demonstrates the inability of the standard exercise stress test to diagnose CAD in a female with significant symptoms plus significant risk factors for CAD. The thallium exercise test was definitive for CAD, intervention by PTCA was performed, and patient was symptom-free after PTCA.

## Summary

- The laboratory tests that are specific to the patient with cardiac dysfunction measure the serum enzymes (particularly troponin and creatine phosphokinase [CPK-MB]), blood lipids (triglycerides and cholesterol), complete blood cell count, coagulation profile (prothrombin time), electrolyte levels, blood urea nitrogen and creatinine levels, and serum glucose levels.

- The markers that are diagnostic of cardiac injury include troponin, CPK-MB isoenzyme, myoglobin, carbonic anhydrase III, cardiac myosin light chains, lactic dehydrogenase (LDH isoenzyme 1), and aspartate aminotransferase.

- The enzymes that are diagnostic of cardiac injury include creatine phosphokinase, lactic dehydrogenase, and aspartate aminotransferase.

- Clinically, an early or a secondary peak in CPK levels followed by a more rapid decline in the CPK-MB levels is strongly suggestive of reperfusion following thrombolytic therapy.

- Sodium, potassium, and $CO_2$ are the most important electrolytes to monitor. Hydration state, medications, and disease can affect the electrolyte levels.

- Indications for use of the Holter monitor include identifying symptoms possibly caused by arrhythmias (e.g., dizziness, syncope, shortness of breath at rest as well as with activity), describing the arrhythmias noted with activity (frequency and severity), and evaluating antiarrhythmia therapy and pacemaker functioning.

- Important information can be obtained from the echocardiogram, including the size of the ventricular cavity, the thickness and integrity of the interatrial and interventricular septa, the functioning of the valves, and the motions of individual segments of the ventricular wall.

- Using an intravenously injected contrast agent with the echocardiogram has improved the diagnostic accuracy of echocardiography in assessing myocardial perfusion and ventricular chambers.

- Positron emission tomography (PET), computed tomography (CT), single photon emission computed tomography (SPECT), electron beam computed tomography (EBCT), multigated acquisition (MUGA) imaging, and magnetic resonance imaging (MRI) are all imaging techniques used for evaluation of coronary artery disease (CAD) and cardiac dysfunction.

- Positron emission tomography is a nuclear assessment technique that provides visualization and direct measurement of metabolic functioning, including glucose metabolism and fatty acid metabolism as well as blood flow of the heart.

- Magnetic resonance imaging is used to evaluate morphology, cardiac blood flow, and myocardial contractility.

- The commonly used agents include thallium-201 and technetium-99m (labeled sestamibi). These agents are taken up by the myocardium based on coronary blood flow.

- The most common agents used in pharmacologic stress testing are dipyridamole, dobutamine, and adenosine.

- Most exercise tests are symptom limited and, as such, are terminated at the request of the patient or when an abnormality is identified in one or more parameters being measured.

- Indications for uses of thallium injection with stress testing include detection of myocardial infarction (MI) and transient myocardial ischemia.

- Low-level exercise testing may be useful for predicting the subsequent course of a MI or bypass surgery as well as for identifying the high-risk patient.

- Exercise-induced ST-segment depression of 2.0 mm or greater on low-level exercise tests has been identified as the single most valuable indicator of prognosis after MI.

- Low-level exercise testing can also provide information useful for optimal medical management after myocardial injury or surgery, including treatment for angina, arrhythmias, or hypertension.

- Although the physical therapist may not actually perform the stress test, obtaining the interpretation of the results provides valuable data for developing an exercise prescription.
- Sensitivity is the measure of the reliability of stress testing to identify the presence of disease. Specificity is the measure of the reliability of stress testing to identify the population without disease.
- Although exercise testing alone is diagnostic for coronary disease, exercise testing with ventilatory gas analysis using a metabolic cart can provide greater information regarding oxygen exchange, breathlessness, etc.
- Digital subtraction angiography is a technique involving the introduction of small concentrations of iodinated contrast material into a vascular bed that is then analyzed by a computer to produce an angiogram without direct injection of contrast material into an artery or cardiac chamber.
- Specific determinations that can be made as a result of cardiac catheterization include (1) severity of CAD (degree of stenosis); (2) left ventricular dysfunction or aneurysm or both; (3) valvular heart disease and the severity of the dysfunction, including aortic valve stenosis or regurgitation, mitral valve stenosis or regurgitation or prolapse, tricuspid valve dysfunction, or pulmonary valve dysfunction; (4) pericardial disease; (5) myocardial disease including cardiomyopathy; and (6) congenital heart disease.
- Ergonovine stimulation is used when coronary spasm is suspected, particularly in a patient with ECG-documented changes during symptoms or with documented ischemic episodes and a normal coronary angiographic study.
- There may be some indication to follow heart rate variability in the asymptomatic at-risk population as well as the post-MI population in the future.
- Samples of the right or left ventricular endomyocardium may be obtained at the time of catheterization to determine myocardial rejection in patients with cardiac transplant.
- PET is a nuclear assessment technique that provides visualization and direct measurement of metabolic functioning including glucose metabolism, fatty acid metabolism, and blood flow of the heart without the patient performing exercise.
- Multigated acquisition imaging or gated pool imaging is a noninvasive technique to calculate left ventricular ejection fraction.

## References

1. Karmazyn M. Reduction of enzyme release from reper-fused ischemic hearts by steroidal and nonsteroidal prostaglandin synthesis inhibitors. Prostaglandins Letikot Med 11:299–315, 1983.
2. Mouzopoulos G, Kouvaris C, Antonopoulos D, et al. Perioperative creatine phosphokinase (CPK) and troponin I trends after elective hip surgery. J Trauma 63:388–93, 2007.
3. Adams JE, Sicard GA, Allen BT, et al. Diagnosis of perioperative myocardial infarction with measurement of cardiac troponin I. N Engl J Med 330:670–4, 1994.
4. Cummins B, Auckland ML, Cummins P. Cardiac-specific troponin-I radio-immunoassay in the diagnosis of acute myocardial infarction. Am Heart J 113:1333–44, 1987.
5. Jaffe AS, Ravkilde J, Roberts R, et al. It's time for a change to a troponin standard. Circulation 102(11):1216–20, 2000.
6. Wu AHB, Apple FS, Gibler WB, et al. National Academy of Clinical Biochemistry Standards of Laboratory Practice: recommendations for the use of cardiac markers in coronary artery diseases. Clin Chem 45(7):1104–21, 1999.
7. Casey PE. Markers of myocardial injury and dysfunction. AACN Clin Issues 15(4):547–57, 2004.
8. Babuin L, Jaffe AS. Troponin: the biomarker of choice for the detection of cardiac injury. CMAJ 173(10):1191–202, 2005.
9. Alpert JS, Thygesen K, Antman E, et al. Myocardial infarction redefined: a consensus document of the Joint European Society of Cardiology/American College of Cardiology committee for the redefinition of myocardial infarction. J Am Coll Cardiol 36(3):959–69, 2000.
10. Lim W, Qushmaq I, Devereaux PJ, et al. Elevated cardiac troponin measurements in critically ill patients. Arch Intern Med 166(22):2446–54, 2006.
11. George EL, Shatzer M. Troponin targets cardiac injury: learn about troponin levels so you can give your patient the best possible care. Nursing 38:15–17, 2008.
12. Piano MR. Serologic markers of ischemia: creatine kinase and the troponins. American Heart Association, 71st Scientific Sessions, November 8, 1998.
13. Katus HA, Rcmppis A, Neumann FJ, et al. Diagnostic efficiency of troponin T measurements in acute myocardial infarction. Circulation 83:902–12, 1991.
14. Polanczyk CA, Lee TH, Cook EF, et al. Cardiac troponin I as a predictor of major cardiac events in emergency department patients with acute coronary care syndromes. J Am Coll Cardiol 32:8–14, 1998.
15. Heeschen C, Goldman BU, Moeller RH, et al. Analytic performance and clinical application of a new rapid bedside assay for the detection of serum cardiac troponin I. Clin Chem 44:1925–30, 1998.
16. Christcnson RH, Azzazy HM. Biochemical markers of the acute coronary syndromes. Clin Chem 44(8 Pt 2):1855–64, 1998.
17. Ohman EM, Armstrong PW, Christenson RH, et al. Cardiac troponin T levels for risk stratification in acute myocardial ischemia. N Engl J Med 335:1333–41, 1996.
18. Selker HP, Zalenski RJ, Antman EM, et al. An evaluation of technologies for identifying acute cardiac ischemia in the emergency department: a report from a National Heart Attack Alert Program Working Group. Ann Emerg Med 29:13–87, 1997.
19. Katus HA, Diedrich KW, Schwartz F, et al. Influence of reperfusion on serum concentrations of cytosolic creatine kinase and structural myosin light chains in acute myocardial infarction. Am J Cardiol 60:440–5, 1987.
20. Hobeig E, Katus HA, Diederich KW, et al. Myoglobin, creatine kinase-B isoenzyme, and myosin light chain release in patients with unstable angina pectoris. Eur Heart J 8:989–94, 1987.
21. Katus HA, Diedrich KW, Hoberg E, et al. Circulating cardiac myosin light chains in patients with angina at rest:

identification of a high risk subgroup. J Am Coll Cardiol 11:487–93, 1988.

22. Jacobs DS, Kasten BL, DeMott WR, et al. Laboratory Test Handbook. Cleveland, Lexicomp, 1988.

23. Smith AM, Theirer JA, Huang SH. Serum enzymes in myocardial infarction. Am J Nurs 73(2):277, 1973.

24. White HD, Cross DB, Williams BF, et al. Safety and efficacy of repeat thrombolytic treatment after acute MI. Br Heart J 64(3):177–81, 1990.

25. Pollock ML, Schmidt DH. Epidemiologic Insights into Atherosclerotic Cardiovascular Disease from the Framingham Study in Heart Disease and Rehabilitation. 2nd ed. New York, John Wiley, 1986.

26. Castelli WP. Cholesterol and lipids in the risk of coronary artery disease—the Framingham Heart Study. Can J Cardiol 4(Suppl A):5A–10A, 1988.

27. National Cholesterol Education Program (NCEP). Second report of the expert panel in detection, evaluation and treatment of high blood cholesterol in adults (Adult Treatment Panel II). JAMA 269:3015–21, 1993.

28. Gordon T, Castelli WP, Hjortlan MC, et al. Diabetes, blood lipids, and the role of obesity in coronary heart disease for women. Ann Intern Med 87:393, 1977.

29. Superko HR, Fogelman A. Lipoproteins and atherosclerosis—the role of HDL cholesterol, Lp(a), and LDL particle size. Paper presented at the American College of Cardiology, 48th Scientific Session, March 7–10, 1999.

30. Cohen J, Wilson WF. Homocysteine, fibrinogen, Lp(a), small dense LDL, oxidative stress, and C. pneumoniae infection: how important are they? Am Coll Cardiol March 7–10, 1999.

31. American Diabetes Association, Inc. Management of dyslipidemia in adults with diabetes, position statement, January 1999. Diabetes Care 22(Suppl 1):56–9, 1999.

32. Anderson JL, Muhlestein JB, Horne BD, et al. Plasma homocysteine predicts mortality independently of traditional risk factors and C-reactive protein in patients with angiographically defined coronary artery disease. Circulation 102(11):1227–32, 2000.

33. Vasan RS, Beiser A, D'Agostino RB, et al. Plasma homocysteine and risk for congestive heart failure in adults without prior myocardial infarction. JAMA 289:1251–7, 2003.

34. Wang TJ, Gona P, Larson MG, et al. Multiple biomarkers for the prediction of first major cardiovascular events and death. N Engl J Med 355:2631–9, 2006.

35. Fallon UB, Ben-Shlomo Y, Elwood P, et al. Homocysteine and coronary heart disease in the Caerphilly cohort: a 10 year follow up. Heart 85:153–8, 2001.

36. Boysen G, Brander T, Christensen H, et al. Homocysteine and risk of recurrent stroke. Stroke 34:1258–61, 2003.

37. Loffredo L, Violi F, Fimognari FL, et al. The association between hyperhomocysteinemia and ischemic stroke in patients with non-valvular atrial fibrillation. Haematologica 90(9):1205–11, 2005.

38. Robinson K, Arheart K, Refsum H, et al. Concentrations: risk factors for stroke, peripheral vascular disease and coronary artery disease. European Comac Group. Circulation 97(5):437–43, 1998.

39. Boushey CJ, Beresford SA, Omenn GS, et al. A quantitative assessment of plasma homocysteine as a risk factor for vascular disease. JAMA 274(13a):1049–57, 1995.

40. Evans RW, Shaten BJ, Hempel JD, et al. Homocysteine and risk of cardiovascular disease in the Multiple Risk Factor Intervention Trial. Arterioscler Thromb Vasc Biol 17(10):1947–53, 1997.

41. MacCallum PK, Cooper JA, Price C, Meade TW. (LEADER: Lower Extremity Arterial Disease Event Reduction Substudy—Effect of Aspirin on the Predictive Value of CRP for MI in Men With LEAD). The predictive value of C-reactive protein (CRP) for myocardial infarction may be affected by aspirin therapy in men with lower extremity arterial disease [Abstract]. Program and abstracts of the XIX Congress of the International Society on Thrombosis and Haemostasis; Birmingham, UK, July 12–18, 2003.

42. Omland T, Sabatine MS, Jablonski KA, et al. Prognostic value of B-Type natriuretic peptides in patients with stable coronary artery disease: the PEACE Trial. J Am Coll Cardiol 50(3):205–14, 2007. Epub 2007 Jun 29.

43. Greenburg AG. Pathophysiology of anemia. Am J Med 101(2A):7S–11S, 1996.

44. Krantz SB. Pathogenesis and treatment of the anemia of chronic disease. Am J Med Sci 307(5):353–9, 1994.

45. Szaflarski NL. Physiologic effects of normovolemic anemia: implications for clinical monitoring. AACN Clin Issues 7(2):198–211, 1996.

46. Hirsh J, Dalen JE, Anderson DR, et al. Oral anticoagulants: mechanism of action, clinical effectiveness, and optimal therapeutic range. Chest 119:8S–21S, 2001. (From the American College of Chest Physicians' 6th Consensus Conference on Antithrombotic Therapy). The sixth (2000) ACCP guidelines for antithrombotic therapy for prevention and treatment of thrombosis. Chest 119:1S–2S, 2001; doi:10.1378/chest.119.1_suppl.1S.

47. Bigger JT, Weld F, Rolnitzky L. Prevalence, characteristics and significance of ventricular tachycardia detected with ambulatory electrocardiographic recording of late hospital phase of acute myocardial infarction. Am J Cardiol 48(5):815, 1981.

48. Epstein AE, Dimarco JP, Ellenbogen KA, et al. ACC/AHA/HRS 2008 Guidelines for Device-Based Therapy of Cardiac Rhythm Abnormalities: a report of the American College of Cardiology/American Heart Association Task Force on Practice Guidelines (Writing Committee to Revise the ACC/AHA/NASPE 2002 Guideline Update for Implantation of Cardiac Pacemakers and Antiarrhythmia Devices) developed in collaboration with the American Association for Thoracic Surgery and Society of Thoracic Surgeons. J Am Coll Cardiol 51(21):e1–62, 2008.

49. Zipes DP, Camm AJ, Borggrefe M, et al. ACC/AHA/ESC 2006 guidelines for management of patients with ventricular arrhythmias and the prevention of sudden cardiac death: a report of the American College of Cardiology/American Heart Association Task Force and the European Society of Cardiology Committee for Practice Guidelines (Writing Committee to Develop Guidelines for Management of Patients With Ventricular Arrhythmias and the Prevention of Sudden Cardiac Death). J Am Coll Cardiol 48(5):e247–346, 2006.

50. Fisher JD, Buxton AE, Lee KL, et al. Designation and distribution of events in the Multicenter UnSustained Tachycardia Trial (MUSTT). Am J Cardiol 100(1):76–83, 2007. Epub 2007 May 11.

51. Caro JJ, Ward A, Deniz HB, et al. Cost-benefit analysis of preventing sudden cardiac deaths with an implantable cardioverter defibrillator versus amiodarone. Value Health 10(1):13–22, 2007.

52. Brodsky MA, McAnulty J, Zipes DP, et al. A history of heart failure predicts arrhythmia treatment efficacy: data from the Antiarrhythmics versus Implantable Defibrillators (AVID) study. Am Heart J 152(4):724–30, 2006.

53. Gentile R. Clinical usefulness of a new echocardiographic window: the transesophageal approach. Medicina (Firenze) 10(4):411–15, 1990.

54. Pedersen WR, Walker M, Olson JD, et al. Value of transesophageal echocardiography as an adjunct to transthoracic echocardiography in evaluation of native and prosthetic valve endocarditis. Chest 100(2):351–6, 1991.

55. Orihashi K, Hong YW, Chung G, et al. New applications of two dimensional transesophageal echocardiography in cardiac surgery. J Cardiothorac Vasc Anesth 5(1):33–9, 1991.

56. Font VE, Obarski TP, Klein AL, et al. Transesophageal echocardiography in the critical care unit. Cleve Clin J Med 58:3315–22, 1991.

57. Labovitz AJ. Embolic stroke and echocardiographic findings—What are the implications? Controversies in Clinical Echocardiography, 72nd Scientific Sessions of American Heart Association, November 9, 1999.

58. Crawford MH. Should transesophageal echocardiogram be performed in all patients with atrial fibrillation? Controversies in Clinical Echocardiography, 72nd Scientific Sessions of American Heart Association, November 9, 1999.

59. Kelly WN. Textbook of Internal Medicine. Philadelphia, JB Lippincott, 1989.

60. Armstrong WF. Treadmill exercise echocardiography methodology and clinical role. Eur Heart J 18(Suppl D):D2–8, 1997.

61. Devereux RB, Pini R, Aurigemmla GP, et al. Measurement of left ventricular mass: methodology and expertise. J Hypertens 15(8):801–9, 1997.

62. De Castro S, Yao J, Pandian NG. Three-dimensional echocardiography: clinical relevance and application. Am J Cardiol 81(12A):96G–102G, 1998.

63. Hung J, Lang R, Flachskampf F, et al. 3D echocardiography: a review of the current status and future directions. J Am Soc Echocardiogr 20(3):213–33, 2007.

64. Shaw, LJ. Impact of contrast echocardiography on diagnostic algorithms: pharmaco-economic implications. Clin Cardiol 20(10 Suppl):I39–48, 1997.

65. P'erez JE. Current role of contrast echocardiography in the diagnosis of cardiovascular diseases. Clin Cardiol 20(10 Suppl):I31–8, 1997.

66. Feinstein SB, Cheirif J, Ten Cate FJ, et al. Safety and efficacy of a new transpulmonary ultrasound contrast agent: initial multicenter clinical results. J Am Coll Cardiol 16:316–24, 1990.

67. Crouse LJ, Cheirif J, Hanly DE. Opacification and border delineation improvement in patients with suboptimal border definition in routine echocardiography: results of the phase III Albunex multicenter trial. J Am Coll Cardiol 22:1494–500, 1993.

68. Gandhok NK, Block R, Ostoic T, et al. Reduced forward output states affect the left ventricular opacification of intravenously administered Albunex. J Am Soc Echocardiogr 10:25–30, 1997.

69. Main ML, Grayburn PA. Clinical applications of transpulmonary contrast echocardiography. Am Heart J 137(1):144–53, 1999.

70. Cheirif J, Desir RM, Bolli R, et al. Relation of perfusion defects observed with myocardial contrast echocardiography to the severity of coronary stenosis: correlation with thallium-201 single-photon emission tomography. J Am Coll Cardiol 19(6):1343–9, 1992.

71. DiCarli MF, Davidson M, Little R, et al. Value of metabolic imaging with positron emission tomography for evaluating prognosis in patients with coronary artery disease and left ventricular dysfunction. Am J Cardiol 73(8):527–33, 1994.

72. Merz CN, Berman DS. Imaging techniques for coronary artery disease: current status and future directions. Clin Cardiol 20(6):526–32, 1997.

73. Maddahi J, Blitz A, Phelps M, et al. The use of positron emission tomography imaging in the management of patients with ischemic cardiomyopathy. Adv Card Surg 7:163–88, 1996.

74. Beller GA, Gibson RS. Sensitivity, specificity and prognostic significance of noninvasive testing for occult or known coronary disease. Prog Cardiovasc Dis 29:241, 1987.

75. Chan SY, Brunken RC, Buxton DB. Cardiac positron emission tomography: the foundations and clinical applications. J Thorac Imaging 5(3):9–19, 1990.

76. Berman DS, Kiat H, Van Train KF, et al. Comparison of SPECT using technetium-99m agents and thallium-201 and PET for the assessment of myocardial perfusion and viability. Am J Cardiol 66(13):72E–9E, 1990.

77. Williams MJ, Odabashian J, Lauer MS, et al. Prognostic value of dobutamine echocardiography in patients with left ventricular dysfunction. J Am Coll Cardiol 27(1):132–9, 1996.

78. Toole JF. The Willis lecture: transient ischemic attacks, scientific method, and new realities. Stroke 22(1):99–104, 1991.

79. May JM, Shuman WP, Strote JN, et al. Low-risk patients with chest pain in the emergency department: negative 64-MDCT coronary angiography may reduce length of stay and hospital charges. AJR Am J Roentgenol 193:150–4, 2009.

80. Graboys TB, Blatt CM. Angina Pectoris: Management Strategies and Guide to Interventions. Cado, OK, Professional Communications, Inc., 1997.

81. Rumberger JA, Sheedy PF, Breen JF, et al. Electron beam computed tomography and coronary artery disease: scanning for coronary artery calcification. Mayo Clin Proc 71:369–77, 1996.

82. Budoff MJ, Georgiou D, Brody A, et al. Ultrafast computed tomography as a diagnostic modality in the detection of coronary artery disease: a multicenter study. Circulation 93:898–904, 1996.

83. Kaufmann RB, Peyser PA, Sheedy PF, et al. Quantification of coronary artery calcium by electron beam computed tomography for determination of severity of angiographic disease in young patients. J Am Coll Cardiol 25:626–32, 1995.

84. Fallovollita JA, Brody AS, Bunnell IL, et al. Fast computed tomography detection of coronary calcification in the diagnosis of coronary artery disease: comparison with angiography in patients <50 years old. Circulation 89:285–90, 1994.

85. O'Malley PG, Taylor AJ, Gibbons RV, et al. Rationale and design of the Prospective Army Coronary Calcium (PACC) Study: utility of electron beam computed tomography as a screening test for coronary artery disease and as an intervention for risk factor modification among young, asymptomatic, active-duty United States Army personnel. Am Heart J 137(5):932–41, 1999.

86. Wang S, Detrano RC, Secci A, et al. Detection of coronary calcification with electron beam computed tomography: evaluation of interexamination reproducibility and comparison of 3 image acquisition protocols. Am Heart J 132:550–8, 1996.

87. Breen JF, Sheedy PF, Shwartz RS, et al. Coronary artery calcification detected with ultrafast CT as an indication of coronary artery disease. Radiology 185:435–9, 1992.

88. Haberl R, Becker A, Leber A, et al. Correlation of coronary calcification and angiographically documented stenoses in patients with suspected coronary artery disease: results of 1764 patients. J Am Coll Cardiol 37:451–7, 2001.

89. Achenbach S, Nomayo A, Couturier G, et al. Relation between coronary calcium and 10-year risk scores in primary prevention patients. Am J Cardiol 92:1471–5, 2003.

90. Arad Y, Goodman KJ, Roth M, et al. Coronary calcification, coronary disease risk factors, c-reactive protein, and atherosclerotic cardiovascular disease events: the St. Francis Heart Study. J Am Coll Cardiol 46:158–65, 2005.

91. Park R, Detrano R, Xiang M, et al. Combined use of computed tomography coronary calcium score and c-reactive protein levels in predicting cardiovascular evens in nondiabetic individuals. Circulation 106:2073–7, 2002.

92. Becker A, Leber A, Becker C, et al. Predictive value of coronary calcifications for future cardiac events in asymptomatic individuals. Am Heart J 155(1):154–60, 2008.

93. Schmermund A, Erbel R, Silber S. Age and gender distribution of coronary artery calcium measured by four-slice computed tomography in 2,030 persons with no symptoms of coronary artery disease. Am J Cardiol 90(2):168–73, 2002.

94. Greenland P, Labree L, Azen SP, et al. Coronary artery calcium score combined with Framingham score for risk prediction in asymptomatic individuals. JAMA 291:210–5, 2004.

95. Ben-David Y, Shefer A, Weiss AT, et al. Early postoperative assessment of coronary artery bypass surgery using nuclear left ventriculography and atrial pacing. Thorac Cardiovasc Surg 31(6):377–81, 1983.

96. Gunnar WP, Martin M, Smith RF, et al. The utility of cardiac evaluation in the hemodynamically stable patient with suspected myocardial contusion. Am Surg 57(6):373, 1991.

97. Yang DC, Jain CU, Patel D, et al. Use of IV radionuclide total body arteriography to evaluate arterial bypass shunts—a new method—a review of several cases. Angiology 41(9 Pt 1):745–52, 1990.

98. Gottlieb SO, Gottlieb SH, Achuff SC, et al. Silent ischemia on Holter monitoring predicts mortality in high risk post infarction patients. JAMA 259:1030, 1988.

99. Carrol CL, Higgins CB, Caputo GR. Magnetic resonance imaging of acquired cardiac disease. Texas Heart Inst J 23(2):144–54, 1996.

100. Colletti PM, Term MR. Magnetic resonance imaging applications to cardiac diagnosis. Biomed Instrum Technol 30(4):354–8, 1996.

101. Fayad ZA, Fuster V, Fallon JT, et al. Human coronary atherosclerotic wall imaging using in vivo high resolution MR. Presented at the American Heart Association 72nd Scientific Sessions, Atlanta, GA; November 7–10, 1999. Abstract 2742, November 9.

102. Kramer CM. Integrated approach to ischemic heart disease. The one-stop shop. Cardiol Clin 16(2):267–76, 1998.

103. Yang PC, Kerr AB, Liu AC, et al. New real-time interactive cardiac magnetic resonance imaging system complements echocardiography. J Am Coll Cardiol 32(7):2049–56, 1998.

104. Sakuma H, Takeda K, Higgins CB. Fast magnetic resonance imaging of the heart. Eur J Radiol 29(2):101–13, 1999.

105. De Roos A, Niezen RA, Lamb HJ, et al. MR of the heart under pharmacologic stress. Cardiol Clin 16(2):247–65, 1998.

106. Cooper KH. The Aerobics Way. New York, Bantam, 1981.

107. McGavin CR, Gupta SP, McHardy GJR. Twelve minute walking tests for assessing disability in chronic bronchitis. Br Med J 1:822–3, 1976.

108. Jones NL, Cambell EJ. Clinical Exercise Testing. 2nd ed. Philadelphia, Saunders, 1982.

109. Blessey RL. Aerobic capacity and cardiac catheterization results in 13 patients with exercise bradycardia [Abstract]. Med Sci Sports Exerc 8:50, 1976.

110. Davidson DM, DeBusk RJ. Prognostic value of a single exercise test 3 weeks after uncomplicated myocardial infarction. Circulation 61:236–42, 1980.

111. Starling MR, Crawford MH, Kennedy GT, et al. Predictive value of early post-myocardial infarction modified exercise testing in multivessel coronary artery disease detection. Am Heart J 102(2):169, 1981.

112. Schwartz K, Turner J, Sheffield L, et al. Limited exercise testing soon after MI (correlation with early coronary and left ventricular angiography). Ann Intern Med 94(6):727, 1981.

113. Fuller C, Razner A, Verani M, et al. Early post myocardial infarction treadmill stress testing. Ann Intern Med 94:734, 1981.

114. Savnamki KI, Anderson D. Early exercise test in the assessment of long term prognosis after acute MI. Acta Med Scand 209:185, 1981.

115. Weld F, Chu K, Bigger J, et al. Risk stratification with low level exercise testing two weeks after acute MI. Circulation 64(2):306–14, 1981.

116. Theroux P, Waters D, Halphen C, et al. Prognostic value of exercise testing soon after myocardial infarction. N Engl J Med 301(7):341, 1979.

117. Firth BG, Lange RA. Pathophysiology and management of primary pump failure. In Gersh BJ, Rahimtoola SH (eds.): Acute Myocardial Infarction. New York, Elsevier, 1991.

118. Ibsen H, Kjoller E, Styperck J, et al. Routine exercise ECG three weeks after acute myocardial infarction. Acta Med Scand 198:463, 1975.

119. Ross J. Hemodynamic changes in acute MI. In The Myocardium Failure and Infarction. New York, HP Publishing, 1974:261.

120. Ericsson M, Granath A, Ohlsen P, et al. Arrhythmias and symptoms during treadmill testing three weeks after myocardial infarction in 100 patients. Br Heart J 35:787, 1973.

121. Ellestad MH. Stress Testing Principles and Practice. Philadelphia, FA Davis, 1986.

122. McIntyre KM, Lewis AJ. Textbook of Advanced Cardiac Life Support. Dallas, American Heart Association, 1983.

123. American College of Sports Medicine. Guidelines for Exercise Testing and Prescription. 4th ed. Philadelphia, Lea & Febiger, 1990.

124. Stuart RJ Jr, Ellestad MH. National survey of exercise stress testing facilities. Chest 77(1):94–7, 1980.

125. Ellestad MH, Wan MKC. Standards for adult exercise testing laboratories. The Exercise Standards Book. Dallas, American Heart Association, 1979.

126. Cahalin LP, Blessey R, Cummer D, et al. The safety of exercise testing performed independently by physical therapists. J Cardiopulm Rehab 7(6):269, 1987.

127. Squires RW, Allison TG, Johnson BD, et al. Non-physician supervision of cardiopulmonary exercise testing in chronic heart failure: safety and results of a preliminary investigation. J Cardiopulm Rehab 19(4):249–53, 1999.

128. Olivotto I, Montereggi A, Mazzuoli F, et al. Clinical utility and safety of exercise testing in patients with hypertrophic cardiomyopathy. G Ital Cardiol 29(1):11–19, 1999.

129. Rodgers GP, Ayanian JZ, Balady G, et al. American College of Cardiology/American Heart Association Clinical Competence statement on stress testing: a report of the American College of Cardiology/American Heart Association/American College of Physicians—American Society of Internal Medicine Task Force on Clinical Competence. J Am Coll Cardiol 36(4):1441–53, 2000.

130. Golding LA, Myers CR, Sinning WE. Y's Way to Physical Fitness. 3rd ed. Champaign, IL, Human Kinetics, 1989.

131. Froelicher VF. Exercise and the Heart. 2nd ed. Chicago, Clinical Concepts, 1987.

132. Diamond GA, Forrester JS. Analysis of probability as an aid in the clinical diagnosis of coronary artery disease. N Engl J Med 300:1350, 1979.

133. Goldschlager H, Selzer Z, Cohn K. Treadmill stress tests as indicators of presence and severity of coronary artery disease. Ann Intern Med 85:277, 1976.

134. Bruce RA, DeRouen T, Peterson DR, et al. Noninvasive predictors of sudden death in men with coronary heart disease. Am J Cardiol 39:833, 1977.

135. Weiner DA, Ryan TJ, McCabe GH, et al. Prognostic importance of a clinical profile and exercise test in medically treated patients with coronary artery disease. J Am Coll Cardiol 3(3):772, 1984.

136. Wong YK, Dawkins S, Grimes R, et al. Improving the positive predictive value of exercise testing in women. Heart 89(12):1416–21, 2003.

137. Higginbotham MB. Cardiopulmonary Exercise Testing: An Interpretation for the Cardiologist. St. Paul, MN, Medical Graphics Corporation, 1993.

138. Hilton TC, Thompson RC, Williams HJ, et al. Technetium-99m sestamibi myocardial perfusion imaging in the emergency room evaluation of chest pain. J Am Coll Cardiol 23:1016–22, 1994.

139. Weissman IA, Dickinson C, Dworkin H, et al. Emergency center myocardial perfusion SPECT: long-term follow-up: cost-effective imaging providing diagnostic and prognostic information [Abstract]. J Nucl Med 36:P88, 1995.

140. Radensky PW, Stowers S, Hilton TC, et al. Cost effectiveness of acute myocardial perfusion imaging with Tc99m sestamibi for risk stratification of emergency room patients with acute chest pain. Circulation 90:1–528, 1994.

141. Bonow RO. The hibernating myocardium: implications for management of congestive heart failure. Am J Cardiol 75(3):17A–25A, 1995.

142. Zaret BL, Wackers FJ. Nuclear cardiology. N Engl J Med 329:775–83, 855–63, 1993.

143. Ritchie J, Bateman TM, Bonow RO, et al. Guidelines for clinical use of cardiac radionuclide imaging. A report of the American Heart Association/American College of Cardiology Task Force on Assessment of Diagnostic and Therapeutic Cardiovascular Procedures, Committee on Radionuclide Imaging, developed in collaboration with the American Society of Nuclear Cardiology. Circulation 91(4):1278–303, 1995.

144. Cerqueira MD, Maynard C, Ritchie JL, et al. Long-term survival in 618 patient from the Western-Washington Streptokinase in Myocardial Infarction Trials. J Am Coll Cardiol 20:1452–9, 1992.

145. Dilsizian V, Bonow RO. Current diagnostic techniques of assessing myocardial viability in hibernating and stunned myocardium. Circulation 87:1–20, 1993.

146. Van der Wieken LR, Kan G, Belfer AJ, et al. Thallium-201 scanning to decide CCU admission in patients with nondiagnostic electrocardiograms. Int J Cardiol 4:285–99, 1983.

147. Van Train KF, Garcia EV, Maddahi J, et al. Multicenter trial validation for quantitative analysis of same-day rest-stress technetium-99m-sestamibi myocardial tomograms. J Nucl Med 35:609–18, 1994.

148. Berman DS, Kiat HS, Van Train KF, et al. Myocardial perfusion imaging with technetium-99m-sestamibi: comparative analysis of available imaging protocols. J Nucl Med 35:681–8, 1994.

149. Beanlands RSB, Dawood F, Wen WH, et al. Are the kinetics of technetium-99m methoxyisobutyl isonitrile affected by cell metabolism and viability? Circulation 82:1802–14, 1990.

150. Piwnica-Worms D, Kronauge JF, Chiu ML. Uptake and retention of hexakis(2-methoxyisobutyl isonitrile) technetium in cultured myocardial cells: mitochondrial and plasma membrane potential dependence. Circulation 82:1826–38, 1990.

151. Kim C, Kwok YS, Heagerty P, et al. Pharmacologic stress testing for coronary disease diagnosis: a meta-analysis. Am Heart J 142(6):934–44, 2001.

152. Ellhendy A, van Domburg RT, Poldermans D, et al. Safety and feasibility of dobutamine-atropine stress echocardiography for the diagnosis of coronary artery disease in diabetic patients unable to perform an exercise stress test. Diabetes Care 21(11):1797–802, 1998.

153. Bouvier F, Hojer J, Hulting J, et al. Myocardial perfusion scintigraphy (SPECT) during adenosine stress can be performed safely early on after thrombolytic therapy in acute myocardial infarction. Clin Physiol 18(2):97–101, 1998.

154. Maseri A. Role of coronary artery spasm in symptomatic and silent myocardial ischemia. J Am Coll Cardiol 9:249, 1987.

155. Igarashi Y, Yamazoe M, Shibata A. Effect of direct intracoronary administration of methylergonovine in patients with and without variant angina. Am Heart J 121(4 Pt 1):1094–100, 1991.

156. Khoshio A, Miyakoda H, Fukuiki M. Significance of coronary artery tone assessed by coronary responses to ergonovine and nitrate. Jpn Circ J 55(1):33–40, 1991.

157. Malik M, Bigger JT, Camm AJ. Heart rate variability: standards of measurement, physiological interpretation, and clinical use. Eur Heart J 17(3):354–81, 1996.

158. Pagani M, Lombardi F, Guzzetti S, et al. Power spectral analysis of heart rate and arterial pressure variabilities as a marker of sympatho-vagal interaction in man and conscious dog. Circ Res 59:178–93, 1986.

159. Frenneaux MP. Autonomic changes in patients with heart failure and in post-myocardial infarction patients. Heart 90:1248–55, 2004.

160. De Jong MJ, Randall DC. Heart rate variability analysis in the assessment of autonomic function in heart failure. J Cardiovasc Nurs 20:186–95; quiz 96–7, 2005.

161. Eckberg DL. Parasympathetic cardiovascular control in human disease: a critical review of methods and results. Am J Physiol 2239:H581–93, 1980.

162. Malliani A, Schwartz PJ, Zanchetti A. Neural mechanism in life threatening arrhythmias. Am Heart J 100:705–14, 1980.

163. Katz A, Liberty IF, Porath A, et al. A simple bedside test of 1-minute heart rate variability during deep breathing as a

prognostic index after myocardial infarction. Am Heart J 138(1):32–8, 1999.

164. Van Ravenswaaij-Arls CA, Kollee LA, Hopman JC, et al. Heart rate variability. Ann Intern Med 118:436–47, 1993.

165. Bernardi L, Valle F, Coco M, et al. Physical activity influences heart rate variability and very-low-frequency components in Holter electrocardiograms. Cardiovasc Res 32(2):234–7, 1996.

166. Roach D, Wilson W, Ritchie D, et al. Dissection of long-range heart rate variability: controlled induction of prognostic measures by activity in the laboratory. J Am Coll Cardiol 43:2271–7, 2004.

167. Osterhues HH, Hanzel SR, Kochs M, et al. Influence of physical activity on 24-hour measurements of heart rate variability in patients with coronary artery disease. Am J Cardiol 80:1434–7, 1997.

168. Glagov S, Weisenberg E, Zarins CK, et al. Compensatory enlargement of human atherosclerotic coronary arteries. N Engl J Med 316(22):1371–5, 1987.

169. Zarins CK, Weisenberg E, Kolettis G, et al. Differential enlargement of artery segments in response to enlarging atherosclerotic plaques. J Vasc Surg 7(3):386–94, 1988.

170. Ross J Jr, Fisch C. Guidelines for coronary angiography. J Am Coll Cardiol 10:935, 1987.

171. Liao L, Kong DF, Shaw LK, et al. A new anatomic score for prognosis after cardiac catheterization in patients with previous bypass surgery. J Am Coll Cardiol 46(9):1684–92, 2005.

172. Andreoli TE, Carpenter CCJ, Plum F, et al. Cecil Essentials of Medicine. Philadelphia, Saunders, 1996.

173. Ibañez B, Badimon JJ, Garcia MJ. Diagnosis of atherosclerosis by imaging. Am J Med 122(1 Suppl):S15–25, 2009.

174. Mintz GS, Nissen SE, Anderson WD, et al. ACC Clinical Expert Consensus Document on Standards for the acquisition, measurement and reporting of intravascular ultrasound studies: a report of the American College of Cardiology Task Force on Clinical Expert Consensus Documents (Committee to Develop a Clinical Expert Consensus Document on Standards for Acquisition, Measurement and Reporting of Intravascular Ultrasound Studies IVUS). J Am Coll Cardiol 37:1478–92, 2001.

175. Komiyama N, Berry GJ, Kolz ML, et al. Tissue characterization of atherosclerotic plaques by in intravascular ultrasound radiofrequency signal analysis: an in vitro study of human coronary arteries. Am Heart J 40:565–74, 2000.

176. Prati F, Arbustini E, Labellarte A, et al. Correlation between high frequency intravascular ultrasound and histomorphology in human coronary arteries. Heart 85:567–70, 2001.

177. Komiyama N, Courtney BK, Toyozaki T, et al. In vivo on-line intravascular ultrasound radio-frequency signal analysis for tissue characterization of coronary atherosclerosis validated by histology of coronary atherectomy tissue specimens [Abstract]. Circulation 104:II–590, 2001.

178. Kawasaki M, Takatsu H, Noda T, et al. In vivo quantitative tissue characterization of human coronary arterial plaques by use of integrated backscatter intravascular ultrasound and comparison with angioscopic findings. Circulation 105:2487–92, 2002.

179. Nair A, Kuban BD, Tuzcu EM, et al. Coronary plaque classification with intravascular ultrasound radiofrequency data analysis. Circulation 106:2200–6, 2002.

180. Ricciardi MJ, Meyers S, Choi K, et al. Angiographically silent left main disease detected by intravascular ultrasound: a marker for future adverse cardiac events. Am Heart J 146(3):507–12, 2003.

181. Patterson RE, Churchwell KB, Eisner RL. Diagnosis of coronary artery disease in women: roles of three dimensional imaging with magnetic resonance or positron emission tomography. Am J Card Imaging 10(1):78–88, 1996.

182. Jaff MR. Diagnostic testing in vascular medicine: the foundation for successful intervention. J Invasive Cardiol 11(10):640–4, 1999.

183. Weitz JI, Byrne J, Clagett GP, et al. Diagnosis and treatment of arterial insufficiency of the lower extremities: a critical review. Circulation 94:3026–49, 1996.

184. Kornitzer M, Dramaix M, Sobolski J, et al. Ankle/arm pressure index in asymptomatic middle-aged males: an independent predictor of ten year coronary heart disease mortality. Angiology 46:211–9, 1995.

185. Newman AB, Siscovick DS, Manolio TA, et al. Ankle-arm index as a marker of atherosclerosis in the cardiovascular health study. Circulation 88:837–45, 1993.

186. MacDonald NR. Pulse volume plethysmography. J Vasc Technol 18:241–8, 1994.

187. Sacks D, Robinson ML, Marinelli DL, et al. Evaluation of the peripheral arteries with duplex US after angioplasty. Radiology 176:39–44, 1990.

188. Bandyk DF. Ultrasonic duplex scanning in the evaluation of arterial grafts and dilatations. Echocardiography 4:251–64, 1987.

189. American Association for Cardiovascular and Pulmonary Rehabilitation. Guidelines for Cardiac Rehabilitation and Secondary Prevention Programs. Champaign, IL, Human Kinetics, 1995.

190. Gardner AW, Poehlman ET. Exercise rehabilitation programs for the treatment of claudication pain: a metaanalysis. JAMA 274(12):975–80, 1995.

191. de Liefde II, Hoeks SE, van Gestel YR, et al. Usefulness of hypertensive blood pressure response during a single-stage exercise test to predict long-term outcome in patients with peripheral arterial disease. Am J Cardiol 102(7):921–6, 2008.

192. Autret A, Saudeau D, Bertrand PH, et al. Stroke risk in patients with carotid stenosis. Lancet 1:888–90, 1987.

193. O'Leary DH, Polak JF, Kronmal RA, et al. Carotid artery intima and media thickness as a risk factor for myocardial infarction and stroke in older adults. N Engl J Med 340:14–22, 1999.

194. Feussner JR, Matchar DB. When and how to study the carotid arteries. Ann Intern Med 109:805–18, 1988.

195. Kirsch JD, Wagner LR, James EM, et al. Carotid artery occlusion: positive predictive value of duplex sonography compared with arteriography. J Vasc Surg 19:642–9, 1994.

196. Spence JD, Eliasziw M, DiCicco M, et al. Carotid plaque area: a tool for targeting and evaluating vascular preventive therapy. Stroke 33(12):2916–22, 2002.

197. Spence JD. Point: uses of carotid plaque measurement as a predictor of cardiovascular events. Prev Cardiol 8(2):118–21; discussion 126, 2005.

198. Gailloud P, Oishi S, Carpenter J, et al. Three-dimensional digital angiography: new tool for simultaneous three-dimensional rendering of vascular and osseous information during rotational angiography. Am J Neuroradiol 25:571–3, 2004.

# CHAPTER 9

# Electrocardiography

*Ellen Hillegass*

## Chapter Outline

Understanding the electrocardiogram (ECG) requires a basic understanding of the electrophysiology and anatomy of the heart and conduction system (see Chapters 1 and 2), an appreciation of the ECG waveforms (both their normal and abnormal presentations in different leads), and a certain amount of practice in the systematic review of 12-lead and single-lead ECG rhythm strips. After reading this chapter the therapist should be able to determine whether an ECG tracing represents a benign or a life-threatening situation and be able to begin to make appropriate clinical decisions based on this determination. Further information regarding the ECG and more advanced arrhythmia detection should be researched in texts devoted entirely to electrocardiography.

One comment should be made about nomenclature before beginning the discussion of electrocardiography. Dysrhythmia is the most accurate term to describe a heart rhythm that is abnormal, because the prefix dys means "bad" or "difficult." However, researchers do not use this term widely but rather favor the term arrhythmia, which means "without rhythm" or "no rhythm." In keeping with current usage, this chapter and text use arrhythmia throughout to refer to abnormal rhythm.

---

**Clinical Tip**

Understanding electrophysiology, and particularly single-lead ECG will help the practitioner when assessing heart rhythm and determining the safety of pursuing interventions in the light of abnormal heart rhythm.

---

## Basic Electrophysiologic Principles

The ECG is inscribed on specially ruled paper. It represents the electrical impulses of the heart and provides valuable information regarding the heart's function. The myocardium is comprised of cells that have different functions, and the ECG is the expression of these cells and their function. The four types of myocytes that compose the muscle include the typical working myocytes, which respond to the electrical stimulus to contract and pump the blood; nodal myocytes, which have the highest rate of rhythmicity but slow impulse-conduction rates; transitional myocytes, which conduct impulses twice as fast as nodal cells; and Purkinje's cells, which have a low rate of rhythmicity yet a high rate of conductivity.

Electrical stimulation makes the cell membrane more permeable to the flow of ions. As there is a predominance of potassium (K+) on the inside of the cell and sodium (Na+) on the outside, the electrical stimulation makes the membrane more permeable to the sodium ions so that they flow inward, creating a change in the resting state of the cells of the cardiac muscle from a negative to a positive charge on the interior. This sodium flow is referred to as the fast channel. The potassium ions then start to flow outward. The potassium flow is referred to as the slow channel. The electrical stimulation of the specialized cells that cause contraction is called depolarization (Fig. 9-1). As the cell becomes positive on the interior, the myocardial cells are stimulated to contract. When the potassium ion flow outward exceeds the

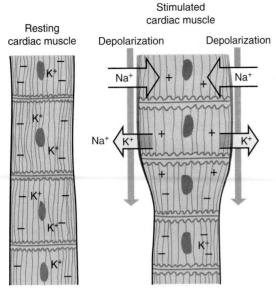

**Figure 9-1** Electrical stimulation to the cardiac muscle cell membrane causes depolarization. With depolarization the membrane is more permeable to sodium ions, allowing them to flow inward and creating a positive charge on the inside.

sodium flow inward, repolarization begins. During repolarization, the myocardial cells return to a negative interior and a positive exterior, and muscle relaxation occurs.[1] When the wave of depolarization is moving toward a positive electrode located on the skin, the ECG records a simultaneous upward deflection (Fig. 9-2).

Cardiac muscle has three unique properties: automaticity, rhythmicity, and conductivity. Cardiac muscle cells are able to discharge an electrical stimulus without stimulation from a nerve, as is typical in all other muscle cells, demonstrating the property of automaticity. Rhythmicity is the regularity with which such pacemaking activity occurs. Cardiac muscle cells can therefore "automatically" discharge an electrical stimulus. This is particularly noticeable in the sinoatrial (SA) node, which is the primary pacemaker and has the most amount of automaticity of the cardiac cells.

However, other cardiac cells may discharge at any time owing to this property of automaticity, creating abnormal rates or rhythms (as in premature beats). The SA node has a normal innate automatic firing rate between 60 and 100 beats per minute. The atrioventricular (AV) node has an inherent firing rate of 40 to 60 beats per minute and begins to act as

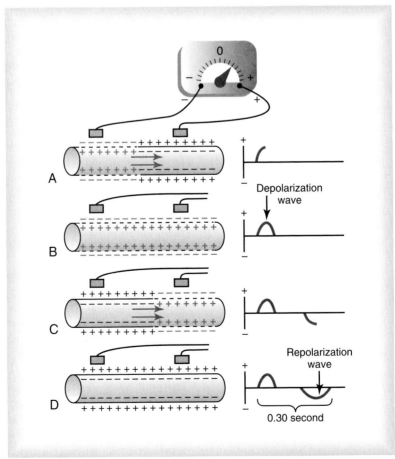

**Figure 9-2** Recording the depolarization wave (**A** and **B**) and the repolarization wave (**C** and **D**) from a cardiac muscle fiber. (From Guyton AC. Textbook of Medical Physiology, ed 11. St. Louis, 2006, Saunders.)

the pacemaker if the SA node is not functioning properly. The His-Purkinje portions of the specialized conduction system have an inherent firing rate of 30 to 40 beats per minute.

Cardiac muscle cells also have the ability to spread impulses to adjoining cells very quickly (the property of conductivity). The rapid spread can be visualized when one considers how fast the cells must depolarize and repolarize at a heart rate of 200 beats per minute. Rapid arrhythmias such as supraventricular tachycardia and slow rates as a result of AV blocks are examples of problems with conductivity. See Chapter 2 for further discussion of the myocytes.

## The Autonomic Nervous System

The autonomic nervous system has a major influence on reflex cardiac activity as a result of two counterbalancing forces: the sympathetic and the parasympathetic divisions. The effects of the two divisions determine the delicate balance between excitation and depression of cardiac activity, which can be altered in favor of one or the other by numerous physiologic and pathologic factors and in a variety of situations. The sympathetic division is equated with acceleration, and the parasympathetic division is equated with deceleration or braking.

### Sympathetic Division

The sympathetic division discharges norepinephrine (noradrenalin) from its terminal nerve branches in the atria and ventricles, resulting in an excitation of the rate of impulse formation and the velocity of impulse propagation and an increase in the force of contractile fibers. The sympathetic division acts on both the SA node and the AV node as well as on the ventricles. In addition, the sympathetic division can stimulate the adrenal gland to secrete norepinephrine and epinephrine into the bloodstream. The direct action of these hormones on the heart is equal to the direct stimulation of the terminal nerve branches in the heart. Increased sympathetic activity increases the heart rate, the conduction velocity throughout the AV node, the contractility of the heart muscle, and the irritability of the heart. In addition, automaticity may increase, which can alter the normal sinus rhythm.

### Parasympathetic Division

The parasympathetic division discharges acetylcholine from the terminal nerve branches. The vagus nerve is the main component of the parasympathetic division in control of the heart, and it acts primarily on the SA node as a general inhibitor on the rate of impulse formation and conduction velocity. Increased parasympathetic activity slows the heart rate and acts to slow the conduction through the AV node. Decreased parasympathetic activity increases the heart rate, the conduction through the AV node, and the irritability of the heart. Therefore, the effect of acetylcholine and the effects of vagal stimulation depress the automaticity and conductivity of the heart. See Chapter 2 for further discussion.

> **Clinical Tip**
> The autonomic system action on the heart can be summarized as parasympathetic input at rest controls heart rate and slows the heart rate. With activity, stress, or any other emotion that would activate the sympathetic system, the parasympathetic input would be withdrawn and the direct sympathetic input would increase the heart rate, increase the conduction velocity, and increase the force of contraction. Individuals with an abnormal autonomic system response (some diabetics and individuals with heart transplants where the nerves are cut) would show different responses.

## The Conduction System

The conduction system is composed of myocytes arranged in a pathway that spreads the electrical activity throughout the four chambers (two atria, two ventricles) (Fig. 9-3). The primary pacemaker that initiates the electrical impulse for the cardiac muscle is the SA node, located in the right atrium near the posterior surface and adjacent to the entry of the superior vena cava. The impulse then spreads throughout the right atrium via intraatrial pathways and to the left atrium via the Bachmann bundle. The wave of atrial depolarization is represented on the ECG as the P wave. Therefore, the P wave represents atrial depolarization electrically and is normally associated with atrial contraction mechanically (Fig. 9-4). Following the spread of depolarization through the atria, the impulse then reaches the AV node, also called the junctional node, which is located near the intraventricular septum in the inferior aspect of the right atrium just superior to the tricuspid valve. The AV node delays the conduction of the electrical impulse from the atria for one-tenth of a second (seen on the ECG as the isoelectric line after the P wave and before the QRS complex), allowing for the

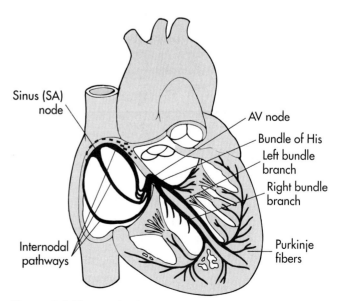

**Figure 9-3** The conduction system. (From Aehlert B. Mosby's Comprehensive Pediatric Emergency Care [Revised]. St. Louis, 2007, Mosby.)

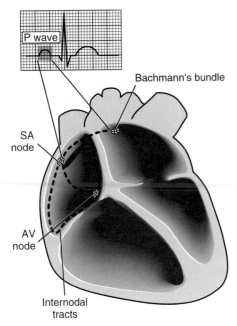

**Figure 9-4** Atrial depolarization is depicted on the electrocardiographic tracing as the P wave. The impulse is spread to the left atrium via the Bachmann bundle.

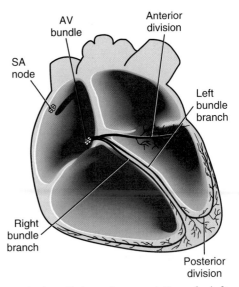

**Figure 9-6** The bundle branches, consisting of a left and right division, are located within the interventricular septum. The left bundle branch has both an anterior and a posterior division.

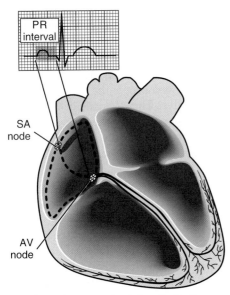

**Figure 9-5** When the spread of depolarization reaches the atrioventricular node, a slight delay occurs. The electrocardiogram records this as the P-R interval.

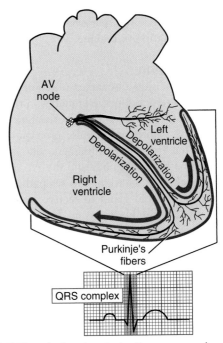

**Figure 9-7** Ventricular depolarization occurs when the electric impulse reaches the Purkinje fibers. The electrocardiogram depicts ventricular depolarization in the QRS complex.

mechanical contraction of the atria to eject blood into the ventricles. This is known as the atrial kick. The ECG depicts this delay as the P-R segment (Fig. 9-5). The P-R segment is also considered to be the isoelectric line. The impulse then passes from the AV node into the His bundle and then to the bundle branches. The bundle branches consist of a left and right division and are located in the interventricular septum (Fig. 9-6).

The right bundle branch is responsible for depolarization of the right ventricle, and the left bundle branch, which has an anterior fascicle and a posterior fascicle, is responsible for the depolarization of the left ventricle. The electrical impulses spread down the bundle branches and terminate in Purkinje fibers, which are numerous and very small. These fibers penetrate the myocardium and stimulate muscle contraction from the apex upward toward the base of the heart in a "wringing" action. The ECG records the electrical stimulus of ventricular depolarization as the QRS complex (Fig. 9-7). The QRS complex represents ventricular depolarization and

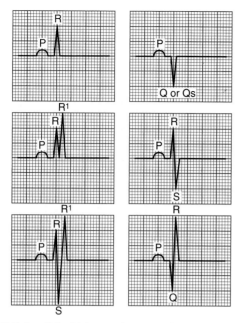

**Figure 9-8** Possible QRS complexes. Each individual's electro-cardiographic tracing is different.

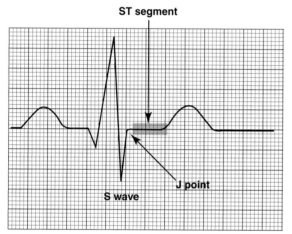

**Figure 9-9** The ST segment on the electrocardiogram tracing begins at the end of the S wave and ends at the beginning of the T wave. Notice the J point, which classically is defined as the point at which the thin line of the QRS tracing turns into a thick line. The J point is also the beginning of the ST segment and is often used as the landmark when the ST segment is aberrant.

is normally followed closely by ventricular contraction. The ECG tracing may demonstrate a variety of QRS waveforms, depending on the pathologic condition or the location of the electrode, but they are generally referred to as the QRS complex regardless of the configuration. Figure 9-8 shows the various forms of QRS complexes that may be seen on an ECG.

Repolarization begins when ventricular contraction ends. Following the QRS complex, a slight pause is noted. This pause is called the ST segment and is defined as the flat piece of isoelectric line that starts at the end of the QRS complex and ends at the beginning of the T wave (Fig. 9-9). The

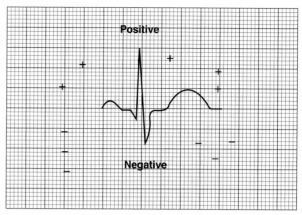

**Figure 9-10** The positive or negative deflections on the electrocardiogram tracing represent voltage. Each small square is 1 mm × 1 mm.

ventricle is initiating repolarization during the ST-segment phase of the ECG. This segment has very important predictive value and is discussed later.

Repolarization is complete with the ending of the T wave. The T wave represents the ventricular repolarization. Because no mechanical contraction is occurring, the T wave is strictly an electrical phenomenon that records the return of potassium inward and that of sodium outward and the change in the polarization of the cell.

## The Electrocardiogram Recording

The electrocardiogram is recorded on ruled graph paper, with the smallest divisions (or squares) being 1 mm long and 1 mm high. The height (positive deflection) or depth (negative deflection) measures the voltage as 0.1 mV/mm (Fig. 9-10). Time is represented on the graph paper by 0.04 second between each small square and 0.2 second between the large squares (Fig. 9-11) when the paper speed is set at 25 mm/second. Exact time is important to note on the ECG to determine the duration of the complexes (e.g., QRS duration) and the intervals (e.g., P-R interval) as well as to identify the heart rates and arrhythmias.

The standard 12-lead ECG consists of tracings from 6 limb leads and 6 chest leads. The six limb leads are I, II, III, aVR, aVL, and aVF. Each limb lead records from a different angle, providing a different view of the same cardiac activity. Therefore, the tracings from the various leads look different because the electrical activity is monitored from different positions. The six chest leads of the ECG are V1, V2, V3, V4, V5, and V6 and are monitored from six electrodes placed on the chest wall. The ECG tracing from the chest leads (V1 to V6) shows gradual changes in all the waves, as seen in Figure 9-12. Leads V1 and V2 are placed over the right side of the heart, and V5 and V6 are placed over the left side of the heart. Leads V3 and V4 are placed over the ventricular septum (Fig. 9-13). Figure 9-14 shows a picture of a standard 12-lead ECG with normal tracings in each of the leads, and the location of the leads on the tracing.

Four elements are specifically assessed on a 12-lead ECG tracing:
- Heart rate
- Heart rhythm
- Hypertrophy
- Infarction

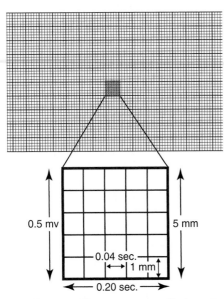

**Figure 9-11** Electrocardiogram paper displays time on the horizontal axis. Each small box represents 0.04 second, and each large box represents 0.20 second. The vertical axis changes are measured in millimeters. Each small box represents 1 mm, each large box represents 5 mm.

A single-lead tracing, often called a rhythm strip, is assessed for heart rate, rhythm, and presence of arrhythmias. If hypertrophy, ischemia, or infarction is suspected, a 12-lead ECG should be obtained.

## Heart Rate

The heart rate can be determined from the ECG recording by a variety of methods, including obtaining a 6-second tracing, measuring specific R waves, and counting the number of large boxes (5 mm or 0.2 second in length).

### Six-Second Tracing

The investigator obtains an ECG recording that is 6 seconds in length (Fig. 9-15). The number of QRS complexes found

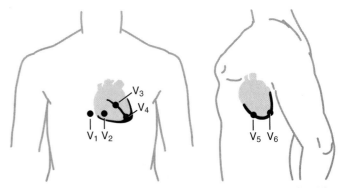

**Figure 9-13** Leads V1 and V2 are placed over the right side of the heart. Leads V3 and V4 are located over the interventricular septum. Leads V5 and V6 demonstrate changes on the left side of the heart.

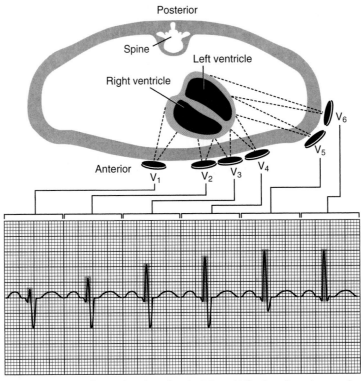

**Figure 9-12** The electrocardiographic tracing from the chest leads (V1 to V6), showing the gradual changes that occur with the R and S waves.

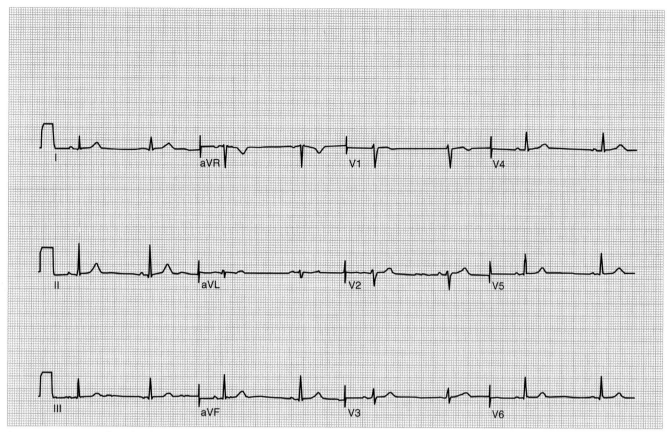

**Figure 9-14** Normal 12-lead electrocardiogram. (From Andreoli T. Andreoli and Carpenter's Cecil Essentials of Medicine, ed 7. Philadelphia, 2008, Saunders.)

in the 6-second recording is then multiplied by 10 to determine the heart rate per minute: number of QRS complexes in a 6-second recording × 10 = heart rate per minute.

### R Wave Measurement

An alternative method of measuring heart rate is by identifying a specific R wave that falls on a heavy black line (large boxline; Fig. 9-16). For each heavy black line that follows this R wave until the next R wave occurs the therapist counts 300, 150, 100, 75, 60, 50. Where the next R wave falls in this counting method gives the actual heart rate. To use this method, one must be able to memorize the specific numbers for the successive dark black lines to determine rapid heart rates from the graph paper. The one problem with R-wave measurement for determining heart rate is that it cannot be used with irregular heart rhythms. For a more accurate estimate, the number of QRS complexes in a 30-second strip must be counted and then multiplied by 2: number of QRS complexes in a 30-second strip × 2 = heart rate per minute.

### Counting Boxes

The third method of obtaining the heart rate from the graph paper is to count the number of large boxes (5 mm or 0.2 second in length) between the first QRS complex and the next QRS complex. The number of large boxes is then divided into 300 to obtain an estimate of the heart rate: 300 ÷ number of large boxes between the next QRS complex and the next QRS complex = heart rate per minute. A more accurate measurement of the heart rate can be made by counting the number of small boxes (1 mm or 0.04 second in length) between the QRS complexes and then dividing this number into 1500. This method requires much greater time to perform heart rate interpretation (Fig. 9-17): number of small boxes between QRS complexes ÷ 1500 = heart rate per minute.

### Heart Rhythm: Assessment of Single-Lead electrocardiogram

The 12-lead ECG is used primarily for determining ischemia or infarction as well as for comparing previous ECG recordings for an individual. However, for simple detection of rate or rhythm disturbances, single-lead monitoring is the appropriate choice. Single-lead monitoring via telemetry is the most common practice in stepdown intensive care units and cardiopulmonary rehabilitation programs. Single-lead monitoring is limited to detection of rate and rhythm disturbances; it cannot detect ischemia owing to the inability to calibrate radiotelemetry. Hardwire systems are frequently used in the intensive care unit or cardiac care unit and should be calibrated appropriately. These systems can record ischemia. Twelve-lead ECG monitoring is used when ischemia is suspect or when a change in condition is noted.

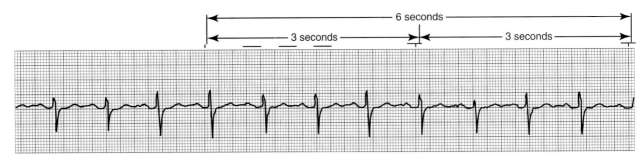

**Figure 9-15** The heart rate can be determined by identifying 6 seconds on the electrocardiogram paper and counting the number of QRS complexes in the 6-second strip. The number of QRS complexes in 6 seconds multiplied by 10 gives the heart rate for 1 minute. The heart rate in this tracing is 84 beats per minute.

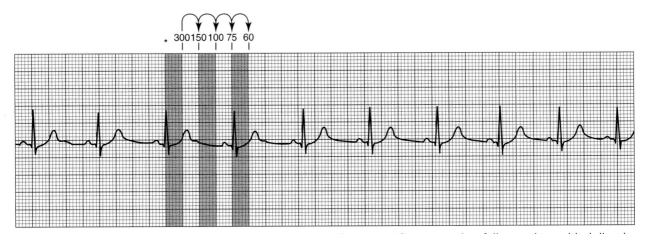

**Figure 9-16** Another method of determining heart rate is to first find a specific R wave that falls on a heavy black line (see *). Then, count off "300, 150, 100, 75, 60, 50" for each heavy black line that follows until the next R wave falls. To find the specific heart rate, determine the difference in rate between the dark lines that encircle the R wave (e.g., 300 − 150 = 150), and divide this number by 5 (the number of small boxes between the dark lines). Between 150 and 300 the distance between each small box is equivalent to 30 beats. Between 100 and 150 the distance between each small box represents 10 beats. This method assists in identifying a more accurate heart rate. The heart rate in this tracing is 72 beats per minute.

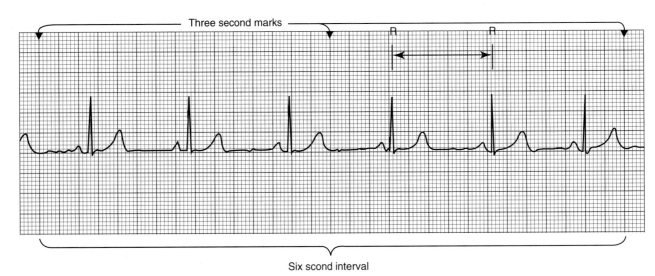

**Figure 9-17** Another method of determining heart rate is to count the number of large boxes between two R waves and divide this number into 300. Or, for greater accuracy, count the number of large boxes between the R waves, multiply this number by 5 (the number of small boxes per large box), and divide this number into 1500. The heart rate in this tracing is 58 beats per minute. (From Wiederhold R. Electrocardiography: The Monitoring Lead. Philadelphia, 1989, Saunders.)

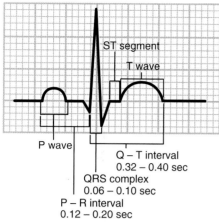

ST segment

T wave

P wave

Q – T interval
0.32 – 0.40 sec

QRS complex
0.06 – 0.10 sec

P – R interval
0.12 – 0.20 sec

**Figure 9-18** The normal electrocardiogram tracing. The P-R interval measures between 0.12 and 0.20 second. The normal duration of the QRS complex is 0.06 to 0.10 second. The normal duration of the Q-T interval is 0.32 to 0.40 second.

## Assessment Approach

To determine heart rate and rhythm from single-lead monitoring, the normal waveforms and intervals must be understood (Fig. 9-18). The waveforms that represent depolarization of the myocardium are labeled P, QRS, T, and U. A systematic approach to waveforms and interval measurement should be undertaken when reviewing cardiac rhythm (Box 9-1).

## Normal Waveforms

The P wave is normally rounded, symmetric, and upright, representing atrial depolarization. A P wave should occur before every QRS complex. The P-R interval is the interval that starts at the beginning of the P wave and ends at the beginning of the QRS complex; the portion following the P wave is also defined as the isoelectric line. The P-R interval is normally 0.12 to 0.20 second (or up to five small squares on the ECG paper). This period of time represents the atrial depolarization and the slowing of electrical conduction through the AV node.

> **Clinical Tip**
> Single-lead monitoring can accurately assess only rate and rhythm; it cannot diagnose ischemia (ST-segment changes) and infarction (Q waves).

The QRS complex follows the P-R interval and has multiple deflections and may have numerous variations, depending on the lead that is being monitored (see Fig. 9-8 for variations in the QRS complexes). The QRS complex begins at the end of the P-R interval and appears as a thin line recording from the ECG stylus, ending normally with a return to the baseline. The QRS duration reflects the time it takes for conduction to proceed to the Purkinje fibers and for the ventricles to depolarize. The normal duration is 0.06 to 0.10 second.

### Box 9-1

#### Assessment of the Cardiac Cycle

A systematic approach to the assessment of the cardiac cycle for rhythm and rate disturbances involves the following:

1. Evaluate the P wave. (Is it normal and upright, and is there a P wave before every QRS? Do all the P waves look alike?)
2. Evaluate the P-R interval. (Normal duration is 0.12 to 0.20 second.)
3. Evaluate the QRS complex. (Do all QRS complexes look alike?)
4. Evaluate the QRS interval. (Normal duration is 0.06 to 0.10 second.)
5. Evaluate the T wave. (Is it upright and normal in appearance?)
6. Evaluate the R-R wave interval. (Is it regular?) (See Fig. 9-19.)
7. Evaluate the heart rate (6-second strip if regular rhythm; normal rate is 60 to 100 beats per minute).
8. Observe the patient, and evaluate any symptoms. (Do the observation, symptoms, or both correlate with the arrhythmia?)

The ST segment follows the QRS complex, beginning where the ECG tracing transforms from a thin line to a thicker line and terminating at the beginning of the T wave. The ST segment should be represented as an isoelectric line along the same line (if measured with a ruler) as the P-R interval or the baseline. The T wave follows the ST segment and should be rounded, symmetric, and upright. The T wave represents ventricular repolarization.

The Q-T interval (from the beginning of the QRS complex until the end of the T wave) normally measures between 0.32 and 0.40 second if a normal sinus rhythm is present. The Q-T interval usually is not measured unless drug toxicity is suspected. Occasionally a U wave may follow the T wave, but its cause and clinical value are essentially unknown.

Finally, the R-R interval is reviewed throughout the rhythm strip to assess regularity of rhythm (Fig. 9-19). Normal rhythm requires a regular R-R interval throughout; however, a discrepancy of up to 0.12 second between the shortest and the longest R-R interval is acceptable for normal respiratory variation. Occasionally single-lead monitoring may be affected, by artifact, such as the following:

- Muscle tremors or movement (including anything from sneezing and coughing to actual physical movement)
- Loose electrodes
- Sixty-cycle electrical interference

In most cases of artifact interference, the R-R interval is regular throughout, and the interference is seen between the R waves (Fig. 9-20).

If the R-R intervals are all regular, a 6-second strip or the counting down from 300 method can be employed to determine heart rate. Normal heart rate is between 60 and 100 beats per minute. If the R-R intervals are irregular (and

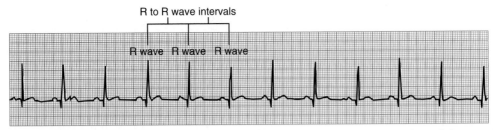

**Figure 9-19** Electrocardiogram tracing demonstrating R to R intervals. R-R intervals are evaluated for regularity of rhythm. The heart rate in this tracing is 68 beats per minute.

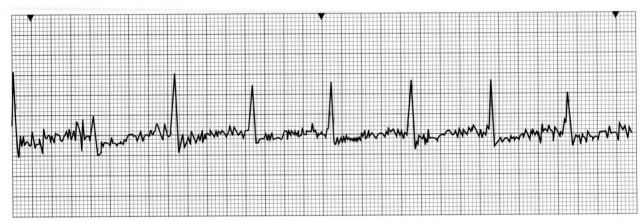

**Figure 9-20** Electrocardiogram tracing of normal sinus rhythm with artifact in between the R waves. (From Wiederhold R. Electrocardiography: The Monitoring Lead. Philadelphia, 1989, Saunders.)

greater than the acceptable range of 0.12 second for respiratory variation), a 30- to 60-second strip may be needed to determine the heart rate and the frequency or seriousness of the arrhythmia, or both.

### Basic Interpretation of Heart Rhythm

The key to the basic interpretation of heart rhythm in the clinical setting involves using the systematic approach as presented earlier, correlating the interpretation with the history and the signs and symptoms of the patient and then deciding if the rhythm is benign or life-threatening. If the decision is that the rhythm is truly benign, then the patient does not require ECG monitoring. If the rhythm is relatively benign, then occasional ECG monitoring may be necessary, or at least physiologic monitoring of the heart rate and blood pressure should be employed. If the arrhythmia is determined to be life-threatening, ECG monitoring as well as physiologic monitoring should be carried out. In some cases, the patient may not be a candidate for any activity or procedure until the arrhythmia is controlled.

For each of the following cardiac rhythms an ECG recording is provided along with a description of the features of each rhythm. In addition, possible etiologic factors as well as signs and symptoms that may be associated with the rhythm are explained. Treatment is discussed only so that the reader may develop an increased understanding of the whole picture of arrhythmias and their control. It should not be inferred that the physical therapist is responsible for the treatment of arrhythmias.

### Normal Sinus Rhythm

The normal cardiac rhythm is termed *normal sinus rhythm* (NSR) and begins with an impulse originating in the SA node with conduction through the normal pathways for depolarization. Parasympathetic stimulation generally slows the rate, and sympathetic stimulation increases the rate. Figure 9-21 illustrates NSR. The characteristics of NSR include the following:

- All P waves are upright, normal in appearance, and identical in configuration; a P wave exists before every QRS complex.
- The P-R interval is between 0.12 and 0.20 second.
- The QRS complexes are identical.
- The QRS duration is between 0.06 and 0.10 second.
- The R-R interval is regular (or if irregular, the difference between shortest and longest intervals is less than 0.12 second).
- The heart rate is between 60 and 100 beats per minute.

### Sinus Bradycardia

Sinus bradycardia differs from NSR only in the rate, which is less than 60 beats per minute (Fig. 9-22). The characteristics of sinus bradycardia include the following:

- All P waves are upright, normal in appearance, and identical in configuration; a P wave exists before every QRS complex.
- The P-R interval is between 0.12 and 0.20 second.
- The QRS complexes are identical.
- The QRS duration is between 0.06 and 0.10 second.

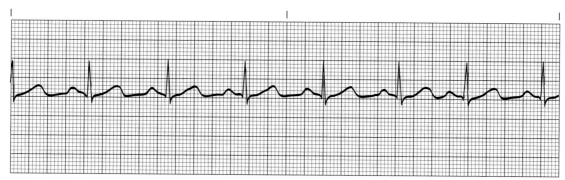

**Figure 9-21** Normal sinus rhythm; heart rate = 80 (6-second strip). (From Atwood S. Introduction to Basic Cardiac Dysrhythmias, ed 4. St. Louis, 2009, Mosby.)

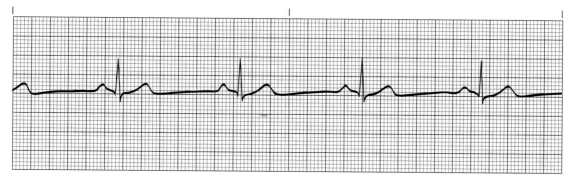

**Figure 9-22** Sinus bradycardia; heart rate = 50 (6-second strip). (From Atwood S. Introduction to Basic Cardiac Dysrhythmias, ed 4. St. Louis, 2009, Mosby.)

- The R-R interval is regular throughout.
- The heart rate is less than 60 beats per minute.

*Signs, Symptoms, and Causes*

Sinus bradycardia is normal in well-trained athletes because of their enhanced stroke volume. It is also common in individuals taking β-blocking medications. Sinus bradycardia may occur because of a decrease in the automaticity of the SA node or in a condition of increased vagal stimulation, such as suctioning or vomiting. Sinus bradycardia has been seen in patients who have traumatic brain injuries with increased intracranial pressures and in patients with brain tumors. Sinus bradycardia may also occur in the presence of second- or third-degree heart block; therefore, close evaluation of the P-R interval and the P-to-QRS ratio is necessary to rule out heart block.

Usually individuals with sinus bradycardia are asymptomatic unless a pathologic condition exists, at which time the individual may complain of syncope, dizziness, angina, or diaphoresis. Other arrhythmias may also develop.

*Treatment*

No treatment is necessary unless the patient is symptomatic. If the patient has symptoms, atropine may be used, and in some cases a temporary pacemaker may be implanted.

## Sinus Tachycardia

Sinus tachycardia differs from NSR in rate only, which is greater than 100 beats per minute (Fig. 9-23). The characteristics of sinus tachycardia include:

- All P waves are upright, normal in appearance, and identical in configuration; a P wave exists before every QRS complex.
- The P-R interval is between 0.12 and 0.20 second.
- The QRS complexes are identical.
- The QRS duration is between 0.06 and 0.10 second.
- The R-R interval is regular.
- The heart rate is greater than 100 beats per minute.

> **Clinical Tip**
> Sinus bradycardia is usually non–life-threatening. The underlying cause should be sought. Some possible causes include beta-blocking medications and second- or third-degree AV block (not benign). Trained athletes with an increased resting and exercise stroke volume may also exhibit bradycardia.

*Signs, Symptoms, and Causes*

Sinus tachycardia is typically benign and is present usually in conditions in which the SA node automaticity is increased (increased sympathetic stimulation). Examples of conditions that induce sinus tachycardia include pain; fear; emotion; exertion (exercise); or any artificial stimulants such as caffeine, nicotine, amphetamines, and atropine. Sinus tachycardia is also found in situations in which the demands for oxygen are increased, including fever, congestive heart failure, infection, anemia, hemorrhage, myocardial injury, and hyperthyroidism. Usually individuals with sinus tachycardia are asymptomatic.

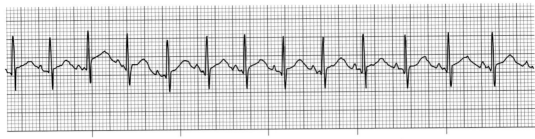

**Figure 9-23** Sinus tachycardia (6-second strip). (From Aehlert B. Mosby's Comprehensive Pediatric Emergency Care [Revised]. St. Louis, 2007, Mosby.)

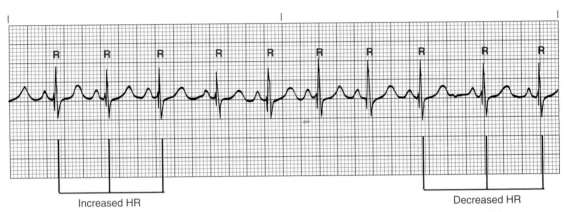

Increased HR                                    Decreased HR

**Figure 9-24** Sinus arrhythmia. Heart rate increases with inspiration and decreases with expiration; overall heart rate = 100 (notice peaked P waves). (From Atwood S. Introduction to Basic Cardiac Dysrhythmias, ed 4. St. Louis, 2009, Mosby.)

---

> **Clinical Tip**
> Sinus tachycardia is considered non–life-threatening. Some causes include exercise, anxiety, hypovolemia, anemia, fever or infection, medications (stimulants), and low cardiac output.

### Treatment

Treatment for sinus tachycardia involves elimination (or treatment) of the underlying cause, or, in some cases, the initiation of β-blocker medication therapy.

## Sinus Arrhythmia

Sinus arrhythmia is classified as an irregularity in rhythm in which the impulse is initiated by the SA node but with a phasic quickening and slowing of the impulse formation. The irregularity is usually caused by an alternation in vagal stimulation (Fig. 9-24). The characteristics of sinus arrhythmia include the following:

- All P waves are upright, normal in appearance, and identical in configuration; a P wave exists before every QRS complex.
- The P-R interval is between 0.12 and 0.20 second.
- The QRS complexes are identical.
- The QRS duration is between 0.06 and 0.10 second.
- The R-R interval varies throughout.
- The heart rate is between 40 to 100 beats per minute.

### Signs, Symptoms, and Causes

The most common type of sinus arrhythmia is related to the respiratory cycle, with the rate increasing with inspiration and decreasing with expiration. This type of arrhythmia is usually found in the young or elderly at rest, and it disappears with activity. The other type of sinus arrhythmia is nonrespiratory and therefore is not affected by the breathing cycle. Nonrespiratory sinus arrhythmia may occur in conditions of infection, medication administration (particularly toxicity associated with digoxin or morphine), and fever.[2]

### Treatment

The respiratory type of sinus arrhythmia is benign and does not require any treatment. The nonrespiratory type should be evaluated for the underlying cause, and then this cause should be treated.

## Sinus Pause or Block

Sinus pause or sinus block occurs when the SA node fails to initiate an impulse, usually for only one cycle (Fig. 9-25). The characteristics of sinus pause and block include the following:

- All P waves are upright, normal in appearance, and identical in configuration; a P wave exists before every QRS complex.
- The P-R interval of the underlying rhythm is 0.12 to 0.20 second.
- The QRS complexes are identical.

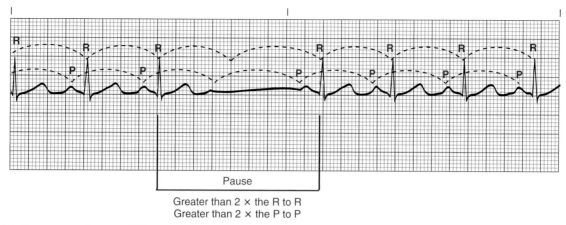

Pause

Greater than 2 × the R to R
Greater than 2 × the P to P

**Figure 9-25** Sinus arrest. Pause will be more than 2 times the previous cardiac cycle of the underlying rhythm; overall heart rate = 70. (From Atwood S. Introduction to Basic Cardiac Dysrhythmias, ed 4. St. Louis, 2009, Mosby.)

Lead II (continuous)

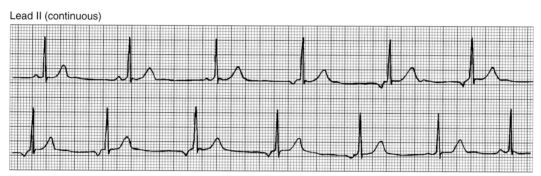

**Figure 9-26** Wandering atrial pacemaker. Continuous strip (lead II). (From Aehlert B. ACLS Study Guide, ed 3. St. Louis, 2007, Mosby.)

- The QRS duration is between 0.06 and 0.10 second.
- The R-R interval is regular for the underlying rhythm, but occasional pauses are noted.
- The heart rate is usually 60 to 100 beats per minute.

### Signs, Symptoms, and Causes

Sinus pause or block can occur for a number of reasons, including a sudden increase of parasympathetic activity, an organic disease of the SA node (sometimes referred to as sick sinus syndrome), an infection, a rheumatic disease, severe ischemia or infarction to the SA node, or a case of digoxin toxicity.[1] If the pause or block is prolonged or occurs frequently, the cardiac output is compromised, and the individual may complain of dizziness or syncope episodes.

### Treatment

Treatment should be initiated when the patient is symptomatic. It involves treatment of the underlying cause, which may include reduction of digoxin, removal of vagal stimulation, and possibly treatment with atropine or implantation of a permanent pacemaker.

## Wandering Atrial Pacemaker

The pacemaking activity in wandering pacemaker shifts from focus to focus, resulting in a rhythm that is very irregular and without a consistent pattern. Some of the impulses may arise from the AV node (Fig. 9-26). The characteristics of wandering pacemaker include the following:

- P waves are present but vary in configuration; each P wave may look different.
- A P wave exists before every QRS complex.
- The P-R intervals may vary but are usually within the normal width.
- The QRS complexes are identical in configuration.
- The QRS duration is between 0.06 and 0.10 second.
- The R-R intervals vary.
- The heart rate is usually less than 100 beats per minute.

### Signs and Symptoms

The cause is usually an irritable focus; however, the discharge of the impulse and the speed of discharge vary within the normal range. This type of arrhythmia is seen in the young and in the elderly and may be caused by ischemia or injury to the SA node, congestive heart failure, or an increase in vagal firing.[3] Usually this arrhythmia does not cause symptoms.

### Treatment

This arrhythmia may lead to atrial fibrillation, which may require treatment; otherwise no treatment is necessary.

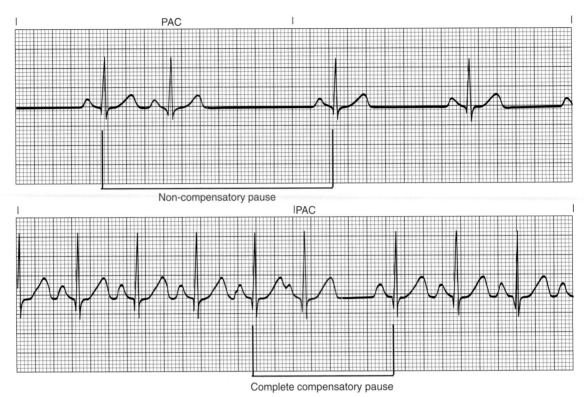

**Figure 9-27** Premature atrial complex with a complete compensatory pause in a sinus rhythm; heart rate = 80 to 90. (From Atwood S. Introduction to Basic Cardiac Dysrhythmias, ed 4. St. Louis, 2009, Mosby.)

## Atrial Arrhythmias

### Premature Atrial Complexes

A premature atrial complex is defined as an ectopic focus in either atria that initiates an impulse before the next impulse is initiated by the SA node (Fig. 9-27). The characteristics of premature atrial complexes include the following:

- The underlying rhythm is sinus rhythm.
- Normal complexes have one P wave and one QRS wave configuration.
- The P wave of the early beat is noticeably different from the normal P waves.
- Depending on the heart rate, the P wave of the early beat may be buried in the previous T wave.
- The QRS complex involved in the early beat should look similar to the other QRS complexes.
- All P-R intervals are 0.12 to 0.20 second.
- All QRS durations are between 0.06 and 0.10 second.
- Often a pause follows the premature atrial complex, but it may not be compensatory.

#### Signs, Symptoms, and Causes

Causes of premature atrial complexes include emotional stress, nicotine, caffeine, alcohol, hypoxemia, infection, myocardial ischemia, rheumatic disease, and atrial damage. There may be no signs or symptoms associated with premature atrial complexes unless the pulse is palpated and the irregularity noticed.

> **Clinical Tip**
> Premature atrial contractions are benign arrhythmias. They are often noticed in patients with chronic obstructive pulmonary disease.

#### Treatment

If the frequency of the premature atrial complexes is low, no treatment is required unless there are hemodynamic consequences. When the frequency is increased, supraventricular tachycardia or atrial fibrillation may develop.[4]

### Atrial Tachycardia

- The definition of atrial tachycardia is three or more premature atrial complexes in a row. Usually the heart rate is greater than 100 and may be as fast as 200 beats per minute (Fig. 9-28). The characteristics of atrial tachycardia include the following:
- P waves may be the same or may look different.
- P waves may not be present before every QRS complex.
- The P-R intervals vary but should be no greater than 0.20 second.
- The QRS complexes should be the same as the others that originate from the SA node.
- The QRS duration is generally between 0.06 and 0.10 second.
- The R-R intervals vary.
- The heart rate is rapid, being greater than 100 and possibly up to 200 beats per minute.

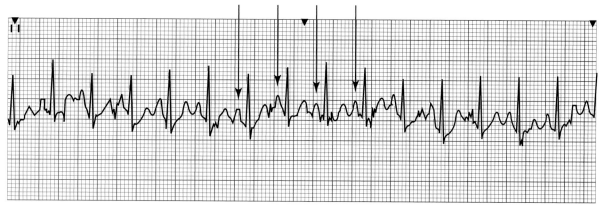

**Figure 9-28** Electrocardiogram tracing showing atrial tachycardia. Note the presence of P waves (*arrows*) despite the fast heart rate (approximately 145 beats per minute).

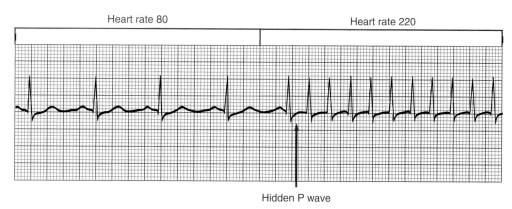

Heart rate 80

Heart rate 220

Hidden P wave

**Figure 9-29** Normal sinus rhythm (NSR) progressing to paroxysmal atrial tachycardia (PAT)/paroxysmal supraventricular tachycardia (PSVT); NSR: heart rate = 80; PAT/PSVT: heart rate = 220. (From Atwood S. Introduction to Basic Cardiac Dysrhythmias, ed 4. St. Louis, 2009, Mosby.)

*Signs, Symptoms, and Causes*

The causes of atrial tachycardia include the causes of premature atrial complexes as well as those of severe pulmonary disease with hypoxemia, pulmonary hypertension, and altered pH. Atrial tachycardia is often found in patients with chronic obstructive pulmonary disease. Symptoms may develop owing to a compromised cardiac output if prolonged, thereby causing dizziness, fatigue, and shortness of breath.[1]

*Treatment*

Treatment for atrial tachycardia involves treatment of the underlying cause (if the patient is hypoxemic or if pH is altered); performance of autonomic maneuvers such as Valsalva, breath holding, and coughing. Medications such as β blockers, verapamil, and digoxin may be prescribed.

## Paroxysmal Atrial Tachycardia

Paroxysmal atrial tachycardia (PAT) or paroxysmal supraventricular tachycardia (PSVT) is the sudden onset of atrial tachycardia or repetitive firing from an atrial focus. The underlying rhythm is usually NSR, followed by an episodic burst of atrial tachycardia that eventually returns to sinus rhythm. The episode may be extremely brief but can last for

hours. The rhythm starts and stops abruptly (Fig. 9-29). The characteristics of PAT include the following:

- P waves may be present but may be merged with the previous T wave.
- The P-R intervals may be difficult to determine but are less than 0.20 second.
- The QRS complexes are identical unless there is aberration.
- The QRS duration is between 0.06 and 0.10 second.
- The R-R intervals are usually regular and may show starting and stopping of the PAT.
- The ST segment may be elevated or depressed, yet the magnitude of change is not diagnostically reliable.
- The heart rate is very rapid, often greater than 160 beats per minute.

*Signs, Symptoms, and Causes*

The causes of PAT can include emotional factors; overexertion; hyperventilation; potassium depletion; caffeine, nicotine, and aspirin sensitivity; rheumatic heart disease; mitral valve dysfunction, particularly mitral valve prolapse; digitalis toxicity; and pulmonary embolus.[1] The clinical description of paroxysmal atrial tachycardia is a sudden racing or fluttering

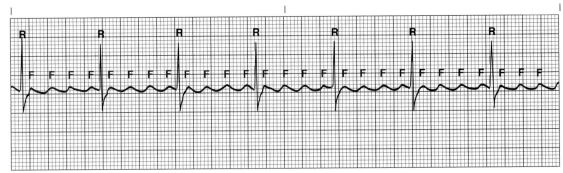

**Figure 9-30** Atrial flutter: atrial heart rate = 280; ventricular heart rate = 70. (From Atwood S. Introduction to Basic Cardiac Dysrhythmias, ed 4. St. Louis, 2009, Mosby.)

of the heart beat. If PAT continues beyond 24 hours, it is considered to be sustained atrial tachycardia. If the rapid rate continues for a period of time, other symptoms may include dizziness, weakness, and shortness of breath (possibly even due to hyperventilation).

> **Clinical Tip**
> PAT or PSVT is often diagnosed on ECG when a patient reports, "all of a sudden my heart was racing away." Initial treatment is to try coughing or breath holding with a Valsalva maneuver. Treatment may require medications.

### Treatment

Treatment includes determining the underlying cause (often in young females this would require evaluation for mitral valve prolapse); discontinuation of medications; performance of autonomic stimulation including Valsalva maneuver, breath holding, and coughing or gagging; and, if prolonged, treatment with medications such as verapamil or β blockers. Carotid massage is often performed, but only in the presence of ECG monitoring.

### Atrial Flutter

Atrial flutter is defined as a rapid succession of atrial depolarization caused by an ectopic focus in the atria that depolarizes at a rate of 250 to 350 times per minute. As only one ectopic focus is firing repetitively, the P waves are called flutter waves and look identical to one another, having a characteristic "sawtooth" pattern (Fig. 9-30). The characteristics of atrial flutter include the following:

- P waves are present as flutter waves having a characteristic "sawtooth" pattern.
- There is more than one P wave before every QRS complex.
- The atrial depolarization rate is 250 to 350 times per minute.
- The QRS configuration is usually normal and identical in configuration, but usually there is more than one P wave for every QRS complex.
- The QRS duration is 0.06 to 0.10 second.

- The R-R intervals may vary depending on the atrial firing and number of P waves before each QRS complex. The conduction ratios may vary from 2:1 up to 8:1.
- The heart rate varies.

### Signs, Symptoms, and Causes

Atrial flutter can be caused by numerous pathologic conditions, including rheumatic heart disease, mitral valve disease, coronary artery disease or infarction, stress, drugs, renal failure, hypoxemia, and pericarditis, to name the most common causes.[5] As the rate of discharge from the ectopic focus is rapid, the critical role is played by the AV node, which blocks all the impulses from being conducted. Consequently, there may be an irregular rhythm associated with atrial flutter. This rhythm is usually not considered to be life-threatening and may even lead to atrial fibrillation. Usually no symptoms are present, and the cardiac output is not compromised unless the ventricular rate is too fast or too slow.

### Treatment

Treatment for atrial flutter includes medications (digoxin, verapamil, or β blockers are the more common drugs of choice) or cardioversion with the defibrillator paddles at 10 to 50 watts.

> **Clinical Tip**
> Atrial flutter is relatively non–life-threatening if the heart rate is below 100 beats per minute at rest. Atrial flutter can be life-threatening at high heart rates. Medical treatment should be initiated if heart rate is elevated above 100 beats per minute at rest.

### Atrial Fibrillation

Atrial fibrillation is defined as an erratic quivering or twitching of the atrial muscle caused by multiple ectopic foci in the atria that emit electrical impulses constantly. None of the ectopic foci actually depolarizes the atria, so no true P waves are found in atrial fibrillation. The AV node acts to control the impulses that initiate a QRS complex; therefore, a totally irregular rhythm exists. Thus, the AV node determines the ventricular response by blocking impulses or allowing them

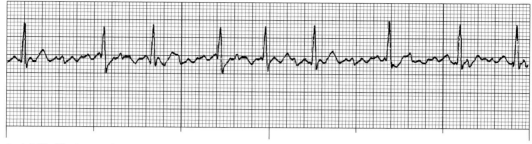

**Figure 9-31** Atrial fibrillation with a ventricular response of 67 to 120 beats per minute (6-second strip). (From Aehlert BJ. ECGs Made Easy, ed 4. St. Louis, 2010, Mosby.)

to progress forward. This ventricular response may be normal, slow, or too rapid (Fig 9-31). The characteristics of atrial fibrillation include the following:

- P waves are absent, thus leaving a flat or wavy baseline.
- The QRS duration is between 0.06 and 0.10 second.
- The R-R interval is characteristically defined as irregularly irregular.
- The rate varies but is called "ventricular response."

*Signs, Symptoms, and Causes*

Numerous factors may play a part in causing atrial fibrillation, including advanced age, congestive heart failure, ischemia or infarction, cardiomyopathy, digoxin toxicity, drug use, stress or pain, rheumatic heart disease, and renal failure. Atrial fibrillation presents problems for two reasons. Without atrial depolarization the atria do not contract. The contraction of the atria is also referred to as the atrial "kick." This atrial kick forces the last amount of volume to flow into the ventricles during diastole. The amount of volume that is forced into the ventricles because of atrial contraction provides up to 30% of the cardiac output. Therefore, without atrial contraction, the cardiac output is decreased up to 30%.[6]

In individuals with atrial fibrillation with heart rates (or ventricular response rates) lower than 100, the decrease in cardiac output is usually not a problem. However, as the individual exercises or if the ventricular response is greater than 100 at rest, the cardiac output may be diminished and signs of decompensation may occur. Atrial fibrillation is therefore considered relatively benign if the ventricular response is less than 100 at rest, but physiologic monitoring should be performed with exercise to assess cardiac output compensation. However, individuals who have atrial fibrillation with a ventricular response greater than 100 at rest should have physiologic monitoring during all activities, and any activity should be engaged in cautiously.

The other problem with atrial fibrillation is the potential for developing mural thrombi because of the coagulation of blood with fibrillating atria. Mural thrombi may lead to emboli (30% of all patients with atrial fibrillation develop emboli), so anticoagulant therapy is usually initiated.

Atrial fibrillation (irregular–irregular heart rhythm) is very common in the older population and is not considered life-threatening unless the heart rate is elevated at rest (above 100 is considered to be uncontrolled). Owing to a lack of

"atrial kick," cardiac output is lower than normal (by 15% to 30%). Because of potential coagulation of blood with this abnormal rhythm, patients should be taking aspirin or Coumadin to prevent the possibility of thrombus formation and potential cerebrovascular accident.

> **Clinical Tip**
> The classic sign of atrial fibrillation is a very irregularly irregular pulse. Symptoms occur only if the ventricular response is too rapid, which causes cardiac output decompensation.

*Treatment*

The treatment for atrial fibrillation usually involves pharmacologic control (e.g., digoxin, verapamil, antiarrhythmic therapy) or cardioversion. If a specific cause is identified, then treatment for that cause should be initiated. All individuals with newly diagnosed atrial fibrillation should be treated immediately with anticoagulants.

## Nodal or Junctional Arrhythmias

### Premature Junctional or Nodal Complexes

Premature junctional complexes are premature impulses that arise from the AV node or junctional tissue. For reasons that are not understood, the AV node becomes irritated and initiates an impulse that causes an early beat. Premature junctional complexes are very similar to premature atrial complexes except for the fact that an inverted, an absent, or a retrograde (wave that follows the QRS) P wave is present (Fig. 9-32). The characteristics of premature junctional complexes include the following:

- Inverted, absent, or retrograde P waves are present.
- The QRS configurations are usually identical.
- The QRS duration is between 0.06 and 0.10 second.
- The R-R interval is regular throughout except when the premature beats arise.
- The heart rate is usually normal (between 60 and 100 beats per minute).

*Signs, Symptoms, and Causes*

Some of the causes of premature junctional complexes include decreased automaticity and conductivity of the SA node or some irritability of the junctional tissue. Pathologic

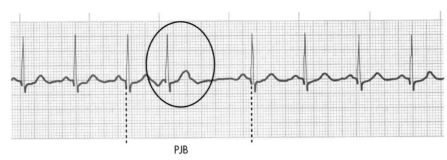

PJB

**Figure 9-32** Sinus rhythm with premature junctional beat; heart rate, 80 beats per minute. (From Monahan FD. Phipps' Medical-Surgical Nursing: Health and Illness Perspectives, ed 8. St. Louis, 2007, Mosby.)

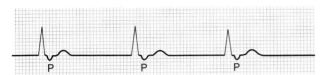

**Figure 9-33** Junctional rhythm. (From Cairo JM. Mosby's Respiratory Care Equipment, ed 8. St. Louis, 2010, Mosby.)

conditions that can cause premature junctional complexes include cardiac disease and mitral valve disease.[2] Usually no symptoms or signs are present.

*Treatment*

Usually no treatment is required because there are no symptoms of clinical significance.

## Junctional (or Nodal) Rhythm

Junctional rhythm occurs when the AV junction takes over as the pacemaker of the heart. Junctional rhythm may be considered an escape rhythm (Fig. 9-33). The characteristics of junctional rhythm include the following:

- Absence of P waves before the QRS complex, but a retrograde P wave may be identified.
- The QRS complex has a normal configuration.
- The QRS duration is between 0.06 and 0.10 second.
- The R-R intervals are regular.
- The ventricular rate is between 40 and 60 beats per minute.

*Signs, Symptoms, and Causes*

Causes of junctional rhythm include a failure of the SA node to act as the pacemaker in conditions such as sinus node disease or increase in vagal tone, digoxin toxicity, and infarction or severe ischemia to the conduction system (typically right coronary artery disease). Symptoms are present only if the heart rate is too slow, which causes a compromise in the cardiac output.

*Treatment*

Treatment consists of identifying the cause and treating it if possible. If the rate becomes too slow (50 beats per minute or less) then the patient may develop symptoms of cardiac output decompensation, dizziness, and fatigue. In the case of

symptoms and slower heart rates, the treatment involves medication to increase the rate (usually atropine or isoproterenol) or pacemaker insertion.

## Nodal (Junctional) Tachycardia

Junctional tachycardia develops because the AV junctional tissue is acting as the pacemaker (as in junctional rhythm), but the rate of discharge is accelerated. The onset of increase in rate of discharge may be sudden, or it may be of long standing (Fig. 9-34). The characteristics of junctional tachycardia include the following:

- P waves are absent, but retrograde P wave may be present.
- The QRS configurations are identical.
- The QRS duration is between 0.06 and 0.10 second.
- The R-R interval is regular.
- The rate is usually greater than 100 beats per minute.

*Signs, Symptoms, and Causes*

Causes of junctional tachycardia include hyperventilation, coronary artery disease or infarction, postcardiac surgery, digoxin toxicity, myocarditis, caffeine or nicotine sensitivity, overexertion, and emotional factors. When the rate is extremely rapid, the individual may experience symptoms of cardiac output decompensation.[1] Symptoms include dizziness, shortness of breath, and fatigue.

*Treatment*

Treatment involves identifying the cause and treating it. Digoxin is given if the underlying cause is not digoxin toxicity. Vagal stimulation may be employed or pharmacologic therapy initiated (verapamil or β blockers).

## Heart Blocks

### First-Degree Atrioventricular Heart Block

First-degree AV block occurs when the impulse is initiated in the SA node but is delayed on the way to the AV node; or it may be initiated in the AV node itself, and the AV conduction time is prolonged. This results in a lengthening of the P-R interval only (Fig. 9-35).

The characteristics associated with first-degree AV block include the following:

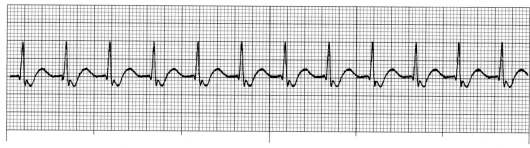

**Figure 9-34** Junctional tachycardia at 120 beats per minute. (From Aehlert BJ. ECGs Made Easy, ed 4. St. Louis, 2010, Mosby.)

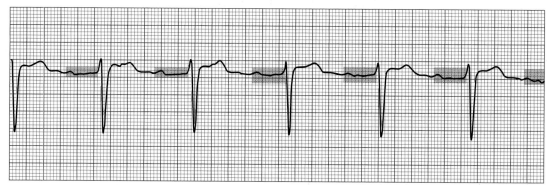

**Figure 9-35** Electrocardiogram tracing of first-degree atrioventricular block (P-R interval measures approximately 0.32 second) with sinus bradycardia. (From Wiederhold R. Electrocardiography: The Monitoring Lead. Philadelphia, 1989, Saunders.)

- A P wave is present and with normal configuration before every QRS complex.
- The P-R interval is prolonged (greater than 0.20 second).
- The QRS has a normal configuration.
- The QRS duration is between 0.06 and 0.10 second.
- The R-R intervals are regular.
- The heart rate is usually within normal limits (60 to 100 beats per minute) but may be lower than 60 beats per minute.

### Signs, Symptoms, and Causes

Causes of first-degree AV block include coronary artery disease, rheumatic heart disease, infarction, and reactions to medication (digoxin or β blockers). First-degree AV block is a relatively benign arrhythmia as it exists without symptoms (unless severe bradycardia exists in conjunction with first-degree AV block); however, it should be monitored over time because it may progress to higher forms of AV block.

### Treatment

Usually treatment is not warranted unless the AV block is a result of reactions to medication, in which case the medication is withheld.

---

*Clinical Tip*
First-degree AV block is relatively benign. The only defining feature is the prolonged P-R interval (>2.0 sec).

---

## Second-Degree Atrioventricular Block, Type I

Second-degree AV block, type I (Wenckebach or Mobitz I heart block) is a relatively benign, transient disturbance that occurs high in the AV junction and prevents conduction of some of the impulses through the AV node. The typical appearance of type I (Wenckebach) second-degree block is a progressive prolongation of the P-R interval until finally one impulse is not conducted through to the ventricles (no QRS complex following a P wave). The cycle then repeats itself (Fig. 9-36).

The characteristics of second-degree type I include the following:
- Initially a P wave precedes each QRS complex, but eventually a P wave may stand alone (conduction is blocked).
- Progressive lengthening of the P-R interval occurs in progressive order.
- As the P-R interval increases, a QRS complex will be dropped.
- This progressive lengthening of the P-R interval followed by a dropped QRS complex occurs in a repetitive cycle.
- The QRS configuration is normal, and the duration is between 0.06 and 0.10 second.
- Because of the dropping of the QRS complex, the R-R interval is irregular (regularly irregular).
- The heart rate varies.

### Signs, Symptoms, and Causes

Causes of Wenckebach heart block include right coronary artery disease or infarction, digoxin toxicity, and excessive

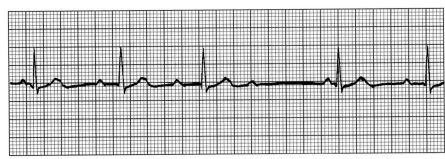

**Figure 9-36** Second-degree atrioventricular block, type I (Wenckebach, Mobitz type I). Note the progressive lengthening of the PR interval until one P wave is not conducted (dropped). (From Copstead-Kirkhorn LC. Pathophysiology, ed 4. St. Louis, 2010, Saunders.)

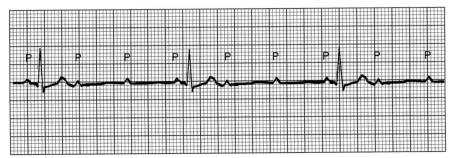

**Figure 9-37** Second-degree atrioventricular (AV) block, type II (Mobitz type II). Every third P wave is followed by a QRS complex. The other P waves are not conducted through the AV node. The PR interval on conducted impulses is constant. (From Copstead-Kirkhorn LC. Pathophysiology, ed 4. St. Louis, 2010, Saunders.)

β-adrenergic blockade; a side effect of the medication. Usually the individual with type I second-degree AV block is asymptomatic.

### Treatment

Treatment is usually unnecessary because the individual usually is without symptoms and without cardiac output compromise. In rare cases, either atropine or isoproterenol have been given, or a temporary pacemaker is inserted.[7] This type of AV block rarely progresses to higher forms of AV block.

Second-degree AV block or Wenckebach heart block may be transient with severe ischemia or infarction. Treatment may include insertion of a temporary pacemaker as well as treatment for any symptoms because of slow heart rate. Rhythm may revert from this AV block with resolution of ischemia.

### Second-Degree Atrioventricular Block, Type II

Second-degree AV block, type II (Mobitz II), is defined as nonconduction of an impulse to the ventricles without a change in the P-R interval. The site of the block is usually below the bundle of His and may be a bilateral bundle branch block (Fig. 9-37).

The characteristics of second-degree AV block type II include the following:
• A ratio of P waves to QRS complexes that is greater than 1:1 and may vary from 2 to 4 P waves for every QRS complex.

• The QRS duration is between 0.06 and 0.10 second.
• The QRS configuration is normal.
• The R-R intervals may vary depending on the amount of blocking that is occurring.
• The heart rate is usually below 100 and may be below 60 beats per minute.

### Signs, Symptoms, and Causes

Second-degree AV block type II occurs with myocardial infarction (especially when the left anterior descending coronary artery is involved), with ischemia or infarction of the AV node, or with digoxin toxicity. Patients may be symptomatic when the heart rate is low and when cardiac output compromise is present.[3]

### Treatment

Treatment usually involves pacemaker insertion, but for immediate relief of symptoms atropine or isoproterenol may be used. The danger with type II second-degree AV block is the possibility of progression to complete heart block (third-degree AV block), which is a life-threatening condition.

### Third-Degree Atrioventricular Block

In third-degree (complete) AV block all impulses that are initiated above the ventricle are not conducted to the ventricle. In complete heart block the atria fire at their own inherent rate (SA node firing or ectopic foci in the atria), and a separate pacemaker in the ventricles initiates all

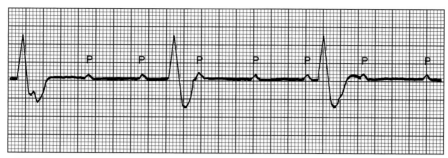

**Figure 9-38** Complete third-degree atrioventricular block. Note that there is no relationship between P waves and QRS complexes because the atria and ventricles are depolarizing independently. (From Copstead-Kirkhorn LC. Pathophysiology, ed 4. St. Louis, 2010, Saunders.)

impulses. However, there is no communication between the atria and the ventricles and thus no coordination between the firing of the atria and the firing of the ventricles, creating complete independence of the two systems (Fig. 9-38).

> **Clinical Tip**
> Second-degree type II AV block requires temporary or permanent pacemaker insertion.

The characteristics of complete heart block include the following:

- P waves are present, regular, and of identical configuration.
- The P waves have no relationship to the QRS complex because the atria are firing at their own inherent rate.
- The QRS complexes are regular in that the R-R intervals are regular.
- The QRS duration may be wider than 0.10 second if the latent pacemaker is in the ventricles.
- The heart rate depends on the latent ventricular pacemaker and may range from 30 to 50 beats per minute.

### Signs, Symptoms, and Causes
The causes of complete heart block usually involve acute myocardial infarction, digoxin toxicity, or degeneration of the conduction system. If a slow ventricular rate is present, then the cardiac output often is diminished, and the patient may complain of dizziness, shortness of breath, and possibly chest pain.

### Treatment
Treatment for complete heart block involves permanent pacemaker insertion, with atropine and isoproterenol injection or infusion used in the acute situation. Complete heart block is a medical emergency.

## Ventricular Arrhythmias

### Premature Ventricular Complexes

Premature ventricular complexes (PVCs) occur when an ectopic focus originates an impulse from somewhere in one

of the ventricles. The ventricular ectopic depolarization occurs early in the cycle before the SA node actually fires. A PVC is easily recognized on the ECG because the impulse originates in the muscle of the heart, and these myocardial cells conduct impulses very slowly compared with specialized conductive tissue. Therefore, the QRS complex is classically described as a wide and bizarre looking QRS without a P wave and followed by a complete compensatory pause (see Fig. 9-38). PVCs may come in patterns (e.g., every third or fourth beat, paired together) or may be isolated. Premature ventricular beats may be identical, or they may look different. All these factors affect the seriousness of the PVCs and also affect the clinical decision-making process and treatment. See illustrations of PVCs: unifocal (Fig. 9-39A), multifocal (Fig. 9-39B), frequent (bigeminy) (Fig. 9-39C), R on T (Fig. 9-39D), paired (Fig. 9-39E), and triplet (Fig. 9-39F).

The characteristics of PVCs include the following:

- An absence of P waves in the premature beat, with all other beats usually of sinus rhythm.
- The QRS complex of the premature beat is wide and bizarre and occurs earlier than the normal sinus beat would have occurred.
- The QRS duration of the early beat is greater than 0.10 second.
- The ST segment and the T wave often slope in the opposite direction from the normal complexes.
- The PVC is generally followed by a compensatory pause.
- The PVC is called bigeminy when every other beat is a PVC, trigeminy when every third beat is a PVC, and so on.
- The PVC is called unifocal if all PVCs appear identical in configuration.
- The PVCs are called multifocal if more than one PVC is present and no two appear similar in configuration.
- The PVC is paired or a couplet if two PVCs are together, a triplet or ventricular tachycardia (VTACH) if three are together in a row.
- The PVC is interpolated if it falls between two normal sinus beats that are separated by a normal R-R interval.

### Signs, Symptoms, and Causes
The causes of PVCs are numerous. Isolated PVCs may be present owing to caffeine or nicotine sensitivity, stress,

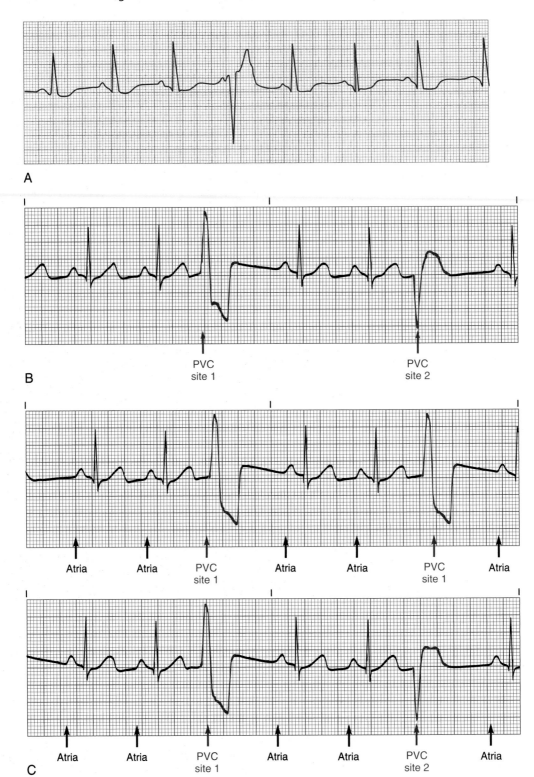

**Figure 9-39** Various Premature ventricular complexes. **A,** Normal sinus rhythm with one end-diastolic premature ventricular contraction. **B,** Sinus rhythm with multifocal premature ventricular complexes; heart rate, 70 (notice peaked P waves). **C,** Trigeminy. Sinus rhythm with an episode of unifocal trigeminy of premature ventricular complexes; heart rate, 60 to 70.

overexertion, or electrolyte imbalance (particularly hypokalemia or hyperkalemia). PVCs are also common in the presence of ischemia; cardiac disease; overdistension of the ventricle, as in congestive heart failure or cardiomyopathy; acute infarction; irritation of the myocardium or its vessels,

as in cardiac catheterization; chronic lung disease and hypoxemia; and as a result of pharmacologic therapy (Procan, quinidine, or digoxin toxicity).

Individuals may experience symptoms with PVCs if they are frequent or more serious in nature because they may

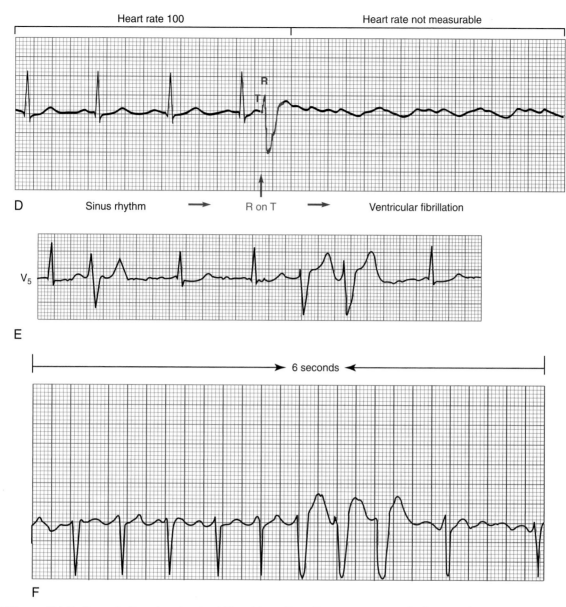

**Figure 9-39, cont'd D,** Sinus rhythm; heart rate, 100, with an R on T premature ventricular complex progressing to ventricular fibrillation (heart rate not measurable). **E,** Atrial fibrillation with ventricular premature beats. F, Electrocardiogram tracing of a triplet, otherwise known as a three-beat ventricular tachycardia. (A from Conover M: Understanding electrocardiography, ed 7, St Louis, 1996, Mosby. B–D from Atwood S. Introduction to Basic Cardiac Dysrhythmias, ed 4. St. Louis, 2009, Mosby. E from Goldberger: Clinical Electrocardiography: A Simplified Approach, ed 7. Philadelphia, 2006, Mosby.)

affect the cardiac output. A skipped beat can be palpated when checking a pulse. A PVC feels like a pause or skip in the regular rhythm that usually is followed by a stronger beat. PVC cannot be diagnosed without seeing the ECG recording; therefore, the individual is placed on telemetry. The PVC may also be felt because of the decreased preload with the PVC beat, which is followed by a long compensatory pause that allows increased filling time of the ventricle and therefore an increased preload for the beat following the premature beat and subsequently an increased stroke volume. This increased stroke volume is usually what is felt in the previously asymptomatic individual and is often a concern. With increased frequency of PVCs, the

filling time of the ventricles decreases, which leads to a decreased preload and subsequently a decreased stroke volume. Symptoms associated with PVCs include anxiety (particularly with a new onset of arrhythmias); however, if the arrhythmias are more frequent, cardiac output may decrease, and therefore shortness of breath and dizziness may occur.

### Treatment

The treatment for PVCs depends on the underlying cause, the frequency and severity of the PVCs, and the symptoms associated with them. The frequency and the type of evidence for them indicate the seriousness of the patient's condition

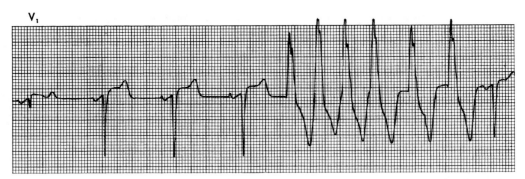

**Figure 9-40** Ventricular tachycardia. (From Conover MB. Exercises in diagnosing ECG tracings, ed 3. St. Louis, 1984, Mosby.)

and help to determine the clinical decision. PVCs are considered to be serious, or possibly life-threatening, when they
- Are paired together (see Fig. 9-39E)
- Are multifocal in origin (see Fig. 9-39B)
- Are more frequent than 6 per minute
- Land directly on the T wave (see Fig. 9-39D)
- Are present in triplets or more (see Fig. 9-39F)

PVCs are considered to be serious or life-threatening because they may indicate increased irritability of the ventricular muscle and may progress to ventricular tachycardia or ventricular fibrillation—two medical emergencies.

Although PVCs may be benign, a full cardiac evaluation should be performed to rule out underlying disease in the individual who demonstrates a sudden onset of PVCs.[6] If the individual has a history of arrhythmias, if the individual with arrhythmias is asymptomatic, and if the frequency or seriousness of the arrhythmias does not change, then treatment is unwarranted. If the arrhythmias produce symptoms or appear to be more frequent either throughout the day or with increased activity, then further evaluation and possibly treatment is warranted. If an individual with chronic lung disease has a new onset of PVCs it may indicate hypoxemia, and supplemental oxygen may be necessary. Otherwise, after all the underlying causes are evaluated, antiarrhythmic medications may be warranted. Caution should be taken when an individual begins antiarrhythmic medication as antiarrhythmic medication therapy is not always effective and can even produce arrhythmias. See Chapter 14 for more information on the pharmacologic management of PVCs.

> **Clinical Tip**
> Premature ventricular contractions, when isolated, without symptoms, and fewer than 6 per minute, are usually considered benign and do not warrant treatment. When PVCs are more frequent than 6 per minute, are paired or multifocal, patients may require closer monitoring or medical treatment. Medical treatment may also cause arrhythmias and may not abate the arrhythmias.

## Ventricular Tachycardia

Ventricular tachycardia is defined as a series of three or more PVCs in a row. Ventricular tachycardia occurs because of a rapid firing by a single ventricular focus with increased automaticity (see Fig. 9-39F and Fig. 9-40). The characteristics of ventricular tachycardia include the following:
- P waves are absent.
- Three or more PVCs occur in a row.
- QRS complexes of the ventricular tachycardia are wide and bizarre.
- Ventricular rate of ventricular tachycardia is between 100 and 250 beats per minute.
- Ventricular tachycardia can be the precursor to ventricular fibrillation.

### Signs, Symptoms, and Causes

Causes of ventricular tachycardia include ischemia or acute infarction, coronary artery disease, hypertensive heart disease, and reaction to medications (digoxin or quinidine toxicity). Occasionally ventricular tachycardia occurs in athletes during exercise (possibly as a result of electrolyte imbalance). Ventricular tachycardia indicates increased irritability as well as an emergency situation because cardiac output is greatly diminished, as is the blood pressure. Symptoms usually involve lightheadedness and sometimes syncope. A weak, thready pulse may be present. The individual may become disoriented if ventricular tachycardia is sustained. Ventricular tachycardia can progress to ventricular fibrillation and death.

### Treatment

Treatment usually is an immediate pharmacologic injection (lidocaine, bretylium tosylate [Bretylol], or procainamide [Pronestyl]) or cardioversion or defibrillation. Ventricular tachycardia is considered a medical emergency.

### Ventricular Tachycardia: Torsade de Pointes

Torsade de pointes is a unique configuration of ventricular tachycardia called the "twisting of the points" (Fig. 9-41). Torsade de pointes is often associated with a prolonged Q-T interval (>0.5 second). The name relates to its presentation by twisting around the isoelectric line. This arrhythmia characteristically occurs at a rapid rate and terminates spontaneously.

### Signs, Symptoms, and Causes

This type of ventricular tachycardia has been identified only in individuals receiving antiarrhythmic therapy and for whom

Increasing amplitude        Decreasing amplitude

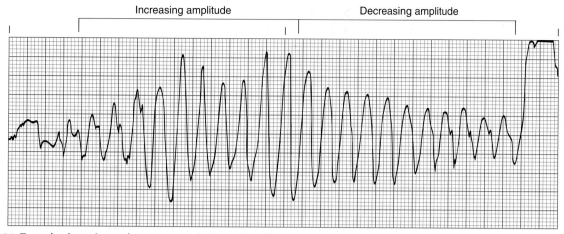

**Figure 9-41** Torsade de pointes; heart rate = 240 to 250. (From Atwood S. Introduction to Basic Cardiac Dysrhythmias, ed 4. St. Louis, 2009, Mosby.)

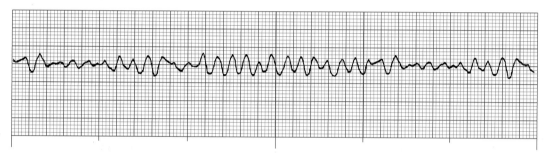

**Figure 9-42** Coarse ventricular fibrillation. (From Aehlert BJ. ECGs Made Easy, ed 4. St. Louis, 2010, Mosby.)

the medication is toxic. As cardiac output is severely diminished and as this arrhythmia often converts to ventricular fibrillation, this condition is considered a medical emergency.[1] The individual who remains conscious with this arrhythmia may be extremely lightheaded or near syncope.

### Treatment
Treatment is usually cardioversion.

### Ventricular Fibrillation

Ventricular fibrillation is defined as an erratic quivering of the ventricular muscle resulting in no cardiac output. As in atrial fibrillation, multiple ectopic foci fire, creating asynchrony. The ECG results in a picture of grossly irregular up and down fluctuations of the baseline in an irregular zigzag pattern (Fig. 9-42).

### Signs, Symptoms, and Causes
The causes of ventricular fibrillation are the same as those of ventricular tachycardia because ventricular fibrillation is usually the sequel to ventricular tachycardia.

### Treatment
Treatment is defibrillation as quickly as possible followed by cardiopulmonary resuscitation, supplemental oxygen, and injection of medications. An example of defibrillation during firing of an Implantable Cardiac Defibrillator (ICD) is shown

in Figure 9-43. However, if the tracing appears to be ventricular fibrillation, and the patient does not have a long-term history of recurrent ventricular tachycardia or ventricular fibrillation, and the patient is able to carry on a conversation, the therapist should assume this is probably only lead displacement creating artifact.

## Other Findings on a 12-Lead Electrocardiogram

### Hypertrophy

Hypertrophy refers to an increase in thickness of cardiac muscle or chamber size. Signs of atrial hypertrophy can be noted by examining the P waves of the ECG for a diphasic P wave in the chest lead V1, or a voltage in excess of 3 mV. Signs of right ventricular hypertrophy are noted by changes found in lead V1 that include a large R wave and an S wave smaller than the R wave. The R wave becomes progressively smaller in the successive chest leads (V2, V3, V4, V5). Hypertrophy of the left ventricle creates enlarged QRS complexes in the chest leads in both height of the QRS (R wave) and depth of the QRS (S wave). In left ventricular hypertrophy a deep S wave occurs in V1 and a large R wave in V5. If when the depth of the S wave in V1 (in mm) is added to the height of the R wave in V5 (in mm) the resulting number is greater than 35, then left ventricular hypertrophy is present (Fig. 9-44).

**ICD: Tiered Therapy**

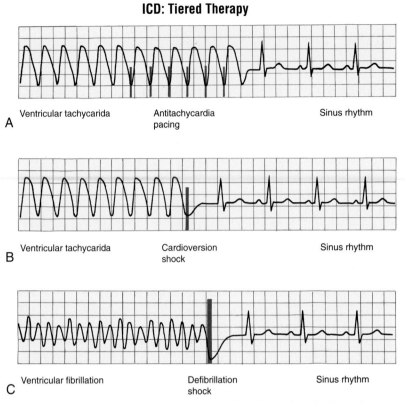

A    Ventricular tachycarida    Antitachycardia    Sinus rhythm
                                pacing

B    Ventricular tachycarida    Cardioversion    Sinus rhythm
                                shock

C    Ventricular fibrillation    Defibrillation    Sinus rhythm
                                 shock

**Figure 9-43** Tiered arrhythmia therapy and implanted cardioverter-defibrillators (ICDs). These devices are capable of automatically delivering staged therapy in treating ventricular tachycardia (VT) or ventricular fibrillation (VF), including antitachycardia pacing (A) and cardioversion shocks (B) for VT, and defibrillation shocks (C) for VF. (From Goldberger: Clinical Electrocardiography: A Simplified Approach, ed 7. St Louis, 2006, Mosby.)

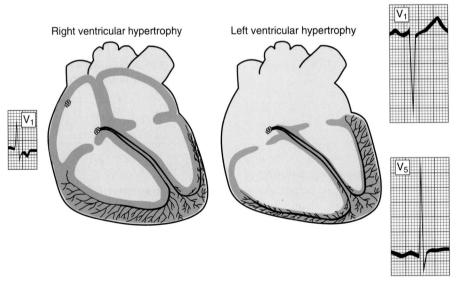

Right ventricular hypertrophy    Left ventricular hypertrophy

**Figure 9-44** Hypertrophy is determined by looking at voltage in V1 and V5. Right ventricular hypertrophy is defined as a large R wave in V1, which gets progressively smaller in V2, V3, and V4; normally there is a very small R wave and a large S wave in V1. Left ventricular hypertrophy is defined as a large S wave in V1 and a large R wave in V5 that have a combined voltage of greater than 35 mV.

## Ischemia, Infarction, or Injury

A review of a 12-lead ECG to detect ischemia, infarction, or injury is performed in a variety of situations, including after any episode of chest pain that brings a patient to the physician's office or to the hospital, during hospitalization, during a followup examination after a cardiac event, or before conducting an exercise test. The difference between ischemia and infarction is covered in detail in Chapter 3. In simplistic terms, ischemia literally means reduced blood

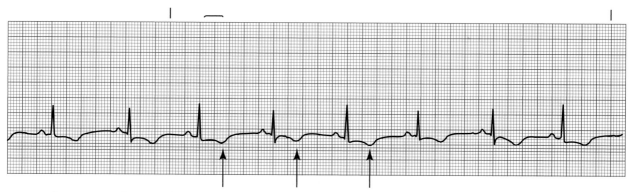

**Figure 9-45** Electrocardiogram tracing showing an inverted T wave, often indicating ischemia (*arrows*).

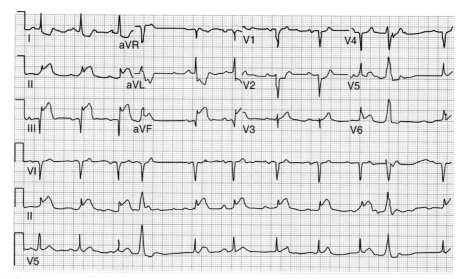

**Figure 9-46** Acute inferior myocardial infarction with ST elevation in the inferior leads. (From Rakel RE. Textbook of Family Medicine, ed 7. Philadelphia, 2007, Saunders.)

and refers to a diminished blood supply to the myocardium. This can occur because of occlusion of the coronary arteries from vasospasm, atherosclerotic occlusion, thrombus, or a combination of the three. Infarction means cell death and results from a complete occlusion of a coronary artery. Injury indicates the acuteness of the infarction. As a result of ischemia, injury, or infarction, conduction of electrical impulses is altered, and therefore depolarization of the muscle changes. As the ECG records the depolarization of the cardiac muscle, changes occur on the ECG in the presence of ischemia, infarction, or injury. The location of the ischemia, infarction, or injury is determined according to the specific leads of the ECG that demonstrate an alteration in depolarization.

Ischemia is classically demonstrated on the 12-lead ECG with T-wave inversion or ST-segment depression. The T wave may vary from a flat configuration to a depressed inverted wave (Fig. 9-45). The T wave is an extremely sensitive indication of changes in repolarization activity within the ventricles.[8] Transient fluctuations in the T wave can be observed in numerous situations and must be associated with the activity and symptoms to determine if the abnormality is

ischemic. For an individual who comes to a physician's office because of an episode of chest pain, T-wave inversion may be the only noticeable abnormality. If the individual took nitroglycerin while at the office and the pain disappeared before the ECG was administered, abnormalities may be absent owing to the resolution of the ischemic event.

The location of the ST segment (that portion of the ECG tracing beginning with the end of the S wave and ending with the beginning of the T wave) is another indication of ischemia or injury. Elevation of the ST segment above the baseline when following part of an R wave indicates acute injury (Fig. 9-46). In the presence of acute infarction, the ST segment elevates and then later returns to the level of the baseline (within 24 to 48 hours).[8] ST-segment elevation may also occur in the presence of a ventricular aneurysm (a ballooning out of the ventricular wall, usually following a large amount of damage to the ventricular wall). The ST-segment elevation with ventricular aneurysm never returns to the isoelectric line, and the configuration differs somewhat. The ST-segment elevation in ventricular aneurysm usually follows a large Q wave and not an R wave of the QRS complex (see Fig. 9-46). If the ECG records the presence of ST-segment

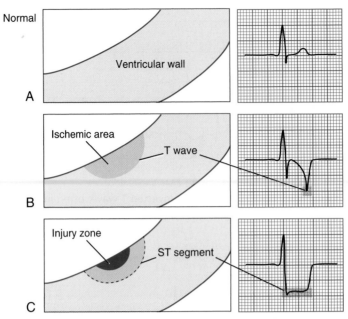

**Figure 9-47** An ST segment on a resting 12-lead ECG often is indicative of subendocardial injury. **A,** Normal tracing and normal ventricular wall. **B,** Subendocardial ischemia with an ECG tracing of T-wave inversion. **C,** Subendocardial injury with ST-segment depression on the ECG.

elevation in the presence of acute onset of chest pain (within hours), a cardiac emergency exists and immediate treatment is indicated.

The ECG may demonstrate ST-segment depression while the patient is at rest in the presence of chest pain or of suspected coronary ischemia. The ST-segment depression in this situation represents subendocardial infarction and also requires immediate treatment. A subendocardial infarct (also called a nontransmural, non–Q-wave infarct or non–ST-segment elevation myocardial infarction [STEMI] infarct) is an acute injury to the myocardial wall, but it does not extend through the full thickness of the ventricular wall. Instead, the injury is only to the subendocardium (Fig. 9-47).

This ECG sign is extremely significant, because it indicates that a transmural (also called STEMI or Q wave) infarction could be pending. Research shows that an individual diagnosed with a subendocardial infarction is at extremely high risk for another infarction (this time transmural) within 6 weeks.[9]

Other situations may precipitate ST-segment depression. ST-segment depression in the absence of suspected ischemia or angina may be caused by digitalis toxicity (see Chapter 14 for discussion of digitalis toxicity). ST-segment depression that develops during exercise, as seen during exercise testing, is defined as an ischemic response to exercise, and following rest it should return to the isoelectric line. This is an abnormal response to exercise that indicates an impaired coronary arterial supply during the exercise. This type of ischemic response should be further evaluated to determine the extent of the coronary artery involvement (see Chapter 8).

During myocardial injury, the affected area of muscle loses its ability to generate electrical impulses, and therefore alterations in the initial portion of the QRS complex occur. The cells are dead and cannot depolarize normally, which results in an inability to conduct impulses. Therefore, as ST-segment elevation or depression is diagnostic for acute infarction, the presence of a significant Q wave (Fig. 9-48) is also diagnostic for infarction, but the date of the infarction is not able to be determined simply by studying the ECG. The date of the infarction is determined by the patient's report of symptoms. The Q wave is the first downward part of the QRS complex (not preceded by anything else), and small Q waves may be present normally in some leads. When the Q wave is 0.06 second in duration wide (one small square on the ECG tracing) or is one-third the size (height and depth included) of the QRS complex, the Q wave is considered to be significant and indicative of a pathologic condition (it persists as a permanent electrocardiographic "scar" from infarction [see Fig. 9-48]). Therefore, any scan of the ECG should include a check for the presence of significant Q waves to identify previous infarction.

The leads that demonstrate the presence of T-wave inversion, ST-segment changes, or Q waves identify the location of the ischemia, injury, or infarction. The presence of significant Q waves in the chest leads, particularly in V1, V2, V3, and V4, indicates an infarction in the anterior portion of the left ventricle. When only V1 and V2 are involved, these infarctions are often called "septal" infarctions because they primarily affect the interventricular septum. Anterior infarctions are easy to recognize if one remembers that the chest leads are placed on the anterior aspect of the left ventricle (Fig. 9-49). Referring back to Chapter 1, remember that because the left anterior descending artery primarily supplies the anterior aspect of the heart, an anterior infarction implies an occlusion somewhere in the left anterior descending artery.

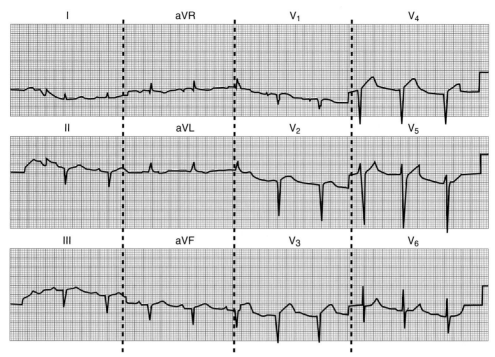

**Figure 9-48** A significant Q wave is defined as a minimum of one small square wide and one-third the height of the QRS. In this electrocardiogram tracing, notice the Q waves in leads II, III, and aVF and in V1, V2, V3, and V4.

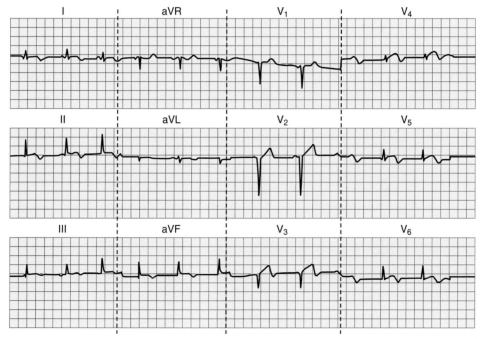

**Figure 9-49** A 12-lead electrocardiogram tracing demonstrating an anterior infarction. Note the significant Q waves in V1, V2, and V3 and the inverted T waves throughout many other leads.

An inferior infarction is identified by significant Q waves in leads II, III, and aVF (Fig. 9-50A). Inferior infarctions are also referred to as diaphragmatic infarctions because the inferior wall of the heart rests on the diaphragm. Given that the right coronary artery primarily supplies the inferior aspect of the myocardium, an inferior infarction implies an occlusion somewhere in the right coronary artery. A lateral infarction demonstrates Q waves in leads I and aVL (Fig. 9-50B). Because the circumflex artery supplies primarily the lateral and posterior aspects of the myocardium, an occlusion of the circumflex artery is suspected in a lateral infarction.

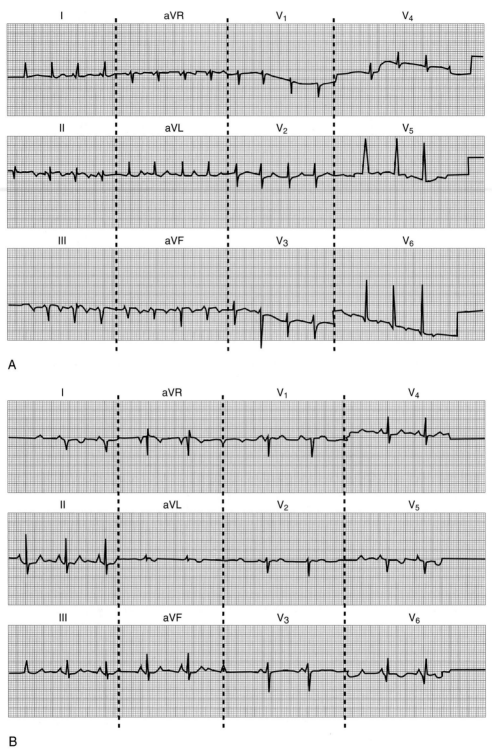

**Figure 9-50 A,** A 12-lead electrocardiogram tracing demonstrating an inferior infarction. Notice the significant Q waves in leads II, III, and aVF. **B,** A 12-lead electrocardiogram tracing demonstrating a lateral infarction. Notice the significant Q waves in I and V5 with inverted T waves in aVL as well.

Probably the most difficult infarction to detect is the posterior infarction because none of the 12 leads is directly measuring the posterior aspect of the heart. Only two leads detect posterior infarcts—V1 and V2—as they measure the direct opposite wall (anterior). Therefore, the direct opposite ECG tracing of an anterior infarction in V1 and V2 should be the ECG tracing of the posterior infarction. An anterior infarction demonstrates a significant Q wave in V1 and V2 with ST-segment elevation. The mirror image of this is seen in Figure 9-51, which demonstrates a large R wave in V1 or V2 and ST-segment depression. Given that the posterior aspect of the myocardium may be supplied by either the right

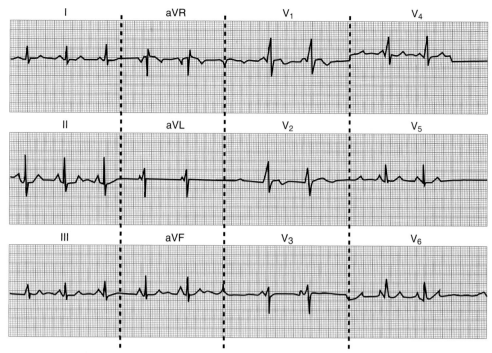

**Figure 9-51** A 12-lead electrocardiogram tracing demonstrating a posterior infarction. Notice the large R waves in V1 and V2 and the inverted T waves in the same leads.

coronary artery or the circumflex artery, a posterior infarction may indicate a problem in either one of these arteries. If changes in the lateral leads (e.g., I, aVL) also exist, then the circumflex artery is probably involved. However, if changes in the inferior leads exist (e.g., II, III, aVR) as well as posterior changes, then the right coronary artery is probably involved.[8]

Caution should be taken when evaluation of an ECG for an infarction is performed in the presence of left bundle branch block.[8] Identification of significant Q waves can be difficult if the conduction is delayed throughout the myocardium on the left side. Conduction may be delayed through the myocardium owing to a dysfunction in the conduction system that is secondary to genetic defect, injury, or infarction. An example of conduction delay with bundle branch block occurs when a block of the impulse occurs in the right or left bundle branch. A bundle branch block creates a delay of the electrical impulse to the side that is blocked, creating a delay in the depolarization of the myocardium that would have received the blocked impulse. When the left and right sides do not depolarize simultaneously, a widened QRS appearance is seen on the ECG tracing and sometimes two R waves. In the case of left bundle branch block, the left side of the myocardium demonstrates delayed depolarization, thereby allowing the right side of the myocardium to depolarize first and hiding any possible significant Q waves coming from the left ventricle (Fig. 9-52).

A systematic review of the 12 lead ECG will improve one's ability to interpret the 12-lead ECG correctly. A systematic approach includes:

- Identify and separate the 12 leads by applying vertical lines between leads I and avR, avR and V1, and V1 and V4.
- Scan all leads to identify if there are any significant Q waves. If so, note which leads demonstrate a significant Q wave.
- Scan all leads to identify if there is any ST elevation or ST depression. If so, note which leads demonstrate ST changes.
- Scan leads V1, V5, and V6 to look for ventricular hypertrophy. A large R in V1 indicates R ventricular hypertrophy and a deep S in V1 with a large R in V5 indicates left ventricular hypertrophy.

Acute pericarditis is a condition that causes ECG changes that differ from those caused by ischemia and infarction. These ECG changes are important to mention because they assist in the diagnosis of the condition. Acute pericarditis, defined as an inflammation of the pericardial sac, is often a complication following myocardial infarction and open heart surgery. Pericardial pain is usually intense but can closely mimic angina in location. The pain is usually aggravated or relieved by respiration and change of position. The ECG findings include ST-segment elevation, P-R interval depression, late T-wave inversion, and atrial arrhythmias (often supraventricular tachycardia) (Fig. 9-53). The symptoms as well as the ECG changes are often all that is needed for diagnosis. In addition, a pericardial rub may be present during auscultation of the heart sounds.

Other abnormalities may exist on the ECG, including pacemaker functioning (Figs. 9-54 and 9-55), which is discussed in Chapter 11, and axis deviation. These abnormalities are beyond the scope of this chapter.

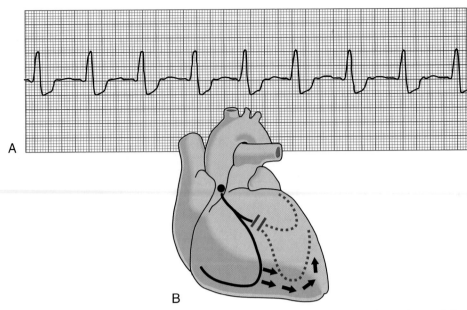

**Figure 9-52 A,** A rhythm strip demonstrating a left bundle branch block. Note the widened QRS interval. **B,** A left bundle branch block.

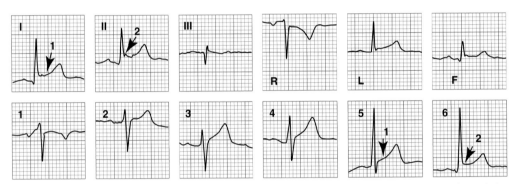

**Figure 9-53** Acute pericarditis. In the first few days, the ECG shows ST elevation, concave upward, with upright T waves in most leads. Classically it is more obvious in lead II than in leads I or III. There are no pathologic Q waves, and the widespread distribution of ST–T changes without reciprocal depression distinguishes acute pericarditis from early myocardial infarction. In the later stages of pericarditis, the T waves become inverted in most leads. The ECG changes in pericarditis are caused by the superficial myocarditis that accompanies it. (From Forbes CD. Color Atlas and Text of Clinical Medicine, ed 3. St. Louis, 2004, Mosby.)

---

### CASE STUDY 9-1

A 68-year-old man has a history of an acute myocardial infarction that occurred 7 months ago. He subsequently underwent coronary artery bypass graft surgery exactly 1 month after the myocardial infarction. It is now 6 months since his surgery, and he is symptom-free. His goal is to return to his previously active lifestyle, so he was referred for an evaluation and exercise program.

On evaluation, his heart rate is 70 beats per minute, blood pressure is 124/84 mm Hg, and ECG is NSR. During the exercise treadmill test, he exercised at 2.5 miles per hour with 12% grade but complained of dizziness at 4.5 minutes of the exercise test. His heart rate was 110 beats per minute and blood pressure was 130/78 mm Hg. The ECG rhythm showed a sudden onset of PVCs and a run of ventricular tachycardia. After the exercise was terminated, his rhythm slowed down to frequent PVCs and then NSR.

#### Discussion

This case demonstrates changes in the heart rhythm with increased activity. PVCs and then ventricular tachycardia occurred with increased activity, corresponding to increased irritability of the myocardium (i.e., probably secondary to ischemia). The individual was symptomatic when the arrhythmias were frequent. This patient should not be exercising to a heart rate of 110 beats per minute and may need further evaluation for the abnormal response with exercise.

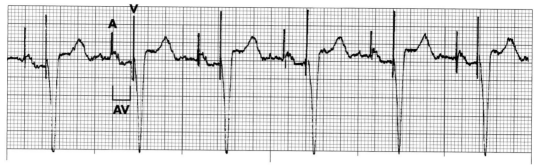

**Figure 9-54** AV sequential pacing. A, Atrial pacing; V, ventricular pacing; AV, AV interval. (From Aehlert BJ: ACLS Study Guide, ed 3. St Louis, 2007, Mosby.)

## Dual-Chamber (DDD) Pacemaker Functions

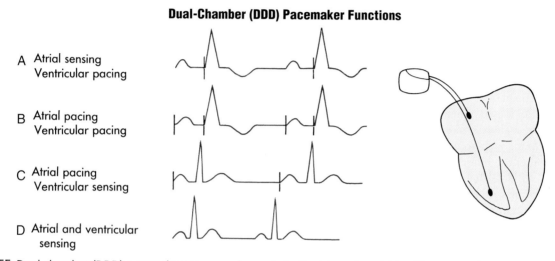

A Atrial sensing
  Ventricular pacing

B Atrial pacing
  Ventricular pacing

C Atrial pacing
  Ventricular sensing

D Atrial and ventricular
  sensing

**Figure 9-55** Dual-chamber (DDD) pacemakers sense and pace in both atria and ventricles. The pacemaker emits a stimulus (spike) whenever a native P wave or QRS complex is not sensed within some programmed time interval. (From Goldberger AL. Clinical Electrocardiography: A Simplified Approach, ed 7. Philadelphia, 2007, Mosby.)

## Summary

- Four cell types exist in the myocardium: working or mechanical cells, nodal cells, transitional cells, and Purkinje cells.
- Depolarization of the cell membrane allows the influx of sodium ions into the cell and the efflux of potassium ions.
- As the cell becomes positive on the interior, the myocardial cells are stimulated to contract (called excitation coupling).
- On the ECG, the wave of depolarization is recorded as an upward deflection when moving toward a positive electrode (located on the skin).
- The cardiac muscle has three properties: automaticity, rhythmicity, and conductivity.
- The autonomic nervous system has a major influence on the cardiac system. Stimulation of the sympathetic division increases the heart rate, conduction velocity, and contractile force, and stimulation of the parasympathetic division (acting primarily via the vagal nerve) slows the heart rate and the conduction through the AV node.

- The conduction system involves the spread of a stimulus via the SA node (primary pacemaker), internodal pathways, AV node, His bundle, bundle branches, and Purkinje fibers.
- The ECG records the electrical activity of the heart on ruled graph paper. Time is represented on the horizontal axis, and each small square is 0.04 second. Voltage is recorded on the vertical axis, and each small square is 1 mm.
- A standard 12-lead ECG consists of 6 limb leads and 6 chest leads, each recording the electrical activity from a different angle and providing a different view of the same activity in the heart.
- The ECG is reviewed to identify four areas that require interpretation: heart rate, heart rhythm, hypertrophy, and infarction.
- Numerous methods can be employed to measure heart rate from the ECG tracing, but often the 6-second strip method is the easiest if the rhythm is regular.
- Hypertrophy is detected on a 12-lead ECG by looking at the waveforms, particularly at the P wave and

QRS complex for the voltage (greater than 3 mV) or configuration.

- Left ventricular hypertrophy is present if the depth of the S wave in V1 plus the height of the R wave in V5 is greater than 35 mm.
- In the presence of acute injury, the ST segment is elevated above the isoelectric line and gradually returns to the level of the isoelectric line over a period of 24 to 48 hours.
- In ventricular aneurysm, the ST segment remains elevated and does not return to the isoelectric line over time.
- ST-segment depression at rest associated with chest pain may indicate acute injury to the subendocardial wall.
- ST-segment depression that develops during exercise is an ischemic response to activity and following rest should return to the baseline.
- The presence of a significant Q wave is diagnostic for an infarction, but the date of the infarction cannot be determined from the ECG.
- A significant Q wave is 1 mm wide or one-third the size of the QRS complex.
- A 12-lead ECG is used primarily for determining ischemia or infarction. Single-lead monitoring is employed for evaluating heart rate or rhythm.
- The location of the infarction is determined by the leads on the 12-lead ECG that demonstrate changes.
- The presence of significant Q waves in V1 through V4 indicates an anterior infarction and probable involvement of the left anterior descending coronary artery.
- The presence of significant Q waves in II, III, and aVF indicates an inferior infarction and probable involvement of the right coronary artery.

- A systematic approach should be taken when evaluating the rhythm strip. All the waveform configurations should be evaluated, as well as the P-R intervals, the QRS intervals, the R-R intervals, and the rate to assess the rhythm disturbance.
- Following identification of the rhythm disturbance, an assessment of signs and symptoms should be undertaken, after which a clinical decision can be made regarding the amount of monitoring the individual will need with activity as well as the safety of activity.

## References

1. Cohen M, Fuster V. Insights into the pathogenetic mechanisms of unstable angina. Haemostasis 20(Suppl 1):102–12, 1990.
2. Schaper J, Schaper W. Time course of myocardial necrosis. Cardiovasc Drugs Ther 2(1):17–25, 1988.
3. Bekn Haim SA, Becker B, Edoute Y, et al. Beat to beat electrocardiographic morphology variation in healed myocardial infarction. Am J Cardiol 68(8):725–8, 1991.
4. Phillips RE, Feeney MK. The Cardiac Rhythms: A Systematic Approach to Interpretation. 3rd ed. Philadelphia, Saunders, 1990.
5. Scheidt S: Basic Electrocardiography: Leads, Axes, Arrhythmias. Summit, NJ, CIBA Clinical Symposia, 1983.
6. Berne RM, Levy MN. Cardiovascular Physiology. 6th ed. St. Louis, Mosby-Year Book, 1992.
7. Grauer K, Curry RW. Clinical Electrocardiography: A Primary Care Approach. 2nd ed. Boston, Blackwell Scientific Publishers, 1992.
8. Abedin Z, Conner RP. 12-Lead ECG Interpretation: The Self-Assessment Approach. Philadelphia, Saunders, 1989.
9. Valle BK, Lemberg L. Non-Q wave versus nontransmural infarction. Heart Lung 19(2):208–11, 1990.

## CHAPTER 10

# Pulmonary Diagnostic Tests and Procedures

*Ana Lotshaw, H. Steven Sadowsky, Ellen Hillegass*

## Chapter Outline

This chapter introduces the reader to several of the diagnostic tests and procedures commonly used in the assessment of patients with pulmonary disease. Although the tests and procedures described in this chapter are not necessarily performed by physical therapists, they nonetheless provide physical therapists with invaluable information. To apply this information to the planning, implementation, and monitoring of patient treatments, physical therapists must have a fundamental understanding of chest imaging, pulmonary function testing, bronchoscopy, arterial blood gas analysis, oximetry, and bacteriologic and cytologic tests. Chapter 17 discusses the incorporation of this information in the evaluative process.

## Chest Imaging

Largely as a result of new technologies, but also because of refinements in older techniques, there are now several imaging options in addition to the standard "plain film" radiograph. It is certainly beyond the scope of this text to present all the abnormal chest findings identifiable by these imaging techniques. Rather, this information is intended to assist in the development of a framework on which to build an understanding of these imaging techniques. A basic knowledge of how these images are produced and what they display can facilitate physician–therapist dialogue and enhance physical therapy treatment planning.

### Chest Radiographs

Despite the availability of newer methods, in most clinical settings the standard radiograph remains the predominant diagnostic test to determine anatomic abnormalities and pathologic processes within the chest, The newer, more technologically advanced imaging techniques are discussed in this chapter in their role to confirm or provide differential diagnostic information that can contribute to information obtained from a chest radiograph.

The standard upright views of the chest are made when a patient is typically placed between an x-ray source and a cassette (Fig. 10-1). When the x-rays penetrate the tissues of the patient, they stimulate the fluorescent screen to emit light that exposes the film. The radiograph thus produced is referred to as a roentgenogram and named after Wilhelm Konrad Roentgen, who received the first Nobel Prize for Physics in 1901 for his work in defining the major properties of x-rays and the conditions necessary for their production. It was Roentgen who coined the term "x-ray."[1-4]

Chest radiographs provide a static view of the anatomy of the chest, and as such, they may be used to screen for abnormalities, to provide a baseline from which subsequent assessments can be made, or to monitor the progress of a disease process or treatment intervention. The principal objects shown on a chest radiograph are air, fat, water, tissue, and bone. Air in the lungs has a very low density and thus allows greater x-ray penetration, resulting in a dark image on the

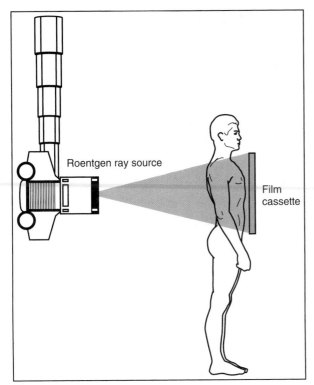

Roentgen ray source

Film cassette

**Figure 10-1** For a standard posteroanterior radiograph the patient stands between the film cassette and x-ray source.

radiograph (radiolucency). At the opposite extreme is bone, which, because it is denser, allows fewer x-rays to penetrate and results in a white image on a radiograph (radiopacity). Depending on the densities and thicknesses of the numerous structures in the chest, the x-rays penetrating a patient are variably absorbed and create "shadows" on the radiographic film. Several other factors also affect the image depicted on a radiographic film, but are beyond the scope of this chapter. The reader is referred to standard radiology texts for more detailed information.

The standard chest radiograph is routinely taken in two views at near total lung capacity: (1) a posteroanterior (PA) view with the patient in the standing position with the front of the chest facing the film cassette (Fig. 10-2) and (2) a left lateral view (Fig. 10-3), unless the pathologic process is known to be present on the right side of the chest (in which case, a right lateral view would be obtained). The lateral view is extremely helpful in localizing the position of an abnormality, because in the PA view, the upper and middle lobes of the lung override portions of the lower lobes. Other views that can be obtained include the following:

- Decubitus views are taken to confirm the presence of an air–fluid level in the lungs or a small pleural effusion. Depending upon the location of the suspected disease, the patient is placed in the supine, prone, or right or left side-lying position.
- The lordotic view is used to visualize the apical or middle (right middle lobe or left lingular segments) regions of the lungs, or specifically to screen for pulmonary tuberculosis, which typically manifests itself

in the apical regions. The x-ray source is lowered and angled upward, and the patient may or may not be tipped slightly backward.

- Oblique views are taken to detect pleural thickening, to evaluate the carina, or to visualize the heart and great vessels. The patient is positioned standing diagonally (at an angle of 45 to 60 degrees to the film) with either the left or right anterior, or the left or right posterior, chest against the film cassette (anterior or posterior oblique views, respectively).
- The anteroposterior (AP) view is taken at the patient's bedside when the patient is unable to travel to the radiology department. AP radiographs are obtained with the patient either supine, semirecumbent, or sitting upright against the film cassette and facing the x-ray machine. When the film is take in the supine position, the abdominal contents tend to elevate the hemidiaphragms, the pulmonary blood flow is redistributed, and the mediastinal structures appear larger (Fig. 10-4).

> **Clinical Tip**
> Positioning for AP views (supine or semirecumbent) often result in a poor inspiratory effort, especially when the patient is critically ill. Clinicians observing AP films must keep this in mind when assessing the film.

The potential interpreter of radiographs is presented with several challenges, among these are the two-dimensional representation of three-dimensional objects and the limited gray-scale "shadow" depiction of the various organs, tissues, and pathologic processes. Although it may be more likely that the clinician will have access to a radiologist's report rather than the actual radiograph, many clinical settings offer the therapist direct access to a patient's chest radiographs. Consequently, therapists should be familiar with the manner in which chest radiographs are assessed.

## Examining Chest Radiographs

Although there is no single "best" method for examining chest radiographs, a systematic approach should be used. One approach entails starting at the center of the film and working outward toward the soft tissues. Another method involves starting with an examination of the bones and soft tissues, including the abdomen; the mediastinum from the larynx to the abdomen; the cardiovascular system; the hila; and finally the lung fields themselves. Independent of the method of examination, the mediastinum and hila are typically assessed for abnormal vasculature or mass lesions, the heart for changes in shape or position, and the lungs for abnormal increased density or lucency. By convention, frontal chest radiographs should be viewed as if the patient's right side was on your left side, as if you were facing each other. The left lateral chest radiograph should be viewed as if the patient's left side was facing you; the reverse is true for the right lateral view.

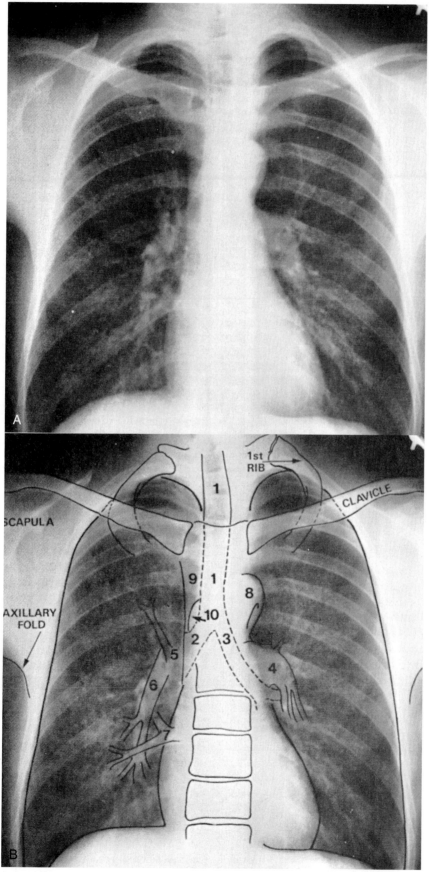

**Figure 10-2  A,** Normal chest radiograph, posteroanterior view. **B,** Same radiograph as in **(A)**, with the normal anatomic structures labeled or numbered: *1,* trachea; *2,* right mainstem bronchus; *3,* left mainstem bronchus; *4,* left pulmonary artery; *5,* pulmonary vein to the right upper lobe; *6,* right interlobular artery; *7,* vein to right middle and lower lobes; *8,* aortic knob; *9,* superior vena cava. (From Fraser RG, Paré JAP. Diagnosis of Diseases of the Chest. Vol. I. 2nd ed. Philadelphia, Saunders, 1977:172, 173.)

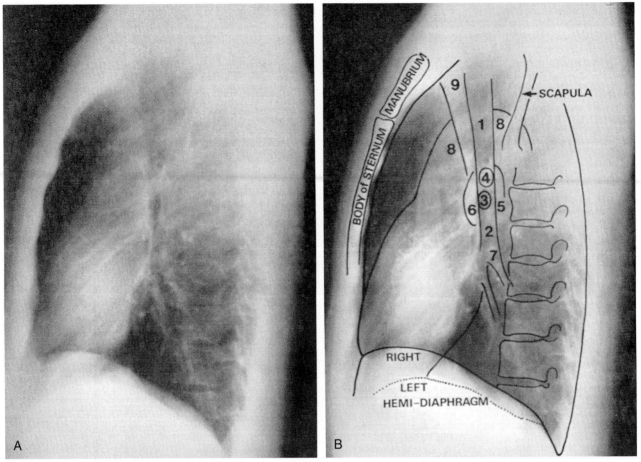

**Figure 10-3 A,** Normal chest radiograph, lateral view. **B,** Same radiograph as in **(A)**, with the normal anatomic structures labeled or numbered: *1,* trachea; *2,* right intermediate bronchus; *3,* left upper lobe bronchus; *4,* right upper lobe bronchus; *5,* left inter-lobar artery; *6,* right interlobar artery; *7,* junction of the pulmonary veins; *8,* aortic arch; *9,* brachiocephalic vessels. (From Fraser RG, Paré JAP. Diagnosis of Diseases of the Chest. Vol. I. 2nd ed. Philadelphia, Saunders, 1977:174, 175.)

---

**Box 10-1**

A systematic approach is essential for interpreting the por-table chest radiograph. The steps are as follows:
- Assess the technical quality of the study.
- Evaluate the location of all catheters, tubes, and support devices.
- Assess the cardiovascular status of the patient.
- Check for abnormal parenchymal opacities.
- Search for evidence of barotrauma.
- Look for pleural effusions.
- Compare with the prior studies; does the patient look the same, better, or worse?

---

Box 10-1 provides a systematic approach to assessment of a portable chest radiograph.

In the body systems approach to examining chest radio-graphs, the overall adequacy of the image should first be addressed. The optimal radiograph should be taken with the patient holding a deep inspiration. Furthermore, the entire chest should be visible on the radiograph (see Fig. 10-2). Then, the following should be considered in turn.

## Bones and Soft Tissues

The size, shape, and symmetry of the bony thorax should be considered; the vertebral bodies should be faintly visible through the mediastinal shadow, and all of the other bones of the thorax should be included on the radiograph.

To determine whether or not the patient is rotated to either side, the medial ends of each clavicle should be checked to see that they are equally distant from the spinous processes of the vertebral bodies (if the patient is rotated, the distances between the medial ends of the clavicles and the spinous processes will be unequal). In a PA film the clavicles often appear to be lower than in an AP film. Because of the position of the shoulders, the medial aspect of the scapulas are typi-cally lateral to and outside the lung fields in a PA film; whereas, in an AP film, the medial borders may appear as vertical or oblique lines within the lung fields.

The various densities of the soft tissues (skin, subcutane-ous fat, and muscle) normally blend together—called the *summation effect.* The width of the intercostal spaces should be considered because widened intercostal spaces may be indicative of increased thoracic volume (the best way to gain an appreciation of the normal intercostal space width is to review normal chest radiographs).

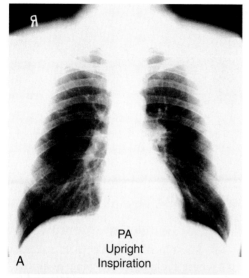

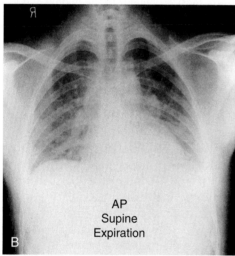

**Figure 10-4** Summation of the effect of position, projection, and respiration. A normal posteroanterior upright chest radiograph with full inspiration **(A)**. Another radiograph was taken of this perfectly healthy college student 1 minute later; it was done in an anteroposterior projection while he was lying supine and during expiration **(B)**. The wide cardiac shadow and prominent pulmonary vascularity could easily trick you into thinking that this individual was in congestive heart failure. (From Mettler FA. Essentials of Radiology. 2nd ed. Philadelphia, Saunders, 2005.)

The two hemidiaphragms should appear as rounded, smooth, sharply defined shadows; the dome of the right hemidiaphragm is normally 1 to 2 cm higher than the left. The diaphragm is said to be elevated if, during a deep inhalation, fewer than nine ribs are visible above the level of the domes; depressed if more than 10 ribs are visible. Where the hemidiaphragms meet the chest wall at their lateral aspects, the costophrenic angles are formed. The costophrenic angles are moderately deep, and they are approximately equal in size on the two sides. Opacification of the costophrenic angle is indicative of either pleural thickening (if the change has occurred over many months or years) or

a pleural effusion (if the change has occurred recently). Medially, the hemidiaphragms normally form a cardiophrenic angle where they meet the borders of the heart.

### Mediastinum, Trachea and Cardiovascular System

The size of the mediastinum varies with body size, ranging from long and narrow in tall, thin persons to short and wide in short, stocky persons.

The borders of the mediastinum are generally as outlined in Figure 1-16 The trachea normally appears as a vertical translucent shadow superimposed on the mediastinal shadow in the midline, overlying the cervical vertebrae. In most cases, tracheal deviation from the midline position suggests that the patient is rotated. However, pathologic conditions can also result in tracheal deviation. For example, a large pneumothorax can push the trachea toward the contralateral side of the chest, or a massive atelectasis can pull the trachea toward the ipsilateral side of the chest. Visualization of the tracheal shadow is particularly important if the patient is intubated (has an endotracheal tube in place), because proper positioning of the endotracheal tube is determined by the proximity of its distal end to the tracheal bifurcation. The tip of a properly placed endotracheal tube should be approximately 2 inches above the carina when the patient's head is in the neutral position.

The heart and great vessels occupy the lower two-thirds of the mediastinum, giving the mediastinum a characteristic profile. There are two distinct curves that should be noted on the right side of the cardiovascular shadow. The first, formed entirely by the right atrium, begins at the right cardiophrenic angle and proceeds superiorly. The inferior vena cava (IVC) can often be seen entering the right atrium, inferiorly. The ascending aorta and the superior vena cava (SVC) form the second curve. On the left side, there are typically four curves of importance. The transverse arch and descending aorta form the first curve before the aorta passes behind the main pulmonary artery, which makes the next curve. The third curve may or may not be visible and denotes the site of the left atrial appendage. The border of the left ventricle extends downward to the diaphragm, forming the fourth curve.

> **Clinical Tip**
> The radiograph of a patient with moderate to severe chronic obstructive pulmonary disease will show widened intercostal spaces, flattened hemidiaphragms, squared off costophrenic angles, and rib angles that approach 90-degree angles.

### The Hila

Formed by the root of the lungs (comprising the pulmonary blood vessels, the bronchi and a group of lymph nodes) the hila are at about the T4-T5 level and appear as poorly defined areas of variable density in the medial part of the central portion of the lung fields. The left hilum is partially obscured by the overlying shadow of the heart and great vessels, and it lies at a slightly higher level than the right hilum.

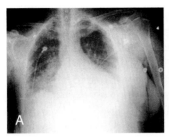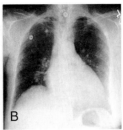

**Figure 10-5** Two chest radiographs of a 77-year-old woman demonstrating rapid clearance of congestive heart failure. The initial chest radiograph **(A)**, obtained when patient was short of breath, demonstrates cardiomegaly, perihilar ground glass densities, vascular indistinctness, Kerley B lines, and bilateral pleural effusions consistent with congestive heart failure. One day later and after diuresis, the chest radiograph **(B)** shows clear lungs without pleural effusions but a persistently enlarged heart. (From Rubinowitz AN, Siegel MD, Tocino I. Thoracic imaging in the ICU. Crit Care Clin 23(3):539–573, 2007.)

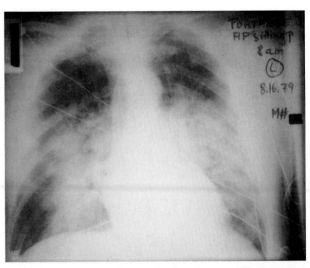

**Figure 10-6** Chest radiograph showing a diffuse alveolar filling pattern, most prominent in the middle and lower lung fields. (From Weinberger SE, Cockrill BA, Mandel J. Principles of Pulmonary Medicine. 5th ed. Philadelphia, Saunders, 2008.)

### The Lung Fields

Although the lobes of the lung cannot normally be distinguished, knowledge of lobar and segmental anatomy is crucial to an assessment of the lung fields. The left and right upper lobes and the right middle lobe lie superiorly and anteriorly within the thoracic cavity, while the lower lobes occupy the posteroinferior aspects. Although the medial segment of the right middle lobe is in contact with the right border of the heart, and the lingular segments of the left upper lobe are in contact with the left border of the heart, the lobes overlap each other considerably, so that a clear localization of each lobe is not possible in the PA or AP view alone. A lateral view is essential in order to delineate accurately the lobes of the lungs and their various bronchopulmonary segments.

The silhouette sign (present when the normal line of demarcation between two structures is partially or completely obliterated) may be used to localize lesions within the lung fields (Fig. 10-5).[5] In the critical care setting, life-support and monitoring equipment can complicate the interpretation of a chest radiograph.

The airways outside the mediastinum are not usually visible on a chest radiograph because of their thin walls and air-filled lumens. However, the pulmonary arteries and veins can frequently be seen as they branch and taper outward toward the periphery until they disappear in the outer third of the lung fields. By observing serial films, these vascular markings can be described as unchanged, increased, or decreased. Increased vascular markings are indicative of venous dilation, whereas decreased vascular markings may indicate hyperinflation of the lungs.

Specific lung lesions are assessed by observing the lung fields for any abnormal density that obliterates the vascular markings or that alters the distribution of the densities within the lung fields. The lung fields should be assessed for any abnormal patterns of radiopacity. If present, these abnormal patterns are typically described as either alveolar patterns or interstitial patterns, and they may be independently localized or diffuse or coexistent. Alveolar patterns are sometimes described as "fluffy infiltrates"; they represent pathologic changes within the distal airways, for example, pulmonary edema or alveolar pneumonia (Fig. 10-6). In contrast, interstitial patterns represent interstitial thickening, for example, inflammation (Fig. 10-7). Interstitial disease may also assume the appearance of fine diffuse nodularity throughout the lungs. If they are of uniform size, they are called *miliary nodules*. The pattern of increased pulmonary vascularity often strongly resembles the interstitial pattern.

> **Clinical Tip**
> Vascular markings that are increased on a chest radiograph are indicative of early left ventricular failure.

The therapist should be able to observe the chest radiograph and distinguish between acute changes and chronic changes. Acute changes would include fluffy infiltrates or increased opacity. Chronic changes include flattened diaphragms, changes in rib angle and intercostal spaces, abnormal lung volumes, and interstitial thickening.

Some neonatal pulmonary diseases have unique radiographic presentations. Nevertheless, the same general principles of radiologic assessment that are used in the assessment of older children and adults apply. To this end, the assessment must determine whether the problem is in the lungs, the heart, the mediastinum (distinct from the heart), or the thoracic wall.

Regardless of the source of the information that details the results of a radiographic chest examination, the data provided can be invaluable to the physical therapist in facilitating the choice and planning of treatment interventions and in the subsequent evaluation of treatment efficacy.

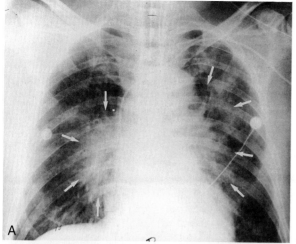

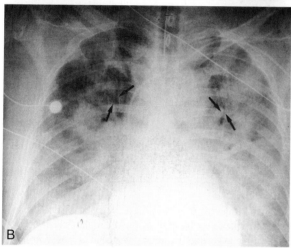

**Figure 10-7** Pulmonary edema. Pulmonary edema, or fluid overload, can be manifested by indistinctness of the pulmonary vessels as they radiate from the hilum **(A)**. This is sometimes termed a "bat wing" infiltrate. As pulmonary edema worsens **(B)**, fluid fills the alveoli, and "air bronchograms" (*arrows*) become apparent. (From Mettler FA. Essentials of Radiology. 2nd ed. Philadelphia, Saunders, 2005.)

Several additional chest-imaging techniques can provide the clinician with information upon which decisions regarding treatment planning or efficacy may be made. several of these techniques are briefly described here.

## Computed Tomography

Computed tomography (CT), or digital chest radiography, involves a narrow beam of x-rays moving across the field of examination in such a way as to define successive adjacent columns of tissue, a process called *translation*. Multiple passes are then made at different angles and each new angle is referred to as a rotation. Each digital image is an array (matrix) of numbers; each number representing a single element of the picture (pixel) and the value of the number defining the degree of brightness or darkness of that particular point in the image. Several digital images are then mathe-

---

**Box 10-2**

**Advantages and Disadvantages of Chest Computed Tomography Compared with Portable Chest Radiography**

| Advantages | Disadvantages |
|---|---|
| • Much more sensitive <br> • Evaluates <br>   • Lungs <br>   • Heart <br>   • Mediastinum <br>   • Pleura <br>   • Chest wall <br>   • Upper abdomen <br> • Localizes disease <br> • Guidance of interventional procedures <br> • Can detect occult pneumothorax or effusions <br> • Evaluates chest tube placement <br> • Can contribute new information <br> • May detect unsuspected abnormalities | • Risk of transporting patient out of the intensive care unit environment <br> • Significant increased radiation <br> • Risks of intravenous contrast (if given) |

From Rubinowitz AN, Siegel MD, Tocino I. Thoracic imaging in the ICU. Crit Care Clin 23(3):539–573, 2007.

matically manipulated to produce a summated image for diagnostic interpretation.

CT scanning of the chest primarily has been used for diagnosis of tumors versus calcifications or nodules. High resolution CT has become the optimal diagnostic method for recognizing parenchymal abnormalities. Contrast enhancement with CT has allowed the assessment of vasculature and lung perfusion. Helical CT was introduced in the 1990s to diagnose for pulmonary embolism (PE) and since that time advances in CT technology (faster scanners and thinner slices) have improved sensitivity and specificity (reported as 90% sensitivity and 96% specificity).[6,7]

With multidetector CT, the entire chest is able to be scanned in 4 to 8 seconds with resultant good visualization and without respiratory movement. The negative predictive value for PE has been defined as 99.1%, therefore a good CT angiogram with a negative conclusion for PE indicates individuals should not have treatment for PE unless the prediagnostic Wells clinical score demonstrated high risk.[8] In contrast, a low clinical risk score but a positive CT report indicates further diagnostic testing (small vessels may be involved).[8]

CT evolves from mere static assessment of morphology into a dynamic and quantifiable tool for regional assessment of the lung. As a result of the improvement in CT imaging of the chest, angiography with CT is now considered the gold standard for diagnosis of PE.[8] Box 10-2 compares the advantages and disadvantages of CT versus chest radiograph.

## Pulmonary Arteriography

Emboli are read on arteriography as one of the following:

- Complete obstruction
- Intraluminal filling defects
- Decrease in flow rate

Although pulmonary arteriography has been considered to be the gold standard for diagnosis of PE, it is a procedure that is invasive, has been thought to have increased morbidity and mortality, associated with complications, and is time-consuming, expensive, and not always available in every facility.[9] Consequently, imaging with CT has become the more widely used diagnostic test because of its excellent specificity and ease of use.

## Magnetic Resonance Imaging

Magnetic resonance imaging (MRI) involves the interaction of stimulated hydrogen nuclei and a strong magnetic field. A MRI scanner produces a gradient magnetic field in the region of the body to be imaged. The hydrogen nuclei tend to align themselves with the magnetic field and resonate at a frequency that is proportional to the strength of the magnetic field. The gradient of nuclear resonance is proportional to the gradient of the magnetic field—magnetic resonance. The patient is then exposed to a radio signal that stimulates those nuclei whose magnetic resonance is the same as the frequency of the radio signal. These stimulated nuclei reemit the radio signal, which is picked up by an antenna in the MRI scanner and digitally recorded by a computer, isolating a "slice of tissue" in much the same manner as that for a CT image. As soon as the reemitted signal is recorded, a new gradient is produced in a perpendicular plane to the original slice and this new slice is stimulated and recorded. The original gradient is then restored. This excitation and retrieval process is repeated many times with the transverse gradient being applied at a slightly different angle each time.[10] The data thus obtained may be mathematically manipulated to produce a final enhanced image for interpretation, an example of which is shown in Figure 10-8. An MRI is primarily indicated for the evaluation of chest wall processes that may involve bone, muscle, fat, or pleura.

Complementary to CT of the lung, MRI of the lung, which previously was handicapped by field inhomogeneity and the lack of protons in lung tissue, is developing its own arsenal for lung assessment in terms of morphology, pulmonary circulation, ventilation, and right heart assessment. It is clear that the inherent advantage of MRI over CT—its lack of ionizing radiation—makes it of primary interest in the field of lung diseases that tend to be chronic with acute exacerbations and require multiple investigations during the life span of the patient. Unfortunately, availability of some of the tools required (such as gas polarizers) or MRI techniques (such as broadband upgrades) is still somewhat limited. However, there is a significant drive toward making access easier, and in many centers, MRI already has become a main diagnostic tool.[11]

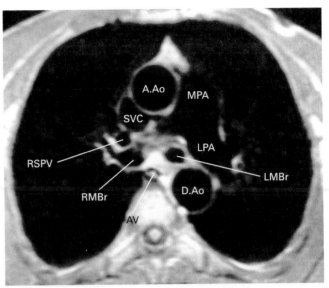

**Figure 10-8** MRI of normal mediastinum and hila 1 cm below the tracheal carina. A.Ao = ascending aorta, AV = azygos vein, D.Ao = descending aorta, LMBr = left main bronchus, LPA = left pulmonary artery; MPA = main pulmonary artery, RMBr = right main bronchus, RSPV = right superior pulmonary vein, SVC = superior vena cava. (From Adam: Grainger & Allison's Diagnostic Radiology, ed 5. Philadelphia, 2008, Churchill Livingstone.)

---

**Clinical Tip**

MRIs may be indicated in individuals with abnormal chest radiographs that show a nodule or mass. An MRI could show an enhanced picture of the mass prior to surgical resection or biopsy, or may be used to enhance the pleural area to distinguish between fibrosis and the presence of nodules.

---

## Ventilation and Perfusion Scans

Several different tests can be used to measure the gas distribution in the lungs. To measure the regional distribution of ventilation in the lungs the patient breathes xenon gas ($^{133}$Xe). The test is usually performed with the patient in a sitting or supine position. The patient is asked to inhale a normal tidal volume from a closed system containing a specific volume or concentration of xenon, and then to hold the breath for several seconds while ventilation scans are made over the lung field. To determine the rate of equilibrium of the gas in the lungs, serial scans are made over a 10- to 15-minute period with the use of a rebreathing technique. Finally, to determine the washout rate of the xenon gas, the patient is returned to atmospheric breathing while serial scans are made.

To measure the regional distribution of pulmonary blood flow in the lungs the patient is injected intravenously with radioactive iodine ($^{131}$I) and serial perfusion scans are made over the lung fields as the blood perfuses the lungs. Although they may be performed as separate tests, ventilation and perfusion scans (V/Q scans) provide the maximum amount of information when used together. Such information describes

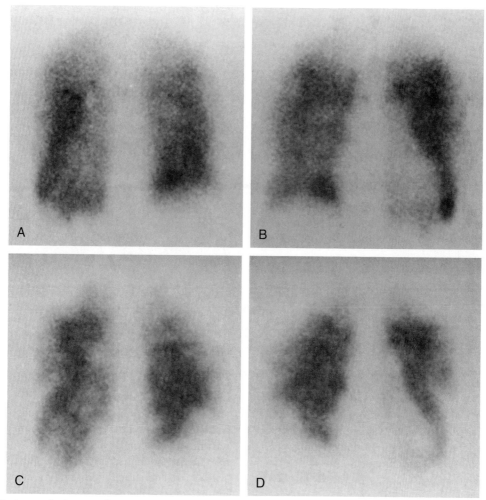

**Figure 10-9** Typical ventilation–perfusion scans in pulmonary arterial hypertension. **A** and **B,** Normal ventilation scans. **C** and **D,** Patchy subsegmental defects on corresponding perfusion scans. (From Albert RK, Spiro SG, Jett JR. Clinical Respiratory Medicine. 3rd ed. Philadelphia, Mosby, 2009.)

how the alveolar ventilation and pulmonary perfusion are matched in the patient. In the normal person, the V/Q scans will show greater ventilation and perfusion in the bases of the lung and less ventilation and perfusion in the apices. Normal and abnormal V/Q scans are shown in Figure 10-9. V/Q scans are described as negative, low, intermediate, and high probability. A negative scan had a less than 5% probability of a PE. A high probability scan has a 96% predictive value in high-risk patients.[12] Yet, most scans are interpreted as low or intermediate probability and thus are nondiagnostic. Consequently, CT scans are considered to have greater reliability than V/Q scans

V/Q scans are usually indicated to rule out pulmonary emboli, particularly in individuals with deep-vein thrombosis. Perfusion defects with normal ventilation strongly suggest PE. However, many V/Q scans are nondiagnostic, which makes V/Q scans less sensitive and specific for PE than CT scans.

## Bronchography

Bronchography is occasionally needed for the evaluation and management of some congenital pulmonary anomalies as well as some acquired diseases, usually of the tracheobronchial tree.[13] Bronchograms permit the study of normal and variant anatomy, and of gross pathologic changes in the bronchial wall and lumen. Contrast bronchography involves the opacification of the bronchial tree by the installation of contrast medium so that the radiographic shadows of the airways may be studied. Figure 10-10 is a bronchogram demonstrating bronchiectasis of the left lower lobe bronchi. Because of the advances in high-resolution CT imaging, CT imaging is identified with increased reliability over bronchography.

## Bronchoscopy

Fiberoptic bronchoscopy has markedly decreased the necessity for contrast bronchography by permitting the direct

> **Clinical Tip**
> Bronchoscopy is indicated to assess for infection that cannot be evaluated from a sample or to assess for malignancy. On occasion, bronchoscopy is used to clear seriously viscous secretions.

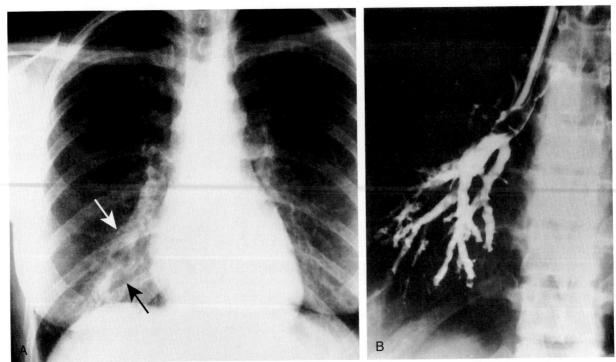

**Figure 10-10** A, Bronchiectasis appearing as prominent, thick bronchial markings in the right paracardiac region of the lung (*arrows*). B, Bronchogram demonstrating ectasia and irregularity of the bronchi. (From Marchiori D: Clinical Imaging, ed 2. St Louis, 2005, Mosby.)

visualization of previously inaccessible areas of the bronchial tree.[14] Figure 10-11 depicts the typical bronchoscopic appearance of the segmental origins within each lobe.

## Pulmonary Function Testing

Pulmonary function tests (PFTs) provide the clinician with information about the integrity of the airways, the function of the respiratory musculature, and the condition of the lung tissues themselves. A thorough evaluation of pulmonary function involves several tests that measure lung volumes and capacities, gas flow rates, gas diffusion, and gas distribution. Based on the results of PFTs, pulmonary diseases may be classified into three basic categories: obstructive, restrictive, or combined. A working knowledge of the principal test and an ability to interpret their findings are essential to the planning and implementation of effective interventions. Table 10-1 defines the most common PFTs and data obtained.

### Tests of Lung Volume and Capacity

Tests of basic lung volumes and capacities are described in Figures 10-12 and 10-13 and include a graphic tracing called a spirogram. Spirometers may be of the traditional manual water-seal type, or they may be electronic computerized devices (e.g., pneumotachometer). In either case, a spirogram of the lung volumes is typically produced to facilitate interpretation of the measurements (Fig. 10-12). Many spirometric measurements can be accurately conducted at the bedside using relatively uncomplicated equipment (Fig. 10-13, A),

although others necessitate the equipment found in a pulmonary function laboratory (see Fig. 10-13, B). In either setting, the patient should be positioned in an upright sitting posture and a nose clip should be used. The patient should breathe normally into the spirometer (or other appropriate instrument) through a tight-fitting mouthpiece until a normal rhythm is established.

### Body Plethysmography

The plethysmograph is an airtight chamber in which the patient sits; pressure transducers measure pressure both at the airway (mouthpiece) and in the chamber. The patient is placed in a plethysmograph, connected to the mouthpiece, and asked to breathe normally. At end-inspiration and end-expiration there is no airflow, and the alveolar pressure is equal to the airway pressure at that time. At a specific time (end-expiration, for example) the shutter is occluded, and the various volume and pressure values are measured. Because the body plethysmography method of functional residual capacity (FRC) determination actually measures the total amount of gas in the thorax, the values obtained may be larger than those from either helium dilution or nitrogen washout techniques (any difference between the measurements is an estimate of the volume of poorly ventilated regions of the lungs).

The total lung capacity (TLC) is the sum of the vital capacity (VC) and the residual volume (RV) and is the only individually diagnostic parameter in spirometry. TLC is always elevated in obstructive lung diseases and reduced in chronic restrictive lung diseases. Certain acute disorders, such as pulmonary edema, atelectasis, and consolidation, also cause a reduction in TLC.

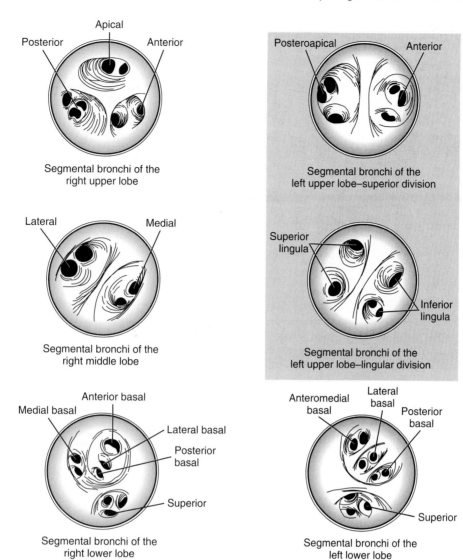

**Figure 10-11** Typical bronchoscopic appearance of the segmental bronchi of each lung.

## Table 10-1 Most Common Pulmonary Function Tests

| Test | Technique | Data Obtained |
| --- | --- | --- |
| Spirometry | Maximal inhalation followed by maximal exhalation, measuring volume of air and time | FVC, FEV$_1$, FEV$_1$/FVC, VC |
| Diffusing capacity of the lung for CO | Inhalation of fixed concentration of CO and helium, breath holding for 10 sec, then expiration with measurement of end-tidal CO and helium | Uptake and diffusing capacity of CO |
| Helium lung volumes | Maximal expiration, then inhalation of a known concentration of helium until steady state is reached | RV, ERV, IRV, TV with calculation of TLC, VC, FRC, IC |

*CO, carbon monoxide; ERV, expiratory reserve volume; FEV$_1$, forced expiratory volume in 1 second; FRC, functional reserve capacity; FVC, forced vital capacity; IC, inspiratory capacity; IRV, inspiratory reserve volume; RV, residual volume; TLC, total lung capacity; TV, tidal volume; VC, ventilatory capacity.*
*From Piccini JP, Nilsson K. The Osler Medical Handbook. 2nd ed. Baltimore, John Hopkins University, 2006.*

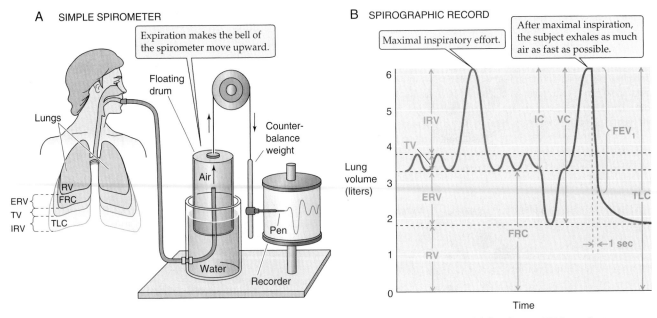

**Figure 10-12** The workings of a simple spirometer. IRV, inspiratory reserve volume; TV, tidal volume; ERV, expiratory reserve volume; RV, residual volume; TLC, Total lung capacity; IC, inspiratory capacity; FRC, functional residual capacity; VC, vital capacity. (From Boron W, Boulpaep EL. Textbook of Medical Physiology, ed 2. St. Louis, 2009, Saunders.)

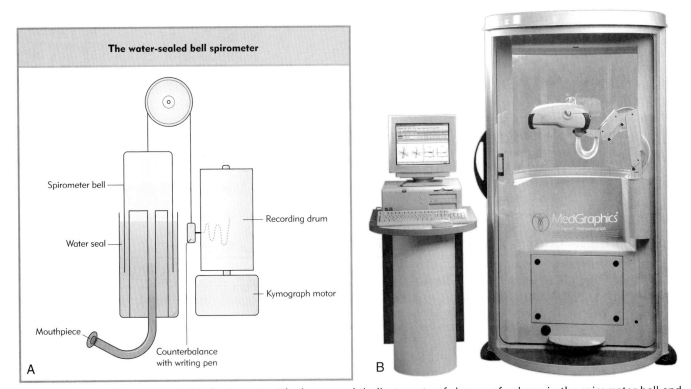

**Figure 10-13 A,** The water-sealed bell spirometer. The kymograph indicates rate of change of volume in the spirometer bell and hence the expiratory and inspiratory flow rates. Hemmings: Foundations of Anesthesia, ed 2. Philadelphia, 2005, Mosby. **B,** Body Plethysmograph. A modern plethysmograph setup, with a highly transparent box, self-contained calibration equipment, and computerized data reduction and display. (Courtesy Medical Graphics, Inc., St. Paul, Minn.)

## Tests of Gas Flow Rates

Tests that measure airflow rates during forced breathing maneuvers provide important information relating to the actual function of the lungs, the degree of impairment, and often the general location (large airways, small airways, etc.)

of the problem. The basic measures of airflow rates include the following:

- Forced vital capacity (FVC) is the maximum volume of gas the patient can exhale as forcefully and as quickly as possible. FVC is measured by having the patient exhale as forcibly and as quickly as possible into a spirometer or

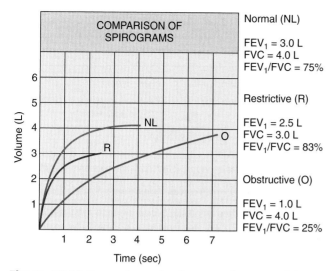

**Figure 10-14** Comparison of spirograms for normal lungs, restrictive lung disease, and obstructive lung disease. FEVI, Forced expiratory volume in 1 second; FVC, forced vital capacity. (From Copstead-Kirkhorn LC: Pathophysiology, ed 4. St Louis, 2010, Saunders.)

pneumotachometer. The patient should breathe in maximally and exhale as quickly as possible. The FVC is highly dependent upon the amount of force used by the patient in early expiration at volumes near TLC. Thus, it may be necessary to coach the patient to achieve the patient's maximum expiratory effort. Figure 10-14 shows a normal spirographic tracing of an FVC. The FVC is generally reduced in both obstructive and restrictive diseases; the primary difference between the curve in the patient with restrictive disease as compared with the patient with obstructive disease is the slope of the curve. The FVC is less than the normal slow VC when airway collapse and air trapping are present. Furthermore, by analyzing the FVC with respect to the volume of air exhaled per unit time and the relationship of expiratory flow to lung volume, inferences may be made about the localization of any problem.

- Forced expiratory volume in 1 second ($FEV_1$) is the volume of air that is exhaled during the first second of the FVC and reflects the airflow in the large airways. The utility of the $FEV_1$ measurement is exemplified by the simple relationship between it and the associated degree of obstruction:
- Little or no obstruction: $FEV_1$ greater than 2.0 L to normal.
- Mild to moderate obstruction: $FEV_1$ between 1.0 and 2.0 L.
- Severe obstruction: $FEV_1$ less than 1.0 L.

This volume may also be expressed as a percentage of the FVC exhaled in 1 second ($FEV_1\%$). Normally, 75% of the FVC should be exhaled within 1 second. An $FEV_1\%$ of more than 80% or 90% indicates restrictive disease, whereas a reduced $FEV_1\%$ indicates airway obstruction. A significant reduction in $FEV_1$ is associated with a higher mortality rate among both sexes, whereas significant declines in $FEV_1\%$ are associated with a higher all-cause mortality rate among male

subjects only.[15,16] Of course, age exerts an influence on both the FVC and the $FEV_1$. The average decline in $FEV_1$ is in the range of 40 mL per year for men and 30 mL per year for women.[17] After the late twenties to mid thirties, a progressive decline in the $FEV_1$ of from 20 to 50 mL per year can be expected in healthy persons, but in adults with chronic obstructive lung disease the decline is as much as 50 to 80 mL per year.

Forced midexpiratory flow ($FEF_{25-75}$), previously called the maximal midexpiratory flow rate, is volume of air exhaled over the middle half of the FVC, divided by the time required to exhale it. The normal $FEF_{25-75}$ is approximately 4 L/sec (240 L/min). Although the $FEF_{25-75}$ has proved to be effective in detecting the presence of changes in lung function, because it depends on the FVC, it has not proved to be a particularly satisfactory parameter for use in quantifying the changes.

> **Clinical Tip**
> Individuals with obstructive defects will demonstrate large lung volumes, but reduced FVC because of inability to get the air out forcefully (as in asthma or emphysema). Individuals with restrictive defects will demonstrate small lung volumes, and possibly reduced FVC because of the lack of muscle strength (as in a patient with pneumonia or severe pulmonary fibrosis).

Numerous additional indices of lung mechanics are frequently presented on PFT reports:
- Forced expiratory flow, 200 to 1200 ($FEF_{200-1200}$) is the average expiratory flow during the early phase of exhalation. Specifically, it is a measure of the flow for 1 L of expired gas immediately following the first 200 mL of expired gas. The normal $FEF_{200-1200}$ is usually greater than 5 L/sec (300 L/min).
- Maximum voluntary ventilation (MVV) is the maximal volume of gas a patient can move during 1 minute (previously called the maximum breathing capacity). The patient is asked to breathe as deeply and rapidly as possible for 10, 12, or 15 seconds, the volume expired is extrapolated to yield the flow rate in L/min. The normal value for adult males is approximately 160 to 180 L/min; it is slightly lower in adult females. Because normal values can vary by as much as 25% to 30%, only major reductions in the values are clinically significant. As a rule of thumb, the MVV is typically described as being about 35 times greater than the $FEV_1$ value.[18]
- Peak expiratory flow (PEF) is the maximum flow that occurs at any point in time during the FVC. Normal peak flows average 9 to 10 L/sec. The reliability of PEF as a clinical tool for evaluation of lung mechanics is limited because of the initial high flows that can occur even in obstructive disorders. Decreased peak flows reflect nonspecific mechanical problems.

The various tests of breathing mechanics are measured again 5 to 20 minutes (the time depends on the specific drug and its dosage) after the administration of a bronchodilator. In normal persons, or in persons with pure restrictive

## Table 10-2 Typical Gas Exchange Variables

| Variable | Symbol | Definition |
|---|---|---|
| Respiratory frequency | f | Number of complete breaths per unit time |
| Tidal volume | VT | Volume of air moved during either inhalation or exhalation over a specific period of time (usually 1 minute) |
| Minute ventilation (expiratory) | VE | Volume of air exhaled per unit time |
| Minute ventilation (inspiratory) | VI | Volume of air inhaled per unit time |
| Carbon dioxide output | $VCO_2$ | Volume of carbon dioxide exhaled per unit time |
| Oxygen uptake | $VO_2$ | Volume of oxygen consumed per unit time |
| Gas exchange ratio | R | Ratio of $CO_2$ to $O_2$ |
| Ventilatory equivalent for carbon dioxide or oxygen | $VE/VCO_2$ or $VE/O_2$ | Ventilatory requirement for a given metabolic rate |
| Oxygen pulse | $VO_2/HR$ | Amount of oxygen consumed per heart beat |

processes, there should be no difference between the before and after bronchodilator measurements. In persons with obstructive disease, bronchodilators are used primarily to measure the reversibility of the obstruction. Airway obstruction is generally said to be reversible when there is 12% or greater increase in the postbronchodilator values for at least two of the following three parameters: FVC, $FEV_1$, and $FEF_{25-75}$.[19] However, the definition of obstruction and reversibility in clinical trials is not uniform. Moreover, at least 11 different criteria can be found in the literature to define obstruction.[20,21]

## Tests of Diffusion

The diffusing capacity of the lung (DL) or diffusing capacity of the lung for carbon monoxide (DLCO) is the amount of gas entering the pulmonary blood flow per unit time and is relative to the difference between the partial pressures of the gas in the alveoli and in the pulmonary blood. The DL is not so much a measure of pulmonary mechanics as it is a measure of the integrity of the functional lung unit. DL is expressed in millimeters per minute per millimeters of mercury (mL/min/mm Hg). Carbon monoxide (CO) is normally employed to measure DL because it has an affinity for hemoglobin nearly 210 times greater than that of oxygen. As long as the patient's hemoglobin is normal, all the alveolar CO should bind to hemoglobin and the partial pressure of CO in the plasma should be zero. The normal diffusing capacity of carbon monoxide is approximately 25 to 30 mL/min/mm Hg. Although there may be many causes for an abnormal DLCO test, they usually can be attributed to three key factors: (1) decreased quantity of hemoglobin per unit volume of blood; (2) increased "thickness" of the alveolar–capillary membrane; and (3) decreased functional surface area available for diffusion. Loss of surface area has been identified as the primary factor. Of the two most often used tests for measuring DLCO, it has been suggested that the single-breath test is of limited value because the results are influenced by unequal

distribution of ventilation and diffusion, although the rebreathing method is not believed to be influenced by such inequalities.[22]

## Additional Tests of Gas Exchange

Table 10-2 presents some of the gas exchange variables that may be helpful in furthering an understanding of the diagnosis of the causes of exertional dyspnea, the extent of functional impairment, or the effect of medical, surgical, or rehabilitative therapy. The reader is warned, however, that without an appreciation of the environmental conditions under which specific gas volumes may have been determined, dramatic errors can be made when interpreting the significance of the volumes. See Chapter 8 for additional information on expired gas analysis.

Expired gas analysis is the reference standard for diagnosis and differentiating between cardiac and pulmonary causes of dyspnea as well as research outcome measures. Readers are encouraged to consult specific texts and positional papers on expired gas analysis for a thorough explanation of the vast array of data acquired in this test.

## Flow-Volume Loop

The flow-volume loop or curve is not so much a pulmonary function test as a way of graphically representing the events that occur during forced inspiration and expiration. The flow-volume procedure simply records flow against volume on an X-Y recorder. Following a period of normal, quiet breathing, the patient is instructed to perform a maximal inspiratory maneuver, to hold the breath for 1 to 2 seconds, to do an FVC maneuver, and then to do another maximal inspiratory maneuver. Figure 10-15 shows a normal flow-volume loop.

The initial portion of the expiratory loop is effort-dependent, however, after the first third of the expiratory curve, the curve is effort independent and reproducible. The highest point on the expiratory curves denotes the peak

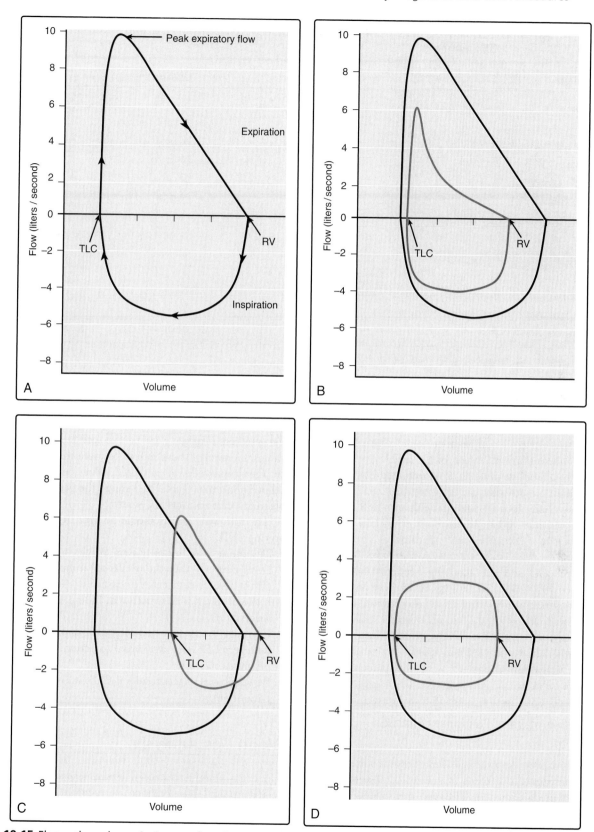

**Figure 10-15** Flow-volume loop. **A,** A normal expiratory and inspiratory flow-volume loop. **B,** A characteristic flow-volume loop as seen in a patient with severe chronic airflow limitation caused by smoking. Notice the deeply scooped-out appearance of the expiratory limb of the curve, reflecting the pronounced flow limitation occurring at low lung volumes (predicted flow-volume loop in the red line). **C,** A characteristic flow-volume loop in a patient with severe lung restriction from pulmonary fibrosis. Notice the patient's relatively small lung volumes. Compared with predicted values, flow rates are relatively increased in relation to lung volume (predicted flow-volume loop in the red line). **D,** A characteristic flow-volume loop in a patient with a fixed tracheal stenosis (predicted flow-volume loop in the red line). TLC, total lung capacity; RV, residual volume. (From Walsh D, Caraceni AT, Fainsinger R, et al: Palliative Medicine. Philadelphia, 2008, Saunders.)

**Table 10-3 Typical Effect of Obstructive and Restrictive Disease on Spirometric and Airflow Volume Measurements**

| Measurement | Obstructive | Restrictive |
|---|---|---|
| Tidal volume (VT) | N or ↑ | N or ↓ |
| Inspiratory capacity (IC) | N or ↓ | N or ↓ |
| Expiratory reserve volume (ERV) | N or ↓ | N or ↓ |
| Vital capacity (VC) | N or ↓ | ↓ |
| Forced vital capacity (FVC) | N or ↓ | ↓ |
| Residual volume (RV) | N or ↑ | N or ↓ |
| Functional residual capacity (FRC) | N or ↑ | N or ↓ |
| Total lung capacity (TLC) | N or ↑ | ↓ |
| Forced expiratory volume in 1 s (FEV1) | ↓ | N |
| Forced expiratory flow rate between 200 and 1200 mL (FEF$_{200-1200}$) | ↓ | N or ↓ |
| Forced expiratory flow rate between 25% and 75% FVC (FEF$_{25-75}$) | ↓ | N or ↓ |
| Maximum voluntary ventilation (MVV) | ↓ | N or ↓ |
| Peak expiratory flow (PEF) | N or ↓ | N or ↓ |

*N, normal; ↑, higher than normal; ↓, lower than normal.*

expiratory flow rate (PEFR). The line that connects the PEFR and the end of expiration at the RV is normally straight. However, both restrictive and obstructive processes alter this effort independent portion. Values for FVC, FEV$_1$, peak flow, and so on, should be the same as those obtained by conventional spirometric methods.

The flow-volume loop of patients with minimal to mild small airway obstructive lung disease look essentially normal except for a slight "scooped out" appearance at the end of expiration. As the disease progresses, the PEFR becomes noticeably reduced and the scooping becomes more pronounced (see Fig. 10-15). The inspiratory portion of the curve is more sensitive to central airway obstruction, whereas the expiratory portion of the curve is more sensitive to peripheral airway obstruction. The restrictive lung disease processes will show near-normal peak expiratory flow volume (FEVt) when compared with the percentage of FVC (%FEVt/FVC).

## Interpretation of Basic Pulmonary Function Test Results

Pulmonary function test results are almost universally formatted to present data in columns of predicted, observed, and percentage of predicted values. The predicted values (derived from a variety of nomograms) are those normally anticipated on the basis of the patient's age (volumes decrease with age), gender (males have larger volumes than females), height (tall individuals have larger volumes than short individuals), weight, and race (American Indians, blacks, and Asians have as much as 12% to 14% lower volumes than whites).[23-26] Children pose a unique challenge to prediction because their development is phasic; thus, specific nomograms are used for

the pediatric population. The observed values are those actually attained by the patient. Dividing the observed value by the predicted value derives the percentage of predicted values. Generally, there should be more than 20% difference between observed and predicted values before they are considered abnormal. Table 10-3 shows the generalized effects of obstructive or restrictive diseases.

The following points should be kept in mind when interpreting PFTs:

- Determine whether or not the results are normal.
- Determine whether the results are indicative of obstructive or restrictive disease.
- If the problem is obstructive in nature, determine its reversibility.
- Consider the history and physical examination along with serial PFTs (if available) to determine disease progression.
- Be suspicious of test results if there are signs of poor patient effort.

## Blood Gas Analysis

Blood gas analysis is crucial to the assessment of problems related to acid–base balance, ventilation, and oxygenation. Samples for blood gas analysis may be obtained from any number of sites representing different regions of the vascular bed: arterial samples are taken from either a needle puncture or an indwelling cannula in a peripheral artery; venous samples are taken from a peripheral venous puncture or catheter; mixed venous samples are taken from a pulmonary artery catheter. Unless otherwise specified, a blood gas sample is presumed to be arterial in origin. Arterial blood gases (ABGs)

## Table 10-4 Normal Ranges (±2 SD) for Arterial Blood Gas Values

|  | pH | PCO$_2$ (mm Hg) | PO$_2$ (mm Hg) | HCO$_3^-$ | BE | % SAT |
|---|---|---|---|---|---|---|
| Normal value | 7.40 | 40 | 97 | 24 | 0 | 97% |
| Normal range | 7.35–7.45 | 35–45 | >80 | 22–28 | ±2 | >95% |

are frequently used to monitor the condition of patients in the critical care setting and to help modify respiratory interventions. A typical report of an ABG analysis contains the following measurements: arterial pH, partial pressures of carbon dioxide (PaCO$_2$) and oxygen (PaO$_2$), oxygen saturation (SaO$_2$), bicarbonate (HCO$_3^-$) concentration, and base excess (BE). Although the immediate utility of ABGs for the physical therapist may have been supplanted by the pulse oximeter, a systematic approach to a more detailed and complete interpretation of acid–base, ventilatory, or oxygenation status should not be overlooked, particularly with respect to patients receiving mechanical and noninvasive mechanical ventilation.

### Normal Values

The laboratory "normal values" for pH and PaCO$_2$ (7.40 and 40 mm Hg, respectively) represent the statistically determined mean values from a large representative sample population. The laboratory "normal range" may vary from institution to institution based on the particular laboratory's established normal range, which may be 1 or 2 standard deviations (SD). The narrower pH range of 7.38 to 7.42 and PaCO$_2$ range of 38 to 42 mm Hg represent 1 SD from the normal values. The wider pH range of 7.35 to 7.45 and PaCO$_2$ range of 35 to 45 mm Hg represent 2 SD from the normal values. For the purposes of this chapter, the normal range for pH is 7.35 to 7.45; for PaCO$_2$, 35 to 45 mm Hg, depending on posture, age, obesity, and other factors. An even broader "clinically acceptable range" has been promoted by some clinicians.[27-30] Table 10-4 presents the normal values and normal ranges for ABG parameters.

In any systematic approach to the interpretation of ABGs, it is advantageous to focus upon three principal categories: the adequacy of alveolar ventilation, the acid–base balance, and the oxygenation status.

### Adequacy of Alveolar Ventilation

The PaCO$_2$ directly reflects the adequacy of alveolar ventilation. Given a normal PaCO$_2$ value of 40 mm Hg, alveolar hyperventilation is indicated by a PaCO$_2$ that is less than normal, and alveolar hypoventilation is indicated by a greater than normal PaCO$_2$. When a patient's PaCO$_2$ is greater than 50 mm Hg, the condition is called *ventilatory failure*. Ventilatory failure can only be diagnosed on the basis of the PaCO$_2$ level, but its severity is determined from the extent of the accompanying acidemia and the rapidity of the change in pH.

Sudden (acute) changes in pH hinder cellular function to a greater degree than do gradual changes, and are more often associated with a loss of alertness and coma than are gradual (chronic) pH changes. When acuity or chronicity is masked by the presence of mixed disorders, the patient's level of alertness should be used as an indicator.

The events leading to ventilatory failure can occur relatively rapidly in patients who are acutely ill, or over a period of days or weeks in patients with chronic lung disease, as they decompensate; that is, become unable to meet the demands for the increased minute ventilation needed to maintain adequate gas exchange. Because there are no reliable means of predicting a patient's ability to avert decompensation with any certainty, monitoring of the ventilatory status is mandatory. Such monitoring consists of ongoing assessment of pH, PaCO$_2$, and the signs and symptoms that suggest an increased work of breathing. To determine the nature and severity of illness with accuracy, an assessment of the relationship between arterial pH and arterial CO$_2$ tension is necessary. Chapters 11 and 13 discuss monitoring equipment.

### Acid–Base Balance

The assessment of blood pH provides insight to the nature and magnitude of respiratory and metabolic disorders. In general terms, the pH describes the balance between blood acids and blood bases. Specifically, it indicates the concentration of hydrogen ions (H+) in the blood. In solution, acids give up hydrogen ions and bases, on the other hand, accept hydrogen ions.

The lungs and the kidneys regulate the two types of acids—volatile and nonvolatile—found in the body. Volatile acids readily alternate from liquid to gaseous states. The lungs regulate volatile acids, primarily represented by carbonic acid in the blood, via the excretion of CO$_2$. Nonvolatile acids (e.g., lactic acid or ketoacid) cannot change to gases and, therefore, must be excreted by the kidneys. The principal source of nonvolatile acids is from dietary intake (organic and inorganic acids), and although the liver is where most of these nonvolatile acids are metabolized, the kidneys regulate their excretion from the body. The kidneys are also primarily responsible for regulation of the major blood base—bicarbonate (HCO$_3^-$). Bicarbonate is responsible for 60% to 90% of the extracellular buffering of nonvolatile acids (buffers act to prevent extreme fluctuations in hydrogen ion concentration so that cellular metabolism will not be hampered). Hemoglobin accounts for approximately 85% of nonbicarbonate buffering action (phosphate and serum proteins are the other nonbicarbonate buffers).

## Henderson-Hasselbalch Equation

By looking at one specific component—the carbonic acid to bicarbonate ion relationship—a complete analysis of acid–base balance is possible, because the amount of hydrogen ion activity resulting from the dissociation of carbonic acid is controlled by the interrelationship of all the blood acids, bases, and buffers. The Henderson-Hasselbalch equation defines pH in terms of this relationship:

$$pH = pK + \log[HCO_3^-]H_2CO_3$$

where pH is the negative log of hydrogen ion concentration $(-\log[H+])$ and pK equals 6.1 (pK is a constant representing the pH at which a solute is 50% dissolved; its mathematical derivation, and that of pH, are beyond the scope of this chapter). In terms of clinically derived variables, the Henderson-Hasselbalch equation can be expressed as follows:

$$pH = pK + \log[HCO_3^-]s \times PaCO_2$$

where s is the solubility coefficient for carbon dioxide, and equals 0.03. In plasma, the concentration of dissolved carbon dioxide $(dCO_2)$ is approximately 1000 times greater than the concentration of carbonic acid because the catalyzing enzyme carbonic anhydrase does not exist in the plasma. Although this total dissolved carbon dioxide in the plasma is a very small portion of the total carbon dioxide content of the blood, it is extremely important because it exerts the pressure that determines the pressure gradient controlling the movement of $CO_2$ into or out of the blood.[27-30] Through these equations, the inverse relationship between pH and $PaCO_2$ is established.[31] This relationship is particularly helpful in clinical decision making regarding the acid–base status of the patient.

## Acid–Base Terminology

Because the "normal" human blood pH is 7.4, a pH of less than 7.4 is defined as acidemia. The process causing the acidemia (whatever it may be) is called *acidosis*. From the Henderson-Hasselbalch equation, there are only two ways in which acidemia can occur: (1) a low $HCO_3^-$ produces metabolic acidosis; or (2) a high $PaCO_2$, which is called respiratory acidosis (synonymous terms are alveolar hypoventilation and hypercapnia). Similarly, a pH greater than 7.4 is defined as alkalemia, and the process causing it is called alkalosis. There are also only two ways in which alkalemia can occur: (1) a high $HCO_3^-$, which is called metabolic alkalosis; and (2) a low $PaCO_2$, which is called respiratory alkalosis (alternatively called alveolar hyperventilation or hypocapnia). These four acid–base states constitute the primary acid–base disorders, and each elicits a compensatory response. For example, if some disease were to cause a decreased $HCO_3^-$ (a primary metabolic acidosis), the body's response would be an attempt to decrease the $PaCO_2$ (a compensatory respiratory alkalosis) to return the pH toward its normal value. In this manner, respiratory compensation for primary metabolic disorders begins in a matter of seconds by means of alveolar hyper- or hypoventilation. The kidneys compensate for primary respiratory disorders by retaining or excreting bicarbonate and hydrogen ions. However, unlike the rapidity with which respiratory compensatory activity exhibits its effect, the renal compensatory process requires 12 to 24 hours to effect significant pH change.

The relationships described in the Henderson-Hasselbalch equation permit us to "quickly" identify any of the four primary disorders based on pH and $CO_2$. If the normal inverse relationship between pH and $PaCO_2$ is maintained, the primary problem is most likely respiratory in nature. On the other hand, if the relationship is not maintained, the primary problem is most likely metabolic. This generalization holds true in most situations, even when combined respiratory and metabolic changes occur at the same time. However, in the face of combined disorders with large $PaCO_2$ changes; one must keep in mind that instead of equally reflecting combined respiratory and metabolic bicarbonate changes, the $PaCO_2$ may preferentially reflect the respiratory component. Because this makes separating metabolic and respiratory components more difficult, an additional parameter that reflects the metabolic component must be considered. The BE is such parameter. The BE is a measure of the deviation of the concentration of nonvolatile acids from normal (defined as a pH of 7.40 and a $PaCO_2$ of 40 mm Hg). As such, BE is a true nonrespiratory measurement that reflects the concentration of bicarbonate in the body. The normal range of BE is $\pm 2$ mEq $\bullet$ L$-1$.

The normal $PaO_2$ is 80 to 100 mm Hg when breathing room air.[27,30,32] The normal newborn infant (range of 40 to 70 mm Hg) and persons older than 60 years of age (in general, for every year older than 60 years of age subtract 1 mm Hg from the normal minimally acceptable $PaO_2$ of 80 mm Hg; this guideline does not apply to persons older than 90 years of age) are exceptions to this rule of thumb. When the arterial oxygen tension is less than normal, a condition called *hypoxemia* is said to exist.

## Interpreting Arterial Blood Gases

The reader cannot expect to interpret very unusual ABG without a great deal of practice and clinical experience. Nonetheless, an orderly approach to the assessment of ABGs will permit the majority of blood gases to be interpreted. Interpretation of ABG data involves just a couple of basic processes:

- Assessment of ventilatory status
- Assessment of oxygenation and hypoxemic status
- Assessing ventilatory status

There are three steps in the assessment of a patient's ventilatory status using the decision tree above:

1. Determine whether the pH value reflects acidemia or alkalemia.
2. Classify the pathophysiologic state of the ventilatory system on the basis of the relationship between the pH

and $PaCO_2$ values. This step determines whether the blood gas values represent a primary respiratory or a primary metabolic disorder. If the normal inverse relationship between pH and $PaCO_2$ is preserved, the primary disorder is likely to be respiratory in nature; if it is not, the primary disorder is probably metabolic.

3. Determine the adequacy of alveolar ventilation on the basis of the $PaCO_2$ value:
   - Less than 30 mm Hg = alveolar hyperventilation.
   - Between 30 and 50 mm Hg = adequate alveolar ventilation.
   - Greater than 50 mm Hg = ventilatory failure.

If the primary problem is metabolic, we classify the problem on the basis of the relationship between the pH and the $PaCO_2$. The problem is classified as "uncompensated" if the reported pH is outside the normal range and the reported $PaCO_2$ is within the normal range; classified as "partially compensated" if both the reported pH and $PaCO_2$ are outside the normal range; or classified as "compensated" if the reported pH is within the normal range and the reported $PaCO_2$ is outside the normal range. For example, in assessment of the second set of pH and $PaCO_2$ values, we concluded that they represented a metabolic alkalosis. The next step is to classify the problem on the basis the relationship between the pH and $PaCO_2$ values. Because the pH is outside the normal range and the $PaCO_2$ is within the normal range, we conclude that the problem is an uncompensated metabolic alkalosis. The extent of the metabolic problem is inferred from the BE/deficit.

Table 10-5 summarizes the classification nomenclature typically used to describe acid–base disorders.

## Assessing Oxygenation and Hypoxemic Status

The oxygenation status of a patient is assessed by determining the extent to which the observed $PaO_2$ is above or below the normal range. Generally, as long as a patient's $PaO_2$ is within the normal range, arterial oxygenation is considered to be acceptable. If a patient's $PaO_2$ is between 60 and 80 mm Hg, the patient is said to be mildly hypoxemic; if it is between 40 and 60 mm Hg, moderately hypoxemic; and if it is less than 40 mm Hg, severely hypoxemic. Hypoxemia is not an absolute indicator of cellular hypoxia—a condition of inadequate cellular oxygenation—because other factors, such as hemoglobin level and capillary circulation, must also be considered. However, hypoxemia strongly suggests tissue hypoxia and necessitates further evaluation.

Quite frequently, patients require supplemental oxygen in the course of their medical treatment. When a patient is receiving supplemental oxygen, the adequacy of arterial oxygenation is assessed on the basis of the fraction of inspired oxygen. As a general rule, the fraction of inspired oxygen ($FIO_2$) multiplied by 500 approximates the arterial oxygen tension expected. If that tension is not present, one may assume that the patient would be hypoxemic. For example, consider two patients, each with a $PaO_2$ of 95 mm Hg. Patient 1 is breathing room air, so we conclude that the $PaO_2$

## Table 10-5 Nomenclature for Evaluating Ventilatory and Metabolic Acid–Base Status

| Acid–Base Status | pH | $PaCO_2$ |
|---|---|---|
| Acute alveolar hyperventilation | >7.50 | <30 mm Hg |
| Chronic alveolar hyperventilation | 7.40–7.50 | <30 mm Hg |
| Compensated metabolic acidosis | 7.30–7.40 | <30 mm Hg |
| Partially compensated metabolic acidosis | <7.30 | <30 mm Hg |
| Metabolic alkalosis | >7.50 | 35–45 mm Hg |
| Normal | 7.35–7.45 | 35–45 mm Hg |
| Metabolic acidosis | <7.30 | 35–45 mm Hg |
| Partially compensated metabolic alkalosis | >7.50 | >50 mm Hg |
| Chronic ventilatory failure | 7.30–7.50 | >50 mm Hg |
| Acute ventilatory failure | <7.30 | >50 mm Hg |

represents adequate oxygenation and no hypoxemia. Patient 2, on the other hand, is receiving supplemental oxygen and has an $FIO_2$, of 0.30 (30% oxygen). If this patient were oxygenating the arterial blood normally, we would anticipate a $PaO_2$ in the neighborhood of 150 mm Hg. Thus, we can reasonably conclude that this patient is hypoxemic.

---

*Clinical Tip*

ABGs are very time dependent, they represent what is occurring at a particular time and under particular circumstances. In the acute care and especially in the critical care settings, ABGs are used to assess current situations as well the response to medical interventions to normalize or stabilize the clinical picture. Therapists working in this environment should remember that once ventilatory support is changed, there might be a change in the ABG.

It is common for ABGs to be drawn after changes in ventilator modes or support. Because changes in respiratory rates can alter ABG results, the therapist working with patients on ventilatory support (mechanical or noninvasive) may need to wait to initiate treatments until after the blood gas is taken. Therapeutic interventions such as exercise, mobility, and airway clearance techniques may affect respiratory rate and therefore the blood gas, possibility distorting the overall values.

Venous blood gases (VBGs) or mixed venous samples, which are obtained from a venous site, peripheral or central, can also provide information on the status of pH and $PaCO_2$. One of the main differences in VBG versus ABG is that the VBG does not provide much information about arterial oxygenation; however, the pH and $PCO_2$ do represent values from the whole body as blood returns to the heart. Generally, the $PCO_2$ from a VBG is 4 to 8 mm Hg greater than the pure arterial sample.[33]

**Table 10-6  Classification of Microbes**

| Taxonomy | Structure | Habitat | Morphology |
|---|---|---|---|
| Viruses | Capsid | Obligate intracellular | Isometric, helical |
| Bacteria | | Extracellular or facultative intracellular | |
| Chlamydias* | Prokaryote | Obligate intracellular | Spherical (cocci), rod-shaped (bacilli), spiral (spirochete) |
| Mycoplasmas* | | Extracellular† | |
| Rickettsias* | | Obligate intracellular | |
| Fungi | Eukaryote | Extracellular or facultative intracellular | |
| Protozoa | | Extracellular, facultative or obligate intracellular | |

*Sometimes classified as bacteria.*
†*Other habitats are possible.*

## Oximetry

Oximetry is a descriptive term for the various technologies available for measuring oxyhemoglobin saturation. The modern pulse oximeter involves a light-emitting diode (LED), a photodiode signal detector, and a microprocessor.[34] The LED alternately emits red and infrared light hundreds of times per second, and the microprocessor compares the signals received by the signal detector and calculates the degree of oxyhemoglobin saturation based on the intensity of transmitted light at the detector. Most units display a digital oxyhemoglobin saturation ($O_2Hb\%$) that updates every few seconds. The reader is referred to Chapter 13 for additional information regarding the clinical interpretation of oximetry values.

The use of the pulse oximetry in the clinical setting has gained great popularity and acceptance for quick and accurate measurements. However the therapist should not always take the readings at face value. Readings can be distorted from a variety of sources from poor circulation and artifact to hemoglobin levels. Therapists should correlate heart rate readings from the oximeter to either electrocardiogram tracings or manual heart rates when presented with "unusual readings" Also remember most pulse oximeters have a +3 error for all readings.

## Cytologic and Hematologic Tests

As part of the diagnostic process, many cytologic and hematologic tests are often performed on patients with pulmonary disease. These tests are helpful in the identification of disease causing organisms and in monitoring the body's responses to them.

Cytologic tests are used to identify specific microorganisms that may cause disease. Several classification schemes, often used simultaneously, describe the various microorganisms identified by cytologic testing: microorganisms are frequently described taxonomically; according to their structure (e.g.,

viruses have a simple central core of DNA or RNA encapsulated by a protein coat; prokaryotes have discrete cell walls, but lack nuclear membranes; eukaryotes have distinct cellular and nuclear membranes); with respect to their habitat (e.g., obligate intracellular parasites require specific cell types or cellular organelles for reproduction; facultative parasites can replicate either outside or inside cells; and extracellular parasites reproduce only outside the cell); or morphologically (e.g., spherical, rod-shaped, spiral). Bacteria are also often categorized on the basis of their staining characteristics (e.g., Gram-negative, Gram-positive, acid-fast) or morphology (Table 10-6).

Numerous microorganisms can normally be found on the skin or mucous membranes of the nasopharynx, oropharynx, and upper airway. Indigenous microbes are often referred to as normal flora. The host organism is said to be colonized if the parasitic microbes cause no injury to the host's cells and is described as infected if the microbes are present below the host cells' external integument. Some parasites share a symbiotic relationship with the host (e.g., vitamin $B_{12}$ is produced by bacteria in the ileum); some are pathogenic, interfering with the host's integrity and function; and some are commensal, having no deleterious effects on a "healthy" host, but becoming opportunistically pathogenic in a compromised host. The extent to which a pathogen interferes with a host's function depends upon the virulence and number of the offending microbes: some organisms are invariably pathogenic, their identification always signifying disease; others are facultative, capable of colonization or infection, depending upon the state of the host's natural chemical and physical barriers.[35] Respiratory infections are typically divided into two groups: upper respiratory tract infection and lower respiratory tract infection. Rhinoviruses account for the majority of upper respiratory infections, although any of the commensal organisms may become pathogenic.

The tracheobronchial tree below the level of the true vocal cords is normally sterile or only minimally colonized. Lower respiratory tract infections are commonly caused by viruses, bacteria, protozoa, and fungi. Table 10-7 lists common

## Table 10-7 Pathogens Commonly Identified in the Lower Respiratory Tract

| Type | Pathogens |
|------|-----------|
| Bacteria | *Streptococcus pneumoniae* |
| | *Staphylococcus aureus* |
| | *Haemophilus influenzae* |
| | Enterobacteriaceae |
| | *Klebsiella pneumoniae* |
| | *Pseudomonas aeruginosa* |
| | *Legionella* (all species) |
| | *Mycoplasma pneumoniae* |
| | *Chlamydia* (all species) |
| Fungi | *Coccidioides immitis* |
| | *Histoplasma capsulatum* |
| | *Blastomyces dermatitidis* |
| | *Aspergillus* (all species) |
| | *Cryptococcus neoformans* |
| | *Candida* (all species) |
| Protozoa | *Pneumocystis carinii* |
| Viruses | Influenza A |
| | Influenza B |
| | Adenoviruses |
| | Respiratory syncytial virus |
| | Parainfluenza viruses |

## Table 10-8 Normal Values for a Complete Blood Cell Count

| Test | Males | Females |
|------|-------|---------|
| Red blood cells | $4.8–6.0 \times 10^6/mm^3$ | $4.1–5.1 \times 10^6/mm^3$ |
| Hemoglobin | 13–16 g/dL or g% | 12–14 g/dL or g% |
| Hematocrit | 40%–54% | 37%–47% |
| White blood cells | 5000–10,000/$mm^3$ | 5000–10,000/$mm^3$ |
| Platelets | 200,000–350,000/$mm^3$ | 200,000–350,000/$mm^3$ |

## Table 10-9 Differential of White Blood Cell Count

| Cell Type | Normal Value |
|-----------|--------------|
| Neutrophils | 50%–75% |
| | Segments: 90%–100% of total neutrophils |
| | Bands: 0%–10% of total neutrophils |
| Eosinophils | 2%–4% |
| Basophils | <0.5% |
| Lymphocytes | 20%–40% |
| Monocytes | 3%–8% |

pathogens of the lower respiratory tract. Microorganisms typically reach the lungs by inhalation, but they are occasionally transported via the blood from another infected site. Unfortunately, many medical treatments and procedures (e.g., immunosuppressive or cytotoxic therapy, intubation, catheterization, and surgical intervention) provide an opportunity for the entry of infectious agents.

Definitive diagnosis of respiratory infections depends on the isolation of specific pathogens from pulmonary secretions or the detection of pathogen-specific antibodies. Microscopic examination and culturing can proceed once appropriate specimens have been collected. Specimens are most often obtained by expectoration, but invasive techniques for specimen collection range from nasotracheal suctioning to open-lung biopsy. Expectorated sputum is the most frequently collected specimen for the diagnosis of pneumonia.[36] The utility of such specimens is controversial because lower respiratory tract secretions are frequently contaminated by upper respiratory tract flora, making interpretation difficult. For this reason, before obtaining an expectorated specimen for culture, it is a good idea to instruct the patient to remove any dentures and to rinse the mouth with water.

Microscopic examination with various stains broadly indicates what sort of organisms are present in the specimen, but culturing is the definitive step. Culturing entails placing the specimen in a variety of cultural media in the presence and absence of oxygen and carbon dioxide, and at different temperatures for varied lengths of time. Antimicrobial therapy is not automatically initiated at the presence of a pathogen-colonization must be distinguished from infection. However, antimicrobial therapy is often initiated when the signs and symptoms of infection are recognized, even before a specific pathogen has been identified. Once a pathogen is identified, its sensitivity to various antimicrobial agents is assessed so that the antimicrobial therapy can be appropriately directed. Refer to Chapter 15 for information regarding pulmonary pharmacologic agents.

Hematologic tests also aid greatly in the assessment of cardiopulmonary disease. Typical tests include ABGs (described previously), electrolyte analysis, complete blood cell (CBC) counts, and coagulation studies. The CBC count imparts information about the number of red blood cells (RBCs), the hemoglobin level, the proportion of the blood that is cells (hematocrit), the number and composition of white blood cells (WBCs), and the platelet count. Coagulation studies evaluate the tendency of the blood to clot.

Tables 10-8 and 10-9 present normal values for the various components of a CBC. A less-than-normal quantity of hemoglobin, a low RBC count, or a low hematocrit is indicative of anemia and suggests that the oxygen-carrying capacity will be decreased. Conversely, an increase in the quantity of hemoglobin, RBC count, or hematocrit is indicative of polycythemia. An increased WBC (leukocytosis) is frequently associated with a bacterial infection, whereas a decreased WBC (leukopenia) may indicate leukemia, although radiation or chemotherapy can also yield this result. An increased neutrophil count is sometimes a first indication of the body's response to inflammation or bacterial infection. An increase in the level of immature neutrophils (bands)—called a *leftward shift of neutrophils*—is an indication of the body's stress response (the greater the shift, the greater the stress). Eosinophilia (an increased number of eosinophils) is usually an indication of an allergic response. Viral infections often result in an increase in the number of lymphocytes. An increased number of monocytes is typical of a chronic infection. An increased number of basophils is frequently associated with some myeloproliferative disorder. Platelets are integral to a normal coagulation process; too few platelets can result in small skin hemorrhages, and too many can increase the likelihood of thrombosis.

In general, four tests are used in an evaluation of the blood's tendency to clot:
1. Bleeding time
2. Platelet count
3. Partial thromboplastin time (PTT)
4. Prothrombin time (PT)

The bleeding time measures the rate of formation of a platelet thrombus; a normal bleeding time is up to 6 minutes. The PTT measures the overall rate of both the intrinsic and common pathways (normal PTT is 32 to 70 seconds), and the PT measures the rate of the extrinsic and common pathways (normal PT is 12 to 15 seconds). Together, the PT and PTT, detect more than 95% of coagulation abnormalities. See Chapter 8 for more information on blood work.

---

### Clinical Tip

The international normalized ratio (INR) is used to adjust for differences in laboratory references between different institutions. Anticoagulation levels are achieved with INR of 2 to 3. Therapists should be aware of the clotting status of patients and refer to individual institution's practice policies regarding activity and mobility of patients with laboratory values outside of reference standards.[37]

---

## CASE STUDY 10-1

HM was admitted to the hospital because of complaints of difficulty breathing. HM has been a cigar smoker for more than 50 years, and has been diagnosed with the respiratory condition emphysema, and chronic obstructive bronchitis, and asthma. His past medical history also includes diabetes, hypertension, arthritis, and prostate cancer. On admission his vital signs included heart rate 106 beats per minute, blood pressure 150/90 mm Hg, respiratory rate 26, temperature 100.5° F. Patient reports a change in sputum production amount and color. His blood counts were normal except an elevated white blood cell count of 19K.

- ABGs: pH 7.29; $PCO_2$ 63.4 mm Hg; $PO_2$ 51 mm Hg; $HCO_3^-$ 30 mEq/L
- During the patient's prior admission his PFTs were recorded as follows:
  - TLC 120% predicted
  - VC 115% predicted
  - RV 130% predicted
- FEV 148% predicted
- FEF 54% predicted
- Chest radiograph showed infiltrates in right lower lobe, hyperinflation, and increased cardiac size.[38]

### Discussion

This case demonstrates the pulmonary diagnostic findings of an individual with chronic lung disease who has an acute event of pneumonia causing him to develop respiratory failure. The patient's ABGs demonstrate an acute respiratory acidosis, with partial compensation that is probably a result of long-standing obstructive lung disease. His PFTs demonstrate severe obstructive airway disease, and the chest radiograph demonstrates chronic lung changes (hyperinflation) with an acute event (infiltrates in right lower lobe). Sputum cultures may be necessary to tailor antibiotic therapies.

---

## Summary

This chapter considered various chest-imaging techniques along with a method for examining chest radiographs. Several tests of pulmonary function and their interpretation were discussed. Finally, cytologic and hematologic tests were covered briefly. This information, together with that in Chapters 13 and 16, will facilitate your interpretation of evaluative findings.

- The standard radiograph is the predominant medium by which anatomic abnormalities arising from pathologic processes within the chest are assessed.
- The standard chest radiograph is typically taken in two views: posteroanterior and left lateral.
- Dark areas on a chest radiograph are termed radiolucent; light areas are radiopaque.
- In a "body systems" approach to the analysis of a chest radiograph, the examiner should examine (1) the bones and soft tissues; (2) the mediastinum, trachea, and cardiovascular system; (3) the hila; and (4) the lung fields.
- A tomogram (sectional radiograph) differs from a standard radiograph because tomography involves the curvilinear movement of the x-ray source and the imaging medium in opposite directions about the patient.

- A magnetic resonance image is produced in much the same manner as a computed tomographic image, except that a gradient magnetic field is used to align the protons of the target tissue and then radio signals are used to stimulate them in order to create an image.
- MRI is currently limited to evaluation of chest wall (bone, muscle, fat, or pleura) processes because the expanded lungs have an insufficient density of protons for the generation of an adequate image from which to evaluate pathologic processes of the parenchyma.
- To obtain a bronchogram, the bronchial tree is opacified by the instillation of a contrast (radiopaque) medium as a radiographic or tomographic image is produced.
- Bronchograms permit the study of gross pathologic changes in the walls and lumina of the bronchial tree.
- V/Q scintillography is used to evaluate the regional distribution of gas and blood flow in the lungs.
- The fiberoptic bronchoscope makes the direct visualization of the bronchial tree clinically possible.
- PFTs provide information about the integrity of the airways, the function of the respiratory musculature, and the condition of the lung tissues themselves. Generally, PFTs involve the assessment of lung volumes and capacities, gas flow rates, diffusion, and gas exchange.
- Pulmonary diseases are classified into three basic categories on the basis of pulmonary function testing: obstructive, restrictive, and combined.
- The three most commonly used methods for the determination of FRC and RV are the helium dilution (closed-circuit) method, the nitrogen washout (open-circuit) method, and body plethysmography.
- When expressed as a percentage of the FVC, the volume of air exhaled in the first second of the maneuver ($FEV_1\%$) is one of the most useful parameters in the assessment of respiratory impairment.
- An $FEV_1\%$ of more than 80% or 90% indicates restrictive disease, whereas an $FEV_1\%$ of 60% or less suggests obstructive disease associated with increased morbidity and mortality rates.
- Blood gas analysis (arterial, venous, or mixed venous) allows the assessment of problems related to acid–base balance, ventilation, and oxygenation. By convention, unless otherwise specified, a blood gas sample is presumed to be arterial in origin.
- The normal pH of the blood is 7.40, a pH of less than 7.40 is defined as acidemia, while a pH of more than 7.40 is defined as alkalemia. Any process that causes acidemia is called an acidosis, and any process that causes an alkalemia is called an alkalosis.
- The adequacy of alveolar ventilation is directly reflected by the $PaCO_2$. Alveolar hyperventilation is indicated by a $PaCO_2$ that is less than normal, and alveolar hypoventilation is indicated by a $PaCO_2$ that is greater than normal. When a patient's $PaCO_2$ is greater than 50 mm Hg, the condition is called ventilatory failure.
- A patient's oxygenation status is assessed by determining the extent to which the observed $PaO_2$ is above or below the normal range (generally accepted as being between 80 to 100 mm Hg, when breathing room air).
- Numerous cytologic tests are used to identify specific microorganisms that may cause disease. A cytologic sample is said to be infected if the parasitic microbes are present below the host cells' integument; it is colonized if the parasitic microbes present cause no injury to the host's cells.
- The CBC count imparts information about the number of RBCs, the hemoglobin level, the hematocrit, the number and composition of WBCs, and the platelet count.

## References

1. Freundlich IM, Bragg DG. A Radiologic Approach to Diseases of the Chest. 2nd ed. Baltimore, Williams & Wilkins, 1997.
2. Meholic A, Ketai L, Lofgren R. Fundamentals of Chest Radiology. Philadelphia, Saunders, 1996.
3. Armstrong P. Imaging of Diseases of the Chest. 2nd ed. St. Louis, CV Mosby, 1995.
4. Lange S, Stark P. Radiology of Chest Diseases. New York, Thieme Medical Publishers, 1990.
5. Evans TJ. AANA Journal Course: Update for nurse anesthetists—Fundamentals of chest radiography. Techniques and interpretation for the anesthetist. AANA J 60:45–62, 1992.
6. Coche E, Verschuren F, Keyeux A, et al. Diagnosis of acute pulmonary embolism in outpatients: comparison of thin-collimation multi-detector row spiral CT and planar ventilation-perfusion scintigraphy. Radiology 229(3):757–65, 2003.
7. Stein PD, Kayali F, Olson RE. Trends in the use of diagnostic imaging in patients hospitalized with acute pulmonary embolism. Am J Cardiol 15;93(10):1316–17, 2004.
8. Gulsun Akpinar M, Goodman LR. Imaging of pulmonary thromboembolism. Clin Chest Med 29(1):107–16, vi, 2008.
9. Johnson MS. Current strategies for the diagnosis of pulmonary embolus. J Vasc Interv Radiol 13(1):13–23, 2002.
10. Rinck PA, Torheim G, Lombardi M. Image postprocessing and contrast agents in clinical MR imaging—An introductory overview. Acta Radiol Suppl 412:7–19, 1997.
11. van Beek E, Hoffman EA. Functional imaging: CT and MRI. Clin Chest Med 29(1):195–vii, 2008.
12. PIOPED Investigators. Value of the ventilation/perfusion scan in acute pulmonary embolism. Results of the prospective investigation of pulmonary embolism diagnosis (PIOPED). JAMA 263(20):2753–9, 1990.
13. Thompson IM, Whittlesey GC, Slovis TL, et al. Evaluation of contrast media for bronchography. Pediatr Radiol 27:598–605, 1997.
14. Borchers SD, Beamis Jr JF. Flexible bronchoscopy. Chest Surg Clin N Am 6:169–92, 1996.
15. Bang KM, Gergen PJ, Kramer R, et al. The effect of pulmonary impairment on all-cause mortality in a national cohort. Chest 103:536–40, 1993.
16. Neas LM, Schwartz J. Pulmonary function levels as predictors of mortality in a national sample of US adults. Am J Epidemiol 147:1011–18, 1998.
17. Ryan G, Knuiman MW, Divitini ML, et al. Decline in lung function and mortality: The Busselton Health Study. J Epidemiol Community Health 53:230–4, 1999.

18. Fulton JE, Pivarnik JM, Taylor WC, et al. Prediction of maximum voluntary ventilation (MVV) in African-American adolescent girls. Pediatr Pulmonol 20:225–33, 1995.

19. Pellegrino R, Viegi G, Brusasco V, et al. Interpretative strategies for lung function tests. Eur Respir J 26(5):948–68, 2005.

20. Quadrelli SA, Roncoroni AJ, Porcel G. Analysis of variability in interpretation of spirometric tests. Respiration 63:131–6, 1996.

21. Pellegrino R, Rodarte JR, Brusasco V. Assessing the reversibility of airway obstruction. Chest 114:1607–12, 1998.

22. Jansons H, Fokkens JK, van der Tweel I, et al. Rebreathing vs single-breath TLCO in patients with unequal ventilation and diffusion. Respir Med 92:18–24, 1998.

23. Hyatt RE, Scanlon PD, Nakamura M. Interpretation of Pulmonary Function Tests: A Practical Guide. Philadelphia, Lippincott-Raven, 1997.

24. Madama VC. Pulmonary Function Testing and Cardiopulmonary Stress Testing. 2nd ed. Albany, NY, Delmar Publishers, 1998.

25. Ruppel G. Manual of Pulmonary Function Testing. 7th ed. St. Louis, Mosby, 1998.

26. Wanger J. Pulmonary Function Testing: A Practical Approach. 2nd ed. Baltimore, Williams & Wilkins, 1996.

27. Shapiro BA, Peruzzi WT, Kozelowski-Templin R. Clinical Application of Blood Gases. 5th ed. St. Louis, Mosby-Year Book, 1994.

28. Cornock MA. Making sense of arterial blood gases and their interpretation. Nurs Times 92:30–1, 1996.

29. Syabbalo N. Measurement and interpretation of arterial blood gases. Br J Clin Pract 51:173–6, 1997.

30. Williams AJ. ABC of oxygen: Assessing and interpreting arterial blood gases and acid-base balance. BMJ 317:1213–16, 1998.

31. DeTurk WE, Cahalin LP. Cardiovascular and Pulmonary Physical Therapy: An Evidenced-Based Approach. New York, McGraw-Hill, 2004.

32. Askin DF. Interpretation of neonatal blood gases. Part II: Disorders of acid-base balance. Neonatal Netw 16:23–9, 1997.

33. Dooley J, Fegley A. Laboratory monitoring of mechanical ventilation. Crit Care Clin 23(2):135–48, vii, 2007.

34. Tallon RW. Oximetry: State-of-the-art. Nurs Manage 27:43–4, 1996.

35. Cotran RS, Kumar V, Collins T, et al. Robbins Pathologic Basis of Disease. 6th ed. Philadelphia, Saunders, 1999.

36. Burton GG, Hodgkin JE, Ward JJ. Respiratory Care: A Guide to Clinical Practice. 4th ed. Philadelphia, Lippincott, 1997.

37. Malone, DJ, Lindsay KLB. Physical Therapy in Acute Care: A Clinician's Guide. Thorofare, NJ, Slack, 2006.

38. Martin TR, Lewis SW, Albert RK. The prognosis of patients with chronic obstructive pulmonary disease after hospitalization for acute respiratory failure. Chest 82(3):310–14, 1982.

## CHAPTER 11

# Cardiovascular and Thoracic Interventions

*Ellen Hillegass, H. Steven Sadowsky*

## Chapter Outline

In addition to the pathologic conditions that were discussed in Chapters 3 through 7, an almost unlimited number of surgical procedures and interventions can have a significant impact on the functioning of and interaction between the cardiovascular and pulmonary systems. Therefore, because an appreciation for the extent and involvement of surgical incisions is beneficial when planning and implementing therapeutic interventions for postoperative patients, the first part of this chapter introduces the reader to the most commonly used thoracic incisions. The second part of the chapter introduces interventions and devices used with patients who have cardiovascular or pulmonary disease.

## Cardiovascular and Thoracic Surgical Procedures

### Cardio-Thoracic Surgical Approaches

Individual surgeons develop preferences for particular surgical approaches based on their particular experiences and training. Thus, posterolateral and lateral thoracotomy incisions are most commonly used for lung resection procedures, although a median sternotomy may be employed occasionally (e.g., when lung resection is combined with a cardiac procedure).[1] Cardiac procedures are performed almost exclusively through a median sternotomy, although the great vessels sometimes are approached via a thoracotomy incision. Procedures that involve the pericardium or epicardium (e.g., pericardial biopsy, epicardial pacemaker insertion) are typically accomplished through a subxiphoid incision. Diaphragmatic procedures are commonly performed through either a lateral thoracotomy or a thoracoabdominal incision.

As surgical procedures continue to advance, surgeons are performing more minimally invasive and video-assisted (and robotic) surgeries with lower number of complications and less healing time.

### Posterolateral Thoracotomy

In preparation for a posterolateral thoracotomy, patients are generally positioned one-quarter turn from prone (operative side elevated) with the uppermost arm elevated forward, flexed at the elbow, and placed beside the head. The typical posterolateral thoracotomy incision extends downward from a point midway between the spine of the fourth thoracic vertebra and the scapula in a gently curving arch around the tip of the scapula to the fifth or sixth intercostal space at the anterior axillary line (Fig. 11-1). The serratus anterior is divided close to its muscular attachment in an effort to preserve its function and to avoid the long thoracic nerve. The pleural space is most often entered via an incision through the intercostal muscles at the fifth intercostal space, although a specific pathologic condition may dictate entry via another intercostal space.

### Anterolateral Thoracotomy

Patients are positioned one-quarter turn from supine (operative side elevated) with the uppermost arm flexed at the elbow and placed beneath the back (retracting the latissimus dorsi muscle) in preparation for an anterolateral thoracotomy. The submammary incision curves from the fourth or fifth intercostal space at the midaxillary line to the midclavicular or parasternal region (Fig. 11-2). The pectoralis major is incised, and fibers of the serratus anterior are separated (with female patients, it is sometimes necessary for the surgeon to reflect the breast superiorly).

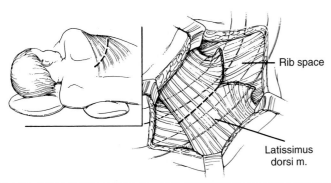

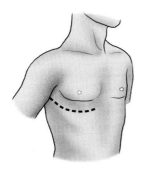

**Figure 11-1** The posterolateral thoracotomy incision. This incision is often used for lung resection procedures or for procedures involving the descending thoracic aorta. (From O'Neill JA, Coran AG, Fonkalsrud E, et al. Pediatric Surgery. 6th ed. St. Louis, Mosby, 2006.)

**Figure 11-2** The anterolateral thoracotomy incision. This incision is not used as often as the posterolateral approach, but it is used for some cardiac procedures, pulmonary resections, and esophageal procedures. (From Watchie J: Cardiovascular and Pulmonary Physical Therapy: A Clinical Manual, ed 2. St Louis, 2010, Saunders.)

> **Clinical Tip**
> Critical therapeutic interventions with individuals who undergo a lateral thoracotomy include segmental breathing to prevent or minimize atelectasis, side bending, and lateral chest wall stretching after surgery.

## Lateral Thoracotomy

Patients are placed in side-lying position, operative side up, with the arm abducted, flexed at the elbow, and rotated in preparation for a lateral thoracotomy (avoiding excessive abduction or rotation, which might cause stretching of the brachial plexus). There are several variations of the lateral thoracotomy incision, although it generally begins near the nipple line and extends toward the scapula (Fig. 11-3). The latissimus dorsi muscle is not incised; instead, it is retracted either anteriorly or posteriorly, and the fibers of either the serratus anterior or the intercostal muscles between the serratus interdigitations are incised to gain access to the appropriate intercostal space (most often the fourth, fifth, or sixth).

Postoperative scapular winging is avoided by careful preservation of the long thoracic nerve.

## Axillary Thoracotomy

An axillary thoracotomy is sometimes used for apical bleb resection or dorsal sympathectomy. Patients are placed in a side-lying position with the arm flexed at the elbow, abducted 90 degrees at the shoulder, and rotated as for a lateral thoracotomy. From the edge of the pectoralis major, anteriorly, the incision extends posteriorly within the second intercostal space to the edge of the latissimus dorsi.

## Median Sternotomy

A median sternotomy is probably the most frequently used incision for cardiothoracic operations.[1,2] In preparation for a median sternotomy, the patient is placed in the supine position. The initial skin incision usually begins in the midline inferior to the suprasternal notch and extends below the xiphoid (Fig. 11-4A). The sternum is divided along its midline in a series of steps, and a sternal retractor is used to hold the incision open (Fig. 11-4B). At the end of the surgical procedure, the sternum is generally closed with stainless steel sutures either through or around the sternum, and the wound is closed in layers (Fig. 11-4C).

## Thoracoabdominal Incisions

A thoracoabdominal incision permits procedures on the diaphragm, esophagus, biliary tract, right lobe of the liver, spleen, adrenal gland, and kidney, as well as placement of portacaval shunts. In preparation, patients are positioned supine with the operative side rotated upward 30 to 45 degrees, the buttocks and back elevated, and the arm on the operative side extended anteriorly as in a posterolateral thoracotomy. The incision usually extends from the eighth or ninth intercostal space at the posterior axillary line to the midline of the abdomen, transecting the latissimus dorsi, serratus anterior, external oblique, and rectus abdominis muscles (Fig. 11-5).

> **Clinical Tip**
> Individuals with a thoracoabdominal incision often have problems with coughing, deep breathing, and thoracic extension. Therefore, therapeutic interventions should be implemented early to prevent pulmonary complications, and forward flexed postures should be avoided.

## Thoracic Surgical Complications

The major causes of perioperative morbidity and mortality in the entire thoracic surgical population are respiratory complications.[3] The respiratory complications include atelectasis, pneumonia and respiratory failure and occur in approximately 15% to 20% of all patients who undergo thoracic surgery.[4] These complications account for approximately 3% to 4% of the postoperative mortality.[4] Pulmonary complications are

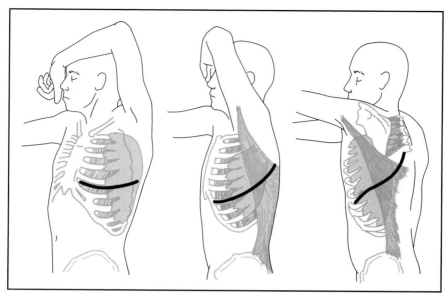

**Figure 11-3** The lateral thoracotomy incision. This incision is often used because it spares the latissimus dorsi (the muscle does not have to be divided) while providing access for pneumonectomy, lobectomy, or wedge resection procedures. (Redrawn with permission from Cooper F [ed.]. The Craft of Surgery. Vol. 1. Boston, Little, Brown, 1964:197.)

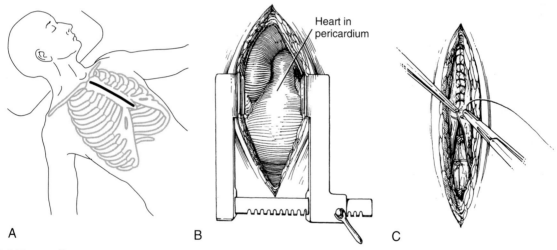

Heart in pericardium

A          B          C

**Figure 11-4** The median sternotomy incision is the most frequently used incision for cardiac procedures. **A,** The incision begins inferior to the suprasternal notch and extends below the xiphoid process. **B,** A sternal retractor maintains the incision open for access to the thoracic contents. **C,** The sternum is approximated and sutured closed with stainless steel sutures through or around the sternum; the wound is then closed in layers. (*B* and *C* from Cooley DA. Techniques in Cardiac Surgery. 2nd ed. Philadelphia, Saunders, 1984:18, 19.)

decreased in thoracic surgical patients who cease smoking for more than 4 weeks before surgery.[3] Carboxyhemoglobin concentrations decrease if smoking is stopped more than 12 hours before surgery.[3] Of course, it is extremely important for patients to avoid smoking postoperatively as smoking affects tissue healing.

Cardiac complications are the second most cause of perioperative morbidity and mortality in the thoracic surgical population and include arrhythmias and ischemia.[4] Cardiac complications occur in approximately 10% to 15% of the thoracic surgical population. For other types of surgery, cardiac and vascular complications are the leading causes of

early perioperative morbidity and mortality.[4] Arrhythmias are most common after pulmonary resection surgery, with the incidence being 30% to 50% of patients in the first week postoperatively.[3] Of these arrhythmias, 60% to 70% are atrial fibrillation. Several factors correlate with an increased incidence of arrhythmias, including extent of lung resection (pneumonectomy, 60%, versus lobectomy, 40%, versus nonresection thoracotomy, 30%), intrapericardial dissection, intraoperative blood loss, and age of the patient.[3] In addition, the development of renal dysfunction after pulmonary resection surgery is associated with a high mortality and has been associated with a history of previous renal impairment,

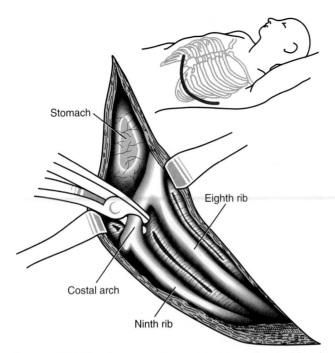

Stomach

Eighth rib

Costal arch

Ninth rib

**Figure 11-5** The thoracoabdominal incision. This incision is used for procedures involving the diaphragm, the upper abdomen, or the retroperitoneal space. (Redrawn from Waldhausen JA, Pierce WS. Johnson's Surgery of the Chest. 5th ed. Chicago, Year Book Medical Publishers, 1985:59.)

diuretic therapy, pneumonectomy, postoperative infection, and blood transfusion.[3]

*Shoulder Pain*
After thoracotomy, up to 80% of patients describe ipsilateral shoulder pain. Shoulder pain occurs after both thoracotomy and video-assisted thoracoscopic surgery (VATS) and is thought to be primarily referred pain of diaphragmatic irritation transmitted by the phrenic nerve afferent.[5,6]

Other factors, including position during operation and major bronchus transection, have been thought to be involved. Several other causes of shoulder pain should be considered when evaluating a patient with shoulder pain postoperatively:

- A chest drain placed too far into the apex of the hemithorax can irritate the parietal pleura and cause shoulder pain. Treatment involves identifying the problem on chest radiograph and withdrawal of chest drain partially.
- The posterior end of a large posterolateral thoracotomy incision may not be blocked by a functioning thoracic epidural block. The epidural analgesia might need to be increased.
- Individuals who have chronic arthralgia of the shoulder may have an exacerbation as a consequence of positioning. Preoperative questioning regarding shoulder problems would alert the surgeon to improved positioning.

Shoulder pain is usually transient and often is resolved completely by the second postoperative day.

Central venous pressure (CVP) monitoring and access is a routine procedure for thoracic surgery in some centers. However, CVP readings in the lateral position with the chest open are unreliable. The CVP is a useful monitor postoperatively, particularly for cases in which fluid management is critical (e.g., pneumonectomies). See Chapter 13 for more details on invasive monitoring.

## Minimally Invasive Approaches
VATS has become the standard procedure for minimally invasive surgery for the treatment of thoracic problems, including lung cancer, pleural problems, and even abdominal surgeries. The advantage of VATS, when compared with open thoracotomy, include (1) reduced hospital length of stay; (2) less blood loss if no mishaps occur; (3) less pain; (4) improvement in pulmonary function when compared with open thoracotomy; (5) early patient mobilization with early recovery and rapid return to work and daily activities; and (6) less inflammatory reaction, as measured by cytokine response in patients undergoing VATS lobectomy compared with open thoracotomy.[7-9]

In addition, patients who undergo VATS lobectomies report less postoperative pain, reduced shoulder dysfunction, decreased time until return to preoperative activities, and higher satisfaction than patients undergoing the conventional thoracotomy.[10] In addition, a lower observed incidence of postoperative confusion is reported in VATS surgery patients, which is an advantage for surgery performed in the older adult.[10] VATS lobectomy also has been demonstrated to be a safe and effective procedure to treat early stage non-small-cell lung cancer.

Thoracoscopic lobectomy is performed with a limited number of ports (one to three) and an access incision of approximately 5 cm in length. The advantage of the VATS technique is that the ribs are not spread and VATS procedures are commonly performed in the lateral decubitus position; however, bilateral VATS procedures, such as bilateral wedge resections or lung volume reduction, can be performed in the supine position.[11]

Kirby and colleagues reported no difference in intraoperative time, blood loss, or length of hospital stay between patients who underwent VATS versus those who underwent thoracotomy, yet the thoracotomy group experienced significantly more postoperative complications, most notably prolonged air leaks.[12] Jaklitsch and colleagues reported that

VATS procedures for patients age 65 years and older resulted in superior 30-day operative mortality and a decreased length of hospital stay, compared with previous reports for standard thoracotomy.[13] Two large series reported lower-than-expected rates of postoperative atrial fibrillation following VATS lobectomy relative to thoracotomy, ranging from 2.9% to 10%.[14]

> **Clinical Tip**
> Anesthesia management with VATS surgeries involves the use of epidural blocks. Epidural blocks are also used in total shoulder surgeries as they they result in less muscle pain and spasm and improve the success rates of postoperative functional outcomes This may be one reason why there is less shoulder pain in VATS surgeries as well.

## Cardio-Thoracic Surgical Interventions

A description of all of the possible cardiovascular or thoracic surgical procedures is well beyond the scope of this chapter. However, because cardiovascular and thoracic surgical procedures are so prevalent, a few procedures deserve attention.

## Percutaneous Revascularization Procedures

As discussed in Chapter 3, coronary arterial atherosclerotic disease can produce occlusive plaques that, in turn, compromise coronary arterial blood flow to such an extent that coronary arterial revascularization procedures become necessary to preserve myocardial integrity. Three procedures are discussed here: angioplasty, arthrectomy, and stenting. Common to each of these procedures is the introduction (under fluoroscopic guidance) of a balloon-equipped catheter, via a peripheral arterial access site (e.g., femoral artery), into the coronary arterial tree to the site of the stenotic lesion. The procedure is successful if the lumen remains patent when the catheter is withdrawn and there is no ensuing angiospasm. The return of blood flow to the distribution of the previously occluded artery is immediately checked by means of an angiogram (or coronary catheterization, see Chapter 8). None of the procedures is completely risk free; the arterial wall can be perforated when the lesion is penetrated, or it can rupture when the balloon is inflated.[15-18] Therefore, it is not uncommon to have a cardiac surgical suite held in reserve for the emergency remediation of any complications. Generally, however, no significant postoperative movement restrictions are associated with the procedure—patients can be ambulatory within a matter of hours following the procedure. Patients are rarely hospitalized for more than 2 to 3 days, if that long. In fact, many patients are tested, on an outpatient basis, to determine the extent of the resolution of preprocedure electrocardiographic ischemic changes and referred for outpatient cardiac rehabilitation within that time frame.

A percutaneous transluminal coronary angioplasty (PTCA) may be performed when a stenotic lesion is not too large; that is, when it does not completely occlude the lumen of the coronary artery. The atherosclerotic lesion is penetrated, and the balloon at the distal aspect of the catheter is

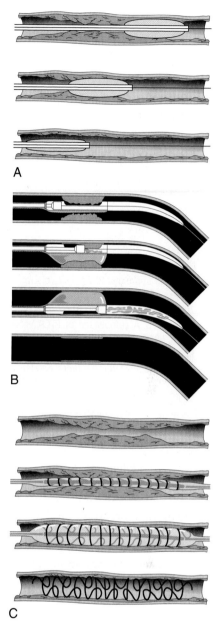

**Figure 11-6** Percutaneous coronary revascularization. **A,** Percutaneous transluminal coronary angioplasty catheters are positioned at the distal end of a stenotic lesion before the balloon is inflated to compress the lesion against the arterial walls. (Redrawn from Greenhalgh RM. Vascular Surgical Techniques—An Atlas. 2nd ed. London, Saunders, 1989:315.) **B,** Atherectomy catheters are positioned so that the cutter housing is held firmly against the atheroma before the cutter is advanced. (Redrawn from Holmes DR, Garratt KN. Atherectomy. Oxford, Blackwell Scientific, 1992:24.) **C,** Intravascular stents are positioned within a stenotic lesion before being expanded. (Redrawn from Roubin GS, King SB, Douglas JS, et al. Intracoronary stenting during percutaneous transluminal coronary angioplasty. Circulation 81[Suppl IV]: IV92–IV100, 1990.)

inflated, compressing the central portion of the lesion outward against the wall of the artery (Fig. 11-6A). This process may be repeated with successively larger catheters to increase the lumen size as much as possible. A directional coronary arthrectomy (DCA) may be performed instead of, or in conjunction with, a PTCA.[19] This procedure involves the introduction of an arthrectomy catheter through the stenotic lesion of a coronary artery. The cutter housing, which is at the distal end of the catheter through the stenotic lesion of a coronary artery, has a longitudinal opening on one side and an inflatable balloon on the other. The opening is positioned so that it faces the atheroma, and the balloon is inflated so that the housing is fixed against the arterial wall, displacing the atheroma into the housing opening. The cutter is then activated and advanced, pushing an excised specimen into the distal part of the housing (Fig. 11-6B). Technologic advances have reached the point that atherectomies may now be performed using laser-tipped catheters also.

---

**Clinical Tip**

The literature reports an approximate 70% success rate with PTCA, of which 30% undergo a repeat PTCA. Of the 30% repeat procedures, approximately 70% are successful. Less-successful outcomes have been reported for women. A comparison of PTCA versus coronary artery bypass graft (CABG) in an entire population was reported by the New York State Cardiac Procedures Registries. On 3-year followup, repeat revascularization was 11 times greater in the PTCA group than in the CABG group (or 37% PTCA vs. 3.3% CABG).[20] In addition the 3-year mortality rate was significantly greater in the PTCA group (43% greater 3-year adjusted mortality rate).[20]

---

The placement of endoluminal stents is another means of coronary revascularization that has gained clinical acceptance.[21] Stents are tiny springlike devices introduced into a stenotic lesion in an effort to increase the intravascular luminal diameter (Fig. 11-6C). Stents have been instrumental in the improvement in the safety and effectiveness of percutaneous coronary interventions. A 40% reduction has been reported in the need for repeat intervention or coronary bypass surgery over a 1-year followup.[22] Also, since the addition of potent antiplatelet agents such as GPIIb/IIIa (glycoprotein) inhibitors and adenosine diphosphate inhibitors, or with thienopyridines, stent placement has improved the angioplasty outcome, particularly for patients at risk for closure (diabetic and repeat stenosis patients).[23–26] Treatment was associated with a lower rate of death, myocardial infarction, and stroke, but with a higher rate of major bleeding.[25,26] A drug-eluting stent (DES) has been used instead of PTCA because of the increased risk of restenosis in PTCA, yet a metaanalysis of a DES versus a bare metal stent did not conclude a mortality benefit for the DES, although there was a decreased incidence of restenosis.[27] The problem with using mortality as the outcome studied in these trials is that oftentimes revascularization is needed in arteries that were not stented in these studies because of the nature of the disease, atherosclerosis being a progressive disease. Therefore, using survival as the outcome, CABG appears to be the main option in patients with multivessel disease and certain subgroups of one- and two-vessel disease.

## Coronary Artery Bypass Graft

When a coronary arterial atherosclerotic lesion progresses to such an extent that the artery becomes completely occluded, or when the lesion is not amenable to percutaneous transluminal coronary angioplasty or DCA, a CABG may have to be performed to revascularize the myocardium. The Coronary Artery Surgery Study (CASS) concluded that surgical revascularization is the optimal choice for management of coronary artery disease when all three vessels are severely obstructed. A reduction in mortality rate was the clinical outcome used in the CASS study when surgical intervention was compared to medical management in patients with severe coronary artery disease and impaired left ventricular function.[28] CABG is now the safest and most reliable method for completely revascularizing the ischemic heart and is associated with excellent medium and long-term outcomes.

Vascular grafts are often procured from either or both of the saphenous veins (Fig. 11-7), but the left internal mammary artery can also be diverted for use in a coronary revascularization procedure. Following a median sternotomy, the site or sites of coronary arterial blockage are located and isolated. When a saphenous vein graft is used, it is cut to the appropriate length and desired shape before being anastomosed above and below the occlusion (Fig. 11-8). If the internal mammary artery is used in the revascularization procedure, it is anastomosed below the level of the occlusive lesion (Fig. 11-9). The use of internal thoracic arteries is preferable for achieving better long-term outcome, because these vessels have proved to be more resistant to graft atherosclerosis (a frequent problem with saphenous graft use).[29,30] Once grafting is completed, the tissue layers are approximated and the wound is closed.

Recent improvements in the surgical approach include the use of smaller incisions with microinstrumentation (termed minimally invasive direct coronary artery bypass, or MIDCAB). MIDCAB involves a small thoracotomy and does not require the use of the heart–lung bypass machine. The procedure is limited, however, to the isolated internal mammary-left anterior descending artery anastomosis, and therefore has not been widely adopted. Postoperative complications and recovery time are reduced, extubation is performed earlier, and patients are mobilized earlier, all potential reasons for improved surgical outcomes.

Other advances in coronary bypass grafting include the use of ultrasound-guided cannulations, which have decreased the incidence of embolic cerebrovascular accidents. Again, patients do not undergo a sternotomy, but are placed on cardiopulmonary bypass by special catheters. Because the procedure is time-consuming and the technique itself is expensive, the surgical community has not adopted this procedure as a standard procedure for bypass.

A third surgical variation for coronary bypass involves a sternotomy, but no cardiopulmonary bypass, called the off-pump coronary artery bypass (OPCAB). The surgeon operates on a beating heart. This procedure has been more accepted than the other procedures mentioned but is not

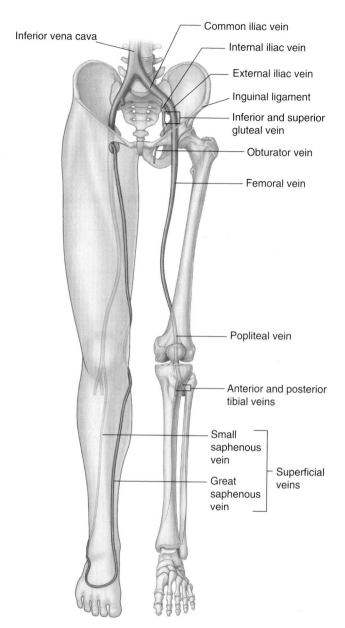

Inferior vena cava

Common iliac vein

Internal iliac vein

External iliac vein

Inguinal ligament

Inferior and superior gluteal vein

Obturator vein

Femoral vein

Popliteal vein

Anterior and posterior tibial veins

Small saphenous vein

Great saphenous vein

Superficial veins

**Figure 11-7** Veins of the lower extremity. (From Aehlert B: ACLS Study Guide, 3rd Edition. St Louis, 2007, Mosby.)

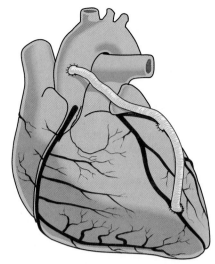

**Figure 11-8** Saphenous vein grafts are anastomosed above and below the level of the occlusive lesion after they are cut to the appropriate length and desired shape.

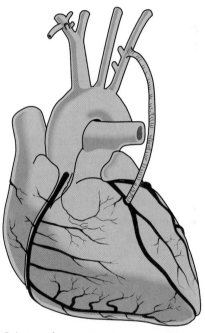

**Figure 11-9** Internal mammary arterial grafts are anastomosed below the level of the occlusive lesion. (Redrawn from Waldhausen JA, Pierce WS. Johnson's Surgery of the Chest. 5th ed. Chicago, Year Book Medical Publishers, 1985:480.)

considered a standard operating procedure at the time of this publication.

Preclinical and clinical studies are now underway to develop and evaluate new methodologies that will make the operation even safer and more effective. This includes use of less-invasive techniques, testing of smaller extracorporeal circulation devices, and developing methods to improve myocardial protection and techniques to enhance graft patency. The less-invasive operative techniques include performing more precise surgery on small and distal vessels. Bypass graft coupling devices under investigation are designed to improve proximal and distal coronary artery graft anastomoses, including interrupted clips, magnetic docking ports, and specialized metallic intracoronary stents. Smaller ven-

tricular assist devices are also under study that may decrease the risk of infection and thromboembolic complications. In addition, current evidence shows a higher incidence of even mild necrosis during the CABG operation (as measured by creatine kinase and creatine kinase-myocardial bound) that is also associated with a decrease in medium- and long-term survival. This has led to interest in developing more effective methods for protecting the heart. One such strategy, which is under intense investigation, is to mimic the phenomenon of ischemic preconditioning pharmacologically. Gene-based therapies may make it possible to transfect human saphenous veins before grafting and to prevent vascular intimal hyperplasia.[31]

### Robotics

Advances in technology have led to the development of robotic CABG. Robotically assisted surgical systems minimize the invasiveness of any coronary artery bypass surgery as well as decrease any surgical tremors.[32] One current system in use is the da Vinci system. Preliminary studies demonstrate safety and equal results to other minimally invasive surgery, but patient candidacy is more limited and fewer surgeons are trained in this technique.[33,34] One multicenter trial also noted that 28% of candidates needed to be converted to nonrobotic surgery.[34] Robotic surgery has the potential to decrease operative complications, and possibly to decrease hospitalization time.

### Thoracic Organ Transplantation

Heart and lung transplantation is performed using a median sternotomy technique and is discussed in detail in Chapter 12.

### Carotid Endarterectomy

Carotid endarterectomy (CEA), although a somewhat controversial surgery from the mid-1980s to mid-1990s, has become more popular since the publication of the North American Symptomatic Carotid Endarterectomy (NASCET) Trial and the Asymptomatic Carotid Atherosclerosis Study (ACAS) trial.[35,36] Both studies provided data on appropriate patient selection, as well as on measuring stenosis (Fig. 11-10).

Candidates for this procedure include:

- The symptomatic patient with carotid artery stenosis of 70% or greater;
- The symptomatic patient with a stenosis of 50% to 69% of the carotid artery (demonstrated only modest benefit); and
- The asymptomatic patient with stenosis of 60% or greater.

The procedure involves a surgical incision along the anterior border of the sternocleidomastoid muscle to allow for maximal exposure of the upper carotid artery (Fig. 11-11A). The common and external carotid arteries are occluded with clamps, an incision is made, and a temporary bypass shunt is inserted (Fig. 11-11B). The plaque is removed (Fig. 11-11C), and the arteriotomy closed with sutures (Fig. 11-11D) as the

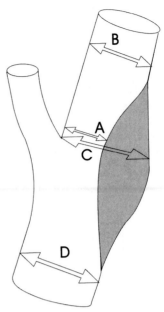

**Figure 11-10** Degree of carotid artery stenosis as measured in the North American Symptomatic Carotid Endarterectomy Trial (NASCET) and the European Carotid Surgery Trial (ECST). NASCET used the distal reference point, measuring the residual lumen (A) in comparison to the normal distal internal carotid artery (ICA) lumen (B). ECST measured the residual ICA lumen (A) compared with the local estimated diameter of the carotid bulb (C). Local degree of stenosis = C − A/C. Distal degree of stenosis = B − A/B. Degree of common carotid artery stenosis = D − A/D. (From Rutherford RB. Vascular Surgery. 6th ed. Philadelphia, Saunders, 2005.)

bypass shunt is removed. The patient is left with an incision scar on the lateral aspect of the neck.[37]

The outcome of carotid endarterectomy, as determined from both the NASCET and ACAS trials, primarily involves a decreased risk of stroke in the vascular distribution "at risk" for many years. The risk of undergoing carotid endarterectomy was shown to increase as the severity of disease increased; therefore, those likely to benefit the most from the surgery were those who had the highest risk in undergoing the operation.[38]

The use of angioplasty in carotid artery disease is not indicated because of the risk of iatrogenic embolization (embolic stroke); however, the use of stents may be indicated for the carotid artery. At present, evidence is not clear whether the results of carotid stenting are in fact equivalent to those of CEA. The Stenting and Angioplasty with Protection in Patients at High Risk for Endarterectomy (SAPPHIRE) trial randomly compared carotid artery stenting to endarterectomy. Analysis of 30-day and 1-year outcomes, including death, stroke, or myocardial infarction, found that carotid stenting was not inferior to CEA.[39] However, the overall results in both arms of this trial were noted to be disturbingly high, with a risk of 12.2% among stenting patients and 20.1% among endarterectomy patients.[39] The Carotid Revascularization Using Endarterectomy or Stenting Systems (CaRESS) trial was a multicenter prospective but

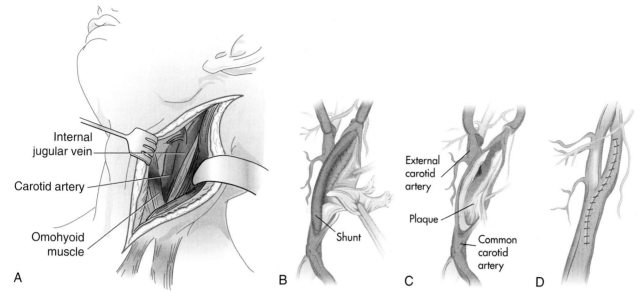

**Figure 11-11** Surgical procedure for carotid endarterectomy to prevent stroke caused by atherosclerotic plaques. **A,** The sterno-cleidomastoid muscle is retracted posteriorly to expose the carotid sheath. **B** through **D,** Carotid endarterectomy is performed to prevent impending cerebral infarction. **A,** A tube is inserted above and below the blockage to reroute the blood flow. **B,** Athero-sclerotic plaque in the common carotid artery is removed. **C,** Once the artery is stitched closed, the tube can be removed. A surgeon may also perform the technique without rerouting the blood flow. (From Lewis SM. Medical-Surgical Nursing: Assessment and Management of Clinical Problems. 7th ed. St. Louis, Mosby, 2008.)

nonrandomized study comparing the two techniques.[40] This study also found that the 30-day and 1-year risks for death, stroke, or myocardial infarction were equivalent between patients undergoing the two procedures. The Carotid and Vertebral Artery Transluminal Angioplasty Study (CAVATAS) trial randomly assigned 504 patients to the two treatments.[41] The incidences of major stroke or death in the 30 days following the procedure did not differ significantly: 6.4% for endovascular treatment and 5.9% for surgery.[41] At 1 year, severe carotid restenosis was noted more frequently in the endovascular group (14% vs. 4%, P < 0.001).[41] An additional Cochrane systematic review of this topic found that no significant differences in the major risks of the treatments were found, but currently there is insufficient evidence to support a widespread change in clinical practice away from recommending CEA as the treatment of choice for appropriate carotid artery stenosis.[42]

## Abdominal Aortic Aneurysmectomy

Thoracic aortic aneurysms (TAAs) are common, with an average incidence of 5.9 per 100,000 person-years, a median age at the time of diagnosis of 65 years, and an incidence of two to four times more frequent in males than females.[43] Common risk factors for thoracic aortic aneurysms include hypertension, hypercholesterolemia, prior tobacco use, collagen vascular disease, or family history of aortic disease.[43] TAAs are classified by location, size, shape, and etiology. Among TAAs, descending thoracic or thoracoabdominal aortic aneurysms are most common, followed by ascending aortic aneurysm, and less often by aortic arch aneurysms.[44,45]

### Indications for Surgery

Patients who are diagnosed with aneurysms greater than or equal to 5 cm or with rapid aneurysm enlargement are considered for surgical repair. A sudden change in the characteristics or the severity of the pain is significant and alerts clinicians to the possibility of rapid aneurysm expansion, leakage, or rupture. Those individuals who have an increased risk of rapid growth rate and risk for rupture include the Marfan patient, as well as patients with inherited collagen vascular disorders or familial patterns of aortic dissection. Individuals with Marfan syndrome have a high incidence of death related to complications of aneurysms or dissections of the aorta (90%).[43]

Patients who undergo abdominal aortic aneurysmectomy elect to have the procedure performed unless the aneurysm has ruptured (at which time the individual must have immediate surgical attention). The procedure involves a midline incision from the xiphoid to the pubis. The aorta is cross-clamped below the renal arteries and above the aneurysm, and two clamps are placed on the iliac arteries (Fig. 11-12A). An incision is made between the renal and iliac vessels, and the atherosclerotic material is removed (Fig. 11-12A). The aneurysm is then cut transversely just distal to the beginning of the aneurysm, and a graft that includes two iliac artery

---

**Clinical Tip**

The clinician should suspect that other vessels, besides the carotid vessels, have atherosclerosis because atherosclerosis is a systemic disease. The other vessels to suspect include the coronary arteries, peripheral vasculature, and possibly the renal vasculature.

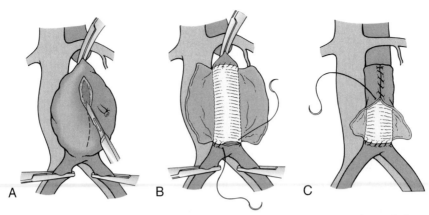

**Figure 11-12** Surgical repair of an abdominal aortic aneurysm. **A,** Incising the aneurysmal sac. **B,** Insertion of synthetic graft. **C,** Suturing native aortic wall over synthetic graft. (From Lewis SM, Heitkemper MM, Dirksen SR [eds]. Medical-Surgical Nursing, Assessment and Management of Clinical Problems. 5th ed. St. Louis, Mosby, 2000.)

extensions is sutured to the aorta, and then to each iliac artery (Fig. 11-12B and C). Following completion of the suturing, the clamps are removed and circulation is evaluated prior to closing the midline incision.[37]

Because of the invasiveness of this procedure throughout the abdomen, patients undergoing this procedure are at high risk for pulmonary complications. Incisional pain and the use of the abdominal musculature in coughing discourage the patient from full inspirations as well as effective forceful huffing or coughing. Appropriate bronchial hygiene techniques are essential for decreasing the incidence of pulmonary complications, especially in patients with chronic pulmonary disease.

Endovascular repair of descending thoracic aortic aneurysm is a less-invasive alternative to traditional open surgery in properly selected patients.[46,47] Early results have been promising, with improved morbidity and mortality, but long-term data are lacking. Technical considerations for thoracic endovascular aortic repair include proximity of aneurysms to arch and visceral vessels, strong hemodynamic forces, large-profile devices, and highly tortuous anatomy. The evolution of branched and fenestrated grafts may make endovascular repairs applicable.

### Peripheral Vascular Interventions

The type of intervention for peripheral vascular disease (surgical intervention vs. percutaneous transluminal angioplasty and possible stenting) is determined based upon the following specific factors:[38]

- Characteristics of the lesions (location, stenosis versus occlusion, lesion length);
- Pattern of arterial occlusive disease (multilevel versus single level, runoff status);
- Patient demographics (gender, presence or absence of diabetes);
- Clinical situation (recurrent disease and indications for intervention); and
- Intraprocedural factors (initial hemodynamic response).

> **Clinical Tip**
> Weight bearing on the affected extremity is a concern with any peripheral vascular intervention; however, exercise and mobility are extremely important. Caution should always be taken to elevate the affected extremity when in the sitting position.

In general, one of the strongest predictors of successful outcome for peripheral vascular intervention involves the clinical symptom of claudication. Patients with claudication pain have better long-term outcomes and require fewer amputations than patients with limb-threatening ischemia.[38] Angioplasty is chosen over surgery in individuals with short- to moderate-length stenotic disease with mild disease in the proximal or distal arterial segments. Stents are used in association with angioplasty.

### Peripheral Vascular Surgery

Surgical bypass and arterial reconstruction interventions can be performed on any vessel peripherally. Some of the more common sites include femoral-popliteal regions, aortofemoral region, infrapopliteal, and axillobifemoral (Fig. 11-13). Candidates for surgical intervention include patients with long lesions (≥0.5 cm), multiple stenoses, a very critical single stenosis in a diffusely irregular segment, or an occlusion.

### Percutaneous Myocardial Revascularization: Use of Lasers

A new technique approved by the Food and Drug Administration (FDA) for the treatment of chronic myocardial ischemia in those who have failed conventional bypass and angioplasty involves laser technology to create small channels in the myocardium using a procedure called transmyocardial laser revascularization (TMR) (Fig. 11-14). The drilled holes do not increase the blood flow, but rather stimulate the myocardium to form small collateral vessels, and this response appears to contribute to relief of chest pain in these patients.[48,49] Studies using thallium injected single photon

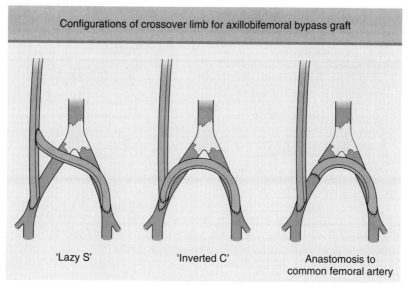

**Figure 11-13** Configurations of crossover limb for axillobifemoral bypass graft. Configurations that minimize low flow in the ipsilateral short femoral limb may be preferable when there is compromised runoff from the short limb. (Adapted from Schneider JR. Extra-anatomic bypass. From Rutherford RB [ed.]. Vascular surgery. 6th ed. Philadelphia, Saunders, 2005 in Hallett. Comprehensive Vascular and Endovascular Surgery. 2nd ed. Philadelphia, Mosby, 2009.)

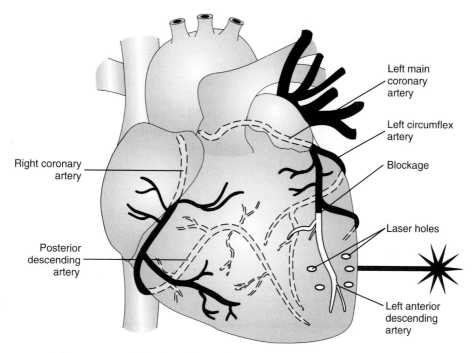

**Figure 11-14** Transmyocardial laser revascularization. (From Linton AD. Introduction to Medical-Surgical Nursing. 4th ed. St. Louis, Saunders, 2008.)

emission computed tomography (TI-SPECT) imaging and positron emission tomography (PET) imaging have failed to show any significant improvement in regional blood flow despite angina relief and this symptom is achieved in 60% to 80% of patients within 6 months of the operation.[50] However, in animal studies using TMR when oxygen tension was measured directly at the tissue level, oxygen tension increased significantly in the ischemic area, indicating a significant effect of TMR on microperfusion and oxygen tension.[51] This

implies that the diagnostic test that is used to measure improvement in regional blood flow with TMR may not be the appropriate test to detect change and that possibly microperfusion is occurring at the site.

Initial transmyocardial channels drilled with a $CO_2$ laser were used as an adjunct to coronary bypass surgery, but are now performed without surgery.[49,52] However, $CO_2$ laser irradiation requires fiberoptic conduits and therefore an open thoracotomy so that the epicardial surface is exposed, placing

**Table 11-1 Three Potential Mechanisms for Biorevascularization**

|  | Gene | Protein | Time |
|---|---|---|---|
| Mechanism | Transfection<br>↓<br>Growth factor<br>↓<br>Angiogenesis | Growth factor<br>↓<br>Angiogenesis | Denervation<br>↓<br>Inflammation<br>↓<br>Growth factors<br>↓<br>Angiogenesis |
| Duration of effect | Weeks | Hours | Weeks |

*The natural angiogenic response initiated in chronically ischemic tissue by hypoxia-responsive growth factors is insufficient to adequately relieve ischemia. Gene transfer of growth factor genes to muscle tissue by either adenovirus, naked DNA, or several other techniques results in transcription, translation, and secretion of the growth factor locally. The growth factor then acts locally on receptors of endothelial cells to stimulate the cell cycle and promote vascular growth. Infusion of growth factor proteins is also effective, but it may require sustained or repeated infusions for maximal effect. Transmyocardial laser revascularization (TMR) uses laser technology to create small channels in the myocardium. It appears that the channels themselves do not remain patent; rather, the inflammatory reaction to the necrotic core created by the laser stimulates an angiogenic response.*
*Modified from Engler RL, Martin J. Joint AHA/ESC Symposium: Biorevascularization. Presented at the American Heart Association 72nd Scientific Sessions, Atlanta, GA, November 7–10, 1999. Plenary Session XI, No. 10.*

patients at similar risk as open thoracotomy bypass surgery. To reduce the risks of open thoracotomy, the technique of percutaneous myocardial revascularization (PMR) was developed.[48] Ultraviolet or infrared laser irradiation is used in PMR and is transmitted along optical fibers without surgical intervention. The thermal effects from the laser may result in local denervation and may be the cause of the decrease in chest pain.[53]

Results have been conflicting with respect to long-term patency following TMR and PMR; however, it has been suggested that angiogenesis plays some role after these procedures. Histologic studies have demonstrated endothelialization and an increase in small capillaries in the laser-treated areas.[54-56]

## Gene Therapy for the Stimulation of Angiogenesis

Recombinant human vascular endothelial growth factor (VEGF) is an agent that shows promise for stimulating the growth of new blood vessels.[57,58] Therapeutic angiogenesis was first successfully demonstrated in humans with critical limb ischemia when gene transfer of naked DNA encoding for VEGF was used for the treatment. Improved blood flow to the ischemic limb was demonstrated on 1-year followup, and patients reported they were symptom-free.[57,59]

The adult heart has been shown to have a reduced ability to produce growth factors and stimulate angiogenesis in response to ischemia. VEGF has several isoforms and is considered to be a potent angiogenic agent because it is endothelial cell specific.[59,60] Currently experimental studies have demonstrated that both VEGF and fibroblast growth factor (FGF) can stimulate small vessel formation, as demonstrated

by angiography; however, clinical benefit for patients has not been demonstrated to date (Table 11-1).[61] There is concern that stimulation of cell proliferation may cause detrimental effects if cell proliferation occurs at the wrong site within a coronary artery (such as at an atherosclerotic plaque, thereby inducing plaque growth), or if a tumorlike hemangioma develops.[61] Consequently, the goal of angiogenesis has been to identify a delivery system targeted to the injured myocardium to improve the local therapeutic efficacy of VEGF and decrease its possible adverse effects.[62] One animal study developed a fusion protein (CBD-VEGF) consisting of VEGF and a collagen-binding domain (CBD). The fusion protein specifically bound to type I collagen *in vitro*. When implanted subcutaneously in rats, collagen membranes loaded with CBD-VEGF were significantly vascularized. After it was injected into rats with acute myocardial infarction, CBD-VEGF was largely retained in the cardiac extracellular matrix, in which collagen I was rich. Four weeks after VEGF or CBD-VEGF was injected into the infarct border zone, cardiac function detected by echocardiography and hemodynamics was preserved in the CBD-VEGF group. Administration of CBD-VEGF also induced reduction of scar size, whereas native VEGF did not have these effects. In addition, a significant increase in the number of capillary vessels in infarcted hearts was found in the CBD-VEGF group. The injection of CBD-VEGF improved cardiac function in rats with induced acute myocardial infarction. This could potentially provide a new treatment option for myocardial infarction.[62]

Another form of gene therapy has involved the transplantation of mesenchymal stem cells (MSCs) has been studied and the effect on the left ventricular function and morphology in rat myocardial infarct hearts. Implanted MSCs showed improvement in cardiac structure and function through the combined effect of myogenesis and angiogenesis.[63] Thus, the

## Table 11-2 Classification of Recommendations

|  | Class I | Class IIa | Class IIb | Class III |
|---|---|---|---|---|
| Benefit: Risk Recommendation | Benefit > > > Risk<br><br>Procedure/ treatment should be performed or administered | Benefit > > Risk<br><br>It is reasonable to perform procedure or administer treatment | Benefit > Risk<br><br>Procedure/ Treatment may be considered | Risk > Benefit<br><br>Procedure/Treatment Should not be performed/ administered; May be harmful |
| Further studies | Not necessary | Additional studies needed with focused objectives | Additional studies with broad objectives needed | No additional studies needed |

*Adapted from Antman EM, Hand M, Armstrong PW, 2007 Focused update of the ACC/AHA 2004 guidelines for the management of patients with ST-elevation myocardial infarction: a report of the American College of Cardiology/American Heart Association Task Force on Practice Guidelines: developed in collaboration With the Canadian Cardiovascular Society endorsed by the American Academy of Family Physicians: 2007 Writing Group to Review New Evidence and Update the ACC/AHA 2004 Guidelines for the Management of Patients With ST-Elevation Myocardial Infarction, Writing on Behalf of the 2004 Writing Committee. Circulation 117(2):296-329, 2008.*

future of possible remodeling of the human heart and blood vessels following damage may be in gene therapy.

## Radiation

Irradiation, which is effective in treating proliferation disorders, has been investigated for the treatment of stent restenosis. When the endothelium is exposed to controlled amounts of radiation emitted from tiny seeds imbedded inside a catheter, the incidence of restenosis of the artery is reduced.[64] Early results have consistently shown a substantial benefit over standard techniques of stent alone. Treatment with radiation may also reduce the risk of restenosis in individuals who undergo angioplasty without stent placement, but again, long-term studies are needed in this area.

## Pacemaker Implantation

A cardiac pacemaker is an electronic pulse generator used to create an artificial action potential for the purpose of controlling some types of cardiac arrhythmias. Pacemakers may be used as a temporary measure to control transient arrhythmias during myocardial infarction or following cardiac surgery when vagal tone (parasympathetic stimulation) is often increased. Chronic arrhythmias (e.g., second- or third-degree heart blocks or recurrent tachyarrhythmias) may require the surgical implantation of a permanent pacemaker. The American College of Cardiology has published guidelines that discuss specific electrocardiographic indications for pacemaker implantation.[65] The published recommendations are separated based upon the benefit of the procedure as compared to the risk, with Class 1 recommendations stating the procedure/treatment *should* be performed/administered, Class IIa stating it is reasonable to perform the procedure/administer the treatment yet additional studies with focused objectives

are needed and IIb stating the procedure/treatment *may* be considered yet additional studies with broad objectives are needed. Table 11-2 lists the recommendations for pacemakers and the class recommendations.

The criteria actually applied for pacemaker indications often vary from institution to institution.[66] Nevertheless, the general indications involve sinoatrial nodal disorders (e.g., bradyarrhythmias), atrioventricular nodal disorders (e.g., complete heart block, Mobitz type II arrhythmia), or tachyarrhythmias (e.g., supraventricular tachycardia, frequent ventricular ectopy) that result in hemodynamic embarrassment (signs and symptoms such as lightheadedness, fainting, blurred vision, slurred speech, confusion, or weakness) as a result of inadequate cardiac output. (See Chapter 9 for more information about cardiac arrhythmias and their appearance on electrocardiogram [ECG].)

Cardiac pacemakers are able to initiate myocardial depolarization by creating an electrical voltage difference between two electrodes, thus initiating an artificial depolarization spike. Chapter 9 provides examples of typical ECG tracings of atrially and ventricularly paced rhythms. Cardiac pacemakers employ electrical conduction configurations that are classified as being either unipolar or bipolar (Fig. 11-15). Unipolar pacing systems use one electrode that is in direct contact with the cardiac tissue; the second, or anodal, electrode is usually the metal housing of the pacemaker, which is located at some point distant to the myocardium. Bipolar pacing systems use two electrodes that are in close proximity to each other where they make contact with the myocardium. Biventricular pacing systems use three leads, including one in the atrium and the two in the two ventricles.

Rechargeable power sources for cardiac pacemakers are no longer employed, and it is highly unlikely that a pacemaker operating from a mercury zinc power source is in operation today. The vast majority of pacemakers in current clinical use operate from lithium-chemistry power sources, although "nuclear" (radioactive plutonium) pacemakers have been available for more than 15 years. On an actuarial basis, the 50% survival point (the battery half-life) of modern lithium–chemistry-powered pacemakers is greater than 6 years. According to Bilitch and coworkers in 1987,[67] 88% of nuclear-powered pacemakers were operational after 12 years of use.

Regardless of the electrode configuration, cardiac pacing leads are of two primary types:
- Endocardial leads are placed inside the right atrium, the right ventricle, or both via a transvenous route.
- Epicardial leads are attached directly to the surface of the right atrium or the right or left ventricle.

No matter which type of electrode is used, the pacing lead is constructed of multiple strands of conductive material so that, unlike monofilament conductors, it can withstand repeated flexure without breaking. The importance of this aspect of pacing lead construction is made abundantly clear when one considers that if a patient's heart is paced at a constant rate of 68 beats per minute, the lead flexes 35,765,280 times per year.

Endocardial lead placement can be made by means of transvenous (technically pervenous because the leads go through the vessel, not across it) insertion via the subclavian, internal jugular, or cephalic venous routes. However, the preferred route of insertion for permanent endocardial leads is via the left cephalic vein, with the impulse generator being placed in an infraclavicular pocket (Fig. 11-16).[68] The tips of these transvenous electrodes are placed in direct contact with the interior surface of either the right atrium or right ventricle, or both. A new kind of pacemaker (experimental at the time of this publication) utilizing three leads has been designed for individuals with severe heart failure. The biventricular pacemaker has two leads that are attached to the right atrium and right ventricle, and the third lead is threaded inside the coronary sinus vein of the left ventricle to resynchronize the ventricles to pump more efficiently (Fig. 11-17). The two primary indications for this pacemaker are left bundle branch block and severe heart failure.

Epicardial implantation is usually accomplished during a cardiac surgical procedure. Sometimes conductive suture electrodes are sewn into the exterior myocardial wall for temporary pacing; however, in most cases electrodes are screwed, hooked, or sewn onto the myocardial surface for permanent pacing. For temporary external pacing, conductive lead wires frequently exit the chest from small subxiphoid incision. For permanent pacing, the impulse generator may be placed in a subxiphoid rectus sheath pocket. If

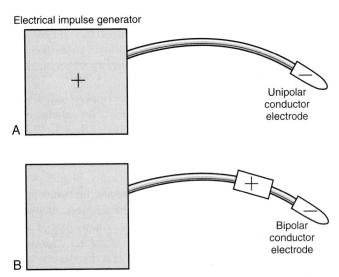

Electrical impulse generator

**Figure 11-15** Pacemaker electrode configurations. **A,** Unipolar electrode. **B,** Bipolar electrode.

---

**Clinical Tip**
The clinician needs to know the type of pacemaker that the patient has in order to understand the ECG tracing that will be displayed, as well as whether or not there are any precautions with exercise.

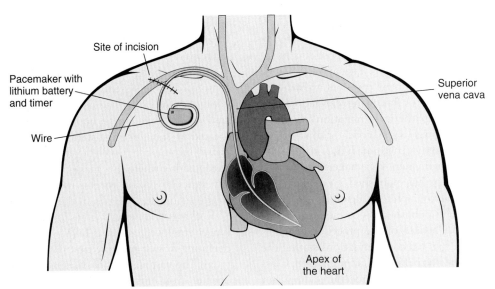

**Figure 11-16** Permanent pacemaker implanted in the chest. The pacemaker may be placed in the right or left side of the chest, or even in the abdomen. (From Chabner DA. The Language of Medicine. 6th ed. Philadelphia, Saunders, 2001.)

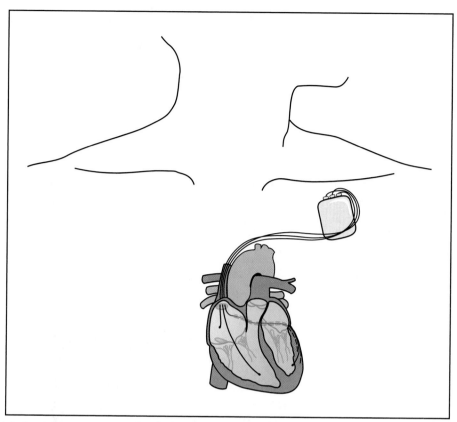

**Figure 11-17** The triple-lead system uses two leads that are threaded into the right atrium and the right ventricle. A third lead goes inside the coronary sinus vein of the left ventricle to resynchronize the ventricles to pump more efficiently.

for some reason (e.g., abdominal infection, primary thoracic entry via median sternotomy) the subxiphoid approach cannot be or is not used, a transthoracic approach may be employed.

The field of cardiac pacing has expanded explosively, creating the need for a uniform means of communicating information regarding the characteristics of a particular device. The capabilities of current pacing devices—which include telemetry; programmability; and antibradyarrhythmia, antitachyarrhythmia, and adaptive-rate pacing—far surpass those of devices from just a few years ago. In response to the need for a simple code to describe such pacing devices, the North American Society of Pacing and Electrophysiology (NASPE) and the British Pacing and Electrophysiology Group (BPEG) collaborated to devise a generic pacemaker code, the NBG Code.[69] The five-position NBG Code has gained widespread clinical acceptance and is summarized in Table 11-3. The first position of the code provides a classification of the possible stimulation sites for antibradyarrhythmia pacing. The second position classifies the pacemaker's ability to "sense" either atrial or ventricular spontaneous depolarizations, or both. The third position indicates what the pacemaker does if it detects a spontaneous depolarization. The fourth position indicates the programmability or rate modulation capabilities of the pacemaker. The fifth position, if used, indicates the pacemaker's ability to prevent tachyarrhythmia. In many instances, however, only the first three positions of the NBG Code are used in clinical conversation. For example, a pacemaker that can stimulate both the atrium and the ventricle

can sense spontaneous depolarizations independently in the atrium and the ventricle, can inhibit a pending stimulus in the chamber in which a spontaneous depolarization was sensed, and at the same time can trigger a ventricular stimulation (after an appropriate interval) in response to sensing a spontaneous atrial depolarization is called a *DDD pacemaker*. Likewise, a pacemaker that stimulates only the ventricle, can sense spontaneous depolarizations only in the ventricle, and can inhibit a pending stimulus when a spontaneous depolarization is sensed is called a *VVI pacemaker*. Clearly, the NBG Code facilitates the exchange of a great deal of information in a very concise format. With a basic understanding of the NBG Code, the physical therapist treating a patient with a pacemaker can anticipate the patient's cardiac response capabilities for myriad situations.

## Implantable Cardioverter Defibrillator

The development and continual refinement of the implantable cardioverter defibrillator (ICD, also known as automatic ICD or AICD) has been one of the most significant improvements in the treatment of life-threatening arrhythmias. An ICD is similar to a pacemaker, but is designed to correct life-threatening arrhythmias. An ICD detects and corrects all tachycardias, ventricular fibrillation, and bradycardia. The ICD is implanted into the patient, much like a pacemaker, and a separate programmer used to change the function of the ICD is kept at the doctor's office for followup care. An

## Table 11-3 The NBG Pacemaker Code

| Pacing Location | | Sensing Location | | Response to Pacing | | Programmability/Modulation | | Antitachyarrhythmia Function | |
|---|---|---|---|---|---|---|---|---|---|
| O = None | No antibradyarrhythmia stimulation | O = None | No bradyarrhythmia detecting capability | O = None | No response | O = None | No programmability; no rate modulation | O = None | No antitachyarrhythmia capability |
| A = Atrium | | A = Atrium | Detects spontaneous atrial depolarizations | I = Inhibited | Inhibits a pending stimulus when a spontaneous depolarization is detected | S = Simple programmable | Capable of either or both rate and output adjustment | P = Pacing | Low-energy stimulus used to interrupt tachyarrhythmia |
| V = Ventricle | | V = Ventricle | Detects spontaneous ventricular depolarizations | T = Triggered | Detection produces an immediate stimulus in the same chamber | M = Multiprogrammable | Can be programmed more extensively | S = Shock | High-energy stimulus used to interrupt tachyarrhythmia (e.g., cardioversion or defibrillation) |
| D = Dual | Atrium and ventricle can be stimulated to control Bradyarrhythmia | D = Dual | Detects spontaneous depolarizations independently in the atrium and the ventricle | D = Dual | Can simultaneously inhibit and trigger a stimulus | C = Communicating | Can be extensively programmed and has some "telemetry" capability | D = Dual | Has both low and high-energy capability |
| S = A or V | Manufacturer's designation to indicate that either chamber is acceptable for pacing by a single-chamber pacemaker | S = A or V | Manufacturer's designation to indicate that either chamber is acceptable for pacing by a single-chamber pacemaker | | R = Rate modulation | Can automatically control rate by measuring one or more other physiologic variables | | | |

Source: Bernstein AD, Camm AJ, Fletcher RD, et al. The NASPE/BPEG generic pacemaker code for antibradyarrhythmia and adaptive-rate pacing and antitachyarrhythmia devices. PACE 10:795, 1987.

ICD may be implanted in conjunction with a pacemaker or may be implanted alone.

Patients with a left ventricular ejection fraction (LVEF) of less than 30% have a threefold to fivefold increase in incidence of sudden death. In addition to ventricular dysfunction, those individuals with frequent or complex premature ventricular complexes or nonsustained ventricular tachycardia have an increased risk for sudden death. The MADIT I (Multicenter Automatic Defibrillator Trial) studies patients with coronary artery disease, low LVEF (an LVEF <35% was used in this trial), and at least one episode of nonsustained ventricular tachycardia. There was close to a 50% reduction in mortality rate of those treated with ICD therapy versus pharmacologic therapy alone.[70–72] Similar results were found in the MADIT II trial but the criteria used was an LVEF criteria <30%.[73] The Multicenter Unsustained Tachycardia Trial (MUSTT), which used a LVEF of less than 40%, provided further evidence supporting the use of the ICD in patients who have not yet had an episode of ventricular tachycardia but who are at high risk for sudden death.[71,72] The current guidelines from the American College of Cardiology/ American Heart Association/Heart Rhythm Society (ACC/ AHA/HRS) use LVEF ≤35%. The Class I through IIb indications for ICD therapy are found in Table 11-2.

## Drainage Tube Placement

Following a thoracic surgical procedure, tubes are typically placed through the chest wall to drain the affected body cavity. Although any tube penetrating the chest wall could be termed a chest tube, this term is generally reserved for the description of intrapleural drainage tubes—tubes that drain the intrapleural space—or mediastinal drainage tubes—tubes that drain the mediastinum. Most chest tubes are multifenestrated, and all are made of an inert material. Like endotracheal tubes, chest tubes have radiopaque markers to facilitate their localization on chest radiographs. Chest tubes and drainage collection systems permit the amount of drainage and intrathoracic blood loss to be monitored, and they provide a means by which the presence of any air leaks can be verified (Fig. 11-18).

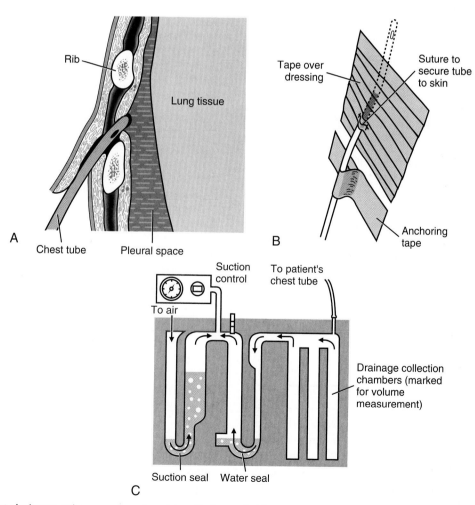

**Figure 11-18** Chest drainage tubes may be placed to eliminate fluids, air, or both from the pleural or mediastinal spaces. **A,** A pleural tube being inserted into the pleural space. **B,** Once positioned, the drainage tube is sutured to the skin and covered with an occlusive dressing. **C,** Chest drainage tubes are typically connected to a collection device that may or may not be attached to suction. (*C,* redrawn from Kersten LD. Comprehensive Respiratory Nursing. Philadelphia, Saunders, 1989:776.)

Whenever a thoracotomy or median sternotomy is performed, the pleural cavity, mediastinum, or both are generally drained by the placement of one or more chest tubes connected to underwater seal or suction. These chest tubes drain pleural or mediastinal fluids and air with expansion of the lung. Intrapleural tubes are inserted into the second or third intercostal space at the midclavicular line to drain air. To drain fluids, they are usually inserted at the fourth or fifth intercostal space at the anterior axillary line (sometimes as low as the eighth or ninth intercostal space at the midaxillary line). The tube's tip is advanced several inches into the pleural space; the distal end of the drainage tube may or may not be attached to a sealed drainage collection system, which may or may not be attached to suction. Posteriorly placed intrapleural tubes are not often used because they are easily kinked; they are also very uncomfortable for the patient. Mediastinal chest tubes are commonly inserted via subxiphoid incisions that are distinct from the sternotomy incision. Chest tubes normally pass obliquely through the chest wall rather than directly through at a right angle (see Fig. 11-18A). The clinician is cautioned against tipping the collection system so as not to compromise the water seal. Because disconnection of intrapleural tubes can result in collapse of the lung, all chest tubes should be treated as if they were intrapleural drainage tubes so that proper precautions are never neglected. Nonetheless, the presence of chest drainage tubes should not preclude the patient's participation in physical therapy activities.

> **Clinical Tip**
> The presence of chest drainage tubes should not preclude the patient's participation in physical therapy activities. Mobility is encouraged unless another complication is a limiting factor.

Much like intrapleural tubes, intraabdominal drainage tubes are used to eliminate air or fluid from the abdominal cavity. Intraabdominal tubes may simply drain into a collection bag by gravity or be connected to a vacuum device (e.g., Jackson-Pratt drainage tubes).

Flexible 19F drains with ridges (Blake), connected to 50cc grenade bulbs and fitted with one-way valves are currently being used for drainage of fluid and blood post thoracic and cardiac surgery in some cases. These Blake drains appear to provide effective drainage following surgical procedures and may provide increased comfort over the traditional drainage tubes (see Fig. 11-18).[74–76]

Bladder drainage tubes are also common in the critical care setting. They are usually attached to "urinary catheter bags," which are also frequently used with general acute care patients as well.

---

## CASE STUDY 11-1

FM is a 56-year-old man who underwent surgical removal of his right lower lobe with a lateral thoracotomy incision after the diagnosis of lung cancer. FM had a 2.5 packs per day history of smoking for the past 36 years. FM works as an automobile mechanic and requires full use of both upper extremities for his job.

Postoperatively, the patient experienced moderate to severe pain and demonstrated a moist nonproductive cough; on the second day after surgery he developed a 100.1° F temperature. Chest radiograph showed atelectasis in the right middle lobe and left lower lobe, and infiltrates in the left lower lobe. The patient was started on incentive spirometry and respiratory breathing treatment of a bronchodilator every 4 hours.

On the fourth postoperative day the nurse's notes documented that the patient was having difficulty feeding himself with his right arm and was using his left arm. He continued to be very inactive, and only got up to the chair with assistance. Physical therapy was ordered for mobility and range of motion to right upper extremity.

### Discussion

This case demonstrates the complications that can develop with a lateral thoracotomy when aggressive bronchial hygiene and range-of-motion activities are not included early in the patient's postoperative recovery.

---

## Summary

- The numerous surgical procedures that may be performed on the cardiovascular or pulmonary systems are generally made via one of three approaches (or modifications thereof): thoracotomy incisions are most commonly used for lung resection procedures; most cardiac procedures are performed through a median sternotomy; procedures involving the diaphragm, pericardium, or epicardium are commonly performed through a thoracoabdominal incision.

- Cardiac revascularization procedures are among the most common of cardiothoracic surgical procedures. They may be performed percutaneously (e.g., angioplasty, atherectomy, stenting) or transthoracically (e.g., bypass graft). Either approach is associated with its own postprocedure movement precautions.

- The CASS study concluded that surgical revascularization is the optimal choice for management of coronary artery disease when all three vessels were severely obstructed.

- The use of internal thoracic arteries is preferable for achieving improved long-term outcome.

- Recent improvements in the surgical approach include the use of smaller incisions with microinstrumentation (MIDCAB) and robotic surgery with fewer complications postoperatively.
- Another surgical variation for coronary bypass involves a sternotomy but no cardiopulmonary bypass and is called the off-pump coronary artery bypass (OPCAB). The surgeon operates on a beating heart.
- A new technique approved by the FDA for the treatment of chronic myocardial ischemia in patients who have failed conventional bypass and angioplasty involves laser technology to create small channels in the myocardium (TMR).
- The risk of undergoing carotid endarterectomy increases as the severity of the disease increases. Those likely to benefit the most from the surgery were those who had the highest risk in undergoing the operation.
- One of the strongest predictors of successful outcome for peripheral vascular intervention involves the clinical symptom of claudication. Patients with claudication pain have better long-term outcomes and require fewer amputations than those with limb-threatening ischemia.
- If, as the result of disease or trauma, the heart is unable to generate an adequate cardiac output, cardiovascular life support equipment is frequently employed to stimulate or augment cardiac function. Pacemaker devices generate an artificial electrical stimulus to supplant or replace the heart's native rhythm of depolarization.
- Chest drainage tubes (e.g., intrapleural or mediastinal) are usually employed following cardiothoracic surgical procedures or chest trauma, or when metabolic disorders so disrupt vascular permeability and osmotic pressures that fluid collects within the thoracic cavity. Their presence should not preclude the patient's participation in physical therapy activities.

## References

1. Kittle CF. Thoracic Incisions. In Baue AE (ed.). Glenn's Thoracic and Cardiovascular Surgery. 5th ed. East Norwalk, CT, Appleton & Lange, 1991.
2. Julian OC, Lopez-Belio M, Dye WS, et al. The median sternal incision in intracardiac surgery with extracorporeal circulation; a general evaluation of its use in heart surgery. Surgery 42(4):753–61, 1957.
3. Slinger PD, Campos JH. Anesthesia for thoracic surgery. In Miller RD, Eriksson LI, Fleisher LA, et al. Miller's Anesthesia. 7th ed. Philadelphia, Churchill Livingstone, 2009.
4. Licker MJ, Widikker I, Robert J, et al. Operative mortality and respiratory complications after lung resection for cancer: impact of chronic obstructive pulmonary disease and time trends. Ann Thorac Surg 81(5):1830–7, 2006.
5. Scawn NDA, Pennefather SH, Soorae A, et al. Ipsilateral shoulder pain after thoracotomy with epidural analgesia: The influence of phrenic nerve infiltration with lidocaine. Anesth Analg 93:260, 2001.
6. Kavanagh BP, Katz J, Sandler AN. Pain control after thoracic surgery: A review of current techniques. Anesthesiology 81:737, 1994.
7. Kaseda S, Aoki T, Hangai N, et al. Better pulmonary function and prognosis with video-assisted thoracic surgery than with thoracotomy. Ann Thorac Surg 70:1644, 2000.
8. Yim AP, Wan S, Lee TW, et al. VATS lobectomy reduces cytokine responses compared with conventional surgery. Ann Thorac Surg 70:243, 2000.
9. McKenna RJ, Houck W, Fuller CB. Video-assisted thoracic surgery lobectomy: Experience with 1,100 cases. Ann Thorac Surg 81:421, 2006.
10. Heerdt PM, Park BJ. The emerging role of minimally invasive surgical techniques for the treatment of lung malignancy in the elderly. Anesthesiol Clin 26(2):315–24, 2008.
11. McKenna Jr RJ, Mahtabifard A, Pickens A, et al. Fast-tracking after video-assisted thoracoscopic surgery lobectomy, segmentectomy, and pneumonectomy. Ann Thorac Surg 84(5):1663–7; discussion 1667–8, 2007.
12. Kirby TJ, Mack MJ, Landreneau RJ, et al. Lobectomy—Video-assisted thoracic surgery versus muscle-sparing thoracotomy. A randomized trial. J Thorac Cardiovasc Surg 109(5):997–1001; discussion 1001–2, 1995.
13. Jaklitsch MT, DeCamp Jr MM, Liptay MJ, et al. Video-assisted thoracic surgery in the elderly. A review of 307 cases. Chest 110(3):751–8, 1996.
14. Park BJ, Zhang H, Rusch VW, et al. Video-assisted thoracic surgery does not reduce the incidence of postoperative atrial fibrillation after pulmonary lobectomy. J Thorac Cardiovasc Surg 133(3):775–9, 2007.
15. RJ Dick, JJ Popma, DW Muller, et al. In-hospital costs associated with new percutaneous coronary devices. Am J Cardiol 68:879–85, 1991.
16. Warner M, Chami Y, Johnson D, Cowley MJ. Directional coronary atherectomy for failed angioplasty due to occlusive coronary dissection. Cathet Cardiovasc Diagn 24:28–31, 1991.
17. Rowe MH, Hinohara T, White NW, et al. Comparison of dissection rates and angiographic results following directional atherectomy and coronary angioplasty. Am J Cardiol 66:49–53, 1990.
18. Mansour M, Carrozza JP, Kuntz RE, et al. Frequency and outcome of chest pain after two new coronary interventions (atherectomy and stenting). Am J Cardiol 69:1379–82, 1992.
19. Hinohara T, Selmon MR, Robertson GC, et al. Directional atherectomy. New approaches for treatment of obstructive coronary and peripheral vascular disease. Circulation 81(Suppl 3):IV79–IV91, 1990.
20. Serruys PW, Ong AT, van Herwerden LA, et al. Five-year outcomes after coronary stenting versus bypass surgery for the treatment of multivessel disease: The final analysis of the Arterial Revascularization Therapies Study (ARTS) randomized trial. J Am Coll Cardiol 46:575–81, 2005.
21. Kuntz RE, Safian RD, Levine MJ, et al. Novel approach to the analysis of restenosis after the use of three new coronary devices. J Am Coll Cardiol 19:1493–9, 1992.
22. Williams DO. Catheter-Based Revascularization Beyond the Stent. Presented at American Heart Association 72nd Scientific Sessions, Atlanta, GA, November 7, 1999. Plenary Session I. Revascularization in the 21st Century.
23. Topol EJ, Byzova TV, Plow EF. Platelet GPIIb-IIIa blockers. Lancet 353(9148):227–31, 1999.
24. Eeckhout E, Kappenberger L, Goy JL. Stents for intracoronary placement: Current status and future directions. J Am Coll Cardiol 27(4):757–65, 1996.

25. Budaj A, Yusuf S, Mehta SR, et al. Benefit of clopidogrel in patients with acute coronary syndromes without ST-segment elevation in various risk groups. Circulation 106:1622–6, 2002.

26. Mehta SR, Yusuf S, Peters RJ, et al. Effects of pretreatment with clopidogrel and aspirin followed by long-term therapy in patients undergoing percutaneous coronary intervention: The PCI-CURE study. Lancet 358(9281):527–33, 2001.

27. Babapulle MN, Joseph L, Belisle P, et al. A hierarchical Bayesian meta-analysis of randomised clinical trials of drug-eluting stents. Lancet 364(9434):583–91, 2004.

28. Ringzvist I, Fisher LD, Mock M, et al. Prognostic value of angiographic indices of coronary artery disease from the Coronary Artery Surgery Study (CASS). J Clin Invest 71(6):1854–66, 1983.

29. Lytle BW, Loop FD, Cosgrove DM, et al. Long-term (5 to 12 years) serial studies of internal mammary artery and saphenous vein coronary bypass grafts. J Thorac Cardiovasc Surg 89(2):248–58, 1985.

30. Bourassa MG, Fisher LD, Campeau L, et al. Long-term fate of bypass grafts: the Coronary Artery Surgery Study (CASS) and Montreal Heart Institute experiences. Circulation 72(6 Pt 2):V71–V78, 1985.

31. Townsend CM. Alternative methods for myocardial revascularization. In Townsend CM, Beauchamp RD, Evers BM, et al. Sabiston Textbook of Surgery. 18th ed. St. Louis, 2008, Saunders.

32. Shennib H, Bastawisy A, Mack MJ, Moll FH. Computer-assisted telemanipulation: An enabling technology for endoscopic coronary artery bypass. Ann Thorac Surg 66:1060–3, 1998.

33. Mohr FW, Falk V, Diegeler A, et al. Computer-enhanced "robotic" cardiac surgery: Experience in 148 patients. J Thorac Cardiovasc Surg 121(5):842–53, 2001.

34. de Cannière D, Wimmer-Greinecker G, Cichon R, Gulielmos V, Van Praet F, Seshadri-Kreaden U, Falk V. Feasibility, safety, and efficacy of totally endoscopic coronary artery bypass grafting: multicenter European experience. J Thorac Cardiovasc Surg 2007;134(3):710–16 (ISSN: 1097–685X).

35. North American Symptomatic Carotid Endarterectomy Trial (NASCET) Collaborators. Beneficial effect of carotid endarterectomy in symptomatic patients with high-grade stenosis. N Engl J Med 325:445–53, 1991.

36. Executive Committee for the Asymptomatic Carotid Atherosclerosis Study. Endarterectomy for asymptomatic carotid stenosis. JAMA 273:1421–8, 1995.

37. Economou SG, Economou TS. Atlas of Surgical Techniques. Philadelphia, Saunders, 1996.

38. Rutherford RB. Vascular Surgery. 5th ed. Philadelphia, Saunders, 2000:1738–9.

39. Yadav JS, Wholey MH, Kuntz RE, for the Stenting and Angioplasty with Protection in Patients at High Risk for Endarterectomy (SAPPHIRE) Investigators, et al. Protected carotid-artery stenting versus endarterectomy in high-risk patients. N Engl J Med 351:1493–501, 2004.

40. Carotid Revascularization Using Endarterectomy or Stenting Systems (CaRESS) Steering Committee. Carotid Revascularization Using Endarterectomy of Stenting Systems (CaRESS) phase I clinical trial: 1-Year results. J Vasc Surg 42:213–9, 2005.

41. Endovascular versus surgical treatment in patients with carotid stenosis in the Carotid and Vertebral Artery Transluminal Angioplasty Study (CAVATAS): A randomised trial. Lancet 357(9270):1729–37, 2001.

42. Coward LJ, Featherstone RL, Brown MM. Safety and efficacy of endovascular treatment of carotid artery stenosis compared with carotid endarterectomy: A Cochrane systematic review of the randomized evidence. Stroke 36:905–11, 2005.

43. Johnston KW, Rutherford RB, Tilson MD, et al. Suggested standards for reporting on arterial aneurysms. Subcommittee on Reporting Standards for Arterial Aneurysms, Ad Hoc Committee on Reporting Standards, Society for Vascular Surgery and North American Chapter, International Society for Cardiovascular Surgery. J Vasc Surg 15(2):456, 1992.

44. Parodi JC, Palmaz JC, Barone HD. Transfemoral intraluminal graft implantation for abdominal aortic aneurysms. Ann Vasc Surg 5:491–9, 1991.

45. Bengtsson H, Sonesson B, Bergqvist D. Incidence and prevalence of abdominal aortic aneurysms, estimated by necropsy studies and population screening by ultrasound. Ann N Y Acad Sci 800:1–24, 1996.

46. Dake MD, Miller DC, Semba CP, et al. Transluminal placement of endovascular stent-grafts for the treatment of descending thoracic aortic aneurysms. N Engl J Med 331:1729–34, 1994.

47. Makaroun MS, Dillavou ED, Kee ST, et al. Endovascular treatment of thoracic aortic aneurysms: Results of the phase II multicenter trial of the GORE TAG thoracic endoprosthesis. J Vasc Surg 41:1–9, 2005.

48. Kim CB, Kesten R, Javier M, et al. Percutaneous method of laser transmyocardial revascularization. Cathet Cardiovasc Diagn 40(2):223–8, 1997.

49. Mihroseini M, Cayton MM, Shelgikar S, et al. Clinical report: Laser myocardial revascularization. Lasers Surg Med 6:456–61, 1986.

50. Bridges CR, Horvath KA, Nugent WC, et al. The Society of Thoracic Surgeons practice guideline series: Transmyocardial laser revascularization. Ann Thorac Surg 77(4):1494–502, 2004.

51. Heidt MC, Sedding D, Stracke SK, et al. Measurement of myocardial oxygen tension: a valid and sensitive method in the investigation of transmyocardial laser revascularization in an acute ischemia model. Thorac Cardiovasc Surg 57(2):79–84, 2009.

52. Mihroseini M, Shelgikar S, Cayton MM. New concepts in revascularization of the myocardium. Ann Thorac Surg 45:415–20, 1988.

53. Kwong KF, Kanellopoulos GK, Schuessler RB, et al. Endocardial laser treatment incompletely denervates canine myocardium. Circulation 96(Suppl I):I–565, 1997.

54. Kohomoto T, Fisher PE, DeRosa C, et al. Evidence of angiogenesis in regions treated with transmyocardial laser revascularization. Circulation 94(Suppl II):294, 1996.

55. Gassler N, Wintzer HO, Stubbe HM, et al. Transmyocardial laser revascularization: Histological features in human non-responder myocardium. Circulation 95:371–5, 1997.

56. Mack CA, Magovern CJ, Hahn RT, et al. Channel patency and neovascularization following transmyocardial laser revascularization utilizing an excimer laser: Results and comparison to non-lased channels. Circulation 94(Suppl I):I–294, 1996.

57. Majesky MW. A little VEGF goes a long way. Therapeutic angiogenesis by direct injection of vascular endothelial growth factor-encoding plasmid DNA. Circulation 94(12):3062–4, 1996.

58. Takeshita S, Pu LQ, Stein LA, et al. Intramuscular administration of vascular endothelial growth factor induces dose-dependent collateral artery augmentation in a rabbit model of

chronic limb ischemia. Circulation 90(5 Pt 2):II228–II34, 1994.

59. Isner JM, Pieczek A, Schainfeld R, et al. Clinical evidence of angiogenesis after arterial gene transfer of ph VEGF 165 in patients with ischemic limb. Lancet 348:370–80, 1996.

60. Isner JM, Walsh K, Symes J, et al. Arterial gene therapy for therapeutic angiogenesis in patients with peripheral artery disease. Circulation 91:2687–92, 1995.

61. Epstein SE. Therapeutic Angiogenesis. Presented at the American Heart Association 72nd Scientific Sessions, Atlanta, GA, November 7, 1999. Plenary Session I. Revascularization in the 21st Century.

62. Zhang J, Ding L, Zhao Y, et al. Collagen-targeting vascular endothelial growth factor improves cardiac performance after myocardial infarction. Circulation 119(13):1776–84, 2009.

63. Tang J, Xie Q, Pan G, et al. Mesenchymal stem cells participate in angiogenesis and improve heart function in rat model of myocardial ischemia with reperfusion. Eur J Cardiothorac Surg 30(2):353–61, 2006.

64. Teirstein PS. Prevention of vascular restenosis with radiation. Tex Heart Inst J 25(1):30–3, 1998.

65. Epstein AE, DiMarco JP, Ellenbogen KA, et al. ACC/AHA/HRS 2008 Guidelines for Device-Based Therapy of Cardiac Rhythm Abnormalities: a report of the American College of Cardiology/American Heart Association Task Force on Practice Guidelines (Writing Committee to Revise the ACC/AHA/NASPE 2002 Guideline Update for Implantation of Cardiac Pacemakers and Antiarrhythmia Devices) developed in collaboration with the American Association for Thoracic Surgery and Society of Thoracic Surgeons. J Am Coll Cardiol 51(21):e1–e62, 2008.

66. Bernstein AD. Classification of cardiac pacemakers. In El-Sherif N, Samet P. Cardiac Pacing and Electrophysiology. 3rd ed. Philadelphia, Saunders, 1991.

67. Bilitch M, Hauser RG, Goldman BS, et al. Performance of implantable cardiac rhythm management devices. Pacing Clin Electrophysiol 10(2):389–98, 1987.

68. Reul GJ. Implantation of permanent cardiac pacemaker. In Cooley DA. Techniques in Cardiac Surgery. 2nd ed. Philadelphia, Saunders, 1984.

69. Bernstein AD, Camm AJ, Fletcher RD, et al. The NASPE/BPEG generic pacemaker code for antibradyarrhythmia and adaptive-rate pacing and antitachyarrhythmia devices. Pacing Clin Electrophysiol 10(4 Pt 1):794–9, 1987.

70. Block M, Breithardt G. The implantable cardioverter defibrillator and primary prevention of sudden death: The Multi-center Automatic Defibrillator Implantation Trial and the Coronary Artery Bypass Graft (CABG)-Patch Trial. Am J Cardiol 83(5B):74D–8D, 1999.

71. Singh B. Sudden Cardiac Death. Presented at the American Heart Association 72nd Scientific Sessions, Atlanta, GA, November 8, 1999.

72. Connolly SJ. ICD Mortality Trials: Results and Practical Implications. Presented at the 20th Annual Scientific Sessions of the North American Society of Pacing and Electrophysiology, May 14, 1999.

73. Moss AJ, Zareba W, Hall WJ, et al. Prophylactic implantation of a defibrillator in patients with myocardial infarction and reduced ejection fraction. N Engl J Med 346;877–83, 2002.

74. Sakopoulos AG, Hurwitz AS, Suda RW, et al. Efficacy of Blake drains for mediastinal and pleural drainage following cardiac operations. J Card Surg 20(6):574–7, 2005.

75. Nakamura H, Taniguchi Y, Miwa K, et al. The 19Fr Blake drain versus the 28Fr conventional drain after a lobectomy for lung cancer. Thorac Cardiovasc Surg 57(2):107–9, 2009.

76. Ehrman WJ, Pike NA, Gundry, Steven R. Cardiac surgery without chest tubes and pleurovacs: A new standard of care. Chest 126:853S, 2004.

## CHAPTER 12

# Thoracic Organ Transplantation: Heart, Heart-Lung, and Lung

*Tamara Versluis Burlis, Anne Mejia Downs, Christen DiPerna*

## Chapter Outline

Organ transplantation has become a common procedure for managing patients with failing organs. Because of the sequelae of the transplantation procedure and alterations in patients' physical performance, physical therapists have become key members of transplantation teams, providing expertise in examination and rehabilitation of transplant recipients both before and after surgery. Although many similarities exist in the treatment of patients undergoing thoracic organ transplantation and other cardiothoracic surgeries, certain differences significantly affect physical therapy intervention and progression of activity.

In addition to a brief historical review of heart, heart-lung, and lung transplantation, this chapter presents an overview of the recipient evaluation process, surgical procedures, frequently used medications, and general complications that affect the management of transplant recipients. The physical therapy management of thoracic organ transplantation recipients, from evaluation to outpatient rehabilitation, is presented with a discussion of the similarities and differences in the treatment of heart and lung transplantation recipients.

## History

In the early 1900s, Carrel and Guthrie[1] first described the techniques for performing extrathoracic transplantation in animal models. Those surgical techniques were not significantly modified until 1933, when Mann[2] proposed a method for heterotopic (donor heart is anastomosed to the native heart without removal of the native heart) cervical cardiac transplantation. For the next 20 years, the cervical anastomosis technique was considered the most suitable method for transplantation in canines. In the 1950s, heterotopic transplantation continued to be the principal technique in the canine model, but orthotopic (replacement of the native heart with a donor heart) transplantation was gaining favor.

During this time, other important aspects of the heart transplantation procedure were also being explored. Marcus and colleagues[3] described the methodology for circulatory loading in a heart transplanted in the cervical position, and Webb and Howard[4] achieved organ viability for up to 8 hours in a previously refrigerated heart using an intrathoracic placement. In 1958, Goldberg and coworkers[5] reported a successful procedure for orthotopic cardiac transplantation using a cuff of the recipient's left atrium, thereby eliminating the need for separate pulmonary venous anastomoses. One year later, Cass and Brock[6] described the use of a right atrial cuff to avoid separate vena caval anastomoses.

In the 1960s, attention turned from the technical surgical aspects of the transplantation procedure toward a consideration of the damage caused to the donor organ by the recipient's intact immune system. Research by Shumway and colleagues[7,8] led the way in studying the problem, and in 1965 they achieved long-term survival in canine transplant recipients with the use of azathioprine and intermittent doses of steroids for immunosuppression.[9]

Following the increased success experienced for heart transplantation in animal models, sufficient information and experience were gained to warrant attempts in humans. The first cardiac transplantation was performed on a human in 1964, when Hardy and colleagues[10] attempted a chimpanzee-to-human heart transplant. Unfortunately, the patient survived less than an hour following the procedure. Three years later, in December of 1967, Christiaan Barnard performed the first successful human-to-human heart transplant, marking the beginning of the modern era of cardiac transplantation.[11] Even though Barnard's transplant recipient survived only 18 days before succumbing to the effects of *Pseudomonas* pneumonitis, the accomplishment led to the subsequent organization of 64 heart transplantation centers in 24 different countries by the end of 1969.[11] The initial optimism, which resulted in the performance of 101 cardiac transplantations within the first year, was tempered by postoperative immunologic difficulties, resulting in an average 1-year survival rate of 30% and a decline in the number of heart transplantation centers over the next few years.[11]

When the first human heart transplantation was performed, the field of lung transplantation was experiencing a parallel development in the research laboratory. Surgeons using the canine model had been focusing on technique, immunosuppression, and effects of pulmonary denervation, prior to clinical trials in humans. In 1963, the first human lung transplantation was performed by Hardy at the University of Mississippi Medical Center.[12] Although the patient died after 18 days because of renal failure, there was no evidence of immunologic rejection of the transplanted lung.[12] Hardy's operation served to demonstrate the technical feasibility of lung transplantation in humans and spurred further research in the field.

During the 1970s and early 1980s, many contributions from a team at Stanford University, directed by Norman Shumway, led to improved survival of transplant recipients by addressing the problems of postoperative care.[13-15] New surgical techniques, instrumentation for tissue sampling, a histologic grading system for tissue samples, and trials of immunosuppressive drugs all served to significantly advance the practice of thoracic transplantation. Most notably, however, the development and use of the immunosuppressant medication, cyclosporin A (now called cyclosporine), in 1980, led to a resurgence of interest and a subsequent increase in the number of thoracic transplantation teams.[11] Cyclosporine therapy improved the outcome of transplant recipients, resulting in fewer immunosuppressive complications compared with previous chemical agents, which were relatively nonspecific in their spectrum of action.

In the realm of heart-lung en bloc transplantation, although earlier experimental animal studies demonstrated the technical feasibility of the procedure, difficulties with donor procurement, immunosuppression, and surgical technique remained.[16-18] In 1980, Reitz and associates[18] performed an extended study on primates that answered many questions concerning heart–lung en bloc transplantation. Instead of the previously used right thoracotomy, Reitz favored a median sternotomy and instituted cardiopulmonary bypass, which also achieved surface hypothermia of the donor organ.[18] Thus, in 1981, the first successful human heart–lung en bloc transplantation was performed by Reitz and colleagues.[16-19]

The introduction of cyclosporine for immunosuppression and the numerous advances in the field of transplantation of other organs paved the way for the success of isolated lung transplantation in humans. In 1983, Joel Cooper and associates,[20] at the University of Toronto, performed the first successful single-lung transplant. Immunosuppression was achieved with cyclosporine, azathioprine, and prednisone, and the patient was discharged from the hospital 6 weeks after surgery.[20] This was followed in 1986 by the first successful isolated double-lung transplant, also by Dr. Cooper and the Toronto Lung Transplant Group.[21] In 1990, while at Stanford University, Starnes[22,23] performed the first lobar lung transplantation from living related donors, introducing an alternative method to expand the donor pool. In addition to the critical status that renders the patient unable to endure the typical waiting time on the list, the recipient's stature must be small enough to function with two donor lobes instead of entire lungs, and two family members must be identified, each of whom are willing and able to undergo a lobectomy to provide donor lobes for the recipient. Survival rate at 1 year for living-donor lobar transplantation was previously reported at 71%, comparable to traditional lung transplantation for some diagnoses.[22,23] The number of living-donor lobar transplantations for patients on the lung transplant list peaked in the 1990s and has decreased significantly in recent years.[24]

Both the impact of cyclosporine and the continued advances in the field of thoracic transplantation have led to an increased number of operations performed throughout the world and increased survival rate of recipients. The number of cardiac transplants increased from 90 in 1981 to more than 3000 performed each year since 1989, at 354 heart transplantation centers.[25-27] The Registry of the International Society of Heart and Lung Transplantation (ISHLT) reported that through June of 2007, there had been 80,106 heart transplantations performed worldwide on adults.[27] The actuarial 1-year survival rate for heart transplant recipients increased from 30% in 1969 to approximately 80% in 1996.[28,29] Currently, the conditional half-life (estimated time point at which 50% of all of the adult recipients who survive to at least 1 year have died) for heart transplant is almost 13 years.[27] With such impressive survival rates, cardiac transplantation is now an accepted treatment for patients with significant heart disease that can no longer be managed medically.

The number of heart–lung en bloc transplantation procedures increased each year between 1982 and 1989 with the peak of almost 230 procedures being reported in 1990.[27,30] However, the number of heart–lung en bloc transplantations started to decline, and by the year 2000, less than 150 were reported worldwide.[27,30] The decline is likely a result of the shortage of heart and lung bloc donors and the more common use of an isolated lung transplantation coupled with a needed cardiac repair. By 1996, actuarial survival rate statistics for 1 year were 60%, but decreased dramatically to less than 20% at 10 years.[30] Currently for adult heart–lung transplantation, the conditional half-life is close to 9 years.[27]

ISHLT data for 1996 indicates that 3194 isolated single-lung transplantations and 1845 double-lung transplantations had been performed to that time, with a survival rate for single-lung transplantation of 70% at 1 year and approximately 70% at 1 year for bilateral (double-) lung transplants.[30] There was an apparent reduction in the survival of recipients who were older than the age of 60 years (60%) compared to those who were younger than 60 years of age (70%) for a 1-year period.[30] The number of single-lung transplantation procedures in adults has stayed fairly steady since 1995, at approximately 700 per year worldwide; however, the number of double-lung transplantations has increased every year, peaking at 2196 procedures in 2005.[27] Currently, the conditional half-life for adult lung transplant recipients is 7.3 years.[27]

# Evaluation

## Candidacy

The primary indication for heart or lung transplantation is a progressive terminal cardiopulmonary disease with a limited life expectancy.[31-36] The majority of patients with end-stage disease show a marked decrease in cardiopulmonary function, require multiple medications and/or supplemental oxygen to carry out activities of daily living, and are no longer able to work or attend school full time. Table 12-1 identifies conditions that may lead to the need for thoracic organ transplantation.

The majority of heart transplantations are performed as a result of coronary artery disease, which leads to myocardial damage and cardiomyopathy.[37] The majority of lung transplantations have been performed in patients who have emphysema.[37] Idiopathic pulmonary fibrosis is the second most frequent indication for lung transplantation after chronic obstructive pulmonary disease.[38] There remains a question as to the ethics of using two lungs for the same patient, considering the donor shortage, when a single lung offers acceptable pulmonary function and satisfactory early and intermediate survival.[39] However, long-term survival data favors bilateral lung transplantation in recipients until approximately age 60 years.[39] These data suggest that double-lung transplantation should be reserved for younger recipients, for those with concomitant or possible chronic infection of the contralateral lung, or cases of marginal donors. A living-related lobar lung procedure is mainly considered for children or very small adults. The timing is based on deteriorating pulmonary function, hypoxia requiring mechanical ventilation, hypercapnia, or increasing antibiotic resistance and the availability of a living related donor. The use of living related donors has not significantly increased the number of transplants performed as originally thought.

Failure of a transplanted organ is also an indication for heart and lung repeat transplantation. The ISHLT reports that in 2007, heart retransplantations made up 4% of total heart transplantations, lung retransplantations made up 5.3%, and heart–lung retransplantations accounted for 1.3% of total heart–lung transplantations.[27]

## Contraindications to Transplantation

Candidate selection criteria vary among transplantation centers. Table 12-2 provides the most commonly accepted relative and absolute contraindications used for keeping an individual off a transplantation waiting list. The ISHLT issued new guidelines in 2006.[40] However, each center retains the freedom to make decisions and place a particular patient on the list at their transplantation center.

## Medical Aspects of Evaluation

The decision to refer a patient to a transplantation center for evaluation is a difficult one. The primary physician must (1) weigh the trend of the health status of the patient against the average time spent on the waiting list, and (2) find a balance between disclosing the complete spectrum of available medical treatments and offering the end-stage treatment of transplantation before a patient is ready to fully acknowledge the gravity of their clinical status. If the decision is made to refer the patient to a transplantation center, the patient must be evaluated by that center for acceptance onto the transplantation list at the center. The evaluation is usually completed as an outpatient; the rare circumstance that requires an inpatient visit for the evaluation is critical illness.

Table 12-3 outlines the laboratory tests and procedures included in the evaluation process. This assessment provides information about the presence of any contraindications to transplantation (see Table 12-2).[41] The candidate is also evaluated by members of the transplantation team. Table 12-4 outlines specific information obtained by each of the team members. The screening evaluation also provides key information about social issues, patient adherence to medical management, and general health that may uncover a relative or absolute contraindication to the transplantation process.

The transplantation candidate must be able to comply with a complicated medical regimen and have sufficient social support to endure the stressors associated with both the pre- and postoperative stages of transplantation.[42,43] The emotional reaction to the transplantation process is complex and intense. Kuhn and colleagues[44] identified stages of emotional adjustment through which a patient progresses in dealing with his or her disease. Kuhn's stages include the pretransplant evaluation, waiting for the organ, perioperative period, in-hospital convalescence, discharge, and postdischarge adaptation. Box 12-1 lists stressors common to these stages.

The patient's style of coping with the stressors inherent in the waiting period for transplantation may predict aspects of quality of life such as depression. An optimistic coping style is related to improved health outcomes, and is seen by patients

## Table 12-1 Indications for Thoracic Organ Transplantation

| Heart Transplantation | Lung Transplantation |
|---|---|
| *Indications for Transplantation* | |
| **End-stage heart disease** | **Chronic obstructive pulmonary disease** |
| Heart failure | BODE index of 7-10 and any of following: |
| Coronary artery disease | Hx of acute hypercapnia |
| Cardiomyopathy | Pulmonary hypertension or cor pulmonale |
| **NYHA Class III-IV despite maximal therapy such as the following:** | $FEV_1$ of 20% and DLCO of 20% |
| Medication | **Idiopathic pulmonary fibrosis** |
| Pacing (CRT) | Evidence of usual interstitial pneumonitis and any of following: |
| Revascularization or valve repair | DLCO of 39% |
| Ventricular remodeling procedure | 10% decrease in FVC |
| Recurrent hospitalization for heart failure | <88% $O_2$ saturation during 6MWT |
| Refractory ischemia and EF <20% | Honeycombing on HRCT |
| **Poor quality of life** | **Cystic fibrosis** |
| Intractable NYHA Class III-IV | FEV1 of 30% and any of following: |
| Intractable angina | Increasing $O_2$ requirements |
| Life-threatening arrhythmia | Hypercapnia |
| $VO_2max$ <10 mL/kg/min | Pulmonary hypertension |
| **Other** | **Idiopathic pulmonary arterial hypertension** |
| Congenital heart disease | Persistent NYHA Class III or IV |
| Cardiac tumors | 350 meters or declining 6MWT |
| | Failing therapy with epoprostenol |
| | Cardiac index of 0.2 $L/min/m^2$ |
| | Right atrial pressure 15 mm Hg |
| | **Sarcoidosis** |
| | NYHA Class III or IV and any of following: |
| | Hypoxemia at rest |
| | Pulmonary hypertension |
| | Right atrial pressure 15 mm Hg |
| *Indications for Repeated Transplantation* | |
| **Repeat heart transplantation** | **Repeat lung transplantation** |
| Severe acute rejection | Bronchiolitis obliterans |
| Transplant coronary artery disease | Graft failure |
| | Intractable airway problems |

*BODE, body mass index, airflow obstruction, dyspnea, and exercise capacity; CRT, cardiac resynchronization therapy; DLCO, diffusing capacity; EF, ejection fraction; $FEV_1$, forced expiratory volume in 1 sec; FVC, forced vital capacity; HRCT, high-resolution computed tomography; NYHA, New York Heart Association; 6MWT, six minute walk test; $VO_2max$, maximum oxygen uptake.*
*Data from Kreider M, Kotloff, RM. Selection of candidates for lung transplantation. Proc Am Thorac Soc 6:20-27, 2009; Novitzky D, Cooper C, Barnard C. The surgical technique of heterotopic heart transplantation. Ann Thorac Surg 36, 476, 1983; Macdonald P. Heart transplantation: Who should be considered and when? Intern Med J 38(12):911-917, 2008; Kirklin JK, McGiffin DC, Pinderski LJ, Tallaj J. Selection of patients and techniques of heart transplantation. Surg Clin North Am 84:257-287, 2004.*

awaiting heart transplantation as the most effective coping strategy.[45] Other strategies have been found to be less effective, including emotive, evasive, and fatalistic styles of coping.[45] Fatalistic coping, in particular, is a predictor of poorer quality of life in heart transplantation candidates,[46] whereas evasive coping is a predictor of more difficulty with

activities of daily living, depression, and poor quality of life in lung transplantation candidates.[47] Patients who had been waiting longer thought that they were coping better, possibly because of strategies learned over time.[47]

Throughout the transplantation process, stress is also experienced by the caregiver.[48] In a study at a midwestern

**Table 12-2 Absolute and Relative Contraindications to Heart and Lung Transplantation**

| Surgery | Absolute Contraindications | Relative Contraindications |
|---|---|---|
| Heart Transplantation | Active malignancy within the past 2 years | Fixed pulmonary hypertension (>15 mm Hg) |
| | Continued abuse of alcohol, tobacco, or narcotics | Severely limited functional status with poor rehabilitation potential |
| | Infection with the human immunodeficiency virus | Morbid obesity (body mass index [BMI] >30 kg/m²) |
| | Untreatable psychiatric condition with inability to comply with regimen | Cardiac amyloidosis (some forms) |
| | Diabetes mellitus with microvascular organ damage | Irreversible renal dysfunction |
| | Severe nonoperable peripheral or cerebrovascular disease | |
| Lung Transplantation | Active malignancy within the past 2 years | Symptomatic osteoporosis |
| | Continued abuse of alcohol, tobacco, or narcotics | Age 65 years or older |
| | Infection with the human immunodeficiency virus | Severely limited functional status with poor rehabilitation potential |
| | Significant chest wall or spinal deformity | Morbid obesity (BMI >30 kg/m²) |
| | Hepatitis B antigen positivity | Mechanical ventilation |
| | Hepatitis C with histologic evidence of liver disease | Colonization with highly resistant bacteria, fungi, or mycobacteria |
| | Limited ability to comply with medical regimen | Critical or unstable clinical condition |
| | Untreatable psychiatric condition with inability to comply with regimen | |
| | Absence of consistent support system | |

*Data from Orens JB, Estenne M, Arcasoy S, et al. International guidelines for the selection of lung transplant candidates: 2006 Update. J Heart Lung Transplant 25(7):745-755, 2006; and Macdonald P. Heart transplantation: Who should be considered and when? Intern Med J 38(12):911-917, 2008.*

---

**Box 12-1**

**Psychosocial Stressors in Transplantation Candidates and Recipients**

- Coping with disabling or life-threatening illness
- Making financial arrangements required for enrollment
- Surgical procedure
- Personal and family expenses
- Postoperative medical and pharmaceutical care
- Travel or moving to area of transplant program
- Changes in medical management and personnel
- Organizing an adequate support system
- Fear of being unsuitable for transplantation
- Onset of medical complications pre- or postoperatively
- Guilt over the donor's life ending to save theirs

Data from Squires R. Cardiac rehabilitation issues for heart transplantation patients. J Cardiopulm Rehabil 10:159-168, 1990; and Craven JL, Bright J, Dear CL. Psychiatric, psychosocial and rehabilitative aspects of lung transplantation. Clin Chest Med 11(2):247–257, 1990.

lung transplantation center, caregivers of patients in the transplantation waiting period reported positive mood, physical health, and general quality of life, but trouble with fatigue, worry, finances, and issues of sexuality.[49] Male caregivers reported significantly more tension than female caregivers.[48] Issues of depression, caregiver general health, financial impact, and lack of family support explained 79% of the quality of life of caregivers.[48] However stressed the caregivers are, lung transplantation candidates continue to experience decreased levels of general health, depression, fatigue, and quality of life from their caregivers.[48]

The results of the evaluation are compiled by the transplantation coordinator and provide the basis for discussion of the patient's candidacy. If accepted, the patient's medical profile is placed on the national patient waiting list for organ transplantation. The patient is not placed on a ranked list at this time. The list of candidates awaiting transplantation is maintained by the United Network of Organ Sharing (UNOS).[24] Upon identification of a potential organ donor, a transplantation coordinator from an organ procurement

## Table 12-3 Laboratory Tests and Procedures for Transplant Examination

| | |
|---|---|
| Laboratory tests | Arterial blood gases |
| | Complete blood cell count |
| | Electrolytes, BUN, creatinine, liver function tests |
| | Chest radiograph |
| | Sputum culture |
| | Urinalysis |
| Pulmonary assessment | Pulmonary function tests |
| | Ventilation/perfusion scan |
| | Computed tomography scan (when indicated) |
| Cardiac assessment | 12-Lead electrocardiogram |
| | Echocardiogram |
| | MUGA scan |
| | Cardiac catheterization |
| | Coronary angiography |
| | Cardiac biopsy (when indicated) |
| Other | Bone density scan (when indicated) |

*BUN, blood urea nitrogen; MUGA, multiple uptake gated acquisition*
*From TM Egan, LR Kaiser, JD Cooper. Lung transplantation. Curr Probl Surg 26:673–752, 1989.*

## Table 12-4 Evaluation by Heart, Lung, and Heart–Lung Transplantation Team Members

| | |
|---|---|
| Transplantation coordinator | Oversees evaluation process and compiles information for team discussion |
| Physicians and medical staff | Medical history |
| | Nature and progression of disease |
| | Social history (smoking, alcohol and drug) |
| | Prior surgery |
| | Medications, including steroid usage |
| | Physical examination |
| Physical therapist | Exercise tolerance test and exercise prescription |
| | Musculoskeletal assessment |
| | Cough/mucociliary clearance |
| Dietitian | Ideal body weight |
| | Caloric intake |
| Social worker or pastoral care | Psychosocial assessment |
| Psychologist/psychiatrist | Psychological testing |

*From TM Egan, LR Kaiser, JD Cooper. Lung transplantation. Curr Probl Surg 26:673–752, 1989.*

organization will access the UNOS database. Each candidate from the organ waiting list is matched with the donor's characteristics and a computer rank orders a candidate waiting list according to the organ allocation policies.[24] Factors affecting ranking include tissue match, blood type, length of time on the waiting list, immune status, and distance between the potential recipient and the donor.[24]

The UNOS policy for the heart transplantation waiting list was revised in July 2006 and gave priority to Status 1A and 1B candidates at transplantation centers within a 500-mile radius of the donor hospital.[49] Consideration was also given to urgent candidates with transplantation centers between 500 and 1000 miles of the donor hospital. A year after implementation of the policy, it was found that death of Status 1A candidates decreased by one-third, and deaths by Status 1B candidates decreased by one-half; Status 2 deaths also declined. Table 12-5 summarizes the priorities for heart transplant recipients. The median waiting time for heart transplantation is currently 50 days for Status 1A, 78 days for Status 1B, and 309 days for Status 2.[50]

Priority on the lung transplantation list is also maintained by UNOS, but unlike the heart transplantation waiting list, recipients 12 years of age or younger are ranked first by ABO blood status and then by the date of placement on the waiting list in each status.[24] For other lung transplantation recipients,

a Lung Allocation Score (LAS) is used to determine priority on the list. Similar to heart recipients, Status 7-identified patients are those who are temporarily unsuitable for transplantation. For example, a patient who develops a significant infection would not be a suitable candidate until the infection is controlled.

The LAS, instituted in 2005, is meant to address the risk of death with and without transplantation as well as factors that may impact survival.[51] Patients are given a score from 0 to 100 and are reassessed every 6 months. Box 12-2 lists the elements used to determine the LAS. The new LAS system versus solely listing a patient by time on the list provides an increased rationale for placing sicker patients on the list and less support for listing patients as early as possible.[51] The new allocation system has resulted in an increased number of organs being distributed to patients with pulmonary fibrosis while fewer are going to patients with chronic obstructive pulmonary disease (COPD).[52] The change has also produced a fewer number of listed patients overall, possibly patients on both ends of the spectrum, those unlikely to survive, and those too well to be offered transplantation.[52] In addition, there has been a decline in wait-list deaths from 14.4 per 100 patient-years, to 11.7 over a 4.5-month period, most likely a

**Table 12-5  Organ Allocation for Heart Transplantation Candidates**

| Status | Criteria for Adults | Criteria for Pediatrics |
|---|---|---|
| 1A (recertified every 14 days) | Admitted to transplant center hospital with mechanical circulatory support:<br>Left or right ventricular assist device<br>Intraaortic balloon pump<br>Extracorporeal membrane oxygenator<br>Mechanical circulatory support with evidence of device-related complication<br>Continuous mechanical ventilation | Requires assistance with a ventilator<br>Requires assistance with a mechanical device, such as extracorporeal membrane oxygenation<br>Requires assistance with an intraaortic balloon pump<br>A candidate younger than age 6 mo with congenital heart disease *and* pulmonary hypertension >50% of systemic level (may be treated with prostaglandin E to maintain patency of ductus arteriosus)<br>Requires infusion of high-dose multiple inotropes<br>Life expectancy of <14 days |
| 1A (recertified every 7 days) | Continuous infusion of single high-dose intravenous inotrope<br>Continuous infusion of multiple intravenous inotropes *and* continuous hemodynamic monitoring of left ventricular filling pressures | |
| 1B | Left and/or right ventricular device implanted<br>Continuous infusion of intravenous inotropes | Requires infusion of low-dose single inotropes<br>Younger than age 6 mos *and* does not meet criteria for Status 1A<br>Growth failure |
| 2 | A candidate who does not meet the criteria for Status 1A or 1B | A candidate who does not meet the criteria for Status 1A or 1B |
| 7 | A candidate who is considered temporarily unsuitable to receive a thoracic organ transplantation | A candidate who is considered temporarily unsuitable to receive a thoracic organ transplantation |

*From UNOS Policy 3.7 Organ Distribution: Allocation of Thoracic Organs, updated 6/20/2008. Available at: www.unos.org.*

**Box 12-2**

**Components of the Lung Allocation Score\***

- Date of birth
- Height and weight
- Lung diagnosis
- Functional status
- Presence of diabetes
- Assisted ventilation
- Supplemental oxygen use
- Percent predicted forced vital capacity
- Pulmonary artery systolic pressure
- Mean pulmonary artery pressure
- Mean pulmonary capillary wedge pressure
- Partial pressure of carbon dioxide
- Six-minute walk distance
- Serum creatinine

*\*To calculate a specific patient's lung allocation score, go to: http://www.unos.org/resources/frm_LAS_Calculator.asp?index=98*

consequence of decreased time spent waiting.[52] Based on data as of July 10, 2009 for patients listed in 2003 to 2004, a median wait-list time for patients with cystic fibrosis was 680 days, with emphysema/COPD 549 days, and with pulmonary fibrosis 445 days.[50]

### Physical Therapy Examination

Physical therapy examination of the potential transplant candidate is similar to that of any cardiopulmonary medical or surgical patient. The physical therapist focuses on the patient's cardiac and pulmonary system limitations while assessing the candidate's musculoskeletal and neuromuscular condition, exercise capacity, ventilatory function, and mucociliary clearance. Refer to Table 12-6 for special considerations about the physical therapy examination.

In the lung transplantation candidate, the efficacy of airway clearance techniques used by the patient should be evaluated by either the respiratory or physical therapist. A careful history and examination of sputum production

## Table 12-6 Physical Therapy Examination

| | Physical Therapy Examination Item | Special Considerations |
|---|---|---|
| Chart review | Mental health and current History<br>Lab results<br>Medical test results<br>Cardiac biopsy<br>Echocardiogram<br>Ejection fraction<br>Pulmonary function tests (PFTs)<br>Arterial blood gases (ABGs)<br>Medication list<br>Baseline vital signs | Typical for the patient to have demonstrated a decline in function over the previous 6-12 mo.<br>Provide overview of the patient's status. If status is critical, before proceeding with the examination it will be important to discuss acceptable limits of activity with physician. |
| Appearance | Skin<br>  Color<br>  Presence of edema<br>Posture<br>Breathing pattern (at rest and with activity)<br>  Use of accessory muscles<br>  Depth of breathing<br>  Areas of decreased chest expansion<br>  Work of breathing<br>Sputum<br>  Color, consistency, amount, odor | |
| Vital signs | At rest and with exercise/activity testing<br>Auscultation of lung and heart sounds | Monitor vital signs and oxygen saturation levels; important to correlate oxygen saturation levels with hematocrit and hemoglobin levels to ensure patient safety. |
| Musculoskeletal | Pain<br>Joint integrity and mobility<br>Muscle performance<br>Bed mobility, transfers, and gait<br>Balance | The musculoskeletal examination is typical of that for other patients, but should emphasize the thoracic area. This part of the examination will be useful to create an individualized strengthening and flexibility program for the patient. |
| Activities of daily living | Function assessment | |
| Anaerobic capacity/ endurance | With activity and exercise<br>Maximal stress test (rarely performed)<br>6-Minute walk test<br>Submaximal treadmill or cycle ergometry | A testing protocol with small increments in workload (Naughton, Balke-Ware) versus a protocol with large increments (Bruce) is better suited to patients with cardiovascular or respiratory disease as it allows for more specificity in determining the patient's capabilities. |

*Data from Biggar DG, Melen JE, Trulock EP, et al. Pulmonary rehabilitation before and after lung transplantation. In Kasaburi R, Petty TL (eds.). Principles and Practice of Pulmonary Rehabilitation. Philadelphia, Saunders, 1993:459–467; and ACSM's Guidelines for Exercise Testing and Prescription. 8th ed. Philadelphia, Lippincott Williams & Wilkins, 1995:112, 218.*

patterns and preferred technique for airway clearance should be performed, noting the effectiveness and ease of techniques used. Auscultation of breath sounds should be included as a part of this examination. The foregoing components of the examination will assist the therapist in counseling the patient

regarding ways to improve current methods and use of alternative techniques for airway clearance.[53]

Assessment of aerobic capacity/endurance with exercise and activity may be achieved in several ways. Complete cardiopulmonary exercise testing, including a maximal stress test, whereby the analysis of expired gases is evaluated, is not routinely performed at this time because exercise testing to this degree is not tolerated well by transplantation candidates. In the small number of studies in which such exercise testing has been reported, heart and lung transplantation candidates exhibit severely reduced aerobic capacities.[54,55] In heart transplantation candidates, Mancini and colleagues[56] demonstrated that patients with a peak oxygen consumption at maximal exercise (VO$_2$max) of 14 mL/kg/min or less were at higher risk for death and should be referred for transplantation, whereas transplantation can be safely deferred in those patients with a VO$_2$max greater than 14 mL/kg/min. More commonly, a baseline exercise examination involves submaximal treadmill or cycle ergometer testing.

The results of the physical therapy examination are used for two purposes; first the results serve as a basis for prescribing an individualized program for the patient and secondly to provide useful information to the transplantation team.[57,58] Exercise may be contraindicated in patients with primary pulmonary hypertension (defined as an increase in normal pulmonary artery pressure, 15 to 18 mm Hg, by 5 to 10 mm Hg) because exercise may aggravate the condition, causing pulmonary artery pressures to rise adversely.[59] Nici and colleagues recommend that a closely supervised activity/exercise program with attention to the intensity of activity/exercise may be useful for treatment addressing functional limitation. Further recommendations include the utilization of low-intensity aerobic exercise, pacing and energy conservation techniques with close monitoring of blood pressure and heart rate, and determination of adequate oxygenation. Telemetry monitoring may be indicated for those patients with known arrhythmias.[60]

## Preoperative Rehabilitation

Research demonstrates that transplantation candidates can achieve significant training effects from long-term rehabilitation programs.[61,62] Most lung transplantation centers require the participation of candidates in a pulmonary rehabilitation program while waiting for the donor organ. The recommendation of cardiac rehabilitation for the heart transplantation candidate is made on an individual basis. The training effects are achieved mainly through peripheral adaptations that provide the patient with an improved functional and exercise capacity. For example, lung transplantation centers have reported improvements of up to 39% in the 6-minute walk test (6MWT) of transplantation candidates participating in preoperative exercise programs.[32,63]

Components of a preoperative rehabilitation program include patient and family education, cardiovascular endurance training, musculoskeletal strength and flexibility training, and breathing retraining. Boxes 12-3 and 12-4 list the American Thoracic and European Respiratory Society's recommendations for pulmonary rehabilitation.

The goal of rehabilitation prior to surgery is to improve or to prevent deterioration of the candidate's physical

---

**Box 12-3**

**Pulmonary Rehabilitation Recommendations**

- Minimum of 20 sessions 3 times/week or 2 times/week plus one home session.
- Encourage high-intensity exercise when possible.
- Interval training may be useful to promote higher intensity levels of exercise.
- Perform both upper extremity and lower extremity training.
- Combine endurance and strength training, especially in patients with muscle atrophy.
- Perform inspiratory muscle training as adjunctive therapy.
- Oxygen supplementation allows for high-intensity training.

From Nici L, Donner C, Wouters E, et al. American Thoracic Society/European Respiratory Society statement on pulmonary rehabilitation. Am J Respir Crit Care Med 173(12):1390-1413, 2006.

---

**Box 12-4**

**Pulmonary Rehabilitation Education Topics**

- Breathing strategies
- Normal lung function
- Pathophysiology of lung disease
- Medication use
- Bronchial hygiene techniques
- Exercise benefits
- Energy conservation
- Nutrition
- Smoking cessation
- Sexuality
- Need for health care

From Nici L, Donner C, Wouters E, et al. American Thoracic Society/European Respiratory Society statement on pulmonary rehabilitation. Am J Respir Crit Care Med 173(12):1390-1413, 2006.

---

condition. Ensuring that candidates are in the best physical condition will increase the likelihood that they will be able to endure the stresses of transplantation. Improving the status of the patients may also play a role in increasing survival of patients on the transplantation waiting list, because a decline in medical status is the most common cause of death for those patients awaiting transplantation.

Typically, the patient waiting for heart transplantation is encouraged to remain as active as possible within the limits of standard hemodynamic guidelines (see Chapter 18). Often the heart transplantation candidates' level of participation in endurance activities will be limited to minimal levels of exertion or solely activities of daily living (ADLs) because of their significantly compromised ejection fraction and cardiac output. Pretransplantation candidates may also demonstrate other unstable hemodynamic symptoms that further compromise oxygen supply to the heart and peripheral body tissues. Examples of unstable hemodynamic abnormalities include hypotension (which limits tissue perfusion), reduced lung volumes and decreased pulmonary perfusion (which may cause ventilation–perfusion mismatch), and increased pulmonary vascular resistance (which is associated with an increased respiratory rate). With increased activity these abnormalities worsen, limiting a candidate's participation in a strengthening or endurance program. If a heart transplantation candidate is suitable for endurance training, the candidate should be monitored closely by individuals trained to recognize inappropriate responses to exercise. The endurance training program often begins in a formal cardiac rehabilitation program and subsequently continues at home or in a community exercise program. When a left ventricular assist device (LVAD) is used to "bridge" the patient to heart transplantation, exercise capacity and functional performance are often improved. LVAD patients are now often the very best candidates for heart transplantation as a result of enhanced physical condition.[64] Other areas to be emphasized in cardiac rehabilitation focus on correct posture, mobility training, and education regarding heart transplantation complications.

Lung transplantation candidates are also encouraged to begin or continue an exercise/activity program and in fact some programs make this a requirement. The exercise may be done at home, in a supervised community program, or in a monitored pulmonary rehabilitation program. Some lung transplantation centers require candidates to relocate close to the center so as to increase exercise participation compliance. Guidelines for pulmonary rehabilitation (see Chapter 19) should be followed in the pretransplantation period. Because of the variable severity of disease, lung transplantation candidates will differ significantly from other participants in a pulmonary rehabilitation program. The likelihood that patients awaiting transplantation will exhibit exercise-induced hypoxemia is increased. Consequently, oxygen saturation should be monitored continuously during exercise sessions, and efforts should be made to maintain oxygen saturation at greater than 90%.[65] A variety of different oxygen delivery systems may be necessary to use during exercise to maintain oxygen saturation at the appropriate level for a given patient. Although lung function may not improve, substantial increases in exercise performance have been reported in patients with end-stage pulmonary disease.[66,67] Most patients are able to participate in 30 to 40 minutes of endurance exercise three to five times per week at 70% to 80% of predicted maximal heart rate while maintaining appropriate oxygen saturation levels.[65]

## Alternative Therapies to Transplantation

Following review by the transplantation team, patient suitability is determined. If the patient is found to be unsuitable for transplantation, this determination may be a result of several factors, including the following:

- The patient did not meet the criteria of organ system failure,
- The presence of contraindications limit the potential success of the surgery,

- There are decreased overall benefits for the patient from the transplantation procedure, or
- The patient opted for more conservative surgical or medical management.

When any of these situations is present, the patient must be managed in other ways. For end-stage pulmonary disease, lung volume reduction surgery (LVRS) or bilevel positive airway pressure (BiPAP) may be used as a replacement for lung transplantation or to improve the patient's status until a transplant is performed. A ventricular assist device (VAD), home pharmacologic management, or cardiac myoplasty may be used for patients with end-stage cardiac disease to improve status or to bridge the time to heart transplantation.

### Alternatives to Lung Transplantation

LVRS is a surgical procedure aimed at reducing the size of the lungs in patients with emphysema (Fig. 12-1). The surgery may be performed prior to a patient being placed on a waiting list to forestall the need for transplantation, or instead of transplantation for those patients who may benefit from this procedure. During the surgical procedure, 20% to 30% of the volume of each lung is removed via a median sternotomy incision. LVRS is performed to improve thoracic distention and chest wall mechanics. Work by Trulock and colleagues[68] demonstrates that improvement is made in both the patient's symptoms and pulmonary function by potentially improving the forced expiratory volume in 1 second ($FEV_1$) by as much as 100%. Carbon dioxide retention is decreased, and oxygen use can often be discontinued owing to the improvement in blood gas values. Benefits of LVRS documented by Sciurba[69] and Criner[70] include clinical improvement of dyspnea and breathing pattern, improved expiratory flow rates, improved lung volumes, and an increase in exercise capacity documented during 6MWT or maximal exercise.[70] Washko and colleagues found that lung volume reduction surgery lessens the frequency of exacerbations of COPD in addition to increasing the time to a patient's first exacerbation.[71]

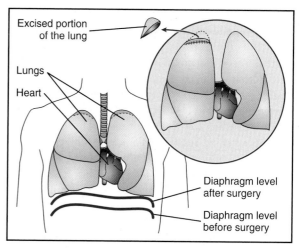

**Figure 12-1** The mechanics of lung volume reduction surgery.

Sciurba,[69] Cooper,[72] and Trulock[68] attribute these improvements to a few possibilities. The first hypothesis suggests that the surgery causes an increase in elastic recoil of the lung, creating a greater efficiency in respiratory muscle and chest wall mechanics. The second hypothesis suggests that there may be a beneficial effect on the mechanical function of the musculoskeletal components of the respiratory system. For example, prior to surgery a patient has hyperinflated lungs and increased functional residual capacity (FRC), which presumably put the respiratory muscles at a mechanical disadvantage. Following surgery, the lung reduction decreases FRC, which might allow for improved function of the respiratory muscles because they are working at a more optimal length for contraction. The third proposed mechanism for improvement is also related to the resultant decrease in lung hyperinflation. With the reduction of lung volume, the restrictive effects caused by lung hyperinflation are ameliorated and normal cardiac filling is possible.[72] Thus, cardiac efficiency is improved and the ventilation-to-perfusion ratio is enhanced.

The National Emphysema Treatment Trial (NETT) was completed to determine the safety and effectiveness of LVRS.[73] The objectives were to document:[73]

- The benefits and risks over long-term followup (5 years),
- The patient-selection criteria that predict the best outcome, and
- The surgical procedure (thoracscopy versus median sternotomy) that is associated with the best outcome.

The NETT found different clinical results for each of four groups:[74]

- Patients with low exercise capacity whose upper lobes were primarily affected had lower mortality with LVRS than with medical treatment.
- Patients with high exercise capacity whose upper lobes were primarily affected had no difference in mortality but had better clinical outcome.
- Patients with low exercise capacity whose lower lobes were primarily affected had similar mortality with LVRS or medical treatment.
- Patients with high exercise capacity whose lower lobes were primarily affected had a higher mortality with LVRS than with medical treatment.

This large, multicenter trial documented a 1 month mortality rate of 16% in patients with an $FEV_1$ less than 20% of predicted, in contrast to an overall mortality rate of 5.2% in the group that excluded "high-risk patients."[75] As the LVRS mortality rate has been reported to be as high as 17%, this improvement in survival supports the practice of patient selection according to specific criteria.[75] This has been challenged, however, by Yusen and colleagues who emphasize the improved clinical picture of patients following LVRS instead of short-term survival, as a few trials have demonstrated improved quality of life for 2 to 5 years following the procedure.[76]

Progressive respiratory failure in the lung transplant candidate may necessitate the use of noninvasive ventilation or BiPAP (see Fig 13-6). This intervention uses a tightly fitting nasal mask to noninvasively deliver positive airway pressure during inspiration as well as on exhalation. It is indicated for patients with signs of respiratory failure despite maximal drug and oxygen therapy in an attempt to avoid intubation. Use of this device at night has resulted in a decrease in work of breathing, headaches, and daytime fatigue, and an increase in quality of sleep and level of activity.[77,78] BiPAP has been useful as an adjunct for patients awaiting transplantation by alleviating symptoms of respiratory failure.[78] It has also been helpful to improve exercise tolerance in patients with severe respiratory failure and may be a useful adjunct during rehabilitation.[79,80]

## Alternatives to Heart Transplantation

Unfortunately, a patient with cardiac muscle dysfunction often demonstrates deterioration in medical status quickly, not leaving adequate time for the surgical or medical procedures that could prevent the need for heart transplantation. In such instances the placement of a left or biventricular assistive device for heart transplantation candidates may be indicated to provide a bridge until a suitable donor organ becomes available for transplantation An LVAD is an implantable electrically powered device that provides permanent support of the systemic circulation in those patients for whom a suitable cardiac donor cannot yet be found (Fig. 12-2).[81] It is indicated for patients with severe hemodynamic compromise for whom maximal drug therapy and other medical interventions have not proven successful. The system allows variability in pump output according to the patient's physiologic demands, allowing the patient to participate in a progressive, monitored exercise program.[82] The ability of the patient to resume ADLs and an exercise program leads to improved conditioning in preparation for

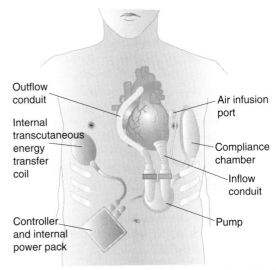

**Figure 12-2** A totally implantable left ventricular assist device (LVAD), the LionHeart Left Ventricular Assist System. (Redrawn from Nemeh H, Smedira N. Mechanical treatment of heart failure: The growing role of LVADs and artificial hearts. Cleve Clin J Med 70:223-234, 2003.)

a heart transplantation. The LVAD has been used successfully as a bridge to transplantation,[82] and it is thought that many more patients could benefit from this therapy. Between 1999 and 2006, 20% of patients listed as Status 1A for heart transplantation died while waiting or were removed from the list without having mechanical cardiac support, leading the author to posit that VAD usage may have improved survival in this patient group.[83]

In patients who are not candidates for heart transplantation and who have less than a 2-year life expectancy, destination VAD therapy is covered by Medicare for patients with New York Heart Association (NYHA) Class IV heart failure under the following conditions:[84]

1. The patient's symptoms have not responded to optimal medical management, including dietary (salt restriction) and pharmaceutical intervention (diuretics, digitalis, β blockers, and angiotensin-converting enzyme inhibitors) for at least 60 days.
2. The patient has a left ventricular ejection fraction less than 25%.
3. The patient has functional limitation with a peak $O_2$ consumption of less than 12 mL/kg/min or has a continued need for intravenous inotropic therapy.
4. The patient has the appropriate body size ($\geq$1.5 m$^2$) to support VAD implantation.

The use of LVAD for destination therapy was compared to medical treatment in those patients not suited for heart transplantation in the Randomized Evaluation of Mechanical Assistance for the Treatment of Congestive Heart Failure (REMATCH) study.[85] Results showed improved survival, 56% in 1 year, in the group of patients who underwent LVAD implantation with in-hospital mortality at 27%, primarily as a consequence of sepsis, right heart failure, and multiorgan failure.[85] Table 12-7 describes examples of LVADs used for end-stage heart disease.

Home intravenous pharmacologic management of the patient with chronic heart failure is becoming more common for patients awaiting heart transplantation as well as for those not suitable for transplantation. Currently, intravenous inotropic therapy is being used at home to improve cardiac output and systemic perfusion.[86] Other desirable aims include the reduction of myocardial oxygen consumption, enhancement of coronary perfusion, slowing of rapid heart rate, restoration of baroreceptor function, reversal of neurohumoral activation, restoration of cardiac size and shape, promotion of cardiac and vascular repair, and enhancement of survival.[87,86] Both dobutamine and milrinone are approved by the Food and Drug Administration for short-term intravenous treatment of acute heart failure, but these medications are also being used longer term for patients on waiting list for heart transplantation.[88] Chronic intravenous milrinone has been used effectively for shorter bridge-to-transplant times (<100 days), with the study authors recommending LVAD placement for longer wait times.[89]

Cardiomyoplasty is a rarely used alternative to heart transplantation. Cardiomyoplasty is a surgical procedure in

## Table 12-7 Characteristics of Left Ventricular Assist Devices

| LVAD Type | General Description | Fill and Drive Mechanism | Indications | Examples |
|---|---|---|---|---|
| Centrifugal pump | Pump is outside the body; spinning motor creates centrifugal force, produces a steady nonpulsatile flow | Filled by gravity; centrifugal force drives blood | Short term use: bridge to recovery; support during percutaneous coronary procedure | TandemHeart PTVA BioMedicus CentriMag VentrAssist |
| Volume-displacement pump | Pump can be implanted or stay outside the body; fill–empty cycle with pulsatile flow | Fill is active or passive; empties by pneumatic or mechanical compression of chamber | Short or long-term use: bridge to transplantation; destination therapy, bridge to recovery | HeartMate XVE Thoratec IVAD Thoratec VAD Novacor Abiomed BVS 5000 |
| Axial flow pump | Helical blades on a central shaft rotating bearings; blood flows through the pump continuously (with pulsatile flow from native heart) | Spinning of the motor draws blood from the ventricles and sends it through the pump and aorta by an outflow graft | Short or long-term use: bridge to transplantation; destination therapy | Jarvik 2000 MicroMed DeBakey Heartmate II Impella |

*From Stahl M, Richards N. Update on ventricular assist device technology. AACN Adv Crit Care 20(1):20-36, 2009.*

## Table 12-8  Criteria for Donors

|  | Absolute Criteria | Marginal Criteria |
|---|---|---|
| Heart donors | Age younger than 40 years<br>No history of cardiac disease<br>No positive test for hepatitis B<br>No evidence of cardiac trauma<br>No prolonged resuscitative efforts applied prior to death | Age up to 65 years<br>Bypassable one- or two-vessel disease, correctable valvular dysfunction by echocardiography, persistent conduction disturbances, elevation of myocardial enzymes<br>History of chest trauma<br>Open cardiac massage |
| Lung donors | Age younger than 35 years<br>Chest radiograph free of infiltrates<br>Arterial $O_2$ tension >300 mm Hg on 100% $O_2$ and 5 cm of positive end expiratory pressure<br>Clear bronchoscopy without evidence of purulent secretions or aspiration<br>No significant chest trauma or pulmonary contusion | Age |
| Both | Size matching<br>Procurement distance<br>Positive HIV status<br>Actively malignancy<br>Current infectious process<br>Evidence of major trauma to the organ | Under- or oversize by more than 20% body weight<br>Long-distance procurement (>1000 miles) |

From UNOS website, www.unos.org, accessed August 28, 2009.

which a fatigue-resistant skeletal muscle, the latissimus dorsi, is wrapped around the patient's heart and is stimulated electrically to contract in synchrony with cardiac systole. It was believed that the contraction of the skeletal muscle during systole would augment ventricular contraction of the failing heart and that structural reinforcement of the myocardium would prevent further dilation of the heart, resulting in an increased ejection fraction.[90,91] Success with this technique has been conflicting, and the procedure is seldom used.[92]

## Donor Selection and Matching Criteria

As waiting lists for thoracic organ transplantation grow as a result of the shortage of suitable donor organs, medical centers are expanding their once more-rigid criteria to allow more organs to be used for transplantation.[93] A suitable organ donor needs to meet the qualifications of brain or cardiac death. When death occurs and organ donation is a possibility, there is a medical examination to determine what organs would be suitable for transplantation. Individual donor and recipient factors are then analyzed on a case-by-case basis and a decision made on whether the donor is appropriate for the recipient.[24] Age, once a major limitation, is now

expanded up to 65 years. A 2006 UNOS data report indicates that the usual organ donor is younger than 59 years of age.[94] Table 12-8 describes the specific criteria applied to heart and lung donors.

## Surgical Techniques

### Cardiac Transplantation

The four methods for performing cardiac transplantation are heterotopic, total transplantation, biatrial, and bicaval techniques.

Heterotopic heart transplantation (HHT), referred to as the "piggyback" technique (Fig. 12-3), is considered to be an alternative technique and is performed less frequently than orthotopic transplantation. Special circumstances that may necessitate use of the heterotopic method are mismatching of size between the donor and recipient or a recipient that has an abnormally high level of pulmonary vascular resistance.[95-97] The heterotopic surgical procedure is performed without the removal of the native heart. The donor heart is connected to the patient's native heart through a median sternotomy incision in the following manner: donor right atrium to recipient right atrium and donor left atrium to recipient left atrium.[95,98-101] The four atria then function

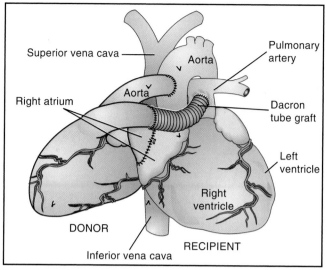

**Figure 12-3** This drawing shows a completed preparation of a heterotopic heart transplant with anastomosis sites indicated by the suture lines. The donor and recipient pulmonary arteries are joined via a Dacron graft.

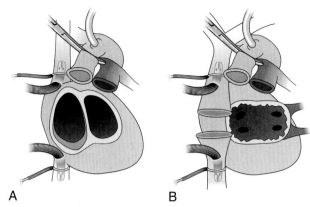

**Figure 12-4** Surgical techniques for cardiac transplantation. **A,** Biatrial technique. The donor heart is anastomosed to the main bulk of the recipient's native right and left atria. **B,** Bicaval technique. The donor left atrium is anastomosed to a single left atrial cuff, including the pulmonary veins, in the recipient. (From Miller RD, Eriksson LI, Fleischer LA, et al. Miller's Anesthesia. 7th ed. Philadelphia, Churchill Livingstone, 2009.)

as two atria. Ascending aortas are anastomosed together, and pulmonary arteries are connected via a Dacron tube graft.[95] Enthusiasm for HHT generally disappeared in the last two decades as more studies showed better survival with orthotopic heart transplant[2-4] and more potential complications with HHT, including pulmonary complications because of compression of right middle and lower lung lobes,[4,5] systemic thromboembolism because of reduced flow through the native left ventricle with increased risk of clot formation,[5] development of mitral and tricuspid regurgitation in the native heart,[3] malignant ventricular arrhythmias, and recurrence of angina in the native heart in patients with ischemic cardiomyopathy.[102]

Total transplantation was described by Web and Neely in 1959, and clinically popularized by Dreyfus and Yacoub in 1991.[13,15,17] The procedure involves complete excision of the recipient atria with complete atrioventricular transplantation, along with separate bicaval and pulmonary venous anastomoses (Fig. 12-4).[18-20] The major disadvantages associated with this technique are the additional time required to complete six anastomoses, as well as increased potential for technical complications, such as bleeding from inaccessible suture lines in the posterior pulmonary veins and twisting or narrowing of the pulmonary veins, causing pulmonary venous anastomotic stenosis. The total technique is infrequently employed (technique of choice in 8% of ISHLT centers), and there is insufficient clinical data describing postoperative outcomes using this technique.[103]

Until most recently, the biatrial anastomotic technique developed and described by Lower and Shumway was used most frequently.[104] The biatrial technique consists of performing biatrial anastomoses whereby donor and recipient atrial cuffs are sewn together (Fig. 12-4A). Although biatrial anastomoses do not require separate caval anastomoses, and

therefore save time, potential problems include atrial dysfunction, sinus node dysfunction, valvular insufficiency, and thrombus formation. In response to these concerns, the bicaval technique (which consists of sewing separate caval anastomoses) was developed and introduced in the early to mid 1990s.[2-6] Studies comparing the two techniques show that the bicaval anastomotic technique leads to improved atrial function,[7,8] lower rate of postoperative arrhythmias,[9] decreased need for permanent pacing,[10] and decreased tricuspid regurgitation,[11-13] and in one series, improved survival.[14] As a result of this perceived superiority, the number of heart transplantations conducted with the bicaval techniques has increased steadily since 1995 and the UNOS database shows that in 2005 in the United States, the bicaval technique is now more popular than the biatrial technique (1083 procedures vs. 806).[105]

Currently, the biatrial technique used for orthotopic heart transplantation leaves the recipient sinoatrial (SA) node intact to avoid the need for venous anastomoses.[106] Despite a loss of blood flow, the SA node remains functional through collateral bronchial circulation, and innervation continues to provide stimulation to the atrial remnants for contraction. Unlike the recipient atrial remnants, the donor heart's SA node is denervated and operates independently of the recipient's. Thus, two separate P waves will be seen on the electrocardiogram (ECG) (Fig. 12-5). One P wave is caused by the recipient SA node and the other is from the donor SA node. The donor's P wave continues to activate the donor heart and a resulting QRST complex occurs, providing total contraction of the donor heart to provide cardiac output. During exercise, periods of anxiety, or other instances of sympathetic stimulation, the rate of the innervated recipient SA node increases according to increases in the intensity of sympathetic stimulation.[106] The donor SA node rate does not

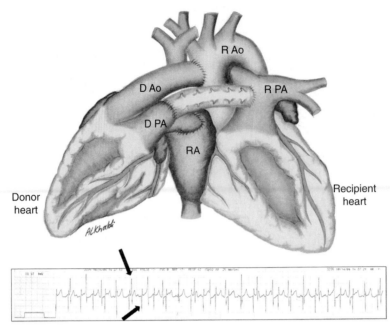

**Figure 12-5** An electrocardiogram from a 22-month-old infant after a heterotopic heart transplant. The separate donor and recipient QRS complexes can be seen (*arrows*). (From Kliegman, RM, Behrman, RE, Jenson, HB, et al. Nelson Textbook of Pediatrics. 18th ed. Philadelphia, Saunders, 2007.)

respond as rapidly with sympathetic stimulation because of its state of denervation.[106]

## Lung Transplantation

The lungs are harvested from the donor in the following manner: the pulmonary veins are detached from the heart along with a cuff from the left atrium; the pulmonary arteries are transected; and the lungs removed en bloc, divided into separate right and left lungs for implantation (Fig. 12-6).[32,107]

Initially, the technique for double-lung transplantation was performed using a tracheal anastomosis and a double-lung bloc. This technique was altered subsequently to use bilateral mainstem bronchial anastomoses through a median sternotomy incision.[108] Currently, the preferred procedure maintains use of mainstem bronchial anastomoses, while progressing to use of bilateral anterior thoracotomies or a transsternal bilateral thoracotomy or "clamshell incision," which provides better exposure than the median sternotomy.[109,110] The anastomoses for double-lung transplantation, more accurately referred to as "bilateral sequential" lung transplantation, include the pulmonary artery anastomosis followed by the bronchial anastomoses. During the surgical procedure, the least-functional lung is removed and transplanted first while the remaining contralateral lung is ventilated (Fig. 12-7). After completion of both lung transplantations, two chest tubes are placed into each pleural space and the chest is closed. The airways are inspected by bronchoscopy. The current techniques decrease the need for cardiopulmonary bypass as opposed to use of a double-lung bloc.[111] The airway anastomoses may be performed using end-to-end anastomoses

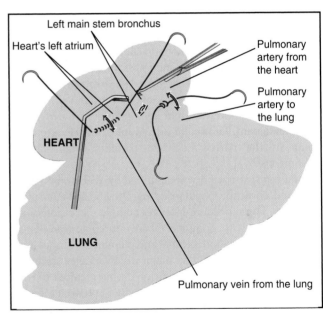

**Figure 12-6** Completed preparation of a single left lung transplant with anastomosis sites designated by suture lines.

or a "telescoping" method whereby the donor or recipient airway is inserted in the opposite airway for a distance of one cartilaginous ring.[112]

Single-lung transplantation is performed similarly, most often using a standard posterolateral thoracotomy incision. In some instances/circumstances, access to the lung may occur through an anterior axillary thoracotomy. The atrial anastomosis is performed first, followed by the pulmonary

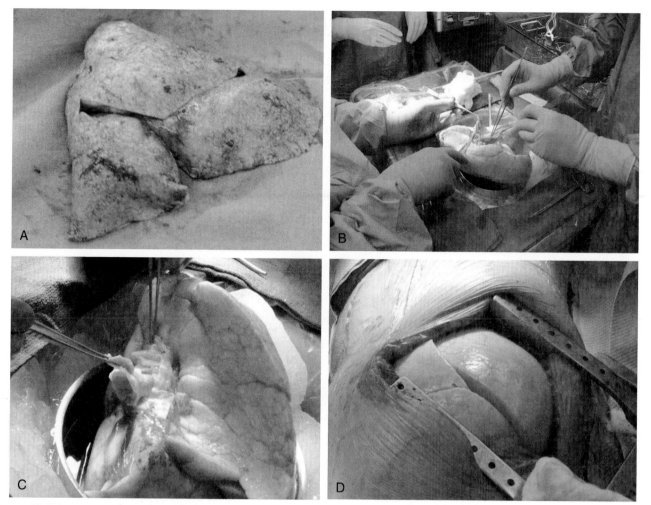

**Figure 12-7** Lung transplantation using bilateral posterolateral thoracotomies. **A,** Diseased lung is removed. **B** and **C,** Donor lung is prepared for transplantation. **D,** Donor lung is inserted.

artery anastomosis and the bronchial anastomosis.[113] For a single-lung transplantation, the side chosen is related to prior surgery, the desire to replace the worst recipient lung, and the best donor side.

## Medications

The majority of medications prescribed for the transplant patient are immunosuppressive agents and drugs used to combat the side effects of these agents.[114,115] The immunosuppressive regimen is necessary to prevent rejection of the donor organ by reducing the normal immune system's response to the foreign tissue. Induction therapy, a strong dose of immunosuppressives given at the time of transplantation, is used in some transplantation centers in the immediate postoperative period, but its efficacy continues to be assessed.[116,117] Induction therapy is thought to reduce acute rejection, allow for later introduction of nephrotoxic calcineurin inhibitors, and decrease the incidence of bronchiolitis obliterans syndrome.[116,117] On the other hand, induction therapy may increase the incidence of malignancy and

infection in addition to the cost of the transplantation. In lung transplantation, a significant reduction in acute rejection was found with induction therapy using an antithymocyte globulin (ATG) compared with induction with an interleukin-2 receptor (IL-2R) or no induction.[116] Recent trends in the use of induction therapy are evident in the ISHLT registry.[117] Use of IL-2R antibodies has been increasing in recent years and antilymphocytic agent use is steady, but there has been a significant reduction in the use of OKT3. In addition, approximately 50% of heart transplantation centers used no induction therapy. The 5-year survival rate of patients who received induction therapy and those with no induction therapy demonstrated no statistically significant difference.

Aliabadi and colleagues[118] point out that as a consequence of the increase in medication options, patients' immunosuppressive regimens are no longer general protocols, but are tailored to the individual. In addition, patient's pharmacologic treatments can be more easily altered depending on treatment sequelae such as hypertension, dyslipidemia, or diabetes.[118] For example, mycophenolate mofetil can be used in the case of nephropathy, and target of rapamycin (TOR)

**Table 12-9 Common Immunosuppressive Agents for Thoracic Organ Transplantation**

| | Drug Class | Trade Name | Mechanism of Action | Significant Adverse Effects |
|---|---|---|---|---|
| Corticosteroids | Prednisone Prednisolone Methylprednisolone | Generic; Deltasone; Pediapred; Prelone; Solu-Medrol; Medrol | Inhibits cytokine synthesis; inhibits interleukin-1 and γ-interferon; inhibits T-cell activation; antiinflammatory agent | HTN, glaucoma, adrenal suppression, cataracts, thinning skin, hyperglycemia, osteopenia, myopathy dyslipidemia |
| Calcineurin inhibitors | Cyclosporine | Gengraf; Neoral; Sandimmune | Inhibits T-lymphocyte proliferation; inhibits interleukin-2 | Nephrotoxicity, HTN, increased infections, gingival hyperplasia, neurotoxicity |
| | Tacrolimus (TAC or FK506) | Prograf | Inhibits interleukin-2; inhibits T-lymphocytes | Nephrotoxicity, hyperglycemia, neurotoxicity, GI disturbances |
| Antiproliferative agents | Azathioprine | Imuran | Probably interferes with DNA synthesis; limits cellular proliferation | Bone marrow suppression, hepatotoxicity, GI distress, skin rash |
| | Mycophenolate mofetil (MMF) | Cellcept | Inhibits synthesis of DNA precursors in T and B lymphocytes | Bone disorders, GI problems, HTN, dysrhythmias |
| Target of rapamycin (TOR) inhibitors | Sirolimus; Everolimus | Rapamycin; Rapamune; Certican | Inhibits function of TOR; decreases growth of T, B cells | Blood disorders, dyslipidemia, delayed postsurgical healing |
| Antithymocyte globulin | | | Selective for antigens that inhibit specific T cells and other lymphocytes | |
| Muromonab-CD3 monoclonal antibody | | Orthoclone OKT3 | Blocks T-cell recognition of antigen | |
| Basiliximab | | Simulect | Blocks interleukin-2 receptor from activating T cells | |

GI, gastrointestinal; HTN, hypertension.
Data from Erbasan O, Kemaloglu C, Bayezid O. Heart transplantation. Anadolu Kardiyol Derg 8(Suppl 2):131-147, 2008; Snell G, Westall G. Immunosuppression for lung transplantation: Evidence to date. Drugs 67(11):1531-1539, 2007; Ciccone C. Pharmacology in Rehabilitation. 4th ed. Philadelphia, FA Davis, 2007.

inhibitors are thought to provide a defense against cancer and graft vasculopathy following cardiac transplantation.[118]

Medications are initiated in the operating room and continue to be part of the patient's daily regimen for life. Doses may be tapered to the lowest level possible to prevent rejection, but some medications are never completely stopped. The ISHLT reports that the most common mediations for maintenance therapy are a calcineurin inhibitor combined with an antiproliferative agent and corticosteroids.[117] The use of azathioprine is in decline in favor of mycophenolate mofetil (MMF), and tacrolimus (TAC) is more commonly used than cyclosporine; patients using TAC and MMF had less rejection in the first postoperative year compared to patients using cyclosporine and MMF.[119] Common immunosuppressive medications and effects are listed in Table 12-9 and in Chapter 14.

## Box 12-5

### Factors Influencing Cardiovascular Resting and Exercise Physiology After Heart Transplantation

- Donor brain death
- Composite atria
- Surgical denervation of donor heart
- Altered ventricular function
- Systolic
- Diastolic
- Drug therapy
- Skeletal muscle changes
- Pretransplantation deconditioning
- Heart failure
- Complications of transplantation
- Rejection
- Accelerated coronary sclerosis
- Hypertension
- Renal impairment
- Anemia
- Steroid side effects (e.g., myopathy)
- Donor–recipient size mismatch

Data from Banner NR, Patel N, Cox AP, et al. Altered sympathoadrenal response to dynamic exercise in cardiac transplant recipients. Cardiovasc Res 23:965–972, 1989; and Banner NR. Exercise physiology and rehabilitation after heart transplantation. J Heart Lung Transplant 11(4):237–240, 1992.

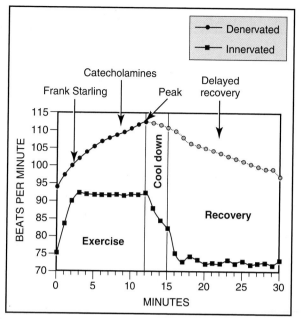

**Figure 12-8** This graph shows the differences in heart rate between an innervated heart and a denervated heart. Note the higher resting heart rate of the denervated heart and its slow acceleration and recovery of heart rate with exercise and rest.

## Postoperative Treatment

### Response to Activity

Following surgery it is important for the physical therapist to note that the patient has undergone a major change in cardiovascular physiology. These changes affect the way that the transplantation team cares for the patient and the way that the physical therapist works with the patient (Box 12-5). Understanding the basics of the change in cardiovascular physiology is important so that proper precautions may be taken during exercise. Typically, there are improvements in hemodynamic function allowing for an increase in aerobic endurance and activity tolerance as compared with prior hemodynamic function. This can be maximized by aerobic training following surgery.

### Changes in Cardiovascular Status

Cardiac denervation initially occurs following heart transplantation and reinnervation may occur in some individuals.[113,120] Denervation is very infrequent following isolated lung transplantation.[113] Bengel and colleagues' research findings demonstrate that sympathetic reinnervation can occur several years (average: 4.4 ± 1.7 years) following heart transplantation.[120] Subjects demonstrating reinnervation had younger donor hearts and had undergone transplantation earlier than the group that remained denervated.[120] The

response of a denervated heart to activity differs from an innervated heart's response. See Table 12-10 and Figure 12-8.

In a patient who has had a HHT, the donor heart responds in the same manner as described for a denervated heart. Because the native heart is still innervated, it continues to respond the way it did before surgery. It is best to monitor both responses by palpation of a peripheral pulse or ECG to see how the donor denervated heart and native innervated heart respond to treatment and activity. Emphasis should be placed on the donor heart when making decisions about treatment and activity tolerance.

The delayed reaction of the denervated heart to the stimulus of activity necessitates an adequate warmup and cooldown period in conjunction with each exercise session.[121] This is to permit accommodation to the change in activity level.[42] Because of the decreased heart rate response to activity, heart rate monitoring will not provide an accurate measure of exercise intensity. As a substitute for measuring heart rate, a scale for rating of perceived exertion (RPE) or ventilatory response can be used as a basis for prescribing and monitoring exercise.

In the heart transplant recipient, blood pressure should be monitored; hypertension is a significant concern because the likelihood of developing ischemia with total loss of perfusion to the heart is increased.[122] Hypertensive episodes can be avoided by employing optimal patient positioning (i.e., placing the patient in upright sitting versus supine position) and by not using long periods of isometric exercise.[122-125] Hypertension has been reported in lung transplant recipients, but does not occur as soon after transplantation and has a

**Table 12-10 Changes in Cardiovascular Status Following Heart Transplantation**

| | Normal Heart | Denervated Heart |
|---|---|---|
| HR at rest | 60-100 bpm | Elevated as high as 90-110 bpm to achieve normal cardiac output |
| Elevation of HR from rest | Up to 120 bpm: Regulated by parasympathetic withdrawal mediated by vagus nerve<br><br>Above 120 bpm: Activation of sympathetic system via sympathetic ganglia | After 5 min of exercise: HR increases due to circulating catecholamines to contribute to increased CO<br><br>Over time: denervation supersensitivity develops (increased sensitivity to endogenous catecholamines such as noradrenaline) |
| HR response to activity | Immediate increase in HR | HR increase has delayed response |
| Initial CV response to exercise | SV and HR provide immediate increase in CO | HR does not change; SV increases to increase CO (Frank-Starling mechanism) |
| Peak HR with exercise | With exercise HR increases 10 bpm per MET | Achieves 70%-80% of normal |
| Stroke volume | 70 mL | Lower than normal |
| LVEF | 50%-65% | Lower than normal |
| Systolic BP | With exercise increases 7-10 mm Hg per MET | At rest: same or higher than before transplantation<br><br>Exercise peak: reduced to 80% of normal |
| Diastolic BP | With exercise: rises gradually (<10 mm Hg), remains the same, or drops slightly (<10 mm Hg) | At rest: elevated because of stiffness of left ventricle myocardium<br><br>With exercise: increases abnormally or may decline (>20 mm Hg) as the result of decreased peripheral resistance, causing patient to become hypotensive |

*BP, blood pressure; bpm, beats per minute; CO, cardiac output; CV, cardiovascular; HR, heart rate; LVEF, left ventricular ejection fraction; MET, metabolic equivalent; SV, stroke volume.*
*From ACSM Exercise Prescription for Patients with Cardiac Disease. 8th ed. p. 218.*

lower incidence than that reported for heart transplant recipients (66% vs. 90%).[126]

## Changes in Pulmonary Status

Although maximum oxygen uptake (VO$_2$max), and subsequently exercise capacity, improves significantly after heart and lung transplantation, it remains well below predicted values.[127-129] Refer to Table 12-11 for additional changes in pulmonary status. The exercise limitation in lung transplant recipients may be attributable to peripheral factors, such as exercise-associated hypertension, muscle atrophy, pretransplantation changes in muscle oxidative capacity, and suboptimal nutritional status, or deconditioning, as greater attention to rehabilitation after transplantation has demonstrated improved exercise capacity with such patients.[54,127-130]

## The Acute Postoperative Inpatient Phase

Postoperatively, patients are evaluated in the intensive care unit (ICU) by the physical therapist once they are medically stable, typically within 12 to 24 hours of surgery. Protective isolation is observed for days to weeks depending on the

transplantation center and the acuteness of the transplant.[131] At the least, a mask should be worn by caregivers and visitors during the first 48 hours after transplantation, and hand washing should be performed before and after each interaction with the patient throughout the hospitalization.[110] Hospital personnel or visitors with a respiratory infection should not be allowed contact with the patient, and this exclusion is also extended for at least 6 weeks to persons who have been given a live vaccine.[110]

Transplant recipients are initially intubated and mechanically ventilated. Multiple medications are infused via intravenous lines and chest drainage tubes, endocardial pacemaker wires, a urinary catheter, and multiple monitoring devices are present. The combination of these elements confronting the physical therapist creates a challenging environment in which to perform the initial postoperative evaluation.

After the initial examination, physical therapy intervention continues until the patient is discharged from the hospital, at which time outpatient rehabilitation provides continuity with inpatient activities. Keeping in mind the ultimate goals of improved function and quality of life, the acute phase of rehabilitation is designed for and focused on increasing functional abilities in self-care and mobility,

## Table 12-11  Changes in Pulmonary Status Following Lung Transplantation

|  | Heart Transplantation | Lung Transplantation |
|---|---|---|
| VO₂max | Limited: between 50% and 70% of gender and age-matched controls. Does not improve with return to pretransplantation activity. | Limited: between 40% and 60% of predicted values. Doesn't improve with return to pretransplantation activity. |
| Ventilatory threshold | 2.5 METS (metabolic equivalents of task) | |
| Anaerobic threshold | Reduced compared to normal. Doesn't improve with return to pretransplantation activity. | Reduced compared to normal. Doesn't improve with return to pretransplantation activity. |
| Respiratory rate | | Mildly elevated at rest. Increases appropriately with exercise. |
| Minute ventilation | | Mildly elevated at rest. No limitations with exercise. |

*From Myers J, Gullestad L, Bellin D, et al. Physical activity patterns and exercise performance in cardiac transplant recipients. J Cardiopulm Rehabil 23(2):100-106, 2003.*

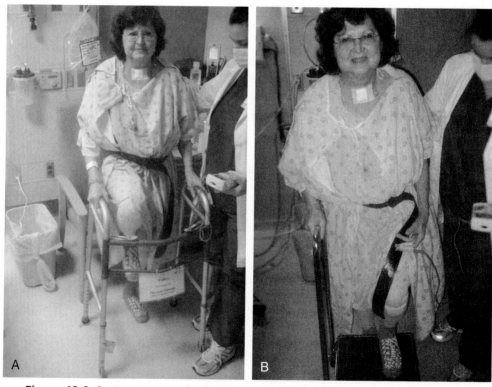

**Figure 12-9** Acute postoperative inpatient rehabilitation with the physical therapist.

including bed mobility, transfers, and ambulation. See Chapter 17 for an extensive discussion of acute care interventions.

## Heart Transplantation

In the ICU, the physical therapist's examination resembles that for any patient following cardiothoracic surgery, but focuses primarily on impaired gas exchange, airway clearance, effects of prolonged static positioning during surgery (screening for nerve injuries), pain, and mobility restrictions. Goals

for this phase include (1) optimizing pulmonary hygiene and chest wall mechanics to facilitate weaning from the ventilator and supplemental oxygen, (2) improving strength and range of motion in the upper extremities and thoracic area, and (3) improving exercise tolerance through ADLs and exercising at a low to moderate intensity (e.g., metabolic equivalent of task, or MET level of 1 to 4).

Exercise should begin in the supine position and progress to sitting and standing (Fig. 12-9). It is essential to monitor vital signs as indicators of cardiovascular status and the patient's response to increases in activity. Although heart

**Table 12-12 Activity Levels for Inpatient Physical Therapy After Cardiac Transplantation**

| Level | Activities |
|---|---|
| Level 1 | Breathing and relaxation techniques |
| | Exercises (15-20 repetitions, supine or seated as appropriate, emphasize proximal muscles) |
| | Shoulder flexion, adduction, horizontal abduction* |
| | Trunk rotation |
| | Hip/knee flexion (seated marching) |
| | Bridging or hip extension |
| | Knee extension |
| | Ankle pumps |
| | Gait: standing pregait activities (mini-squats, weight shifting, single-leg stance) |
| | Up in a chair at least 30–60 minutes |
| Level 2 | Exercises (15-20 repetitions, standing, emphasize proximal muscles) |
| | Shoulder exercises* |
| | Lunges |
| | Marching in place |
| | Mini-squats, weight shifting, single-leg stance |
| | Toe raises |
| | Gait: ambulate in room ad lib, ambulate in the hall, as tolerated |
| | Up in a chair ad lib |
| Level 3 | Exercises (15-20 repetitions, standing, emphasize proximal muscles) |
| | Head and shoulder exercises: progress to wrist weights (1 lb)* |
| | Toe raises (progress to single leg as able) |
| | Dynamic balance exercises |
| | Gait: progress ambulation to 10-15 min continuously |
| | Stair stepping |
| | Add cooldown stretches for lower extremities |
| Level 4 | Exercise per Level 3 |
| | Progress ambulation to <20 min continuously |
| | Stationary cycle: progress to 10-20 min at mild resistance (include 2-3-min slower warmup and cooldown) |

*See discussion of sternal precautions within this lung transplantation section of the chapter.
From Braith RW, Welsch MA, Mills RM, et al. Resistance exercise prevents glucocorticoid-induced myopathy in heart transplant recipients. Med Sci Sports Exerc 30(4):483-489, 1998.

rate should be monitored, it should not be used as the primary indicator of the patient's response.[121] Because the heart is denervated, blood pressure, ventilatory index, and RPE should be monitored along with signs and symptoms of fatigue (such as extreme changes in pallor, flushing, or excessive sweating) for making decisions during treatment. The physical therapist should also remember to allow time for patients to warm up adequately and adapt to changes in position before continuing with an activity.[123,132] A proper warmup is needed to increase stroke volume and catecholamine stimulation so that the patient's cardiac output is increased enough to meet the physical demands of the activity.

After the patient has been moved out of the ICU (typically 24 to 48 hours) or is able to increase the MET level used for activities, conventional postcardiac surgery guidelines may be followed. Table 12-12 presents an example of a protocol that shows a normal progression of activity used with the cardiac transplantation patient population (see also Chapter 18). Once the patient has been transferred out of the ICU, treatment focuses on achieving independence with ADLs, and increasing endurance with activities such as stationary cycling, stair climbing, and ambulation, musculoskeletal activities for posture and strengthening, and development of a home exercise program in preparation for discharge. Strengthening activities should focus on musculoskeletal deficiencies, weight-bearing exercises for osteoporosis prevention, and increasing strength of proximal muscle groups that are more likely to be affected by the complications of steroid therapy.

**Table 12-13 Guidelines to Use When Determining If Exercise Is Appropriate to Begin and When Progression or Termination of Exercise Is Needed**

| Guidelines at Rest | Guidelines to Determine Progression or Termination | Guidelines for use at Rest and With Exercise |
|---|---|---|
| HR >120 bpm | HR that increases >40 bpm above the resting level with exercise | Dyspnea index >15 |
| SBP >190 mm Hg | SBP increases >40 mm Hg with exercise | Excessive fatigue |
| | SBP decreases >10 mm Hg below the resting level with exercise | Vertigo |
| DBP >110 mm Hg | DBP increases >15 mm Hg above the resting level with exercise | Claudication |
| ECG abnormalities that impair perfusion | ECG abnormalities that worsen and impair perfusion | Mental confusion or dizziness |
| RPE >13/20 or 4/10 (somewhat hard) | RPE that increases to ≥15/20 or 5/10 (hard) with exercise | |

bpm, Beats per minute; DBP, diastolic blood pressure; HR, heart rate; RPE, rating of perceived exertion; SBP, systolic blood pressure.
Data from Niset G, Hermans L, Depelchin P. Exercise and heart transplantation: A review. Sports Med 12(6):359–379, 1992; and Kavanagh T, Yacoub MH, Mertens DJ, et al. Cardiorespiratory responses to exercise training after orthotopic cardiac transplantation. Circulation 77:162–171, 1988.

Following transplantation, the patient should be educated on topics related to safety and the correct performance of exercise and activity including: proper techniques for bed mobility and transfers using sternal precautions, self-monitoring of heart rate and RPE, aerobic exercise guidelines including contraindications and progression, and signs and symptoms of the development of complications. For example, patients who required VADs prior to transplantation should pay attention to the site of the drive line for signs of infection. Table 12-13 provides guidelines to be used for an exercising cardiac transplant patient. Each patient will progress at a different rate, and complications that affect an individual patient will alter the progression of rehabilitation.

A variety of complications can affect the heart transplant recipient in the acute inpatient phase of recovery, such as bacterial infections, nonspecific graft failure, and acute rejection.[133] Within the first 30 days, the leading cause of death (27%) is primary graft failure, or failure of the allograft without an obvious anatomic or immunologic source.[134] The next most common causes of death are acute rejection and infection.[30]

Bacterial infections are common in the first 30 days, and treatment focuses on prevention through the use of barriers (personal protective equipment) to reduce the incidence of opportunistic infections and insistence on good hand washing procedures for hospital staff and visitors. In addition, antibiotics are used both prophylactically and therapeutically.

Acute rejection is characterized by either the presence of preformed antibodies or infiltrates of mononuclear cells, which lead to myocyte necrosis.[30] This invasion of mononuclear cells represents the inability of the immunosuppressive regimen to prevent activation of immune effector cells.[99] When the immune system functions properly (instead of being adequately immunosuppressed), the donor organ is not

**Box 12-6**

**Signs and Symptoms of Acute Rejection**

- Low-grade fever
- Increase in resting blood pressure
- Hypotension with activity
- Myalgia
- Fatigue
- Decreased exercise tolerance
- Ventricular dysrhythmias

From Hunt SA, Haddad F. The changing face of heart transplantation. J Am Coll Cardiol 52(8):587-598, 2008.

able to maintain cardiac output because of a loss in cardiac compliance and reduced coronary vasodilation. As a result, the myocardium is at risk for ischemia because of an increased demand for oxygen with exercise and activity.[135] Acute rejection is often suspected as a complication when the patient is exhibiting signs and symptoms of exercise and activity intolerance and is then confirmed via endomyocardial biopsies. Box 12-6 lists the signs and symptoms of acute rejection. In some cases, however, rejection may occur in the absence of signs and symptoms. Reversal of the rejection process is achieved by increasing dosages of immunosuppressive medications.

Progression of self-care activity and exercise may be limited by acute rejection. Rejection may be labeled as mild, moderate or severe based on histologic classifications. If the rejection episode is mild to moderate, exercise and activity are rarely altered. However, if the rejection episode is moderate to severe, as demonstrated clinically by new dysrhythmias, hypotension, or fever, exercise and activity should be reduced to unresisted, symptom-limited modes of activity or discontinued until the patient's status improves, as evidenced by reduction or reversal of symptoms.

## Lung Transplantation

Rehabilitation of the lung transplant patient also begins when the patient is medically stable, usually on the first postoperative day in the ICU. Treatment, including cardiopulmonary conditioning, may be initiated when the patient is hemodynamically stable in the ICU. The problems and goals in this period are similar to those of the heart transplant recipient, with attention given to the changes in the lungs caused by pulmonary denervation. Decreased mucociliary clearance, ventilation–perfusion imbalance, and ineffective cough have been demonstrated in denervated lungs.[41,111,136] The initial postoperative examination should include the effectiveness of pulmonary hygiene, including optimal positioning, mobilization, and enhancement of cough effort.[137]

Clearance of pulmonary secretions often requires a combination of techniques, depending on the requirements for mechanical ventilation, the level of discomfort the patient is experiencing, and the airway clearance techniques with which the patient was familiar prior to surgery. Several airway clearance techniques are effective in the mobilization of secretions, including postural drainage and percussion (avoiding Trendelenburg positioning), shaking, and manual hyperinflation, the active cycle of breathing, and use of the flutter valve.[53] As the transplanted lung is denervated, the patient may not be able to sense the need to cough and should be taught to cough on a regular schedule (directed coughing techniques). Breathing retraining, focusing on lower costal breathing and decreased use of accessory muscles of ventilation, should also be included.

The aforementioned guidelines for exercising heart transplant patients are also applicable to the lung transplant patient population. Although the heart rate provides an accurate measure of exercise intensity, it is helpful to use the ventilatory index, RPE scale, and respiratory rate for additional information to guide ADLs and activity progression from bed mobility, to sitting up in a chair, and finally to ambulation. In the intensive care setting, mobilization of the lung transplant recipient may be accomplished by providing a wheelchair or cardiac walker to accommodate necessary equipment such as the chest drainage tube collection boxes, portable suction unit, oxygen cylinder, and pulse oximeter. The patient then walks behind the wheelchair or walker, using it for support (Fig. 12-10). Supplemental oxygen should be titrated as needed to keep oxygen saturation levels above 90%.

After the patient is moved out of the intensive care setting, usually in 2 to 4 days, rehabilitation continues to focus on ventilation and airway clearance for optimal oxygen transport. Thoracic mobility exercises should be added to the rehabilitative process even though the patient may be averse to moving because of pain.[138] Breathing exercises should be incorporated into all aspects of treatment, including thoracic mobility and the cardiovascular exercise regimens, as well as

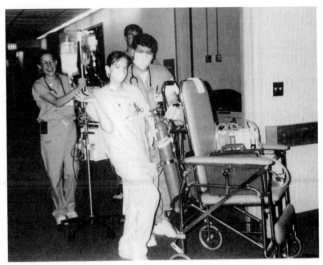

**Figure 12-10** Progression of patient ambulation after leaving ICU using a wheelchair for support.

coughing and airway clearance maneuvers. A stationary bicycle may be used to progress the patient's cardiopulmonary endurance; this precludes the need to mobilize all of the patient's medical equipment for exercise. The incision type used affects whether a 5- to 10-lb. weight restriction for up to 6 weeks should be imposed.

The goals for discharge from the hospital should include independence in self-care and secretion clearance if needed, increased thoracic mobility, general strength and endurance, and the ability to participate in a home exercise program. Many centers have patients perform a 6MWT prior to discharge. Patients who participated in pulmonary rehabilitation in the pretransplantation phase are expected to maintain or better their preoperative distance. Assisted airway clearance and supplemental oxygen are usually no longer necessary at the time of discharge.

In the acute postoperative period, complications include infection, ischemia–reperfusion injury, acute graft failure, and acute rejection. The number of intraoperative complications, as well as problems of airway dehiscence, has been greatly reduced by advances in surgical technique and increasing experience in the field of isolated lung transplantation.[139,140] McCue and colleagues[141] reviewed the effects of the adoption of the LAS on 90-day mortality and complications in lung transplant recipients and found no significant effect on rates of pneumonia, reintubation, tracheostomy, mean days in the ICU, and mean hospital stay.

The most common complication in the lung transplant recipient is infection, usually bacterial; this complication is the primary cause of death after single- or double-lung transplantation within the first 6 months.[110,139,140] The effects of infections include prolonged requirement for mechanical ventilation, pneumonia, sepsis, or increased incidence of acute rejection.[110]

Another complication in the immediate posttransplantation period is ischemia–reperfusion injury.[110] Identified risk factors for this injury are advanced donor age, more than 10 pack-year smoking history, and high pulmonary artery pressure in the recipient.[110] Causes of ischemia–reperfusion injury are thought to be poor graft preservation, longer ischemic time, and donor lung aspiration, and the consequences include impaired oxygenation, hypotension, elevated pulmonary arterial pressures, and pulmonary infiltrates.[110] In some cases, this injury can progress to diffuse alveolar damage, a primary cause for acute graft failure.[110]

The incidence of primary graft dysfunction in lung transplant recipients is 10.2%, but of those who died within the first 30 days, 43% had primary graft dysfunction.[142] Among the recipients who survived at least 1 year after transplantation, primary graft failure resulted in worse survival, even after adjusting for bronchiolitis obliterans syndrome.[142] This points to the role of primary graft dysfunction in almost half of the acute mortality of lung transplant patients, with continued negative consequences after 1 year after transplantation.[142]

Acute rejection, determined from histologic examination of lung tissue obtained by biopsy, is another complication in the lung transplant recipient that can develop in up to 50% of patients within the first month after transplantation, but does not appear to be a major cause of death in the acute period.[110,140] It should be noted, however, that lung transplantation carries the highest rate of acute rejection of all solid-organ transplantations.[110] Treatment of rejection episodes consists of augmentation of the immunosuppressive regimen.

Symptomatically, infection and acute rejection are both manifested by low-grade fever and leukocytosis.[139] With activity, these complications are manifested by a decrease in arterial oxygen saturation and exercise tolerance. This finding demonstrates the importance of close monitoring by the physical therapist during exercise periods.

In an effort to eliminate dehiscence of the incision, sternal precautions are commonly applied to patients postoperatively. Sternal precautions vary greatly by surgeon preference, institution, and type of surgery performed. The instructions vary from a 5- to 10-lb limit of sternal pressure for as long as 8 weeks after surgery and a limitation of shoulder range of motion initially to 90 degrees, to surgeons who allow patients to progress at their own pace to perform whatever activities they are comfortable with. The sternal precautions can be applied to heart transplant recipients after a median sternotomy or double-lung transplantation after a bilateral thoracosternotomy. Some research has identified comorbidities that contribute to dehiscence such as diabetes, infection, or excessive coughing, but there does not seem to be consensus on screening for particular factors.

## The Postoperative Outpatient Phase

The postoperative phase begins when the patient is discharged from the hospital and continues until the patient is discharged from a formal rehabilitation program. This time frame lasts up to 6 weeks and is very similar to phase II cardiac rehabilitation.[132,138] Research promotes the use of formal supervised exercise programs versus the patient utilizing only a home exercise program to improve exercise and functional capacity and quality of life.[143,144] Discharge from the supervised exercise program should occur when the patient's functional capacity has improved to allow them to return to normal activities, such as work or school. In addition the patient should have achieved all goals, be competent with self-monitoring, and be independent with a home exercise program.

If a thorough evaluation was completed as an inpatient and the patient is at the same facility, no further evaluation will be performed, excluding an exercise stress test. Depending on the previous type of exercise evaluation performed or on the level of function of the patient, the stress test may be a 6MWT or a formal symptom-limited treadmill or cycle ergometer test. From the results of the stress test, the patient's exercise prescription will be determined using a combination of heart rate (not useful in heart transplant recipients), RPE, MET level, and other limiting symptoms.[42,138] However, at 1 year post-heart transplantation, nearly one-third of recipients demonstrate a more normal heart rate response during exercise, making an exercise prescription based on heart rate more feasible.[121]

Physical therapy goals during this phase may include strengthening large proximal skeletal musculature, continued aerobic conditioning, attention to and resolution of any musculoskeletal problems, independence with a progressive exercise program, understanding and independence with all areas of education, and self-monitoring.[42,138]

Frequent complications that occur as an outpatient include the following: chronic rejection (30% to 50% at 5 years), cytomegalovirus (CMV) infection, renal dysfunction (25.5% at 1 year, 37.8% at 5 years), hypertension (50% to 60% at 1 year, 85.6% at 5 years) neuromuscular dysfunction (5% in first 6 weeks), steroid myopathy, pleural effusion (85% in 1 year), type II diabetes (24.3% at 1 year, 33.5% at 5 years), osteoporosis (18% to 35% fracture rate reported in patients post-heart transplantation within 1 year),[145] hyperlipidemia (20.5% at 1 year and 52.2% at 5 years), anemia, malignancy (3.7% in 1 year, 12.4% in 5 years and 25% in 10 years), and gastrointestinal complications (43%).[30,42,132,135] Hosenpud[30] reports that late in the posttransplantation period, the three most common causes of death are cardiac allograft vasculopathy, malignancy (accounts for 9.3% of deaths beyond 1 year), and acute rejection.

In heart transplant recipients, chronic rejection, also known as transplant allograft vasculopathy, develops as a form of coronary atherosclerosis.[42,135,146] This form of coronary atherosclerosis is different from atherosclerosis in a native heart, as transplant allograft vasculopathy is defined angiographically to be a diameter stenosis greater than 50%. In addition, it presents with diffuse intimal hyperplasia and concentrically within the lumen.[42,114,132,147] Transplant allograft vasculopathy often is undetectable noninvasively, as denervation of the myocardium prevents signs of ischemia from being present. Manifestations of transplant allograft vasculopathy include myocardial infarction, congestive heart failure, and sudden cardiac death. The understanding of transplant allograft vasculopathy has progressed significantly over the past 10 years; however the exact cause of transplant allograft vasculopathy is unknown. Several immune (donor/recipient mismatches, recurrent cellular rejection, cytomegalovirus infection) and nonimmune (hyperlipidemia, hypertension, diabetes mellitus, older donor age) risk factors have been identified and are thought to be linked to development and progression of transplant allograft vasculopathy.[146] Treatment includes management of risk factors, use of proliferation signal inhibitors (sirolimus) and statin therapy, percutaneous revascularization for focal lesions and repeat transplantation.[42,56,135]

In lung transplant recipients, bronchiolitis obliterans (BO) is thought to be a manifestation of chronic rejection.[139,147-149] A persistent decline in measurements of small airway function is a predictor for the development of BO, but it must be histologically proven with specimens from a transbronchial biopsy.[147,148,150,151] Prevalence of BO has been reported at 26% to 50% for isolated lung and heart–lung transplant recipients, with a reported mortality rate of 40% to 56%.[147-149] As with transplant allograft vasculopathy following a heart transplantation, BO in lung transplant recipients is associated with CMV infection.[148] Bronchiolitis obliterans syndrome and non-CMV infection account for the major causes of death after the first year.

The current management of BO includes augmentation of immunosuppression and reinstitution of cytolytic therapy.[147,149] Valentine[147] reported a median survival time from the diagnosis of BO in bilateral lung and heart–lung transplant recipients of nearly 3 years with minimal limitation in quality of life. However, in general, long-term survival after lung transplantation is limited primarily by BO and its complications.

The medications necessary after transplantation often produce significant adverse effects, as seen in Table 12-9. Cyclosporine is thought to cause hypertension through alterations in the renin–angiotensin system and an increase in sympathetic neural activity.[152] In addition, cyclosporine does impair mitochondrial function, resulting in an inability of working muscle to utilize oxygen, leading to earlier glycolytic metabolism and limited exercise capacity.[153] Tacrolimus, which is also a calcineurin inhibitor and used similarly to cyclosporine for many lung recipients, may have similar effects.[153] New research with rats shows calcineurin inhibitors inhibit bone resorption and thus may increase the risk for osteoporosis.[145]

Morrison and colleagues[152] report that 60% to 90% of transplant patients require medications to combat hypertension. Steroid myopathy and osteoporosis may occur in patients who require a higher dose of steroids for adequate immunosuppression or in patients who have frequent bouts of rejection necessitating repeated bolusing with steroids.[145] Steroid myopathy presents with a weakness of the proximal muscles of the extremities and may be characterized by a patient's inability to climb stairs, rise from low surfaces such as a toilet seat, or increased reliance on the upper extremities when rising from a crouched or seated position. The process may be worsened by inactivity or avoidance of difficult activities. Treatment of steroid myopathy should focus on specific strengthening exercises of proximal muscle groups, especially the lower extremities necessary for weight-bearing activities. The patient should also be encouraged to continue activity and exercise at whatever level is possible.

Several studies suggest that resistance exercise therapy should be initiated prior to transplantation or very early following transplantation to prevent steroid-induced muscle wasting and weakness. Treatment should focus on resistance exercise training at least 2 days/wk beginning with 50% of 1 repetition of maximum performance for 10 to 15 repetitions. Progression of resistance occurs versus increasing repetitions striving to have the individual use the greatest resistance possible to complete 15 repetitions. Special attention should be given to exercising proximal muscle groups and precautions taken to ensure adequate warmup prior to resistance training and maintenance of blood pressure in preload-dependent cardiac denervated heart transplant recipients.[154,155]

## Future Trends in Transplantation Care

Increases in the number and types of thoracic organ transplantations are currently constrained by the availability of donor organs.[30] As a result of the discrepancy between the number of donor organs available and the number of donor organs needed, alternative techniques and donation harvested from a non–heart-beating organ donor are being used. This method of organ procurement has raised ethical concerns and the development of stringent definitions of cardiac death and acceptable practices for the end-of-life care.[156] In addition, advances in donor allocation and selection and support systems must be enhanced and/or developed to "bridge the gap" between being placed on a transplantation waiting list and actually receiving a replacement organ. Other possible solutions to the donor shortage problem include perfecting the surgical technique to reduce complications and increasing the success rate of current transplantations so that recipients do not return to the list as candidates for repeat transplantation.

The trends demonstrate that there continues to be a need for research and monies to support the clinical application of mechanical circulatory support systems that are used to manage the patient until transplantation. The use of circulatory support systems has enabled some very critically ill patients to survive long enough to receive organ transplantation. Now investigators are examining the feasibility of using these support systems as long-term definitive devices. As a result, VADs may not be a bridge but a final treatment. If successful, the number of individuals placed on transplant waiting lists could be reduced substantially.

The use of cadaveric organ transplants is being studied. Because respiration of lung tissue occurs directly across a gas interface, respiration at the cellular level can be accomplished in the absence of vascular perfusion. It has been hypothesized that pulmonary tissue may remain viable for a sufficient period of time post mortem to be useful for transplantation.[157] To test the feasibility of cadaver lung use, Egan and associates[157] transplanted canines with lungs of canine donors that were postmortem up to 4 hours prior to lung harvest. Recipient animals were forced to survive solely on the transplanted lung and were able to do so for up to an 8-hour observation period; the animals with the shorter postmortem donor time survived the longest. It was concluded that if the desirable period of ischemia can be increased so that reliable gas-exchange function is observed for longer periods, then it may be realistic to consider eventually expanding the pulmonary donor pool using cadaver lungs as a resource.

Research is also ongoing to address the immunologic factors present in transplantation using a different species, or xenotransplantation. Although primate-to-human xeno-transplantation has been attempted, study of the use of porcine donor organs has increased, owing to the large number of pigs available and their appropriate size and low cost.[158] Hyperacute rejection is a barrier to clinical xenotransplantation, occurring almost invariably when donor and recipient are of phylogenetically different species.[158] Lin and Platt[158] outlined new strategies for interfering with antibody–antigen interaction and the development of animals more genetically suited for transplantation, averting the occurrence of hyperacute rejection; this still leaves the recipient susceptible to more chronic forms of rejection. The recognition of the barriers to xenotransplantation at the cellular level is leading to the development and testing of therapeutic solutions in the realm of clinical xenotransplantation.[158]

Advances in medication for transplantation continue to be made. In the early 1980s, the introduction of cyclosporine as the mainstay of immunosuppressive regimens was followed. Since then other immunosuppressive agents have been introduced and are being studied to determine the best regimen. Early induction therapy for all thoracic transplantations and delayed initiation of calcineurin inhibitors in those with renal failure are now being studied to determine the best immunosuppressive care that allows for the least chance of complications, for example, the development of lymphoproliferative disorders and allograft vasculopathy. Other changing trends related to immunosuppression include study to develop the ideal immune-monitoring strategy. Currently, biopsy, drug-level monitoring, and specific organ tests are used. Although useful, patients still present with rejection, infection, and organ toxicity. In the future, the ideal strategy may be noninvasive, reliably allow discrimination between presence and absence of rejection, and detect a state of overimmunosuppression.[115]

The care provided for heart and lung transplant patients is also evolving at a rapid pace. In the early 1990s, the initial evaluation process was performed on an inpatient basis and took 5 to 7 days. Today, the majority, if not all, of the evaluation is performed on an outpatient basis and only takes 2 to 3 days. Compared to a few years ago, the patient placed on the waiting list today may be able to stay at home longer and participate in a preoperative program at a local facility on an outpatient basis instead of immediately moving to the city of

the transplantation facility and participating in preoperative rehabilitation at the transplantation facility. Another major change in the course of care is the length of the hospital stay following transplantation. Initially, a patient was hospitalized as long as 1 to 2 months following surgery. This has been significantly shortened to an average length of stay of 1 to 2 weeks, with patients being followed as outpatients after discharge.

For the rehabilitation staff, fewer days in the hospital means that the number of physical therapy visits is decreased and the goals must be accomplished more quickly than in the past. As a result, physical therapy extenders (physical therapist assistants and aides or technicians) often participate in the transplant patient's rehabilitation treatment under the supervision of a physical therapist.

According to Hertz and colleagues, from 1983 through June 2008, data has been collected for more than 117,000 heart, heart–lung, and lung transplantations performed worldwide.[159] Recently, the pace of thoracic transplantation has increased; 5276 transplants from more than 225 centers were added.[159] Table 12-14 summarizes the numbers of thoracic organ transplantations that have been performed in the United States since 1988.

### Table 12-14 Thoracic Organ Transplantations Performed in the United States

| Year | Heart | Lung | Heart/Lung |
|------|-------|------|-----------|
| 1988 | 1558 | 32 | 63 |
| 1989 | 1552 | 90 | 60 |
| 1990 | 1887 | 194 | 46 |
| 1991 | 1866 | 372 | 41 |
| 1992 | 1936 | 498 | 38 |
| 1993 | 2025 | 631 | 46 |
| 1994 | 2077 | 693 | 56 |
| 1995 | 2091 | 805 | 57 |
| 1996 | 2081 | 767 | 29 |
| 1997 | 2016 | 870 | 57 |
| 1998 | 2083 | 807 | 38 |
| 1999 | 1936 | 847 | 40 |
| 2000 | 1926 | 908 | 40 |
| 2001 | 1929 | 1020 | 21 |
| 2002 | 1867 | 998 | 27 |
| 2003 | 1770 | 1038 | 23 |
| 2004 | 1724 | 1118 | 34 |
| 2005 | 1811 | 1352 | 30 |
| 2006 | 1879 | 1350 | 24 |
| 2007 | 1882 | 1416 | 28 |
| 2008 | 1797 | 1433 | 21 |
| 2009 (1/1-7/1/09) | 438 | 405 | 6 |

*From UNOS website, http://www.unos.org. Accessed 7/1/09.*

## Table 12-15 Survival of Thoracic Organ Recipients in the United States

|  | HEART TRANSPLANTATION | | LUNG TRANSPLANTATION | | | |
|---|---|---|---|---|---|---|
|  | Male | Female | Male | Female | Single | Double |
| 1-Year survival | 87.5% | 85.5% | 82.5% | 82.6% | 82.9% | 82.2% |
| 3-Year survival | 78.8% | 76.0% | 61.0% | 62.3% | 59.7% | 63.9% |
| 5-Year survival | 72.3% | 67.4% | 45.4% | 46.1% | 43.3% | 48.6% |

*Data from UNOS website, http://www.unos.org. Accessed 7/1/09.*

Thoracic organ transplantation has evolved from an experimental procedure into an accepted mode of treatment for individuals with end-stage cardiac and pulmonary disease. The 20th century has been witness to the prolongation of survival following transplantation from a period of survival of only 18 days after the first successful heart transplantation to the current 1-year survival rate approaching 88% for heart transplantation and 83% for lung transplantation.[30,115,146] Table 12-15 provides the survival rates for the United States. The current half-life, or median survival, for all heart transplant recipients (transplanted from January 1982 to June 2007) has increased to 10 years, and for those that survive the first year, the median survival is 13 years.[146] The survival rate for patients undergoing repeat heart transplantation is much lower, but improving: median survival between 1982 and 1991 was 1.6 years, but from 1992 to 2007, it increased to 6 years.[160] Worldwide survival of lung transplant recipients has been tracked from January 1994 to June of 2007.[160] Median survival for all lung transplantations is currently 5.4 years, and improves to 7.4 years for those recipients surviving to 1 year.[160] Mortality after heart–lung transplant recipients is most likely to occur during the first year, but survivors after 1 year have a median survival of 9.2 years.[160]

As increasing numbers of patients with end-stage disease are offered thoracic transplantation as a therapeutic option, the importance of keeping abreast of new developments in this evolving field cannot be overstated. Tremendous advances have been made in surgical technique, medications, and the surveillance and management of complications. As members of the healthcare team, physical therapists are challenged to use high-level skills of examination, evaluation, and intervention so as to contribute to a successful outcome for this select group of patients.

## CASE STUDY 12-1

MA is a thin 35-year-old man with end-stage cystic fibrosis, characterized by lower-respiratory-tract infections often requiring hospitalization, pancreatic insufficiency, airway obstruction, chest wall hyperinflation, thoracic kyphosis, digital clubbing, and oxygen desaturation with activity. Patient has thick, tenacious secretions and is prescribed repeated bouts of antibiotics to treat his infections. Patient lives approximately 1.5 hours away from the transplantation center.

MA has been attending a pulmonary rehabilitation program for exercise in his hometown for the past year, although inconsistently. Airway clearance (postural drainage and percussion) is performed by the physical therapist after exercise sessions, but patient admits to not doing additional airway clearance at home other than coughing. MA wears supplemental oxygen only during exercise. Patient's hobby is collecting rare and antique books and he reads the *Bible* regularly.

Crackles and wheezes on auscultation, especially in upper lobes bilaterally. At rest, patient uses accessory muscles, with respiratory rate 24, SpO$_2$ 92%, and heart rate 89 beats per minute.

Activity: During a 6-minute walk test performed according to ATS Guidelines, MA walked 1932 feet without resting, required 5 L of O$_2$ to maintain SpO$_2$ at 90% or higher, with a heart rate of 110 to 142 beats per minute, and an RPE of 17/20.

### Pretransplantation Period

MA was placed on the waiting list for a double-lung transplantation after completing an evaluation by the transplantation team, which included the physical therapist. The patient agreed to attend pulmonary rehabilitation three times a week and to perform airway clearance at least twice daily. The patient also started coming to the transplantation center every other month for an exercise reevaluation and to attend the lung transplantation support group. During this time, the physical therapist instructed MA in the use of a positive expiratory pressure device for airway clearance, reviewed exercises for chest mobility, and increased supplemental oxygen use to continuous, as his resting SpO$_2$ percentage was in the low 80s. The patient continued to be hospitalized at times of severe exacerbation. MA's 6-minute walk distance increased by almost

## CASE STUDY 12-1—cont'd

100 feet in the first year but then showed a decrease as the patient's condition worsened. The last 6-minute walk prior to transplantation was 1762 feet with 8 L of $O_2$ required to maintain $SpO_2$ at 90% or more, with a heart rate of 132 to 162 beats per minute, and an RPE of 18/20.

### Posttransplantation Period

MA received a double-lung transplant 2 years and 7 months after being placed on the list. Physical therapy treatment began within 24 hours and included turning and positioning, airway clearance maneuvers, breathing exercises, chest mobility exercises, and pregait activities. MA was weaned from the ventilator as well as supplemental oxygen, and progressed to walking 800 feet with assistance required only for equipment such as chest tubes and IV pole. At this point, MA resumed exercise on the treadmill and

bicycle ergometer while still an inpatient. His discharge from the hospital was delayed because of gastrointestinal problems, and he was discharged home 2.5 weeks after transplantation.

MA returned to the transplantation center outpatient clinic 1 week posttransplantation and the physical therapist performed a 6-minute walk test at that time: MA covered 1946 feet on room air with an $SpO_2$ of 95 to 98%, a heart rate of 120 to 148 beats per minute, and an RPE of 14/20. He continued to attend outpatient pulmonary rehabilitation in his hometown for another 6 weeks after discharge. At the time of discharge from pulmonary rehabilitation, MA was walking on the treadmill at 4.0 mph at a 10% grade for 30 minutes, and was able to use the bicycle ergometer or stepper for a 30-minute continuous exercise. The 6-minute walk was 2415 feet on room air with $SpO_2$ of 95 to 98%, a heart rate of 116 to 150 beats per minute, and an RPE of 16/20.

## Summary

- The primary indication for heart or lung transplantation is a terminal cardiopulmonary disease.
- The availability of donor organs dictates the pace of transplantation.
- Priority on transplant waiting lists is maintained by UNOS.
- Candidates for transplantation are evaluated by transplantation team members and must meet certain eligibility criteria.
- The physical therapist assesses the patient's cardiac and pulmonary system limitations as well as musculoskeletal condition, exercise capacity, ventilatory function, and mucociliary clearance.
- The preoperative rehabilitation program includes patient and family education, cardiovascular endurance training, musculoskeletal strength and flexibility training, and breathing retraining.
- The goal of preoperative rehabilitation is to improve or prevent deterioration of the candidate's physical condition.
- A candidate who is better conditioned prior to transplantation has a better chance postoperatively of improving physical capacity and function.
- Alternatives to thoracic organ transplantation to "bridge the gap" while waiting for a suitable donor or to replace transplantation include LVRS, BiPAP, VAD, and pharmacologic management.
- Donor organs are selected and matched to the recipient on the basis of blood type and organ size.
- Heart transplantation is usually performed orthotopically using the bicaval or biatrial technique. These techniques

result in heart denervation, and the ECG may demonstrate two separate P waves.
- Lung transplantation is performed using a single-lung or bilateral sequential (double) lung technique resulting in lung denervation.
- Medications are used to prevent rejection and infection. Additional medications are used to combat the side effects of immunosuppressive medication.
- Special adherence to universal precautions should be followed with the transplant patient.
- When exercising a patient following heart transplantation, it is critical to have a sufficient warmup and cooldown period to permit the denervated heart to accommodate the change in activity level and maintain cardiac output. This accommodation occurs in the warmup by an increase in stroke volume provided by the contracting muscles and increases in catecholamine release.
- For all thoracic transplant patients, the following vital signs should be monitored: heart rate, blood pressure, respiratory rate, RPE, and $SpO_2$. The heart rate of a heart transplant recipient will not increase linearly with activity progression secondary to denervation.
- The transplant patient should be assessed postoperatively within 12 to 24 hours.
- Inpatient treatment and goals focus on improving or correcting impaired gas exchange and ineffective airway clearance; patient positioning; pain reduction; and reducing mobility restrictions.
- Outpatient treatment and goals focus on strengthening large skeletal musculature, weight-bearing exercise, continued aerobic conditioning, resolution of any musculoskeletal problems, the home exercise program, education, and independence with self-monitoring.

- Frequent complications of the transplant patient include rejection, infection, steroid myopathy, osteoporosis, and malignancy.
- The physical therapist should be alert for transplant complications, which can often manifest themselves initially in the exercise response. For example, rejection may be noted in a lung transplant patient by a decrease in $SpO_2$ and reduced exercise tolerance during a rehabilitation session.
- Future trends in transplant care include new operative techniques, xenograft transplantations, cadaver organ transplantations, and advances in pharmacologic management.

## References

1. Carrel A, Guthrie CC. The transplantation of veins and organs. Am Med 10:1101–2, 1905.
2. Mann FC, Priestly JT, Markowitz J, Yater WM. Transplantation of the intact mammalian heart. Arch Surg 26:219–24, 1933.
3. Marcus E, Wong SNT, Luisada AA. Homologous heart grafts: Transplantation of the heart in dogs. Surg Forum 2:212–17, 1951.
4. Webb WR, Howard HS. Restoration of function of the refrigerated heart. Surg Forum 8:302, 1957.
5. Goldberg M, Berman EF, Akman LC. Homologous transplantation of the canine heart. J Int Coll Surg 30:575–86, 1958.
6. Cass MH, Brock R. Heart excision and replacement. Guys Hosp Rep 108:285–90, 1959.
7. Lower RR, Shumway NE. Studies of orthotopic homotransplantation of the canine heart. Surg Forum 11:18–19, 1960.
8. Dong E, Hurley EJ, Lower RR, Shumway NE. Isotopic replacement of the totally excised canine heart. J Surg Res 2:90–4, 1962.
9. Lower RR, Dong E, Shumway NE. Long-term survival of cardiac homografts. Surgery 58:110–19, 1965.
10. Hardy JD, Chavez CM, Kurrus FD, et al. Heart transplantation in man. JAMA 188:1132–40, 1964.
11. McGregor CGA. Evolution of heart transplantation. Cardiol Clin 8:3–10, 1990.
12. Hardy JD, Webb WR, Dalton ML, et al. Lung homotransplantation in man. JAMA 186:1065–74, 1963.
13. Caves PK, Schulz WP, Dong EJ, et al. New instrument for transvenous cardiac biopsy. Am J Cardiol 33:264–7, 1974.
14. Morris RE, Dong EJ, Struthers CM, et al. Immunological detection of human cardiac rejection. Surg Forum 25:282–4, 1974.
15. Griepp RB, Stinson EB, Dong EJ, et al. Use of antithymocyte globulin in human heart transplantation. Circulation 45(Suppl 1):147–53, 1972.
16. Kirklin JK. Heart-lung transplantation [editorial]. Am J Med 85:3, 1988.
17. Hutter JA, Despins P, Higenbottam T, et al. Heart-lung transplantation: Better use of resources. Am J Med 85:4–21, 1988.
18. Reitz BA, Burton NA, Jamieson SW, et al. Heart and lung transplantation: autotransplantation and allotransplantation in primates with extended survival. J Thorac Cardiovasc Surg 80:360–72, 1980.
19. Reitz BA, Wallwork JL, Hunt SA, et al. Heart-lung transplantation. N Engl J Med 306:557–64, 1982.
20. The Toronto Lung Transplant Group. Unilateral lung transplantation for pulmonary fibrosis. N Engl J Med 314:1140–5, 1986.
21. Cooper JD, Patterson GA, Grossman R, et al. Double-lung transplant for advanced chronic obstructive lung disease. Am Rev Respir Dis 139:303–7, 1989.
22. Starnes VA, Burr ML, Schenkel FA, et al. Cardiopulmonary physiology in adult and pediatric lobar transplantation recipients: One year follow-up [abstract]. J Heart Lung Transplant 15(1), 1996.
23. Yankaskas JR, Mallory GB. Lung Transplantation in Cystic Fibrosis: Conference Consensus Statement. Chest 113:217–36, 1998
24. UNOS website www.unos.org. How the Transplant System Works: Matching Donors and Recipients. Last updated April 15, 2009.
25. Kaye MP, Elcombe SA, O'Fallon WM. The International Heart Transplantation Registry: The 1984 report. J Heart Transplant 4:290–2, 1985.
26. Solis E, Kaye MP. The Registry of the International Society for Heart Transplantation: Third official report—June 1986. J Heart Transplant 5:2–5, 1986.
27. ISHLT Quarterly Data Report. Available: www.ishlt.org. Accessed 7/8/09.
28. Hosenpud JD, Novick RJ, Breen TJ, Daily OP. The Registry of the International Society for Heart and Lung Transplantation: Eleventh official report—1994. J Heart Lung Transplant 13:561–70, 1994.
29. Kaye MP. The Registry of the International Society for Heart and Lung Transplantation: Tenth official report—1993. J Heart Lung Transplant 12:541–8, 1993.
30. Hosenpud JD, Novick RJ, Bennett LE, et al. The registry of the international society for heart and lung transplantation: Thirteenth official report—1996. J Heart Lung Transplant 15:655–74, 1996.
31. Egan TM, Detterbeck FC, Mill MR, et al. Improved results of lung transplantation for patients with cystic fibrosis. J Thorac Cardiovasc Surg 109:224–35, 1995.
32. Egan TM, Westerman JH, Lambert Jr CJ, et al. Isolated lung transplantation for end-stage lung disease: A viable therapy. Ann Thorac Surg 53:590–6, 1992.
33. Levine SM, Anzueto A, Peters JI, et al. Single lung transplantation in patients with systemic disease. Chest 105:837–41, 1994.
34. Low DE, Trulock EP, Kaiser LR, et al. Lung transplantation of ventilator-dependent patients. Chest 101:8–11, 1992.
35. Fisher JD. New York Heart Association classification. Arch Intern Med 129:836, 1972.
36. Young JB, Naftel DC, Bourge RC, et al. Matching the heart donor and heart transplant recipient: Clues for successful expansion of the donor pool—A multivariable, multiinstitutional report. The Cardiac Transplant Research Database Group. J Heart Lung Transplant 13:353–65, 1994.
37. Hosenpud JD, Novick RJ, Breen TJ, et al. The Registry of the International Society for Heart and Lung Transplantation: Twelfth official report—1995. J Heart Lung Transplant 14:805–15, 1995.
38. Rinaldi M, Sansone F, Boffini M, et al. Single versus double lung transplantation in pulmonary fibrosis: A debated topic Transplant Proc 40(6):2010–12, 2008.

39. Meyer DM, Bennett LE, Novick RJ, Hosenpud JD. Single vs bilateral, sequential lung transplantation for end-stage emphysema: Influence of recipient age on survival and secondary end-points. J Heart Lung Transplant 20(9):935–41, 2001.

40. Orens JB, Estenne M, Arcasoy S, et al. International Guidelines for the Selection of Lung Transplant Candidates: 2006, Update. J Heart Lung Transplant 25(7): 745–55, 2006.

41. Egan TM, Kaiser LR, Cooper JD. Lung transplantation. Curr Probl Surg 26:673–752, 1989.

42. Squires R. Cardiac rehabilitation issues for heart transplantation patients. J Cardiopulm Rehabil 10:159–68, 1990.

43. Craven JL, Bright J, Dear CL. Psychiatric, psychosocial and rehabilitative aspects of lung transplantation. Clin Chest Med 11(2):247–57, 1990.

44. Kuhn WF, Davis MH, Lippman SB. Emotional adjustment to cardiac transplantation. Gen Hosp Psychiatry 10:108–13, 1988.

45. Jalowiec A, Grady K, White-Williams C. Predictors of perceived coping effectiveness in patients awaiting a heart transplant. Nurs Res 56(4):260–8, 2007.

46. Grady KL, Jalowiec A, White-Williams C, et al. Predictors of quality of life in patients with advanced heart failure awaiting transplantation. J Heart Lung Transplant 14:2–10, 1995.

47. Myaskovsky L, Dew MA, McNulty ML, et al. Trajectories of change in quality of life in 12-month survivors of lung or heart transplant. J Heart Lung Transplant 6(8):1939–47, 2006.

48. Lefaiver C. Quality of Life: The Dyad of Caregivers and Lung Transplant Candidates [e-book]. Chicago, Loyola University Chicago, 2006.

49. From: (2008, March 1). Heart Transplant Waiting List Mortality Decreases Following UNOS Policy Change The Free Library. (2008). Retrieved July 13, from

50. UNOS. Organ Procurement and Transplantation Network. Median Waiting Times For Registrations Listed: 1999–2004. Based on OPTN data as of December 4, 2009. www.unos.org. Accessed 12/10/09.

51. Kreider, Maryl, Kotloff, Robert M. Selection of candidates for lung transplantation. Proc Am Thorac Soc 2009, 6: 20–7.

52. McCue JD, Mooney J, Quail J, et al. Ninety-day mortality and major complications are not affected by use of lung allocation score. J Heart Lung Transplant 27(2):192–6, 2008.

53. Downs AM. Clinical application of airway clearance techniques. In DL Frownfelter, E Dean (eds.). Principles and Practice of Cardiopulmonary Physical Therapy. 3rd ed. St. Louis, Mosby-Year Book, 1996.

54. Howard DK, Iademarco EJ, Trulock EP. The role of cardiopulmonary exercise testing in lung and heart-lung transplantation. Clin Chest Med 15(2):405–20, 1994.

55. Ross DJ, Waters PF, Waxman AD, et al. Regional distribution of lung perfusion and ventilation at rest and during steady-state exercise after unilateral lung transplantation. Chest 104:130–5, 1993.

56. Mancini DM, Eisen J, Kussmaul W, et al. Value of peak exercise oxygen consumption for optimal timing of cardiac transplantation in ambulatory patients with heart failure. Circulation 83:778–86, 1991.

57. ATS statement: Guidelines for the six-minute walk test. Am J Respir Crit Care Med 166(1):111–17, 2002.

58. Lotshaw A, Coleman A, Luthye B, et al. The predictive value of the six-minute walk test and lung transplant survival. Cardiopulm Phys Ther J 17(4):143, 2006.

59. Steele B. Timed walking tests of exercise capacity in chronic cardiopulmonary illness. J Cardiopulm Rehabil 16:25–33, 1996.

60. Nici L, Donner C, Wouters E, et al. American Thoracic Society/European Respiratory Society statement on pulmonary rehabilitation. Am J Respir Crit Care Med 173(12):1390–413, 2006.

61. Malen JF, Boychuk JE. Nursing perspectives on lung transplantation. Crit Care Nurs Clin North Am 1:707–21, 1989.

62. Janicki JS, Weber KT, Likoff MJ, et al. Exercise testing to evaluate patients with pulmonary vascular disease. Am Rev Respir Dis 129:593, 1984.

63. Stevenson LW, Steimle AE, Fonarow G, et al. Improvement in exercise capacity of candidates awaiting heart transplant. J Am Coll Cardiol 25(1):163–70, 1995.

64. Miller L. The impact of mechanical circulatory support on post-transplant survival a different view. J Am Coll Cardiol 53(3):272–4, 2009.

65. Sullivan MJ, Higginbotham MB, Cobb FR.Exercise training in patients with severe left ventricular dysfunction: Hemodynamic and metabolic effects. Circulation 81:78, 1990.

66. The Toronto Lung Transplantation Group. Experience with single-lung transplantation for pulmonary fibrosis. JAMA 259:2258–62, 1988.

67. Moser KM, Bokinsky GE, Savage RT, et al. Results of a comprehensive rehabilitation program: Physiologic and functional effects on patients with chronic obstructive pulmonary disease. Arch Intern Med 140:1596–601, 1980.

68. Trulock EP, Cooper JD. Reduction pneumoplasty for COPD [abstract]. Chest 106:52s, 1994.

69. Sciurba FC, Rogers RM, Keenan RJ, et al. Improvement of pulmonary function and elastic recoil after lung reduction surgery for diffuse emphysematous lung. N Engl J Med Apr 25;334(17):1095–9, 1996.

70. Criner G, Belt P, Sternberg A, et al. Effects of lung volume reduction surgery on gas exchange and breathing pattern during maximum exercise. Chest 135(5):1268–79, 2009.

71. Washko G, Fan V, Ramsey S, et al. The effect of lung volume reduction surgery on chronic obstructive pulmonary disease exacerbations. Am J Respir Crit Care Med 177(2):164–9, 2008.

72. Cooper J. Technique to reduce air leaks after resection of emphysematous lung. Ann Thorac Surg 57:1038–9, 1994.

73. MacIntyre NR, Tapson V, Davis RD, et al. Clinical Centers for Lung Volume Reduction Surgery for Emphysema: A Multicenter Assessment and Prospective Patient Registry. Proposal for NHLBI RFP-HR-97-02, August 19, 1996.

74. National Emphysema Treatment Trial Research Group. A randomized trial comparing lung-volume-reduction surgery with medical therapy for severe emphysema. N Engl J Med 348: 2059–73, 2003.

75. Hillerdal G, Löfdahl C, Ström K, et al. Comparison of lung volume reduction surgery and physical training on health status and physiologic outcomes: a randomized controlled clinical trial. Chest 128(5):3489–99, 2005.

76. Yusen R, Littenberg B. Integrating survival and quality of life data in clinical trials of lung disease: the case of lung volume reduction surgery. Chest 127(4):1094–6, 2005.

77. Padman R, Von Nesson S, Goodill J, et al. Noninvasive mechanical ventilation for cystic fibrosis patients with end stage disease. Pediatr Pulm A 232:297, 1992.

78. Hill AT, Edenborough EP, Cayton RM, et al. Nasal intermittent positive pressure ventilation in cystic fibrosis: More than a bridge to transplantation? Pediatr Pulm A 285:259, 1995.

79. Schonhofer B, Wallstein S, Wiese C, Kohler D. Noninvasive mechanical ventilation improves endurance performance in patients with chronic respiratory failure due to thoracic restriction. Chest 119(5):1371–8, 2001.

80. Garrod R, Mikelsons C, Paul EA, Wedzicha JA. Randomized controlled trial of domiciliary noninvasive positive pressure ventilation and physical training in severe chronic obstructive pulmonary disease. Am J Respir Crit Care Med 162:1335–41, 2000.

81. McCarthy PM, Portner PM, Tobler HG, et al. Clinical experience with the Novacor ventricular assist system: Bridge to transplantation and the transition to permanent application. J Thorac Cardiovasc Surg 102:578–87, 1991.

82. Maddocks RM. Case study: Novacor left ventricular assist system in end-stage cardiac dysfunction. Phys Ther Pract 1(4):62–9, 1992.

83. Miller L. The impact of mechanical circulatory support on post-transplant survival a different view. J Am Coll Cardiol 53(3):272–4, 2009.

84. Lietz K, Miller L. Patient selection for left-ventricular assist devices. Curr Opin Cardiol 24(3):246–51, 2009.

85. Lietz K, Long J, Kfoury A, et al. Outcomes of left ventricular assist device implantation as destination therapy in the post-REMATCH era: Implications for patient selection. Circulation 116(5):497–505, 2007.

86. Armstrong PW, Moes BW. Medical advances in the treatment of congestive heart failure. Circulation 6:7941–52, 1988.

87. Stevenson LW. Advanced congestive heart failure. Postgrad Med 5:97–116, 1994.

88. Levine B. Intermittent positive inotrope infusion in the management of end-stage, low-output heart failure. J Cardiovasc Nurs 14(4):76–93, 2000.

89. Assad-Kottner C, Chen D, Jahanyar J, et al. The use of continuous milrinone therapy as bridge to transplant is safe in patients with short waiting times. J Card Fail 14(10):839–43, 2008.

90. Chiu RCJ. Dynamic cardiomyoplasty: An overview. Pacing Clin Electrophysiol 14(1):577–83, 1991.

91. Chachques J, Grandjean P, Carpentier A. Patient management and clinical follow up after cardiomyoplasty. J Card Surg 6(1 Suppl):89–99, 1991 Mar.

92. Nicolini F, Gherli T. Alternatives to transplantation in the surgical therapy for heart failure. Eur J Cardiothorac Surg 35(2):214–28, 2009.

93. Orens JB, Boehler A, de Perrot M, et al. A review of lung transplant donor acceptability criteria. J Heart Lung Transplant 22(11):1183–200, 2003 Nov.

94. Steinbeck R. Organ donation. N Engl J Med 352:209–13, 2007.

95. Novitzky D, Cooper C, Barnard C. The surgical technique of heterotopic heart transplantation. Ann Thorac Surg 36:476, 1983.

96. Novitzky D, Cooper DK, Rose A. The value of recipient heart assistance during severe acute rejection following heterotopic cardiac transplantation. J Cardiovasc Surg (Torino) 25(4):287–95, 1984.

97. Bourge RC, Naftel DC, Costanzo-Nordin MR, et al. Pretransplantation risk factors for death after heart transplantation: A multi-institutional study—The Transplant Cardiologists Research Database Group. J Heart Lung Transplant 12:549–62, 1993.

98. Bolman RM. Cardiac transplantation: The operative technique. Cardiovasc Clin 20:133–45, 1990.

99. Hakim MG, Gill SS. Heart transplantation: Operative techniques and postoperative management. J La State Med Soc 145:233–40, 1993.

100. Yacoub M, Mankad P, Ledingham S. Donor procurement and surgical techniques for cardiac transplantation. Semin Thorac Cardiovasc Surg 2:153–61, 1990.

101. Frazier O, Okereka O, Cooley D. Heterotopic heart transplantation in three patients at the Texas Heart Institute. Tex Heart Inst J 12:221, 1985.

102. Al-Khaldi A, Reitz BA, Zhu H, Rosenthal D. Heterotopic heart transplant combined with postoperative Sildenafil use for the treatment of restrictive cardiomyopathy. Ann Thorac Surg 81(4):1505–7, 2006.

103. Morgan JA, Edwards NM. Orthotopic cardiac transplantation: comparison of outcome using biatrial, bicaval, and total techniques J Card Surg 20(1):102–6, 2005.

104. Jacob S, Sellke F. Is bicaval orthotopic heart transplantation superior to the biatrial technique? Interact Cardiovasc Thorac Surg 9(2):333–42, 2009.

105. Weiss ES, Nwakanma LU, Russell SB, et al. Outcomes in bicaval versus biatrial techniques in heart transplantation: an analysis of the UNOS database J Heart Lung Transplant 27(2):178–83, 2008.

106. Calhoon JH, Grover FL, Gibbons WJ, et al. Single lung transplantation: Alternative indications and technique. J Thorac Cardiovasc Surg 101:816–25, 1991.

107. Griffith BP, Hardesty RL, Armitage JM, et al. A decade of lung transplantation. Ann Surg 218(3):310–20, 1993.

108. Patterson GA. Double lung transplantation. Clin Chest Med 11(2):227–33, 1990.

109. Khaghani A, Tadjkarimi S, Al-Kattan K, et al. Wrapping the anastomosis with omentum or an internal mammary artery pedicle does not improve bronchial healing after single lung transplantation: Results of a randomized clinical trial. J Heart Lung Transplant 13:767–73, 1994.

110. Carlin B, Lega M, Veynovich B. Management of the patient undergoing lung transplantation: an intensive care perspective. Crit Care Nurs Q 32(1):49–57, 2009.

111. Egan TM, Cooper JD. Surgical aspects of single lung transplantation. Clin Chest Med 11(2):195–205, 1990.

112. Craig CR, Stitzel RE. Modern Pharmacology. 4th ed. Boston, Little, Brown, 1994.

113. Schaefers JH, Frost AE, Waxman MB, et al. Cardiac innervation following double lung transplantation [abstract]. Am Rev Respir Dis 137:245, 1988.

114. Niset G, Hermans L, Depelchin P. Exercise and heart transplantation: A review. Sports Med 12(6):359–79, 1992.

115. Hunt SA, Haddad F. The changing face of heart transplantation. J Am Coll Cardiol 52(8):587–98, 2008.

116. Snell G, Westall G. Immunosuppression for lung transplantation: Evidence to date. Drugs 67(11):1531–9, 2007.

117. Erbasan O, Kemaloglu C, Bayezid O. Heart transplantation. Anadolu Kardiyol Derg. 2008 November 02;8:131–47, Available from: CINAHL, Ipswich, MA. Accessed July 17, 2009.

118. Aliabadi A, Zuckermann A, Grimm M. Immunosuppressive therapy in older cardiac transplant patients. Drugs & Aging [serial online]. 2007 November;24(11):913–32. Available from: CINAHL, Ipswich, MA. Accessed July 17, 2009

119. Erbasan O, Kemaloglu C, Ö B. Heart transplantation. Anadolu Kardiyol Derg 8:131–47, 2008.

120. Bengel F, Ueberfuhr P, Schiepel N, et al. Effect of sympathetic reinnervation on cardiac performance after heart transplantation. N Engl J Med 345(10):731–8, 2001.
121. ACSM's Guidelines for Exercise Testing and Prescription, ed 8. Philadelphia, 2010, Lippincott, Williams & Wilkins.
122. Hausdorf G, Banner NR, Mitchell A, et al. Diastolic function after cardiac and heart-lung transplantation. Br Heart J 62:123–32, 1989.
123. Rudas L, Pflugfelder PW, Kostuk WJ. Comparison of hemodynamic responses during dynamic exercise in the upright and supine postures after orthotopic cardiac transplant. J Am Coll Cardiol 16:1367, 1990.
124. Paulus WJ, Bronzwaer JG, Felice H, et al. Deficient acceleration of left ventricular relaxation during exercise after heart transplantation. Circulation 86:1175, 1992.
125. Kao AC, Van Trigt PR, Shaeffer-McCall GS, et al. Central and peripheral limitations to upright exercise in untrained cardiac transplant recipients. Circulation 89:2605–15, 1994.
126. DJ Ross, PF Waters, Z Mohsenifar, et al. Hemodynamic responses to exercise after lung transplantation. Chest 103:46–53, 1993.
127. Orens JB, Becker FS, Lynch JP, et al. Cardiopulmonary exercise testing following allogeneic lung transplantation for different underlying disease states. Chest 107:144–9, 1995.
128. Levy RD, Erns P, Levine SM, et al. Exercise performance after lung transplantation. J Heart Lung Transplant 12:27–33, 1993.
129. Sadeghi AM, Guthaner DF, Wexter L, et al. Healing and revascularization of the tracheal anastomosis following heart-lung transplantation. Surg Forum 33:236–8, 1982.
130. Mathur S, Reid W, Levy R. Exercise limitation in recipients of lung transplants. Phys Ther 84(12):1178–187, 2004.
131. Egan TM, Cooper JD. The lung following transplantation. In Crystal RG, West JB (eds.). The Lung. New York, Scientific Foundations, 1991:2205–15.
132. Fick AW, Holloway V. Rehabilitation of the postsurgical cardiac patient. In Payton OD. Manual of Physical Therapy. New York, Churchill Livingston, 1989.
133. Holden DA, Stelmach KD, Curtis PS, et al. The impact of a rehabilitation program on functional status of patients with chronic lung disease. Respir Care 35(4):332–41, 1990.
134. Marasco SF, Esmore DS, Negri J, et al. Early institution of mechanical support improves outcomes in primary cardiac allograft failure. J Heart Lung Transplant 24(12):2037–42, 2005.
135. Badenhop DT. The therapeutic role of exercise in patients with orthotopic heart transplant. Med Sci Sports Exerc 277:975–85, 1995.
136. Dolovich M, Rossman C, Chambers C, et al. Mucociliary function in patients following single lung or lung heart transplantation [abstract]. Am Rev Respir Dis 135:363, 1987.
137. Downs AM. Physical therapy in lung transplantation. Phys Ther 76:626–42, 1996.
138. Butler BB. Physical therapy in heart and lung transplantation. In Irwin S, Tecklin JS (eds.). Cardiopulmonary Physical Therapy. 3rd ed. St. Louis, Mosby-Year Book, 1995.
139. Chaparro C, Maurer JR, Chamberlain D, et al. Causes of death in lung transplant recipients. J Heart Lung Transplant 13:758–66, 1994.
140. Bando K, Paradis IL, Komatsu K, et al. Analysis of time-dependent risks for infection, rejection, and death after pulmonary transplantation. J Thorac Cardiovasc Surg 109:49–59, 1995.
141. McCue JD, Mooney J, Quail J, et al. Ninety-day mortality and major complications are not affected by use of lung allocation score J Heart Lung Transplant 27(2):192–6, 2008.
142. Christie J, Kotloff R, Ahya V, et al. The effect of primary graft dysfunction on survival after lung transplantation. Am J Respir Crit Care Med 171(11):1312–16, 2005.
143. Karapolat H, Eyigor S, Zoghi M, et al. Comparison of hospital-supervised exercise versus home-based exercise in patients after orthotopic heart transplantation: effects on functional capacity, quality of life and psychological symptoms. Transplant Proc 39(5):1586–8, 2007.
144. Muno PE, Holland AE, Bailey M, et al. Pulmonary rehabilitation following lung transplantation. Transplant Proc 41(1):292–5, 2009.
145. Stein E, Ebeling P, Shane E. Post-transplantation osteoporosis. Endocrinol Metab Clin North Am 36(4):937, 2007.
146. Taylor DO, Stehlik J, Edwards LB, et al. Registry of the International Society for Heart and Lung Transplantation: Twenty-sixth official adult heart transplant report—2009. J Heart Lung Transplant 28:1007–22, 2009.
147. Valentine BG, Robbins RC, Berry GJ, et al. Actuarial survival of heart-lung and bilateral sequential lung transplant recipients with obliterative bronchiolitis. J Heart Lung Transplant 15:317–83, 1996.
148. Keller CA, Cagle PT, Brown RW, et al. Bronchiolitis obliterans in recipients of single, double, and heart-lung transplantation. Chest 107:973–80, 1995.
149. Sundaresan S, Trulock EP, Mohanakumar T, et al. Prevalence and outcome of bronchiolitis obliterans syndrome after lung transplantation. Ann Thorac Surg 60:1341–7, 1995.
150. Yousem SA, Berry GJ, Cagle PT, et al. Revision of the 1990, working formulation for the classification of pulmonary allograft rejection: Lung rejection study group. J Heart Lung Transplant 15:1–15, 1996.
151. Nathan SD, Ross DJ, Belman MJ, et al. Bronchiolitis obliterans in single lung transplant recipients. Chest 107:967–72, 1995.
152. Morrison RJ, Short HD, Noon GP, et al. Hypertension after lung transplantation. J Heart Lung Transplant 12:928–31, 1993.
153. Mathur S, Reid W, Levy R. Exercise limitation in recipients of lung transplants. Phys Ther 84(12):1178–87, 2004.
154. Braith RW, Welsch MA, Mills RM, et al. Resistance exercise prevents glucocorticoid-induced myopathy in heart transplant recipients. Med Sci Sports Exerc 30(4):483–9, 1998.
155. Braith RW, Magyari PM, Pierce GL, et al. Effect of resistance exercise on skeletal muscle myopathy in heart transplant recipients. Am J Cardiol 95(10):1192–8, 2005.
156. Steinbrook R. Organ donation after cardiac death. N Engl J Med. 357: 209, 2007.
157. Egan TM, Lambert Jr CJ, Reddick R, et al. A strategy to increase the donor pool: Use of cadaver lungs for transplantation. Ann Thorac Surg 52:1113–21, 1991.
158. Lin SS, Platt JL. Immunologic barriers to xenotransplantation. J Heart Lung Transplant 15:547–55, 1996.
159. Hertz MI, Aurora P, Christie JD, et al. Scientific Registry of the International Society for Heart and Lung Transplantation: Introduction to the 2009 annual reports. J Heart Lung Transplant 28:989–92, 2009.
160. Christie JD, Edwards LB, Aurora P, et al. The Registry of the International Society for Heart and Lung Transplantation: Twenty-sixth official adult lung and heart-lung transplantation report—2009. J Heart Lung Transplant 28:1031–49, 2009.

## CHAPTER 13

# Monitoring and Life Support Equipment

*Rohini Chandrashekar and Christiane Perme*

## Chapter Outline

**Monitoring Equipment**
Noninvasive Monitoring Equipment
Invasive Monitoring Equipment
**Temperature Monitoring**
**Intracranial Pressure Monitoring**

**Life Support Equipment**
Noninvasive Ventilatory Devices
Invasive Ventilatory Devices
**Summary**
**References**

---

This chapter discusses equipment commonly used for monitoring and supporting the lives of critically ill patients. Although it is true that much of the monitoring and life support equipment is often restricted to the confines of the intensive care unit (ICU), this equipment is making its way ever more frequently into long-term and outpatient rehabilitation, as well as into home care settings. With this in mind, it has become increasingly important for the clinician to recognize the reason for presence of the equipment, interpret the settings and the readouts, and have the ability to assimilate the information available so as to provide a safe and effective intervention.

Monitoring and life support equipment may be noninvasive or invasive. Descriptions of commonly seen apparatus around patients who are in need of vigilant care are provided in this chapter. They may be seen in scenarios of primary cardiovascular or pulmonary compromise, as well as in comorbid situations involving multiorgan dysfunction.

## Monitoring Equipment

The physiologic monitoring equipment commonly found in ICUs primarily addresses the concerns involving the cardiovascular, pulmonary, and neurologic systems. Much of the equipment is electronic and consists of some or all of the following basic components: (1) a device to detect the physiologic event of interest, (2) an amplifier to increase the magnitude of the signal from the sensor, and (3) a recorder or meter to display the resultant signal. The method of detection may be invasive or noninvasive.

### Noninvasive Monitoring Equipment

#### Electrocardiogram

The electrocardiogram (ECG) is a graphic representation of the electrical activity of the heart. An electrocardiographic tracing demonstrates depolarization and repolarization of the atria and ventricles. The position of the positive (recording) electrode in relation to the spread of the electrical impulse is referred to as the lead. In the critical care unit, patients are routinely monitored using only one or two of several possible leads for heart rate and rhythm.

> **Clinical Tip**
> An electrocardiogram monitors two things: heart rate and heart rhythm.

A single-channel ECG monitor with an oscilloscope, strip recorder, and digital heart rate display is typically located above the patient at bedside in the ICU (Fig. 13-1). The ECG can often also be observed at a central monitoring console, where the ECGs of all patients in the ICU can be observed simultaneously.

The ECG monitor allows for continuous surveillance of the patient. Heart rates above or below the preset ranges will trigger an alarm. Electrodes are positioned on the chest to provide optimal information regarding changes in rhythm and heart rate and thereby ensure close patient monitoring. Problems with the monitor usually result from faulty technique, electrical interference, or movement artifact. An erratic signal often results from coughing and movement. The cause of any irregularity must be explained and untoward changes in electrical activity of the myocardium ruled out.[1] When treating patients requiring continuous ECG monitoring it is important to know the reasons for monitoring, the baseline rhythm, and have the ability to recognize rhythm changes and implications. Box 13-1 outlines some of the changes in rhythm that would indicate caution with physical therapy intervention. For details of cardiac dysrhythmia see Chapter 9.

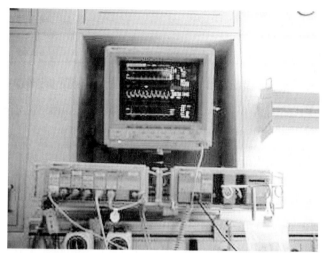

**Figure 13-1** ECG monitor. (From Frownfelter D, Dean E. Cardiovascular and Pulmonary Physical Therapy: Evidence and Practice. 4th ed. St. Louis, Mosby, 2006.)

---

**Box 13-1**

### Some Indications of Declining Cardiac Status

- ST change (elevation or depression)
- Onset, increase, or change of foci of premature ventricular contractions (PVCs)
- Onset of ventricular tachycardia or fibrillation
- Onset of atrial flutter or fibrillation
- Progression of heart block
- Loss of pacer spike

Modified from Paz JC, West MH. Acute Care Handbook for Physical Therapists. 3rd ed. St. Louis, Saunders, 2009.

---

*Clinical Tip*

It is important for physical therapists to be capable of recognizing medical emergencies that require immediate treatment. Knowledge about cardiac dysrhythmia and the correlating clinical picture is essential for providing safe interventions in the critical care setting. Physical therapists must be capable of identifying the cause of an alarm and taking appropriate measures to correct the problem before silencing it during a treatment.

---

## Pulse Oximetry

Noninvasive measurement of arterial oxygen saturation ($SaO_2$) by pulse oximetry provides continuous, safe, and instantaneous measurement of blood oxygenation. Pulse oximeters compute $SaO_2$ by measuring differences in the visible and near infrared absorbances of fully oxygenated and deoxygenated arterial blood. The measurement is expressed as a percentage of oxygen that is bound to hemoglobin. Pulse oximetry is based on two physical principles: (1) the presence of a pulsatile signal generated by arterial blood, which is relatively independent of nonpulsatile arterial, venous, and capillary blood and other tissues; and (2) the fact that oxyhemoglobin ($O_2Hb$) and reduced hemoglobin (Hb) have different absorption spectra.[2] In ICU patients, a probe is attached

---

**Box 13-2**

### Inaccuracies in Pulse Oximetry Readings

Inaccuracies in the pulse oximetry readings may be seen in:
- Low perfusion states, such as low cardiac output, vasoconstriction, and hypothermia, may impair peripheral perfusion and may make it difficult for a sensor to distinguish a true signal from background noise
- Anemia
- Abnormal HbHb
- Jaundice
- Arrhythmias, including atrial fibrillation
- Intravascular dyes such as methylene blue
- Dark nail polish
- Fluorescent light
- Motion artifact
- Dark skin pigmentation

Data from Jubran A. Pulse oximetry. Crit Care 3(2):R11-R17, 1999; and Frownfelter D. Arterial blood gases. In Frownfelter D. Cardiovascular and Pulmonary Physical Therapy: Evidence and Practice. 4th ed. St. Louis, Mosby, 2005.

---

to the patient's finger, forehead, or earlobe, and the reading is displayed continuously on the monitor. For physical therapists the pulse oximeter provides valuable information regarding the adequacy of available oxygen before, during, and after exercise. The recommendation is to keep the $O_2$ saturation above 90% during exercise unless otherwise ordered by the physician. Supplemental oxygen can be titrated to keep the $O_2$ saturation within the appropriate range according to hospital guidelines (Box 13-2).[3]

## Blood Pressure Monitoring

Arterial blood pressure is the result of the rate of flow of blood (cardiac output) through and against the resistance of the circulatory system (systemic vascular resistance [SVR]). Manual assessment of the blood pressure can be performed with a sphygmomanometer and a stethoscope when the Korotkoff sounds are auscultated over the brachial artery. When the pressure within the sphygmomanometer cuff is increased above arterial blood pressure, the arteries under the cuff are occluded and no pulse can be palpated distal to the cuff. As the cuff pressure is gradually released, the systolic peaks of pressure finally exceed cuff pressure, and blood spurts into the arteries below the cuff, producing palpable pulses at the wrist. The sudden acceleration of blood below the cuff produces vibrations that are audible through a stethoscope. As cuff pressure is diminished, the sounds increase in intensity and then rather suddenly become muffled at the level of diastolic pressure where the arteries remain open throughout the entire pulse wave. At still lower pressures, the sounds disappear completely when laminar flow is reestablished. The sounds auscultated over the artery are called *Korotkoff sounds* (Table 13-1).[4]

In critical care units arterial blood pressure is monitored noninvasively by the oscillometric technique and displayed

## Table 13-1 Korotkoff Sounds

| Phase | Sound | Indicates |
|---|---|---|
| 1 | First sound heard, faint tapping sound with increasing intensity | Systolic pressure (blood starts to flow through compressed artery). |
| 2 | Start swishing sound | Because of the compressed artery, blood flow continues to be heard while the sounds change as a result of the changing compression on the artery. |
| 3 | Sounds increase in intensity with a distinct tapping | Blood flow is increasing as artery compression is decreasing. |
| 4 | Sounds become muffled | Diastolic pressure in children younger than 13 years of age and in adults who are exercising, pregnant, or have hyperthyroidism (see phase 5). |
| 5 | Disappearance | Diastolic pressure in adults; occurs 5-10 mm Hg below phase 4 in normal adults. In states of increased rate of blood flow, it may be >10 mm Hg below phase 4. In these cases, the phase 4 sound should be used as diastolic pressure in adults. |

*From Paz JC, West MH. Acute Care Handbook for Physical Therapists. 3rd ed. St. Louis, Saunders, 2009.*

---

**Clinical Tip**
Blood pressure monitoring provides digital measurements of systolic and diastolic blood pressures, and mean arterial pressures.

---

on the bedside monitor. An inflatable cuff is attached to a pressure monitoring device. Oscillometric blood pressure is determined based on arterial wall pulsations. The reentry of blood into the arteries occluded by the cuff makes the wall of the arteries expand or "pulse." These pulsations travel through the soft tissue to the surface of the limb where they are detected by the cuff and analyzed by the microprocessor. This analysis provides systolic, diastolic, and mean arterial pressure readings along with heart rate. Typically, it is strapped on proximal to the antecubital space in the upper extremity to assess the pressures in the brachial artery. If this area is not accessible, it may be placed over the distal lower extremity to assess the pressures in the tibial artery. The ICU monitor may be set to assess the pressures at preset times for updates or can be assessed as needed with the push of the appropriate button. The systolic blood pressure, or the maximum systolic left ventricular pressure, reflects the compliance of the large arteries and the total peripheral resistance. The diastolic blood pressure is the lowest point of declining pressure resulting from the runoff of blood from the proximal aorta to the peripheral vessels, and it reflects the velocity of the runoff and the elasticity of the arterial system. Because the duration of the diastolic period of the cardiac cycle is directly related to the heart rate, the longer the period of diastole, the more the diastolic pressure falls. In the normal adult, resting systolic blood pressure is acceptable at approximately 120 mm Hg and the resting diastolic blood pressure is acceptable at a range of 60 to 80 mm Hg (Table 13-2).

## Table 13-2 Normal Adult Ranges for Cardiopulmonary Values at Rest

| Value | Normal Range |
|---|---|
| Heart rate | 50-100 beats per minute |
| Systolic blood pressure | 85-140 mm Hg |
| Diastolic blood pressure | 40-90 mm Hg |
| Respiratory rate | 12-20 breaths per minute |
| Oxygen saturation | >95% on $FIO_2$ (fraction of inspired oxygen) |

### Respiratory Rate

The respiratory rate of a patient in the ICU is typically monitored as a waveform produced as a result of the ECG electrodes and is displayed on the bedside monitor. If a patient is mechanically ventilated the number of breaths are also displayed on the ventilator screen.

Respiratory rates vary by age and condition of the patient (Table 13-3). Normal adult respiratory rates during quiet breathing are between 12 and 18 breaths per minute. A rate above this range is termed *tachypnea* and a rate below this range is termed *bradypnea* (Box 13-3).[5] Along with the rate, the pattern and depth of breathing should be assessed (Box 13-4).

### Level of Consciousness

A bispectral index sensor (BIS) is used in patients to assess level of consciousness and thereby monitor sedation levels in the ICU. There is minimal evidence suggesting that it also might be useful in assessing pain.[6] The BIS measures the muscular and cortical activity using a single, small, flexible

### Table 13-3 Pulse and Respiratory Rates by Age

| Age | Pulse (beats per minute) | Respiratory Rate (breaths per minute) |
|---|---|---|
| Newborn | 90-170 | 35 to 45-70 with excitement |
| 1 Year | 80-160 | 25-35 |
| Preschool | 80-120 | 20-25 |
| 10 Years | 70-110 | 15-20 |
| Adult | 60-100 | 12-20 |
| Athlete | ≅50 | 12-20 |

*From Wilkins RL. Clinical Assessment in Respiratory Care. 6th ed. St. Louis, Mosby, 2010.*

---

### Box 13-3

#### Causes of Tachypnea and Bradypnea

| Tachypnea | Bradypnea |
|---|---|
| Exercise | Head injuries |
| Atelectasis | Sedation |
| Fever | Drug overdose |
| Hypoxemia | |
| Anxiety | |
| Pain | |

---

### Box 13-4

#### Indications of Respiratory Distress

- Increased respiratory rate
- Nasal flaring
- Intercostal and sternal retractions
- Visible expression of distress
- Increased use of neck accessories
- Paradoxic breathing

---

sensor that is applied to the forehead and temporal region.[7] The sensor provides rapid feedback for quick titration of medication and an objective score. A value is produced every 15 seconds that ranges from 0 (no cortical electrical activity and full suppression) to 100 (awake, aware, no suppression).[8] In the ICU, protocols have been developed for titrating sedatives to maintain a BIS value within set parameters (usually 60 to 70) that correspond with the manufacturer's guidelines for light-to-moderate sedation.[9]

## Invasive Monitoring Equipment

### Arterial Line

Hemodynamic monitoring generally involves observing or calculating and then assessing some specific cardiovascular parameter. In invasive monitoring, a pressure transducer, pressure transmission (connective) tubing, and a pressure monitor or recorder are used.

An arterial line is most commonly inserted through the radial artery but can also be inserted through the femoral artery. Less commonly, it can be inserted into the brachial, axillary, ulnar, or dorsalis pedis arteries. It allows for continuous measurement of arterial blood pressure and allows blood draw access for arterial blood gas measurements.

In the severely ill patient with hemodynamic compromise, a low stroke volume and excessive peripheral vasoconstric-

tion may make Korotkoff sounds impossible to hear and arterial pulsations difficult to detect. Patients on more than a small amount of any vasoactive drip usually have an arterial line for continuous blood pressure management. Consequently, in addition to a blood pressure cuff, an intraarterial catheter frequently connects a monitoring device to a pressure transducer. A typical pressure transducer is a disposable, solid-state piezoelectric device (Fig. 13-2) that can be mounted easily on the patient's bed or an IV pole. The piezoelectric pressure transducer is similar to a strain gauge in principle; the piezoelectric crystal creates a change in voltage when it is strained. When pressure is applied to a piezoelectric crystal its shape is distorted, causing a reorientation of electrical charges within the crystal. The distortion causes a displacement of the positive and negative charges within the crystal, producing surface changes in opposite polarity on opposite sides of the crystal. The resultant voltage is amplified and converted into a graphic or numeric image on a monitor. The transducer, the connective tubing, and an indwelling catheter are typically filled with a saline solution, producing a continuous fluid column. When calibrated in relation to the standard anatomic reference level at which the catheter tip is assumed to rest (the phlebostatic point), this fluid-filled monitoring system should be accurate to within 1 mm Hg.[10,11]

The monitoring via the arterial line provides and displays a continuous measurement of systolic, diastolic, and mean arterial pressures. Figure 13-3 shows a normal arterial pressure tracing and its relation to the cardiac cycle. The mean arterial pressure (MAP) is the average pressure tending to push blood through the circulatory system, and it reflects the tissue perfusion pressure. The MAP is the same in all parts of the cardiovascular system when the patient is supine.[11]

The MAP is closer to the diastolic than the systolic pressure because the duration of diastole is greater than that of systole. The MAP is not, therefore, a true arithmetic mean of systolic and diastolic pressures, but rather slightly less than

---

*Clinical Tip*
The MAP reading does not vary significantly with motion artifact or movement on the catheter site.[11] It is useful clinically because it yields one number that relates to cardiac output and the SVR. A MAP of less than 60 mm Hg may indicate inadequate tissue perfusion.

Pressurized, heparinized
saline solution

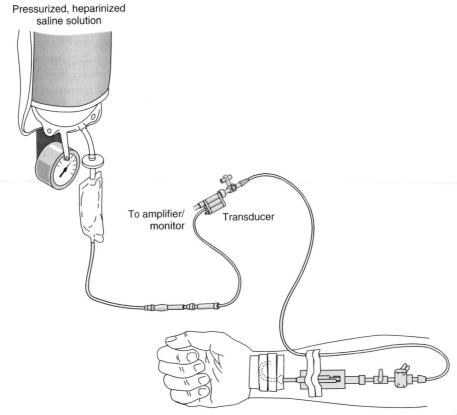

To amplifier/
monitor

Transducer

**Figure 13-2** Typical transducer for continuous monitoring of arterial blood pressure. For perspective on the size, consider that the actual transducer is smaller than the diameter of a U.S. quarter.

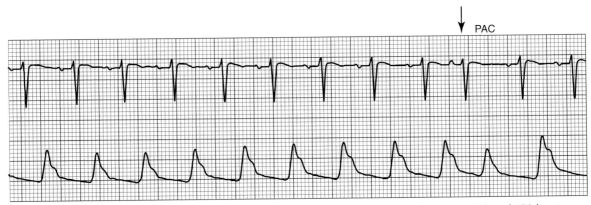

PAC

**Figure 13-3** Electrocardiogram and arterial pressure tracings (sinus tachycardia at a rate between 110 and 120 beats per minute). The tenth ECG complex is a premature atrial complex (PAC); note the resultant decrease in the area of the tenth arterial pressure wave.

the average of the two pressures. The acceptable MAP varies between 70 and 110 mm Hg.

Table 13-4 shows the commonly adhered to parameters for hemodynamic pressures.

Often, critically ill patients need frequent measurement of arterial blood gases to assist in the assessment of ventilatory efficacy. An indwelling arterial catheter reduces the need for repeated invasive needle sticks required to draw blood (Box 13-5). So, in addition to measuring arterial pressures, the arterial line provides a convenient route of access for arterial blood sampling.

## Central Line

The central line is a central venous catheter inserted most commonly through the subclavian or jugular vein; however, the femoral access is also used at times. The catheter is placed by a physician and is advanced to rest in the proximal superior vena cava allowing central venous pressures to be measured directly. It also allows IV access for medication administration and other procedures.

The central venous catheter allows for the continuous monitoring of central venous pressure (CVP) or right atrial pressure (RAP) to assess cardiac function and intravascular

**Table 13-4 Common Hemodynamic Parameters**

| Parameter | Common Acronym | Normal Values |
|---|---|---|
| Arterial blood pressures | BP | |
| Systolic | SBP | 90-140 mm Hg |
| Diastolic | DBP | 60-80 mm Hg |
| Right atrial pressure | RAP | 0-8 mm Hg (mean) |
| Right ventricular pressures | RV | |
| Systolic | RVs | 15-30 mm Hg *or* |
| End-diastolic | RVEDP | 0-8 mm Hg |
| Pulmonary artery pressures | PAP | |
| Systolic | Pas | 15-30 mm Hg |
| Diastolic | Pad | 5-15 mm Hg |
| Pulmonary artery wedge pressure | PWP, PCWP | 4-15 mm Hg (mean) |
| Left atrial pressure | LAP | 4-12 mm Hg (mean) |
| Left ventricular pressures | | |
| Systolic | LVs | 100-140 mm Hg |
| End-diastolic | LVEDP | 4-12 mm Hg |
| **Calculated Values** | | |
| Mean arterial pressure | MAP | 70-110 mm Hg |
| Mean PAP | | 8-20 mm Hg |
| Systemic vascular resistance | SVR | 800-1200 dynes·sec$^{-1}$ cm$^{-1}$ |
| Pulmonary vascular resistance | PVR | <100 dynes·sec$^{-1}$ cm$^{-1}$ or 1/6 SVR |

---

**Box 13-5**

**Precautions for an Arterial Line**

- The transducer for an arterial line should be positioned at the level of the right atrium to assure accurate pressure values[2]
  - If transducer is too low: BP will read higher
  - If transducer is too high: BP will read lower
- If an arterial line is dislodged accidentally, apply pressure immediately and notify nursing staff

---

*Clinical Tip*
Elevations in CVP may result from fluid overload, right ventricular failure, tricuspid insufficiency, or chronic left ventricular failure. Low CVP may be indicative of hypovolemia and dehydration.

---

fluid status. Additionally, the catheter may be used as a route for medication or fluid administration, blood sampling, or emergency placement of a temporary pacemaker.

For patients requiring a prolonged placement of a central line, a peripherally inserted central catheter (PICC or PIC line) or a tunneled catheter is commonly used for intravenous access. These catheters are considered a safe alternative to the temporary catheters, which have higher rates of infection and complications.

---

*Clinical Tip*
A PIC line is inserted in a peripheral vein such as the cephalic vein, basilic vein or brachial vein, and then advanced through increasingly larger veins, toward the heart until the tip rests in the distal superior vena cava.

---

Tunneled catheters are long-term catheters that are tunneled under the skin prior to entering a central vein. They are generally placed in the operating room or in the interventional radiology department. The tunneled catheters can last for months if working properly. These catheters are typically associated with a lesser rate of infections since the skin provides a natural barrier to infection. In addition, the cuff around the catheter under the skin leads to fibrin and collagen deposition, which, in turn, stabilizes the catheter in place and provides a second internal barrier against infection. Box 13-6 provides information about associated risks.

**Pulmonary Artery Catheter (Swan-Ganz Catheter)**

The pulmonary artery catheter can only be placed by a physician. It is introduced via a central venous access point (e.g.,

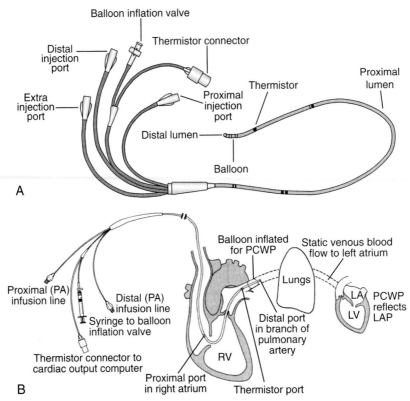

**Figure 13-4** Quadruple-channel pulmonary arterial catheter. **A,** Typical multilumen pulmonary artery catheter. **B,** The pulmonary artery catheter passes through the right atrium and ventricle to rest in the pulmonary artery. (*A* from Wilkins RL. Egan's Fundamentals of Respiratory Care. 9th ed. St. Louis, Mosby, 2009. *B* from Kersten LD. Comprehensive Respiratory Nursing: A Decision-Making Approach. Philadelphia, Saunders, 1989.)

---

**Box 13-6**

**Risks Associated with Central Venous Access**

| Risks Associated During Insertion of Central Venous Access | Delayed Risks Associated with Central Venous Access |
| --- | --- |
| Pneumothorax (a chest radiograph should be done to rule this out prior to mobilization) | Infection |
| | Catheter fracture |
| | Catheter dislodgement |
| Bleeding | Catheter occlusion |
| Arrhythmias | Air in the catheter |
| Arterial entry | |

---

internal jugular or subclavian vein), passing from the vena cava into the right atrium, through the right atrioventricular (tricuspid) valve into the right ventricle, through the pulmonary valve, and into the pulmonary artery (Fig. 13-4).

The pulmonary artery catheter permits:
- Direct measurement of RAP,
- Direct measurement of pulmonary arterial pressure (PAP) and pulmonary capillary wedge pressure (PCWP),
- Indirect measurement of left atrial pressure (LAP),
- Determination of mixed venous oxygen saturation ($SvO_2$) and cardiac output (CO),
- Calculation of systemic and pulmonary vascular resistance (PVR),
- Pacing of the atrium and ventricles.

There are two ports in the catheter toward its tip that are placed distal and proximal to a small balloon that can be inflated with air. These ports are connected to pressure transducers. The distal port connection measures the PAP and the proximal port measures the RAP.

When treating patients with a pulmonary arterial catheter, recognition of the "normalcy" of the potential waveforms is key to deciding whether or not it is advisable to perform physical therapy. A RAP waveform should be recognizable when RAPs are being monitored; likewise, it should be possible to recognize a pulmonary arterial waveform when PAPs are being monitored. Figure 13-5 shows normal wave configurations for RAP, right ventricular, PAP, and PCWP. Box 13-7 lists possible complications of the pulmonary artery catheter.

### Pulmonary Capillary Wedge Pressure

The LAP is the outflow or venous pressure for the pulmonary circulation and the left ventricular end-diastolic pressure (LVEDP) reflects the PVR and is the primary indicator of left ventricular performance. Measurement of the LAP reflects the value of the LVEDP. Although left-heart pressures could

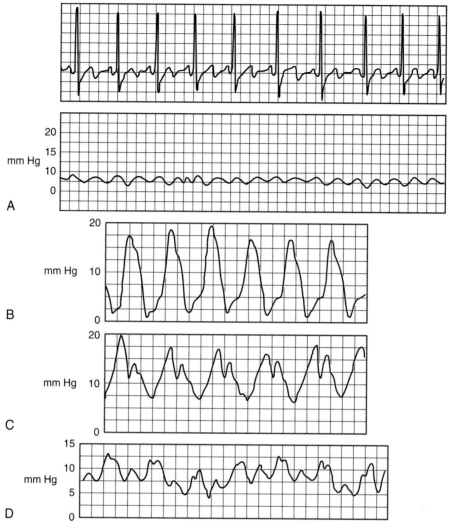

**Figure 13-5** Normal pressure tracings of the right side of the heart. **A,** Electrocardiogram and concurrent right atrial pressure tracings. **B,** The right ventricular pressure waveform normally is observed only when the catheter is initially being inserted. **C,** Pulmonary arterial pressure waveform. **D,** Capillary wedge pressure waveform.

**Box 13-7**

**Possible Complications of the PA Catheter**

Complications of insertion and dislodgement of the PA catheter include[13]:
- Malignant arrhythmias
- Pulmonary artery rupture
- Pulmonary valve tear
- Infection

For these reasons it is recommended that mobilization, if essential, only be undertaken by an experienced clinician after it has been determined that the patient is hemodynamically stable.

Data from Parillo JE, Dellinger JE. Critical Care Medicine: Principles of Diagnosis and Management in the Adult. 3rd ed. Philadelphia, Mosby, 2008.

be directly measured by angiography during coronary catheterization it is difficult to measure continuously for clinical monitoring.

Because there are no valves in the pulmonary venous system, the pressures in the pulmonary veins, the pulmonary capillaries, and the pulmonary artery are also equal at the end of diastole. Thus, the pulmonary artery end-diastolic pressure is essentially equal to the LVEDP (normally less than 12 mm Hg), in the absence of any pathology in the vascular system, between the tip of the catheter and the left ventricle. Monitoring the PCWP intermittently will provide the information needed regarding the left atrial and ventricular end-diastolic pressures (Box 13-8).

To measure the PCWP, the balloon at the tip of the pulmonary catheter is inflated with air, thus "wedging" the catheter into a branch of the pulmonary artery and effectively occluding it. When this occurs, the pressure in the distal port rapidly falls, and reaches a stable value after several seconds that is very similar to LAP (normally approximately 8 to

---

**Box 13-8**

**Reasons to Measure PCWP**

- Assess severity of left ventricular failure
- Assess mitral and aortic valve dysfunction
- Assess and treat pulmonary edema (PCWP >20 mm Hg)
- Assess pulmonary hypertension
- Assess and treat hypovolemic states

---

10 mm Hg) because the occluded vessel, along with its distal branches that eventually form the pulmonary veins, acts as a long catheter that measures the blood pressures within the pulmonary veins and left atrium. The balloon is then deflated.[12]

## Cardiac Output

The same catheter can be used to measure CO by the thermodilution technique. The amount of blood pumped by the heart per unit of time is termed the *cardiac output* (Q), and unless an intracardiac shunt is present, the output of both the right and left ventricles is essentially the same. The normal resting is 4 to 8 L/min. The amount of blood ejected with each contraction of the heart is called the stroke volume (SV) and the normal SV ranges from 55 to 130 mL.[13,14] CO is generally determined clinically by the thermodilution method. A cold bolus of saline is injected into the right atrium via the proximal lumen of the pulmonary artery line. The resultant temperature change is sensed by a thermistor near the tip of the catheter located in the pulmonary artery. A temperature–time curve is constructed and calculated.[15] The mean SV is calculated by dividing the CO by the ventricular rate over a specific period of time. CO measurements do not take into account an individual's specific needs with respect to actual body size. For this reason, the CO per square meter of body surface area, the cardiac index is often reported. The normal cardiac index for adults is approximately 3.0 L/min/m².

Conditions such as an arteriovenous fistula, anoxia, and Paget disease may ultimately decrease the PVR and increase CO by increasing venous return to the heart. Conversely, conditions that result in decreased blood volume will reduce the venous return to the heart, decreasing CO.

---

*Clinical Tip*

Cardiogenic shock is a condition in which the blood supply to the body tissues is insufficient because of inadequate CO. A cardiac index of less than 2.2 L/min/m² is considered diagnostic of cardiogenic shock.[15]

---

## Mixed Venous Oxygen Saturation

The supply of oxygen to the tissues depends on CO, Hb level, and $SaO_2$. The partial pressure of arterial oxygen in the blood ($PaO_2$) is normally just about 100 mm Hg at the arteriolar end of the capillary bed and approximately 5 mm Hg at the cellular level. Because of this pressure gradient, dissolved

oxygen diffuses out of the capillaries and into the cells. There is depletion of oxygen at the venous end of the capillary bed and the partial pressure of venous oxygen ($PvO_2$) is approximately 40 mm Hg. The amount of oxygen returning to the heart is called the venous oxygen reserve. $SvO_2$ is the direct measurement of the venous oxygen reserve and is expressed as a percentage of oxygen left combined with Hb after the tissues have extracted the oxygen needed. The value is calculated from a blood sample drawn from the right ventricle through the pulmonary artery port of the Swan-Ganz catheter. Under normal conditions, the $SvO_2$ is in the range of 60% to 80%.[16,17]

$SvO_2$ demonstrates the balance between oxygen delivery and oxygen demand. Because changes in oxygen saturation are prompted by changes in the $PaO_2$, and because venous saturation is decreased only when oxygen supply fails to meet the demand, the $SvO_2$ can be a sensitive indicator of oxygen supply or demand status.

---

*Clinical Tip*

A high $SvO_2$ indicates inadequate tissue perfusion despite a high CO, signaling a poor demand status. A low $SvO_2$ indicates high tissue oxygen consumption and a low CO, signaling a poor supply status. The information can be used to assess the patient's ability to perform or sustain a desired level of activity.

---

## Temperature Monitoring

A rectal thermometer may be used invasively in patients whose body temperature cannot be measured orally, such as comatose, intubated, or confused patients.

---

*Clinical Tip*

To trend temperature over time, the same site and same device must be used for each temperature measurement.

---

## Intracranial Pressure Monitoring

Alterations in intracranial pressure (ICP) result from neurologic insults resulting from a head injury, hypoxic brain damage, aneurysm, hemorrhage, cerebral tumor, or brain surgery.[11] There are a number of ways in which the ICP may be monitored (Table 13-5) to provide direct measurement of the cranial pressure. A hollow screw is positioned through the skull into the subarachnoid space. The screw is attached to a Luer-Lok, which is connected to a transducer and oscilloscope for continuous monitoring. The normal range of the ICP is 0 to 10 mm Hg for adults and 0 to 5 mm Hg for patients younger than 6 years of age. In a normal brain, the ICP may transiently reach 50 mm Hg, but typically returns to baseline levels quickly. In patients with brain injury, a high ICP correlates with a low cerebral perfusion pressure. Extra care must be exercised during routine management and therapy (Box 13-9). When the ICP readings are elevated, observing changes in ICP during nursing procedures or by

## Box 13-9

### Activities That May Increase ICP

- Isometric exercise
- Valsalva maneuver
- Extreme hip flexion
- Lateral neck flexion
- Coughing
- Prone position
- Head position below 15 degrees horizontal (ideal position for venous drainage: HOB >30 degrees)
- Occlusion of the tube
- Pain

Data from Batavia M. Contraindications in Physical Rehabilitation: Doing No Harm. Philadelphia, 2006, Saunders.

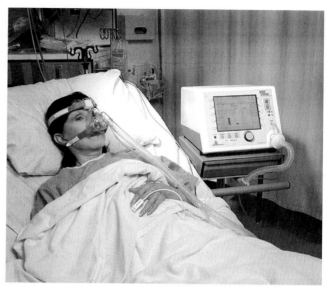

**Figure 13-6** BiPAP Vision Face Mask in use. (Courtesy Respironics Inc., Murrysville, PA.)

titrating small degrees of movement or position change and observing the rate at which the ICP returns to baseline following the removal of the challenge can help establish whether a patient will tolerate a treatment that requires movement. Rapid return to baseline minimizes the risk of reduced cerebral perfusion pressure caused by the increased ICP. A slow return to baseline or sustained elevation of ICP is consistent with poor cerebral compliance and indicates that treatment should be modified or possibly not performed at all.[1]

---

### Clinical Tip

Patients with an elevated ICP may be mechanically hyperventilated with a manual resuscitator bag to keep arterial partial pressure of carbon dioxide at low levels, because hypercapnia dilates cerebral vessels and hypocapnia constricts them. Physical therapist involvement in the presence of a persistently elevated ICP may only include an assessment. Further interventions should be withheld until cerebral compliance improves.

---

## Life Support Equipment

### Noninvasive Ventilatory Devices

#### Noninvasive Positive-Pressure Ventilation

Noninvasive positive-pressure ventilation is a form of mechanical ventilation that uses a mask instead of an artificial airway. The purpose is to assist the patient with the ventilatory needs when short-term ventilatory support is needed.

Continuous positive airway pressure (CPAP) and bilevel positive airway pressure (biPAP) ventilation (Fig. 13-6) are increasingly being used to provide noninvasive ventilatory support in the management of obstructive sleep apnea, chronic ventilatory failure, and acute respiratory failure for infants, children, and adults. CPAP is currently the treatment of choice in cases of obstructive sleep apnea syndrome.[18] It

has been suggested that biPAP improves ventilation and vital signs more rapidly than CPAP in patients with acute pulmonary edema.[19]

### Manual Resuscitators

A patient requires ventilatory assistance by use of a manual resuscitator

- In an emergency response situation.
- When there is a need to disconnect the patient from the mechanical ventilator for a prolonged period of time (e.g., transfer or ambulation training, endotracheal suctioning).
- To stimulate or mimic a cough and/or to augment tidal volume and supplement oxygen for intubated and nonintubated patients.

Manual resuscitation bags (Fig. 13-7) are self-inflating. When compressed, they deliver a volume of gas to the patient by means of a one-way valve. The flow of gas then opens the inhalation valve, permitting gas to flow to the patient. When flow from the bag ceases and exhalation begins, exhaled gas from the patient pushes the inhalation valve closed and opens the diaphragm, allowing gas to flow out the exhalation ports. The bag intake port may be fitted with an oxygen reservoir system to deliver oxygen-enriched breaths.

### Oxygen Delivery Devices

#### Nasal Cannula

The nasal cannula is the most commonly used delivery device. It is generally intended to be used with oxygen flow rates between 1 and 6 L/min for adults, and as low as $\frac{1}{16}$ L in neonates (Fig. 13-8). Whether or not a humidifier is used in conjunction with a nasal cannula may depend on individual physician preference. However, at flows exceeding 3 or 4 L/min the nasal mucosa may become dried and irritated with sustained use of nonhumidified gas.[20,21] An accurate

## Table 13-5 Intracranial Pressure (ICP) Monitors

| Device | Description |
| --- | --- |
| Epidural sensor | • Purpose:<br>  ○ To monitor ICP.<br>• Consists of:<br>  ○ A fiberoptic pneumatic flow sensor. It is placed in the epidural space (i.e., superficial to the dura) and connects to a transducer and monitor.<br>• Clinical implications:<br>  ○ The transducer does not need to be adjusted (releveled) with position changes.<br>  ○ Fair to good reliability. |
| Subarachnoid bolt | • Purpose:<br>  ○ To directly monitor ICP.<br>• Consists of:<br>  ○ A hollow bolt or screw placed in the subarachnoid space through a burr hole.<br>• Clinical implications:<br>  ○ The physician will determine the level to which the transducer should be positioned. This is documented in the chart and posted at the bedside.<br>  ○ The transducer must be repositioned to the appropriate level with position changes.<br>  ○ Poor reliability and decreased accuracy at high ICP readings.<br>  ○ Complications include infection and blockage of the bolt by clot or brain tissue. |
| Intraventricular catheter (ventriculostomy) | • Purpose:<br>  ○ To directly monitor ICP and provide access for the sampling and drainage of CSF. Occasionally used to administer medications or to instill air or contrast agent for ventriculography.<br>• Consists of:<br>  ○ A small catheter that is placed in the anterior horn of the lateral ventricle through a burr hole. The catheter connects to a transducer and to a drainage bag, where CSF collects.<br>• Clinical implications:<br>  ○ The nondominant hemisphere is the preferable insertion site.<br>  ○ There are two different types of drainage systems: intermittent and continuous.<br>  ○ The intermittent system allows the nurse to drain CSF for 30-120 seconds by momentarily opening a stopcock when the ICP exceeds the parameters set by the physician.<br>  ○ A continuous system allows the drainage of CSF to occur against a pressure gradient when the collection bag is positioned (leveled) above the foramen of Monro. This is usually 15 cm above the external auditory meatus (EAM).<br>  ○ The transducer must be repositioned to the appropriate level with position changes.<br>  ○ Very reliable.<br>  ○ Complications can include infection, meningitis, ventricular collapse, or catheter occlusion by blood or brain tissue. |
| Fiberoptic transducer-tipped catheter | • Purpose:<br>  ○ To monitor ICP. Can also be used in conjunction with a CSF drainage device (if the catheter is placed in the parenchyma).<br>• Consists of:<br>  ○ A fiberoptic transducer-tipped catheter. It is placed in the ventricle, within the parenchyma, in the subarachnoid or subdural space, or under a bone flap.<br>• Clinical implications:<br>  ○ The transducer does not need to be adjusted (releveled) with position changes.<br>  ○ Very reliable. |

*CSF, Cerebrospinal fluid.*
*Data from Smeltzer SC, Bare BG, Hinkle JL, et al. (eds). Management of Patients with Neurologic Dysfunction. In Brunner & Suddarth's Textbook of Medical-Surgical Nursing (11th ed). Philadelphia: Lippincott Williams & Wilkins, 2007.*

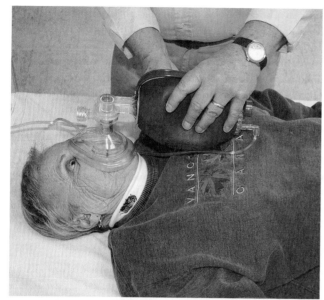

**Figure 13-7** Demonstration using a resuscitation device (Ambu bag). (From Pierson FM. Principles & Techniques of Patient Care. 4th ed. St. Louis, Saunders, 2008.)

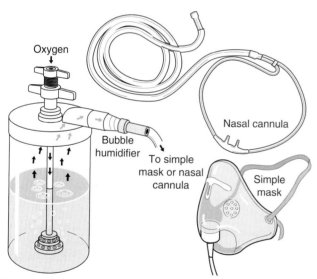

**Figure 13-8** Low-flow supplemental oxygen delivery devices and flow-by humidifier. (Redrawn from Kersten LD. Comprehensive Respiratory Nursing. Philadelphia, WB Saunders, 1989:608, 609.)

### Table 13-6 Approximate FIO₂ Achieved with Different Oxygen Delivery Devices

| Device | Oxygen Flow Rate | FIO₂ |
|---|---|---|
| Nasal cannula (estimated FIO₂, assuming normal minute ventilation) | 1 L/min | 0.24 |
| | 2 L/min | 0.28 |
| | 3 L/min | 0.32 |
| | 4 L/min | 0.36 |
| | 5 L/min | 0.40 |
| | 6 L/min | 0.44 |
| Simple mask | 5-6 L/min | 0.35 |
| | 6-7 L/min | 0.45 |
| | 7-10 L/min | 0.55 |
| Aerosol mask | 10-12 L/min | 0.35-1.0 (depends on setting) |
| Venturi mask (O₂ flow rates are minimums to be used with specific-sized orifice for desired FIO₂) | 4 L/min | 0.24* |
| | 4 L/min | 0.28* |
| | 6 L/min | 0.31 |
| | 8 L/min | 0.35* |
| | 8 L/min | 0.40* |
| | 10 L/min | 0.50 |
| Partial nonrebreather mask | Lower | 40%-60% |
| Nonrebreather mask | Higher | 60%-80% |

*FIO₂ depends on the size of the orifice or the entrainment ports; these vary among manufacturers.*

Fig. 13-8) is designed to provide a flow of gas into a face piece that fits over the patient's nose and mouth. Some simple masks also include a diluter to add room air and thus increase the total gas flow as the oxygen flows into the mask. The oxygen percentage that can be delivered with a simple mask ranges from 35% to 55%, at flow rates of 5 to 10 L/min (for adults). As is true with nasal cannulas, whether or not a humidifier is used in conjunction with a simple mask depends on individual physician preference. However, at oxygen concentrations exceeding 30%, the nasal and oral mucosa may become dried and irritated with sustained use of nonhumidified gas.

### Aerosol Mask
The aerosol mask (Fig. 13-9) was originally designed for the administration of aerosolized medications. However, these masks are widely used for the administration of controlled percentages of oxygen at flow rates slightly greater than those for simple masks (10 to 12 L/min), to exceed the patient's inspiratory demand. Typically, aerosol masks are used in conjunction with a nebulizer to humidify the gas. The FIO₂ is regulated between 35% and 100% by means of an adjustable

fraction of inspired oxygen (FIO₂) cannot be delivered with a nasal cannula because respiratory rate, tidal volume, and anatomic dead space are so variable among patients.[22] Nonetheless, as Table 13-6 shows, we assume that the approximate FIO₂ is increased by 4% with each 1 L/min increase in oxygen flow rate when the patient is breathing regularly.

### Simple Mask
Patients who are breathing through their mouths will often not receive the benefit of an increased flow rate through a nasal cannula. These patients may benefit from using a mask to improve oxygenation in the blood. The simple mask (see

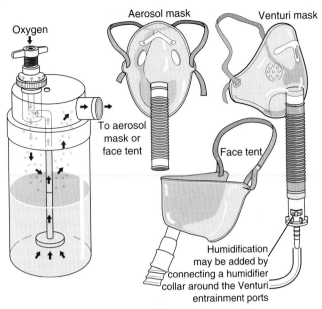

**Figure 13-9** High-flow supplemental oxygen delivery devices and aerosol nebulizer. (Redrawn from Kersten LD. Comprehensive Respiratory Nursing. Philadelphia, WB Saunders, 1989:581, 585.)

air entrainment port on the nebulizer. Increasing the $FIO_2$ setting closes the entrainment port and decreases the dilution of the oxygen.

### Venturi Mask

The Venturi mask (see Fig. 13-9) generally provides a greater flow of gas to a patient by entraining room air through a side port. The $FIO_2$ is selected by changing either the size of the orifice through which oxygen is delivered or the size of the entrainment ports, and adjusting the oxygen flow rate. Venturi masks operate by application of the Bernoulli principle: oxygen enters the larger flexible tubing via a narrowed orifice, creating a relative negative pressure within the tubing, which pulls room air through the entrainment ports. These masks may or may not be humidified. Table 13-6 details the oxygen flow rates and $FIO_2$ delivered by Venturi masks. It is important to note that different manufacturers may provide different $FIO_2$ values for the same color; consequently, a clinician must follow the information on the device that indicates the $FIO_2$ provided by the color as well as the flow required.

### Nonrebreather Masks

These types of oxygen delivery devices consist of a mask and a reservoir and are used to allow a high percentage of oxygen to be delivered. Humidification is not used with these methods, as it would alter the percent of oxygen delivered.[23-25]

The partial rebreather mask covers the nose and the mouth and is held in place by an elastic strap. The mask has holes for ventilation on either side and is attached to a reservoir bag. In a typical, adult partial-rebreathing mask, the reservoir bag has a volume capacity of approximately 300 to 500 mL. Gas flow from the oxygen source is directed into the

mask and the reservoir via small-bore tubing that connects at the junction of the mask and bag.[26] Approximately two-thirds of the bag is filled with oxygen from a supplemental source and room air flowing in from the exhalation ports. During exhalation the first third of the exhaled gas fills the reservoir bag, and the last two-thirds of the exhaled gas are vented into the room through the exhalation ports. The exhaled volume that fills the reservoir bag represents gas that has not participated in gas exchange, and therefore has a high partial pressure of oxygen ($PO_2$) and a low partial pressure of carbon dioxide ($PCO_2$). This oxygen-rich air mixture is inhaled with the next breath, thereby allowing some rebreathing of air. The $FIO_2$ provided with this system is 40% to 60% (see Table 13-6).[25,26]

The nonrebreather mask looks similar to the partial rebreather mask but does not allow for rebreathing of any exhaled air. The mask has one-way valves at the ventilation ports, which prevent room air from entering during inhalation and allow all of the air to exit during exhalation. There is another one-way valve located between the reservoir bag and the base of the mask. During inspiration this valve allows the flow of supplemental source from the wall to distend the bag fully and the air in the bag is inhaled.[25,26]

Theoretically, nonrebreathing masks can deliver 100% oxygen, assuming that the mask fits snugly on the patient's face and the only source of gas being inhaled by the patient is derived from the oxygen flowing into the mask-reservoir system. In actual practice, disposable nonrebreathing masks are usually supplied with one of the exhalation valves removed. The valve is removed as a precaution so that the patient can still inhale room air if there is an interruption in supplemental source gas flow.[26] The $FIO_2$ provided with this system is 60% to 80% (Fig. 13-10).

---

**Clinical Tip**
Reservoir bag should remain one-third to one-half full on inspiration. Oxygen saturation needs to be closely monitored during physical therapy interventions if the patient requires a high amount of supplemental oxygen to maintain adequate saturation.

---

### Pediatric Delivery Devices

In the pediatric setting, oxygen tents, hoods, or incubators are frequently used. In an oxygen tent, the $FIO_2$ attained depends on the incoming gas flow, the canopy volume, and the degree to which the tent is sealed. Tents generally envelop the patient's upper torso or entire body. Continuous oxygen monitoring is necessary because patient care requires entering the tent. This, therefore, alters the $FIO_2$. Ice reservoirs are often incorporated for temperature control. An oxygen hood, a small plastic enclosure placed over the patient's head, permits nursing care or other treatment without hindering oxygen therapy. An incubator may be used for similar reasons as an oxygen tent, but it generally provides for warming instead of cooling of the environment. Chapter 20 provides more detailed information on pediatric equipment.

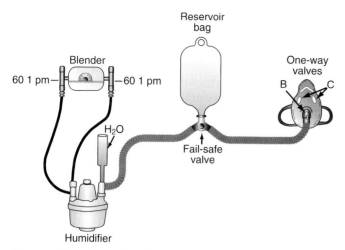

**Figure 13-10** Nonrebreathing reservoir circuit with a valved face mask. Reservoir bag in combination with high-flow (0 to 100 L/min) flowmeters ensures delivery of set FIO$_2$. (From Foust GN, Potter WA, Wilons MD, et al. Shortcomings of using two jet nebulizers in tandem with an aerosol face mask for optimal oxygen therapy. Chest. 1991 Jun;99(6):1346-51.)

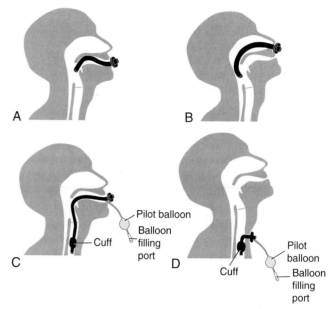

**Figure 13-11** Airway adjuncts. **A,** Oral pharyngeal tube. **B,** Nasal pharyngeal tube. **C,** Oral endotracheal tube. **D,** Tracheostomy tube. (Redrawn from Kersten LD. Comprehensive Respiratory Nursing. Philadelphia, Saunders, 1989:630.)

## Invasive Ventilatory Devices

### Airway Adjuncts

An oral pharyngeal airway (Fig. 13-11A) is a semirigid tube of plastic or rubber shaped to fit the natural curve of the soft palate and tongue. It is used to hold the tongue away from the back of the throat and maintain airway patency. The oral airway may also be used as a bite block.

The nasal pharyngeal airway (see Fig. 13-11B) is a soft latex or rubber tube inserted through one of the nares. It follows the wall of the nasopharynx and oropharynx to the base of the tongue. The nasal airway is generally better tolerated because it is less likely to stimulate a gag reflex in the semiconscious or alert patient. Both the oral and the nasal airways provide a pathway to the hypopharynx, which may reduce mucosal trauma caused by the need for frequent suctioning.

> **Clinical Tip**
> When nasal airways are left in place for prolonged periods of time, interference with normal sinus drainage may occur.

An endotracheal tube (see Fig. 13-11C), an artificial airway inserted into the trachea, is a disposable silicone rubber or polyvinyl chloride tube. An oral endotracheal tube is inserted via the mouth, and a nasal endotracheal tube is inserted via the nose; the specific rationale for using each type of tube may vary regionally. Regardless of the route, endotracheal intubation is usually undertaken as a last resort when other means of airway management have or are likely to fail.

There are four primary reasons for employing endotracheal intubation:

- Upper airway obstruction,
- Inability to protect the lower airway from aspiration,

- Inability to clear secretions from the lower airways,
- Need for positive-pressure mechanical ventilatory assistance.

A radiopaque line extending the length of the tube, or a marker at the distal end of the tube, facilitates location of the endotracheal tube by radiography. Endotracheal tubes are beveled at their distal ends, and they are usually labeled near their proximal ends with the manufacturer's name, tube type, and internal diameter in millimeters.

The adult endotracheal tube typically has a low-pressure, large-volume inflatable cuff at its distal end. Inflating the cuff stabilizes the endotracheal tube and seals the airway.

Neonatal and pediatric endotracheal tubes generally do not have cuffs. A standard 15-mm adapter or universal adapter is attached at the proximal end of the endotracheal tube to facilitate connection to mechanical ventilators, manual resuscitation bags, or other respiratory modalities.

> **Clinical Tip**
> In patients who are endotracheally intubated, the location of the tube should be noted prior to initiation of any physical therapy intervention. It is also important to observe the location of the tube at the end of the physical therapy session and notify the nurse and/or respiratory therapist if any changes are noted.

A tracheostomy is an airway opening that is surgically created directly over the trachea (see Fig. 13-11D). Although it is usually an elective procedure, it occasionally needs to be performed emergently in patients in whom it is difficult to establish an airway through the nose or mouth. In the critical care setting, a tracheostomy usually follows prolonged endotracheal intubation and is performed to minimize tracheal or

Metal tubes are not routinely used in the ICU, but are commonly seen in some patients with long-standing tracheostomies. Metal tubes can be made of either stainless steel or sterling silver and are composed of three parts: an outer cannula that fits into the tracheal incision, an inner cannula that fits into the outer cannula, and an obturator that facilitates insertion of the tube. These three parts comprise a tracheostomy set and are not interchangeable with any other set.[27]

> **Clinical Tip**
> Two important things to note in the care of metal tracheostomy tubes is that (1) sterling silver tubes can be easily dented, and (2) the inner cannula may come out with a forceful cough or exhalation if it is not locked into position.

Plastic tracheostomy tubes were developed for the following three important reasons:
- Minimize crusting and adherence of secretions,
- Greater ease in attaching a safe, dependable, permanent inflatable cuff,
- Lower costs allow the tube to be disposable.

Plastic tubes come with and without cuffs.[27] The cuffed tracheostomy tube is primarily used in conjunction with a positive-pressure ventilator to form a closed system. It is also used to reduce the possibility of aspiration because of absent, protective laryngeal, and pharyngeal reflexes. Although most adult tracheostomy tubes are cuffed, there are many situations in which the cuff is deflated. For example, when assessing the patient's ability to protect the lower airway during swallowing, the cuff may be deflated. When the cuff is inflated, the only route for air exchange is through the patient's tracheostomy tube; consequently, careful observation of the patient for any signs of respiratory distress is essential.[27]

Some tracheostomy tubes have a removable inner cannula to facilitate cleaning of the tube. There are several types of special tracheostomy tubes, and the clinician should be aware of the type of tube being used with the patient so that any special precautions are noted.

A tracheostomy button or a Passy-Muir valve (Fig. 13-13) may be used as an intermediate step between mechanical ventilation and spontaneous breathing in the process of weaning a patient from mechanical ventilatory support. The tracheostomy button permits the upper airway to be used for spontaneous ventilation, while providing a means of maintaining the tracheostomy stoma as a direct access route to the lower airway until the patient no longer requires assistance to clear bronchial secretions.[28] Both devices allow the patient to vocalize.

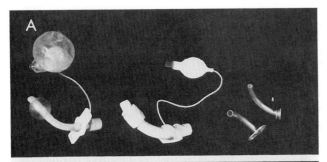
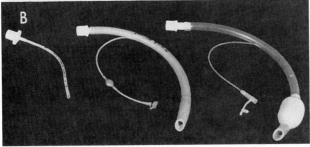

**Figure 13-12** **A**, Cuffed adult tracheostomy tubes, uncuffed pediatric tracheostomy tube (*far left*). **B**, Cuffed adult endotracheal tubes, uncuffed pediatric endotracheal tube (*far left*). (From Frownfelter D, Dean E. Cardiovascular and Pulmonary Physical Therapy: Evidence and Practice, ed 4. St. Louis, 2006, Mosby.)

vocal cord injury. Box 13-10 identifies some possible complications of a tracheostomy.

A tracheostomy tube (Fig. 13-12) is an artificial airway inserted into the trachea, via a tracheostomy, below the level of the vocal cords. The tracheostomy tube is short (2 to 6 inches long), but otherwise similar to an endotracheal tube except that it is not beveled at its distal end. An external flange near the proximal end of the tube is usually labeled with the manufacturer's name and internal or external diameter in millimeters. The flange serves to stabilize the tube in the trachea and as a base from which the tube may be secured to the patient's neck. Tracheostomy tubes are of two basic types: metal and polyvinyl chloride (hard and soft).

> **Clinical Tip**
> A Passy-Muir valve is a one-way valve. The tracheostomy cuff *must* be deflated before valve is applied. Some patients may not be able to tolerate increased levels of activity with the valve in place.

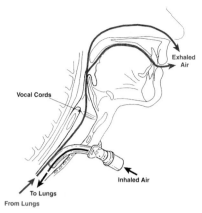

**Figure 13-13** The Passy-Muir Valve. This valve attaches to a standard 15-mm tracheostomy adapter. The adaptor allows **(A)** inspiration through the valve. Expiration **(B)** must occur through the upper airway to allow speech. (Courtesy Passy-Muir, Irvine, CA.)

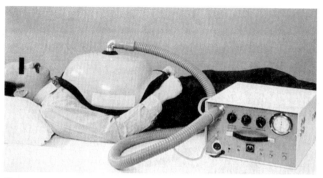

**Figure 13-14** Chest cuirass attached to a negative pressure generator. (From Albert RK, Spiro SG, Jett JR. Clinical Respiratory Medicine. 3rd ed. Philadelphia, Mosby, 2008.)

## Mechanical Ventilation

Mechanical ventilation is an emergent intervention for patients who are unable to maintain the demands of their respiratory system on their own. Such patients are typically in the intensive care unit and mechanical ventilation may be necessary for a few hours. If the need extends beyond a few days, it is considered to be prolonged mechanical ventilation.[29] Patients requiring extended periods of mechanical ventilation may be transferred to facilities equipped to take care of the multiple needs of the patient and to assist in weaning the patient off the ventilator. If the patient is unable to wean off the ventilator, the patient may go home and be ventilator-dependent for life.

The use of ventilators allows for mechanical ventilatory support so as to:

- Meet physiologic needs in acute respiratory failure indicated by failure of the respiratory system to maintain an adequate balance of pH, $PaO_2$, and/or $PaCO_2$
- Protect the airway and lung parenchyma (drug overdose, cerebrovascular accident, head or spinal cord injury)
- Relieve upper airway obstruction (tumor, allergic reaction, edema)
- Improve pulmonary toilet in patients with excessive secretions or inability to successfully clear secretions by coughing

Mechanical ventilators are generally classified according their cycling mechanism, that is, the method used to stop the inspiratory phase and initiate the expiratory phase. Negative pressure ventilators are rarely in use in critical care units. The cuirass (Fig. 13-14) is a rigid shell that encloses the patient's anterior thorax so that subatmospheric pressure can be exerted within the shell. A vacuum-cleaner-like pump generates the negative pressure. The shells are usually custom made for each patient, although prefabricated shells are available. The cuirass is probably not more widely used because (1) it tends to be noisy, (2) provision of patient care may be hampered, and (3) regulation of inspiratory/expiratory ratios is difficult. These units are useful, however, for providing augmentation to spontaneously breathing patients with weakened respiratory musculature. Additionally, ventilatory mechanics are more physiologic than they are with positive-pressure machines, and many patients do not require a tracheostomy. Patients requiring intermittent or periodic ventilatory assistance (e.g., patients with Guillain-Barré syndrome or amyotrophic lateral sclerosis) may benefit from such ventilators. The "iron lung" made famous during the poliomyelitis epidemics of the 1940s and 1950s is still in use by some patients today. In fact, it is often used at night by patients so that they can rest sufficiently to assume the task of spontaneous ventilation during the daytime.

Positive-pressure ventilators are used almost exclusively for mechanical ventilatory assistance in critical care units. The positive pressure from the ventilator provides the force that delivers gas into the patient's lungs by increasing intrathoracic pressure to expand the chest wall. The termination of gas flow allows the chest wall to recoil to the resting position, thus exhaling the gas.

Knowledge of the basic components and terminology (Table 13-7) associated with the mechanical ventilator will assist the clinician in being better prepared to monitor the mechanically ventilated patient. The tubing that connects the patient to the ventilator is called the circuit. The circuit generally consists of wide-bore tubing and valves that attach either to a mask or mouthpiece, or directly to an endotracheal or tracheostomy tube. An additional port in the terminal end of the circuit can be added to allow suctioning while maintaining the integrity of the circuit without the need to disconnect the endotracheal tube from the circuit.

Table 13-8 provides guidelines for initial ventilator settings for various clinical indications. In addition, Box 13-11 provides parameters for traditional ventilation.

---

> **Clinical Tip**
> Several parameters should be noted on the ventilator screen: (1) Mode of ventilation, (2) $FIO_2$, (3) PEEP (positive end-expiratory pressure [mm of $H_2O$]), (4) respiratory rate (breaths per minute), (5) tidal volume (milliliters), (6) minute volume (mL/min), and (7) alarm settings.

## Table 13-7 Ventilator Terminology

| | |
|---|---|
| Assist control (A/C) | Nonweaning mode |
| | Rate and tidal volume are set to deliver a minimum minute ventilation |
| | Patient can generate as many breaths as needed by triggering the ventilator |
| | On each spontaneous respiratory effort generated by the patient, the machine delivers the preset tidal volume |
| | Patients usually tolerate increased demands during physical therapy if medically stable |
| | *Main disadvantage* is in patients breathing at a rate greater than set respiratory rate as each breath triggers a full tidal volume (VT). This can lead to respiratory alkalosis or in patients with airway obstruction breath stacking and hyperinflation. Hyperinflation can lead to barotraumas, pneumothorax or severe decrease in venous return (autoPEEP) |
| Synchronized intermittent mandatory ventilation (SIMV) | Weaning mode |
| | Rate and tidal volume are set to deliver a minimum minute ventilation |
| | Patient is able to breath spontaneously between ventilator breaths |
| | Each spontaneous breath receives a VT that depends on the patient's effort |
| | Often used with in conjunction with PSV |
| | Good mode for respiratory muscle exercise |
| | *Main disadvantage* is that it may increase the work of breathing, therefore may need to switch patient to A/C or pressure support if patient shows signs of fatiguing |
| Continuous positive airway pressure (CPAP) | Spontaneous mode of ventilation |
| | Weaning mode |
| | CPAP maintains positive pressure continuously in the airways |
| | Pressure support is be added to augment patient's tidal volume |
| | When used with a mask is considered noninvasive ventilation |
| Positive end-expiratory pressure (PEEP) | Positive pressure applied at the end of expiration during ventilation |
| Pressure support ventilation (PSV) | Applies to spontaneous breaths only |
| | May be applied to a patient's spontaneous breathing during SIMV or CPAP |
| | Once the patient triggers the ventilator, the preset positive pressure is delivered |
| | Volume is not preset; pressure support augments the VT |
| | The patient controls respiratory rate and inspiratory time |
| | Helps to decrease work of breathing and allows for more patient comfort |
| | *Main disadvantage* is there is no guaranteed ventilation. If patient stops breathing for any reason (such as fatigue) ventilation ceases and often alarms are triggered |
| Tube compensation (TC) | Not a mode, but a spontaneous breath type |
| | Accurately overcomes the imposed work of breathing through an artificial airway |
| | The flow compensates for the size and diameter of tube |
| | Used to determine if patient is ready for extubation |

*Data from Piccini JP, Nilsson K. The Osler Medical Handbook, ed 2. Baltimore, 2006, Saunders.*

## Other Modes (Nontraditional) of Mechanical Ventilation

- Pressure control ventilation (PCV): peak inspiratory pressure (PIP) is set by clinician and not exceeded by the ventilatory system in effort to reduce barotraumas, air leaks and development of chronic lung disease.
- High-frequency oscillatory ventilation (HFOV): uses extremely high respiratory rate (180 to 300 breaths/minute) with tidal volumes that are low (and at this date not well defined). Used to treat refractory hypoxemia especially when associated with acute lung injury. HFOV lowers peak airway pressure, recruits atelectatic alveoli and prevents lung injury. Importantly, HFOV provides active expiration. Disadvantages include risk of dynamic hyperinflation and hemodynamic compromise. Patients require heavy sedation and possibly paralytics when on HFOV.

## Table 13-8 Guidelines for Initial Ventilator Settings for Various Clinical Indications

| Clinical Setting | Clinical Objectives | Tidal Volume (mL/kg) | Target pH/ PaCO$_2$ | Target PaO$_2$ | Positive End-Expiratory Pressure (cm H$_2$O) |
|---|---|---|---|---|---|
| Routine (e.g., postoperative, drug overdose) | Prevent atelectasis | 7-10 | Normal | Normal | 0-5 |
| Obstructive lung disease (e.g., chronic obstructive pulmonary disease, asthma) | Unload ventilatory muscles, prevent hyperinflation | 5-7 | Permissive hypercapnia | Normal | 0-5 or more if autopositive end-expiratory pressure present |
| Acute lung injury (e.g., acute respiratory distress syndrome) | Prevent further lung injury, support oxygenation | 5-7 | Permissive hypercapnia | If severe, may tolerate 50-60 mm Hg | Usually 8-15 |
| Focal or unilateral pulmonary disease (e.g., lobar pneumonia) | Avoid barotrauma, support oxygenation | 7-10 | Normal | Normal | Avoid or use cautiously |
| Acute brain injury (e.g., head trauma) | Maintain cerebral perfusion pressure | 7-10 | Normal or respiratory alkalosis | Normal | Avoid |

*Modified from Albert R, Spiro S, Jett J. Comprehensive Respiratory Medicine. St. Louis, Mosby, 1999.*

### Box 13-11

#### Parameters of Traditional Ventilation

- Minute ventilation (VE) = Respiratory rate (RR) – Tidal volume (Vt).
- VE = Alveolar ventilation(VA)* + Dead space ventilation (VD).
- Positive end-expiratory pressure (PEEP)† minimizes atelectasis and decreases intrapulmonary shunting.
- Plateau pressure (Pplat) is a static pressure measured at end-inspiration and is related to respiratory system compliance (CRS) = Vt/(Pplat – PEEP).
- Peak airway pressure (Ppk) depends on CRS, Vt, and airway resistance, (Raw) = (Ppk – Pplat)/Inspiratory flow rate.

*PaCO$_2$ is inversely proportional to VA.
†Oxygenation may be improved by increasing FIO$_2$ or PEEP.
From Albert R, Spiro S, Jett J. Comprehensive Respiratory Medicine. St. Louis, Mosby, 1999.

- High-frequency jet ventilation (HFJV): produced by ventilators that deliver a high-velocity jet of gas directly into the airway.
- Pressure control-inverse ratio ventilation (PC-IRV) involves increasing the inspiratory time to change the inspiratory to expiratory ratio of >1 to improve oxygenation. At this time there are no studies that demonstrate the benefit of this type of ventilation.
- Bilevel positive airway pressure (BiPAP) ventilation is a noninvasive technique used to provide ventilatory support to a spontaneously, but insufficiently, breathing patient using a face mask or nasal mask. BiPAP cycles between two levels of CPAP. Used in adults with respiratory failure such as pneumonia, chronic obstructive pulmonary disease, and pulmonary edema. Results in shorter duration of ventilation, less need for sedation, and fewer complications than intubation and positive-pressure ventilation.
- Airway pressure release ventilation (APRV) involves the application of CPAP with regular release of this pressure at a defined respiratory rate to permit ventilation. Patients may also breathe spontaneously at any time in ventilatory cycle. This results in lower airway pressures and may improve hemodynamics.
- Pressure regulated volume control (PRVC) combines volume control and pressure control. PRVC is a pressure limited time cycled mode that the pressure is adjusted on previous four-breath average. Can be switched to volume support mode when trying to wean patient from ventilator.
- Extracorporeal support (ECMO): Currently beneficial effects have not been confirmed, but considered only for patients with severe hypoxemia and hypercapnia unresponsive to optimal management. Inflates lungs to moderate pressures to maintain functional residual capacity while CO$_2$ removal occurs via low-flow partial venovenous bypass.[30]

> **Clinical Tip**
> AutoPEEP or intrinsic PEEP (PEEPi): When alveolar pressure remains positive at the end of expiration causing a dynamic hyperinflation or air trapping. This occurs when the time available for expiration is shorter than the time required for passive emptying to individual's functional residual capacity (FRC).

## Portable Ventilators

Portable, battery-powered mechanical ventilators provide the ventilatory support needed during patient transport and ambulation outside the room. Clinicians should become thoroughly familiar with the equipment utilized by their patients.

> **Clinical Tip**
> It is *always* important to know ventilator settings, respiratory rate, and oxygen saturation prior to starting the therapy session.

## Innovative Ventilation System

Neurally adjusted ventilatory assist (NAVA) is not available on current ventilators, but has clinical promise. The NAVA system measures electrical activity of the diaphragm via an electrode inserted into a nasogastric tube that is placed in lower esophagus to sense diaphragmatic activity. The signal from diaphragm triggers the ventilator to assist patient's inspiratory effort in proportion to diaphragmatic effort. Therefore, the respiratory drive controls the assisted positive breaths in all phases of ventilatory cycle.[31]

## Chest Tubes

Chest tubes are large catheters placed in the thoracic cavity and connect to a graduated collection reservoir at bedside.[32] Chest tubes are used to remove and prevent the reentry of air or fluid from the pleural or mediastinal space and provide negative intrapleural pressure.[25]

Reasons for insertion of a chest tube include:

- Thoracotomy
- Pleural effusion
- Pneumothorax, hemothorax, or chylothorax
- Empyema
- Chemical pleurodesis

In nonsurgical situations, chest tubes are commonly inserted in the sixth intercostal space in the mid or posterior axillary line. After thoracic surgery, mediastinal chest tubes are placed to drain the pericardium and exit the chest through the surgical incision. Apical chest tubes drain air, which typically collects in the apices of the pleural spaces. If fluid needs to be drained, the chest tube is placed inferiorly in the thoracic cavity as fluid tends to collect near the bases of the lungs.[25]

The collection system is designed to seal the drainage site from the atmosphere. Immersing the end of the collection tube in water and creating an underwater seal accomplishes this. A single-reservoir system in which the reservoir serves as both the collection receptacle and the underwater seal offers a greater resistance to the fluid and air leaving the chest and in order to decrease an additional reservoir is included. A third reservoir, which connects to wall suction, may be added to the system to serve as a pressure regulator. Tubes may be connected to a small one-way valve (Heimlich valve) that allows air or fluid to escape from the pleural space while preventing reentry.[25] Figure 13-15 shows a typical chest tube drainage and collection system.

The more elaborate drainage systems are used for precise measurement of fluid loss in patients after thoracic and cardiovascular surgery. The presence of a chest tube is *not* a contraindication to mobilization. Careful mobilization can assist with drainage (Box 13-12). Changes in the quantity and quality of exudates should be noted by the physical therapist before, during, and after changes in position and therapeutic interventions.

## Invasive Cardiac Device

**Pacemakers.** Implantation of a cardiac pacemaker involves placing unipolar or bipolar electrodes on the myocardium for chronic rhythm disorders that require long-term control. For details of cardiac pacemaker implantation, see Chapter 11. When mobilizing patients with a temporary pacemaker, be aware of the location of the pacemaker and the wires, monitor the patient continuously when being mobilized, keep the area around the pacemaker dry, and check with RN/MD regarding restrictions because of underlying pathology.

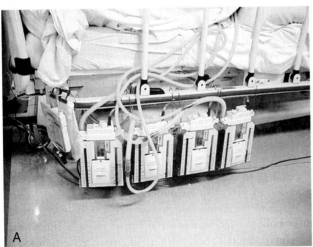
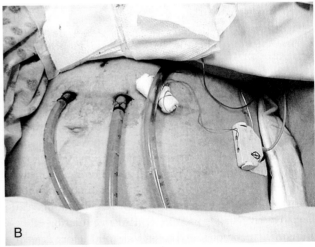

**Figure 13-15 A,** Chest tube drainage. **B,** Anterior view; mediastinal drains. (From Frownfelter D, Dean E. Cardiovascular and Pulmonary Physical Therapy: Evidence and Practice. 4th ed. St. Louis, Mosby, 2006.)

**Box 13-12**

**Effective Mobilization**

For effective mobilization:
• Ensure that the patient is premedicated for pain.
• Always keep chest tube drainage system below the chest level.
• Check for air leaks (air bubbles will be present in the underwater seal compartment if air leaks are present).
• Always discuss with MD/RN prior to disconnecting suction.
• A portable suction device may be used when indicated.
• After the chest tube is removed hold therapy until radiography rules out pneumothorax.

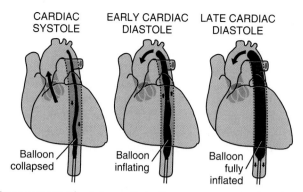

**Figure 13-16** The intraaortic balloon counterpulsation device is positioned in the descending aorta just below the orifice of the left subclavian artery. (Redrawn from Waldhausen JA, Pierce WS. Johnson's Surgery of the Chest. 5th ed. Chicago, Year Book Medical, 1985:273.)

Temporary pacemakers provide temporary cardiac pacing:
• Emergency treatment of arrhythmias with severe hemodynamic compromise
• Status postcardiac surgery
• Status postmyocardial infarction
• Dysrhythmias that would not likely require permanent pacing
  Before placing a permanent pacemaker
• The pacemaker is classified according to its location:
  • Epicardial
  • Transvenous
  • Transcutaneous
  • Permanent

**Automatic implantable cardiac defibrillator.** An automatic implantable cardiac defibrillator (AICD) is used to manage uncontrollable, life-threatening ventricular arrhythmias by sensing the heart rhythm and defibrillating the myocardium as necessary to return the heart to a normal rhythm. If prescribing activity intensity using heart rate for patients with an AICD, the exercise target heart rate should be 20 to 30 beats below the threshold rate on the defibrillator.[33] Indications for AICD include ventricular tachycardia and ventricular fibrillation.[34] See Chapter 11 for more in-depth information.

**Intraaortic balloon pump.** The intraaortic balloon pump (IABP) is indicated in pathologies that cause a patient to be hemodynamically unstable. It assists the circulation of blood through the body and reduces myocardial oxygen consumption by:
• Augmenting flow of blood through coronary arteries
• Increasing CO
• Lowering systolic blood pressure
• Decreasing heart rate

It can also be used to assist weaning a patient from the cardiopulmonary bypass machine and to provide perioperative circulatory support during high-risk cardiac or general surgical procedure.[35] Intraaortic balloon counterpulsation (IABC) via the IABP is used to augment the diastolic blood pressure and to increase coronary blood flow. The balloon catheter is usually inserted into one of the femoral arteries and advanced until its tip is in the thoracic aorta just distal to the left subclavian artery (Fig. 13-16; IABP is also discussed in Chapter 4).

When activated, the balloon is inflated during diastole as soon as the aortic valve closes. The increase in intraaortic and diastolic pressure forces the blood in the aortic arch to flow in a retrograde direction into the coronary arteries. Through this diastolic augmentation the oxygenation to the myocardium is greatly improved. When the balloon is deflated during left ventricular systole it lowers the left ventricular systolic pressure and the afterload by forcing the blood to move from an area of higher pressure to one of lower pressure and enhances the CO.[36] The alteration in the systolic and diastolic arterial pressure is accompanied with little change in the MAP.

When mobilizing patients on IABP, the following precautions should be taken:
• No hip flexion is allowed in the leg in which the catheter is inserted. The patient may be log rolled for turning in bed.
• Patients are on strict bed rest but they can usually participate in therapeutic activities with an IABP catheter in place. Out-of-bed activities are contraindicated until the IABP catheter is removed.

**Pulmonary artery balloon counterpulsation.** Pulmonary artery balloon counterpulsation (PABC) differs from IABP in that it is inserted into the pulmonary artery rather than the thoracic aorta. It may be used in conjunction with the IABP in treatment of right ventricular or biventricular failure that is resistant to inotropic drugs or the use of the IABP alone.

**Ventricular assistive device.** A ventricular assist device (VAD) is a mechanical device that augments the pumping capability of the heart, providing the circulatory support necessary to sustain life. It could be used to assist the right ventricle, left ventricle, or both ventricles. The most commonly used device is the left ventricular assist device (LVAD). This device is implanted in patients with end-stage heart failure as:
• A bridge to recovery until the clinical condition improves.

- A bridge to transplantation while waiting for a donor heart.
- A destination therapy for patients who are not eligible for a cardiac transplantation.

Optimal function of the left ventricle is essential for an effective CO. Heart failure can result from a structural or functional disorder that affects the pumping ability of the ventricles. The stages of ventricular dysfunction failure can range from patients being asymptomatic with relatively normal activity tolerance to those who are severely symptomatic and unable to tolerate any level of exertion. The implantation of a LVAD can aid in restoring adequate CO and help the patient recover from secondary organ dysfunction.

The basic components of an LVAD include a prosthetic left ventricle, an inflow cannula, an outflow cannula, and an external source of power. The prosthetic left ventricle is the pump that is implanted within the abdominal wall or in the peritoneal cavity. The inflow cannula enters the apex of the left ventricle and the outflow cannula is connected to the ascending aorta. There are many types of LVAD devices that are currently used. The pump can be driven by air (pneumatic) or with a battery. Typically, the LVAD has an external electronically powered console at the patient's bedside. A battery backup is provided in such a device with an external battery pack that is held in place by a shoulder harness, allowing for greater portability and mobility.[37]

> **Clinical Tip**
> Evidence shows that patients who receive an LVAD do tolerate early activity. A progressive physical therapy program can be initiated early in the patient's ICU stay. The focus is on mobilization out of bed and ambulation so as to minimize the effects of additional deconditioning and assist in functional recovery.

### Extracorporeal Membranous Oxygenation

The extracorporeal membranous oxygenation (ECMO) is an external circulatory assist device, that can provide direct oxygenation of the blood and assist in removal of carbon dioxide. The primary indication for ECMO is cardiac or respiratory failure that is not responding to maximal medical therapy and conventional mechanical ventilation. The pediatric population with respiratory failure seems to benefit from this therapy the most; however, the successful use of ECMO in the adult population is improving.[38,39]

> **Clinical Tip**
> Mobilization of a patient who is on ECMO is typically not recommended.

### Hemodialysis

This process is a treatment that replaces the function of the kidneys. The blood is removed from the body and filtered through a membrane called a dialyzer which performs the function of the kidney (Fig. 13-17). The blood is then

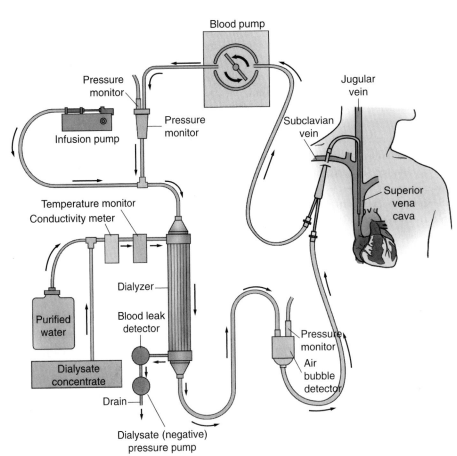

**Figure 13-17** Schematic representation of hemodialysis. (From Thompson JM, McFarland GK, Hirsch JE, et al. Mosby's Clinical Nursing, ed 3. St. Louis, 1993, Mosby.)

returned to the body. Hemodialysis is used when an existing metabolic condition causes acute or chronic renal failure. There are three types of vascular access for hemodialysis: arteriovenous (AV) fistula, AV graft, and central venous catheter. Hemodialysis may be intermittent where the patient receives dialysis two to three times a week or continuously. Continuous renal replacement therapy (CRRT) is a slower continuous mode of dialysis. It is beneficial in patients in the critical care setting to help stabilize them without the adverse effects of hypotension that can occur with hemodialysis. Continuous arteriovenous hemofiltration (CAVH) uses the femoral artery and vein as common sites for vascular access. In critically ill patients who experience frequent episodes of hypotension, the pressure gradients between the artery and the vein are too weak to create a significant driving pressure necessary to achieve adequate filtration rates. In this patient population, continuous venovenous hemofiltration (CVVH) uses the internal jugular vein or subclavian vein as access sites along with a mechanical pump and an external filter for blood exchange. When a dialysate solution is used to help waste products diffuse out of the bloodstream the process is known as continuous venovenous hemodialysis (CVVHD).[40,41]

Indications for CRRT include[25]:

- Cardiovascular instability
- Parenteral nutrition
- Cerebrovascular or coronary artery disease
- Acute renal failure with multiple organ failure
- Inability to tolerate hemodialysis
- Azotemia
- Sepsis

As long as the patient is hemodynamically stable, physical therapy on dialysis days (either pre- or postdialysis) is not contraindicated. Of patients receiving dialysis, vital signs must be closely monitored, along with symptoms to assess for cardiovascular stability during physical therapy. When measuring blood pressure in dialysis patients, care must be taken to avoid using the arm with an arteriovenous fistula (see Chapter 7).

## Summary

- Physical therapists face a difficult challenge when working with critically ill patients in ICUs. It is important for the clinician to recognize the monitoring and life support equipment surrounding a patient and understand the reason for its presence. The physical therapist must have the knowledge and the ability to interpret large amounts of information in order to provide a safe and effective therapeutic intervention.
- The physiologic monitoring equipment commonly found in critical care units primarily addresses the cardiovascular, pulmonary, and neurologic systems.
- The method of detection may be invasive or noninvasive. The various parameters being monitored must be observed and recorded before, during, and after any therapeutic intervention to ensure patient safety.
- Life support equipment can range from noninvasive ventilatory and cardiac devices to invasive airway adjuncts, mechanical ventilation, and maximal cardiovascular and renal support. It is important for physical therapists to be able to differentiate between medical emergencies that require immediate treatment and inaccuracies that may be caused by extraneous factors unrelated to the physiologic status of the patient.
- A physical therapy program should be designed according to the patient population and should assist the patient in functional recovery. The presence of numerous lines, tubes, and monitoring and life support equipment should not be a contraindication to mobilization. Interdisciplinary involvement is important to ensure a safe therapeutic intervention.
- To provide safe and effective care for critically ill patients, the therapist must use strong critical thinking skills and understand:
  - Basic anatomy and pathophysiology of cardiovascular and pulmonary systems.
  - Medical interventions provided in the critical care setting.
  - Mechanical ventilatory support.
  - Pharmacology prescribed for the patient.
  - Function of the equipment present and its impact on therapeutic interventions.
  - Emergency procedures.

## References

1. Dean E, Perme C. Monitoring systems in the intensive care unit. In Frownfelter D, Dean E (eds.). Cardiovascular and Pulmonary Physical Therapy: Evidence and Practice. 4th ed. St. Louis, Mosby, 2006.
2. Fearnley SJ. Update in Anesthesia: Practical Procedures. Issue 5, (1995) Article 2.
3. Frownfelter D. Arterial blood gases. In Frownfelter D, Dean E (eds.). Cardiovascular and Pulmonary Physical Therapy: Evidence and Practice. 4th ed. St. Louis, Mosby, 2006.
4. Rushmer RF. Cardiovascular Dynamics. 3rd ed. Philadelphia, Saunders, 1970.
5. Wilkins RL. Clinical Assessment in Respiratory Care. 5th ed. St. Louis, Mosby, 2006.
6. Gambrell M. Using the BIS monitor in palliative care: A case study. J Neurosci Nurs 37(3):140–3, 2005.
7. Barbato M. Bispectral index monitoring in unconscious palliative care patients. J Palliat Care 17(2):102–8, 2001.
8. De Deyne C, Struys M, Decruyenaere J, et al. Use of continuous bispectral EEG monitoring to assess depth of sedation in ICU patients. Intensive Care Med 24(12):1294–8, 1998.
9. Kelley SD. Monitoring Level of Consciousness During Anesthesia and Sedation: a Clinician's Guide to the Bispectral Index. Norwood, MA, Aspect Medical Systems, 2004.
10. Gardner RM. Accuracy and reliability of disposable pressure transducers coupled with modern pressure monitors. Crit Care Med 24(5):879–82, 1996.
11. Darovic GO. Hemodynamic Monitoring: Invasive and Noninvasive Clinical Application. 2nd ed. Philadelphia, Saunders, 1995.
12. Klabunde RE. Cardiovascular Physiology Concepts. Baltimore, Lippincott Williams & Wilkins, 2005.
13. Daily EK, Schroeder JS. Techniques in Bedside Hemodynamic Monitoring. 5th ed. St. Louis, Mosby, 1994.

14. Baird MS. Manual of Critical Care Nursing: Nursing Interventions and Collaborative Management. 5th ed. St. Louis, Mosby, 2006.

15. Lehmann KG, Platt MS. Improved accuracy and precision of thermodilution cardiac output measurement using a dual thermistor catheter system. J Am Coll Cardiol 33(3):883–91, 1999.

16. Cathelyn JL, Samples DA. $SvO_2$ monitoring: Tool for evaluating patient outcomes. Dimens Crit Care Nurs 17(2):58–63; quiz 64–6, 1998.

17. Ahrens T. Technology utilization in the cardiac surgical patient: $SvO_2$ and capnography monitoring. Crit Care Nurs Q 21(1):24–40, 1998.

18. Resta O, Guido P, Picca V, et al. Prescription of nCPAP and nBIPAP in obstructive sleep apnoea syndrome: Italian experience in 105, subjects. A prospective two centre study. Respir Med 92(6):820–7, 1998.

19. Mehta S, Jay GD, Woolard RH, et al. Randomized, prospective trial of bilevel versus continuous positive airway pressure in acute pulmonary edema. Crit Care Med 25(4):620–8, 1997.

20. Branson RD, Hess D, Chatburn RL. Respiratory Care Equipment. 2nd ed. Philadelphia, JB Lippincott, 1998.

21. Campbell EJ, Baker MD, Crites-Silver P. Subjective effects of humidification of oxygen for delivery by nasal cannula. A prospective study. Chest 93(2):289–93, 1988.

22. Redding JS, McAfee DD, Gross CW. Oxygen concentrations received from commonly used delivery systems. South Med J 71(2):169–72, 1978.

23. Cairo JM. Administering medical gases: Regulators, flowmeters, and controlling devices. In Cairo JM, Pilbeam SP (eds.). Mosby's Respiratory Care Equipment. 7th ed. St. Louis, Mosby, 2004.

24. Arata L, Farris L. Oxygen delivery devices. In George-Gay B, Chernicky CC (eds.). Clinical Medical Surgical Nursing. Philadelphia, Saunders, 2002.

25. Paz JC. Acute Care Handbook for Physical Therapists. 3rd ed. St. Louis, Saunders, 2009.

26. Cairo JM. Mosby's Respiratory Care Equipment. 7th ed. Philadelphia, Mosby, 2004.

27. Frownfelter D, Mendelson LS. Care of the patient with an artificial airway. In Frownfelter D, Dean E (eds.). Cardiovascular and Pulmonary Physical Therapy: Evidence and Practice. 4th ed. St. Louis, Mosby, 2006.

28. Kacmarek RM. The Essentials of Respiratory Care. 4th ed. St. Louis, Mosby, 2006.

29. Perme C, Chandrashekar R. Managing the patient on mechanical ventilation in ICU. early mobility and walking program. Acute Care Perspect 17(1):10–15, 2008.

30. West M. The medical record. In Paz J, West M (eds.). Acute Care Handbook for Physical Therapists. 3rd ed. St. Louis, Saunders, 2009.

31. Grasso S, Mascia L, Ranieri VM. Respiratory care. In Miller RD, Eriksson LI, Fleisher LA (eds.). Miller's Anesthesia. 7th ed. Philadelphia, Churchill Livingstone, 2009.

32. Phipps WJ, Long BC, Woods NF (eds.). Medical-Surgical Nursing: Concepts and Clinical Practice. 7th ed. St. Louis, Mosby, 2000.

33. Wegener NK. Rehabilitation of the patient with coronary heart disease. In Schlant RC, Alexander RW (eds.). Hurst's The Heart. 8th ed. New York, McGraw-Hill, 1994.

34. Collins SM, Cahalin, LP. Acute care physical therapy in patients with pacemakers. Acute Care Perspect 14(5):9–14, 2005.

35. Darovic GO. Handbook of Hemodynamic Monitoring. 2nd ed. Philadelphia, Saunders, 2004.

36. Massie B, Conway M, Yonge R, et al. Skeletal muscle metabolism in patients with congestive heart failure: Relation to clinical severity and blood flow. Circulation 76(5):1009–19, 1987.

37. Perme C, Chandrashekar R. Early mobilization and ambulation of patients with left ventricular assist devices (LVAD) who require long-term mechanical ventilation: clinical and therapeutic implications. Yearbook of Respiratory care clinics and applied technologies 2009, Editor in Chief Esquinas Rodríguez, Antonio Matías MD PhD. FCCP.

38. Kaplon, RJ, Smedira, NG. Extracorporeal membrane oxygenation in adults. In Goldstein DJ, Oz MC (eds.). Cardiac Assist Devices. Armonk, NY, Futura, 2000.

39. Mulroy J. Acute respiratory distress syndrome. In Bucher L, Melander S (eds.). Critical Care Nursing. Philadelphia, Saunders, 1999.

40. Paz JC. Genitourinary system. In Paz JC, West M (eds.). Acute Care Handbook for Physical Therapists. 3rd ed. St. Louis, Saunders, 2009.

41. Dirkes S, Hodge K. Continuous renal replacement therapy in the adult intensive care unit: History and current trends. Crit Care Nurse 27(2):61–6, 68–72, 74–80; quiz 81, 2007.

## CHAPTER 14

# Cardiovascular Medications

*Meryl Cohen, Kate Grimes, Wolfgang Vogel*

## Chapter Outline

"Pharmacology can be broadly defined as the science dealing with interactions between living systems and ... chemicals introduced from outside the system. ... A drug [is] any small molecule that, when introduced into the body, alters the body's function by interactions at the molecular level."[1] A drug is then biologically defined as any chemical that causes mostly a beneficial or therapeutic effect within the body although some interactions can also produce unwanted or adverse results. However, not all such chemicals can be used as drugs because their use is governed by legal considerations. Thus, a drug is now any chemical that the Food and Drug Administration (FDA) allows medical professionals to prescribe or use in order to diagnose, prevent, or treat diseases. This permission is only granted after the pharmaceutical company has demonstrated that the drug is both efficacious (therapeutically effective) and relatively safe (acceptable toxicity) or that the therapeutic effects must outweigh the adverse reactions. Although heroin is an excellent analgesic fulfilling the biological definition, it is not allowed today to be medically used (because the FDA does not allow its use).

Although medications have significantly broadened the management of cardiovascular dysfunction, "a drug cannot impart a new function to a cell ... it modulates ongoing function."[2] The impact of pharmacologic management for the patient with a cardiovascular disorder cannot be underestimated. The responsibility of the physical therapist in treating any individual is to understand the effects and potential side effects of the individual's drug regimen as well as the drugs' influence on the outcome of the physical therapy intervention. This chapter presents the pharmacologic clinical management of the most common cardiovascular dysfunctions.

To appreciate the impact and complexity of drug management, a few supportive concepts should be introduced. Drugs have two names: a generic and a trade name. The generic name is the scientific description of the drug whereas the brand name is the name that the individual drug company assigns to its own product. Thus, a drug has only one generic name but can have many brand names if manufactured by different companies (e.g., Advil, Nuprin, and Motrin are different brand names of the same drug ibuprofen). In this chapter, the generic name appears first, the brand or trade name or names follow in parentheses; for example, verapamil (Calan, Isoptin). In addition, there are brand name and generic drugs available. A brand name drug is a drug that is manufactured by the company and solely sold by this company (under its brand name with its specific generic name) as long as it has the patent for the drug. After the patent has expired, any company can now manufacture and sell this drug (under its own brand name or often under its generic name), which is now referred to as a generic drug. Both of these drug preparations contain the same active ingredient and must be shown to be clinically equally effective—which is often not or only poorly understood by many patients. Thus, they can be used interchangeably and the pharmacist is allowed to dispense the generic drug version even if the physician did prescribe the brand name drug (unless specifically prohibited by the physician). Generic drugs are much less expensive and some insurance companies will only pay for this preparation.

> **Clinical Tip**
> Inform patient that a brand name drug and its equivalent generic drug contain the same medication and should work the same in spite of the fact that they may look different in shape and color and are less expensive.

The goal of drug therapy is to prescribe the appropriate medication for the individual's needs with the expectation that the medication is delivered to the site of action in adequate strength (therapeutic level) to elicit the appropriate clinical response. The foundation of this goal rests on two broad concepts, pharmacokinetics and pharmacodynamics.[3] Pharmacokinetics addresses how the drug is absorbed, how the drug is distributed (distribution), how much of the drug is delivered to the target site or sites (bioavailability), and how the drug is metabolized and excreted (clearance). Pharmacodynamics addresses two components: the mechanism of drug action and the relationship between drug concentration and clinical effect (Fig. 14-1).[4] It must be added that drugs used are defined and fixed parameters whereas individuals can show differences in the way they interact with them. Although most individuals will show only minor, pharmacologically insignificant differences, some individuals will indeed show major differences that can result in unexpected and sometimes dangerous clinical situations. Unfortunately, such major differences cannot be predicted and manifest themselves only after drug exposure.

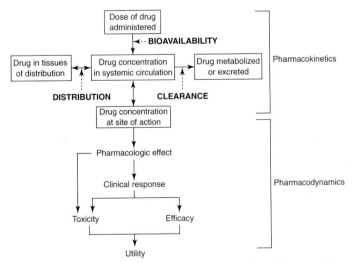

**Figure 14-1** Schematic representation of the pharmacokinetic and pharmacodynamic processes. (From Katzung BG [ed]. Basic and Clinical Pharmacology. 5th ed. East Norwalk, CT, Appleton & Lange, 1992:29.)

# Pharmacokinetics

Pharmacokinetics describes the fate of a drug in the body. Drugs may be administered to the body through different access routes; the two most common are by mouth or by injection. By mouth (oral, or p.o.) is also known as enteral, indicating that the drug enters the gastrointestinal system before it enters the circulation. Parenteral routes bypass the absorption within the gastrointestinal system. Injection is one form of parenteral administration, a nongastrointestinal (i.e., nonenteral) route. See Table 14-1 for examples of drug routes.

## Bioavailability

The route of administration affects the bioavailability of the drug, the onset of drug action, and its duration of action. Drugs taken by mouth are absorbed from the stomach and intestine and then pass through the liver (portal circulation) before reaching the systemic circulation. Some drugs cannot be taken orally. They can be destroyed in the gastrointestinal tract like insulin. They may be inactivated in the liver when they pass through this organ the first time. This is known as the first-pass effect. The greater the first-pass effect, the less is the bioavailability of the drug. These drugs, such as morphine, must then be given at very small doses or by other routes.

> **Clinical Tip**
> When working with patients with liver dysfunction, remember that the first-pass effect may not occur and therefore the effects of the medications the patients are taking may be increased.

Parenterally given drugs by definition bypass the gastrointestinal system; therefore, the bioavailability is usually greater and the onset of action is mostly faster with the parenteral routes than with enteral routes. Because of their fast onset of action, parenteral medications, particularly those using the intravenous and sublingual routes, are a key component in the management of hemodynamic instability in emergency and critical care settings. Drugs administered through sublingual routes enter the circulation through the systemic veins that drain the highly vascular oral mucosa and do not pass through the gastrointestinal system or portal circulation. Nitroglycerin is perhaps the most widely used sublingual medication.

## Distribution

Although drugs are not distributed exclusively into body tissues and organs via the circulatory system, it is by far the most common route. Drug distribution may be general or restricted, depending on the ability of the drug to pass through particular cell membranes and on the permeability of the capillaries for the particular drug. Differential distribution

## Table 14-1 Common Routes of Drug Administration

| Route | Comments |
| --- | --- |
| Parenteral | No gastrointestinal absorption |
| | Fast acting |
| Injection | Valuable in emergencies |
| | May cause pain and tissue damage at injection site |
| Intravenous (IV) | May deliver a high concentration of drug quickly |
| Subcutaneous (SQ) | May be self-administered |
| Intramuscular (IM) | |
| Intrathecal (spinal) | |
| Intraperitoneal | |
| Buccal (sublingual) | Quick onset |
| Inhalation | Quick delivery of drug to bronchi and alveoli for local effect |
| | Gaseous anesthetic |
| | Useful with drugs that vaporize quickly |
| Enteral | Absorbed through the gastrointestinal system |
| By mouth (p.o.) | Convenient |
| Tablets or capsules | Most common |
| Enteric coated | Effective absorption |
| Sustained release | Usually most economical |
| Chewable | |
| Liquid | Effective with children |
| Oral solutions | |
| Elixir | |
| Rectal | May have local or systemic effects |
| | Effective when gastrointestinal upset precludes use of oral |
| Transdermal | Slowly absorbed; prolongs blood levels |

Adapted from Gilman AG, Goodman LS, Rall TW, Murad F (eds.). Goodman and Gilman's The Pharmacologic Basic of Therapeutics. 7th ed. New York, Macmillan, 1985:3-10; and Katzung BG (ed.). Basic and Clinical Pharmacology. 4th ed. East Norwalk, CT, Appleton & Lange, 1989.

may occur as a result of one of the following situations: drug binding to proteins (especially plasma protein), difficulty of drugs crossing the blood–brain barrier of the central nervous system, or storage of drugs within body tissues (particularly adipose and muscle tissues). Drugs bind to proteins both in the tissues and in the plasma; the most common plasma proteins are albumin and $\alpha_1$-acid-glycoprotein. Although protein–drug binding is a reversible and dynamic process, it may temporarily limit drug distribution.

> **Clinical Tip**
> The recommended drug dose might have to be increased in very heavy individuals because the volume of distribution is much greater and the drug is much more diluted in their bodies.

## Clearance

"Clearance of a drug is the rate of elimination by all routes relative to the concentration of drug in any biologic fluid."[3] There are the major routes of drug metabolism in the liver and excretion in the kidney as well as some minor routes as through the pulmonary system and the biliary tract.

Lipophilic (fat-soluble) drugs are chemically transformed in the liver by a family of enzymes referred to as p450 enzymes or mixed-function oxidases into more hydrophilic (water-soluble) metabolites. This is called drug metabolism or drug biotransformation. These drug reactions are divided into Phase I and II reactions and include oxidations, reductions, hydrolysis, and conjugation. They can render the metabolites pharmacologically inactive, or the metabolites can maintain their therapeutic activity. This can terminate the therapeutic activity or can prolong it. In a few instances, tissues other than the kidney can also perform such biotransformations. Some drugs called prodrugs are pharmacologically inactive and are only activated in the body by these reactions. Most individuals metabolize within a narrow range but some can be high or low metabolizers, which can affect the therapeutic and toxic responses of drugs and the doses must be adjusted accordingly either higher or lower. In addition, multiple drugs can compete for the same enzyme and overwhelm its capacity leading to the accumulation of one or both drugs, resulting sometimes in dangerous drug interactions.

Hydrophilic drugs (the kidney cannot excrete lipophilic drugs or compounds) or metabolites are then excreted by the kidney into the urine. This occurs mostly in that the drugs or metabolites are filtered by glomerular filtration from the blood into the nephron. A few drugs can also be actively secreted into the nephron per se. Most healthy individuals excrete within a narrow range.

These processes of drug clearance are influenced by genetic and environmental factors, nutritional habits, weight of the person, exercise, and age, with very young and older individuals having less capacities. Furthermore, a dysfunction of any of these clearance routes caused by diseases or an inadequate circulatory system to distribute the drug can also interfere with the normal clearance of the drug from the body. Liver problems can slow biotransformation, and kidney malfunction can reduce excretion—both leading to potential drug overdose effects unless the doses have been adjusted accordingly.

## Half-Life

The elimination of most drugs follows first-order kinetics, and the time it takes for the plasma concentration of the drug to be reduced by 50% is known as the half-life. Half-life reflects the rate at which the drug is eliminated from the body. It takes about 4 to 5 half-lives until a drug is eliminated from the body. It also serves as a rough indicator of the length of time the effects of the medication will last; the longer the half-life, the longer the effect of the drug. The half-life determines the frequency of the administration of medication. Some medications must be taken four times a day (q.i.d.) to be most effective; others may be taken only once (q.d.), twice (b.i.d.), or three times a day (t.i.d.).

Patients should not try to manipulate the timing of their medications because medications need to be taken at regular intervals; a delay in taking the medication, for example, waiting until after a physical therapy appointment, only delays the onset and effectiveness of the medication. In some instances, once a medication schedule has been interrupted, such as a delay in taking pain medications, the prescribed dosage may be insufficient for patient comfort or desired action. An example of different half-lives can be seen with two commonly used cardiac medications, digoxin (Lanoxin) and propranolol (Inderal). The half-life of digoxin is 36 hours; that of propranolol is only 3 to 6 hours.

## Dosage

In deciding the appropriate dosage of a drug, the drug to be used, the disease to be treated, the possible presence of other diseases and their drug treatments, and the constitution of the patient considered.[3] Based on the clinical condition or disease, it must be decided if the drug is to be used intermittently or continuously. Medications given at certain time intervals throughout the day by any route are examples of intermittent doses. Here, the drug can be given as the regular preparation or a sustained-release preparation that allows for longer drug action and reduced dosings. Infusions by the intravenous (nitroglycerin given temporarily during the acute stages of myocardial ischemia) or subcutaneous (insulin pumps) routes, and use of patches on the skin are examples of continuous administration. Chronic drug treatment requires the administration of the drug at the half-life intervals so that a drug with a short half-life has to be given more frequently than a drug with a long half-life. It must here also be recognized that the full effect occurs only after the fourth dose. If the full effect is required immediately as in emergency and critical care situations, then the drug is started with an initial high loading dose to achieve a therapeutic level more quickly. Following the loading dose, a lower maintenance dose, is given. In steady state, a balance is achieved between effective drug availability and drug elimination. The goal of dosing is to give the minimal amount of drug needed for the desired effect.

Effective drug management is complex and multidimensional; it is strongly influenced by metabolic processes, the functioning of the liver, kidneys, lungs, heart, and circulatory systems. Impairment in any of these may result in ineffective drug therapy or drug therapy that requires more vigilance. Drug clearance may be impaired in kidney or liver failure, resulting in a greater amount of drug within the system; if the drug dose is not adjusted to accommodate the impaired clearance, drug overdose or toxicity may result. Exercise enhances metabolism, systemically and/or locally. In situations where the drug may be administered locally (e.g., IM injections, transdermal, subcutaneous insulin), exercise may enhance the distribution of the drug into circulation faster than planned. In the case of insulin, patients need to be aware of this, plan accordingly, and watch for signs and symptoms of hypoglycemia.

## Pharmacodynamics

Pharmacodynamics describes the interaction of drugs with tissue receptors and the resulting pharmacologic effects. These drug receptors are located throughout the body, and the drug affects all the receptors specific to the drug's structure. This results in both therapeutic and adverse reactions. Drug receptors are located outside and inside our cells and are mostly cellular proteins. The best identified protein receptors are those that interact with certain neurotransmitters, hormones, and autocoids. Other common drug receptors are located on various enzymes as well as on nucleic acids.

The drug and its receptor form a specific complementary relationship, as a key fits into a lock. This interaction is either brief as in most cases but can also be irreversible.

$$\text{Drug} + \text{Receptor} \rightarrow \text{Drug-Receptor} + \text{Effect} \rightarrow \text{Drug} + \text{Receptor}$$

Receptors may have different biochemical functions common to many cells such as opening electrolyte channels or affecting second messenger systems. Receptors for the same drug can be located on various tissues or organs and, as a result, no drug produces a single effect or affects only a specific tissue. This accounts for their therapeutic as well as adverse effects. Digoxin is one of the earliest drugs discovered to be effective for some cardiac disorders. It has widespread effects on many types of tissue, a variety of side effects, and a low threshold for toxicity. Digoxin may not only have the desired direct cardiac effects, such as decreased conduction through the A-V node and increased myocardial contractility, but it may also have gastrointestinal effects (nausea, anorexia, diarrhea), central nervous system (CNS) effects (blurred or yellow vision, confusion, headache), and undesired cardiac effects (ventricular tachycardia, ventricular fibrillation, cardiac toxicity).

Drugs are selective regarding the type of receptor to which they are attracted and which they are affecting. They can be roughly divided into agonists that stimulate a receptor and enhance a physiological effect or antagonists that inhibit a receptor and decrease a physiological effect. A drug may be a complete or partial agonist or antagonist in that they can be either agonistic or antagonistic depending on the state of the system.

### Autonomic Nervous System and Its Receptors

Understanding the autonomic nervous system requires a thorough review of its anatomy; please refer to Chapter 1 for more detail. The autonomic nervous system contains two divisions: the sympathetic and the parasympathetic. One of the distinctions between the two is their postganglionic neurotransmitter substance: acetylcholine in the parasympathetic system and norepinephrine in the sympathetic system. As a result of their neurotransmitters, the receptors of the parasympathetic nervous system are known as cholinergic, and the receptors of the sympathetic system are known as adrenergic. The cholinergic receptors are classified as muscarinic receptors whereas the adrenergic receptors have two subdivisions, the α-adrenergic and β-adrenergic adrenoceptors. Both α- and β-receptors are further subclassified into $\alpha_1$ and $\alpha_2$ and $\beta_1$ and $\beta_2$ receptors. The cholinergic receptors at the autonomic ganglia are classified as nicotinic. In addition, the vascular bed and heart contains dopaminergic receptors. The sensitivity of each receptor to its neurotransmitter differs depending on the location and action of each receptor. When α-receptors in the vascular smooth muscle are stimulated, contraction occurs; when β-receptors are stimulated in the vascular smooth muscle, relaxation occurs.

Although drug receptors are found in many cells of the body, the most common sites for cardiac drug–receptor interactions are the autonomic nervous system (Table 14-2), the kidneys, and the vascular smooth muscle. Other sites such as the central nervous system for the management of hypertension and the blood cells for their role in clotting and lysis are also critically important for achieving cardiovascular stability.

## Autonomic Drugs

Adrenergic agonists are also known as sympathomimetics. The sympathomimetics are a group of drugs that mimic the activity of the endogenous catecholamines epinephrine, norepinephrine, and dopamine. They are roughly divided into $\alpha_1$ and $\alpha_2$ and $\beta_1$ and $\beta_2$ agonists. Adrenergic antagonists are also known as sympatholytics or drugs that reduce the action of the sympathetic nervous system. They again can be roughly divided into $\alpha_1$ and $\alpha_2$ and $\beta_1$ and $\beta_2$ antagonists. A well-known group of adrenergic antagonists are the β-adrenergic antagonists (β-blockers), which has formed a cornerstone in the management of coronary artery disease for the past more than 30 years.

Cholinergic drugs that simulate parasympathetic activity are known as parasympathomimetic or cholinergic agonists; conversely, drugs that block cholinergic activity are known as parasympatholytic or cholinergic antagonists. They can be classified based on their specific action, that is, into

## Table 14-2 Autonomic Receptors

| Type | Tissue | Actions |
|---|---|---|
| $\alpha_1$ | Most vascular smooth muscle (innervated) | Vasoconstriction |
| | Pupillary dilator muscle | Contraction (dilates pupil) |
| | Pilomotor smooth muscle | Erects hair |
| | Heart | Increase force of contraction |
| | Platelets | Aggregation |
| | Some vascular smooth muscle (noninnervated) | Vasoconstriction |
| | Fat cells | Inhibition of lipolysis |
| $\beta_1$ | Heart: myocardium and SA node | Increase force and rate of contraction |
| | Fat cells | Activate lipolysis |
| $\beta_2$ | Respiratory, uterine (pregnant), and vascular smooth muscle | Bronchodilation |
| | | Uterine relaxation |
| | | Vasodilation |
| | Skeletal muscle | Increased strength |
| | Human liver | Glycogenolysis |
| Muscarinic | Heart: atria; AV node; SA node; smooth muscle cells | Decreased contractility; decreased heart rate; decreased peripheral vascular resistance |
| Nicotinic | Sympathetic and parasympathetic post ganglionic neurons | Increased vascular constriction: arterial and venous |
| | | Heart rate: may decrease |
| Dopaminic | Vascular smooth muscle | Vasodilation |
| | Heart | Increased contractility |

*Adapted from Guyton AC, Hall JH. Textbook of Medical Physiology, ed 11. Philadelphia, 2006, Saunders; Katzung BG (ed). Basic and Clinical Pharmacology, ed 4. East Norwalk, CT, 1989, Appleton & Lange.*

muscarinic and nicotinic agonists or antagonists. Muscarinic drugs usually have a better-defined mode of action whereas nicotinic drugs affect both systems via their autonomic ganglionic action. Generally, agonists cause vasoconstriction and antagonists vasodilatation, with decrease in blood pressure and reduced venous return.

## Kidney

Drug receptor sites within the kidneys are found within the proximal tubule, collecting tubule and ducts, and Henle loop. Refer to the section on antihypertension drugs and to Figure 14-7 for a discussion of the site of action and the effect of specific drugs.

## Vascular Smooth Muscle

Cardiac drug receptors within vascular smooth muscle are primarily adrenoceptors; they include the subtypes of $\alpha_1$-, $\alpha_2$-, and $\beta_2$-adrenoceptors. In addition, other receptors (e.g., histamine, prostaglandin, angiotensin) and electrolytes (e.g., sodium, calcium) affect blood vessel dynamics.

## General Considerations of Pharmacologic Management

Management of cardiac dysfunction often involves the prescription of a multifaceted drug regimen that must be dynamic in its ability to respond to individual's needs. Long-term use of certain drugs may cause an alteration of receptor responses in that agonists can downregulate and antagonists upregulate receptors, leading to tolerance or physical dependence. In the case of tolerance, the dosage may need to be increased, the drug replaced, or an additional drug prescribed to supplement the initial drug. In the case of physical dependence, the drug should never be discontinued suddenly because this can lead to a withdrawal syndrome that can range from unpleasant to outright dangerous. Slow reduction of the dose over a period of time can avoid this problem. β-Blockers are an example, whose long-term use should not be terminated abruptly but be slowly discontinued. Drug effectiveness may also be decreased as a result of a systemic illness, gastrointestinal upset, or a change in drug metabolism in that some drugs can increase their own (and that of other drugs as well) biotransformation.

The cost of drugs often influences which drug (generic or brand name) or class of drugs is prescribed when a choice is available. Patient compliance is also influenced by drug cost; some patients choose to decrease the frequency of their medications "to save money" or avoid taking the drug at all. Patients are often unaware of the consequences of self-regulation of medications.

The awareness by all health care professionals that a drug cannot work effectively unless it is taken as prescribed should sensitize prescribers of drugs to the issues that contribute to noncompliance: cost of drug, difficulty in following a complicated drug regimen, poorly tolerated side effects, and undesirable interactions with other prescribed medications are just a few examples. Solid explanations and good instructions by the prescriber to the patient can minimize these problems.

Although drug prescription is looked at across broad populations, it would be remiss to ignore the individual's response to a drug or category of drug. Drugs do not have the same universal effect on all individuals within a population. Genetic background, environmental factors, habits (e.g., smoking), race, age, and gender have been shown to influence drug response and therefore will influence drug choice. Within the 21st century, the ongoing roles of pharmacogenetics and stem cell research in understanding an individual's cellular and genetic makeup will help to streamline and identify the best treatment options for the individual.

## Ischemic Heart Disease

### Antiischemic Drugs

Dramatic changes took place during the latter part of the 20th century in the pharmacologic management of ischemic heart disease. With the introduction of β-blockers, calcium-channel blockers, thrombolytic agents, and the critical care regimen of vasopressors and positive inotropics, hemodynamic stability was able to be established in many individuals who formerly might have led the lifestyle of the "cardiac cripple" at best or faced death at worst. As understanding of atherosclerosis increased, the impact of inflammation, lipid metabolism, and cellular physiology on the development of atherosclerosis led the way to the development of new drugs with improved and earlier drug management. As the understanding was enhanced of the time course and cellular events that take place in the development of a myocardial infarction from an ischemic condition, the clinical syndrome of acute coronary syndrome (ACS) was established. ACS is a constellation of clinical presentations and myocardial tissue changes that occur when myocardial ischemia cannot be readily resolved with rest and minimal routine intervention. The emergent drug and interventional management of the patient with ACS involves eliminating the coronary thrombosis as quickly as possible, decreasing myocardial oxygen demand, identifying the culprit lesion, and enhancing myocardial oxygen supply. Emergent management of ACS may result in an aborted myocardial infarction (ideal outcome) or a smaller infarction than would have happened without intervention and therefore preserved left ventricular or LV function.

> **Clinical Tip**
> If a patient has undesired side effects of a drug, another drug in the same class may often be substituted, with acceptable clinical effects and less troublesome side effects. If a patient develops drug tolerance, drug substitution or a change in dosage will occur.

Primary prevention became an active goal in drug (and lifestyle) management for those with risk factors for atherosclerosis, and secondary prevention took on even more importance for those already diagnosed. As science and technology developed, interventions to reduce the impact of atherosclerosis on myocardial tissue as well as to augment LV function also developed. Minimally invasive coronary artery bypass graft (CABG), percutaneous coronary interventions (PCIs) such as angioplasties and stents, biventricular pacemakers, and newer categories of automatic implantable cardioverter–defibrillators (AICDs) led to aggressive management of atherosclerosis and its sequelae (see Chapter 3). Although coronary artery disease continues to hold the distinction of being the number one cause of death in the United States, the overall mortality trend has declined steadily since 1980.[5] The 21st century sees the partnering of drugs, technology, stem cell research, genetics, and lifestyle changes (including nutrition, exercise, and stress management) toward minimizing or eliminating the impact of atherosclerosis on society.

### Physiology

The heart is an oxygen-dependent organ whose energy needs are met by aerobic metabolism. Oxygen is delivered to the myocardium and conducting tissues via the coronary arteries. Adequate myocardial oxygen supply is dependent on many factors, most particularly the coronary blood flow, the oxygen-carrying capacity of blood, and the anatomy of coronary arteries (e.g., lumen diameter). When myocardial oxygen demand is increased, it is satisfied by an increase in coronary blood flow.

Multiple factors determine the demand for myocardial oxygen, such as afterload, systolic wall tension, wall thickness, contractile state, preload, heart rate, and left ventricular volume and diameter. Although many factors influence myocardial oxygen demand, $MVO_2$ may be clinically assessed as the product of heart rate and systolic blood pressure. This clinical method for $MVO_2$ assessment is called the double product or rate–pressure product (RPP).

Demand is increased under conditions that increase heart rate, blood pressure, or both: exercise; increased systemic vascular resistance; high-output states such as pregnancy, fever, and increased thyroid function; anemia; emotional stress; and anxiety are but few examples.

### Pathophysiology

Unlike striated muscle, the myocardium can function without adequate oxygen for only a relatively short period of time. Inadequate oxygenated blood to the myocardium may result from either inadequate blood flow (ischemia) or inadequate arterial oxygenation (hypoxemia). Coronary blood flow is the prime mechanism for supplying oxygenated blood to the myocardium. When coronary blood supply is inadequate to meet the myocardial oxygen demands, the myocardium becomes ischemic. Pathologically, the most common cause of decreased myocardial oxygen supply is coronary artery disease or CAD. The atherosclerotic plaque

associated with coronary artery disease reduces the lumen size and therefore reduces blood flow. Lumen diameter may also be decreased as a result of spasm of the smooth muscle within the endothelium of the coronary artery; spasm may occur in the presence or absence of coronary artery disease, as in the case of Prinzmetal angina. In these cases, the patient experiences chest fullness and severe pain or angina pectoris. It must here also be mentioned that similar symptoms can be experienced by other conditions, for example, esophageal spasm.

In an acute myocardial infarction, a thrombus may form at the site of the atherosclerotic lesion and further occlude the lumen. Three steps are necessary for thrombus formation[6]:

- A conducive surface (such as damaged intravascular endothelium) on which the thrombus can form
- A sequence of platelet-mediated events: platelet adhesion, followed by platelet aggregation, followed by release of agents further stimulating platelet aggregation and vasoconstriction
- Activation of the clotting mechanism and the formation of fibrin

A clot is made up of insoluble fibrin filaments and platelets that join together to form a durable mesh. Clot formation occurs through a series of complex interactions involving platelets, tissue thromboplastin, clotting factors, prothrombin, fibrinogen, and fibrin. Fibrin is derived from the protein fibrinogen that is produced in the liver and present in the plasma. Fibrinogen is a stable structure and converts to fibrin only under the influence of thrombin.

Prothrombin, a naturally occurring plasma protein, is converted to thrombin, in the setting of injury to specific blood components. Injury activates and accelerates the formation of thrombin. The formation of thrombin from prothrombin requires a highly complex, integrated network. Adequate calcium, vitamin K, phospholipids, and at least seven plasma proteins (factor V, factor VIII, and factors IX to XIII) are necessary for thrombin formation. Thromboplastin is also required; at the time of injury, injured tissue releases thromboplastin and therefore makes it available to interact with factor X (Fig. 14-2).[7] Although clotting is essentially one multistep process, it may be viewed as two concurrent, interactive, and somewhat overlapping processes that converge at a common site, the prothrombin activator, factor X. The two pathways are the extrinsic pathway that is initiated by an injury to the vascular wall and adjacent tissue and the intrinsic pathway, which is activated by injury to the blood cells, which subsequently results in increased platelet aggregation and adherence.

Once clot formation has occurred, the process of clot lysis occurs. Under normal conditions, this occurs a few days after the bleeding site has been stabilized. Naturally occurring tissue plasminogen activator (t-PA) is slowly released from the injured tissue and converts plasminogen, a plasma protein (also present in the thrombus), into plasmin.[8] Plasmin actively lyses the thrombus, resulting in the formation of fibrin fragments and the dissolution of the clot (Fig. 14-2B).

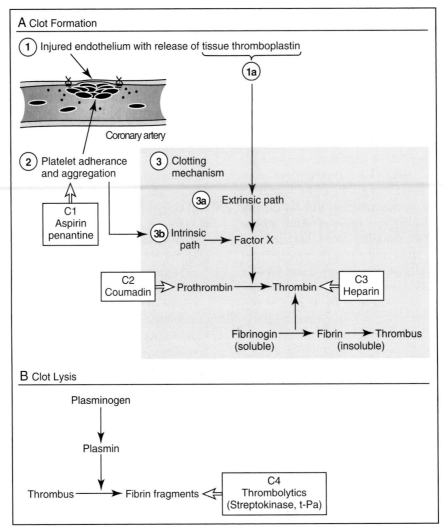

**Figure 14-2  A,** Clot formation. **1,** At the site of an atherosclerotic lesion, injured endothelium releases tissue thromboplastin **(Ia).** **2,** As a result of the exposed endothelial surface, platelets begin to adhere to its surface and aggregate. **3,** The clotting mechanism is very complex and is presented here in simplified form. **3a,** With the release of thromboplastin, the extrinsic clotting cascade begins. **3b,** The intrinsic clotting cascade begins in response to the injured endothelium and influenced by platelets. The common point for both the intrinsic and extrinsic pathways is factor X, which facilitates the eventual formation of fibrin from fibrinogen by activating thrombin from prothrombin. **B,** Clot lysis can be achieved through the antiplatelet agents aspirin and Persantine **(C1),** the anticoagulant Coumadin (warfarin, **C2),** the anticoagulant heparin **(C3),** or thrombolytics (e.g., streptokinase and t-PA, **C4),** which activate plasminogen into plasmin at the site of action of these specific drugs.

### Pharmacologic Intervention

Pharmacologic management of myocardial ischemia involves the reestablishment of a balance between myocardial oxygen supply and myocardial oxygen demand. This can be accomplished by decreasing oxygen demand or by increasing oxygen supply. Drugs that decrease either the heart rate or systemic blood pressure decrease the myocardial oxygen demand. Drugs that increase arterial lumen size by decreasing either coronary arterial spasm or thrombus increase myocardial oxygen supply. At present, no drug exists that acutely and emergently dissolves the fixed atherosclerotic plaques in the coronary vessels. Reduction of risk factors for coronary artery disease and aggressive lipid management with or without the use of drugs have been shown in controlled settings to result in a slow regression of coronary plaque.[9]

Clinical diagnoses associated with myocardial oxygen supply–demand imbalance are myocardial ischemia, acute coronary syndrome, and myocardial infarction. As a result of an imbalance in myocardial supply–demand, ventricular arrhythmias and acute heart failure may also occur in

> **Clinical Tip**
> Myocardial ischemia is a reversible process. Myocardial infarction is irreversible and involves permanent tissue death. ACS is a temporary condition that results in either a myocardial infarction or an aborted myocardial infarction or MI. Pharmacologic management at each phase of the continuum from ischemia to infarction is driven by the pathophysiologic conditions, patient's hemodynamic stability, and patient comfort.

addition to tissue injury. Pharmacologic management of these conditions is also imperative to establish hemodynamic stability.

## Drugs That Decrease Myocardial Oxygen Demand

Current medications used to decrease $MVO_2$ are β-blockers, which decrease heart rate and contractility; calcium-channel blockers, which inhibit coronary vasospasm and dilate coronary blood vessels; and nitrates, which decrease both peripheral vascular resistance and venous return or preload.

### β-Blockers

β-Adrenergic antagonists compete with the catecholamines epinephrine and norepinephrine for β-receptor–binding sites. β-Adrenergic antagonists therefore block catecholamines from binding and limiting their effects. β-Antagonist activity may be complete (blocking all catecholamine stimulation) or partial (some catecholamine stimulation). Of the two β subtypes, $β_1$-receptors are found primarily in the myocardium and have an equal affinity for epinephrine and norepinephrine. $β_2$-Receptors have a higher affinity for epinephrine than norepinephrine; they are also found in the myocardium, especially the atria, but the majority of receptor sites are found within the peripheral circulation and bronchi. Inhibition of catecholamine stimulation by β-blockers affects the heart by decreasing heart rate, decreasing contractility, decreasing cardiac output, and decreasing blood pressure. These reduce the oxygen demand of the heart.

Drugs that block both $β_1$ and $β_2$-receptors are referred to as nonselective whereas drugs that block $β_1$-receptors more preferentially are referred to as cardioselective or $β_1$-selective. Patients with disease processes involving the sites of $β_2$-receptors, especially the bronchi, (e.g., asthma), and to a lesser degree the peripheral circulation, pose a challenging problem in drug management when they require β-adrenergic blockade for management of their cardiovascular disease. In that case, use of a nonselective β-blocker would not only decrease myocardial oxygen cost by decreasing heart rate and blood pressure but also have the unfortunate effect of enhancing bronchospasm. Therefore, $β_1$-selective drugs rather than a nonselective β-blocker are usually prescribed for patients with chronic obstructive pulmonary disease or peripheral vascular disease to avoid the unwanted $β_2$-antagonist effects. Because no $β_1$-selective antagonist is able to completely avoid interactions with $β_2$-receptors, caution should be exercised in prescribing β-blockers for patients with pulmonary disease.

β-Blockers may also have α-adrenergic blocking activity (Table 14-3). This combination results in a decrease in systemic vascular resistance without a compensatory increase in heart rate. The α-blocking component causes vasodilation and thus results in decreased systemic vascular resistance or SVR. A decrease in SVR would normally be accompanied by a compensatory increase in heart rate. The β-blocking component suppresses the compensatory rise in heart rate that would be expected with α-blockade alone, thereby limiting the increase in $MVO_2$. Another category of β-blockers is that

### Table 14-3 β-Adrenergic Antagonists: β-Blockers

| Category | Generic (Trade) |
| --- | --- |
| Nonselective | Propranolol (Inderal) |
| | Timolol (Blocadren) |
| | Nadolol (Corgard) |
| | Sotalol (Betapace, Sorin) |
| $β_1$ Selective | Metoprolol (Lopressor) |
| | Atenolol (Tenormin) |
| | Acebutolol (Sectral) |
| | Esmolol (Brevibloc) |
| | Bisoprolol (Zebeta) |
| | Nebivolol (Bystolic) |
| $β_2$-Selective | Butoxamine |
| α- And β-antagonists | Labetalol (Normodyne, Trandate) |
| | Carvedilol (Coreg) |
| β-Blockers with intrinsic sympathomimetic activity | Penbutolol (Levatol) |
| | Pindolol (Visken) |

of β-blockers with both antagonistic and agonistic properties. They are β-antagonists with intrinsic sympathomimetic activity or ISA. These drugs block high β-receptor activity while stimulating these receptors during periods of low activity.

**Side effects of β-blockers.** The potential side effects associated with the use of β-blockers are varied. "Three major mechanisms … (of side effects) … are through (1) central nervous penetration (sedation), (2) smooth muscle spasm (bronchospasm and cold extremities), and (3) exaggeration of the cardiac therapeutic actions (bradycardia, orthostatic hypotension, heart block, excess negative inotropic effect with heart failure)."[10] $β_1$-Selective drugs such as atenolol (Tenormin) should have fewer peripheral side effects of bronchospasm, cold extremities, worsening claudication, and sexual dysfunction than nonselective drugs like propranolol (Inderal). β-Blockers also may cause fatigue, insomnia, depression, masking of symptoms, of hypoglycemia (e.g., tachycardia) in diabetic patients, impaired glucose tolerance, hypertriglyceridemia, and decreased high-density lipoprotein (HDL) cholesterol. Serious adverse reactions like agranulocytosis are rare.

Their actions can be decreased by use of barbiturates and increased by cimetidine. The antihypertensive effect can be increased by a number of herbal preparations, such as mistletoe, kelp, black cohosh, and dandelions.

The popularity of β-blockers as part of an antiischemic regimen cannot be disputed. β-Blockers, however, have also been used in the treatment of the following conditions: hypertension; congestive heart failure (CHF); cardiac arrhythmias; glaucoma; hyperthyroidism; mitral valve prolapse; and various neurologic disorders, such as migraine headaches, alcohol withdrawal, and anxiety. Awareness of the potential side effects of β-blockade for these patient populations is certainly clinically relevant. As with patients with peripheral vascular disease and chronic obstructive pulmonary disease, the use of β$_1$-selective drugs may also be preferred for patients with diabetes. β$_2$-Receptors of the liver activate glycogenolysis; however, a nonselective β-blocker suppresses this action. Use of a β$_1$-selective drug minimizes the suppression of this critical function. Poor tolerance of one β-blocker does not mean that all β-blockers will be poorly tolerated; experimentation and trial and error are credible clinical tools in assessing the compatibility of the patient–drug interaction.

> **Clinical Tip**
> β-Blockers may mask the symptoms of hypoglycemia. Caution should be taken during exercise with patients who have diabetes and who are also taking β-blockers. Awareness to the signs and symptoms of hypoglycemia and a quick and appropriate intervention are imperative.

Although β-blockers are negative inotropes, they have been used successfully in the clinical management of patients with impaired LV function (e.g., when ejection fraction is less than 35%). Improved management of this patient population has also been found when β-blockers with α-blocking activity, such as carvedilol (Coreg), is used. It has been well described in controlled clinical trials that carvedilol administered twice daily improves the LVEF in patients with ischemic or nonischemic heart failure. If a patient on a β-blocker, regardless of the reason that he or she was initially put on the drug, begins to complain of new-onset dyspnea, ankle or extremity edema, and breathing problems such as orthopnea, or there are other signs/symptoms of heart failure, the appropriate physical therapy intervention is to defer treatment and discuss these findings with the physician before continuing with treatment. Once the patient has stabilized and is medically cleared to continue with physical therapy, treatment should begin slowly, patient tolerance should be assessed on an ongoing basis, and the appropriate physical therapy examination to rule out edema and hemodynamic instability should be conducted.

β-Blockers decrease both resting and exercise heart rates. Before prescribing aerobic exercise based on heart rate for a patient on β-blockers, it is necessary to know the heart rate response and results of the patient's performance on an exercise tolerance test given with the same drug and dosage that the patient is presently taking. There does not appear to be a reliable relationship between heart rate response and drug dosages among individual drugs. A patient who was changed from propranolol (Inderal) to metoprolol (Lopressor) has a different exercise heart rate response on each drug and may therefore need a new exercise prescription, a new exercise tolerance test, or both. Prescribing exercise by RPE (rate of perceived exertion) is a reasonable alternative to exercise prescription by heart rate; however, the physical therapist must document the physiologic response at the desired RPE.

A potentially interesting relationship may exist between weight control and β-blockers. Fat cells have β$_1$-receptors, which, when stimulated, activate lipolysis. With β-blockade, lipolysis is inhibited. Clinical observation has been that patients on β-blockers have a difficult time achieving weight loss. Whether this is owing to decreased metabolism, fatigue, lipocyte inhibition, or some other factor or combination of factors remains to be seen.

**Calcium-channel blockers.** Calcium-channel blockers do not fit exclusively into either category of decreasing myocardial oxygen demand or increasing myocardial oxygen supply; they influence both. They decrease myocardial oxygen demand by decreasing arterial blood pressure and may increase supply by facilitating vascular smooth muscle relaxation. Calcium-channel blockers are discussed in detail under the section regarding increasing myocardial oxygen supply; its effects on myocardial oxygen demand as well as supply are discussed at that time.

### Nitrates

First synthesized in 1846, nitroglycerin and its analogues are perhaps one of the oldest antiischemic medications. Nitrates are converted in the vessels to nitric oxide (NO is also an endogenous endothelial relaxing factor), which increases the action of the secondary messenger cyclic guanosine monophosphate or cGMP. This seems to stimulate a kinase enzyme that decreases the sensitivity of the contractile proteins to calcium and relaxes the blood vessels. This group of drugs is unusually selective in that it almost exclusively acts on smooth muscle cells, in particular on vascular smooth muscle. Nitroglycerin acts physiologically in at least three ways[11]:

- As a venodilator, thus decreasing venous return (preload)
- As an arteriodilator, thus decreasing afterload
- As a relaxant for coronary artery smooth muscle, thus possibly increasing coronary blood supply

These factors decrease myocardial oxygen demand, specifically in their ability to decrease venous return and left ventricular filling pressures. Besides their use for antiischemia, nitrates may also be prescribed for the management of congestive heart failure by decreasing preload and for the control of diastolic hypertension. Many different preparations of nitrates are available. Routes of administration and duration of action vary widely among the preparations, from the immediate- and short-acting sublingual nitroglycerin to the slow-release, longer-acting transdermal patch (Table 14-4).

Perhaps the side effect of nitrate therapy that is most troublesome to patients is headache, particularly with the short-acting sublingual tablet and during the "adjustment" stage when a long-acting transdermal patch is started. Other potential side effects resulting from the vasodilator action are as follows:

- Hypotension and dizziness
- Reflex tachycardia
- Flushing of the skin
- Nausea and vomiting

Because hypotension may accompany the use of nitrates, it is recommended that when taking nitroglycerin for the first

## Table 14-4 Nitrate Preparations

| Generic Name | Trade or Common Name | Duration and Comments |
|---|---|---|
| Amyl nitrate inhalation | Aspiryl, Vaporole | 10 sec–10 min |
| Nitroglycerin (glyceryl trinitrate) | Nitro-Bid, Nitrostat, Nitro Bid, Nitrol, others | |
| Sublingual | | 1½ min–1 hr peak: 2 min |
| Spray | | Effects apparent in 5 min: duration unknown |
| Percutaneous ointment | | 3–4 hr |
| Oral, sustained relief | | 8–12 hr |
| Intravenous | | During infusion and 30 min after infusion |
| Transdermal patch | Nitro-Dur | Suggest wearing patch 12–14 hr: remove after 10–12 hr |
| | Transderm-Nitro | |
| | Nitrodisc | |
| | Deponit | |
| | Minitran | |
| Isosorbide dinitrate | Isordil, Sorbitrate, Isonate | |
| Sublingual | | 5–60 min |
| Oral | | 15 min–4 hr |
| Chewable | | 2 min–2½ hr |
| Oral, sustained release | ISMO | Reported 2–6 hr free from angina |
| Isosorbide mononitrate | ISMO, Imdur, Monoket | |
| Pentaerythritol tetranitrate | | |
| Sublingual | Peritrate | 10–30 min |
| Oral | Pentrinitrol | 30 min–12 hr |
| | Pentafin | 4–5 hr |
| Sustained release | Vasitol | 30 min–12 hr |
| Erythrityl tetranitrate | | |
| Oral | Tetranitrol | 30 min–4 hr |
| | Erythrol tetranitrate | 30 min–2–4 hr |
| Sublingual | Cardilate | 5 min–2–4 hr |

*Adapted from Opie LH (ed). Drugs for the Heart, ed 2. Philadelphia, 1987, Saunders; Hahn AB, Barkin RL, Oestrrich, SJK. Pharmacology in Nursing, ed 15. St. Louis, 1982, Mosby.*

time, the patient should be seated. If a patient in the physical therapy clinic takes a sublingual nitroglycerin tablet either before or as a result of a physical therapy intervention, it is important to reevaluate both the intervention and the patient (e.g., heart rate, blood pressure) before making a decision to continue with the planned treatment. Use of prophylactic sublingual nitroglycerin is sometimes recommended before exercise, but this decision must be by physician order and cannot be decided by the physical therapist and patient. Patients should store nitroglycerin in a dark container, keep it tightly closed, and avoid moisture. Once the jar is opened the tablets begin to lose their potency. Unused sublingual nitroglycerin should be discarded according to the manufacturer's recommendation, often within 3 to 6 months of opening. Active sublingual nitroglycerin gives a burning sensation when placed under the tongue. If the nitroglycerin does not "burn," the effect of the drug may be substantially reduced. Nitroglycerin is also available in the form of a lingual spray, which has a longer shelf-life than the sublingual preparations.

> **Clinical Tip**
> Use of one to three nitroglycerin tablets usually terminates an attack of angina quickly. If discomfort and pain persist, then this might be the sign of a heart attack, and the physical therapist should call 911 immediately.

Long-acting nitrates may cause a nitrate tolerance to develop, such that the drug receptors become desensitized. Use of interval dosage, with nitrate-free times (often at night), may prolong receptor site sensitivity. Patients must be informed that they are not to alter their prescribed drug

## Table 14-5 Antithrombotic Agents[a]

| Parmacologic Agent | Action | Generic (Trade) Name |
| --- | --- | --- |
| Thrombolytic agents | Facilitate the conversion of plasminogen to plasmin | Alteplase recombinant t-PA (Activase) |
| | | Anistreplase (Eminase) |
| | | Drotrecogin alfa (Xigris) |
| | | Reteplase (Retavase) |
| | | Streptokinase (Streptase) |
| | | Tenecteplase (TNKase) |
| | | Urokinase (Abbokinase) |
| Antiplatelet drugs | Decrease platelet aggregation | Abciximab (ReoPro) |
| | | Acetylsalicylic acid (aspirin) |
| | | Cilostazol (Pletal) |
| | | Clopidogrel (Plavix) |
| | | Dipyridamole (Persantine) |
| | | Eptifibatide (Integrilin) |
| | | Prasugrel (Effient) |
| | | Ticlopidine (Ticlid) |
| | | Tirofiban (Aggrastat) |
| | | Treprostini (Remodulin) |
| Anticoagulants | Thrombin inhibitor | Heparin sodium (Heparin): unfractionated heparin |
| | | LMWH: Low molecular weight heparin |
| | | Dalteparin Sodium (Fragmin) |
| | | Enoxaparin Sodium (Lovenox; Clexane) |
| | | Tinzaparin sodium (Innohep) |
| | | Argatroban (Acova) |
| | | Bivalirudin (Angiomax) |
| | | Desirudin (Iprivask) |
| | | Fondaparinux Sodium (Arixtra) |
| | | Lepirudin (rDNA) (Refludan) |
| | | Warfarin sodium (Coumadin) |

[a]*See Figure 14-2.*

schedule without consulting their health care provider. Nitrates must be given along their prescribed route; for example, taking sublingual nitroglycerin orally markedly decreases its effectiveness.

Drug interactions occur with other antihypertensive medications that enhance their hypotensive effects. Drugs used for erectile dysfunction, such as sildenafil and others, can cause severe hypotensive episodes combined with fainting and should not be used with these drugs.

## Drugs That Increase Myocardial Oxygen Supply

Pharmacologic interventions to increase myocardial oxygen supply in coronary artery disease are limited. Although calcium-channel blockers and nitrates may have secondary effects because of coronary vasodilation, and calcium-channel blockers can decrease coronary artery spasm, no direct pharmacologic way exists to increase coronary blood flow in the presence of ischemic heart disease. The prevention of an impending acute myocardial infarction includes the emergent use of thrombolytic or fibrinolytic and antiplatelet agents as part of acute coronary syndrome management.

For an outline of thrombolytic agents, antiplatelet agents, and anticoagulants, please see Table 14-5.

### Thrombolytic Agents

The purpose of these drugs is to acutely destroy (lyse) or decrease the blood clot (thrombus) formation that occurs within the coronary artery at the time of plaque rupture. In doing so, some coronary blood flow within the affected area is maintained, and reduction in infarction size may be possible. Thrombolytic agents work by slightly different mechanisms, but all facilitate the conversion of plasminogen to plasmin, and therefore clot lysis can occur quickly rather than over a period of days that would naturally occur.

To achieve the goal of increasing coronary blood flow, medical decisions need to be made regarding the acute management of the patient with ruptured plaque and thrombus formation, who presents with cardiac symptoms and ST elevation on ECG (Chapter 3). The American College of Cardiology (ACC) and American Heart Association (AHA) suggest the following recommendations[12]: If the patient is a candidate for PCI (percutaneous coronary intervention), then the goal is to perform the angioplasty within 90 minutes of presenting to the emergency room ("door to balloon" interval). If the patient presents to a facility that does not perform PCIs or cannot be transferred to a facility and have the procedure performed within 90 minutes, then the use of thrombolytics is warranted ("door to needle"). The suggested goal is to treat with fibrinolytics within 30 minutes of hospital presentation[12]; however, when that time frame is not possible, "[the writing group believes] that every effort should be made to reduce the time … from first medical contact to fibrinolytic therapy when that is considered the appropriate reperfusion strategy."[12] The American College of Cardiology and the American Heart Association (ACC/AHA) guidelines state that the overall goal in treatment of this patient population is to keep total ischemic time less than 120 minutes from onset of symptoms to reperfusion, either via PCI or thrombolytics.[12]

In the consideration of thrombolytics, a history of bleeding abnormalities, cerebral vascular events, or uncontrolled hypertension may be contraindications. Risks associated with thrombolytic use include systemic bleeding. An agent such as streptokinase (Kabikinase, Streptase) is not fibrin specific and has the potential to produce systemic lysis; in contrast, t-PA is fibrin-specific, thereby causing fewer systemic effects than streptokinase.

Although thrombolytic agents may limit the amount of myocardial tissue damage, the use of these agents is not without risk. Thrombolytic agents are not absolutely tissue-specific; therefore, systemic bleeding may occur as well as lysis of the coronary thrombus. Potential undesirable side effects include the following:
- Cerebrovascular accidents
- Genitourinary bleeding
- Gastrointestinal bleeding

In addition, these medications are used for acute cerebral ischemic attacks if the cerebral ischemic attack is not from a hemorrhagic stroke.

Ventricular arrhythmias are common within the acute time frame following thrombolysis and are believed to be in response to tissue reperfusion and do not therefore require prolonged antiarrhythmic management. Care must be taken with thrombolytic agents to avoid situations of potential tissue trauma such as venipunctures, manual shaving, high-intensity resistive exercises, or soft tissue injury because the patient's blood clotting ability is markedly altered during this period. Cardiac rehabilitation physical therapy, including progressive ambulation and strength training, may proceed within established acceptable guidelines.

Rethrombosis can occur following thrombolysis, and therefore anticoagulants are usually coadministered and continued after thrombolytic therapy for a period of time.

### Antiplatelet Agents
As a strategy for both primary and secondary prevention, antiplatelet agents are given prophylactically to prevent thrombus formation. By decreasing the platelets' ability to adhere and aggregate at the site of the injury, the first step for thrombus formation is deterred. Commonly used agents for this purpose are salicylic acid (aspirin, ASA) and dipyridamole (Persantine) (Fig. 14-2).

Advances in the understanding of clot formation have led to the development of two additional groups of platelet inhibitors. Glycoprotein IIb/IIIa (gp2b/3a) inhibitors block platelet receptors from binding to fibrinogen, consequently limiting platelet aggregation. Abciximab (Reapro) and eptifibatide (Integrelin) are commonly used gp2b/3a inhibitors. These drugs are given intravenously during the management of acute coronary syndrome (ACS). A second group of antiplatelet agents interfere with the adenosine diphosphate (ADP) activator, decreasing the available energy source for platelet aggregation processes. Clopidogrel (Plavix) and ticlopidine (Ticlid) are common drugs that act in this way.[13]

The American Heart Association recommends the use of low-dose aspirin (81 mg) for men with cardiovascular problems only but not necessarily for those who have no predisposing risk factors or past cardiovascular problems. The AHA recommends use of aspirin of an increased dose (325 mg) for women. The use of aspirin may also prevent ischemic but not or might even enhance hemorrhagic strokes[12]

### Anticoagulants
Anticoagulants are used prophylactically to prevent blood clot formation. These agents inhibit the formation of thrombin and thereby prevent the influence of thrombin on fibrinogen. Anticoagulants may also be used when a thrombus is already formed to prevent emboli. Commonly used agents are heparin sodium (Heparin, Liquaemin Sodium), enoxaparin sodium (low-molecular-weight heparin [LMWH]; Clexane, Lovenox), and warfarin (Coumadin).

### Calcium-Channel Blockers
There are two sources of calcium within the body:
- Intracellular calcium, stored within the sarcoplasmic reticulum
- Extracellular calcium, stored within the plasma

Different tissue types have an affinity for the different sources of calcium. Smooth muscle, located within the coronary arteries and peripheral vascular system as well as within the sinoatrial and atrioventricular nodes of the heart, is more dependent on extracellular calcium; striated muscle, myocardium, and coronary veins have a primary affinity for intracellular calcium.

Calcium plays a key role in muscular contraction. The process of muscular contraction requires the availability of actin, myosin, troponin, tropomyosin, and calcium. In order

## Table 14-6 Calcium-Channel Blockers

| Generic (Trade) | Common Usage[a] | Side Effects Common to All |
|---|---|---|
| Amlodipine (Lotrel, Norvasc) | Blood pressure control | Cough reflex[b] |
| Bepridil (Vascor) | Chronic stable angina | Tremor, dry mouth[c] |
| Diltiazem (Cardizem) | Ischemic heart disease | Constipation[d] |
| Felodipine (Plendil) | Blood pressure control | Pharyngitis |
| | | Ankle edema |
| Isradipine (Dyna-Circ) | Similar to nifedipine but may have less reflex tachycardia | Dizziness |
| Nicardipine (Cardene) | Blood pressure control | Headache |
| Nifedipine (Procardia, Adalat) | Blood Pressure Control | Orthostatic hypotension[e] |
| Nimodipine (Nimotop) | | GI upset |
| Nisoldipine (Sultar, Solar) | Blood pressure control | Peripheral edema |
| Verapamil (Isoptin, Calan) | Supraventricular arrhythmias | Flushing |

[a]Prevention of coronary spasm is common to all.
[b]Especially amlodipine.
[c]Especially bepridil.
[d]Especially verapamil and diltiazem.
[e]Especially nifedipine and nicardipine.

for actin and myosin to form cross bridges, calcium must bind with troponin. Troponin, when not bound to calcium, inhibits coupling of actin and myosin. In the absence of calcium, troponin is free to inhibit the actin–myosin interaction, thereby reducing or inhibiting contraction. Calcium-channel blockers block the entrance of calcium into the cell from the extracellular stores. Calcium-channel blockers therefore relax systemic and coronary blood vessels (i.e., coronary spasm).

Calcium-channel blockers were initially used as part of an antiischemic regimen[14]; the ability to decrease vasospasm and facilitate vasodilatation contributes to improved oxygenated blood flow (Table 14-6).

In addition to that primary role, specific calcium-channel blockers are now also used for

- Arrhythmia control, particularly supraventricular tachycardia
- Blood pressure control
- Reducing the incidence of reinfarction in patients with non–Q-wave infarcts

(See the subsequent sections on drug management of hypertension and arrhythmia for further discussion.)

Myocardial ischemia causes an influx of calcium ions into the cell. This increase in intracellular calcium elevates the cellular metabolic rate, which in turn elevates myocardial oxygen demand. Decreasing intracellular calcium may therefore decrease myocardial oxygen demand.

Although calcium-channel blockers are relatively safe drugs with few serious side effects, these medications may have negative inotropic properties at high doses; therefore clinical observation for heart failure is warranted. Orthostatic hypotension often occurs in the initiation and regulation of dosages of nifedipine (Procardia), so the clinician should be

sensitized to watching for orthostatic signs and symptoms when initiating an increase in activity orders or when assisting the patient out of bed for the first time. New onset of symptoms such as peripheral edema and persistent cough should be thoroughly investigated before deciding that they are primarily due to the use of calcium-channel blockers. Additional side effects include headache, drowsiness, and flushing.

Actions are increased by other antihypertensive drugs, and some drugs can decrease the effectiveness of lithium. Grapefruit juice and several herbal products can increase their hypotensive effects.

### Heart Failure

Heart failure is a neurohormonal disorder that includes not just the left ventricle but other body systems as well (see Chapter 4). The clinical presentation varies according to the pathophysiology of LV dysfunction and how well the disease is compensated; it may present as well compensated with minimal impact on function, easily managed by oral medications over a period of years or in extreme cases it may be acute and life-threatening, requiring the use of parenteral medications to maintain an adequate cardiac output and tissue perfusion. As the understanding of the disease process, progression, symptomatology and neurohormonal characteristics has evolved, so too have the classification stages. This system now includes Stages A and B for patients without clinical signs and symptoms of heart failure but who are at risk for its development and includes Stage C, patients who have presented with clinical symptoms and Stage D, patients who require advanced management (Chapter 4). Recommendations for pharmacologic

## Table 14-7 Stages of Heart Disease

| Stage A | Stage B | Stage C | Stage D |
|---|---|---|---|
| No structural heart disease | Structural heart disease | Symptomatic heart disease | Severely symptomatic |
| Treat underlying medical conditions (e.g., HTN) | As in Stage A | As in Stage A and B | |
| Encourage therapeutic lifestyle changes or TLC (e.g., smoking cessation) | | | |
| Consider[a] ACE inhibitor or ARB | Consider[a] ACE inhibitor or ARB | Diuretics | See critical care |
| | Consider[a] β-blockers | ACE inhibitor | |
| | | β-Blockers | |
| | | Consider[a] | |
| | | Aldosterone antagonist | |
| | | ARBs | |
| | | Digitalis | |
| | | Nitrates/hydralazine | |

[a]*In appropriate patients.*
*Adapted from ACC/AHA 2005 Guideline Update for the Diagnosis and Management of Chronic Heart Failure in the Adult—summary article: a report of the American College of Cardiology/American Heart Association Task Force on Practice Guidelines (writing committee to update the 2001 guidelines for the evaluation and management of heart failure): developed in collaboration with the American College of Chest Physicians and the International Society for Heart and Lung Transplantation: Endorsed by the Heart Rhythm Society. Circulation 112:1825-1852, 2005; Hunt SA, Abraham WT, Chin MH, et al.*
*ACE, angiotensin-converting enzyme; ARB, angiotensin-receptor blocker; HTN, hypertension; TLC, therapeutic lifestyle changes.*

management of heart failure are influenced by the stage of the disease (Table 14-7). Pharmacologic management is a dynamic variable that takes into consideration the systemic as well as the cardiovascular effects of the disease. Effective pharmacologic management is most successful when close patient monitoring occurs and an easy system exists for dynamic, ongoing reevaluation and aggressive pharmacologic intervention as determined by the degree of hemodynamic compromise.

In general, the following categorizes the drugs that are commonly used for LV and systemic management of CHF: sympathetic antagonists with β-blockers, preload reduction with diuretics, angiotensin-converting enzyme (ACE) inhibitors, angiotensin-receptor blockers (ARB), or aldosterone antagonists. In critical care situations, management may expand to include increased inotropy with cardiac glycosides, sympathomimetics, or bipyridines; afterload reduction with arteriodilators, calcium-channel blockers, ACE inhibitors, or ARBs.

### Physiology

For a more complete review of cardiovascular physiology, please refer to Chapter 2. This discussion will serve only as a brief review of key concepts influential in the drug management of heart failure.

The heart is a pump, the function of which is to provide oxygenated blood to all parts of the body. The amount of blood that the heart is able to pump per minute is called the cardiac output. Cardiac output is directly affected by

stroke volume (the amount the left ventricle pumps out with each heart beat) and the heart rate (the number of heart beats per minute). The factors that influence stroke volume are preload, afterload, and contractility (Table 14-8). Drugs that increase myocardial contractility are known as positive inotropes and drugs that decrease contractility as negative inotropes.

### Pathophysiology

Heart failure occurs when the heart is unable (i.e., fails) to provide sufficient cardiac output to serve the metabolic needs of the body. Heart failure occurs, therefore, because of impairment in heart rate, stroke volume, or both or, more specifically, because of failure of their components: rhythm, preload, afterload, and/or contractility. There are a variety of situations that may induce heart failure, such as the following[15]:

- Significant loss of contractile tissue as a result of a myocardial infarction
- Arrhythmias (especially if cardiac output is impaired as a result)
- Increased preload associated with fluid overload
- Increased afterload as seen with hypertension
- Significant decrease in contractility as a result of ischemia, cardiac muscle dysfunction, or cardiomyopathy

The most common cause of CHF is coronary artery disease (CAD), particularly for those patients who have had a previous MI. There are many degrees of heart failure, from mild, in which the symptoms of decreased cardiac output are

## Table 14-8 Factors that influence Stroke Volume

| Factors | Definition | Influenced by/ Dependent on |
|---------|-----------|------------------------------|
| Preload | Filling pressure of the left ventricle (left ventricular end-diastolic pressure) | Venous return<br>Distention of the left ventricle |
| Afterload | Resistance against which the left ventricle contracts | Arterial pressure<br>Resistance across the aortic valve |
| Contractility (inotropy) | Ability of the myocardial muscle to contract | Adequate amounts of sodium, potassium, and calcium to facilitate cellular depolarization and actin–myosin interaction |

apparent only with moderate activity, to severe, in which the heart fails to provide adequate cardiac output even at rest. Heart failure is a chronic disease with systemic effects requiring dynamic, ongoing reevaluation and aggressive pharmacologic intervention as determined by the amount of hemodynamic compromise.

## Pharmacologic Intervention

Drug management of heart failure attempts to address the underlying contribution to the failure and to maintain an adequate cardiac output. Initial treatment of mild heart failure involves regulating fluids and salt intake, decreasing preload, decreasing afterload, decreasing sympathetic stimulation, and improving contractility through oral medications. As the hemodynamic compromise progresses and the clinical picture declines (progressing from Stage A to Stage D), medical management broadens to include parenteral medications, oxygen, and sedation (to decrease anxiety and metabolic energy) Categories of drugs commonly used during the management of the various stages of heart failure are (Table 14-9):

- Diuretics
- β-Blockers
- ACE/ARB
- Calcium-channel blockers
- Vasodilators
- Positive inotropes

Morphine and oxygen are used in critical care management and stabilization of the patient in Stage D heart failure (see Critical Care section). Morphine reduces anxiety and discomfort associated with pulmonary edema but also has a

vasodilatation effect reducing preload. There are no exclusive drug categories for the treatment of diastolic dysfunction. Optimizing filling pressures and blood pressure control as well as optimally treating any comorbidities is part of the overall comprehensive management plan.

### Diuretics

Diuretics can be used alone but mostly in combination with other drugs. In these cases, drugs can be given separately but combination products are also available like lisinopril and hydrochlorothiazide (Prinzide, Zestoretic) or metoprolol/hydrochlorothiazide (Lopressor HCT). As a first-line drug for the management of heart failure, diuretics decrease circulating blood volume, thereby decreasing preload. Diuretics encourage diuresis and influence water and electrolyte balance by inhibiting sodium and water reabsorption.[16] The influence on diuresis is dependent on the site of action of the drug within the kidneys. The strongest diuretics are those that act at Henle loop (loop diuretics); the milder diuretics are those that act on the proximal tubules and the collecting tubules and ducts. The most common diuretic for symptomatic heart failure is the loop diuretic furosemide (Lasix), which, besides sodium inhibition, also inhibits the movement of potassium and chloride across the plasma membrane of the ascending Henle loop.

Diuretics reduce preload with resultant improvement in the ventricular length–tension relationship. This improved mechanical advantage optimizes contractility and reduces myocardial oxygen demand.

Spironolactone (Aldactone, Alatone) is a comparatively weak diuretic in relation to Lasix. It is used in the management of heart failure, not for its diuretic effect but for its secondary effect of suppression of aldosterone. Aldosterone is a key component in the rennin–angiotensin–aldosterone system (RAAS), and suppression of aldosterone favorably decreases the adverse effect of the RAAS on the management of heart failure.

The subsequent section on antihypertension drugs provides an expanded list of diuretics and their sites of action (see Fig. 14-7; Table 14-10).

### β-Blockers

In their review of multiple controlled studies regarding the efficacy of the use of β-blockers in patients with heart failure (HF), the ACC/AHA in 2009 jointly stated that the "long-term treatment with beta blockers can lessen the symptoms of HF, improve the clinical status of patients, and enhance the patient's overall sense of well-being. ... In addition, like ACE inhibitors, beta blockers can reduce the risk of death and the combined risk of death or hospitalization. These benefits of beta blockers were seen in patients with or without coronary artery disease and in patients with or without diabetes mellitus, as well as in women and black patients. The favorable effects of beta blockers were also observed in patients already taking ACE inhibitors, which suggests that combined blockade of the 2 neurohormonal systems can produce additive effects."[17]

## Table 14-9 Pharmacologic Management of Heart Failure

| | Category | Generic (Trade) Name | | Side Effects |
|---|---|---|---|---|
| Diuretics | Thiazide | Chlorothiazide (Diuril) Hydrochlorothiazide | | Headache, nausea, muscle cramps, hypokalemia, agranulocytosis (severe adverse reactions with aconite) |
| | Thiazide-like | Chlorthalidone (Thalitone) Indapamide (Lozol) Metolazone (Zaroxolyn) | | See above |
| | Loop | Bumetanide (Bumex) Ethacrynic acid (Edecrin) Furosemide (Lasix) Torsemide (Demadex) | | See above (plus jaundice, renal failure, Steven–Johnson syndrome) |
| | Potassium sparing | Amiloride (Midamor) Triamterene (Dyrenium) Eplerenone (Inspra) Spironolactone (Aldactone) | | See above (hyperkalemia, and foods high in potassium can contribute) |
| | Osmotic | Mannitol Urea | | |
| Positive inotropes | Cardiac glycosides | Digitalis | Digitoxin (Crystodigin) Digoxin (Lanoxin) Deslanoside (Cedilanid-DIV) | Toxicity common |
| | Sympathomimetics | $\beta_1$ | Dobutamine (Dobutrex)[a] Prenalterol | Arrhythmias |
| | | Nonselective $\beta$ | Epinephrine (Adrenalin Chloride)[a] Isoproterenol (Isuprel)[a] | Tachycardia |
| | | Dopaminergic | Dopamine (Intropin, Dopastat)[a] | Myocardial ischemia similar to $\beta$ |
| | | Mixed $\alpha$ and $\beta$ | Norepinephrine (Levophed)[a] | May cause dangerous decrease in peripheral blood flow owing to peripheral and visceral vasoconstriction. |
| | Bipyridines | | Amrinone (Inocor)[a] | Nausea and vomiting Thrombocytopenia Ventricular ectopy Liver abnormalities |
| Vasodilators | Venodilators Nitrates Arteriolar | See Table 14-4 Hydralazine (Apresoline) Minoxidil (Loniten) Milrinone (Primacor)[a] Enoximone (Perfan) (investigational)[a] | | Hydralazine: tachycardia Palpitations, orthostatic hypotension, rebound hypotension Fluid retention Both hydralazine and minoxidil should be used with a $\beta$-blocker and diuretic. |

*Continued*

## Table 14-9 Pharmacologic Management of Heart Failure—cont'd

| Category | | Generic (Trade) Name | Side Effects |
|---|---|---|---|
| Vasodilators (cont'd) | | Vesnarinone (investigational) | Minoxidil is useful when renal failure accompanies heart failure. |
| | | Nifedipine (Procardia) | See Table 14-6 |
| | | Diazoxide (Hyperstat IV) | |
| | Combined arteriolar and venodilator | Sodium nitroprusside (Nipride) | Rapid onset of action, delivery via infusion pump |
| | | | May result in excess hypotension, metabolic acidosis, and arrhythmias |
| Angiotensin-converting | Enzyme inhibitors | Captopril (Capoten) | Hypotension |
| | | Enalapril (Vasotec) | Renal failure |
| | | Lisinopril (Prinivil, Zestril) | Neutropenia |
| | | | Skin rashes |
| | | | Taste disturbances |
| Analgesic | | Morphine sulfate (Morphine, MS Contin) | Used in acute pulmonary edema |

[a]Parenteral.

Three β-blockers have been shown to be effective in reducing the risk of death in patients with chronic HF: two β₁-selective receptors—bisoprolol (Zebeta) and sustained-release metoprolol succinate (Toprol XL)—and a nonselective β-blocker with α₁ antagonist properties—carvedilol (Coreg).[18] The choice of which drug to use is multifactorial, including the patient's symptoms and etiology of heart failure. The FDA has approved the use of carvedilol for mild to severe classes of heart failure based upon the results of the COPERNICUS study.[19] Metoprolol succinate has FDA approval for the mild–moderate heart failure based on the results of the MERIT-HF trials.[20]

In discussing the overall use of β-blockers with variable populations, the ACC/AHA position states: "they (beta blockers) are not utilized in a substantial portion of eligible HF patients, possibly because physicians are unsure of the safety and benefit of beta-blockers in special populations (women, the elderly, African Americans, patients with diabetes, and patients with atrial fibrillation). The current standard of care is to treat all heart failure (HF) patients according to the recommendations for the overall population. A review of the clinical trial data reveals that there is no evidence that one evidence-based beta-blocker is preferential over the others in women or in the elderly with HF. In contrast, carvedilol may confer greater benefit in HF patients with diabetes and atrial fibrillation as well as in African American patients."[18] In recent clinical trials, carvedilol has shown improved LVEF and possible remodeling in patients with heart failure.[21]

### Drugs Affecting the Renin–Angiotensin–Aldosterone System

Inhibition of the renin–angiotensin–aldosterone system can take place at multiple sites: at the level of the enzyme that converts angiotensin I to angiotensin II, at the angiotensin receptor, or at the receptor for aldosterone, which is under control of both the renin–angiotensin system and other systemic and local influences (aldosterone antagonists).[17]

**Angiotensin-converting enzyme inhibitors.** When cardiac output is decreased, such as with symptomatic heart failure, perfusion of the renal artery is also decreased. Decreased renal perfusion stimulates the release of renin from the afferent arteriole of the glomerulus. Renin, along with a renin substrate, forms angiotensin I, which converts into angiotensin II (see Fig. 14-8). "This reaction is catalyzed by angiotensin converting enzyme (ACE), which is located in many organs, including the lung, the luminal membrane of vascular epithelial cells, and the juxtaglomerular apparatus itself."[22] Angiotensin II has two key effects: an increase in systemic vascular resistance owing to its effects as a vasoconstrictor and an increase in extracellular volume owing to renal sodium and water retention via aldosterone stimulation.[22] When the conversion of angiotensin I to angiotensin II is inhibited, the clinical effects of angiotensin II are significantly reduced and limited. Inhibitors of the ACE are used in the management of HF in order to decrease the excess intravascular volume that occurs as a result of sodium and water retention and to decrease the afterload due to arterial vasoconstriction. A decrease in volume decreases preload. A

## Table 14-10 Antihypertensive Agents

| Category | | Generic (Trade Name) | Comments |
|---|---|---|---|
| Diuretics | High ceiling (loop) | Bumetanide (Bumex, Burinex) | Mild to severe hypokalemia may occur with diuretics, necessitating $K^+$ supplementation. |
| | | Ethacrynic acid (Edecrin) | |
| | | Furosemide (Lasix, Furomide, Dryptal) | |
| | | Torsemide (Demadex) | |
| | Sulfonamide (thiazide and thiazide-like) | Hydrochlorothiazide[a] (HydroDIURIL, Esidrix, Oretic, Dirame) | |
| | | Chlorothiazide (Diuril, Saluric) | |
| | | Quinethazone (Hydromox, Aquamox) | |
| | | Bendroflumethiazide (Naturetin) | |
| | | Methyclothiazide (Duretic, Enduron, Aquatensen) | |
| | | Polythiazide (Renese) | |
| | | Trichlormethiazide (Naqua, Metahydrin) | |
| | | Metolazone (Zaroxylin, Mykrox, Diulo) | |
| | | Indapamide (Lozol, Natrilix) | |
| | | Chlorthalidone[a] (Hygroton) | |
| | Carbonic anhydrase inhibitors | Acetazolamide (Diamox) | |
| | | Dichlorphenamide (Daranide) | |
| | | Methazolamide (Neptazane) | |
| | Potassium-sparing (aldosterone-receptor blocker; aldosterone antagonist) | Spironolactone (Aldactone, Alatone) | Hyperkalemia may occur with $K^+$-sparing agents. |
| | | Triamterene (Dyrenium, Dytac) | |
| | | Amiloride (Midamor) | |
| | | Eplerenone (Inspra) | |
| | Osmotic combination diuretics | Mannitol (Osmitrol) | |
| Sympathetic nervous system inhibition | Central nervous system acting | Clonidine (Catapres) | May have side effects of sedation, mental depression, and sleep disturbances |
| | | Methyldopa (Aldomet) | |
| | | Guanabenz (Wytensin) | |
| | | Guanfacine (Tenex) | |
| | Ganglion blocking | Trimethaphan (Arfonad) | |
| | Postganglion blocking | Guanethidine (Ismelin Sulfate) | May cause hypotension that is increased with exercise and upright posture |
| | | Guanadrel (Hylorel) | |
| | $\alpha_1$-adrenergic blocking | Prazosin (Minipress) | Prazosin is both a venous and an arterial dilator. |
| | | Terazosin (Hytrin) | |
| | | Doxazosin mesylate (Cardura) | |

*Continued*

## Table 14-10 Antihypertensive Agents—cont'd

| Category | | Generic (Trade Name) | Comments |
|---|---|---|---|
| Sympathetic nervous system inhibition (cont'd) | $\alpha_1$- and $\alpha_2$-adrenergic blocking | Phenoxybenzamine (Dibenzyline) Phentolamine (Regitine) | Useful in treating pheochromocytoma hypertension; decreases peripheral vascular resistance; increases cardiac output |
| | β-Adrenergic blocking | See β-blockers, Table 14-3 | |
| Vasodilators | Venodilators Arteriolar dilators | Nitrates (see Table 14-4) Hydralazine (Apresoline) Minoxidil (Loniten) Diazoxide (Hyperstat IV) Calcium-channel blockers (see Table 14-6) | Hydralazine and minoxidil are used for outpatient, long-term therapy, whereas nitroprusside and diazoxide are parenteral agents, used in emergent conditions; $Ca^{2+}$-channel blockers are used in both acute and chronic conditions. |
| | Combination arteriolar and venodilator | See $\alpha_1$-adrenergic blockers, above Nitroprusside (Nipride) | Nitroprusside is preferred over intravenous $\alpha_1$-adrenergic blockers. |
| Angiotensin-converting enzyme inhibitor | | Captopril (Capoten) Enalapril (Vasotec) Lisinopril (Zestril, Prinivil) Quinapril HCL (Accupril) Fosinopril sodium (Monopril) Benazepril (Lotensin) Ramipril (Altace) Moexipril (Univasc) Perindopril (Aceon) Trandolapril (Mavik) | Severe hypotension in some patients who are hypovolemic due to diuretics, salt restriction, or gastrointestinal fluid loss. Dry hacking cough in 15% to 20% of patients |
| Angiotensin II–receptor antagonist (angiotensin-receptor blocker, ARB) | | Losartan (Cozaar) Candesartan cilexetil (Atacand) Irbesartan (Avapro) Telmisartan (Micardis) Valsartan (Diovan) Eprosartan (Teveten) Olmesartan (Benicar) | Additive effects with hydrochlorothiazide; may be better tolerated than ACE inhibitors; side effects of dizziness, insomnia, leg cramps, gastrointestinal symptoms, upper respiratory effects |

aDiuretic agents most commonly used and least expensive.

decrease in preload in a failing heart decreases myocardial oxygen demand and may improve contractility (refer to sections on diuretics and antihypertensive drugs). Commonly used ACE inhibitors for heart failure are as follows:

- Captopril (Capoten)
- Enalapril (Vasotec)
- Lisinopril (Zestril)

Angiotensin-converting enzyme inhibitors are also used in patients with suppressed LV dysfunction but without signs of overt heart failure. The findings of Studies of Left Ventricular Dysfunction (SOLVD), in which asymptomatic patients with ejection fractions of 35% or less were treated with enalapril, showed a significant reduction in the incidence of symptomatic heart failure and the rate of related hospitalizations.[23]

Pfeffer et al.[24] reported an improvement in survival and reduced morbidity and cardiovascular mortality rates in asymptomatic patients with an ejection fraction of 40% or less who were treated with captopril following an MI. The mechanism of action of the ACE inhibitors in these cases is complex and not fully understood, but they may play a favorable role in limiting adverse ventricular remodeling and ventricular dilatation after MI.[24]

**Angiotensin-receptor blockers.** Angiotensin-converting enzyme inhibitors remain the first choice for inhibition of the renin–angiotensin system in chronic HF, but angiotensin-receptor blockers that inhibit the action of angiotensin II at the vasoconstrictor receptor or ARBs can now be considered a reasonable alternative. Candesartan improved outcomes in patients with preserved LVEF who were intolerant of ACE inhibitors in the Candesartan in Heart Failure Assessment of Reduction in Mortality and Morbidity (CHARM) Alternative trial.[25]

**Aldosterone antagonist.** Spironolactone is the most widely used aldosterone antagonist. In the study reported by Pitt et al.,[26] in which they added low-dose spironolactone to an ACE inhibitor for the management of NYHA Class III and IV CHF patients, the risk of death was reduced from 46% to 35% over 2 years, along with a 35% reduction in HF hospitalization and an improvement in functional class. Although hyperkalemia is a side effect of spironolactone, cautious monitoring of potassium levels has allowed this drug to have an effective role in the management of heart failure.

**Calcium-channel blockers.** According to the ACC/AHA guidelines,[27] calcium-channel blockers are not routinely recommended for Stage C heart failure patients with reduced ejection fraction (EF) and present or past symptoms of heart failure. They further state that in Stage B patients (i.e., those who have not developed symptoms of heart failure but have structural abnormalities), calcium-channel blockers with negative inotropic properties may be harmful in asymptomatic patients after an MI.

The use of positive inotropes (except oral digoxin), h-BNP, vasodilators, and morphine is usually used in the critical care management of patients in Stage D heart failure (see section on Cardiac Drugs in Critical Care.

**Positive inotropes.** Three categories of drugs increase contractility: cardiac glycosides, sympathomimetics, and phosphodiesterase inhibitors (bipyridines). Positive inotropes, nesiritide (which is a human brain natriuretic peptide or h-BNP), vasodilators, and morphine are most often used for Stage D heart failure and critical care management of the decompensated patient. Some drugs within these categories (e.g., digoxin) may be used in special cases in Stage C (refer to the section on Critical Care Management).

**Cardiac glycosides.** One of the oldest classes of cardiac medications, cardiac glycosides is represented by the drug digitalis. Digitalis is available in several preparations, the most common of which are digitoxin (Crystodigin) and digoxin (Lanoxin, Lanoxicaps). Digoxin appears to be the more commonly used of the two preparations, perhaps owing to its comparatively shorter half-life and therefore

decreased risk of toxicity. Digitalis increases contractility by inhibiting the sodium–potassium–ATPase enzyme, which normally provides the energy for the sodium–potassium pump ($NA^+$–$K^+$ pump). The $Na^+$–$K^+$ pump expels $Na^+$, accumulated during depolarization, from the cell and brings in $K^+$ during repolarization. By binding to the enzyme, digitalis inhibits the active transport of sodium and potassium, thereby increasing intracellular sodium. An increase in intracellular sodium results in an ionic exchange of intracellular sodium for extracellular calcium ($Ca^{2+}$). The resultant increase in intracellular calcium stimulates large quantities of calcium to be released from the sarcoplasmic reticulum and to be available for excitation–contraction. Myocardial contractility is therefore increased as a result of increased calcium.

In the setting of heart failure, particularly with ventricular dilation, myocardial contraction is often inefficient and results in an increase in myocardial oxygen demand. Besides its positive inotropic effects, digitalis also has both negative chronotropic (decreased heart rate) and negative dromotropic (conduction delay) action, the dromotropic effect being primarily on the atrioventricular conduction system. The bradycardic and delayed atrioventricular node conduction effect of digitalis allow it to be considered for use in the treatment of atrial fibrillation (see Dysrhythmias section).

Digitalis toxicity may occur for a variety of reasons. The more common causes are the following:
- The interaction of digitalis with other drugs
- Decreased renal function
- Altered gastrointestinal absorption

Examples of drugs known to interact with digitalis are quinidine (various preparations and trade names, Duraquin, Cardioquin), amiodarone (Cordarone), verapamil (Calan, Isoptin), potassium-sparing diuretics, sympathomimetic drugs, and some antibiotics. Antacids, a high-fiber diet, and chemotherapeutic agents may decrease the bioavailability of digitalis. Herbal preparations like mistletoe, Siberian ginseng, and aconite are also effective. The typical patient with digitalis toxicity is usually elderly, in atrial fibrillation, with underlying heart disease of many years, abnormal renal function, and concomitant pulmonary disease.

Signs and symptoms of digitalis toxicity include:
- Gastrointestinal problems
  - Anorexia
  - Nausea
  - Vomiting
  - Diarrhea
- Neurologic problems
  - Malaise
  - Fatigue
  - Vertigo
  - Colored vision (especially green or yellow halos around lights)
  - Insomnia
  - Depression
  - Facial pain

- Cardiologic problems
  - Palpitations
  - Arrhythmias
  - Syncope
- Hematologic problems
  - High digoxin levels, especially with low potassium
  - Altered blood urea nitrogen (BUN) and creatinine

> **Clinical Tip**
> As a result of increased risk of digitalis toxicity in individuals with decreased renal function, individuals who have decreased renal function are usually prescribed half-strength dosages of digoxin/Lanoxin. The recommended dosage for individuals with decreased renal function is 0.125 Lanoxin or digoxin rather than the regular dosage of 0.25.

Although patients in chronic heart failure who experience limited hemodynamic compromise have been successfully managed with digitalis in the past, the ACC/AHA 2009 recommendations for management of heart failure suggest that the use of digoxin be lowered to a Class IIb recommendation instead of its former class I recommendation (Table 14-11). Concern was expressed that blood plasma levels of digoxin in the suggested therapeutic range may have deleterious effects with long-term use, even though they may be well tolerated in the short term.[17]

**Sympathomimetics.** Drugs that bind to adrenoceptors and partially or fully mimic the actions of epinephrine or norepinephrine are known as sympathomimetics. The use of sympathomimetics, given parenterally in the treatment of heart failure to optimize cardiac output, is reserved for hemodynamically compromised patients within a critical care setting.

Stimulation of $\beta_1$ adrenoceptors of the myocardium results in an increased calcium influx into myocardial cells with resultant electrical and mechanical influences: increased sinus node firing, enhanced atrioventricular conduction, and increased myocardial contractility. Stimulation of $\beta_2$ adrenoceptors causes dilation of smooth muscles of the bronchi and blood vessels. Pharmacologic stimulation of both $\beta_1$- and $\beta_2$-agonist receptors in a failing heart therefore increases contractility and decreases afterload by its peripheral arterial vasodilatory effect. Use of these drugs is limited to acute interventions in a critical care setting because prolonged use of beta stimulators may lead to receptor desensitization and decreased inotropy. Unwanted ventricular arrhythmias may develop in response to the increased myocardial oxygen cost from pharmacologically induced improved contractility. Increased myocardial oxygen cost may further aggravate ischemia.

Examples of $\beta$-agonist adrenoceptors are the following:
- Selective $\beta_1$:
  - Dobutamine (Dobutrex),
  - Norepinephrine (Levophed),
- Nonselective $\beta_1$ and $\beta_2$:
  - Epinephrine (Adrenalin Chloride),
  - Isoproterenol (Isuprel).

Relatively selective $\beta_2$ agonists are used primarily in the management of respiratory dysfunction.

Another category of sympathomimetic agonists is dopamine (Intropin). Dopamine stimulates $\beta_1$-myocardial receptors, D-1 (dopamine) vascular receptors, and $\alpha$-vascular receptors. Dopamine is used when heart failure is accompanied by systemic hypotension because it acts as both a positive inotrope (via $\beta_1$-receptors) and a vasopressor (via $\alpha$-receptors). The combined $\beta$ and $\alpha$ effect increases cardiac output through increased contractility and increases blood pressure through both peripheral vascular vasoconstriction and increased cardiac output. At low doses, dopamine (via its D-1 receptors) causes selective vasodilation and therefore increased blood flow to the renal, cerebral, coronary, and mesenteric arterial beds.

## Table 14-11 Classification of Recommendations

| | Class I | Class IIa | Class IIb | Class III |
|---|---|---|---|---|
| Benefit: Risk Recommendation | Benefit >>> Risk <br> Procedure/treatment should be performed or administered | Benefit >> Risk <br> It is reasonable to perform procedure or administer treatment | Benefit > Risk <br> Procedure/Treatment may be considered | Risk > Benefit <br> Procedure/Treatment Should not be performed/administered; May be harmful |
| Further studies | Not necessary | Additional studies needed with focused objectives | Additional studies with broad objectives needed | No additional studies needed |

*Adapted from Antman EM, Hand M, Armstrong PW, 2007 Focused update of the ACC/AHA 2004 guidelines for the management of patients with ST-elevation myocardial infarction: a report of the American College of Cardiology/American Heart Association Task Force on Practice Guidelines: developed in collaboration With the Canadian Cardiovascular Society endorsed by the American Academy of Family Physicians: 2007 Writing Group to Review New Evidence and Update the ACC/AHA 2004 Guidelines for the Management of Patients With ST-Elevation Myocardial Infarction, Writing on Behalf of the 2004 Writing Committee. Circulation 117(2):296-329, 2008.*

Dopamine (Intropin) and its analogue dobutamine (Dobutrex) are often used together in the management of heart failure with accompanying hypotension. Although both are potent β-adrenergic agonists, dobutamine has no α-adrenergic stimulation and therefore does not increase blood pressure through vasoconstriction, whereas dopamine is able to do so. Moderate doses of both drugs, when given together, have been demonstrated to maintain arterial blood pressure, decrease pulmonary artery wedge pressure, and increase contractility (see section on Cardiac Drugs used in Critical Care).

**Bipyridines/phosphodiesterase inhibitors.** As a group, phosphodiesterase inhibitors (bipyridines) act as positive inotropes and vasodilators. They are often recommended for the treatment of heart failure that has failed to respond to other drug management. The inotropic effect of these drugs differs from that of the previous two drugs in that bipyridines increase myocardial contractility without altering the Na$^+$–K$^+$ pumping mechanism (as does digoxin) or stimulating the adrenoceptors (as does dopamine). Bipyridines increase intracellular calcium influx by inhibition of the cyclic nucleotide phosphodiesterase. Amrinone/Inamrinone (Inocor) was the first drug in this category approved for use with patients with severe CHF not responding adequately to digitalis, diuretics, or vasodilators. Amrinone/Inamrinone is relatively specific for myocardial and vascular smooth muscle because its vasodilatory effects are balanced between preload and afterload. Overall effects are an increase in cardiac output, reduction in preload, and decrease in afterload. In preload reduction, as measured by decreased pulmonary artery wedge pressure, amrinone/inamrinone is more effective than dopamine (Intropin) or dobutamine (Dobutrex); as a positive inotrope and vasodilator, it is intermediate between nitroprusside (Nipride) and dobutamine. Milrinone (Primacor) has a mechanism of action similar to that of amrinone/inamrinone and is used primarily for the short-term management of acute heart failure. Milrinone however has also been used intravenously in outpatient settings for Class IV CHF patients refractory to oral medications and as a bridge to transplantation.[28]

**h-BNP.** Nesiritide or h-BNP is a new drug for patients with acute decompensatory heart failure who have dyspnea at rest or with minimal activity. Nesiritide (Natrecor)[29] is used intravenously to decrease pulmonary capillary wedge pressure (PCWP) with the goal of improving hemodynamics and increasing cardiac output.

**Vasodilators.** Both arterial and venous vasodilators are used in the management of heart failure as afterload and preload reducers, respectively. Arterial vasodilators are useful only when arterial hypotension is not present. Arterial vasodilators decrease afterload, which decreases left ventricular myocardial oxygen demand. Reduction in preload may also decrease myocardial oxygen demand by decreasing ventricular volume, thus improving the length–tension relationship of the myocardial fibers. The improvement allows for a greater actin–myosin interaction and more effective contractility.

Myocardial oxygen demand may be reduced as the efficiency of the contraction improves.

Drugs that exhibit vasodilator properties are the following:
- Smooth muscle relaxants such as nitroglycerin, nitroprusside (Nipride), and hydralazine (Apresoline)
- Calcium-channel blockers
- Morphine
- ACE inhibitors

**α-adrenergic antagonists.** Alpha antagonists are primarily used for the management of hypertension rather than heart failure. Reflex tachycardia and a compensatory increase in blood volume with long-term use have been identified as potential detrimental side effects of alpha antagonists. Prazosin (Minipress) and terazosin (Hytrin) are examples of α$_1$-antagonists.

**Venodilators.** Nitrates reduce preload via venodilation. Nitrates are available in many forms, including topical, sublingual, and oral. Please refer to the previous section on antiischemic drugs for further discussion.

**Arteriodilators.** Hydralazine (Apresoline) and minoxidil (Loniten) decrease afterload by decreasing arterial resistance. Because there is a potential increase in side effects when hydralazine is used alone, it is commonly used in combination with a diuretic and a β-blocker. Please refer to the section on antihypertension drugs and Table 14-10 for further discussion.

**Combined arteriolar and venous dilators.** Nitroprusside (Nipride) affects both arterial resistance and venous capacitance. When it is given parenterally, it has a rapid onset of action and is effective in the treatment of severe heart failure with or without cardiogenic shock. An increase in venous capacitance results in a decrease in preload and therefore in left ventricular end-diastolic pressure and decreases myocardial oxygen demand; an increase in arterial resistance decreases afterload and thereby decreases myocardial oxygen demand.

**Morphine.** The use of morphine in the treatment of severe heart failure has proved invaluable for both its analgesic and its hemodynamic effects. Morphine decreases preload via marked venodilation and exhibits mild arterial vasodilation. The anxiety and effort of dyspnea associated with severe heart failure appear to improve with the administration of morphine.

The importance of recognizing the side effects of all drugs has previously been stated and yet bears repetition. In the case of digoxin (Lanoxin), for example, the side effects may be perceived initially by the patient as "just not feeling well"; the correlation of those feelings to the specific drug may go unnoticed. Many patients seen by physical therapists for noncardiac reasons are taking digoxin. Any new patient complaint should be evaluated in light of its relationship to digoxin and reported to the physician. If patients are on digoxin because of atrial fibrillation, the physical therapist must recognize that they will have an irregular pulse. In addition, atrial fibrillation with a ventricular response at rest greater than 110 beats per minute warrants evaluation before continuing with an exercise program. Resting pulses should be taken for a full minute when atrial fibrillation or any other rhythm disturbance is present owing to the irregularity of the rhythm.

## Signs and Symptoms of Impending Heart Failure

For the therapist who is seeing a patient on an outpatient basis, the signs and symptoms of impending heart failure may be subtle, developing over a period of days; therefore, the therapist should be alerted to any complaints of dyspnea, ankle swelling, weight gain (1 to 2 lb in 2 days), or the presence of an S3 heart sound or lung crackles. If these symptoms are present, the patient should not be exercised until a physician is contacted and the situation clarified or remedied. In the case of severe heart failure warranting parenterally delivered vasopressors and positive inotropes to maintain an appropriate cardiac output at rest, progressive exercise is not recommended until the patient is hemodynamically stable. As the patient becomes hemodynamically stable, appropriate treatment interventions may include the following: techniques to maintain good alveolar expansion and gas exchange, education regarding energy conservation techniques (e.g., arms supported on pillows for activities of daily living to decrease upper extremity energy requirements), and initiation of low-level activity. As stroke volume decreases, heart rate compensatorily rises to prevent cardiac output from falling further. Therefore, when the patient has tachycardia at rest, it is inappropriate to begin an exercise program without evaluation of the etiology and clear direction and mutual understanding of treatment goals from all members of the health care team.

Patients on diuretics may become dehydrated and have alteration in their blood levels of potassium. Their complaints may be of lightheadedness, weakness, fatigue, or an irregular pulse. Symptoms may be more pronounced when standing as compared with sitting or lying down. Clinical signs may be resting tachycardia and postural hypotension. Patients should not participate in an exercise regimen until the situation has been stabilized and the patient has appropriately rehydrated (and replaced electrolytes if needed) under a physician's guidance.

### Dysrhythmias

Disturbances in cardiac rhythm are known as dysrhythmias, which are usually called arrhythmias (although this actually means "no rhythm"). They are the result of irregularities in heart pacemaker or conduction tissue function. Arrhythmias present a broad spectrum of clinical consequences: they may be benign and remain undetected throughout life or prove fatal on initial presentation (e.g., sudden cardiac death). Arrhythmias are recognized clinically as irregularities in the rhythm of the heartbeat on palpation, auscultation, or electrocardiographic (ECG) tracing. They are labeled according to the anatomic origin of the abnormal beat (e.g., atrial, nodal, or ventricular), their frequency (e.g., tachycardia or bradycardia), and their relationship to the previous beat (e.g., premature or late).

Numerous cardiac pathologies including coronary artery disease, heart failure, cardiomyopathy, and congenital heart disease can be responsible for the production of arrhythmias. Noncardiac causes, including electrolyte imbalances, drug toxicity, excessive nicotine or caffeine ingestion, emotional stress, hyperthyroidism, or mitral valve prolapse syndrome, can also produce arrhythmias. On correction of these conditions, persistent cardiac rhythm disturbances that are hemodynamically significant require drug therapy. The focus of antiarrhythmic therapy, therefore, is to maintain adequate cardiac output in the presence of pacemaker or conduction tissue disease.

Physical therapists must be alert to the etiology and presence of arrhythmias, their hemodynamic consequences, and the efficacy of the antiarrhythmic agent prescribed. Drugs suppress arrhythmias (abnormal impulse formation or conduction) by altering cell membrane permeability to specific ions, for example, sodium and calcium. Although exercise may be responsible for production of arrhythmias, electrolyte imbalances and toxic level of antiarrhythmic drugs are other nondisease states that may be arrhythmogenic.

### Physiology

To understand how antiarrhythmic agents suppress rhythm disturbances, it is necessary to review the unique characteristics of normal myocardial pacemaker and conduction system functioning. See Chapter 9 for an in-depth discussion of cardiac arrhythmias. Inherent myocardial properties of automaticity, excitability, and conduction depend on the resting polarity of pacemaker (nodal) and myocardial conduction tissue (Purkinje fibers). Refer to Chapter 2 for further information. This specialized conduction system is able to initiate, respond to, and conduct a stimulus as long as an adequate transmembrane potential exists. Resting cell polarity depends on two factors:

- The membrane permeability to sodium, calcium, potassium, and chloride ions
- The duration between action potentials (diastole)

The cardiac action potential is thought to result from an orderly and sequential change in membrane permeability to various ions. The characteristic time course has been described by phases and separated into "fast" and "slow" responses (Fig. 14-3). Whereas membrane permeability to sodium alone is felt to be responsible for the rapid upstroke of phase 0 depolarization found in normal atrial and ventricular contractile cell action potential, membrane permeability to both calcium and sodium is responsible for the slow phase 0 depolarization of sinus and atrioventricular nodal cell action potential. Repolarization via the "fast" channels can be described by three phases:

- Phase 1 is the early rapid phase and depends on membrane permeability to chloride.
- Phase 2 is the plateau phase affected by calcium and potassium movement across the membrane.
- Phase 3 is the final rapid phase of repolarization primarily influenced by membrane permeability to potassium.

FAST CHANNEL

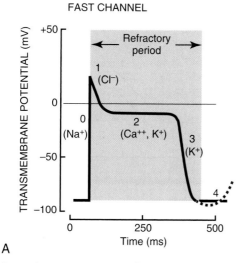

SLOW CHANNEL

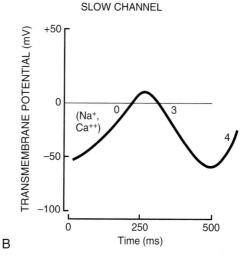

A                          B

**Figure 14-3** Schematic representation of phases of action potential (AP) in fast and slow depolarization. The primary ion movement responsible for AP is noted at each phase. **A,** Fast response AP (*black line*) begins with a relatively greater negativity and has a rapid rate of depolarization and a plateaued repolarization. This AP is found in ordinary atrial, ventricular, and Purkinje fibers. Purkinje fibers demonstrate a fast depolarization phase (0) but also have similar phase 4 diastole characteristics of self-excitation as in the slow channel (*red dotted line*). **B,** Slow response AP (*red line*) begins with a less negative voltage and has a slower depolarization phase (0). Repolarization lasts longer and exhibits a slow, spontaneous depolarization during phase 4 diastole. This AP is found in sinoatrial and atrioventricular nodal cells.

These three phases of repolarization cannot be distinguished clearly in cells with slower action potentials (see Fig. 14-3B). Phase 4 is the period of diastole and is constant in many atrial and ventricular contractile cells that rest indefinitely until stimulated. However, sinus node, atrioventricular node, and Purkinje fibers have a unique ability to spontaneously depolarize and self-excite as a result of altered cell membrane permeability to sodium. This slow "leak" of sodium causes these fibers to achieve a threshold at which more rapid depolarization occurs.

Both myocardial contractile and conduction tissue are refractory to restimulation when the cell membrane is still depolarized. When the membrane is partially repolarized (phase 3), excitation becomes possible but not usual, and the cell is in a "relative" refractory state (see Fig. 14-3).

### Pathophysiology
The action potential and the diastolic interval between action potentials are affected by changes in the
- maximum diastolic potential,
- slope of phase 4 depolarization, and
- threshold potential required to depolarize the cell.[30]

Figure 14-4 demonstrates slowing of the heart rate by changes in any of these three action potential parameters. Numerous cardiac conditions, including cell hypoxia, ischemia, scarred tissue, and medications, can alter these parameters and can cause some cardiac cells that normally have fast action potentials to become faster or much slower, and slow action potentials to respond faster or slower than normal. When any of these alterations in the action potential occur, slow, fast, or escape rhythms may become manifest. For example, if sinoatrial node cells have an excess of potassium (hyperkalemia), the resting polarity is greater than normal (more negativity).

Consequently, more sodium has to enter the cell to fully depolarize the membrane, and more sodium has to leave the cell to complete repolarization. This excess of sodium and potassium creates a longer interval before the occurrence of another action potential, as illustrated in Figure 14-4A. Each heart beat reflects the mechanical event triggered by the electrical conduction of an action potential. Hence, a longer period between action potentials is seen clinically as a slower heart rate. In addition, if the interval is long enough, pacemaker cells in the atrioventricular node may depolarize spontaneously, producing an "escape" action potential or a premature nodal heart beat. Similarly, if normal cell membrane integrity is disturbed and sodium permeability increases, cells may depolarize and repolarize more rapidly, causing an increase in heart rate.

In addition to the changes in the action potential, variability in the duration of the refractory period of the action potential can cause arrhythmias. In certain conditions, diseased myocardial cells repolarize and conduct slower than neighboring healthy myocardial cells, enabling "reentry" to occur. Reentry, a common cause of rhythm disturbances, occurs when one impulse reenters and excites areas of the heart that have already been stimulated (and partially repolarized) by the original impulse (Fig. 14-5).

For reentry to occur, there must be
- some obstacle blocking normal impulse conduction,
- another "avenue" for the impulse to be conducted through the tissue (unidirectional block), and
- sufficient time for the impulse to travel via this alternative "avenue" (i.e., long enough so that after the impulse passes through this tissue, the surrounding tissue will have repolarized and will be able to "accept" the impulse).

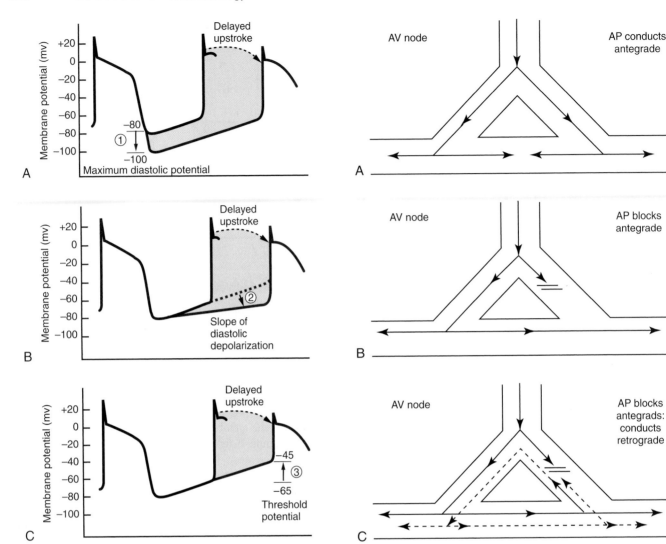

**Figure 14-4** Determinants of action potential rate and diastolic interval, as seen in Purkinje fibers. The rate can be slowed (and the interval lengthened; shaded area) by three diastolic mechanisms: more negative maximum diastolic potential (**A**), reduction of the slope of diastolic depolarization (**B**), or more positive threshold potential (**C**). (Adapted from Katzung BG [ed.]. Basic and Clinical Pharmacology. 5th ed. East Norwalk, CT, Appleton & Lange, 1992:169.)

**Figure 14-5** Mechanism of reentry arrhythmias. **A,** Reentry requires two conduction pathways that may be anatomically or physiologically distinct, such as an AV node and an accessory pathway (AP). **B,** Conduction block may occur in one pathway, such as an accessory pathway, with slow conduction over the other pathway, the AV node. **C,** If this slowly conducted impulse travels retrograde over the previously blocked pathway, it will reenter the circuit and then initiate a regular tachycardia by repetitively circling the path. As an example of accessory pathway–mediated tachycardia, the circuit would be antegrade unidirectional block in the accessory pathway with slow antegrade conduction over the AV node to the ventricle and return to the atrium due to retrograde conduction over the accessory pathway. (From Nichols: Critical Heart Disease in Infants and Children, ed 2. Philadelphia, 2006, Mosby.)

When these three conditions exist, the single or repetitive conduction of a "secondary" pacemaker occurs and is manifested clinically as a premature beat or a series of premature beats. Disease conditions such as myocardial ischemia with resultant hypoxia can cause partial depolarization and "unidirectional" block, providing the setting for reentrant rhythms. The slower repolarization rate of such disease tissue slows the reentrant impulse so that healthy surrounding tissue is no longer refractory and can respond to stimulation by this "secondary" pacemaker, subsequently making the healthy tissue refractory to the primary pacemaker.

Reentry is probably responsible for many cardiac arrhythmias, including atrial and ventricular flutter and fibrillation, supraventricular tachycardia involving accessory pathway or nodal reentry, and many ventricular tachycardias.[31]

Electrophysiologic testing enables precise identification of the origin and physiology of the reentrant rhythm. With this knowledge, physicians can plan treatment and more accurately prescribe pharmacologic alteration of the action potential.

### Pharmacologic Intervention

Suppression of arrhythmias by pharmacologic intervention can be complex. Although antiarrhythmic agents can reverse lethal rhythms, it is unclear that these drugs promote longevity. They can depress cardiac inotropy and may even produce arrhythmias per se owing to their effect on the action potential (arrhythmogenic). Antiarrhythmic agents act to inhibit abnormal impulse formation or conduction by altering cell membrane permeability to specific ions. The exact interaction of antiarrhythmics with various ionic channels is complex and beyond the scope of this text. Simply stated, activation and inactivation "gates" exist that control the flow of sodium, calcium, potassium, and chloride ions depending on stimulation. Classification of antiarrhythmic drugs according to their effects on the action potential of myocardial and pacemaker cell gates is found in Table 14-12. Significant overlapping of drug properties exists across all categories. In addition, two classes of antiarrhythmics, β-blockers (Class II) and calcium-channel blockers (Class IV), not only are effective in the treatment of arrhythmias but also are primary antiischemic and antihypertensive agents (as is discussed elsewhere in this chapter).

> **Clinical Tip**
> Caution: Some antiarrhythmic drugs may actually induce arrhythmias in some individuals (prorhythmic effect).

### Membrane stabilizers

CLASS 1 DRUGS. Class 1 drugs primarily block the fast sodium channels (acting like local anesthetics) and reduce the inflow of sodium ions. Subclasses A, B, and C all significantly block the sodium channel of depolarized cells, but vary in the degree of sodium-channel block in normal cells. Similarly, class 1 drugs prolong the refractory period of depolarized cells but vary in their effect on normal cells. Prolongation of the refractory period of diseased tissue inhibits reentry by creating bidirectional block in these cells (see Fig. 14-5). Lidocaine (Xylocaine), a class IB agent, facilitates propagation of the original (sinoatrial) stimulus by shortening the refractory period of normal cell action potentials while slowing or completely blocking the potential reentrant stimulus in diseased tissue. Lidocaine is a very effective drug for ventricular arrhythmia

In general, class 1 drugs are very effective in the treatment of ventricular tachycardia (VT). They may be useful in the treatment of supraventricular tachycardia (SVT), with classes 1C (and III) being the most effective for pharmacologic cardioversion of atrial fibrillation.[32,33] The ECG of a patient on a class 1 antiarrhythmic drug may exhibit a prolongation of the QRS duration, with a normal or prolonged P-R interval.

CLASS 2 DRUGS. Class 2 antiarrhythmic agents (Table 14-12)—β-blockers—do not directly affect the cell membrane. They indirectly alter the action potential by blocking sympathetic excitation of the heart to control cardiac rhythm disturbances. They are especially indicated for the treatment of supraventricular and ventricular arrhythmias that occur in the post–myocardial infarction period and arrhythmias that occur during exercise. β-Blockers, used in patients with heart failure, also improve outcomes in this population owing to their antiarrhythmic properties.[32] Of note, β-blockers are prescribed cautiously owing to their negative inotropic activity. Patients taking β-blockers may have a prolongation of the P-R interval on their ECG tracing.

CLASS 3 DRUGS. The class 3 drugs act primarily to prolong the refractory period of cardiac tissue, thereby slowing repolarization and making it more difficult for myocardial cells to respond to stimulation. They may be effective in both SVT and VT. Amiodarone (Cordarone), one of several drugs currently in this class, has properties of class 1A, 2, 3, and 4 agents. Amiodarone may adversely affect a variety of bodily systems making patient compliance challenging. It can cause any the following side effects: exacerbation of arrhythmias, sinus bradycardia, photosensitivity, hepatotoxicity, hypothyroidism or hyperthyroidism, pulmonary fibrosis, skin pigmentation, corneal deposits, peripheral neuropathy, and general malaise.[29] Patients on amiodarone should be monitored for increased weakness, fatigue, and shortness of breath as this may indicate toxicity (pulmonary).

CLASS 4 DRUGS. Class 4 drugs primarily block the slow calcium channel. Like class 1 drugs, they prolong the refractory period and decrease pacemaker activity of depolarized cells. The ECG of a patient on calcium-channel blockers may show a prolonged P-R interval and no effect on the QRS complex. Verapamil (Isoptin, Calan) demonstrates the most antiarrhythmic properties in this class and is significantly more effective in the treatment of SVT than of VT.

**Digitalis.** Digitalis, not found in the preceding classification, is a cardiac glycoside that may also be used in arrhythmia management. In the healthy heart, it directly enhances vagal tone (parasympathetic nervous system), whereas in the failing heart, it depresses adrenergic action (sympathetic nervous system); both actions result in slowing the heart and depressing conduction through the atrioventricular node. Hence, digitalis can be used to prevent conduction of atrial arrhythmias into the ventricles. Digitalis administration, however, can predispose an individual to arrhythmias, owing to its action on the electrophysiologic properties of the heart. Used in the treatment of congestive heart failure, digitalis "poisons" (inhibits) the sodium–potassium pump (review previous section on Heart Failure in this chapter). This causes excessive calcium to accumulate in the cell, along with intracellular sodium. Although this increased calcium enhances myocardial cell contraction, thereby ameliorating heart failure, the increased sodium causes a decrease in intracellular potassium. As intracellular potassium falls, maximal diastolic membrane potential decreases (less negativity), and the slope of phase 4 depolarization increases (see Fig. 14-4). The resultant increase in automaticity and ectopic activity can increase the likelihood of arrhythmias. Hence, whether prescribed for heart failure or management of rapid atrial heart rates, serum digitalis concentration and electrolyte levels should be monitored carefully.

Pharmacologic management of arrhythmias is most successful when approached in a systematic fashion.[34] First, adequate documentation of the arrhythmia is made by

**Table 14-12  Classification of Antiarrhythmic Drugs**

| Category | Physiological Effect[a] | Drug: Generic (Trade Name) | Comments |
|---|---|---|---|
| **Class 1** Membrane depressants (sodium-channel blockers) | Depolarized cells<br>↑ Na$^+$ channel block<br>↑ Refractory period<br>↓ Pacemaker activity | | |
| IA | Normal cell<br>↑ Na$^+$ channel block<br>↑ Refractory period | Quinidine (Biquin, Cardioquin)<br>Disopyramide (Norpace, Rythmodan)<br>Procainamide (Pronestyl) | Gastrointestinal side effects<br>Myocardial depressant<br>Urinary retention effect<br>Myocardial depressant<br>Lupus erythematosus |
| IB | Normal cell<br>No effect | Lidocaine (Xylocaine)<br>Mexiletine (Mexitil)<br>Tocainide (Tonocard)<br>Phenytoin (Dilantin)<br>Moricizine (Ethmozine)[b] | Signs of central nervous system abnormality (tremors, nausea may indicate toxicity)<br>Anticonvulsant; effective with digoxin-induced arrhythmias; acts as IC |
| IC | Normal cell<br>↑↑ Na$^+$ channel block<br>Ø, ↑ Refractory period | Flecainide (Tambocor)<br>Propafenone (Rythmol) | Primarily for ventricular arrhythmias; effective with PVCs; arrhythmogenic during exercise; defibrillation problems |
| **Class 2** β-Adrenoceptor blockers | Depolarized cells<br>Ø Effect on Na$^+$ channel<br>↑ Refractory period<br>Normal cell<br>Variable effect | See β-blocker (Table 14-3)<br>Sotalol | Effective with ventricular and supraventricular arrhythmias |
| **Class 3** Refractory period alterations | ↑↑↑ Refractory period<br>↓ Pacemaker activity<br>Sympatholytic | Amiodarone (Cordarone)<br>Bretylium tosylate (Bretylol)<br>Ibutilide fumarate (Covert) | Class 1A, 2,4 properties; useful with ventricular and supraventricular arrhythmias; may transiently increase pacemaker activity |
| **Class 4** Calcium-channel Blockers | All cells ↑↑↑ Ca$^{2+}$ channel blockade<br>Depolarized cells<br>↑ Na$^+$ channel block<br>↑ Refractory period<br>↓ Pacemaker activity<br>Sympatholytic | See calcium-channel blocker (Table 14-6) | Verapamil (Isotopin, Calan) is most effective in this group for treatment of supraventricular tachycardia |

[a]General effect on action potential; individual agents may differ slightly.
[b]Controversial classification; acts like IC as well.
↑ Slight increase, ↑↑ Moderate increase, ↑↑↑ Significant increase, ↓ Decrease, Ø No change.

clinical evaluation, electrocardiogram, Holter monitor, or electrophysiologic study. Assessment of hemodynamic compromise, consequences, and symptom prevalence in an emergency or long-term-care setting is considered. Second, once a drug is chosen, its efficacy is evaluated by clinical and electrocardiographic observation with possible electrophysiologic study. Third, the adequacy of the dosage is measured by determination of drug concentration in the blood. Intolerance to antiarrhythmic agents and drug toxicity are common problems. Current prescription of antiarrhythmics is empirical, and several agents may need to be tried before one is found that is both effective and well tolerated by the patient. Rapid advances in electrophysiologic study and testing have helped verify the effectiveness of certain agents. In addition, as this technology progresses, new combinations of drugs are developed (see Table 14-12).

Health professionals responsible for monitoring the exercise response of patients on antiarrhythmic agents should understand the basis of arrhythmia production and suppression. Exercise is commonly the culprit in the production of arrhythmias (Box 14-1). However, abnormal electrolyte levels or toxic levels of a drug may be responsible for cardiac rhythm disturbances. A medication prescribed to inhibit arrhythmias can in fact become arrhythmogenic if therapeutic serum levels are exceeded. Arrhythmias, regardless of their etiology, must be interpreted by the health care provider. The hemodynamic effects and potential consequences of the arrhythmia dictate subsequent patient management and program planning.

**Miscellaneous drugs.** In addition, adenosine and atropine are sometimes used. Adenosine is given intravenously and slows conduction in the reentry pathway through the atrioventricular (AV) node; it is used to treat supraventricular tachycardia. Atropine blocks cardiac muscarinic receptors and is used to treat bradydysrhythmias; it causes the typical anticholinergic adverse reactions.

## Hypertension

Although surveys vary, an estimated 25% of adult Americans have hypertension when defined as >140/90 mm Hg. Another 25% of the population is considered to have prehypertension, defined as a systolic blood pressure of 120 to 139 mm Hg or a diastolic blood pressure of 80 to 89 mm Hg.[35] Of those who obtain medical treatment, most are prescribed diet or exercise or drug therapy, or a combination of these. The goal of hypertensive therapy is to prevent the negative effects of chronic blood pressure elevation. Sustained hypertension results in increased morbidity and mortality rates associated with renal failure, coronary disease, and stroke. Unfortunately, hypertension does not cause any noticeable signs or symptoms to the patients and is often not recognized and treated early enough. It has been labeled the "silent killer." Similarly, the absence of symptoms of poorly controlled hypertension and the numerous side effects of available drug agents result often in noncompliance with therapy. This is often enhanced frequently because of the use of multiple drugs to control blood pressure.

## Physiology

A number of physiologic factors combine to establish and maintain normotension in the cardiovascular system. At any one moment, several mechanisms interact to maintain adequate pressure in the circulation to allow vital systems to function properly. Carotid baroreceptors and kidney sensors detect changes in blood pressure and trigger appropriate physiological responses in cardiac output and peripheral vascular resistance to maintain normotension. Here, increases in blood pressure reduce heart rate and cardiac output whereas decreases in blood pressure increase heart rate and cardiac output. These alterations are regulated at three anatomic sites: the arterioles, the postcapillary venules, and the heart. A fourth site, the kidneys, acts to control blood pressure by regulating intravascular volume (cardiac preload). The sympathetic nervous system and humoral mechanisms, that is, the renin–angiotensin–aldosterone system, continuously control the various sites and cause compensatory mechanisms among them (Fig. 14-6).

## Pathophysiology

In the majority of individuals with hypertension, the threshold of stimulation of both the baroreceptors and the renal blood volume–pressure control systems is "set" too high.[36,37] This causes a delay in the initiation of central and peripheral changes involved in the maintenance of normotension. Once baroreceptors are stimulated, the sympathetic nervous system and the kidneys usually respond normally. However, just as in normotensive individuals, if one anatomic site is "blocked" for some reason (e.g., disease, drug), other sites compensate to maintain a blood pressure level that no longer stimulates the baroreceptors. When this baseline

---

**Box 14-1**

### Associations of Arrhythmias with Exercise

- Normal cardiovascular system
- Coronary artery disease
- Mitral valve prolapse
- Left ventricular trabeculations
- Digitalis
- Hypokalemia
- Cardiomyopathy
- Left ventricle outflow obstruction
- Aortic stenosis
- Hypertrophic cardiomyopathy
- Long–Q-T interval syndromes
- Idiopathic
- Quinidine induced
- Phenothiazine induced
- Proarrhythmias due to antiarrhythmic drugs (Flecainide)
- Pulmonary disease

From Froelicher V, Marcondes G: Manual of Exercise Testing. St. Louis, MO, Mosby, 1989.

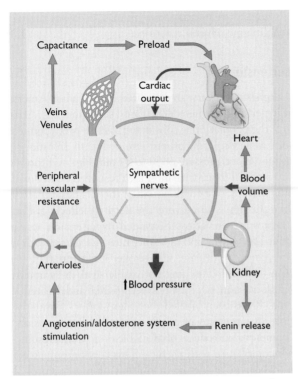

**Figure 14-6** Factors involved in blood pressure control. Determinants of blood pressure are cardiac output, determined by heart rate and stroke volume. Cardiac output depends on the amount of blood returning to the heart, which in turn depends on vein and venule capacitance (preload) and blood volume (under the control of the kidneys). Peripheral vascular resistance is determined by the arterioles. (From Page C, Curtis MJ, Sutter MC, Walker MJ, Hoffman BB [eds.]. Integrated Pharmacology. 2nd ed. Philadelphia: Mosby, 2002.)

blood pressure level is pathologically elevated, another of the remaining three anatomic sites of blood pressure regulation warrants blocking.

## Pharmacologic Intervention

Classification of antihypertensive drugs is related to their primary receptor site and mode of action.

- Diuretics, which act on kidneys to reduce volume
- Drugs, which act to limit sympathetic nervous system activity to cause vasodilation (arterial and venous) and to reduce cardiac output
- Drugs, which act on the renin–angiotensin–aldosterone system at the kidney to reduce volume and cause vasodilation

At present, no drug has been found effective and safe in directly altering baroreceptor activity. Some drugs affect only one site whereas other drugs can act on more than one site. Similarly, drugs with different actions are often combined. This allows for a reduction in the dose of each drug, minimizing adverse reactions. Recently, drugs have been combined into one tablet. For example, a diuretic and β-blocker, or diuretic and ACE inhibitor, may be combined into one pill or tablet to facilitate patient self-management

(Table 14-13). Of note, extensive research has been done in attempts to "tease" out which antihypertensive agent is most appropriate for the treatment of hypertension associated with specific pathologies, for example, primary or secondary prevention of heart failure or coronary artery disease, diabetes, or chronic renal failure.[35,38] Similarly, identification of optimal hypertensive therapy for women, minority, pediatric, and elderly populations has also been rigorously investigated. The American Heart Association frequently summarizes and publishes updates of best evidence recommendations resulting from comprehensive analysis of these studies, and the interested reader is encouraged to review these updates.[35,38,39]

### Diuretics

Alterations in intravascular blood volume have a significant effect on blood pressure. Diuretics, one of the most commonly prescribed antihypertensive agents, act to reduce circulating volume and thereby lower blood pressure by reducing preload and contractility via Starling's law. Acting at various sites along the renal tubule or Henle loop, diuretics alter the reabsorption of sodium, consequently affecting the retention of water (Fig. 14-7). Furosemide (Lasix), a "loop" diuretic, acts on the medullary ascending limb of Henle loop and has the greatest diuresing effect. Carbonic anhydrase inhibitors, acting on the proximal tubules, and potassium-sparing diuretics, acting on the collecting tubules and ducts, are the mildest diuretics. The sulfonamide diuretics (thiazides and thiazide-like drugs) have moderate diuretic effects. These act on the cortical ascending limb of Henle loop and the distal tubule. Thiazides are a frequently prescribed diuretic; however, they have been associated with hypokalemia and glucose intolerance.[40] In addition, some diuretics after a while are posited to reduce intracellular sodium and cause some vasodilation reducing peripheral resistance.

The physician may choose to prescribe diuretic therapy from a long list of agents (Table 14-10). The choice of diuretic depends on the severity of the hypertension and the drug's side effects. The potency of the drug is dependent on its site of action in the nephron (see Fig. 14-7). Combinations of diuretics can be prescribed to treat hypertension. Caution should be used when patients taking diuretics are encouraged to participate in aerobic exercise. Volume reduction and electrolyte disturbances can predispose the exercising individual to hypotension and arrhythmias, respectively. Hypokalemia can be a serious consequence of diuretic therapy when potent agents are prescribed. Usually potassium supplementation is prescribed to prevent a potentially unstable electrolyte environment. Hyperkalemia may occur with potassium-sparing diuretics.

### Drugs Acting on the Sympathetic Nervous System

Blood pressure is influenced by sympathetic nervous system regulation of cardiac output and peripheral vascular resistance. Pharmacologic agents can be used to alter sympathetic nervous system activity to control blood pressure in the following ways:

**Table 14-13 Combination Antihypertensive Agents**

| Drug Group | Drug Combination | Trade Name |
|---|---|---|
| Diuretic and Diuretic | Amiloride–hydrochlorothiazide | Moduretic |
| | Spironolactone–hydrochlorothiazide | Aldactazide |
| | Triamterene–hydrochlorothiazide | Dyazide, Maxzide |
| ACE inhibitors and diuretics | Benazepril–hydrochlorothiazide | Lotensin HCT |
| | Captopril–hydrochlorothiazide | Capozide |
| | Enalapril–hydrochlorothiazide | Vaseretic |
| | Fosinopril–hydrochlorothiazide | Monopril/HCT |
| | Lisinopril–hydrochlorothiazide | Prinzide, Zestoretic |
| | Moexipril–hydrochlorothiazide | Uniretic |
| | Quinapril–hydrochlorothiazide | Accuretic |
| ARBs and diuretics | Candesartan–hydrochlorothiazide | Atacand HCT |
| | Eprosartan–hydrochlorothiazide | Teveten HCT |
| | Irbesartan–hydrochlorothiazide | Avalide |
| | Losartan–hydrochlorothiazide | Hyzaar |
| | Olmesartan medoxomil–hydrochlorothiazide | Benicar HCT |
| | | Micardis HCT |
| | Telmisartan–hydrochlorothiazide | Diovan HCT |
| | Valsartan–hydrochlorothiazide | |
| β-Blockers and diuretics | Atenolol–chlorthalidone | Tenoretic |
| | Bisoprolol–hydrochlorothiazide | Ziac |
| | Metoprolol–hydrochlorothiazide | Lopressor HCT |
| | Nadolol–bendroflumethiazide | Corzide |
| | Propranolol LA–hydrochlorothiazide | Inderide LA |
| | Timolol–hydrochlorothiazide | Timolide |
| Centrally acting drug and diuretics | Methyldopa–hydrochlorothiazide | Aldoril |
| | Reserpine–chlorthalidone | Regroton |
| | Reserpine–chlorothiazide | Diupres |
| | Reserpine–hydrochlorothiazide | Hydropres |
| ACE inhibitors and calcium-channel blockers | Amlodipine–benazepril hydrochloride | Lotrel |
| | Enalapril–felodipine | Lexxel |
| | Trandolapril–verapamil | Tarka |
| α-Blockers and β-blockers | Carvedilol | Coreg |
| | Labetalol | Normodyne, Trandale |

*Adapted from Chobanian AV, Bakris GL, Black HR, et al. Seventh report of the Joint National Committee on Prevention, Detection, Evaluation, and Treatment of High Blood Pressure. Hypertension. 42:1206-1252, 2003.*

- Centrally acting compounds reduce neural transmission from vasopressor centers in the brainstem, inhibiting vasoconstriction.
- Ganglionic blockers block cholinergic transmission at sympathetic ganglia which reduces norepinephrine release from postganglionic nerves causing vasodilatation.
- Postganglionic cardiac blockers block the action of norepinephrine on β-receptors and reduce cardiac output.

- Blocking α-adrenoceptors in arterioles and venules prevents the action of norepinephrine and reduces peripheral vascular resistance.
- Blocking β-adrenoceptors on juxtaglomerular cells responsible for the release of renin limits vasoconstriction.

*Drugs Acting on Other Sites*

Angiotensin-converting enzyme inhibitors, ARBs, and calcium-channel blockers are common second drug groups

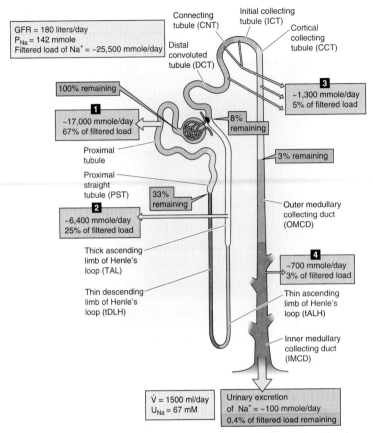

GFR = 180 liters/day
$P_{Na}$ = 142 mmole
Filtered load of $Na^+$ = ~25,500 mmole/day

Connecting
tubule (CNT)

Initial collecting
tubule (ICT)

Cortical
collecting
tubule (CCT)

Distal
convoluted
tubule (DCT)

100% remaining

**1**
~17,000 mmole/day
67% of filtered load

8%
remaining

**3**
~1,300 mmole/day
5% of filtered load

Proximal
tubule

3% remaining

Proximal
straight
tubule (PST)

33%
remaining

**2**
~6,400 mmole/day
25% of filtered load

Outer medullary
collecting duct
(OMCD)

Thick ascending
limb of Henle's
loop (TAL)

**4**
~700 mmole/day
3% of filtered load

Thin descending
limb of Henle's
loop (tDLH)

Thin ascending
limb of Henle's
loop (tALH)

Inner medullary
collecting duct
(IMCD)

$\dot{V}$ = 1500 ml/day
$U_{Na}$ = 67 mM

Urinary excretion
of $Na^+$ = ~100 mmole/day
0.4% of filtered load remaining

**Figure 14-7** Renal handling of $Na^+$ along the nephron. The numbered boxes indicate the absolute amount of $Na^+$—as well as the fraction of the filtered load—that various nephron segments reabsorb. The pink boxes indicate the fraction of the filtered load that remains in the lumen at these sites. PNa, plasma sodium concentration; UNa, urine sodium concentration. (From Boron WF: Medical Physiology. Updated ed. Philadelphia, Saunders, 2005.)

used to control hypertension when a mild diuretic alone is insufficient. If these drugs cannot be prescribed because of intolerance, vasomotor center-acting agents like clonidine typically can be used. "Compelling indications," frequency of drug administration, and potential side effects of different agents are also considered in making decisions about the appropriate therapy for hypertension. Compelling indications are those benefits that have been identified from outcome studies or clinical guideline recommendations for hypertensive therapies.[38]

The Seventh Report of the Joint National Committee on Prevention, Detection, Evaluation, and Treatment of High Blood Pressure (JNC 7) was published in 2003.[38] Included in the extensive review of landmark studies regarding pharmacologic management of high blood pressure, the committee identified high-risk conditions with "compelling indications" for recommending the use of certain antihypertensive agents.

For individuals with hypertension associated with
- Heart failure: diuretics, β-blockers, ACE inhibitors, ARBs, and aldosterone antagonists are recommended.
- Post–myocardial infarction: β-blockers, ACE inhibitors, and aldosterone antagonists are recommended.
- High coronary disease risk: diuretics, β-blockers, ACE inhibitors, and calcium-channel blockers are recommended.

- Diabetes mellitus: diuretics, β-blockers, ACE inhibitors, ARBs, calcium-channel blockers are recommended.
- Chronic kidney disease: ACE inhibitors and ARBs are recommended.

**Vasodilators.** This group of antihypertensive drugs acts directly on vascular smooth muscle cells to reduce peripheral vascular resistance (arterial dilation) or venous return to the heart (venous dilation). Systolic hypertension can be treated effectively with arterial dilators. Hydralazine (Apresoline), minoxidil (Loniten), and diazoxide (Hyperstat IV) are examples of arterial dilators. Calcium-channel blockers reduce blood pressure by inhibiting actin and myosin coupling within vascular smooth muscle, thereby promoting smooth muscle dilation (discussed earlier in this chapter). Venodilators are especially effective in the treatment of diastolic hypertension because they reduce cardiac preload and end-diastolic pressure (see Table 14-10). Sodium nitroprusside (Nipride) is both a venous and arterial dilator. Many vasodilators can be administered either orally or intravenously; the latter is the route of choice for rapid treatment of malignant systemic hypertension.

In response to vasodilation, compensatory sympathetic activation such as tachycardia, reflex vasoconstriction, increased aldosterone, and elevated plasma renin often occurs. For these reasons, in the management of hypertension, vasodilators are usually used in combination with β-blocking or other sympathetic nervous system–inhibiting drugs. In addition, simultaneous diuretic therapy can limit fluid retention caused by the compensatory increase in aldosterone associated with the use of vasodilators.

Several newer groups of drugs with vasodilating properties have been used in acute management of pulmonary hypertension and with critically ill patients. These include prostacyclin and inhaled nitric oxide (see discussion in the section Cardiac Drugs Used in Critical Care).

### Drugs Acting on the Renin-Angiotensin System

Three of the stimulants for renin production by the renal cortex are (1) a drop in renal artery pressure, (2) sympathetic nervous system stimulation, and (3) sodium reduction. Renin reacts to form angiotensin I, and in the presence of a converting enzyme (ACE), angiotensin I forms angiotensin II (Fig. 14-8). This latter substance is a potent vasoconstrictor that influences aldosterone production and subsequent sodium retention, all factors that result in blood pressure elevation. Unlike vasodilators, ACE inhibitors do not result in reflex sympathetic nervous system activity. Studies provide strong evidence of the efficacy of ACE inhibitors in blood pressure management in patients with depressed ejection fraction, further accounting for their frequent use (see Table 14-10).[41]

Another class of antihypertensive agents that block the angiotensin II receptor are vasoconstrictive (angiotensin-receptor blockers, ARBs). As a result, vasoconstriction and aldosterone secretion are reduced. Blood pressure is lowered by decreased vascular tone and decreased water and sodium retention (see Table 14-10).[42] Both ACE inhibitors and ARBs are equally effective in controlling blood pressure; however, the cough found in about 20% of individuals taking ACE inhibitors is not a side effect of ARBs.

### Centrally Acting Drugs

A number of drugs reduce central sympathetic outflow, of which clonidine (Catapres Duraclon) is the most important one. It inhibits the vasomotor center in the brain and reduces peripheral resistance and cardiac output. It can cause some nausea, drowsiness, palpitations, and in rare cases CHF.

## Lipid Disorders

In 1985, a turning point occurred in the awareness and management of lipid disorders in the United States. In that year the National Institutes of Health Consensus Conference concluded what many practitioners had believed for years: elevated blood cholesterol levels, especially low-density lipoprotein (LDL), were associated with premature coronary heart disease and, most important for clinical practice, lowering the LDL levels decreased the risk of developing coronary heart disease. The panel recommended guidelines for treatment, including dietary and pharmacologic interventions as well as screening programs to identify persons at risk. Since that time, people have become familiar with the

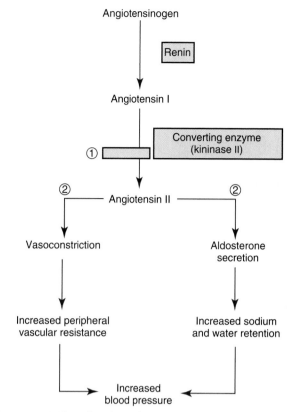

**Figure 14-8** Site of action of captopril (Capoten) blockade at 1 and angiotensin II–receptor blockade at 2. (Adapted from Katzung BG [ed.]. Basic and Clinical Pharmacology. 5th ed. East Norwalk, CT, Appleton & Lange, 1992.)

terms *good cholesterol* (HDL), *bad cholesterol* (LDL), and *saturated fat*, not only from the medical establishment but also from the media, food corporations, and consumer activism. Early detection and awareness of lipid abnormalities has improved over the past quarter century because of advances within the scientific community and heightened consumer knowledge.

The 21st century has brought lipid management into a new arena based on the contributions of technological advances, genetics, and expanded understanding of lipid metabolism and subclasses of HDL and LDL.

Cholesterol is a naturally occurring fat-like substance that is found within various tissues of the body: cell membranes, hormones, and plasma. Approximately 93% of all cholesterol is found in cell membranes, and the other 7% circulates within the blood plasma. A relatively small amount of the circulating cholesterol is used by the adrenals and gonads for hormone synthesis, and another small proportion is used by peripheral cells in building and maintaining membranous structures.

Cholesterol is transported in the blood within a lipid molecule, which in turn is carried by a protein. This complex is called a lipoprotein. Therefore, assessment of cholesterol abnormalities involves lipoprotein assessment. Three major lipoproteins carry blood cholesterol:

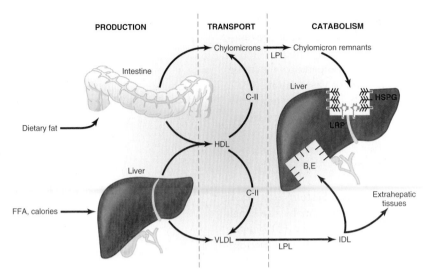

**Figure 14-9** Lipid metabolism: Dietary fat is hydrolyzed by pancreatic lipase, absorbed by intestinal mucosal cells and secreted as chylomicrons. Liver transforms plasma free fatty acids (FFAs) (when excess calories are ingested) into triglycerides (TGs) and also secretes additional very-low-density lipoprotein (VLDL). High-density lipoprotein (HDL) is secreted by both liver and intestines. HDL increases the availability of apolipoprotein C II (apo C-II) for chylomicrons and VLDL degradation. apo C-II is an important factor for lipoprotein lipase (LPL). LPL catabolizes the breakdown of chylomicrons into chylomicron remnants and VLDL into intermediate-density lipoproteins (IDLs). After hydrolysis of VLDL and chylomicrons, any excess phospholipids, apoproteins, or cholesterol is taken up by HDL. HDL mass may increase. IDLs are partly converted to cholesterol rich LDL (low density lipoprotein) particles and taken up by the LDL receptors on the liver (apo B and apo E) or on the receptors of extrahepatic tissue. Chylomicrons are taken up by receptors on the liver: LDL receptor–related protein (LRP) and heparin sulfate proteoglycans (HSPG). HDL scavenges cholesterol from extrahepatic tissue and transports it back to the liver for processing.

- Low-density lipoproteins
- High-density lipoproteins
- Very-low-density lipoproteins (VLDL)

Triglycerides, a glycerol molecule with three fatty acid chains, make up about 80% of VLDL with the remaining 20% being cholesterol (Fig 14-9).

The liver is the major site of cholesterol metabolism.[11] The liver obtains cholesterol from three major sources: (a) the intestines, in the form of chylomicrons, (b) from LDL, and (c) and via de novo synthesis. The liver exports cholesterol as bile acids and as VLDL.[11]

As understanding of the complex nature of lipoproteins has advanced, lipid management has become more targeted toward specific populations and pathologies. In general, recommendations for optimal lipid management include the following: total cholesterol <200 mg/dL; HDL >40 mg/dL; and LDL <100 mg/dL. However specific lipid profile recommendations for any individual is strongly influenced by age, gender, the amount of atherosclerotic risk factors present, as well as the medical conditions of diabetes, metabolic syndrome, and known atherosclerotic disease, such as peripheral vascular disease, abdominal aortic aneurysm, vessel inflammatory processes, and carotid stenosis.[43]

## Drugs for Lipid Disorders

Therapeutic intervention for dyslipidemia begins with LDL-c control.[44] The first recommended treatment approach to decrease LDL-C is therapeutic lifestyle changes (TLCs) for 12 weeks including a diet with reduced saturated fat, reduced cholesterol, increased soluble fiber, increased plant sterols, weight loss, increased physical activity. Initiation of drug therapy is appropriate after that time, if the response is inadequate to achieve the LDL-C treatment goal within a reasonable time frame.[44] Target levels of LDL-C are influenced by the existence of cardiovascular disease (CVD) risk factors, already existing coronary heart disease (CHD), diabetes, metabolic syndrome, and atherogenic dyslipidemia, which consists of low HDL-C, elevated triglycerides, and increased apo B lipid protein (small, dense LDL-C) (Table 14-14).

Although in general drug interventions and target guidelines are directed toward reduction in LDL-C, non-HDL values are used instead of LDL in the patient population with elevated triglycerides (>200): "non-HDL-C more accurately reflects the cholesterol concentration in all atherogenic lipoproteins."[45] Drug management for lipid control is often multidimensional. In general, the primary goal is to reduce LDL, usually with the use of "statin drugs." Addition of niacin, fish oils, fibrates and bile acid sequestrants may be added based on an individual's medical profile and response to the side effects of the drugs (Table 14-15).

### Side Effects

Some of the more common side effects include the following: gastrointestinal distress (e.g., constipation, diarrhea, and nausea), liver function abnormalities, skin rashes and flushing (especially with niacin), increased bleeding time (especially with fish oils), slight increase in gallstone formation (gemfibrozil), increased blood glucose levels (niacin),

## Table 14-14 Lipid Goals per Populations

| LDL-C Goal | Non-HDL Goal (When Triglycerides > 200) | Population |
|---|---|---|
| <70 | <100 | Metabolic syndrome |
| | | ACS |
| | | Known CV disease |
| | | Diabetes + 1 major CV risk factor (smoking, HTN, family history) |
| <100 | <130 | Poorly controlled CV risk factors |
| | | CHD or CHD risk equivalents |
| | | Diabetes, no other major CV risk |
| | | 2+ CV risk factors (but no diabetes) |
| <130 | <160 | 2+ risk factors for CVD |

*ACS, acute coronary syndrome; CHD, coronary heart disease; CV, cardiovascular; CVD, cardiovascular disease; HDL, high-density lipoprotein; HTN, hypertension; LDL-C, low-density lipoprotein cholesterol.*
*Data from Brunzell JD, Davidson M, Furberg CD, et al. Lipoprotein management in patients with cardiometabolic risk: consensus statement from the American Diabetes Association and the American College of Cardiology Foundation. Diabetes Care. 2008 Apr;31(4):811-22.; and Grundy SM, Cleeman JI, Merz CN, et al. Implications of recent clinical trials for the National Cholesterol Education Program Adult Treatment Panel III guidelines. Circulation. 2004 Jul 13;110(2): 227-39.*

and potential to worsen glucose levels in diabetes patients (niacin).

Lovastatin may contribute to headaches, sleep disturbances, decreased sleep duration, fatigue, and muscle cramping. Pravastatin, another 3-hydroxy-3-methylglutaryl–coenzyme A (HMG-CoA) reductase inhibitor, does not cross the blood–brain barrier, as does lovastatin, and therefore may have less effect on the central nervous system.

One of the most common adverse effects concerns the skeletal muscles. Resting muscle pain in the first few weeks after starting a statin medication usually indicates toxicity to the medication and can lead to muscle breakdown and in extreme cases rhabdomyolysis (dark urine and kidney failure from protein processing by the kidney). The medication should be discontinued when this symptom occurs and the effects are usually reversible.

Adverse side effects are more likely with combinations of drug therapy rather than single agent management; for example, HMG-CoA reductase agents (statins), when combined with niacin, increases the risk of liver toxicity; stains

with gemfibrozil or niacin may provoke myositis, muscle tenderness, and fatigue. Caution must be observed in prescribing fibric acids for patients who are on oral anticoagulants, as their anticoagulation effect may be potentiated.

Because of the potential for worsening glucose levels, niacin is not generally recommended for the diabetic patient; if deemed medically necessary, there must be very tight glucose monitoring. Liver enzyme levels should be checked within the first 6 weeks and again at 3- and 6-month intervals as needed for patients on lovastatin, niacin, and gemfibrozil. General fatigue, achiness, and abdominal discomfort may accompany elevated lipid levels. Patients who exercise and take lovastatin often complain of muscle achiness and should be evaluated for possible drug-induced side effects and exercise intolerance.

It is imperative to have blood liver enzyme determinations done, in particular during early therapy with statins. Early detection of liver problems and discontinuation of the drug usually reverses adverse hepatic pathology.

## Cardiac Drugs Used in Critical Care

Many pathologic conditions warrant observation and management in the critical care setting. The hemodynamic instability caused by an underlying pathologic condition often requires quick responsiveness by the medical staff. Administration of appropriate pharmacologic agents and close monitoring of their effects can significantly alter the outcome of therapy. Numerous cardiovascular conditions may be responsible for systemic compromise. Common etiologies include the following:

- Acute myocardial ischemia or infarct
- Congestive heart failure and pulmonary edema
- Cardiac structural abnormalities
- Cardiac conduction system disease

Clinical presentations of these cardiac dysfunctions may include the following:

- Hypoxia
- Pain
- Alterations in blood pressure (e.g., hypertension or hypotension)
- Shock
- Alterations in heart rate
- Heart rhythm abnormalities

Whenever possible, drug therapy is directed at correction of the underlying pathologic condition, for example, thrombolysis (discussed elsewhere in this chapter). In addition to providing the patient with oxygen to help reverse hypoxia, pharmacologic therapy may focus on the manipulation of the autonomic nervous system to favorably alter hemodynamics. Drug agonists and antagonists of the parasympathetic and sympathetic nervous systems are used to induce changes in vasomotor tone, cardiac inotropy, and chronotropy. Cardiac output may be further improved by the administration of antihypertensive agents (those acting independent of the autonomic nervous system) and antiarrhythmic drugs.

## Table 14-15 Lipid Management

| Primary Goal | Drug Class | Drug name | Action | Major Adverse Side Effects |
|---|---|---|---|---|
| Decrease LDL | HMG-CoA Reductase Inhibitor/ "STATINS" | Atorvastatin (Lipitor) Cerivastatin (Baycol) Fluvastatin (Lescol) Lovastatin (Mevacor) Pravastatin (Pravachol) Rosuvastatin (Crestor) Simvastatin (Zocor) | Increases LDL-receptor activity Inhibits cholesterol synthesis | Myopathy Liver problems with elevated blood liver enzymes |
| | Anion exchange resins/bile acid sequestrants | Cholestyramine (Questran) Colestipol (Colestid) Colesevelam (WelChol) | Binds intestinal bile, causing fecal excretion of bile acids Increase LDL-receptor activity | GI distress Decreased absorption of other drugs and vitamins May increase triglycerides |
| | Inhibit intestinal absorption of cholesterol | Ezetimibe (Zetia) | | |
| Increase HDL | Nicotinic acid Immediate release Extended release Sustained release Nicotinic acid combined w statin | Niacin | Increases HDL Reduces hepatic synthesis of VLDL Decreases plasma levels of free fatty acids | Flushing; upper GI distress; increase blood sugar |
| Decrease triglycerides and increase HDL | Fibrates | Fenofibrate Gemfibrozil (Lopid) Clofibrate (Atromid-S) Fenofibric acid delayed release (Trilipix Oral) | Reduces ability of free fatty acids to form triglycerides Increases intravascular breakdown of VLDL | Dyspepsia; gallstones; myopathy |
| | Inhibit intestinal absorption of cholesterol | Ezetimibe (Zetia) | | GI distress; myalgia; arthralgia |
| Decrease triglycerides | Fish oils/ Omega-3 fatty acid | Many over-the-counter varieties | | GI distress; fishy aftertaste; increased bleeding time |
| | Nicotinic acid | | | |

*GI, gastrointestinal; HMG-CoA, 3-hydroxy-3-methylglutaryl-coenzyme A; HDL, high-density lipoprotein; LDL, low-density lipoprotein; VLDL, very-low-density lipoprotein.*
*Adapted from Rakel R: Conn's Current Therapy 1999. Philadelphia, WB Saunders, 1999:570.*

Elimination of pain, induction of sedation, and prevention of the complications of bedrest may also be addressed with drug therapy in the critical care setting.

Pharmacologic management of the patient in the cardiac critical care setting is often guided by invasive measurement as well as by symptoms. For example, when prescribing a vasodilator, the physician must closely monitor left ventricular filling pressures (preload) and cardiac output. Patients with dyspnea and high filling pressures might benefit from venodilators to reduce preload, whereas patients with fatigue and low cardiac output might benefit from arteriodilators to improve forward output.[46]

**Table 14-16 Suggested Therapeutic Interventions in Relation to Hemodynamic Indices Found in Acute Myocardial Infarction**

| Hemodynamic Category | Cardiac Output | Left Ventricular Filling Pressure | Suggested Therapy |
|---|---|---|---|
| Normal | Normal | Normal | Observation |
| Hypovolemia | Decreased | Decreased or normal | Volume replacement |
| Pulmonary congestion Left ventricular failure | Normal | Raised | Diuretics |
| Moderate | Decreased | Raised | Afterload-reducing agents, with or without diuretics |
| Severe (cardiogenic shock) | Markedly decreased | Raised | Circulatory assist (counterpulsation) Afterload-reducing agents Use of inotropic agents if other measures do not increase cardiac output[a] |

[a]*For example, dopamine (Intropin, Dopastat), dobutamine (Dobutrex).*
*Adapted from Sokolow M, McIlroy M, Cheitlin M. Clinical Cardiology. 5th ed. East Norwalk, CT, Appleton & Lange, 1990.*

Table 14-16 categorizes hemodynamic indices found in acute myocardial infarction and suggests guidelines for use of pharmacologic agents in this setting.

## Oxygen

Although oxygen is not frequently thought of as a drug, it should be thought of as a drug, and it warrants a brief discussion in the context of pharmacologic considerations in cardiac critical care. Tissue hypoxia caused by disturbances in cardiac output can rarely be improved by the administration of oxygen. However, oxygen therapy is usually beneficial when concomitant hypoxemia exists.[47] Pulmonary edema, often a finding with congestive heart failure, can hinder oxygen diffusion in the lung, thereby decreasing arterial oxygen content. The administration of oxygen may help limit the severity of hypoxemia and consequent tissue hypoxia. In addition, when hemoglobin concentration is reduced, as in anemia or in conditions that cause hemoglobin to desaturate, the administration of oxygen is considered beneficial. Oxygen delivery systems are discussed in Chapter 10.

## Drugs that Affect the Autonomic Nervous System

The autonomic nervous system (ANS) exerts significant control over cardiovascular function. A complex system of feedback loops coordinates reflex responses of the sympathetic and the parasympathetic nervous systems. Transmission of impulses from the autonomic portion of the central nervous system to the effector organ to be stimulated occurs via neurotransmitter substances. As discussed in the introduction, most preganglionic fibers, and all parasympathetic nervous system postganglionic fibers, release acetylcholine. Most sympathetic nervous system postganglionic fibers release

norepinephrine (noradrenaline). These substances can be partially or completely mimicked by pharmacologic agents (e.g., sympathomimetics, parasympathomimetics, or sympathetic or parasympathetic nervous system agonists). Similarly, receptors in the effector organ can be partially or completely blocked by pharmacologic agents (e.g., adrenoceptor or cholinoceptor blocking agents or sympathetic or parasympathetic nervous system antagonists).

When negative alterations in mean arterial blood pressure are sensed, adrenoceptors and cholinoceptors are stimulated. Appropriate modification of peripheral vascular resistance and cardiac output are orchestrated (Fig. 14-10). In a critically ill cardiac patient, pharmacologic agents can act on the autonomic nervous system receptors to help bring about a hemodynamic stability and an effective cardiac output. By fine manipulation of the degree of vasodilation, vasoconstriction, or cardiac inotropy, an adequate mean arterial blood pressure can be established with drug therapy. Table 14-17 lists drugs that act as agonists or antagonists to the sympathetic and parasympathetic nervous systems to control blood pressure in the critical care setting. Because of the reflex nature of the feedback "loop" of the autonomic nervous system, the effects of these agents must be monitored closely. Although some drugs are receptor selective, most act on multiple receptor sites. Often drugs are used in combinations in an attempt to reduce or augment certain hemodynamic responses, which further emphasizes the importance of medical observation. Epinephrine (Adrenalin Chloride), for example, is both an α-adrenergic agonist and a β-adrenergic agonist.

## Non-ANS Vasodilator and Inotropic Agents

In addition to manipulating the autonomic nervous system with drugs to manage arterial blood pressure in critical

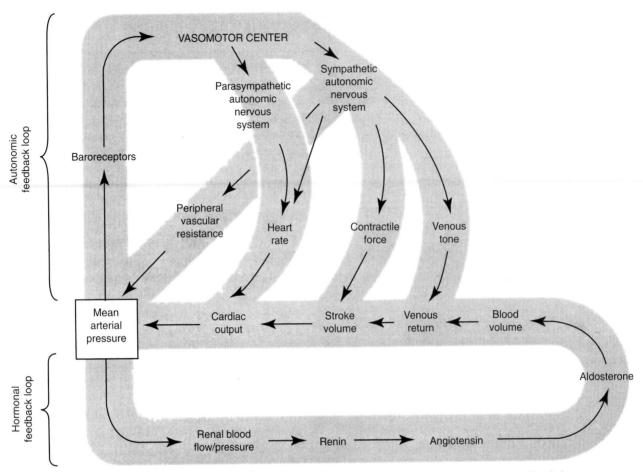

**Figure 14-10** Autonomic and hormonal control of cardiovascular function. Note that at least two feedback loops are present: the autonomic nervous system loop and the hormonal loop. In addition, each major loop has several components. Thus, the sympathetic nervous system directly influences four major variables: peripheral vascular resistance, heart rate, force, and venous tone. The parasympathetic nervous system directly influences heart rate. Angiotensin II directly increases peripheral vascular resistance (not shown), and the sympathetic nervous system directly increases renin secretion (not shown). Because these control mechanisms are designed to maintain normal blood pressure, the net feedback effect of each loop is negative in that it tends to compensate for the change in arterial blood pressure that evoked the response. Thus, decreased blood pressure due to blood loss would be compensated for by increased sympathetic outflow and renin release. Conversely, elevated pressure due to the administration of a vasoconstrictor drug would cause reduced sympathetic outflow and renin release and increased parasympathetic (vagal) outflow. (From Katzung BG [ed.]. Basic and Clinical Pharmacology. 5th ed. East Norwalk, CT, Appleton & Lange, 1992:76.)

care, physicians can also prescribe other antihypertensive and/or vasodilating agents. Sodium nitroprusside (Nipride), a potent peripheral vasodilator, and intravenous nitroglycerin are frequently used.[33] The intravenous nitroglycerin produces a slightly greater reduction in preload and a slightly lesser reduction in afterload as compared with those of sodium nitroprusside.[48] Although both agents are effective in reducing blood pressure, the intravenous nitroglycerin is the emergency drug of choice in the treatment of congestive heart failure associated with ischemic heart disease. Sodium nitroprusside is the parenteral treatment of choice for hypertension emergencies. Nesiritide (Natrecor) is a recombinant form of human brain natriuretic peptide, and is a potent vasodilator. Its use is typically reserved for symptomatic relief of acute decompensated heart failure when initial therapy (diuretics and nonparenteral nitrates) is not effective.[49]

As discussed earlier in this chapter, diuretics act to reduce central venous pressures by decreasing venous return. Furosemide (Lasix) is a potent, rapidly acting diuretic often administered parenterally in the emergency treatment of pulmonary congestion in the presence of left ventricular dysfunction.

Phosphodiesterase inhibitors are positive inotropic agents that are used cautiously in the treatment of acute decompensated heart failure. Milrinone (Primacor) and inamrinone (Inocor; previously amrinone) belong to this group of inotropes. They are used short term, parenterally administered, and have severe side effects that may result in increased mortality when compared to similarly acting agents. Patients awaiting heart transplantation are frequently managed on one of these drugs.[50]

Direct pharmacologic treatment of pulmonary hypertension has not been available until recently. Potent vasodilators

## Table 14-17 Drugs Affecting the Autonomic Nervous System: Agents Commonly Used in Critical Care

| Autonomic Nervous System Receptor | Action | Agonist Generic (Trade) Name | Antagonist Generic (Trade) Name |
|---|---|---|---|
| **Adrenoceptor** | | | |
| $\alpha_1$ | Contraction of vascular smooth muscle | Phenylephrine (Neo-Synephrine) | See antihypertensives (Table 14-10) ($\alpha_1$ blockers) |
| | | Methoxamine (Vasoxyl) | |
| $\alpha_2$ | Contraction of vascular smooth muscle | Clonidine (Catapres) | Tolazoline (Priscoline) |
| | Platelet aggregation | $\alpha$-methyl-norepinephrine | Yohimbine (Yohimex) |
| Combined $\alpha_2$ and $\alpha_2$ | | Epinephrine[a] (Adrenalin Chloride) | Phentolamine (Rogitine) |
| | | Norepinephrine[b] (Levophed) | |
| $\beta_1$ | Increased force and rate of cardiac contraction | Norepinephrine[b] (Levophed) | See $\beta$-blockers (Table 14-3) |
| | | Dobutamine (Dobutrex) | |
| $\beta_2$ | Relaxation of vascular, respiratory smooth muscle | Albuterol (Proventil, Ventolin) | See $\beta$-blockers (Table 14-3) |
| | | Terbutaline (Brethine) | |
| | | Metaproterenol (Alupent, Metaprel) | |
| Combined $\beta_1$ and $\beta_2$ | | Isoproterenol[c] (Isuprel) | See $\beta$-blockers (Table 14-3) |
| | | Epinephrine[a] (Adrenalin Chloride) | |
| Dopaminic | Vasodilation | Dopamine (Intropin) | |
| **Cholinoceptor** | | | |
| Muscarinic | Decreased rate and force of atrial contraction | Acetylcholine (Miochol) | Atropine (Isopto Atropine) |
| | Decreased peripheral vascular resistance | Edrophonium[d] (Tensilon) | |

[a]Epinephrine is also called adrenalin; it acts primarily as a $\beta$-agonist.
[b]Norepinephrine is also called noradrenalin or levarterenol.
[c]Isoproterenol is also called isoprenaline.
[d]This is not a direct-acting agonist; rather it acts indirectly by inhibiting acetylcholinesterase, thereby increasing acetylcholine.

including prostacyclin (and prostacyclin analogues) and nitric oxide have shown hemodynamic and symptomatic benefits in certain patients. A number of these agents, with variable routes of administration (inhaled, oral, subcutaneous), are in research trials and have demonstrated improvement in functional status.[33,50] Currently, prostacyclin (PGI2; epoprostenol; Flolan) is administered via central line into a continuous ambulatory infusion system; nitric oxide (INOmax) is inhaled. The latter has been used to treat pulmonary HTN associated with respiratory distress syndrome.[49]

### Antiarrhythmic Agents

Life-threatening arrhythmias are commonly treated in cardiac critical care units. In addition to electrical cardioversion of unstable rhythms, pharmacologic intervention is the mainstay of medical treatment. Lidocaine (Xylocaine) and amiodarone (Cordarone) are the primary agents used to suppress ventricular ectopy in critically ill patients.[33] If the patient is stable, lidocaine may be used prophylactically for patients with acute myocardial ischemia and therapeutically for patients suffering ventricular tachycardia or fibrillation. In emergencies, either drug is delivered as a bolus injection that is followed by a subsequent continuous intravenous infusion. When lidocaine (Xylocaine) or amiodarone (Cordarone) is unable to control ventricular arrhythmias, procainamide (Pronestyl) may be useful.

Verapamil (Isoptin, Calan), a calcium-channel blocker (class 4 antiarrhythmic), has been used in the management of supraventricular tachycardia not requiring cardioversion.

Acute management of new-onset paroxysmal supraventricular tachycardia (PSVT) is often treated with adenosine, a naturally occurring endogenous purine nucleoside. Adenosine (Adenocard) is very effective in terminating PSVT when a reentry pathway involving either the sinus node or AV node is involved, including the tachycardias associated with Wolff–Parkinson–White syndrome. Adenocard is given as a rapid IV bolus; its peak effect occurs within seconds.

Finally, digitalis may be used to control the ventricular response rate to atrial flutter or fibrillation. Unfortunately, it may cause significant toxicity and adverse drug interactions in critically ill patients. Although digitalis may successfully convert paroxysmal supraventricular tachycardia to normal sinus rhythm, it may alternatively convert atrial flutter to atrial fibrillation. Digitalis's effects on contractility are less potent than those of sympathomimetic parenteral inotropes, such as dobutamine (Dobutrex) or norepinephrine (Levophed) and therefore digitalis typically is not used for this purpose in critical care.

## Other Pharmacologic Agents Used in Critical Care

Other pharmacologic agents frequently used in critical care include anticoagulants, such as heparin (Liquaemin Sodium), sedatives to reduce agitation and anxiety, and analgesics. Morphine sulfate, included in this last group, is the drug of choice for management of myocardial ischemic pain.

However, it is also very useful in the treatment of acute cardiogenic pulmonary edema. It is a potent vasodilator and acts to increase venous capacitance as well as to relieve pulmonary congestion. Electrolyte replacement is also a common occurrence in the management of the critically ill patient. Imbalances of potassium, sodium, or magnesium often occur as a result of compromised renal function and/or excess fluid administration.

Advances in the management of acute coronary syndromes have facilitated the growth of specialized critical care units. Patients who undergo percutaneous coronary interventions typically receive protocol-driven pharmacologic therapies and require close monitoring and specific management. These patients are at high risk for excessive bleeding owing to the inherent thrombolytic, fibrinolytic, antiplatelet, and anticoagulant properties of many of the agents used to reverse the blockage responsible for the initial coronary event (Table 14-5). In conclusion, as patients become hemodynamically stable, the prescription of many of the potent drugs described in this section is discontinued and replaced by oral medications. Readers interested in additional information regarding drugs used in critical care are encouraged to refer to the *Textbook of Advanced Cardiac Life Support* published by the American Heart Association.

## Cardiac Pharmacology in the Geriatric Population

All drugs, not just those prescribed for cardiac problems, may have altered pharmacokinetics and pharmacodynamics in the elderly. Normal aging involves changes in body composition

### Table 14-18 Average Changes in Body Composition and Function with Age

| Area of Change | Change from Age 20 To Age 80 (%) |
| --- | --- |
| Body fat/total body weight | +35 |
| Plasma volume | −8 |
| Plasma albumin | −10 |
| Plasma globulin | −10 |
| Total body water | −17 |
| Extracellular fluid (from age 20 to age 65) | −40 |
| Conduction velocity | −20 |
| Cardiac index | −40 |
| Glomerular filtration rate | −50 |
| Vital capacity | −60 |
| Cardiac output | −30–40 |
| Splanchnic and renal blood flow | −40 |

*From Kalant H, Roschlau W, Sellers M. Principles of Medical Pharmacology. 4th ed. New York, Oxford University Press, 1985:68.*

and function (Table 14-18). Specifically, decreases in renal function, reduced liver metabolism, and altered blood flow (as in coronary artery disease and congestive heart failure) are responsible for adverse or suboptimal reactions to cardiac drugs. The elderly also exhibit increased sensitivity to the toxic effects of cardiac drugs, such as antiarrhythmics, digitalis, or β-blockers. Other disease states such as kidney, liver, or nutritional deficiencies, which often accompany aging, can alter the effectiveness of cardiac drug therapy. In addition, numerous socioeconomic and practical considerations can affect the degree of compliance by the elderly with these drug regimens.

## Alteration in Pharmacokinetics

Elderly patients may have difficulty with absorption, distribution, or metabolism of cardiac drugs. Effective drug elimination is dependent on adequate hepatic and renal function. The typical age-related decline in kidney competency significantly increases the likelihood of drug accumulation and subsequent toxicity. This problem of drug accumulation is especially relevant with regard to the older patient's cardiac conduction system. The elderly are more susceptible to arrhythmias. Positive inotropes, such as digitalis, and antihypertensive agents, such as diuretics, can be particularly dangerous. These drugs alter electrolytes involved in conduction tissue depolarization. Inadequate drug elimination and consequent accumulation can cause cardiac irritability and a higher incidence of arrhythmias. Evidence from the Atrial Fibrillation Follow-up Investigation of Rhythm Management (AFFIRM)[51] trial demonstrated that older individuals in atrial fibrillation have better cardiovascular outcomes when using medications that control cardiac rate (β-blockers, diltiazem, verapamil) than on medications that control rhythm (antiarrhythmics)

"Specific drugs" that are poorly tolerated by older persons include class IB antiarrhythmics (see Table 14-12). These drugs tend to be associated with mental confusion in this population. The antihypertensives methyldopa, reserpine, and clonidine can decrease mental acuity and produce sedation at increased doses in geriatric individuals (see Table 14-10). In addition, propranolol, a nonselective β-adrenergic antagonist, can cause confusion, sleep disturbance, and depression in older persons. Postural hypotension can result from certain antihypertensive drugs (e.g., Prazosin initiation) as well as ACE inhibitors used in conjunction with diuretics.[52] The combination of sensitivity to these drugs, and the blunted baroreceptor responsiveness in geriatric patients, enables postural hypotension to occur occasionally. There is evidence that when used to treat hypertension in the elderly, diuretics have less morbidity than ACE inhibitors or calcium-channel blockers.[53] However, evidence shows that when used to treat CHF in the elderly, ACE inhibitors are safer than digoxin. This is especially true when treating elderly women (mean 85 years old) with systolic heart failure.[54,55]

Another problem in the elderly is the presence of noncardiac diseases as well as the use of multiple drugs for all conditions increasing the risk of unwanted drug interactions. It is imperative for the physician and pharmacist to pay special attention to such problems because a sophisticated selection of medications can easily reduce or even prevent detrimental drug interactions.

## Therapeutic Indications

Cardiovascular drugs are used for treatment of the same conditions in the elderly as in other age groups.[56] Evidence from the Heart Protection Study and the Prospective Study of Pravastatin in the Elderly at Risk (PROSPER) study demonstrate that lipid lowering with statins reduces cardiovascular deaths (vs. no medications), and that this effect on cardiovascular mortality is especially significant in secondary prevention in the elderly with known cardiovascular disease.[57,58] Results from additional randomization in the Heart Protection Study revealed no cardiovascular benefit from vitamins E or C or β-carotene in the elderly. Ott and colleagues were able to demonstrate that diuretic use in the elderly had no negative effect on blood lipids.[59]

Although not specifically considered cardiovascular pharmacologic therapy, it is important to address the role of hormone replacement therapy in the prevention of cardiovascular disease in women. Until the results of the Women's Health Initiative (WHI) were released, the use of estrogen in postmenopausal women was considered cardioprotective.[60] Although the results of the WHI have been controversial, it appears that hormone replacement therapy may have negative cardiac effects if started in women 10 years after menopause and after 65 years of age.

Elderly patients often demonstrate difficulty with full compliance with drug prescriptions. Patients may get confused and forget a dose. When elderly patients feel good, they may choose to discontinue taking the drug, or the side effects themselves may discourage patients from taking the drug. Although these issues may occur in younger age groups, the elderly are especially susceptible to these problems. Dementia or physical inability may also hamper adequate utilization of cardiovascular drugs. Seemingly simple items such as reading drug labels, removing bottle caps, or distinguishing pill color can present major obstacles to visually impaired or physically disabled elderly patients. Drug holders with the day of the week written on each compartment may improve compliance with medications. There are also pill containers with alarms that help with compliance. These patients are also confused when they obtain their generic drugs in different colors and shapes during different refills. Here it is the duty of the pharmacist to explain carefully that it is indeed the correct drug just manufactured by different pharmaceutical producers.

Safe and effective use of cardiovascular agents in the geriatric population can be enhanced by knowledgeable health care providers and educated patients and family members. Drug regimens should be simplified whenever possible, with small initial doses and progressive titration until a therapeutic response is reached. In addition, when working with the older patient, the medical team should remain alert to adverse drug reactions and interactions, taking care to avoid provoking a drug reaction that would be worse than the disease itself.

In addition, socioeconomic factors will play a role. Lower-socioeconomic groups might have difficulty obtaining proper health care and might not be financially able to afford the medications or to save on the use of medications by skipping doses. These patients should be alerted that there are special governmental as well as industrial programs available that might help in getting the proper drugs either free or at a greatly reduced rate. Educational status also plays a role in that less-educated patients do not understand the seriousness of their illnesses or the need to take drugs as prescribed.

## Cardiac Pharmacology in the Neonate and Pediatric Populations

Although many pharmacologic agents used to treat adult cardiac conditions are also used to treat neonate and pediatric patients, the younger population's response may again demonstrate significant clinical differences. The immature organism can demonstrate unpredictable responses because of the unique pharmacokinetic and pharmacodynamic reactions found during each stage of development. In addition, most cardiac drug activity has been studied in adults, and the paucity of controlled research on the immature patient causes further concern regarding optimal drug therapy in this population. Of note, when evidence of drug efficacy is available in this population, oftentimes there is a lack of evidence regarding the long-term use of these agents on growth and development, including during transition through puberty and adolescence.

## Alteration in Drug Eliminations

Newborns and infants show different pharmacokinetics. Adequate plasma concentrations of a drug can be influenced by administration and absorption of the agent. Newborns absorb drugs more slowly than children, whereas children may have difficulty swallowing medicines. Drugs delivered intravenously bypass the absorption process; however, choosing the intravenous route increases the risks of fluid overload. The relative intolerance of infants to the volumes of fluid needed to carry a drug warrants slower rates of infusion and at times negligible concentrations if the drug is eliminated at the same rate. As the infant develops, changes in body composition and plasma protein-binding capacity affect the distribution of a drug. Total body water decreases as adipose tissue increases and fluid shifts between body compartments. Drugs are less avidly bound to plasma proteins in neonates and infants than in children and adults. Development of the liver and kidneys affects metabolism and elimination of a drug, with both organs showing decreased function at birth. However, infants and young children may metabolize some drugs faster than adults.

Similarly, infants and young children exhibit different pharmacodynamics. The ability of the infant or child to respond to adequate concentrations of a cardiac drug is influenced by structural concerns that are unique to the developing organism.[61,62] Although not well studied in humans, fetal and newborn puppies and lambs exhibit (1) stiffer, less compliant ventricles; (2) smaller myocardial cells (adjusted for weight and size); and (3) a higher proportion of noncontractile to contractile tissue (e.g., mitochondria to myofilaments) as compared with the adult. Sympathetic nervous system innervation of the heart and periphery are decreased at birth and continue to develop during the first few months of life. Infants and young children have a higher baseline heart rate; this, in combination with a lower stroke volume, which has a limited ability to increase, means that the ways to improve cardiac output with drugs may be impaired.

## Therapeutic Indications

Cardiac conditions in pediatric populations that warrant pharmacologic intervention usually include heart failure, blood pressure and lipid abnormalities, and arrhythmias. Digoxin (Lanoxin), a commonly used inotrope, is better tolerated in infants and young children than in adults, and usually achieves a satisfactory response at lower doses (normalized for weight and size). Other inotropes frequently used include isoproterenol (Isuprel), dopamine (Intropin, Dopastat), and dobutamine (Dobutrex). Because the immature heart is limited in its ability to increase stroke volume, inotropic agents may be less effective in it than in an adult heart. Therefore, increases in cardiac output may depend on drug-induced increases in heart rate. Of note, a recent study documented the safety of outpatient parenteral inotropic therapy in six of seven children waiting for heart transplantation at home.[63]

Patients with severe congestive cardiomyopathy and post–cardiac surgery patients are often treated with vasodilators such as sodium nitroprusside (Nipride) and nitroglycerin (Nitro-Bid, Nitrostat, and others). They are used with special caution in newborns owing to the immature peripheral vascular resistance mechanisms of the sympathetic nervous system and the consequent enhanced risks of hypotension.

Treatment of ambulatory high blood pressure (BP) in children should focus on lifestyle modification. However, if the response is unsuccessful, antihypertensive drug therapy is indicated.[64] Normal BP values in children are calculated according to age and gender, and are standardized to height percentiles. When a child's BP is above the calculated 95th percentile, pharmacologic therapy is indicated with the goal of reducing BP to <95th percentile. If comorbid conditions exist, then the BP goal of drug therapy is <90th percentile. Diuretics and β-blockers have a long history of safe and effective use; short-term efficacy studies document the utility of ACE inhibitors, ARBs, and calcium-channel blockers. Studies comparing the ability of different drug groups or specific agents within a drug group to control BP have not been rigorously studied in children.

Advances in the detection of lipid abnormalities and the obesity epidemic in children have caused the medical and scientific communities to examine current drug therapy in these groups of children and adolescents.[39] At this time, drug therapy is not recommended in the management of hyperlipidemia that results from obesity. However, those children with familial hypercholesterolemia and/or a family history of coronary artery disease are considered to be at high risk for cardiovascular diseases and are candidates for pharmacologic therapy if rigorous lifestyle modification is not successful. Evidence shows that drug therapy should begin in these children when they are >10 years of age; the initial drug of choice in these children is a statin. There is preliminary evidence that statins are safe for children who are 8 years old, and they are able to safely remain on the drug for 4.5 years.[65]

Drug therapy for pediatric patients parallels therapy for adults. The same agents are typically used for the same physiologic abnormalities. The immature heart, lungs, and systemic vascular structures require individualized therapeutic regimens. Understanding the progressive nature of the organism's development and the exact stage of maturity greatly influences the clinical efficacy of cardiac pharmacotherapy for this population.

It is a rule of thumb that in this patient group (as well as in the geriatric group discussed above) drug therapy usually starts with one half or one third of the adult dose and then is adjusted according to the clinical response.

## Pharmacologic Management of Diabetes

Pharmacologic management for the diabetic patient includes the use of insulin and non-insulin antihyperglycemic agents (Tables 14-19 and 14-20). Diabetes mellitus is roughly distinguished into type I (complete lack of insulin) and type II

## Table 14-19 Oral Hypoglycemic Agents used in Diabetic Management

| Category | Generic Name | Trade Name | Action |
|---|---|---|---|
| Sulfonylureas | | | Stimulates pancreatic insulin secretion |
| First generation | Tolbutamide | Orinase | |
| | Chlorpropamide | Diabinese | |
| | Tolazamide | Tolinase | |
| | Acetohexamide | Dymetor | |
| Second generation | Glyburide | Micronase, Diabeta | |
| | Micronized glyburide | Glynase | |
| | Glipizide | Glucotrol | |
| | Glipizide GTS | Glucotrol XL | |
| | Glimepiride | Amaryl | |
| Non-sufonylurea meglitinides | Repaglinide | Prandin | Stimulates pancreatic insulin secretion |
| d-Phenylalanine derivatives | Nateglinide | Starlix | Stimulates pancreatic insulin secretion |
| Biguanides | Metformin | Glucophage | Suppresses hepatic glucose production |
| | Metformin extended release | Glucophage XR; Fortamet; Glumetzal | |
| α-Glycosidase inhibitors | Acarbose | Precose | Impairs carbohydrate absorption |
| | Miglitol | Glyset | |
| Thiazolidinediones "TZDs" | Rosiglitazone pioglitazone | Avandia Actos | Enhances insulin sensitivity at peripheral muscle |
| DPP-IV inhibitors "gliptins" | Sitagliptin | Januvia | Suppresses glucagon levels; slows gastric emptying; stimulates insulin secretion |
| | Vildagliptin | Galvus | |
| Bile acid sequestrant | Colesevelam | Welchol | |
| Fixed combinations | Metformin + glipizide | Metaglip | |
| | Metformin + glyburide | Glucovance | |
| | Metformin + pioglitazone | Actoplus met | |
| | Pioglitazone + glimepiride | Duetact | |
| | Rosiglitazone + glimepiride | Avandaryl | |
| | Rosiglitazone + metformin | Avandamet | |
| | Sitagliptin + metformin | Janumet | |
| | Repaglinide + metformin | PrandiMet | |

*Adapted from Rakel R. Conn's Current Therapy 1999. Philadelphia, WB Saunders, 1999:545-546, Nathan DM. Finding New Treatments for Diabetes—How Many, How Fast, How Good? N Engl J Med 356(5), 2007; Perspective www.nejm.org.*
*Joslin Diabetes Center & Joslin Clinic. Clinical Guideline for Pharmacological Management of Type 2 Diabetes.*

(reduced insulin levels or insulin-receptor responses). Type I patients need insulin. Patients with type II and with impaired insulin production, insulin resistance, or both who initially present with only mild symptoms, negative urine ketones, and A1C <7.5 are counseled to appropriate nutrition and physical activity guidelines. If these behavioral interventions fail to reach blood glucose target levels within 6 to 8 weeks or if on entrance the A1C level is >7.5% and the patient is believed to have moderate disease, oral agents are begun in addition to ongoing nutritional and exercise interventions. If these fail to control glucose levels, insulin might have to be added.[66]

One of the important components of a safe exercise program is avoidance of exercise-induced hypoglycemia, which occurs mostly with insulin therapy. Signs and symptoms of hypoglycemia include the following:

- Weakness
- Diaphoresis

## Table 14-20 Types of Insulin

| Insulin Type | Trade Name | Onset[a] | Peak Action[a] (Hours) | Duration[a] |
|---|---|---|---|---|
| Rapid-acting | | | | |
|   Insulin lispro analog | Humalog | 10-30 min | 30 min-3 hr | 3-5 hr |
|   Insulin glulisine analog | Apidra | | | |
|   Insulin aspart analog | NovoLog | | | |
|   Inhaled | Exubera | Taken before meals | | |
| Short-acting | | | | |
|   Human regular | Humulin R | 30-60 min | 2-5 hr | Up to 12 hr |
|   Semilente | Novolin R | 1-1.5 hr | 3-8 hr | 8-16 hr |
| Intermediate-acting | | | | |
|   Human NPH insulin | Humulin N | 90 min-4 hr | 4-12 hr | Up to 24 hr |
|   Lente | Novolin N | 1-2.5 hr | 6-14 hr | 18-28 hr |
| Long–Acting | | | | |
|   Insulin detemir | Levemir | 45 min-4 hr | Minimal | Up to 24 hr |
|   Insulin glargine | Lantus | | | |
|   Ultralente | | 4-8 hr | None | 24-36 hr |
| Non-insulin synthetics | | | | |
|   Pramlintide | Symlin | | | |
| Incretin mimetics | | | | |
|   Exenatide | Byetta | | | |

Adapted from Joslin Diabetes Center & Joslin Clinic. Clinical Guideline for Pharmacological Management of Type 2 Diabetes, January 9, 2009. Rakel R (ed). Conn's Curent Therapy 1999. Philadelphia, WB Saunders, 1999:551.

- Mental confusion
- Muscle rigidity
- Tachycardia

For patients with coronary artery disease, angina, or an anginal equivalent may occur. In insulin-dependent diabetics, hypoglycemia may occur during or immediately following the exercise session or hours after the session has ended as the muscles are replenishing their energy stores. Knowledge of the type of insulin that a person is taking and avoidance of exercise during its peak effect is crucial to avoid augmentation of exercise-induced hypoglycemia (see Table 14-20 and further discussion in Chapter 7). During the beginning days of an exercise program, insulin-dependent patients should monitor their blood glucose both before and after exercise to understand their individualized response to exercise. Patients should make certain that their blood sugar is appropriate before starting exercise (usually in the 120 to 160 mg/dL range) and may need to take a supplemental snack within the 60 to 90 minutes before beginning (Table 14-21). Patients should be encouraged to carry a readily available carbohydrate source, for example, hard candy or jelly beans, and to meet with a nutritionist for specific diet instruction. It is prudent for any physical therapy department that treats insulin-dependent patients to have easy access to juice, sugar,

and long-term glucose management snacks such as peanut butter.

Patients whose blood glucose level is greater than 250 mg/dL should not exercise until cleared by a physician who knows their metabolism. This elevation in plasma blood sugar may indicate an inability of glucose to enter the cell as a result of inadequate insulin. Insulin deficiency results in increased levels of FFA (free fatty acids) from the breakdown of adipose tissue. Oxidation of FFA by the liver produces ketones; ketones are used as an energy source in the absence of sufficient glucose. When the rate that ketones bodies are formed exceeds the rate at which they are being used as fuel, ketonuria may result.[67] Metabolic ketoacidosis may result from the increased levels of ketone production and inadequate urinary excretion. Therefore, the presence of ketone bodies in the urine with an elevated blood sugar >250 mg/dL is a worrisome condition that needs immediate medical consultation before exercise may continue.

Patients should be reminded not to inject insulin into muscle but into subcutaneous tissue. Exercise of a limb that has received an insulin injection should be avoided for at least 60 to 90 minutes or until the peak effect of the insulin has been reached. Exercising the limb sooner than that may cause the insulin effect to peak prematurely because the

**Table 14-21 General Guidelines for Making Food Adjustments for Exercise**

| Type of Exercise and Examples | If Blood Glucose Is: | Increase Food Intake by: | Suggestions of Food to Use |
|---|---|---|---|
| Exercise of short duration and of low to moderate intensity (walking a half mile or leisurely bicycling for less than 30 minutes) | Less than 100 mg/dL | 10 to 15 g of carbohydrate per hour | 1 fruit or 1 starch/bread exchange |
| | 100 mg/dL or above | Not necessary to increase food | |
| Exercise of moderate intensity (1 hr of tennis, swimming, jogging, leisurely bicycling, golfing, etc.) | Less than 100 mg/dL | 25 to 50 g of carbohydrate before exercise, then 10 to 15 g per hour of exercise | 1/2 meat sandwich with a milk or fruit exchange |
| | 100 to 180 mg/dL | 10 to 15 g of carbohydrate | 1 fruit or 1 starch/bread exchange |
| | 180 to 300 mg/dL | Not necessary to increase food | |
| | 300 mg/dL or above | Do not begin exercise until blood glucose is under better control | |
| Strenuous activity or exercise (about 1 to 2 hours of football, hockey, racquetball, or basketball games; strenuous bicycling or swimming; shoveling heavy snow) | Less than 100 mg/dL | 50 g of carbohydrate, monitor blood glucose carefully | 1 meat sandwich (2 slices of bread) with a milk and fruit exchange |
| | 100 to 180 mg/dL | 25 to 50 g of carbohydrate, depending on intensity and duration | 1/2 meat sandwich with milk or fruit exchange |
| | 180 to 300 mg/dL | 10 to 15 g of carbohydrate | 1 fruit or 1 starch/bread exchange |
| | 300 mg/dL or above | Do not begin exercise until blood glucose is under better control | |

*From Franz MJ. Norstrom RD, Norstrom J. Diabetes Actively Staying Healthy [DASH]: Your Game Plan for Diabetes and Exercise, Minneapolis, International Diabetes Center. Wayzata, MN, DCI Publishing, 1990:112-113.*

increased blood flow associated with exercise facilitates the entry of insulin into the blood. As with all patients, adequate fluid intake is important before, during, and after exercise beyond 30 minutes in duration.

Awareness that blisters from ill-fitting footwear may lead to prolonged healing and may develop complications is sufficient reason to instruct patients to choose footwear wisely. Within the physical therapy department, avoiding situations that may bruise the patient is very important for all patients but particularly for diabetic patients. Patients with diabetic retinopathy should avoid any head-down position or situation that would cause a blood pressure reading of greater than 180 mm Hg systolic. Peripheral neuropathy may make walking on uneven surfaces unsafe for the patient, and routine activities of daily living may be cumbersome and difficult.

Hypoglycemia may also occur in the non–insulin-dependent diabetic patient, although this is not seen as frequently as in insulin-dependent patients.[67]

## Heart Transplantation

Survival after orthotopic heart transplantation has improved dramatically since the first procedure was performed in 1967. Advances in drug therapy that reduced rejection reactions have played a major role in the current 1-year survival rate, nearing 90% and a median survival of 10 years.[68] Rejection and infection have been the primary precursors of early death in this population. A combination of improved techniques used to monitor and detect early rejection and newer immunosuppressive pharmacologic agents and the availability and use of a wide variety of antimicrobial drugs may account for this reduction in morbidity and mortality rates. Clinical and laboratory research continues in an attempt to identify agents that act on specific components of the immune system while leaving other parts of this system unaffected. Thus far, no one drug satisfies this goal. Another goal of pharmacologic therapy in these individuals is to achieve "immune tolerance," whereby the immune system is "shut down" just enough to control organ rejection yet not shut down enough to affect the individual's ability to fight infection or develop cancer. Thus far, no combination of drugs satisfies this goal. Of note, future study to achieve these goals may include the use of donor stem cells, as preliminary studies of recipients of kidney ($n = 2$) and liver ($n = 1$) transplants have been able to totally discontinue immunosuppressive therapy for 5 years.[69]

## Immune Mechanism

The immune system is a complex network of humoral and cellular functions that protect human beings from foreign substances (antigens), microbes, and origination of cancer cells. This system is stimulated when an organ like a heart is implanted in a patient with end-stage heart disease, because the recipient's immune system recognizes the donor heart as foreign and tries to destroy it.

Lymphocytes, mononuclear cells that circulate in the blood and lymph, interact with foreign substances to protect the body from invasion. Two types of lymphocytes, T cells and B cells, mediate cellular and humoral immunity, respectively. Cytokines, inflammatory proteins, are involved in the activation of lymphocytes. Current immunosuppressive therapy limits organ rejection by interfering with lymphocyte development, activation, and proliferation, and cytokine expression.

Four types of rejection have been identified.[70] Institutions vary in their approach with regards to dosing and timing of medications used to treat each rejection type. Hyperacute rejection occurs in the perioperative period (minutes to hours) and occurs in response to preformed antibodies that remain in the recipient's body. Acute cellular rejection is T-cell mediated and can occur anytime, usually in the first 3 to 6 months after transplantation. Acute humoral or vascular rejection occurs days to weeks after transplantation and is an antibody-associated form of rejection. The fourth type, chronic rejection, which appears as a cardiac allograft vasculopathy (CAV) can occur any time after the first year and is due to both humoral and cellular responses.

Typical immunosuppression regimens combine drugs specific to the type of rejection and phase of recovery (perioperative also known as the induction period, and maintenance periods). Some agents are initiated in the immediate postoperative period and continued indefinitely, whereas others may be quickly discontinued or slowly tapered. Rescue agents are those medications that are used specifically during acute

(cellular or humoral) episodes of rejection. Finally, a number of agents may be used acutely and/or chronically to address the medical complications that commonly occur over the lifetime of the transplant recipient.

Patients on such immunosuppressive medications are at a high risk of contracting an infection and care must be taken to avoid contact with individuals suffering from an infection.

## Pharmacologic Intervention

### Corticosteroids

Corticosteroids were the first group of drugs to be recognized as having lympholytic properties. Prednisone is the most commonly used immunosuppressor in this drug class. It is cytotoxic to certain subsets of T cells and further suppresses antibody, prostaglandin, and leukotriene synthesis, all important components of the immune system. Lymphocyte formation may be diminished because precursor lymphoid cells (stem cells) are sensitive to prednisone. Unfortunately, long-term use of steroids has deleterious sequelae such as osteoporosis, muscle wasting, impaired healing, ocular effects (cataracts and glaucoma), fat shifting (moon face and buffalo hump), and steroid-induced diabetes. The development of additional immunosuppressive agents (as discussed later) has enabled heart transplant recipients to be maintained on lower doses of steroids, or even have their steroids totally discontinued, thereby reducing the incidence of their negative side effects. However, 63% of patients were still prescribed steroids 1 year after transplant in the literature as recent as 2007.[70]

### Calcineurin Inhibitors

These medications inhibit calcineurin, a phosphatase enzyme important for the production of cytokines. The calcineurin inhibitors (CIs) have had a major impact on the success of immunosuppressive therapy in these patients. Prior to the use of cyclosporine (Sandimmune), the first CI to be used for patients undergoing heart transplantation, the 1-year survival rates were at best 65%.[27] Cyclosporine use, either alone or in combination with prednisone, has resulted in a lower incidence of rejection and infection in this population.[71] This agent appears to act at an early stage in stem cell differentiation to block the activation of T cells, which are significantly involved in rejection reactions. It does not appear to affect already converted lymphoblasts. The lymphocytes that are affected recover their normal function after the drug is eliminated from the system.

Although cyclosporine appears to be impressive as a highly selective agent that is effective against a subpopulation of lymphocytes, it has a considerable number of side effects. Besides promoting lymphoma, cyclosporine causes nephrotoxicity and consequently hypertension. Elevated blood pressure due to cyclosporine is usually well controlled by one or two agents, such as ACE inhibitors and β-blockers.[72] A newer CI, tacrolimus (Prograf), has been shown to be as effective as cyclosporine with less nephrotoxicity.[70]

Another group of drugs also found to inhibit T and B lymphocyte proliferation and having similar action to CIs are the target of rapamycin inhibitors (mTOR inhibitors). Two of these, sirolimus (Rapamune) and everolimus (Afinitor), are showing promise since they show less renal toxicity.[70]

## Anti-Proliferative Agents Azathioprine

Azathioprine (AZA, Imuran) and mycophenolate mofetil (MMF, CellCept) are two antiproliferative agents that are routinely used to interfere with lymphocyte proliferation that occurs after the antigen stimulates the immune system. These agents are especially effective against T cells but can also block humoral immune responses. Toxicity to azathioprine results in bone marrow depression and hepatic dysfunction. Gastrointestinal (GI) disorders may occur at higher doses. At 1 year posttransplant, 76% of patients are taking MMF as it appears to have slightly less bone marrow depression than AZA.[70] A newer coated MMF also shows promise in GI tolerance to higher doses of this agent.

> **Clinical Tip**
> Keep in mind that all drugs have indications for use and side effects when used alone. However, with multiple drug regimens that are prescribed, there exists the chance of interaction of drugs, and possibly increased side effects—some being negative or counterproductive. When in doubt, consult the pharmacist about the drug–drug interactions as well as the effect or side effects that are observed.

## Antilymphocyte Antibodies

These preparations, antilymphocyte globulin and antithymocyte globulin (Thymoglobulin), are routinely being used during the perioperative/induction period for immunosuppression. Injection of an animal (e.g., horse, rabbit) with human lymphocytes provokes the animal's immune mechanism to form antibodies to human lymphocytes. The animal's antilymphocytic globulin can then be injected into the transplant recipient, which ultimately causes cytotoxic destruction of the recipient's lymphocytes. Using these agents does increase the risk of cancer, however, because of the suppression of the normal defense system against carcinogens. Another antibody, OKT3 (Muromonab, orthoclone, a monoclonal antibody as indicated by the last three letters -*mab*), has been found effective in blocking both cytotoxic activity of human T cells and the generation of other T-cell function. It is not being used as often as the antithymocyte globulins as there is an increased incidence of severe allergic reactions to these agents.[70]

Newer, anticytokine antibodies are beginning to replace the antilymphocytic preparations. Two of these, daclizumab and basiliximab, are synthetic, humanized monoclonal preparations that appear to have fewer side effects than the antilymphocytic agents. When used with cyclosporine, these agents seem to offer greater protection from the nephrotoxicity that is commonly seen with cyclosporine.[70]

## Maintenance Therapy

Although the use of certain agents is considered to be standard therapy, medical centers vary considerably in their pharmacologic protocols for the heart transplant population.

Most institutions use a triple-drug immunosuppressive drug regimen for their first-year survivors of heart transplantation. This includes an antiproliferative agent, a calcineurin inhibitor, and a steroid. The addition of other medications to this regimen is typically guided by the occurrence of acute or chronic rejection, or other medical complications that occur. Acute rejection is typically managed with augmented drug-induced immunosuppression, including higher doses of maintenance drugs with the addition of an antilymphocytic or anticytokine agent.

Cardiac allograft vasculopathy (CAV) often presents as a diffuse atherosclerosis and is found in about 50% of patients by 5 years after transplantation.[73] The use of some of the newer immunosuppressive agents may have a positive impact in reducing CAV in part by reducing the associated hypertension and hyperlipidemia. The HMG-CoA reductase inhibitors (statins) are often routinely prescribed in these patients to effectively lower cholesterol and possibly modulate the immune and inflammatory responses. Of note, although statin use has shown benefits related to CAV, a consequent drug–drug interaction of rhabdomyolysis has been documented. Antiplatelet agents, primarily aspirin, has been commonly prescribed because of its usefulness in the management of nontransplanted patients with coronary artery disease and the likely role that platelets have in CAV.

Reduction in the use and/or dosage of cyclosporine (and increased use of the CI tacrolimus) has reduced the occurrence of hypertension and chronic renal insufficiency and failure. The availability and potential use of antibacterial, antiviral, and antifungal agents has reduced the occurrence and severity of infections, a common consequence of profound immunosuppression. In an effort to prevent osteoporosis, a common adverse effect of chronic steroid use, individuals taking >5 mg/day of prednisone for 3 months are treated with the bone-forming drug bisphosphonate and calcium and vitamin D, as well as regular weight-bearing exercise.

## Cardiovascular Medications for Pulmonary Function

### Pulmonary Arterial Hypertension

Pulmonary arterial hypertension (PAH) is an uncommon lung disorder in which the arteries that carry blood from the right heart to the lungs become narrowed, making the blood flow through the vessels difficult. This often results in less volume of blood reaching the lungs for gas exchange and subsequently less volume returning to the left heart to be sent out to the periphery. Increased work is placed on the right ventricle; right ventricular dysfunction or failure sometimes follows. Pulmonary hypertension is often treated with medications which lower the pressure in the pulmonary arteries through vasodilation (Table 14-22).

## Table 14-22 Drugs Used in the Treatment of Pulmonary Arterial Hypertension

| Medications | Effects |
| --- | --- |
| Isordil (Isosorbide dinitrate) | Vasodilation |
| Revatio (sildenafil) | Relaxes pulmonary smooth muscle cells |
| Tracleer (Bosentan) | Blocks endothelin (which results in vasodilation) |
| Remodulin (Treprostinil) | Dilates pulmonary arteries |
| Flolan (Epoprostenol) | Dilates pulmonary arteries |
| Ventavis (Iloprost) | Dilates pulmonary arteries |
| Tyvaso (Treprostinil) (inhalation only) | A synthetic form of prostacyclin |
| Letairis (Anbrisentan) | Endothelin receptor antagonist |
| Adcirca (Tadalafil) | Phosphodiesterase-5 (PDE-5) inhibitor |

## References

1. Katzung BG. Basic and Clinical Pharmacology. 8th ed. East Norwalk, CT, Appleton & Lange, 1989.
2. Ross EM, Gilman AG. Pharmacodynamics: Mechanisms of drug action and the relationship between drug concentration and effect. In Gilman AG, Goodman LS, Rall TW, et al. (eds.): Goodman and Gilman's The Pharmacologic Basis of Therapeutics. 7th ed. New York, Macmillan, 1985.
3. Benet LZ. Pharmacokinetics: absorption, distribution and elimination. In Katzung BG (ed.): Basic and Clinical Pharmacology. 8th ed. East Norwalk, CT, Appleton & Lange, 1989.
4. Blaschke TF, Nies AS, Mamelok RD. Principles of therapeutics. In Gilman AG, Goodman LS, Rall TW, et al. (eds.): Goodman and Gilman's The Pharmacologic Basis of Therapeutics. 7th ed. New York, Macmillan, 1985.
5. Heron M, Hoyert DL, Murphy SL, et al. Deaths: final data for 2006. Natl Vital Stat Rep 57(14):1–134, 2009.
6. Opie LH, Gersh BJ. Antithrombotic agents: platelet inhibitors, anticoagulants, and fibrinolytics. In Opie LH (ed.): Drugs for the Heart. 2nd ed. Philadelphia, Saunders, 1987.
7. Conley CL. Hemostasis. In Mountcastle VB (ed.): Medical Physiology. 13th ed. St. Louis, Mosby, 1974.
8. Andreoli T. Andreoli and Carpenter's Cecil Essentials of Medicine. 7th ed. Philadelphia, Saunders, 2008.
9. Haskell WL, Alderman EL, Fair JM, et al. Effects of intensive multiple risk factor reduction on coronary atherosclerosis and clinical cardiac events in men and women with coronary artery disease. The Stanford Coronary Risk Intervention Project (SCRIP). Circulation 89(3):975–90, 1994.
10. Opie LH, Sonnenblick EH, Frishman W, Thadini U. Beta-blocking agents. In Opie LH (ed.): Drugs for the Heart. 2nd ed. Philadelphia, Saunders, 1987.
11. Boron WF. Medical Physiology. Philadelphia, Saunders, 2005.
12. Antman EM, Hand M, Armstrong PW, et al. 2007 Focused update of the ACC/AHA 2004 guidelines for the management of patients with ST-elevation myocardial infarction: a report of the American College of Cardiology/American Heart Association Task Force on Practice Guidelines: developed in collaboration With the Canadian Cardiovascular Society endorsed by the American Academy of Family Physicians: 2007 Writing Group to Review New Evidence and Update the ACC/AHA 2004 Guidelines for the Management of Patients With ST-Elevation Myocardial Infarction, Writing on Behalf of the 2004 Writing Committee. Circulation 117(2):296–329, 2008.
13. Cannon CP. Expanding the treatment paradigm for acute myocardial infarction with GP IIb/IIIa inhibitors. New Era of Reperfusion 3:1–12, 1999.
14. Koeppen BM. Berne & Levy Physiology. 6th ed. Philadelphia, Mosby, 2009.
15. Rich MW. Epidemiology, pathophysiology, and etiology of congestive heart failure in older adults. J Am Geriatr Soc 45(8):968–74, 1997.
16. Levy MN. Berne & Levy Principles of Physiology. 4th ed. Philadelphia, Mosby, 2006.
17. Hunt SA, Abraham WT, Chin MH, et al. 2009 focused update incorporated into the ACC/AHA 2005 guidelines for the diagnosis and management of heart failure in adults: a report of the American College of Cardiology Foundation/American Heart Association Task Force on Practice Guidelines developed in collaboration with the International Society for Heart and Lung Transplantation. J Am Coll Cardiol 53(15):e1–e90, 2009.
18. Fonarow GC. A review of evidence-based beta-blockers in special populations with heart failure. Rev Cardiovasc Med 9(2):84–95, 2008.
19. Fowler MB. Carvedilol prospective randomized cumulative survival (COPERNICUS) trial: carvedilol in severe heart failure. Am J Cardiol 693(9A):35B–9B, 2004.
20. Effect of metoprolol CR/XL in chronic heart failure: Metoprolol CR/XL Randomised Intervention Trial in Congestive Heart Failure (MERIT-HF). Lancet 353(9169):2001–7, 1999.
21. Greenberg BH, Mehra M, Teerlink JR, et al. COMPARE: comparison of the effects of carvedilol CR and carvedilol IR on left ventricular ejection fraction in patients with heart failure. Am J Cardiol. 2006 Oct 2;98(7A):53L–59L.
22. Rose BD. Pathogenesis of essential hypertension. In Rose BD (ed.): Pathophysiology of Renal Disease. 2nd ed. New York, McGraw-Hill, 1987:475–6.
23. Effect of enalapril on mortality and the development of heart failure in asymptomatic patients with reduced left ventricular ejection fractions. The SOLVD Investigators. N Engl J Med 327(10):685–91, 1992.
24. Pfeffer MA, Braunwald E, Moyé LA, et al. Effect of captopril on mortality and morbidity in patients with left ventricular dysfunction after myocardial infarction: results of the Survival and Ventricular Enlargement trial. The SAVE Investigators. N Engl J Med 327(10):669–77, 1992.
25. Young JB, Dunlap ME, Pfeffer MA, et al. Mortality and morbidity reduction with Candesartan in patients with chronic heart failure and left ventricular systolic dysfunction: results of the CHARM low-left ventricular ejection fraction trials. Circulation 110(17):2618–26, 2004.

26. Pitt B, Zannad F, Remme WJ, et al., for the Randomized Aldactone Evaluation Study Investigators. The effect of spironolactone on morbidity and mortality in patients with severe heart failure. N Engl J Med 341:709–17, 1999.

27. Hunt SA, Abraham WT, Chin MH et al. ACC/AHA 2005 guideline for the diagnosis and management of chronic heart failure in the adult: a report of the American College of Cardiology/American Heart Association Task Force on Practice Guidelines (writing committee to update the 2001 guidelines for the evaluation and management of heart failure): Developed in collaboration with the American College of Chest Physicians and the International Society for Heart and Lung Transplantation: endorsed by the heart rhythm society. Circulation 112:1825–54, 2005.

28. Zewail AM, Nawar M, Vrtovec B, et al. Intravenous milrinone in treatment of advanced congestive heart failure. Tex Heart Inst J 30(2):109–13, 2003.

29. Mosby's Drug Consult 2004. St. Louis, Mosby, 2005.

30. Hondeghen L, Mason J. Agents used in cardiac arrhythmias. In Katzung BG (ed.): Basic and Clinical Pharmacology. 4th ed. East Norwalk, CT, Appleton & Lange, 1989.

31. Katzung B, Scheinman M. Drugs used in cardiac arrhythmias. In Katzung BG (ed.): Basic and Clinical Pharmacology. 4th ed. East Norwalk, CT, Appleton & Lange, 1989.

32. Fuster V, Rydén LE, Cannom DS, et al. Guidelines for the management of patients with atrial fibrillation. Executive summary. Rev Esp Cardiol 59(12):1329, 2006.

33. Tierney LM, McPhee SJ, Papadakis MA. 2008 Current Medical Diagnosis and Treatment. New York, McGraw-Hill Medical, 2009.

34. Zipes DP, Camm AJ, Borggrefe M, et al. ACC/AHA/ESC 2006 guidelines for management of patients with ventricular arrhythmias and the prevention of sudden cardiac death: a report of the American College of Cardiology/American Heart Association Task Force and the European Society of Cardiology Committee for Practice Guidelines (writing committee to develop guidelines for management of patients with ventricular arrhythmias and the prevention of sudden cardiac death). J Am Coll Cardiol 48(5):e247–e346, 2006.

35. Rosendorff C, Black HR, Cannon CP, et al. Treatment of hypertension in the prevention and management of ischemic heart disease: a scientific statement from the American Heart Association Council for High Blood Pressure Research and the Councils on Clinical Cardiology and Epidemiology and Prevention. Circulation 115(21):2761–88, 2007.

36. Zsoter T. Pharmacotherapy of hypertension. In Kalant H, oschlau W, Sellers E (eds.): Principles of Medical Pharmacology. 4th ed. New York, Oxford University Press, 1985.

37. Benowitz M, Bourne H. Anti-hypertensive agents. In Katzung BG (ed.): Basic and Clinical Pharmacology. 4th ed. East Norwalk, CT, Appleton & Lange, 1989.

38. Chobanian AV, Bakris GL, Black HR, et al. The seventh report of the Joint National Committee on Prevention, Detection, Evaluation, and Treatment of High Blood Pressure: the JNC 7 report. JAMA 289(19):2560–72, 2003.

39. McCrindle BW, Urbina EM, Dennison BA, et al. Drug therapy of high-risk lipid abnormalities in children and adolescents: a scientific statement from the American Heart Association Atherosclerosis, Hypertension, and Obesity in Youth Committee, Council of Cardiovascular Disease in the Young, with the Council on Cardiovascular Nursing. Circulation 115(14):1948–67, 2007.

40. Zillich AJ, Garg J, Basu S, et al. Thiazide diuretics, potassium, and the development of diabetes: a quantitative review. Hypertension 48(2):219–24, 2006.

41. O'Gara PT, Dec WG, Curfman GD. Acute myocardial infarction. In Rakel R (ed.): Conn's Current Therapy. Philadelphia, Saunders, 1991.

42. Weir MR. Angiotensin-II receptor antagonists: a new class of antihypertensive agents. Am Fam Physician 53(2):589–94, 1996.

43. Grundy SM, Cleeman JI, Merz CN, et al. The National Heart, Lung, and Blood Institute; American College of Cardiology Foundation; American Heart Association. Implications of recent clinical trials for the National Cholesterol Education Program Adult Treatment Panel III Guidelines. Circulation 110(2):227–39, 2004.

44. National Cholesterol Education Program (NCEP) Expert Panel on Detection, Evaluation, and Treatment of High Blood Cholesterol in Adults (Adult Treatment panel III). Third report of the National Cholesterol Education Program (NCEP) Expert Panel on Detection, Evaluation, and Treatment of High Blood Cholesterol in Adults (Adult Treatment Panel III) final report. Circulation 106(25):3143–421, 2002.

45. Atherogenic Dyslipidemia, A Pocket Guide. Comprehensive Lipoprotein Management to Reduce Residual CVD Risk. Pri-Med Institute, Winter, 2008:11. http://pri-med.com/PMO/Activity.aspx?activity=127286

46. Katzung B, Parmley W. Cardiac glycosides and other drugs used in congestive heart failure. In Katzung BG (ed.): Basic and Clinical Pharmacology. 4th ed. East Norwalk, CT, Appleton & Lange, 1989.

47. Albert J, Rippe J. Manual of Cardiovascular Diagnosis and Therapy. 3rd ed. Boston, Little, Brown, 1988

48. Textbook of Advanced Cardiac Life Support. Dallas, American Heart Association, 1987.

49. Barnes S, Shields B, Bonney W, et al. The Pediatric Cardiology Pharmacopoeia: 2004 update. Pediatr Cardiol 25:623–46, 2004.

50. Ciccone CD. Pharmacology in Rehabilitation. 4th ed. Philadelphia, PA, F A Davis, 2007:339.

51. The Atrial Fibrillation Follow-up Investigation of Rhythm Management Investigators. A Comparison of Rate Control and Rhythm Control in Patients with Atrial Fibrillation. N Engl J Med 347(23):1825–33, 2003.

52. Sullivan GM, Korman LB. Drug-associated confusional states in older persons. Topics Geriatr Rehab 8(4):14–26, 1993.

53. Wing LM, Reid CM, Ryan P, et al. A comparison of outcomes with angiotensin-converting enzyme inhibitors and diuretics for hypertension in the elderly. N Engl J Med 348(7):583–92, 2003.

54. Gambassi G, Lapane KI, Sgadari A, et al. Effects of angiotensin-converting enzyme inhibitors and digoxin on health outcomes of very old patients with heart failure. Arch Intern Med 160:53–60, 2000.

55. Rathore SS, Wang Y, Krumolz HM. Sex-based differences in the effect of digoxin for the treatment of heart failure. N Engl J Med 347(18):1403–11, 2002.

56. Linnebur SA. What's new about old drugs: implications for the care of older adults. J Gerontol Nurs 30(1):4–11, 2004.

57. Heart Protection Study Collaborative Group. MRC/BHF heart protection study of cholesterol lowering with simvastatin in 20,536 high-risk individuals: a randomized placebo-controlled trial. Lancet 360(9326):7–22, 2002.

58. Shepherd J, Blauw GJ, Murphy MB, et al. Pravastatin in elderly individuals at risk of vascular disease (PROSPER): a randomised controlled trial. Lancet 360(9346):1623–30, 2002.

59. Ott SM, LaCroix AZ, Ichikawa LE, et al. Effect of low-dose thiazide diuretics on plasma lipids: results from a double-blind, randomized clinical trial in older men and women. J Am Geriatr Soc 51(3):340–7, 2003.

60. Rossouw JE, Anderson GL, Prentice RL, et al. Risks and benefits of estrogen plus progestin in healthy postmenopausal women: principal results from the Women's Health Initiative randomized controlled trial. JAMA 288(3):321–33, 2002.

61. Notterman D. Pediatric pharmacology. In Chernow B (ed.): Essentials of Critical Care Pharmacology. 2nd ed. Baltimore, Williams & Wilkins, 1989.

62. MacLeod S, Radde I. Textbook of Pediatric Clinical Pharmacology. Littleton, MA, PSG Publishing, 1985.

63. Price JF, Towbin JA, Dreyer WJ, et al. Outpatient continuous parenteral inotropic therapy as bridge to transplantation in children with advanced heart failure. J Card Fail 12(2):139–43, 2006.

64. US Department of Health and Human Services, NIH, NHLBI. The Fourth Report on the Diagnosis, Evaluation, and Treatment of High Blood Pressure in Children and Adolescents (NIH Publication No. 05-5267). Washington, DC, USDHHS, 2005:26–33.

65. Rodenburg J, Vissers MN, Wiegman A, et al. Statin treatment in children with familial hypercholesterolemia: the younger, the better. Circulation. 116(6):664–8, 2007.

66. Joslin Diabetes Center & Joslin Clinic. Clinical guideline for pharmacological management of type 2 diabetes. www.joslin.org.

67. Kumar V. Robbins' Basic Pathology. 8th ed. Philadelphia, Saunders, 2008.

68. Hunt SA, Haddad F. The changing face of heart transplantation. J Am Coll Cardiol 52(8):587–98, 2008.

69. Starzl TE. Immunosuppressive therapy and tolerance of organ allografts. N Engl J Med 358(4):407–11, 2008.

70. Sulemanjee NZ, Merla R, Lick SD, et al. The first year post-heart transplantation: use of immunosuppressive drugs and early complications. J Cardiovasc Pharmacol Ther 13(1):13–31, 2008.

71. Salmon S. Immunopharmacology. In Katzung BG (ed.): Basic and Clinical Pharmacology. 4th ed. East Norwalk, CT, Appleton & Lange, 1989.

72. Copeland J. Teaching Conference in Clinical Cardiology, University of Miami, School of Medicine, February 19–22, 1991.

73. Lindenfeld J, Page RL 2nd, Zolty R, et al. Drug therapy in the heart transplant recipient, Part III: Common medical problems. Circulation 111(1):113–17, 2005.

# CHAPTER 15

# Pulmonary Medications

*Kelley Crawford, Susan Butler McNamara,*
*Wolfgang Vogel, H. Steven Sadowsky*

## Chapter Outline

The rationale for prescriptions of pulmonary medications can be divided into the following categories[1-6]:

1. Bronchodilation and/or alleviation of bronchoconstriction;
2. Facilitation of mucociliary/secretion clearance;
3. Increased alveolar ventilation and/or improved oxygenation; and
4. Improved control of the breathing pattern.

Which medication is used depends on the specific disease process and the presenting respiratory signs and symptoms. Consequently, pulmonary medications are presented in terms of their principal desired effects: bronchodilators, antiinflammatory agents, decongestants, antihistamines, antitussives, mucokinetics, respiratory stimulants and depressants, paralyzing drugs, and antimicrobial agents.

## Physiology

For this chapter, the bronchi, bronchioles, and alveoli are most important. The first two consist basically of an outer layer of cartilage, an inner layer of smooth muscle, and an inner layer of mucus membrane, and they regulate the flow of air. The last has a thin membrane where the exchange of oxygen and carbon dioxide from the blood occurs.

Diseases involving the first two are mostly characterized by bronchoconstriction or a narrowing of the lumen of the bronchi. Thus, bronchodilators are the most frequently used drugs in the treatment of pulmonary disease.[4,5] The bronchial smooth muscle fibers of the lungs involuntarily constrict in response to various types of irritation. The resultant bronchoconstriction plays a major role in the pathophysiology of most obstructive pulmonary diseases. Bronchoconstriction can be attributed to any, or all, of three primary pathologic factors: abnormal bronchomotor tone (bronchospasm), inflammation, and mechanical obstruction. With the elimination of overt mechanical obstruction, the control of bronchomotor tone and inflammation become the components of airway management for patients with pulmonary disease. Only after constricted airways are dilated can mucociliary transport, removal of secretions, and subsequent alveolar ventilation and oxygenation take place.[7]

## Bronchomotor Tone

Normal bronchomotor tone, an equilibrium point between constrictive and dilatational stimuli, is mostly the result of a balance between adrenergic and cholinergic influences (Fig. 15-1).[8-11] When something (i.e., disease, allergy) disrupts the normal bronchomotor tone balance, bronchospasm results. The characteristic findings in acute bronchospasm are smooth muscle constriction, mucus production, vascular engorgement, and submucosal inflammatory edema. The mechanisms of bronchospasm are most clearly demonstrated when asthma is used as a model. In asthma, a predominant parasympathetic influence increases bronchomotor tone and results in narrowing of bronchial and bronchiolar passages.[12]

Other receptors in the connective tissues of the airways (e.g., mast cells) and the blood are also stimulated to release mediator substances. This response is called *inflammation*, and it plays a central role in the production of bronchospasm in the vast majority of respiratory disorders.[13-15] The mediator substances originate from the plasma, adjacent cells, or from

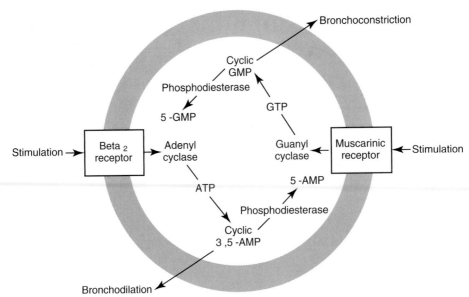

**Figure 15-1** Normal bronchomotor tone is the result of a balance between adrenergic and cholinergic influences mediated through the intracellular nucleotides cyclic adenosine 3′,5′-monophosphate (cAMP) and cyclic guanosine monophosphate (cGMP). Adrenergic stimulation of the appropriate receptor catalyzes (via adenyl cyclase) the conversion of adenosine triphosphate (ATP) to cAMP, eliciting relaxation of the affected bronchial smooth muscle. cAMP is metabolized by phosphodiesterase. Cholinergic stimulation of the appropriate receptor catalyzes (via guanyl cyclase) the conversion of guanosine triphosphate (GTP) to cyclic GMP, eliciting contraction of the affected bronchial smooth muscle. CGMP is metabolized by phosphodiesterase.

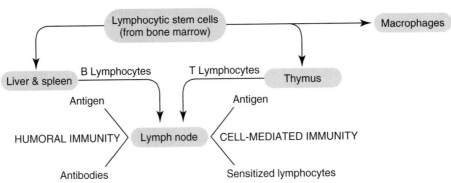

**Figure 15-2** In acquired immunity, the formation of antibodies (immunoglobulins) results from the interaction of antigens with B lymphocytes and initiates the humoral immune response. The formation of lymphokines results from the interaction of antigens with T lymphocytes and initiates the cell-mediated immune response.

the damaged tissue, and are associated with at least eight major events[13,16,17]:

1. Changes in vascular flow and caliber,
2. Changes in vascular permeability,
3. Leukocytic (e.g., neutrophils, monocytes, eosinophils, lymphocytes, and basophils) exudation,
4. Clustering of leukocytes along the capillary endothelial cells at the site of injury (margination),
5. Adherence of the leukocytes to the endothelial surface at the site of injury (sticking),
6. Leukocytic insinuation between endothelial cells (emigration),
7. Unidirectional migration of polymorphonuclear leukocytes from the bloodstream to the site of injury in response to released attractants (chemotaxis), and
8. Phagocytosis.

Although macrophages, leukocytes, and neutrophils assist in the elimination of invading pathogens by means of phagocytosis, it is the action of the lymphocytes that is probably most significant.[18,19]

Invading organisms (e.g., antigens on bacteria or viruses) or other irritants (e.g., allergens) elicit an immune response. Antigens stimulate the different types of lymphocytes stored in the lymph nodes to produce two mediator substances: antibodies or sensitized lymphocytes (Fig. 15-2). Antibodies are produced by the interaction of antigens and B lymphocytes in a process referred to as humoral immunity. Antibodies are also called immunoglobulins, because many reside in the gammaglobulin fraction of the blood. Antibodies are generally grouped into five major classes: immunoglobulin (Ig) A, IgE, IgG, IgM, and IgD; the first four of these have been identified in respiratory secretions.[20] Sensitized lymphocytes (also called *lymphokines*) are produced through the interaction of antigens with T lymphocytes in a process referred to as cell-mediated immunity.

Lymphokines are responsible for a variety of immunologic actions, including the activation of macrophages (by the production and release of macrophage-activating factor), inhibition of leukocyte migration (by the production and release of leukocyte inhibitory factor), and destruction of susceptible target cells (lymphotoxic effect).[21]

The allergic or immunologic responses to allergens can be divided into four types, two of which are of importance here. The type I sensitivity reaction occurs immediately and is related to IgE antibody activity on mast cells, which in response release large amounts of histamine. This reaction is manifested by redness, itching, and hives within 10 to 20 minutes. In the most severe case, an anaphylactic reaction occurs, which is characterized by life-threatening bronchoconstriction and hypotension. The type IV sensitivity reaction takes approximately 48 hours to develop (often referred to as delayed allergic reaction) and is most likely caused by

the macrophagic release of specific enzymes that produce inflammation (but not histamine). This delay makes it often difficult to determine the offending allergen. Typically for these reactions is that they do not occur at first exposure but only thereafter and that they are dose-independent in that minuscule amounts can precipitate an anaphylactic reaction and death. Generally, type I reactions are treated with antihistamines or corticosteroids, whereas the type IV reactions are treated only with corticosteroids.

## Rationale for Bronchodilators

The primary purpose for bronchodilator therapy is to influence the autonomic nervous system receptors via two opposing nucleotides: cyclic adenosine monophosphate (cAMP) and cyclic guanosine monophosphate (cGMP; Fig. 15-3). These two substances are often referred to as second messengers (where the neurotransmitter or drug is the first messenger that causes the formation of these second messengers,

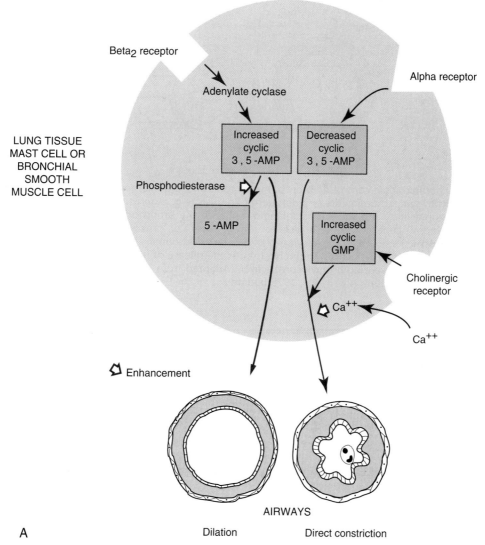

**Figure 15-3 A,** Factors influencing adrenergic and cholinergic mediation of bronchomotor tone.

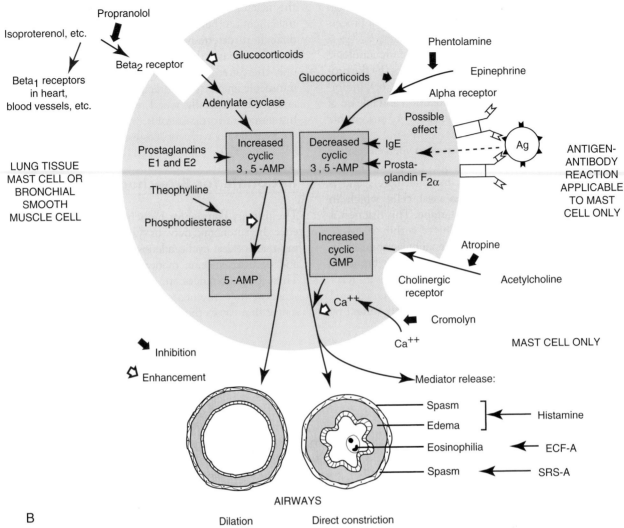

**Figure 15-3, cont'd B,** Pharmacologic control of bronchomotor tone and the allergen-induced release of chemical mediators. Stimulation of $\beta_2$ receptors by sympathomimetics or $\beta$-adrenergic agonists (e.g., isoproterenol) facilitates dilation. Glucocorticoids, methylxanthines (e.g., theophylline), and some prostaglandins enhance the bronchodilator effect of $\beta_2$-adrenergic stimulation. However, glucocorticoids and $\alpha$ sympatholytics or $\alpha$ receptor antagonists (e.g., prazosin, phentolamine) inhibit the $\alpha$-adrenergic contribution to bronchoconstriction. Similarly, parasympatholytics or anticholinergic or cholinergic antagonists (e.g., atropine) inhibit cholinergic bronchoconstrictive influences. Cromolyn retards the release of mediators by inhibiting calcium ion movement into unstable mast cells, thereby preventing bronchoconstriction. (Adapted from Townley RG. Pharmacologic blocks to mediator release: Clinical applications. Adv Asthma Allergy 2:7, 1975 update.)

which are the actual physiologically active substances). cAMP facilitates smooth muscle relaxation and inhibits mast cell degranulation causing bronchodilation. cGMP facilitates smooth muscle constriction and may enhance mast cell release of histamine and other mediators causing bronchoconstriction. Within the lungs, the effects of cAMP and/or cGMP can be attributed to either of the following:

- Muscarinic receptor stimulation, which increases cGMP and enhances bronchoconstriction,
- Adrenergic $\beta_2$ receptor stimulation, which produces an increase in cAMP and bronchodilation (whereas $\alpha_1$ receptor stimulation results in a decrease in cAMP and facilitates bronchoconstriction).[22,23]

The effect of parasympathetic activity (heart rate slowing, bronchial constriction, and increased exocrine gland secretion) can be deleterious to a patient with pulmonary disease. $\beta$-Adrenergic agonists, some prostaglandins, corticosteroids (although not technically bronchodilators), and methylxanthines may be given to increase cAMP and thereby promote bronchodilation. $\alpha$-Adrenergic antagonists, corticosteroids, cholinergic antagonists, and cromolyn or nedocromil may be given to inhibit cGMP or enhance cAMP.

Because asthma is the model being used for bronchoconstriction, we will rely upon the recommendations promulgated by the National Asthma Education and Prevention Program and the National Institutes of Health in describing the medications used to control bronchoconstriction.[24] The principal drug groups recommended by the National Heart Lung and Blood Institute are listed in Table 15-1 and discussed in the following section.

## Table 15-1 Pharmacotherapy for the Treatment of Bronchoconstriction

| | | |
|---|---|---|
| Long-term control medications | Antiinflammatory/antiallergic agents | Corticosteroids |
| | | Cromolyn sodium |
| | | Nedocromil |
| | Immunomodulators | Omalizumab |
| | Leukotriene modifiers | Leukotriene receptor antagonists |
| | | Montelukast |
| | | Zafirlukast |
| | | 5-Lipoxygenase inhibitors |
| | | Zileuton |
| | Long-acting β₂-adrenergic receptor agonists | Salmeterol |
| | | Formoterol |
| | Methylxanthines | Theophylline |
| Quick-relief medications | Anticholinergics | Ipratropium bromide |
| | | Tiotropium |
| | Short-acting β₂-adrenergic receptor agonists | Albuterol |
| | | Levalbuterol |
| | | Pirbuterol |
| | Systemic corticosteroids | Various |

## Bronchodilators

Medications that stimulate the adrenergic receptors are frequently referred to as sympathomimetics or adrenergic agonists. Those that inhibit adrenergic receptors are referred to as sympatholytics or adrenergic antagonists. Similarly, medications that stimulate the cholinergic receptors at end organs are referred to as parasympathomimetics or muscarinic agonists. Those that inhibit these cholinergic receptors are called parasympatholytics or muscarinic antagonists.

The actions and adverse effects of the main bronchodilators, specifically the autonomic active agents (adrenergic sympathomimetics and parasympatholytics) and methylxanthines are reviewed next.

### Sympathomimetic Agents or Adrenergic Agonists

Sympathomimetic drugs may be selective or nonselective in their action. Selective medications react directly with one specific receptor type. Nonselective medications increase the release of or prevent the reuptake of norepinephrine. This increase in synaptic norepinephrine occurs on all receptors and they react on all adrenergic receptors. The response from sympathomimetic agents is dependent on their affinity to the receptor, the route of administration, and the dosage of the particular drug.[3,6,23]

α Receptors are distributed within peripheral and bronchial smooth muscle, the myocardium, and mucosal blood vessels. They are most abundant in the peripheral vascular smooth muscles.

β₁ Receptors are mostly in cardiac tissue but are also found in mucosal blood vessels.

β₂ Receptors predominate in the bronchial smooth muscles but also are found in peripheral smooth muscle and skeletal muscle.

Epinephrine (adrenaline) acts directly on all receptor types and ephedrine increases norepinephrine synaptic concentrations again on all receptor types and are classified as general, nonselective sympathomimetics. Epinephrine has a short duration of action, demonstrating moderate α receptor activity, strong β₁ receptor activity, and moderate β₂-receptor activity.[3,6,23] Ephedrine has a long duration of action, exhibiting mild α-receptor activity and moderate β₁ and β₂ activity. Thus, when used in the relief of bronchoconstriction, α- and β₁-receptor stimulation may induce peripheral vascular constriction and can accelerate cardiac responses. Other side effects include agitation, sweating, headache, and nausea. In addition, the route by which a particular medication is administered may significantly influence the extent of any adverse reactions.[3,6,23] For example, inhaled sympathomimetic medications generate less-profound deleterious side effects than administered systemically.

> **Clinical Tip**
> Intramuscular or subcutaneous epinephrine is the drug of choice for treating acute bronchospasm as well as acute anaphylactic reaction because of its quick short-acting response.

## Table 15-2 Long-Acting and Short-Acting β₂-Adrenergic Agonists

| Generic Name | Brand Name | Route of Administration | Onset of Action (min) | Time to Peak Effect (hr) | Duration of Action (hr) |
|---|---|---|---|---|---|
| Epinephrine | | Inhalation | 3–5 | – | 1–3 |
| | | Intramuscular | Variable | – | <1–4 |
| | | Subcutaneous | 6–15 | 0.3 | <1–4 |
| Formoterol | Foradil | Inhalation | 1–3 | – | 12 |
| Isoetharine | Bronkosol | Inhalation | 1–6 | 0.25–1 | 1–4 |
| Isoproterenol | Medihaler-Iso | Inhalation | 2–5 | – | 0.5–2 |
| | Isuprel | Intravenous | Immediate | – | <1 |
| | | Sublingual | 15–30 | – | 1–2 |
| Metaproterenol | Alupent | Inhalation | 1 | 1 | 1–5 |
| | | Oral | 15–30 | 1 | <4 |
| Pirbuterol | Maxair | Inhalation | 5 | 0.5–1 | 5 |
| Salbutamol | Albuterol | Inhalation | 5–15 | 1–1.5 | 3–6 |
| | Ventolin | Oral | 15–30 | 2–3 | 8+ |
| Salmeterol | Serevent Diskus | Inhalation | 10–20 | 3–4 | 12 |
| Terbutaline | Brethaire | Inhalation | 15–30 | 1–2 | 3–6 |
| | Brethine tablet | Oral | 60–120 | 2–3 | 4–8 |
| | Bricanyl tablet | Parenteral | 15 | 0.5–1 | 1.5–4 |
| Albuterol | AccuNeb Proventil VoSpire | Inhalation Oral | 5–30 | 30–120 | 3–6 |
| Arformoterol | Brovana | Inhalation | 5 | 60–90 | 4–6 |
| Levalbuterol | Xopenex | Inhalation | 5–15 | 60–90 | 4–6 |

*Adapted from Ciccone CD. Pharmacology in Rehabilitation, ed 4. Philadelphia, 2007, FA Davis.*

Ideally, a drug with a more specific β₂-receptor action with no α- and β₁-receptor activities would be the most preferred for bronchodilator therapy. Unfortunately, no pure β₂-specific sympathomimetic medications have yet been identified. Nevertheless, drugs with relatively selective stimulation of β₂ receptors that would only affect the lungs without affecting the β₁ receptors of the heart are now available. These β₂-specific agents produce bronchiolar dilation by relaxing the bronchial smooth muscle through facilitation of increased cAMP levels. The recommended β₂ agonists are considered either long- or short-acting (Table 15-2). The adverse effects of the currently available β₂-specific sympathomimetics are less intense than those of the nonspecific β-receptor sympathomimetics. However, this selectivity breaks down when high doses are used or in certain cardiac sensitive individuals. These adverse effects include tremor, palpitations, headache, nervousness, dizziness, nausea, hypertension as well as inotropic (enhanced myocardial contractility) and chronotropic (enhanced heart rate) effects.

Short-acting β₂-adrenergic agonists (SABAs) work quickly (generally within 3 to 5 minutes), but last for relatively short periods of time (4 to 6 hours). SABAs are often prescribed as quick-reliever medications because of their fast relief from symptoms of shortness of breath. SABAs are also used to prevent or decrease symptoms of bronchospasm that are known to be triggered by specific situations, such as exercise or cold weather. SABAs are recommended for use as rescue therapy to treat the breakthrough symptoms of bronchospasm in diseases of the airway, that is, reactive airway diseases (asthma). Long-acting β₂-adrenergic agonists (LABAs) usually take longer to work (3 to 20 minutes) but last for longer periods of time (up to 12 hours). Because of their long-acting features, LABAs are considered maintenance drugs. The 12-hour protection from symptoms of LABA drugs is an important feature in providing stable airways on a day-to-day basis. Some people with chronic obstructive pulmonary disease (COPD) sleep better at night or find they need to use their "reliever" medication less frequently because of this benefit.

In 2006, the Salmeterol Multicenter Asthma Research Trial was published, showing a small, but statistically significant increase in respiratory-related and asthma-related deaths and combined asthma-related deaths or life-threatening experiences in the total population receiving salmeterol.[25] As a result of these finding both the U.S. Food and Drug Administration (FDA) and the U.S. National Asthma Education and Prevention Program (NAEPP) recommend using LABAs only as an addition to inhaled corticosteroids.[24,26]

The reader is referred again to Table 15-2 for commonly used $\beta_2$-adrenergic agonists. $\beta_2$-Adrenergic drugs can be administered through a variety of methods: orally, subcutaneously, or by inhalation. Inhalation is the preferred route of administration as it allows the drug to be delivered directly to the respiratory tissues while bypassing the systemic circulation and minimizing systemic side effects. In addition, because of its direct delivery, the onset of action is more rapid with inhalation over subcutaneous or oral administration. Prolonged use of $\beta_2$-adrenergic agonists may increase bronchial response to allergens or irritants, causing airway irritation and bronchospasm.

There are two methods of providing medications by inhalation: the metered dose inhaler (MDI) and nebulizer.

A MDI is a device that delivers a specific amount of medication to the lungs, in the form of a short burst of aerosolized drug that is inhaled by the patient. The inhaler consists of three major components: the canister, where the drug is stored; the metering valve, which allows a metered quantity of the drug to be dispensed with each actuation; and a mouthpiece that allows the patient to operate the device and directs the aerosol into the patient's lungs. To use the inhaler the patient presses down on the top of the canister, with his or her thumb supporting the lower portion of the actuator. Actuation of the device releases a single metered dose of the formulation that contains the medication either dissolved or suspended in the propellant. Breakup of the volatile propellant into droplets, followed by rapid evaporation of these droplets, results in the generation of an aerosol consisting of micrometer-sized medication particles that are then inhaled.

A MDI contains enough medication for a certain number of actuations (or puffs), which is printed on the canister. Even though the inhaler may continue to work beyond that number of uses, the amount of medication delivered may not be accurate. It is important to keep track of the number of times an inhaler was used, so that it can be replaced after its recommended number of uses. MDIs are convenient because of their small size and portability; however, they require a certain amount of coordination to time delivery of the medication with a proper inspiratory effort.[27-29] MDIs are sometimes used with add-on devices referred to as holding chambers or spacers, which are tubes attached to the inhaler that act as a reservoir or holding chamber and reduce the speed at which the aerosol enters the mouth. They serve to hold the medication that is sprayed by the inhaler. A spacer device holds the medicine in a chamber after you squeeze the canister, allowing you to inhale slowly and deeply once or twice. This makes it easier to use the inhaler and helps ensure that more of the medication gets into the lungs instead of just into the mouth or the air. With proper use, a spacer can make an inhaler somewhat more effective in delivering medicine. Spacers can be especially helpful to adults and children who

find a regular MDI hard to use. People who use corticosteroid inhalers should use a spacer to prevent getting the medicine in their mouth, where oral yeast infections and dysphoria can occur.[30,31]

A nebulizer is a device used to administer medication in the form of a mist inhaled into the lungs. There are different types of nebulizers, although the most common are the jet nebulizers. Jet nebulizers are connected by tubing to a compressed air source that causes oxygen to blast at high velocity through a liquid medicine to turn it into an aerosol, which is then inhaled by the patient over the course of 10 minutes. As a general rule, physicians most commonly prescribe MDIs for their patients, largely because they are more convenient and portable than nebulizers. However, jet nebulizers are commonly used in hospital settings for patients who have difficulty using inhalers, such as in serious cases of respiratory disease or severe asthma attacks. Nebulizers accept their drugs in the form of a liquid solution, which is loaded into the device upon use. Usually, the aerosolized drug is inhaled through a tubelike mouthpiece, similar to that of an inhaler. The mouthpiece, however, is sometimes replaced with a face mask for ease of use with young children or the elderly, although mouthpieces are preferable if patients are able to use them as face masks result in reduced lung delivery because of aerosol losses in the nose.[29]

## Sympatholytic Agents or Adrenergic Antagonists

Because $\alpha$-receptor stimulation produces both vasoconstriction and bronchoconstriction, the pharmacologic reduction of $\alpha$-adrenergic activity in the bronchi via $\alpha$-adrenoceptor antagonists can be useful for patients with pulmonary disease. $\alpha$ Antagonists prevent the decrease of cAMP, which can be associated with an antigen–antibody reaction and cause bronchodilation. Nausea, fall in blood pressure, and dizziness are the most common side effects associated with $\alpha$ antagonists.[3,6,23]

## Parasympatholytic Agents or Muscarinic Antagonists

The vagus nerve (10th cranial nerve) supplies the lungs with a rich supply of parasympathetic innervation.[32] Cholinergic receptors can be divided into nicotinic (skeletal muscles, autonomic ganglia) and muscarinic (end-organ) receptors. The receptors on the smooth muscles of the bronchi are muscarinic in nature.

Blockade of muscarinic receptors prevents the increase in cGMP which would ordinarily be caused by activation of these receptors.[6] This tips the balance in favor of $\beta$-receptor activation and causes an increased action of cAMP resulting in bronchial smooth muscle relaxation. The most commonly used agent had been atropine. However, atropine is readily absorbed into the systemic circulation and has been frequently associated with a number of adverse reactions. Some of these side effects are dry mouth and skin, headache, confusion, dizziness, tachycardia, blurred vision, rash, delirium (elderly patients), and decreased gastrointestinal activity.[3,6,23]

Because an increased vagal tone and acetylcholine release are important factors that mediate bronchoconstriction in emphysema and chronic bronchitis, muscarinic antagonists that reduce vagal influence are integral to the management of bronchoconstriction in COPD. Airway inflammation, rather than an increase in vagal tone and acetylcholine release, is the hallmark in reactive airway disease/asthma. Therefore, muscarinic agonists are not typically prescribed to treat the underlying cause of asthma but may be used to assist antiinflammatory medications in treating acute episodes of moderate to severe asthma. Common medications include ipratropium (Atrovent) and tiotropium (Spiriva). These drugs are given by inhalation and not absorbed as well into the systemic circulation. There are fewer systemic adverse reactions. These may include dry mouth, tachycardia, blurred vision and constipation.[33,34]

## Methylxanthines

The intracellular level of cAMP can be enhanced if its degradation process by the enzyme phosphodiesterase (PDE) can be inhibited. By blocking the inactivation of cAMP, its action is enhanced and prolonged, resulting in bronchodilation. The group of drugs that most significantly inhibits PDE is the methylxanthines.[3,6,23] Methylxanthines may also facilitate bronchodilation by means of prostaglandin inhibition, adenosine receptor blockade, enhancement of endogenous catecholamine levels, inhibition of cGMP, and enhancement of the translocation of intracellular calcium.[3,6,23] Methylxanthines are also stimulatory to the central nervous system and skeletal muscle. Therefore, there is an improved diaphragmatic contractility plus a decrease in diaphragmatic fatigue in patients with chronic lung disease. In turn, trouble breathing or dyspnea is reduced and exercise tolerance improved.[35-42] The most commonly used methylxanthines are theophylline (Bronkodyl, Theo-Dur, Slo-Phyllin) and aminophylline (Aminophyllin, Cardophyllin), which are associated with a variety of side effects, including increased myocardial work load, heightened susceptibility to ventricular and supraventricular dysrhythmias, and possibly diuresis. The identification and functional characterization of different PDE isoenzymes have led to the development of various pulmonary-specific isoenzyme inhibitors as potential antiasthma drugs. Because the isoenzymes PDE3 and PDE4 are found in airway smooth muscle and inflammatory cells, selective inhibitors of these isoenzymes may add to the therapy of chronic airflow obstruction with less-adverse reactions. The development of "second-generation" selective drugs has produced promising clinical results not only for the treatment of bronchial asthma but also for the treatment of COPD.[43]

## Corticosteroids

Corticosteroids are drugs that are similar to the human hormone cortisol except that they are longer acting and have more pronounced immune suppressive or antiinflammatory activity. They are not routinely regarded as primary bronchodilators. But because bronchoconstriction is basically an inflammatory response, corticosteroids reduce the inflammatory response, decrease mucosal swelling, and increase bronchial lumen and airflow.[44,45] The following effects of corticosteroids result in an increase in bronchial intraluminal diameter:[6,23,33,42,44,45]

- Inhibition of the migration of lymphocytes, eosinophils, and mast cells,
- Reduction of stickiness and margination of polymorphonuclear leukocytes,
- Potentiation of β-receptor activity with increase in cAMP,
- Suppression of kinin activity, resulting in constriction of the vasculature within the bronchial mucosa,
- Inhibition of IgE action and stabilization of mast cell membranes with decreased release of histamine and other bronchoconstrictor mediators,
- Reduction of PDE activity with increased cAMP activity,

Because of their profound antiinflammatory actions, corticosteroids are considered to be the drugs of first choice for both the long-term and quick relief of asthma.

Although it influences all medications, the route of administration of corticosteroids is of particular importance because of the tremendous impact it plays in the incidence of side effects. During episodes of severe bronchoconstriction, corticosteroids are usually administered intravenously. However, for prolonged use, an oral or inhalational route of administration is used.[33] The inhalational route is preferred because it is associated with fewer side effects.

Most of the adverse effects of corticosteroid therapy are dose dependent and take a few days or weeks to manifest themselves. However, some side effects are unavoidable and reactions span the spectrum from merely unpleasant to dangerous. The primary side effects associated with high dose and long-term steroid therapy include immunosuppression with increased risk of infections; gastrointestinal disturbance; emotional lability (vacillation between euphoria and depression); insomnia; osteoporosis; retardation of growth; muscle weakness and atrophy (particularly of pelvic and shoulder girdle musculature); hyperglycemia; sodium and water retention; increased incidence of glaucoma and cataracts; and shift of body fats to face ("moon" face) and back ("buffalo back").[6,23,33] Table 15-3 lists the most often recommended steroids for long-term and quick relief.

## Mast Cell Stabilizers

Research in England in the 1960s on an extract of a Mediterranean plant resulted in the discovery of cromolyn sodium (Intal). A similar, nonsteroidal antiinflammatory drug, nedocromil sodium (Tilade) is also available.[42,46,47] They stabilize mast cells and prevent the release of histamine and other inflammatory mediators. However, this mechanism is probably not why it works in asthma.[6] It is more likely that they inhibit the response of sensory C fibers to the irritant capsaicin, inhibiting local axon reflexes involved in asthma, and the release of preformed T-cell cytokines and other inflammatory mediators involved in asthma.[42,48,49] They also have been shown to inhibit chloride and calcium channels.[50] They need time to do so and for this reason are used mostly prophylactically in cases of chronic asthma.[6] However, they can

**Table 15-3 Long-Term Control and Quick-Relief Steroids**

| | Drug Generic | Brand Name | Route of Administration |
|---|---|---|---|
| Long-term control steroids | Budesonide | Pulmicort, Turbuhaler | Inhaled |
| | Flunisolide | AeroBid | Inhaled |
| | Fluticasone | Flovent | Inhaled |
| | Triamcinolone | Azmacort | Inhaled |
| | Methylprednisolone | Medrol | Oral |
| | Prednisone | Prednisone, Deltasone, Orasone, Prednisone Intensol | Oral |
| | Prednisolone | Prelone, Pediapred | Oral |
| Quick-relief steroids | Prednisone | Prednisone, Deltasone, Orasone, Prednisone Intensol | Oral |
| | Prednisolone | Prelone, Pediapred | Oral |

prevent the late-phase reaction in an acute asthma episode (which can cause severe airway obstruction 4 to 6 hours after initial bronchoconstriction).[48,49] Both cromolyn and nedocromil have few side effects, as they are poorly absorbed. These are minor and usually occur at the site of deposition. Symptoms may include dry mouth, cough, and throat irritation. Although these drugs are unlikely to eliminate the use of inhaled corticosteroids in patients with more significant obstructive airway disease, they have the potential benefit of steroid-sparing effects.

## Leukotriene Inhibitors

Leukotrienes are strong inflammatory mediators that promote neutrophil–endothelial interactions, induce bronchoconstriction, and increase airway hyperresponsiveness. Leukotrienes are formed from membrane lipids via the enzyme phospholipase $A_2$ to yield arachidonic acid. This compound is converted by the enzyme lipoxygenase into different leukotrienes that act on special leukotriene receptors. They are synthesized in response to many triggers, including receptor activation, antigen–antibody interaction, physical stimuli such as cold, and any stimulation that increases intercellular calcium.[32] They also cause smooth muscle hypertrophy, mucus hypersecretion, and the influx of eosinophils into airway tissues. Therefore, inhibition of the action of leukotrienes potentially plays an important role in the treatment of asthma and other allergic conditions such as allergic rhinitis, atopic dermatitis, and chronic urticaria.[34] There are two ways to achieve this goal. Zileuton (Zyflo) causes inhibition of 5-lipoxygenase and reduces or prevents leukotriene synthesis. Montelukast (Singulair) and Zafirlukast (Accolate) inhibit leukotriene $B_4$ ($LTB_4$) from binding to its receptor on target tissues. In both cases, smooth muscle constriction is reversed. These leukotriene inhibitors are taken orally and are combined with other drugs ($\beta_2$ agonists or corticosteroids). Side effects of leukotriene inhibitors include hepatic impairment, headaches, fatigue, nausea, and vomiting.

## Anti-IgE Monoclonal Antibodies

Allergies are triggered by allergens. These can be large molecules like proteins but can also be very small molecules called *haptens*, which then bind to body-own proteins, altering their structure and converting them into allergens. After first exposure to such an allergen in a sensitive person, only IgE, which is a member of one class of antibodies, starts to multiply and to bind to mast cells and other cells such as basophils. Renewed exposure to these allergens causes a combination of these allergens with the IgEs and a massive release of inflammatory substances such as histamine, leukotrienes, prostaglandins, and interleukins. These mediators cause vasodilation, mucosal swelling, and secretion and constriction of the bronchi. Omalizumab (Xolair) is an anti-IgE monoclonal antibody. Monoclonal antibodies (name ending in *mab* or *moab*) are laboratory-created antibodies toward a particular substance. In this case, omalizumab binds specifically to IgE antibodies and prevents their action. Because of its high cost, omalizumab is generally prescribed to patients with severe, persistent asthma, which cannot be controlled with high doses of corticosteroids. Side effects of omalizumab include itching, headaches, injection site pain, or, in severe cases, anaphylaxis.[35]

## New Drug Development

Protease inhibitors and inhibitors of neutrophil elastase, cathepsins, and matrix metalloproteases are in the clinical development pipeline as possible new antiinflammatory treatments.

## Ancillary Pulmonary Medications

In addition to the aforementioned medications, several other drug groups are frequently used in the treatment of respiratory

## Table 15-4 Common Decongestants

| Drug Generic | Brand Name | Route of Administration |
|---|---|---|
| Ephedrine | Rynatuss*, Primatene Tablets* | Oral |
| Epinephrine | Primatene Mist | Nasal spray |
| Oxymetazoline | Neo-Synephrine 12-Hour Afrin, Dristan*, Vicks Sinex*, and Mucinex Full Force | Nasal spray |
| Phenylephrine | Neo-Synephrine | Nasal spray |
| Pseudoephedrine | Sudafed, Dimetapp Decongestant | Oral |

*Decongestant combined with other ingredients.*

disorders: decongestants, antihistamines, antitussives, muco-kinetics, respiratory stimulants and depressants, paralyzing drugs, and antimicrobial agents. The drug grouping may provide clues regarding the nature of the problem for which it was taken, or vice versa. For example, a patient experiencing mucosal edema may complain of congestion and take an over-the-counter decongestant or antihistamine.

## Decongestants

The common cold, allergies, and many respiratory infections have in common the symptoms of "runny nose and stuffy head." These are caused by vasodilation and "leaky" blood vessels leading to mucosal swelling and fluid leaks. The most common decongestants are $\alpha$-adrenergic sympathomimetics, specifically $\alpha_1$ agonists.[51,52] These medications stimulate $\alpha$ receptors and cause vasoconstriction reducing or preventing the underlying pathology.

Decongestants are frequently combined with other ingredients (e.g., antihistamines) as constituents of commercially available, nonprescription, over-the-counter preparations (Table 15-4). When used appropriately, these medications can be safe and effective. However, if a patient has a specific sensitivity or if the decongestant medication is improperly used, adverse effects may arise. Primary side effects include headache, dizziness, nausea, nervousness, insomnia, hypertension, and cardiac irregularities (e.g., palpitations).

The use of $\alpha$-agonist-containing nasal sprays should be limited to a few days only as long-term use can lead to a "rebound" effect (nasal congestion gets progressively worse) and can also cause nasal ulcers.

## Antihistamines

Treatment of the respiratory allergic responses associated with seasonal allergies (e.g., hay fever) is one of the most common uses of antihistamines. Histamines interact with two specific receptor types referred to as $H_1$ and $H_2$ receptors.[23] The $H_2$ receptors are located in the stomach and are involved in acid secretion. The $H_1$ receptors, primarily located in vascular, respiratory, and gastrointestinal smooth muscle, are specifically targeted for blockade by antihistamines in the treatment of asthma.[53] $H_1$-antagonists decrease the mucosal

## Table 15-5 Common Antihistamines

| Drug Generic | Brand Name | Route of Administration |
|---|---|---|
| Brompheniramine | Dimetapp* | Oral |
| Chlorpheniramine | Chlor-Trimeton,* Sudafed,* Coricidin* | Oral |
| Cetirizine | Zyrtec | Oral |
| Desloratadine | Clarinex | Oral |
| Dexbrompheniramine | Drixoral* | Oral |
| Dimenhydrinate | Dramamine | Oral |
| Diphenhydramine | Benadryl | Oral |
| Loratadine | Claritin* | Oral |
| Pheniramine | Triaminic* | Oral |
| Phenyltoloxamine | Sinutab* | Oral |
| Triprolidine | Actifed* | Oral |

*Antihistamine combined with other ingredients.*

congestion, irritation, and discharge caused by inhaled allergens. Antihistamines may also reduce the coughing and sneezing often associated with common colds.

Table 15-5 lists some of the antihistamines commonly used to treat the symptoms of hay fever and other hay fever-like allergies. The adverse effects most often attributable to antihistamines include sedation, fatigue, dizziness, blurred vision, loss of coordination, and gastrointestinal distress. Antihistamines are frequently combined with other ingredients, such as $\alpha$-adrenergic sympathomimetics or $\alpha$ agonists.

## Antitussives

Cough is a common symptom of respiratory problems so that there a fair number of prescription drugs available for the treatment of coughs.[54] Cough can be divided into a productive cough, which removes mucus from the airway and increases airflow, and an unproductive cough, which is not useful and causes discomfort to the patient. Drugs should be

## Table 15-6 Common Antitussives

| Drug Generic | Brand Name | Classification/Action |
|---|---|---|
| Benzonatate | Tessalon | Local anesthetic |
| Codeine* | Many brand names | Increases threshold in cough center |
| Dextromethorphan* | Many brand names | Increases threshold in cough center |
| Diphenhydramine | Benadryl | Antihistamine |
| Hydrocodone | Triaminic Expectorant DH | Increases threshold in cough center |
| Hydromorphone | Dilaudid Cough | Increases threshold in cough center |

*Frequently combined with other ingredients (i.e., expectorants, decongestants).*

used to only suppress the ineffective, dry hacking cough associated with minor throat irritations and the common cold. Cough-suppressive drugs, or antitussive agents, act either to block the overly active receptors or to increase the threshold of the cough center in the medulla portion of the brain. They are generally indicated for only short-term use (often at night) and are not indicated for coughs caused by retained secretions.

Antitussives may be classified as topical anesthetics (e.g., benzonatate, Tessalon), nonnarcotics (e.g., dextromethorphan, Congespirin for Children, Mediquell, Pertussin), and narcotics (e.g., codeine, morphine). The primary adverse effect of nonnarcotic and narcotic antitussive agents is sedation. However, gastrointestinal distress, nausea, and constipation, as well as dizziness, may also occur. Table 15-6 lists common antitussives.

## Mucoactive Agents

Drugs that promote the mobilization and removal of secretions from the respiratory tract are called *mucoactive drugs*. There are four basic types of mucoactive agents: mucolytics, expectorants, wetting agents, and surface-active agents.

Mucolytic drugs disrupt the chemical bonds in mucoid and purulent secretions, decreasing the viscosity of the mucus and promoting expectoration. Administered by inhalation, acetylcysteine (Mucomyst) was the principal mucolytic drug used previously. It supposedly "opens" disulfide linkages in mucus and makes it more fluid. However, it is used infrequently today. Acetylcysteine's primary adverse effects include mucosal irritation, coughing, bronchospasm (especially in those with a reactive airway component) and nausea.

Dornase alfa (Pulmozyme) is a highly purified solution of recombinant human deoxyribonuclease I (rhDNase). This enzyme selectively cleaves and hydrolyses DNA present in sputum/mucus and reduces viscosity in the lungs promoting improved clearance of secretions. Its primary use is in patients with cystic fibrosis who culture positively for *Pseudomonas aeruginosa*. However, dornase alfa has been shown to be effective in treating patients with non-cystic fibrosis bronchiectasis, that is, primary ciliary dyskinesia. Dornase alfa is administered via nebulizer.[55,56]

Expectorants are described as medications that facilitate expectoration of respiratory secretions by increasing hydration of the airway or the volume of secretions. Examples of the most prevalent expectorants are simple hydration (via aerosol, i.e., 3% saline or orally, iodinated glycerol, and glyceryl guaiacolate [guaifenesin]). Guaifenesin can be found in the over-the-counter expectorants of Mucinex and Robitussin, and its efficacy seems to be minimal.[55,56]

Wetting agents that humidify and lubricate the secretions make sputum expectoration easier for the patient. Half normal saline (0.45% NaCl) had been the agent of choice for sputum induction. It was delivered by either continuous aerosol or intermittent ultrasonic nebulization. However, this practice is infrequently performed clinically at this time. Inhaled hypertonic saline (7% NaCl) has been found to increase mucociliary clearance by increasing sputum volume. Anecdotally, the effect of hypertonic saline was discovered by Australian surfers with cystic fibrosis; they told clinicians that sea water helped their secretion clearance. Subsequent studies have, in short-term trials, demonstrated improved lung function in people with cystic fibrosis.[55-58]

Surface-active agents, or surfactant, may stabilize aerosol droplets and thereby enhance their efficacy as carrier vehicles for nebulized drugs. However, the usefulness of these agents is still under study.[6,23,33]

## Respiratory Stimulants and Depressants

A drug that stimulates the central respiratory centers is considered a respiratory stimulant. Noxious stimuli, such as pain, may result in central nervous system excitation and thus elicit enhanced respiratory center activity. Some medications, such as certain sympathomimetics and methylxanthines, also stimulate respiratory center activity and induce an increase in ventilation. Drugs that have a specific ability to cause central respiratory excitation with subsequently increased respiratory activity are called *analeptics*. Unfortunately, analeptic drugs elicit dose-dependent levels of central stimulation that can ultimately result in convulsions. Thus, the clinical use of analeptic medications is not without controversy. However, when respiratory failure has been aggravated by a potentially

**Table 15-7 Common Neuromuscular Blocking Agents**

| Drug Generic | Brand Name | Type | Usual Duration of Effect (minutes) | Adverse Reactions |
|---|---|---|---|---|
| Atracurium | Tracrium | Nondepolarizing | Up to 30 | Hypotension |
| Gallamine | Flaxedil | Nondepolarizing | 60 to 120 | Tachycardia |
| Pancuronium | Pavulon | Nondepolarizing | Up to 180 | Tachycardia |
| Vecuronium | Norcuron | Nondepolarizing | Up to 50 | Mild hypertension, mild tachycardia |
| Succinylcholine | Suxamethonium, Anectine | Depolarizing | About 5 | Vagal and sympathetic stimulation; associated fasciculations may cause muscle pain |

harmful intervention (e.g., oxygen, narcotics), respiratory stimulants serve a purpose.[6,23,33]

> **Clinical Tip**
> Prescription of β-blocking medications in patients who have a history of bronchospasm or asthma should be done with caution. Some β-blocking medications may actually have a slight effect on $\beta_2$ receptors, blocking $\beta_2$ stimulation.

Doxapram (Dopram) it thought to stimulate chemoreceptors in the carotid arteries and/or cortical and spinal neurons,[58] which, in turn, stimulate the respiratory center in the brainstem. It increases tidal volume and respiratory rate and is one of the most widely accepted analeptics. Administered intravenously, its use serves to prevent a rise in partial pressure of arterial carbon dioxide ($PaCO_2$) with oxygen therapy in acute ventilatory failure.[59] It is also used to prevent respiratory depression in high-risk postoperative patients.[60,61]

Some drugs (e.g., sedatives, tranquilizers, narcotic analgesics) are, to varying degrees, respiratory depressants. In general, patients with pulmonary disease should avoid the use of these drugs because they suppress the ventilatory drive. However, in some instances intravenous morphine, midazolam (Versed), propofol (Diprivan), or diazepam (Valium) is given to mechanically ventilated patients if anxiety or agitation is contributing to an increased work of breathing and hindering mechanical ventilation. The antipsychotic drug haloperidol (Haldol) may be prescribed for spontaneously breathing patients to control agitation because it has less respiratory depressant action than other tranquilizers or sedatives.[62] Many of the drugs used in the treatment of psychiatric disorders have varying degrees of sedative effect, depressing the central nervous system and possibly leading to respiratory depression in some patients. Some other antipsychotic drugs are associated with significant parasympatholytic or anticholinergic effects, causing some bronchodilation but also dry mouth, blurred vision, constipation, and urinary retention. The latter are more pronounced in geriatric patients.

## Neuromuscular Blocking Drugs

Although muscle relaxants can relieve muscle spasm, they do not prevent volitional muscle activity. To completely ablate muscular tone during general anesthesia, the level of anesthesia must be profound, a situation that is not wholly desirable. Consequently, anesthetists and anesthesiologists usually opt for lighter general anesthesia in conjunction with muscle-paralyzing agents to produce the desired degree of immobilization. Neuromuscular blocking drugs are also used to facilitate endotracheal intubation, to control laryngeal spasm, to treat diseases that cause neuromuscular hyperactivity (e.g., tetanus, severe intractable seizure activity), and, occasionally, to prevent struggling, fighting, or excessive tachypnea in patients being mechanically ventilated. A long-acting agent (botulinus toxin) is used to treat localized muscle spasms (and cosmetically to remove wrinkles). Table 15-7 presents the short-term neuromuscular blocking agents most frequently used clinically.

## Antimicrobial Agents

Drugs used to combat unicellular organisms (e.g., bacteria, viruses, fungi) that invade the body are often called antimicrobial agents or, if derived from natural sources, antibiotics. Because individuals often suffer from infections caused by pathogenic microorganisms, it is quite likely that many patients receiving physical therapy will be taking one or more antimicrobial drugs. Unfortunately, antimicrobial agents not only retard the growth or kill the microbes, but are also toxic to the host cells.[23,33] Antimicrobial agents (Table 15-8) act by different mechanisms with some examples following. The penicillins, the cephalosporins, polypeptides, the antifungal polyenes, and the monobactams inhibit cell wall synthesis and function. The aminoglycosides, the macrolides, the tetracyclines and lincomycins inhibit microbial protein synthesis. The quinolones and some antiviral drugs interfere with the synthesis of microbial DNA.

Antibacterial drugs may be classified as bactericidal (killing or destroying bacteria) or bacteriostatic (limiting growth and proliferation of bacteria). The bactericidal or

## Table 15-8 Common Antimicrobial Medications

| Group | | Drug Name | Brand Name | Indication for Specific Antimicrobial Use |
|---|---|---|---|---|
| Aminoglycosides* | | Amikacin | Amikin | |
| | | Gentamicin | Apogen, Garamycin | |
| | | Kanamycin | Kantrex, Klebcil | |
| | | Netilmicin | Netromycin | |
| | | Streptomycin | | |
| | | Tobramycin | Nebcin | |
| Cephalosporins† | First generation | Cefadroxil | Duricef, Ultracef | |
| | | Cefazolin | Ancef, Kefzol | |
| | | Cephalexin | Keflex | |
| | Second generation | Cefaclor | Ceclor | |
| | | Cefamandole | Mandol | |
| | | Cefonicid | Monocid | |
| | | Ceforanide | Precef | |
| | | Cefotetan | Cefotan | |
| | Third generation | Cefoperazone | Cefobid | |
| | | Cefotaxime | Claforan | |
| | | Cefoxitin | Mefoxin | |
| | | Ceftazidime | Fortaz, Tazicef | |
| | | Ceftibuten | Cedax | |
| | Fourth generation | Cefepime | Maxipime | |
| | | Cefpirome | Cefrom | |
| Macrolides | | Erythromycin | ERYC, E-Mycin, Ilosone, EES, Pediamycin, Ilotycin, Erythrocin, Erypar, Ethril | |
| | | Troleandomycin | TAO | |
| Monobactams | | Aztreonam | Azactam | |
| | | Loracarbef | Lorabid | |
| Lincomycins | | Clindamycin | Cleocin | |
| | | Lincomycin | Lincocin | |
| Penicillins | Natural penicillins | Penicillin G | Bicillin, Crysticillin, Permapen, etc. | |
| | | Penicillin V | V-Cillin, Pen-Vee, Penapar VK, etc. | |
| | Penicillinase-resistant penicillins | Cloxacillin | Cloxapen, Tegopen | |
| | | Dicloxacillin | Dynapen, Pathocil | |
| | | Methicillin | Staphcillin | |
| | | Nafcillin | Unipen | |
| | | Oxacillin | Bactocill, Prostaphlin | |
| | Aminopenicillins | Amoxicillin | Amoxil, Polymox | |
| | | Ampicillin | Amcill, Omnipen, Polycillin, etc | |
| | | Bacampicillin | Spectrobid | |
| | Wide-spectrum penicillins | Azlocillin | Azlin | |
| | | Carbenicillin | Geocillin, Geopen, Pyopen | |

*Continued*

## Table 15-8 Common Antimicrobial Medications—cont'd

| Group | Drug Name | Brand Name | Indication for Specific Antimicrobial Use |
|---|---|---|---|
| Penicillins (cont'd) | Mezlocillin | Mezlin | |
| | Piperacillin | Pipracil | |
| | Ticarcillin | Ticar | |
| Quinolones | Ciprofloxacin | Cipro | |
| | Lomefloxacin | Maxaquin | |
| | Ofloxacin | Floxin | |
| Sulfonamides | Sulfadiazine | Silvadene | |
| | Sulfamethoxazole | Gantanol, Methoxanol | |
| | Sulfisoxazole | Gantrisin | |
| Tetracyclines | Chlortetracycline | Aureomycin | |
| | Doxycycline | Doxychel, Vibramycin, etc. | |
| | Oxytetracycline | Terramycin | |
| | Tetracycline | Achromycin V, Sumycin, etc. | |
| Others | Aminosalicylic acid | PAS, Teebacin | |
| | Bacitracin | Bacitracin ointment | |
| | Chloramphenicol | Chloromycetin, Amphicol, etc. | |
| | Cycloserine | Seromycin | |
| | Sulfamethoxazole/ Trimethoprim | Bactrim, Septra | |
| | Vancomycin | Vancocin IV, Vancoled | |
| Antituberculosis drugs | Capreomycin | Capastat | |
| | Isoniazid | INH, Nydrazid, etc. | |
| | Pyrazinamide | PZA | |
| Antiviral drugs | Acyclovir | Zovirax | Herpes (especially simplex-related) infections |
| | Amantadine | Symadine, Symmetrel | Influenza A infections |
| | Ribavirin | Tribavirin, Virazole | Respiratory syncytial infections |
| | Vidarabine | Vira-A | Herpes simplex, cytomegalovirus, varicella zoster infections |
| | Zidovudine | Retrovir | To slow HIV progression |
| | Ganciclovir | Cytovene | To slow HIV progression |
| Antifungal drugs | Amphotericin B | Fungizone | Aspergillosis, blastomycosis, candidiasis, coccidioidomycosis, cryptococcosis, histoplasmosis |
| | Flucytosine | Ancobon | Candidiasis, cryptococcosis, aspergillosis |
| | Nystatin | Mycostatin, Nilstat | Oropharyngeal candidiasis |
| | Fluconazole | Diflucan | Oropharyngeal candidiasis |
| | Itraconazole | Sporanox | Pulmonary blastomycosis |

## Table 15-8 Common Antimicrobial Medications—cont'd

| Group | Drug Name | Brand Name | Indication for Specific Antimicrobial Use |
|---|---|---|---|
| Antiprotozoal drugs | Chloroquine | Aralen | Malaria |
| | Hydroxychloroquine | Plaquenil | Malaria |
| | Metronidazole | Flagyl | Amebiasis, giardiasis, trichomoniasis |
| | Pentamidine | Pentam | Pneumocystis carinii |

*Often used as supplements to the penicillins.
†Cephalosporins generally serve as alternatives to penicillins if they prove ineffective or are poorly tolerated by the patient.

bacteriostatic characteristics of a drug may depend upon the dosage of the drug: some drugs (e.g., erythromycin) are bacteriostatic at low doses and bactericidal at higher doses. Bacteria can be divided according to their *in vitro* staining as Gram-negative or Gram-positive staining bacteria. They can also be divided if they need (aerobes) or do not need oxygen (anaerobes).

Penicillins are a mainstay in the treatment of respiratory infections. The semisynthetic penicillins have a broader spectrum of antibacterial activity than the natural penicillins and are also orally effective.[23,33] The principal disadvantage to the use of penicillins are allergic reactions, which manifest as skin rashes, hives, bronchoconstriction, or even an anaphylactic reaction.

Cephalosporins are generally considered as alternatives to the penicillins when penicillins are not tolerated by the patient or when they are ineffective. These drugs are divided according to their introduction into medicine as different generation drugs. First-generation cephalosporins are used in the treatment of Gram-positive cocci and some Gram-negative bacteria. Second-generation cephalosporins are similar in effectiveness against Gram-positive cocci and are generally thought to be more effective against Gram-negative bacteria. Third-generation cephalosporins are effective against the greatest number of Gram-negative bacteria, but they are of limited effectiveness against Gram-positive cocci. Cephalosporins may elicit stomach cramps, diarrhea, nausea, and vomiting. In addition, some patients may exhibit allergic reactions similar to those of the penicillins.

Aminoglycoside drugs have a wide spectrum of antibacterial activity. They are active against many aerobic Gram-negative bacteria, some aerobic Gram-positive bacteria, and many anaerobic bacteria.[6,23,33] Unfortunately, this wide spectrum of activity is associated with more toxicity. Nephrotoxicity and ototoxicity are the primary toxic manifestations, especially in patients with particular susceptibility (elderly, patients with liver or renal failure). The erythromycins also exhibit a broad spectrum of antibacterial activity, being effective against many Gram-positive and some Gram-negative bacteria.[6,23,33] The most common side effect of erythromycin administration is gastrointestinal distress (stomach cramps, nausea, vomiting, and diarrhea).

When the tetracyclines were first introduced, they were effective against many Gram-positive and Gram-negative bacteria, as well as organisms such as *Chlamydia*, *Rickettsia*, and *Spirochaeta*. However, because tetracyclines are generally bacteriostatic, many bacterial strains have developed resistance to tetracycline and its derivatives.[6,23,33] Because these drugs can interfere with tooth and bone growth, they should not be used in children or teenagers.

Monobactams are a new class of synthetic antibiotics. These drugs are effective against Gram-negative and Gram-positive aerobes and anaerobes. Currently, there are a number of quite effective antiviral and antifungal drugs available and their use is becoming more common to treat successfully infections from these microorganisms.

The determination of the causative factor in an acute respiratory infection is often difficult because clinical signs are often quite similar. Specimens of transoral sputum for microbiologic analysis are easily contaminated, yielding mixtures of multiple organisms on culture. Nevertheless, the organisms *Streptococcus pneumoniae* and *Haemophilus influenzae* are generally thought to be the primary cause of infection of the respiratory mucosa in patients with chronic pulmonary disease.[63] Often treatment based on clinical observations suffices but in nonresponding infections a precise diagnosis generally requires that sputum samples are obtained by transtracheal aspiration, bronchoscopy, or transpulmonary aspiration. Treatment is then based on the findings of the clinical laboratory.

## Other Agents

Oxygen is considered a drug when inhaled concentrations are higher than those found in atmospheric air. Regardless of its etiology, arterial hypoxemia (partial pressure of oxygen in arterial blood [$PaO_2$] less than 60 mm Hg) is the most common indication for oxygen therapy. The therapeutic administration of oxygen can elevate the arterial oxygen tension and increase the arterial oxygen content (which shifts the oxyhemoglobin dissociation curve to the right), improving peripheral tissue oxygenation. Additionally, the constriction of the central pulmonary vascular beds associated with hypoxia can be reduced or reversed.[64]

Supplemental oxygen is most commonly administered via nasal tubes at flow rates between 1 and 6 L/min. Systems for such low gas flow rates are generally prescribed on the assumption that the patient is breathing at a relatively constant rate and depth (minute ventilation). However, when breathing patterns deviate from the norm, patients cannot be assured of receiving the intended $FIO_2$ (fraction of inspired oxygen). Therefore, when higher gas flow rates are indicated (e.g., respiratory rate greater than 30 per minute), or more accurate titrations of $FIO_2$ are required, oxygen is typically delivered by any one of several types of moderate- and high-flow face masks (providing oxygen concentrations of 40% to 60% or more).[65] Care must be exercised so as to avoid the potential for depression of the hypoxic drive to breathe in patients with chronically elevated $PaCO_2$ levels primarily in patients with COPD.[66,67] See Chapter 13 for more information on oxygen-delivery devices.

When used judiciously, oxygen therapy has few side effects. However, depending upon the oxygen concentration and its duration of administration, oxygen toxicity can occur. In general, the pathologic changes in the lungs associated with oxygen toxicity can be described in three phases: exudative, proliferative, and recovery.[68–70] In the exudative phase, damage to the alveolar–capillary membrane results in an increased permeability to water, electrolytes, and protein. Secondarily, the capillaries become plugged with platelets and the interstitium is invaded by polymorphonuclear leukocytes. As lung damage progresses, the inflammatory response is intensified. In the proliferative phase, fibroblasts and type II epithelial cells proliferate in conjunction with interstitial collagen deposition. The recovery phase may result in complete healing or areas of fibrosis.

Since the discovery of the important role the vascular endothelium plays in the regulation of vascular smooth muscle tone, the identification of endothelium-derived relaxing factor (EDRF) and the fact that EDRF is indistinguishable from nitric oxide (NO), numerous articles regarding the actions and effects of NO have been published.[71–74] NO is widely distributed in the body and plays an important role in the regulation of the blood circulation. In the body, NO is derived from L-arginine in a reaction catalyzed by NO synthase. Once produced, NO diffuses to the vascular smooth muscle cells where it activates the enzyme guanylate cyclase, which synthesizes more cGMP and which causes vascular smooth muscle relaxation. Other potential therapeutic roles of NO include the treatment of endotoxic shock, adult respiratory distress syndrome, and hypertension in various disease states, such as atherosclerosis and chronic renal failure.[75–77]

Although the side effects of NO are incompletely understood, the marked oxidizing effects of nitrogen dioxide ($NO_2$, the product of NO and oxygen) are known to:[66]

- Decrease alveolar permeability,
- Decrease $PaO_2$ and the diffusing capacity of lung for carbon monoxide,
- Cause pulmonary edema,
- Cause loss of cilia and disintegration of bronchiolar epithelium, and
- Decrease pulmonary function tests (i.e., forced expiratory volume in 1 second).

The few studies investigating the toxic effects of NO have shown that at concentrations of NO greater than 15 to 20 ppm, $PaO_2$ decreased 7 to 8 mm Hg, and airway resistance increased.[5,78,79]

---

**Clinical Tip**

Herbal medications now appear to be playing a role in the treatment of acute and chronic pulmonary dysfunction. The current availability of herbal medicines without prescription in the United States contributes to their use. Research data are not available to support or refute the use of herbal medicines. Also, little is known of the potential drug–drug interactions. More research is needed before their use can be recommended.

---

## CASE STUDY 15-1

An 89-year-old white woman was admitted to the hospital with complaints of shortness of breath, productive sputum, and nausea. Up to 2 weeks prior to admission, the patient was independently active in the community and around her own home. However, 3 days prior to admission, the patient required a walker to get around because of weakness and shortness of breath. A diagnosis of an upper respiratory tract infection was made and treated with Biaxin (clarithromycin). However, a dry cough persisted. On hospital admission, she was diagnosed with mild congestive heart failure. She was started on diuretics and digoxin was continued. While she was in intensive care unit, her daughter noticed an increase in thick, gray-yellow sputum. She also had abdominal discomfort, but denied indigestion. Other complaints included low back pain with radicular signs thought to be aggravated by her coughing. Currently she is on 3 L of supplemental $O_2$.

Social history: The patient lives alone, but has a supportive, family. She denies smoking or alcohol use.

Past medical history:

Cholecystectomy, 1993

Polynephritis

Atrial fibrillation

Congestive heart failure

Arteriosclerotic cardiovascular disease

Hypertensive cardiovascular disease

## CASE STUDY 15-1—cont'd

Medications:

Ascorbic acid, 500 mg PO twice daily

Biaxin (clarithromycin), 250 mg PO twice daily

Fosamax (alendronate sodium), 10 mg every morning

Lasix (furosemide), 80 mg PO every 12 hours

Prilosec (omeprazole), 20 mg PO every 4 hours or when needed

Digoxin, 125 mg PO

Ativan (lorazepam), as needed (PRN)

Azmacort inhaler (triamcinolone acetonide), daily

Phenergan with codeine, 5 to 10 mL PO every 4 to 6 hours, as needed (PRN) for cough

---

## Summary

- This chapter covered the principal groups of drugs used in the treatment of pulmonary dysfunction and their potential effects on exercise performance:

- Bronchoconstriction is the result of abnormal or increased bronchomotor tone (bronchospasm), inflammation, or mechanical obstruction.

- The primary goal of bronchodilator therapy is to manipulate the influences of the autonomic nervous system.

- Decongestants are used to constrict blood vessels and treat the mucosal edema and increased mucus production often associated with common colds, allergies, and many respiratory infections.

- Antihistamines are used to block the vasodilatory effects of histamine and control the production of mucus and the mucosal edema and irritation commonly associated with respiratory allergic responses.

- Antitussives are used to suppress the ineffective, dry, hacking cough associated with minor throat irritations and the common cold.

- Mucoactives promote the mobilization and removal of secretions from the respiratory tract.

- Analeptics are used to stimulate the central nervous system and enhance respiratory center activity.

- Neuromuscular blocking agents are used to ensure immobility in patients during surgical procedures, to facilitate endotracheal intubation, and to reduce the work of breathing in some mechanically ventilated patients.

- Antimicrobial agents are used to combat microorganisms that invade the body, either by killing them or by limiting their growth and proliferation.

- Oxygen is considered a drug when it is administered in concentrations higher than those found in the atmospheric air.

- NO is used for the treatment of pulmonary hypertension.

## References

1. Popa V. Respiratory pharmacology. Beta-adrenergic drugs. Clin Chest Med. 1986 Sep;7(3):313–29, 1986.

2. Ziment I, Popa V. Respiratory pharmacology. Clin Chest Med 7:313–29, 1986.

3. III Baltic Meeting on Pharmacology. Physiology and Pharmacology of the Respiratory System. Symposium proceedings. Copenhagen, Denmark, August 15–16, 1992. Pharmacol Toxicol 72:1–55, 1993.

4. Drain CB, Robinson SE. The pharmacology of respiratory disorders related to anesthesia. CRNA 7:193–9, 1996.

5. Leff AR. Pulmonary and Critical Care Pharmacology and Therapeutics. New York, McGraw-Hill, 1996.

6. Rau JL. Respiratory Care Pharmacology. 5th ed. St. Louis, Mosby, 1998.

7. Deitmer T. Physiology and pathology of the mucociliary system. Special regards to mucociliary transport in malignant lesions of the human larynx. Adv Otorhinolaryngol 43:1–136, 1989.

8. Marek W. Chronobiology of the bronchial system. Pneumologie 51(Suppl 2):430–9, 1997.

9. Morrison JF, Pearson SB. The effect of the circadian rhythm of vagal activity on bronchomotor tone in asthma. Br J Clin Pharmacol 28:545–9, 1989.

10. Leff AR. Endogenous regulation of bronchomotor tone. Am Rev Respir Dis 137(5):1198–216, 1988.

11. Widdicombe JG. Pulmonary and respiratory tract receptors. J Exp Biol 100:41–57, 1982.

12. van der Velden VH, Hulsmann AR. Autonomic innervation of human airways: Structure, function, and pathophysiology in asthma. Neuroimmunomodulation 6:145–59, 1999.

13. Pearlman DS. Pathophysiology of the inflammatory response. J Allergy Clin Immunol 104:S132–7, 1999.

14. Bjornsdottir US, Cypcar DM. Asthma: An inflammatory mediator soup. Allergy 54:55–61, 1999.

15. Carter PM, Heinly TL, Yates SW, et al. Asthma: The irreversible airways disease. J Investig Allergol Clin Immunol 7(6):566–71, 1997.

16. Rossi GL, Olivieri D. Does the mast cell still have a key role in asthma? Chest 112:523–9, 1997.

17. Marney Jr SR. Pathophysiology of reactive airway disease and sinusitis. Ann Otol Rhinol Laryngol 105:98–100, 1996.

18. Leung DY. Molecular basis of allergic diseases. Mol Genet Metab 63:157–67, 1998.

19. Wills-Karp M. Immunologic basis of antigen-induced airway hyperresponsiveness. Annu Rev Immunol 17:255–81, 1999.

20. Chin JE, Hatfield CA, Winterrowd GE, et al. Preclinical evaluation of anti-inflammatory activities of the novel pyrrolopyrimidine PNU-142731A, a potential treatment for asthma. J Pharmacol Exp Ther 290(1):188–95, 1999.

21. Oda N, Yamashita N, Minoguchi K, et al. Long-term analysis of allergen-specific T cell clones from patients with asthma treated with allergen rush immunotherapy. Cell Immunol 190(1):43–50, 1998.

22. Dent G, Giembycz MA. Phosphodiesterase inhibitors: Lily the Pink's medicinal compound for asthma? Thorax 51:647–9, 1996.

23. Dahan A, vanBeek JHGM. Physiology and Pharmacology of Cardio-respiratory Control. Boston, Kluwer Academic, 1998.

24. National Heart, Lung, and Blood Institute. Guidelines for the diagnosis and management of asthma: Expert panel report 3. In NIH publication no. 08-4051. Bethesda, MD, U.S. Dept. of Health and Human Services, Public Health Service, National Institutes of Health, National Heart, Lung, and Blood Institute, 2007.

25. Nelson HS, Weiss ST, Bleecker ER, et al. The Salmeterol Multicenter Asthma Research Trial. Chest 129:15–26, 2006.

26. Levenson M. Long-acting beta-agonists and adverse asthma events meta-analysis: Statistical briefing package for joint meeting of the Pulmonary-Allergy Drugs Advisory Committee, Drug Safety and Risk Management Advisory Committee, and Pediatric Advisory Committee on December 10–1, 2008.

27. Hickey AJ. Pharmaceutical Inhalation Aerosol Technology. 2nd ed. New York, Marcel Dekker, 2004.

28. Swarbrick J. Encyclopedia of Pharmaceutical Technology. 3rd ed. London, Informa Health Care, 2007.

29. Finlay WH. The Mechanics of Inhaled Pharmaceutical Aerosols: An Introduction. London, Academic Press, 2001.

30. Togger DA, Brenner PS. Metered dose inhalers. Am J Nurs 101(10):26–32, 2001.

31. Hickey AJ. Inhalation Aerosols: Physical and Biological Basis for Therapy. 2nd ed. London, Informa Healthcare, 2007.

32. Salvi SS, Krishna MT, Sampson AP, et al. The anti-inflammatory effects of leukotriene-modifying drugs and their use in asthma. Chest 119:1533–46, 2001.

33. Ciccone CD. Pharmacology in Rehabilitation. 4th ed. Philadelphia, FA Davis, 2007.

34. Drazen JM, Israel E, O'Byrne PM. Treatment of asthma with drugs modifying the leukotriene pathway. N Engl J Med 340(3): 197–206, 1999.

35. Holgate ST, Chuchalin A, Herbert J, et al. Efficacy and safety a recombinant anti-immunoglobulin E antibody (omalizumab) in severe allergic asthma. Clin Exp Allergy 34:632–8, 2004.

36. Sparrow MP, Weichselbaum M, McCray PB. Development of the innervation and airway smooth muscle in human fetal lung. Am J Respir Cell Mol Biol 20:550–60, 1999.

37. Lu CC. Bronchodilator therapy for chronic obstructive pulmonary disease. Respirology 2:317–22, 1997.

38. Gauthier AP, Yan S, Sliwinski P, et al. Effects of fatigue, fiber length, and aminophylline on human diaphragm contractility. Am J Respir Crit Care Med 152:204–10, 1995.

39. Krzanowski JJ, Polson JB. Mechanism of action of methylxanthines in asthma. J Allergy Clin Immunol 82:143–5, 1988.

40. Murciano D, Aubier M, Curran Y, et al. Action of aminophylline on the strength of contraction of the diaphragm in patients with chronic obstructive respiratory insufficiency. Presse Med 16:1628–30, 1987.

41. Church MK, Featherstone RL, Cushley MJ, et al. Relationships between adenosine, cyclic nucleotides, and xanthines in asthma. J Allergy Clin Immunol 78:670–5, 1986.

42. Katzung BG, Masters SB, Trevor AJ. Basic and Clinical Pharmacology. New York, McGraw-Hill, 2009.

43. Schmidt D, Dent G, Rabe KF. Selective phosphodiesterase inhibitors for the treatment of bronchial asthma and chronic obstructive pulmonary disease. Clin Exp Allergy 29(Suppl 2):99–109, 1999.

44. Kelly HW. Comparative potency and clinical efficacy of inhaled corticosteroids. Respir Care Clin N Am 5:537–53, 1999.

45. Cave A, Arlett P, Lee E. Inhaled and nasal corticosteroids: Factors affecting the risks of systemic adverse effects. Pharmacol Ther 83:153–79, 1999.

46. Krawiec ME, Wenzel SE. Inhaled nonsteroidal anti-inflammatory medications in the treatment of asthma. Respir Care Clin N Am 5:555–74, 1999.

47. Haahtela T. Advances in pharmacotherapy of asthma. Curr Probl Dermatol 28:135–52, 1999.

48. Aswania OA, Corlett SA, Chrystyn H. Relative bioavailability of sodium cromoglycate to the lung following inhalation, using urinary excretion. Br J Clin Pharmacol 47:613–18, 1999.

49. Furukawa C, Atkinson D, Forster TJ, et al. Controlled trial of two formulations of cromolyn sodium in the treatment of asthmatic patients > or = 12, years of age. Intal Study Group. Chest 116(1):65–72, 1999.

50. Fanta CH. Asthma. N Engl J Med 360(10):1002–14, 2009.

51. Fireman P. Pathophysiology and pharmacotherapy of common upper respiratory diseases. Pharmacotherapy 13(6 Pt 2):101S–9S; discussion 143S–6S, 1993.

52. Hornby PJ, Abrahams TP. Pulmonary pharmacology. Clin Obstet Gynecol 39:17–35, 1996.

53. Slater JW, Zechnich AD, Haxby DG. Second-generation antihistamines: A comparative review. Drugs 57:31–47, 1999.

54. Zemp E, Elsasser S, Schindler C, et al. Long-term ambient air pollution and respiratory symptoms in adults (SAPALDIA study). The SAPALDIA Team. Am J Respir Crit Care Med 159:1257–66, 1999.

55. Rubin BK. Mucolytics, expectorants and mucokinetic medications. Respir Care 52:859–65, 2007.

56. Gadson B. Pharmacology for Physical Therapists. St. Louis, Saunders, 2006.

57. Elkins MR, Robinson M, Rose BR, et al. A controlled trial of long-term inhaled hypertonic saline in patients with cystic fibrosis. N Engl J Med 354(3):229–40, 2006.

58. Casaburi R. Pharmacological modulators of respiratory control. Monaldi Arch Chest Dis 53:287–93, 1998.

59. Kerr HD. Doxapram in hypercapnic chronic obstructive pulmonary disease with respiratory failure. J Emerg Med 15:513–15, 1997.

60. Bjork L, Arborelius Jr M, Renck H, Rosberg B. Doxapram improves pulmonary function after upper abdominal surgery. Acta Anaesthesiol Scand 37:181–8, 1993.

61. Huon C, Rey E, Mussat P, et al. Low-dose doxapram for treatment of apnoea following early weaning in very low birthweight infants: A randomized, double-blind study. Acta Paediatr 87:1180–4, 1998.

62. Kersten LD. Comprehensive Respiratory Nursing: A Decision-Making Approach. St. Louis, Saunders, 1989.

63. Sethi S. Infectious exacerbations of chronic bronchitis: Diagnosis and management [see comments]. J Antimicrob Chemother 43(Suppl A):97–105, 1999.

64. Hillier SC, Graham JA, Hanger CC, et al. Hypoxic vasoconstriction in pulmonary arterioles and venules. J Appl Physiol 82:1084–90, 1997.

65. Burkhart Jr JE, Stoller JK. Oxygen and aerosolized drug delivery: Matching the device to the patient. Cleve Clin J Med 65:200–8, 1998.

66. Hida W. Role of ventilatory drive in asthma and chronic obstructive pulmonary disease. Curr Opin Pulm Med 5:339–43, 1999.

67. Dunn WF, Nelson SB, Hubmayr RD. Oxygen-induced hypercarbia in obstructive pulmonary disease. Am Rev Respir Dis 144:526–30, 1991.
68. Capellier G, Maupoil V, Boussat S, et al. Oxygen toxicity and tolerance. Minerva Anestesiol 65:388–92, 1999.
69. Beckett WS, Wong ND. Effect of normobaric hyperoxia on airways of normal subjects. J Appl Physiol 64:1683–7, 1988.
70. Bryan CL, Jenkinson SG. Oxygen toxicity. Clin Chest Med 9:141–52, 1988.
71. Barst RJ. Diagnosis and treatment of pulmonary artery hypertension. Curr Opin Pediatr 8:512–19, 1996.
72. Weitzenblum E, Kessler R, Oswald M, Fraisse P. Medical treatment of pulmonary hypertension in chronic lung disease. Eur Respir J 7:148–52, 1994.
73. Roger N, Barbera JA, Roca J, et al. Nitric oxide inhalation during exercise in chronic obstructive pulmonary disease. Am J Respir Crit Care Med 156:800–6, 1997.
74. Wanstall JC, Jeffery TK. Recognition and management of pulmonary hypertension. Drugs 56:989–1007, 1998.
75. Shah AM, Prendergast BD, Grocott-Mason R, et al. The influence of endothelium-derived nitric oxide on myocardial contractile function. Int J Cardiol 50:225–31, 1995.
76. Paulus WJ, Kastner S, Pujadas P, et al. Left ventricular contractile effects of inducible nitric oxide synthase in the human allograft. Circulation 96:3436–42, 1997.
77. Watkins DN, Jenkins IR, Rankin JM, Clarke GM. Inhaled nitric oxide in severe acute respiratory failure—Its use in intensive care and description of a delivery system [see comments]. Anaesth Intensive Care 21:861–6, 1993.
78. Okamoto K, Hamaguchi M, Kukita I, et al. Efficacy of inhaled nitric oxide in children with ARDS. Chest 114:827–33, 1998.
79. Young JD, Dyar O, Xiong L, Howell S. Methaemoglobin production in normal adults inhaling low concentrations of nitric oxide. Intensive Care Med 20:581–4, 1994.

# CHAPTER 16

# Examination and Assessment Procedures

*Ellen Hillegass*

## Chapter Outline

**Elements of Patient Management**
**Preferred Physical Therapist Practice Patterns**
**Patient History**
**Medical Chart Review**
    Diagnosis and Date of Event
    Symptoms
    Other Medical Problems and Past Medical History
    Medications
    Risk Factors for Heart Disease
    Relevant Social History
    Clinical Laboratory Data
    Radiologic Studies
    Oxygen Therapy and Other Respiratory Treatment
    Surgical Procedures
    Other Therapeutic Regimens
    Electrocardiogram and Serial Monitoring
    Pulmonary Function Tests
    Arterial Blood Gases
    Cardiac Catheterization Data

    Vital Signs
    Hospital Course
    Nutritional Intake
    Occupational History
    Home Environment and Family Situation
**Interview with the Patient and the Family**
**Systems Review**
**Physical Examination**
    Inspection
    Auscultation of the Lungs
    Auscultation of the Heart
    Palpation
    Mediate Percussion
    Activity Evaluation
**Evaluation**
**Case Study**
**Summary**
**References**

---

Optimal rehabilitation depends on a thorough examination of the entire patient to evaluate the extent of dysfunction that may affect future performance. In this chapter, the examination procedures, used to provide information regarding specific cardiopulmonary-system diseases are described. The examination includes a systems review prior to an entire examination as well as a battery of tests and measures. While performing the initial examination, objective information can be obtained from a thorough review of the medical record, an interview with the patient, and an assessment of the patient at rest (including observation and inspection, palpation, auscultation, mediate percussion, general muscle strength, and joint range of motion) and during activity. In addition, the physical therapist must also have a good understanding of other therapeutic regimens and concomitant problems and be able to recognize them. On conclusion of the examination, the therapist should be able to interpret the evaluative findings appropriately to make a decision regarding therapeutic interventions.

## Elements of Patient Management

The process involved in determining the most appropriate interventions to address and ultimately achieve the desired outcomes for the patient involves six elements (Fig. 16-1):

- Examination: A comprehensive patient screening of history and a systems review as well as specific tests and measures to collect data on the patient.
- Evaluation: Evaluation of the data from the examination to make a clinical judgment
- Diagnosis: Determining the impact of a condition on function at the level of the system and the level of the individual. This diagnosis classifies a patient within a specific practice pattern and indicates the primary dysfunctions to guide the therapist toward interventions that should be addressed initially. These are not to be confused with medical diagnoses.
- Prognosis: Determining the patient's predicted level of optimal function as well as the estimated length of time to achieve expected improvement. A plan of care is developed based on the prognosis, which includes anticipated goals and expected outcomes.
- Intervention
- Outcomes

Once the elements have been performed, a plan of care is established. Re-examination begins, implementing the process of performing tests and measures to evaluate the patient's progress with subsequent modifications to

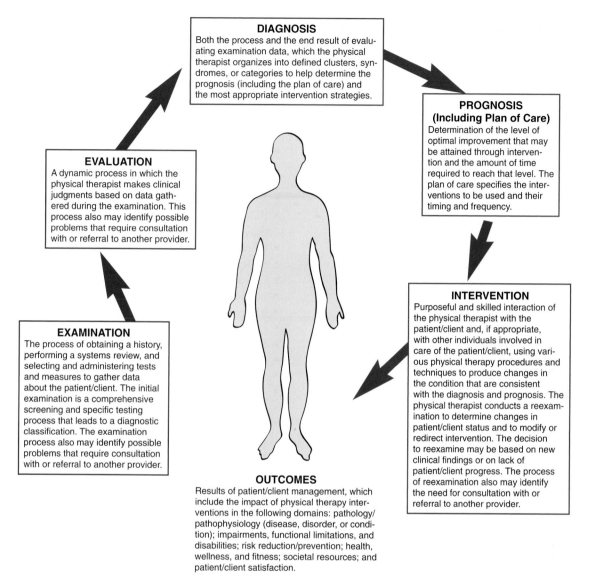

**DIAGNOSIS**
Both the process and the end result of evaluating examination data, which the physical therapist organizes into defined clusters, syndromes, or categories to help determine the prognosis (including the plan of care) and the most appropriate intervention strategies.

**EVALUATION**
A dynamic process in which the physical therapist makes clinical judgments based on data gathered during the examination. This process also may identify possible problems that require consultation with or referral to another provider.

**PROGNOSIS**
**(Including Plan of Care)**
Determination of the level of optimal improvement that may be attained through intervention and the amount of time required to reach that level. The plan of care specifies the interventions to be used and their timing and frequency.

**EXAMINATION**
The process of obtaining a history, performing a systems review, and selecting and administering tests and measures to gather data about the patient/client. The initial examination is a comprehensive screening and specific testing process that leads to a diagnostic classification. The examination process also may identify possible problems that require consultation with or referral to another provider.

**INTERVENTION**
Purposeful and skilled interaction of the physical therapist with the patient/client and, if appropriate, with other individuals involved in care of the patient/client, using various physical therapy procedures and techniques to produce changes in the condition that are consistent with the diagnosis and prognosis. The physical therapist conducts a reexamination to determine changes in patient/client status and to modify or redirect intervention. The decision to reexamine may be based on new clinical findings or on lack of patient/client progress. The process of reexamination also may identify the need for consultation with or referral to another provider.

**OUTCOMES**
Results of patient/client management, which include the impact of physical therapy interventions in the following domains: pathology/pathophysiology (disease, disorder, or condition); impairments, functional limitations, and disabilities; risk reduction/prevention; health, wellness, and fitness; societal resources; and patient/client satisfaction.

**Figure 16-1** The elements of patient management leading to optimal outcomes. Screening takes place anywhere along this pathway. (From American Physical Therapy Association. Guide to Physical Therapist Practice. 2nd ed. Baltimore, APTA, 2003.)

the intervention. Throughout the episode of care, anticipated goals and expected outcomes determined at initial evaluation are reviewed and assist the clinician with assessing the impact of the intervention on patient physical, social, and psychological domains.

## Preferred Physical Therapist Practice Patterns

Patients with cardiopulmonary dysfunction can be grouped into eight practice patterns that describe the five elements of patient management for each specific diagnostic classification. The patterns describe inclusion and exclusion criteria for each pattern as well as examination findings that help to describe the patients that appropriately fall into that category. The eight practice patterns are listed in Table 16-1 and the full description of each practice pattern as well as practice

patterns from the other three groupings (musculoskeletal, neuromuscular and integumentary) can be found in the *Guide to Physical Therapist Practice.*[1]

## Patient History

Information is obtained on the patient's current symptoms and medical problems as well as past medical history from a history and data form, medical chart, patient/family interview, and/or other members of the team treating the patient (Fig. 16-2). The data obtained provide the initial information to begin to identify impairments and functional limitations that may be identified during a physical examination, as well as provide information identifying areas that may require intervention or education to prevent additional health problems. The history taking is a very critical part of the examination, and according to a McMaster study is a key distinctive

**Table 16-1 Preferred Physical Therapist Practice Patterns: Cardiovascular/Pulmonary**

| Practice Pattern | Description of Pattern |
|---|---|
| 6A | Primary prevention/risk reduction for cardiovascular/pulmonary disorders |
| 6B | Impaired aerobic capacity/endurance associated with deconditioning |
| 6C | Impaired ventilation, respiration/gas exchange and aerobic capacity/endurance associated with airway clearance dysfunction |
| 6D | Impaired aerobic capacity/endurance associated with cardiovascular pump dysfunction or failure |
| 6E | Impaired ventilation and respiration/gas exchange associated with ventilatory pump dysfunction or failure |
| 6F | Impaired ventilation and respiration/gas exchange associated with respiratory failure |
| 6G | Impaired ventilation, respiration/gas exchange and aerobic capacity/endurance associated with respiratory failure in the neonate |
| 6H | Impaired circulation and anthropometric dimensions associated with lymphatic system disorders |

*From American Physical Therapy Association. Guide to Physical Therapist Practice.*

difference between novice clinicians and experienced clinicians.[2] According to the McMaster study, experienced clinicians are much better history takers than the novice clinician and this may be related to the value the experienced clinicians have found over the years they have practiced.

As not all patients present to the physical therapist with a full medical chart, much information must be obtained from other sources than the chart, such as the patient/family/friends as well as other members of the team. In the absence of the medical chart, the physical therapist must gather as much of the information discussed in the following sections as possible. In the future, possibly all patients will be presenting to physical therapy with their medical chart on a memory stick to share with all medical providers.

## Medical Chart Review

The purpose of the medical chart review is to extract pertinent information to develop a database on the patient. Based on the information obtained, the physical therapist performs the appropriate physical assessment and develops an optimal treatment plan. In the event the patient does not present with a medical record, the therapist must try and obtain similar information as best as possible. The therapist should focus the review of the medical record by identifying the following significant information:

- Diagnosis and date of event
- Symptoms on admission and after the patient's admission
- Other significant medical problems in the past medical history
- Current medications
- Risk factors for cardiovascular and pulmonary disease
- Relevant social history, including smoking, alcohol and drug use, lifestyle, support mechanisms
- Clinical laboratory data
- Radiologic studies
- Oxygen therapy and other respiratory treatment
- Surgical procedures
- Other therapeutic regimens
- Electrocardiogram and telemetry monitoring
- Pulmonary function tests
- Arterial blood gases
- Cardiac catheterization data
- Other diagnostic tests
- Vital signs
- Hospital course since admission, particularly in the patient with cardiac injury to determine whether it has been a complicated or an uncomplicated course
- Nutritional intake
- Occupational history
- Home environment assessment

### Diagnosis and Date of Event

The physical therapist needs to know and understand the primary diagnosis as well as any additional diagnoses made since the hospital admission or referral to rehabilitation to determine the appropriateness of treatment and the need for monitoring of the patient's responses. Often a patient's primary diagnosis may have been the reason for admission (e.g., a fractured hip), yet a secondary diagnosis may be the reason for referral for physical therapy (e.g., pneumonia postoperatively). Any diagnosis that begins "Rule out—" requires a thorough review of the chart to see if the diagnosis was confirmed or rejected.

The date of the event is significant, because it determines the acuteness of the situation. The date of the primary event or diagnosis is often documented in the physician's history and physical examination report; however, reviewing the physician's progress notes or orders may discover the date of the secondary diagnosis or subsequent events.

### Symptoms

Both cardiovascular and pulmonary symptoms need to be evaluated. Cardiac ischemic symptoms are those that occur anywhere above the waist; they are typically expressed on, or

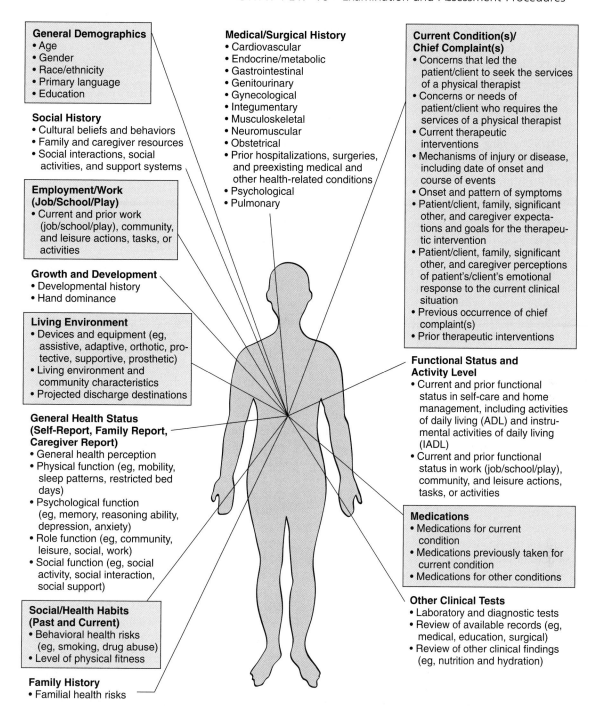

**General Demographics**
- Age
- Gender
- Race/ethnicity
- Primary language
- Education

**Social History**
- Cultural beliefs and behaviors
- Family and caregiver resources
- Social interactions, social activities, and support systems

**Employment/Work (Job/School/Play)**
- Current and prior work (job/school/play), community, and leisure actions, tasks, or activities

**Growth and Development**
- Developmental history
- Hand dominance

**Living Environment**
- Devices and equipment (eg, assistive, adaptive, orthotic, protective, supportive, prosthetic)
- Living environment and community characteristics
- Projected discharge destinations

**General Health Status (Self-Report, Family Report, Caregiver Report)**
- General health perception
- Physical function (eg, mobility, sleep patterns, restricted bed days)
- Psychological function (eg, memory, reasoning ability, depression, anxiety)
- Role function (eg, community, leisure, social, work)
- Social function (eg, social activity, social interaction, social support)

**Social/Health Habits (Past and Current)**
- Behavioral health risks (eg, smoking, drug abuse)
- Level of physical fitness

**Family History**
- Familial health risks

**Medical/Surgical History**
- Cardiovascular
- Endocrine/metabolic
- Gastrointestinal
- Genitourinary
- Gynecological
- Integumentary
- Musculoskeletal
- Neuromuscular
- Obstetrical
- Prior hospitalizations, surgeries, and preexisting medical and other health-related conditions
- Psychological
- Pulmonary

**Current Condition(s)/Chief Complaint(s)**
- Concerns that led the patient/client to seek the services of a physical therapist
- Concerns or needs of patient/client who requires the services of a physical therapist
- Current therapeutic interventions
- Mechanism of injury or disease, including date of onset and course of events
- Onset and pattern of symptoms
- Patient/client, family, significant other, and caregiver expectations and goals for the therapeutic intervention
- Patient/client, family, significant other, and caregiver perceptions of patient's/client's emotional response to the current clinical situation
- Previous occurrence of chief complaint(s)
- Prior therapeutic interventions

**Functional Status and Activity Level**
- Current and prior functional status in self-care and home management, including activities of daily living (ADL) and instrumental activities of daily living (IADL)
- Current and prior functional status in work (job/school/play), community, and leisure actions, tasks, or activities

**Medications**
- Medications for current condition
- Medications previously taken for current condition
- Medications for other conditions

**Other Clinical Tests**
- Laboratory and diagnostic tests
- Review of available records (eg, medical, education, surgical)
- Review of other clinical findings (eg, nutrition and hydration)

**Figure 16-2** Types of data that may be generated from a client history. In this model, data about the visceral systems is reflected in the medical/surgical history. The data collected in this portion of the patient history is not the same as information collected during the Review of Systems (ROS). It has been recommended that the ROS component be added to this figure. (From American Physical Therapy Association. Guide to Physical Therapist Practice. 2nd ed. Baltimore, APTA, 2003.)

exacerbated by, exertion and are relieved with rest. Each patient may describe these symptoms differently. Classically, any discomfort, such as chest pain, tightness or pressure, shortness of breath, palpitations, indigestion, and burning, should be considered a cardiac symptom unless cardiac dysfunction has been ruled out. Reviewing the patient's symptoms on admission and during hospitalization provides the therapist with an awareness of those symptoms that are to be assessed as cardiac or noncardiac. During activity, the therapist may be trying to reproduce those symptoms as well as observe for new ones. Ischemic-related symptoms may also be present in other vasculature of the body, and they too should be assessed (such as claudication discomfort in lower extremities indicate peripheral arterial disease). Angina is discussed in greater detail later in this chapter under abnormal responses during activity evaluation.

Classic pulmonary symptoms are described as shortness of breath, dyspnea on exertion, audible wheezing, cough, increased work of breathing, and sputum production. The symptoms and their severity as well as the means of reproducing these symptoms are important to identify. Changes in these symptoms (e.g., worsening of symptoms vs. improvement) assist the therapist in developing a plan of care that meets the patient's changing needs.

## Other Medical Problems and Past Medical History

The patient's past medical history, including other medical problems, may have a bearing on the evaluation or the plan of treatment proposed by the therapist. Diagnoses other than cardiovascular and pulmonary may include orthopedic, neurologic, psychological, or integumentary, and these diagnoses may affect the optimal treatment plan proposed. For example, an attempt to increase the activity level of a patient with a history of rheumatoid arthritis may be limited by an orthopedic (joint) dysfunction rather than by a cardiovascular or pulmonary condition.

## Medications

The medications the patient is currently taking are usually listed in the chart (often in the physician's orders). In the inpatient setting, a comprehensive listing can be found on the nurse's medication chart. Knowledge of the patient's medications can provide information about the patient's present or recent-past medical history and may include clues regarding treatment for hypertension, heart failure, angina, bronchospasm, infection, and the like. In the outpatient setting, the patients should always be asked to bring either a listing of their current prescribed as well as over-the-counter medications and herbal supplements or the actual medication containers, and these medications should be documented in their outpatient chart.

Because certain medications may affect the patient's responses to exercise, the physical therapist must become familiar with the broad categories of cardiac and pulmonary medications, understand the indications for their use, and know their general side effects. For further discussion of medications and their indications and side effects, see Chapters 14 and 15.

## Risk Factors for Heart Disease

From the history and physical examination, one usually can determine whether the patient has any of the following major risk factors for heart disease[3]:

- Hypertension
- Smoking
- An elevated serum cholesterol or a diet high in cholesterol
- A family history of heart disease
- Stress (anger and hostility; personality factors)
- A sedentary lifestyle

- Older age
- Male gender
- Obesity
- Diabetes

An awareness of the patient's risk factors enables the therapist to develop realistic goals for the patient's long-term treatment, to identify other rehabilitation team members to whom the patient should be referred, discuss a plan for prevention, and most important, to decide on precautions to and monitoring of increased activity, depending on the risk for heart disease. Detailed information on the risk factors can be obtained from Chapter 3.

## Relevant Social History

Self-abusive social habits, such as excessive drinking of alcohol, smoking, and use of illicit drugs, can affect the cardiopulmonary system and could affect rehabilitation. Therefore, knowledge of the patient's habits, including the length of time involved in the habit and the degree of intake, is an important component of the evaluation. Some of this information can be obtained from the history and physical examination, but often this information is obtained from the patient or the family.

Heavy alcohol consumption has been associated with the development of cardiomyopathy, and long-term cigarette smoking has been associated with the development of chronic obstructive lung disease and also affects wound healing. Drug use is one habit that may not be readily acknowledged but that may be suspected from the individual's behavior (e.g., extreme nervousness), history of sleeplessness, muscle twitching, anorexia, and nasal irritation. For example, cocaine has serious effects on the cardiovascular system, particularly on the coronary arteries. Cocaine is known to cause severe coronary artery spasm and in some cases can precipitate acute myocardial infarction.[4-6] Cocaine use (especially crack cocaine) has been associated with an increased incidence of severe arrhythmias and in some cases sudden death.

The physician or other medical personnel treating the patient may be unaware of the patient's heavy alcohol consumption or drug addiction. Either of these conditions could prove to be an extreme problem early in the patient's hospitalization because of the symptoms and side effects of sudden withdrawal from these substances.

## Clinical Laboratory Data

Laboratory data provide important objective information regarding the clinical status of the patient with cardiopulmonary dysfunction. The seriousness of the dysfunction may also be inferred from the magnitude of deviation of the values from normal. The laboratory data specific to the patient with cardiopulmonary dysfunction include the values for cardiac enzymes (troponin, creatine phosphokinase, lactate dehydrogenase, aspartate aminotransferase), blood lipids (cholesterol and triglycerides), complete blood cell count (specifically hemoglobin, hematocrit, white blood cell count), BUN and creatinine, arterial blood gases, and culture and sensitivity, as well as the results of coagulation studies, electrolyte screening panels, and glucose tolerance tests. These are discussed in greater detail in Chapters 8 and 10.

## Radiologic Studies

In most situations the therapist reviews the radiologic report and not the actual study films because of lack of access. The radiologic reports that are routinely reviewed for patients with cardiopulmonary dysfunction include chest radiographs, computed tomography (CT) scan, magnetic resonance imaging (MRI), and scintigraphy.

The chest radiographs provide a general static assessment of pathologic conditions of the lungs and chest wall, including changes in functional lung space, pleural space, chest wall configuration, presence of fluid, heart size, and vascularization of the lungs. Information about the extent of heart failure or cardiomyopathy as well as pneumonia, restrictive lung disease, pleural effusion, and the like can be obtained from the chest radiograph.

In addition to baseline chest radiographs, patients with heart failure and acute pulmonary dysfunction can be followed with serial radiographs to monitor disease progression, effectiveness of treatment, or both. Therefore, it is important to note the date of the radiograph (particularly if the patient's status is fluctuating). Also the orientation of the chest radiograph is important to identify. The ideal chest radiograph is a posterior-anterior (PA) film taken at a distance of approximately 6 feet with the patient in an upright position and performing a maximal inspiration. Portable equipment utilizing the anteroposterior (AP) orientation is used to take chest films of patients who are too sick or unstable to be transported to the radiology department for a standard PA film. The quality of the film taken with portable equipment and using the AP orientation is generally poorer than a PA film owing to the position of the patient and the patient's inability to cooperate or to perform a maximal inspiration. The therapist should keep these limitations in mind when evaluating the findings of a portable AP chest radiograph.

## Oxygen Therapy and Other Respiratory Treatment

The use of supplemental oxygen should be noted along with its method of delivery (e.g., nasal cannula, face mask, tracheostomy collar, blow-by ventilator, or mechanical ventilator), as well as the actual breathing performed by the patient with the oxygen in use. If a patient is a mouth breather and is given supplemental oxygen via nasal cannula, the patient will not obtain the maximal benefit from the supplemental oxygen. The physical therapist must also know the amount of oxygen being delivered (e.g., 60% via mask or 2 L via cannula). This information should be correlated with arterial blood gas analysis or hemoglobin saturation data to determine if the patient is adequately oxygenated before beginning any therapy. Depending on the arterial blood gas or oxygen

saturation information, the therapist may need to use oxygen or to increase the amount of oxygen while exercising the patient (e.g., during formal exercise, activities of daily living, gait). Any patient with a resting $PO_2$ of less than 60 mm Hg on room air or an oxygen percentage saturation of less than 90% should be considered for supplemental oxygen. If a patient has a low $PO_2$ but one not below 60 mm Hg on room air or a low $PO_2$ on oxygen, the patient may require supplemental oxygen with exercise to prevent hypoxemia during exercise. Chapter 10 presents a method of assessing the degree of hypoxemia when patients are receiving supplemental oxygen.

Other respiratory treatments (e.g., aerosols, bronchodilator treatments, inspirometers) that are prescribed should be noted because these treatments can improve the patient's exercise performance if they are administered before exercise; however, they may also be extremely fatiguing to the patient and may necessitate limitations on activity immediately following treatment. The necessity for the coordination of physical therapy and respiratory treatments to optimize rehabilitation should be readily apparent. If the patient is being ventilated mechanically, the mode of ventilator assistance, the set rate, the set volume, the peak inspiratory pressure, the fraction of inspired oxygen, the spontaneous rate, and the like should be identified. A full description of ventilators is found in Chapter 13.

## Surgical Procedures

An understanding of specific surgical approaches and procedures, as well as knowledge of the anatomy of the chest wall, is integral to the chart review process. Knowledge of the approach or procedure may be helpful in defining the physical therapy diagnosis and extent of the problem and in identifying limitations or precautions to any therapeutic procedures being planned (see Chapter 11).

It is important to understand the number of and placement of the bypass grafts as well as any complications that occurred during the procedure (e.g., whether a pacemaker was inserted) in patients who have undergone coronary artery bypass surgery. For the patient who has undergone bypass surgery with numerous vessels requiring bypass grafts or requiring left main or left main equivalent bypass, one might assume that the patient was more limited in activity before surgery. With extensive disease, patients usually have more symptoms with activity and may have had restrictions with low levels of exertion. In addition, the patient who experiences complications (such as a perioperative myocardial infarction or stroke) during or following the surgery usually has a slower recovery and may require increased activity supervision and may make slower progress.

In the patient who has undergone pulmonary surgery, the amount of lung tissue that was operated on is significant to note (e.g., wedge resection, lobectomy, or pneumonectomy), as well as the location of the incision. The greater the amount of lung tissue that was removed, the smaller the amount of lung space that is available (one would expect) to actively diffuse oxygen and carbon dioxide and therefore the greater the impairment in performance of activities.

## Other Therapeutic Regimens

As a result of the patient's primary or secondary diagnoses or subsequent surgical procedures, additional therapeutic interventions could have an impact on the proposed treatment. Identification of these interventions (e.g., pacemaker implantation, intravenous or intraarterial drug administration, parenteral nutrition, electrolyte replacement, or bedrest limitations) helps the physical therapist develop an appropriate treatment plan with appropriate precautions.

## Electrocardiogram and Serial Monitoring

The electrocardiogram (ECG) provides valuable information regarding the state of the heart muscle and the rhythm of the heart at the time of the ECG. The ECG is used to define previous as well as current myocardial injury, hypertrophy of the heart muscle, pericardial involvement, or delays in the generation of the depolarization impulse. Serial ECG monitoring provides a historic record of the patient's cardiac injury and rhythm disturbances and allows the correlation of the history of rhythm disturbances with changes in medications or medical status. ECGs do not predict the future and cannot give medical information of coronary anatomy. Details of the ECG and rhythm disturbances are discussed in Chapter 9.

## Pulmonary Function Tests

A pulmonary function test (PFT) is an essential component of the assessment process because abnormal PFTs indicate the effects of the pathologic condition and may provide clues regarding the patient's motivation. Measurement of PFTs is done via spirometry. PFTs can measure static and dynamic properties of the chest and lungs as well as gas exchange. Static measurements assess the lung volumes and capacities (e.g., tidal volume, vital capacity, inspiratory reserve volume) and determine mechanical abnormalities, whereas dynamic measurements provide data on the flow rates of air moving in and out of the lungs. The dynamic properties reflect the nonelastic components of the pulmonary system and include the forced expiratory flows and volumes.

Values for PFTs are used primarily to identify a baseline of pulmonary dysfunction as well as to follow the progression of altered respiratory mechanics in chronic lung and musculoskeletal diseases. Chapter 10 explains PFTs in greater detail.

Values for PFTs may be described as abnormal owing to the static values (volumes and capacities), the dynamic values (flow volumes and rates), or both. When patients demonstrate decreased volumes and capacities, they are exhibiting restrictive lung dysfunction. They therefore have less lung space for active diffusion of oxygen into the circulatory system and carbon dioxide out of the system. Patients with decreased dynamic values often have limitations on exercise owing to an inability to actively move large volumes of air rapidly. Treatment planning requires modifications, possibly including supplemental oxygen for patients with extremely low lung volumes or bronchodilator medication before exercise for patients with decreased flow rates or volumes.

## Arterial Blood Gases

Arterial blood gases are a measurement of the acid–base and oxygenation status of patients via arterial blood sampling. Blood gas determinations can identify the effectiveness of a treatment designed to improve airway clearance and ventilation. Therefore, serial arterial blood gases are often measured to provide feedback on the therapeutic regimen to the medical personnel. Arterial blood gases are discussed in greater detail in Chapter 10.

## Cardiac Catheterization Data

Cardiac catheterization, which is an invasive diagnostic procedure, provides information about the anatomy of the coronary arteries and can provide a dynamic assessment of the cardiac muscle. In addition, information on hemodynamic measurement (e.g., estimates of ejection fraction or systolic and diastolic pressures) as well as valvular function can be obtained. Cardiac catheterizations are performed to visualize the cardiac dysfunction and to assist in the decision-making process regarding medical versus surgical management. Repeat cardiac catheterizations also provide information on the progression or, in rare cases, regression of coronary disease or valvular dysfunction. See Chapter 8 for more detailed information.

## Vital Signs

Daily recordings of vital signs are often kept in the graphics section of the chart. Vital signs such as heart rate, temperature, blood pressure, and respiration are important to review for trends as well as for the establishment of a baseline. For example, pulmonary patients with infection who are being monitored for improvement can be followed by checking temperature and in some cases respirations and heart rate. Hypertension and treatment for hypertension can be monitored daily by viewing the blood pressure recordings (keeping in mind that these have been recorded at rest and usually in the supine position).

## Hospital Course

A thorough review of the medical record, including physicians' and other caregivers' notes, and the order sheets should reveal pertinent information regarding the patient's clinical course since admission. For example, patients with serious complications within the first 4 days of a myocardial infarction have a higher incidence of later serious complications or death. Criteria for a complicated postmyocardial infarction hospital course as defined by McNeer and coworkers include the following[7]:

- Ventricular tachycardia and fibrillation
- Atrial flutter or fibrillation
- Second- or third-degree atrioventricular (AV) block
- Persistent sinus tachycardia (more than 100 beats per minute)
- Persistent systolic hypotension (lower than 90 mm Hg)
- Pulmonary edema
- Cardiogenic shock
- Persistent angina or extension of infarction

Patients who are characterized as "uncomplicated" have significantly lower morbidity and mortality rates following their initial cardiac events. A prolonged or complicated hospital course can affect an individual's activity progression owing to the effects of inactivity or bedrest.

## Nutritional Intake

Identifying nutritional intake is especially important in individuals who are under or over-weight, yet all patients should be evaluated for intake during the time of rehabilitation. Patient may be receiving enteral (providing food through tube in nose, stomach, or intestine) or parenteral (intravenously; bypassing eating and digestion) feedings or simply by mouth. If the patient is feeding himself or herself, then nutritional intake needs to be verified by interview with patient and family as to how well the patient is eating. Without proper intake of carbohydrates and proteins, the patient may be limited in exercise performance.

## Occupational History

Identifying the type of work the patient currently performs allows for the setting of realistic goals and for developing a plan for return to work, if possible. For example, a patient who has experienced a massive complicated myocardial infarction may not be an appropriate candidate for returning to a job requiring heavy lifting and may need a referral for vocational rehabilitation. The earlier the referral is made, the less the chance of financial or emotional distress. In addition, if a patient requires job modifications or will be delayed in returning to work, referrals can be made to appropriate team members to assist the employer in making the changes necessary or to assist the patient with financial planning.

## Home Environment and Family Situation

A supportive family is important to the success of the rehabilitation of any patient. A support system can improve a patient's ability to respond to disease, whereas a negative home environment can deter the patient's rehabilitation.[8] In addition, if the patient requires a great deal of care, the family's ability to supply this care and its financial resources should be assessed. Early assessment of the family situation and home environment as well as involvement of the family in the patient's rehabilitation provides for optimal transition to home.

## Interview with the Patient and the Family

After a thorough chart review, the interview with the patient and the family is the next step in the physical therapist's initial evaluation. The purpose of this interview is to gather important information about the patient's present complaint, history of medical problems, report of symptoms, risk factors, perception and understanding of the problem, family situation, readiness to learn, and goals for rehabilitation (both occupational and leisure).

Important components of the interview are the establishment of effective communication and rapport with the patient and family. Simple, open-ended questions using language easily understood by the patient and family should elicit the answers needed. For example, the therapist might ask, "What did your discomfort feel like when you were admitted to the hospital?" or "How long have you had this breathing problem?" Listening is essential for learning about the patient's problems, as well as the patient's understanding of and reaction to them. The therapist must remember that a patient with pulmonary dysfunction may have difficulty with phonation owing to shortness of breath and may have to take breaths frequently between words. Table 16-2 provides some sample descriptors and questions for assessing cardiac symptoms.

### Table 16-2 Differentiation of Nonanginal Discomforts from Angina

| Stable Angina | Nonanginal Discomfort (Chest Wall Pain) |
|---|---|
| Relieved by nitroglycerin (30 sec to 1 min) | Nitroglycerin generally has no effect |
| Comes on at the same heart rate and blood pressure and is relieved by rest (lasts only a few minutes) | Occurs any time; lasts for hours |
| Not palpable | Muscle soreness, joint soreness, evoked by palpation or deep breaths |
| Associated with feelings of doom, cold sweats, shortness of breath | Minimal additional symptoms |
| Often seen with ST-segment depression | No ST-segment depression |

From Irwin SI, Techlin JS. *Cardiopulmonary Physical Therapy.* 2nd ed. St. Louis, MO, Mosby, 1990.

## Systems Review

The systems review is a brief examination of all systems that would affect the ability of the patient to "initiate, sustain, and modify purposeful movement for the performance of actions, tasks or activities that are important for function" (p. 34).[1] The systems review is a limited examination performed prior to the full examination and used as a screening of all the major systems. The systems review includes the assessment of the following:

- Communication ability, affect, cognition, language, and learning style
- The cardiovascular and pulmonary systems, with an examination of the heart rate, respiratory rate, blood pressure, and presence of edema
- The musculoskeletal system, with an examination of gross symmetry, gross range of motion, gross strength, height, and weight
- The neuromuscular system, including an examination of gross movement involving balance, gait, locomotion, transfers, and transition as well as motor control and motor learning
- The integument system, including examination of pliability (texture), presence of scar formation, skin color, and skin integrity

The results of the systems review should be documented in the chart. Following the systems review the therapist is able to utilize an extensive battery of tests and measures to further define limitations or problems.

The rest of the physical examination requires the physical therapist to use select tests and measures that are appropriate to examine the impairments and functional limitations of the patient (Box 16-1).

In patients with cardiopulmonary dysfunction, the skills of inspection, palpation, percussion, auscultation, and activity assessment are the most common procedures utilized to assess the impairments and functional limitations, so these are the ones that will be discussed in this chapter. These components are found under the categories aerobic capacity/endurance, circulation, and ventilation and respiration/gas exchange. After the entire assessment is performed, documentation of the findings should be made of all components that were examined.

## Physical Examination

The physical examination is the third step in the initial evaluation of the patient. Prior to the full examination, a systems review should be performed on all patients.

### Inspection

Inspection (observation) is a key component in the assessment of any patient, but it is extremely important in patients with cardiopulmonary dysfunction. The patient's physical appearance may change slightly as the clinical state changes.

---

**Box 16-1**

### Guide Categories for Tests and Measures

- Aerobic capacity/endurance
- Anthropometric characteristics
- Arousal, attention, and cognition
- Assistive and adaptive devices
- Circulation (arterial, venous, lymphatic)
- Cranial and peripheral nerve integrity
- Environmental, home, and work (job/school/play) barriers
- Gait, locomotion, and balance
- Integumentary integrity
- Joint integrity and mobility
- Motor function (motor control and motor learning)
- Muscle performance (including strength, power, and endurance)
- Neuromotor development and sensory integration
- Orthotic, protective, and supportive devices
- Pain
- Posture
- Prosthetic requirements
- Range of motion (including muscle length)
- Reflex integrity
- Self-care and home management (including activities of daily living and instrumental activities of daily living)
- Sensory integrity
- Ventilation and respiration/gas exchange
- Work (job/school/play), community, and leisure integration or reintegration (including instrumental activities of daily living)

From American Physical Therapy Association. Guide to Physical Therapist Practice. 2nd ed. Baltimore, APTA, 2003.

---

Recognition of these slight changes is essential to the day-to-day management and therapeutic treatment of patients with cardiopulmonary dysfunction. Inspection should be performed in a systematic manner, starting with the head and proceeding caudally (until the therapist has developed a degree of proficiency). In addition to the general appearance, the other specific areas that should be noted on inspection include facial expression, effort to breathe through nose or mouth, the neck, the chest in both a resting and a dynamic situation, phonation, cough and sputum production, posture and positioning, and finally the extremities.

### General Appearance

The patient's level of consciousness, body type, posture and positioning, skin tone, and need for external monitoring or support equipment should be considered in an assessment of "general appearance." Obviously, a patient's level of consciousness (e.g., alert, agitated, confused, semicomatose, comatose) may have a direct impact on whether the treatment plan is understood. A comatose patient may require constant attention for positioning and prevention of pulmonary dysfunction, whereas a confused patient may not be able to follow a therapist's instructions without help. Observation

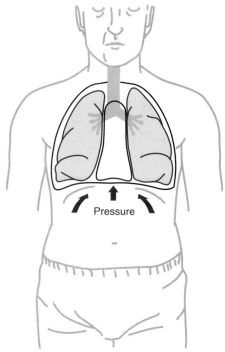

**Figure 16-3** The increased size of the abdomen in obesity (or pregnancy) restricts the full downward movement of the diaphragm during inspiration and restricts lung tissue at rest, therefore creating a restrictive effect on the lung.

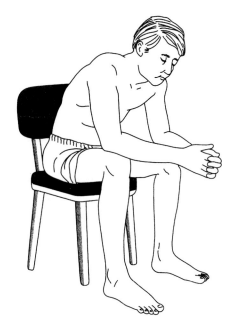

**Figure 16-4** The professorial position provides stabilization of the thorax and arms to increase the effectiveness of accessory muscles during breathing.

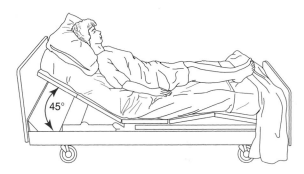

**Figure 16-5** Semi-Fowler's position. Patients with cardiopulmonary dysfunction often require the head of the bed elevated.

of body type (e.g., obese, normal, cachectic) is a routine aspect of assessment that gives an indirect measure of nutrition and in some cases an indication of level of exercise tolerance. For example, a patient who is markedly obese may demonstrate a decreased exercise tolerance and an increased work of breathing owing to the restrictive effects of an excessively large abdomen pushing against the diaphragm (Fig. 16-3). By contrast, cachectic patients may also demonstrate a decreased exercise tolerance and an increased work of breathing with exercise because of weakness from muscle wasting.

Body posture and position should also be assessed to determine their impact on the pulmonary system. Kyphosis and scoliosis are two postures that functionally limit vital capacity and may therefore affect exercise tolerance. In addition, if a patient is assuming the professorial position (leaning forward on knees or on some object; Fig. 16-4) and demonstrating increased effort with breathing and increased use of accessory muscles, one might begin to assume the patient has chronic obstructive disease. Most patients with cardiopulmonary dysfunction cannot tolerate lying on a bed with the head flat and often are found lying either in the semi-Fowler's position in bed (Fig. 16-5) or sitting over the side of the bed or in a chair.

Skin tone may indicate the general level of oxygenation and perfusion of the periphery. An individual who has a general cyanotic look (bluish color most noticeably at lips and fingernail beds) may have a low $PO_2$ and may be in need of supplemental oxygen.

Finally, the presence of all equipment used in managing the patient, including monitoring or support equipment, should be noted. In addition, an assessment should be made of whether the equipment is being used correctly by the patient. For example, a patient who requires supplemental oxygen may be breathing through the mouth and therefore not inhaling the oxygen appropriately. As a result, the patient may be in a confused state, which can result in an unstable clinical situation. This patient's general appearance may be cyanotic, when in fact the most recent blood gas values recorded on the chart with the patient on the oxygen are normal. However, if the patient forgot to put the oxygen mask on or happened to pull the mask off because of "feelings of suffocation" and became confused and agitated as well as cyanotic, the acute change the therapist may note on entering the patient's room may be reversed by simply observing that the oxygen is not being used appropriately. Quick action

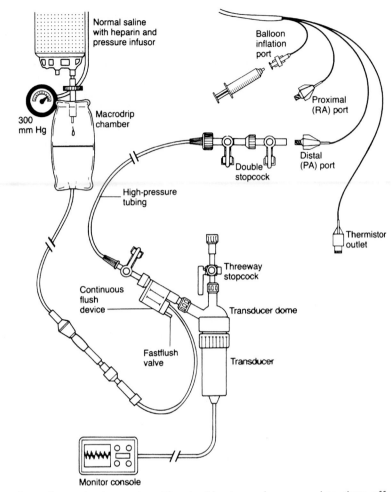

**Figure 16-6** Invasive hemodynamic monitoring system. The double stopcocks are used to close off the tubing system or sample blood from the patient. This then connects to the distal port of the pulmonary artery catheter. This same monitoring system can be used with an arterial catheter for continuous-pressure monitoring and blood sampling. (From Oblouk DG. Hemodynamic Monitoring. Philadelphia, Saunders, 1987.)

by the therapist may solve this unstable clinical situation. In addition, the use of a cardiac monitor, pulmonary artery catheter, or intraaortic balloon pump indicates a more seriously ill patient who may have rhythm or hemodynamic disturbances (Fig. 16-6).

## Facial Characteristics

Facial expression and effort to breathe are two characteristics that can be observed easily; both give important information for the clinical evaluation of the patient. Facial expressions of distress or fatigue may indicate a need for change in the therapeutic treatment. Facial signs of distress include nasal flaring, sweating, paleness, and focused, or enlarged pupils. The effort to breathe can be evaluated not only by the facial expression of distress but also by the degree of work put forth from the musculature of the face and neck and the movement of the lips to breathe. Pursed-lip breathing is a clinical sign of chronic obstructive lung disease, is performed to alleviate the trapping of air in the lungs and to improve gas exchange, and is characterized by the patient breathing out against lips that are mostly closed and shaped in a circular fashion (Fig. 16-7).

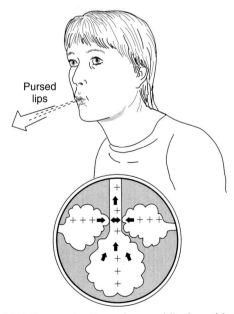

**Figure 16-7** Demonstration of pursed-lip breathing and its effects in patients with emphysema. The weakened bronchiole airways are kept open by the effects of positive pressure created by the pursed lips during expiration.

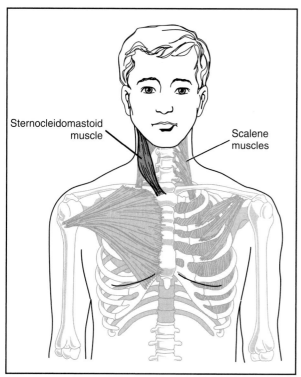

**Figure 16-8** The sternocleidomastoid muscles often hypertrophy in chronic obstructive pulmonary disease owing to increased work of the accessory muscles to assist with breathing.

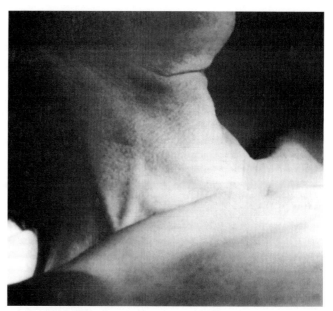

**Figure 16-9** Photograph of jugular venous distention. (From Daily EK, Schroeder JP. Techniques in Bedside Hemodynamic Monitoring. 4th ed. St. Louis, Mosby, 1981.)

## Evaluation of the Neck

The activity of the neck musculature during breathing and the appearance of the jugular veins should be a part of the standard patient assessment. The presence of hypertrophy or adaptive shortening of the sternocleidomastoid muscles may indicate a chronic pulmonary condition. (The sternocleidomastoid muscle is a very important accessory respiratory muscle that often hypertrophies when used excessively for breathing; Fig. 16-8). In addition, because of a chronic forward-bent posture of the head and trunk typically assumed to improve the efficiency of the breathing effort, the sternocleidomastoid muscle may adaptively shorten, and the clavicles may appear more prominent. Breathing efforts during activity may elicit more work from the neck accessory muscles to lift the chest wall up and assist in breathing during rest.

The presence of jugular venous distention should be assessed with the patient sitting or recumbent in bed with the head elevated at least 45 degrees. Jugular venous distention is said to be present if the veins distend above the level of the clavicles. It is an indication of increased volume in the venous system and may be an early sign of right-sided heart failure (cor pulmonale) (Fig. 16-9). In addition, the patient may have left-sided heart failure (congestive heart failure), but this distinction requires auscultation of the lungs, arterial pressure measurements, and possibly a chest radiograph.

## Evaluation of the Chest: Resting and Dynamic

The resting chest is evaluated for its symmetry, configuration, rib angles, and intercostal spaces and musculature. Checking symmetry between sides and comparing anteroposterior (AP) and transverse diameters provide information regarding the chronicity of the cardiopulmonary dysfunction as well as any present pathologic condition. For example, a patient with chronic obstructive disease may have a hyperinflated chest, which increases the AP diameter (more barrel-like). The normal AP diameter is one half the size of the transverse diameter (measured as shoulder to shoulder). In the chronically hyperinflated chest wall, the AP diameter may be equal to the transverse diameter (Fig. 16-10). An individual with scoliosis has asymmetry from side to side when observed from either the front or the back. Scoliosis also rotates the lungs as the scoliotic curve progresses throughout life. In addition, an individual who undergoes thoracic surgery with a lateral incision may have developed asymmetry due to pain and splinting or due to actual lung or rib loss from the surgical procedure (see Fig. 5-22). Symmetry of the chest wall is also assessed dynamically with palpation of the spinous processes, ribs, and clavicles, comparing the motion from side to side and from top to bottom, anteriorly, laterally, and posteriorly.

Some congenital defects such as pectus excavatum (funnel chest) or pectus carinatum (pigeon chest) are important to observe, although they often have little effect on pulmonary function unless they are a severe deformity (see Figs 5-18 and 5-19). Pectus excavatum can have an impact on the cardiac function. Rib angles and intercostal spaces should be observed for abnormalities that might suggest the presence of chronic disease. Normally, rib angles measure less than 90 degrees (Fig. 16-11), and they attach to the vertebrae at approximately 45-degree angles. The intercostal spaces are normally

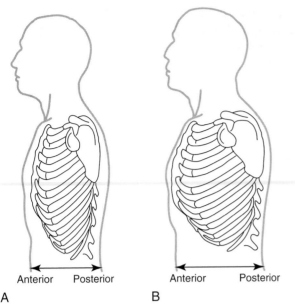

**Figure 16-10 A,** A normal anteroposterior (AP) diameter. **B,** The increased AP diameter in a chronically hyperinflated chest.

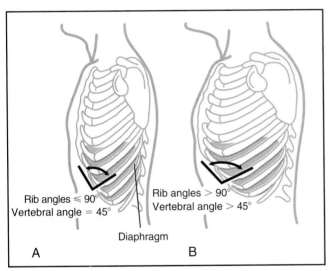

**Figure 16-11** Rib angles. **A,** Normal: measuring less than 90 degrees and attaching at the vertebrae at approximately a 45-degree angle. **B,** Abnormal: rib angles greater than 90 degrees and attaching to the vertebrae with angles greater than 45 degrees in the hyperinflated chest. Also note that the position of the diaphragm is flattened.

broader posteriorly than anteriorly, but chronic hyperinflation causes the rib angles to increase and the intercostal spaces to become broader anteriorly. Consequently, an increased stretch is placed on the diaphragm muscle, and it adapts by becoming flatter and thus less effective (see Fig. 16-11).

Other respiratory accessory muscles may hypertrophy as a result of chronic obstructive pulmonary disease because of the demand placed on them owing to the diminished capacity of the diaphragm muscle. The scalenes, trapezius, and

| Age | Respiratory Rates (Breaths/Minute) |
|---|---|
| Infant: Birth-1 year | 30–60 |
| Toddler 1–3 years | 24–40 |
| Preschooler 3–6 years | 22–34 |
| Elementary school age 6–12 years | 18–30 |
| Adolescent 12–18 years | 12–16 |
| Adult 18+ years | 12–20 |

**Table 16-3 Respiratory Rates for Infants Through Adults**

intercostals work harder than normal when their contribution to normal resting or exercise breathing is increased. Ultimately, the muscles make adaptive changes to the increased workloads by becoming hypertrophied.

> **Clinical Tip**
> Patients with rigid chest walls or the diagnosis of diffuse pulmonary fibrosis usually demonstrate a complete lack of lateral costal expansion. Therefore, the chest wall goes up and down, but there is no outward expansion.

Just as the resting chest wall must be evaluated, so must the dynamic or moving chest wall. Observations of breathing patterns, rates (Table 16-3), inspiratory to expiratory ratios, and symmetry of chest wall motion must all be made. Abnormal breathing patterns should be noted with descriptive terminology, as is presented in Table 16-4. The normal adult respiratory rate is 10 to 20 breaths per minute and can be assessed by counting the respirations for 1 full minute. Observation and palpation of the moving chest are the recommended methods, but one problem with assessing the respiratory rate is the fact that patients are often aware that respirations are being counted, and therefore they may subconsciously alter the rate.

The ratio of inspiration to expiration during the normal breathing cycle is an important consideration. The normal inspiration-to-expiration ratio is 1:2; however, in individuals with chronic obstructive pulmonary diseases, particularly with asthmatics, the ratio may be reduced to 1:4 owing to their inability to get rid of air in the lungs. Also, the pattern of breathing should be noted: paradoxical breathing occurs because of an impairment of the respiratory center's control over breathing (often found in chronic respiratory disease or neurologic insult). An example of paradoxical breathing is the individual with chronic obstructive pulmonary disease and air entrapment who must actively contract the abdominal musculature during expiration to decrease the air trapped in the lungs. The same sort of paradoxical breathing is found in an infant in respiratory distress.

**Table 16-4 Breathing Patterns Commonly Encountered in the Assessment of Patients with Respiratory Problems**

| Pattern of Breathing | Description |
|---|---|
| Apnea | Absence of ventilation |
| Fish-mouth | Apnea with concomitant mouth opening and closing; associated with neck extension and bradypnea |
| Eupnea | Normal rate, normal depth, regular rhythm |
| Bradypnea | Slow rate, shallow or normal depth, regular rhythm; associated with drug overdose |
| Tachypnea | Fast rate, shallow depth, regular rhythm; associated with restrictive lung disease |
| Hyperpnea | Normal rate, increased depth, regular rhythm |
| Cheyne-Stokes (periodic) | Increasing then decreasing depth, period of apnea interspersed; somewhat regular rhythm; associated with critically ill patients |
| Biot's | Slow rate, shallow depth, apneic periods, irregular rhythm; associated with central nervous system disorders like meningitis |
| Apneustic | Slow rate, deep inspiration followed by apnea, irregular rhythm; associated with brainstem disorders |
| Prolonged expiration | Fast inspiration, slow and prolonged expiration yet normal rate, depth, and regular rhythm; associated with obstructive lung disease |
| Orthopnea | Difficulty breathing in postures other than erect |
| Hyperventilation | Fast rate, increased depth, regular rhythm; results in decreased arterial carbon dioxide, tension; called "Kussmaul breathing" in metabolic acidosis; also associated with central nervous system disorders like encephalitis |
| Psychogenic dyspnea | Normal rate, regular intervals of sighing; associated with anxiety |
| Dyspnea | Rapid rate, shallow depth, regular rhythm; associated with accessory muscle activity |
| Doorstop | Normal rate and rhythm; characterized by abrupt cessation of inspiration when restriction is encountered; associated with pleurisy |

*Adapted from Irwin SI, Techlin JS. Cardiopulmonary Physical Therapy. 2nd ed. St. Louis, MO, Mosby, 1990.*

## Phonation, Cough, and Cough Production

Evaluation of a patient's speech also is an assessment of shortness of breath at rest. When speech is interrupted for breath, an individual is described as having dyspnea of phonation. Confusion exists in the literature as well as in the clinic, because shortness of breath and dyspnea are often used interchangeably. The definition of dyspnea is "the patient's subjective report of discomfort with breathing." Shortness of breath is thus the actual symptom observed. Therefore, the description of dyspnea of phonation is made by identifying how many words can be expressed before the next breath. For example, one-word dyspnea would mean that speech is interrupted for a breath between every word. Voice control can also be used to assess shortness of breath as well as strength of the musculature used in speaking and breathing, because poor voice control often indicates weak musculature in both breathing and speaking.

The strength of the patient's cough needs to be assessed, as well as the production of any secretions from the cough (if they are present). Several characteristics of the cough are essential to evaluate, including the effectiveness of the cough (strength, depth, and length of cough). For example, an individual with weak respiratory accessory muscles (e.g., one who

has a high spinal cord injury) would have a very weak and therefore ineffective cough. In addition, an individual with bronchospasm may have a very long, drawn out spasmodic cough that is just as ineffective.

The secretions should be assessed and described with regard to quantity, color, smell, and consistency (Table 16-5). Normally, persons may raise 100 mL of mucus (clear to white) per day and not notice it.

In addition to the sputum odor, the individual's breath odor should be assessed. Foul-smelling breath may indicate an anaerobic infection of the mouth or respiratory tract, whereas an acetone breath may indicate diabetic ketoacidosis.

## Appearance of Extremities

Observation of the fingers and toes and the calves of the legs should indicate whether long-term problems with circulation and oxygenation are present. Digital clubbing of the fingers and toes indicates chronic tissue hypoxia and is found in many instances of hypoxemia-producing disease (Fig. 16-12). Cyanosis (blueness) of the nail beds may also indicate cardiopulmonary dysfunction, but cyanosis can be an indication of decreased circulation to these areas because of cold,

## Table 16-5 Guidelines for Evaluating Cough

| Cough Characteristics | Associated Features | Interpretation |
|---|---|---|
| Nonspecific | Sore throat, runny nose, runny eyes | Acute lung infection; tracheobronchitis |
| Productive | Preceded by an earlier, painful, nonproductive cough associated with an upper respiratory tract infection | Lobar pneumonia |
| Dry or productive | Acute bronchitis | Bronchopneumonia |
| Paroxysmal; mucoid or bloodstained sputum | Flu-like syndrome | *Mycoplasma* or viral pneumonia |
| Purulent sputum | Sputum formerly mucoid | Acute exacerbation of chronic bronchitis |
| Productive for more than 3 months consecutively and for at least 2 years | | Chronic bronchitis |
| Foul-smelling, copious, layered purulent sputum | Long-standing problem | Bronchiectasis |
| Blood-tinged sputum | Month long | Tuberculosis or fungal infection |
| Persistent, nonproductive | | Pneumonitis, interstitial fibrosis, pulmonary infiltrates |
| Persistent, minimally productive | Smoking history, injected pharynx | "Smoker's cough" |
| Nonspecific; minimal hemoptysis | Long-standing | Neoplastic disease |
| Nonproductive | Long-standing; dyspnea | Mediastinal neoplasm |
| Brassy | | Aortic aneurysm |
| Violent cough | Sudden; onset at the same time as signs of asphyxia; localized wheezing | Aspiration of foreign body |
| Frothy sputum | Worsens in supine position; dyspnea | Heart failure, pulmonary edema |
| Hemoptysis | Sudden; simultaneous dyspnea; pleural effusion | Pulmonary infarct |

*Adapted from Fishman AP. Pulmonary Disease and Disorders. Vol. 1. New York, McGraw-Hill, 1980.*

vasospasm, peripheral vascular disease, or decreased cardiac output. The calves of the legs should be observed for skin color changes of blue or purple. This may be indicative of peripheral vascular insufficiency.

### Auscultation of the Lungs

Auscultation is an evaluation technique used to confirm the findings of chart assessment and inspection as well as to rule out other cardiopulmonary dysfunction. Auscultation is also an excellent tool for reassessment of an individual's ventilation following treatment techniques to improve bronchial hygiene or regional ventilation.

Auscultation requires appropriate equipment (the stethoscope) as well as appropriate instructions to the patient and proper positioning. It is recommended that the physical therapist invest in a personal stethoscope, because stethoscopes fit different people in different ways owing to the types, sizes, and positions of the earpieces. The most appropriate choice is a stethoscope that comes with adjustable earpieces, with adequate but not excessive tubing, and with both a

diaphragm (the flat side) and a bell, including a valve to turn toward either the diaphragm or the bell. Auscultation of lung sounds is performed with the diaphragm of the stethoscope preferably in a quiet environment (Fig. 16-13). Auscultation of heart sounds requires both the diaphragm and the bell and, again, a quiet environment.

For auscultation of the lung sounds, the optimal position is for the patient to be sitting to permit auscultation of the entire lung space, including both the anterior and posterior chest wall. In addition, optimal auscultation involves removal of bed clothes to expose the bare skin while the individual breathes deeply through an open mouth. Unfortunately, some of the more seriously ill patients can neither tolerate the sitting position at the time of initial visit nor perform adequate deep breaths for auscultation.

Auscultation should be performed over the entire lung space, with at least one breath auscultated in each bronchopulmonary segment. The intensity, pitch, and quality of the breath sounds should be compared between right and left and in the craniocaudal direction. Auscultation should be performed in a systematic manner, anteriorly and then

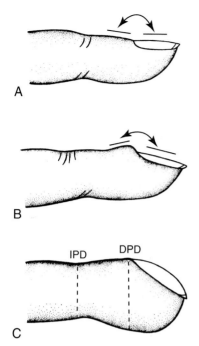

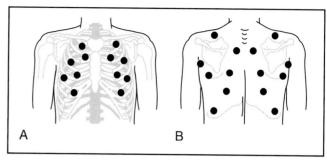

**Figure 16-14** One method of auscultating the chest. **A,** The chest. **B,** The back. (Redrawn from Buckingham EB. A Primer of Clinical Diagnosis. 2nd ed. New York, Harper & Row, 1979.)

- Maintain appropriate draping of the patient, particularly females.
- If auscultation reveals very faint or distant sounds, remind the patient to take deep breaths and to breathe in and out through the mouth so that a recheck can be done.

**Figure 16-12** Normal digit configuration (**A**) and digital clubbing (**B**). Note that the angle between the nail and the proximal skin exceeds 180 degrees. **C,** Also note that the distal phalangeal depth (DPD) is greater than the interphalangeal depth (IPD). (From Wilkins RL, Krider SJ. Clinical Assessment in Respiratory Care. St. Louis, Mosby, 1985.)

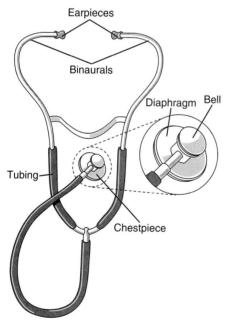

**Figure 16-13** A stethoscope, showing the diaphragm (*flattened side*) and the bell.

posteriorly (or vice versa) (Fig. 16-14). Precautions that should be taken during auscultation are the following:
- Prevent the patient from falling if weak or if poor balance is noted.
- Prevent the patient from becoming dizzy secondary to hyperventilation by auscultating slowly between pulmonary segments.

## Lung Sound Definitions

Disagreement exists regarding the terms used to identify the auscultated lung sounds.[9] Nonetheless, lung sounds may be divided into two types: normal breath sounds and adventitious breath sounds. Normal breath sounds are the normal noises of breathing that can be heard with a stethoscope. They are described as vesicular and are soft, low-pitched sounds heard primarily during inspiration. During expiration low, vesicular sounds are minimal and occur only during the initial one third of exhalation. Expiratory sounds flow directly from inspiratory sounds, without a break in the sounds.

Different breath sounds are auscultated over different portions of the tracheobronchial tree, which are also normal. Bronchial breath sounds, described as tubular sounds, are loud, high-pitched sounds with approximately equal inspiratory and expiratory duration. Also a pause occurs between the inspiratory and expiratory components. A third type of "normal" breath sound is heard over the junction of the mainstem bronchi with the segmental bronchi, called bronchovesicular. Bronchovesicular breath sounds are a softer version of bronchial sounds but differ only in that they are continuous between inspiration and expiration. Posteriorly the bronchovesicular sounds are normally heard only between the scapulae (Fig. 16-15). Table 16-6 provides a list of errors of auscultation to avoid.

> **Clinical Tip**
> To understand what are bronchial breath sounds, take your stethoscope and listen to breathing over the anterior chest right near the trachea over the sternum (near the sternal notch). The breath sounds are loud. Then, listen to breathing posteriorly at the bottommost part of the lungs. If the sounds heard anteriorly near the sternal notch are found posteriorly in any of the segments of the lungs, or anteriorly at the middle and lower parts of the ribs, these are abnormal breath sounds.

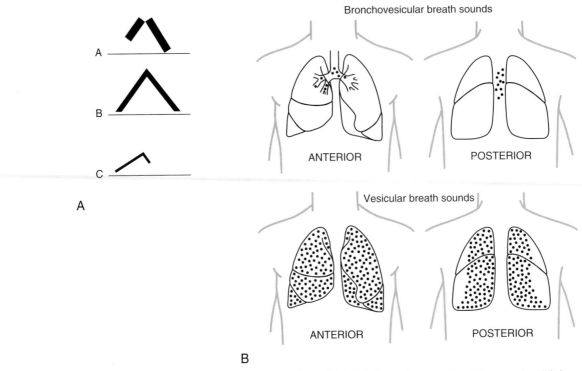

**Figure 16-15 A,** Breath sound diagrams: normal tracheobronchial (A); bronchovesicular (B): vesicular (C) breath sounds. The upstroke represents inspiration and the downstroke expiration. The thickness of the line indicates intensity. **B,** The positions on the anterior and posterior chest walls at which normal vesicular and bronchovesicular breath sounds are identified. (Redrawn from Wilkins RL, Hodgkin JE, Lopez B. Lung Sounds: A Practical Guide. St. Louis, Mosby, 1988.)

### Table 16-6 Errors of Auscultation to Avoid

| Errors | Correct Technique |
|---|---|
| Listening to breath sounds through the patient's gown | Placing bell or diaphragm directly against the chest wall |
| Allowing tubing to rub against bed rails or patient's gown | Keeping tubing free from contact with any objects during auscultation |
| Attempting to auscultate in a noisy room | Turning television or radio off |
| Interpreting chest hair sounds as adventitious lung sounds | Wetting chest hair before auscultation if thick |
| Auscultating only the "convenient" areas | Asking alert patient to sit up; rolling comatose patient onto side to auscultate posterior lobes |

These normal sounds are produced from the turbulence of airflow in the airways. The belief is that the inspiratory component of vesicular sounds is produced regionally within each lung and possibly within each lobe.[10] The expiratory component is believed to be produced in the larger airways. The fact that airflow is directed away from the chest wall during expiration might explain the fading away of the sound during expiration and the reason why only approximately the first third of expiration can be heard.

A pathologic condition in the lungs can change the transmission of the sounds. An increase in lung tissue density causes increased sound transmission. This is the reason one may hear bronchial breath sounds in areas other than the mainstem bronchi when a pathologic condition that causes consolidation exists. A decrease in lung tissue density, as in the emphysematous lung, would cause decreased sound transmission. Decreased sound transmission also occurs if only shallow breaths are taken or if distance of transmission between the airways and the stethoscope is increased (as in obesity, pleural effusion, or barrel chest).

When a pathologic condition of the lung is suspected because of increased or decreased transmission sounds, then further evaluative measures must be taken. Egophony, bronchophony, and whispering pectoriloquy are three techniques to further evaluate the abnormal transmission of sound. Asking a patient to say "99" or "E," or to whisper are three techniques that can be employed to assess the abnormally transmitted sounds. Egophony is demonstrated when a patient is asked to say "E" aloud, but the sound that is auscultated over the chest is "A." Bronchophony is demonstrated when a patient is asked to say "99," and the words are auscultated clearly over the entire chest. Whispering pectoriloquy is evident when a patient is asked to whisper, and the whispered words are clearly and distinctly heard through the stethoscope. The relative strengths of each of the sounds auscultated when using these techniques suggest the degree of consolidation or hyperinflation of the underlying lung; stronger, louder sounds are heard in the presence of consolidative pathology, whereas weaker, softer sounds are heard in the presence of hyperinflation.

### Adventitious Lung Sounds

Adventitious lung sounds are the abnormal noises heard only with a stethoscope. These can be divided into two categories: continuous and discontinuous lung sounds. The American Thoracic Society and the American College of Chest Physicians (ATS-ACCP) Ad Hoc Subcommittee on Pulmonary Nomenclature further clarified the continuous sounds as wheezes (previously defined as rhonchi) and the discontinuous adventitious lung sounds as crackles (previously called rales).[11]

**Wheezes.** Wheezes are continuous adventitious lung sounds with a constant pitch and varying duration. These sounds are most frequently heard on exhalation and are associated with airway obstruction. Some clinicians still advocate using the term rhonchi to describe low-pitched continuous adventitious lung sounds. The ATS-ACCP, however, recommends referring to all continuous adventitious sounds as wheezes and specifying whether they are high-pitched or low-pitched. When describing the wheeze it is extremely important to document the time of its occurrence (inspiration or expiration) because this may help to differentiate pathologic conditions.

Wheezes on expiration are most common and are often associated with airway constriction as is found in bronchospasm or when secretions are narrowing the airway. The wheeze on inspiration is not very common and indicates a more severe obstruction of the airway.[12] Wheezes may diminish or change in pitch as a result of bronchodilator treatments. The monophonic, continuous adventitious sound heard over the upper airways of a patient with upper airway obstruction (as when a peanut is lodged in a bronchus or when epiglottic interference occurs) is called stridor and differs from the normal wheeze in intensity and pitch.

**Crackles.** Crackles are discontinuous adventitious lung sounds that sound like brief bursts of popping bubbles. Crackles are more commonly heard during inspiration and may be associated with restrictive or obstructive respiratory disorders because they can be produced via several mechanisms.[12-14] They may result from the sudden opening of closed airways[10-16] (Fig. 16-16) or as the result of the movement of secretions during inspiration and expiration.[17] Some clinicians still use the term *rales* for what are now called crackles.

Peripheral airways can collapse owing to atelectasis, pulmonary edema, fibrosis, or compression from pleural effusion, and often crackles auscultated with these pathologic conditions are in the latter half of inspiration. Crackles occurring in the early half of inspiration often result from the popping open of more proximal airways.[16] The closure of proximal airways may result from the weakening of bronchial and broncheolar support structures as occurs in the latter stages of chronic obstructive pathologic diseases such as bronchitis

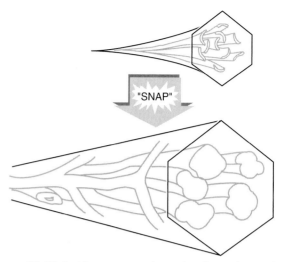

**Figure 16-16** Sudden reexpansion of collapsed peripheral airways. (Redrawn from Murphy RLH. Lung sounds. Basics of respiratory disease. Am Thor Soc 8(4):1–6, 1980.)

or emphysema. Crackles due to the movement of fluid or secretions within the lungs are often described as low-pitched and may be found on either inspiration or expiration or both.

**Pleural rub.** Another abnormal sound that should be checked by auscultation in the lower lateral chest areas (both right and left) is a pleural (friction) rub, which may be an indication of pleural inflammation. The pleural rub sounds like two pieces of leather or sandpaper rubbing together, and it occurs with each inspiration and expiration.[12]

Evaluation of breath sounds via auscultation should be systematic, beginning with an initial description as vesicular, bronchovesicular, bronchial, diminished, or absent. With bronchial and bronchovesicular sounds found in peripheral lung tissue, further definitive techniques such as egophony, bronchophony, and whispering pectoriloquy should be employed. If adventitious sounds are heard, they first must be defined as continuous or discontinuous. Following this distinction, descriptors such as pitch, intensity, duration, and portion of the respiratory cycle in which they occur should be used to further define the sounds. On completion of the auscultatory assessment, the therapist can interpret the sounds with regard to what they may indicate (Table 16-7).

## Auscultation of the Heart

Auscultation of heart sounds requires a quiet environment and a stethoscope with a diaphragm and bell. The diaphragm is placed firmly on the skin and is used to auscultate initially the topographic areas on the chest wall, identifying high-pitched sounds. The bell accentuates lower-frequency sounds, including atrial and ventricular gallops, filtering out the high-pitched sounds. Care must be taken to place the bell lightly on the skin and not to press firmly, because increased pressure causes the skin to act like a diaphragm so that low-frequency sounds cannot be heard.

**Table 16-7 Guidelines for the Documentation and Interpretation of Lung Sounds Auscultation**

| Type of Sound | Nomenclature | Interpretation |
|---|---|---|
| Breath sound | Normal | Normal, air-filled lung |
| | Decreased | Hyperinflation in chronic obstructive pulmonary disease |
| | | Hypoinflation in acute lung disease, e.g., atelectasis, pneumothorax, pleural effusion |
| | Absent | Pleural effusion |
| | | Pneumothorax |
| | | Severe hyperinflation |
| | | Obesity |
| | Bronchial | Consolidation |
| | | Atelectasis with adjacent patent airway |
| | Crackles | Secretions, if biphasic |
| | | Deflation, if monophasic |
| | Wheezes | Diffuse airway obstruction, if polyphonic |
| | | Localized stenosis, if monophonic |
| Voice sound | Normal | Normal, air-filled lung |
| | Decreased | Atelectasis |
| | | Pleural effusion |
| | | Pneumothorax |
| | Increased | Consolidation |
| | | Pulmonary fibrosis |
| Extrapulmonary adventitious sounds | Crunch | Mediastinal emphysema |
| | Pleural rub | Pleural inflammation or reaction |
| | Pericardial rub | Pericardial inflammation |

*From Irwin SI, Techlin JS. Cardiopulmonary Physical Therapy. 2nd ed. St. Louis, Mosby, 1990.*

---

> **Clinical Tip**
> Auscultation of heart sounds is a clinical skill that can be learned only by practice with auscultation on individuals with different heart sounds. The entry-level practitioner should not be expected to be competent in auscultation of all heart sounds. However, an entry-level practitioner should be able to perform a competent systematic auscultation of the heart and be able to note normal heart sounds and blatantly abnormal heart sounds (e.g., loud murmurs and loud atrial or ventricular gallops).

Auscultation of the heart requires selective listening for each component of the cardiac cycle while placing the stethoscope over the five main topographic areas for auscultation (Fig. 16-17).

The five areas where sounds are best heard are
- The aortic area: auscultated best in the second intercostal space close to the sternum on the right of the sternum
- The pulmonary area: auscultated best at the second intercostal space to the left of the sternum
- The third left intercostal space: murmurs of both aortic and pulmonary origin are best heard here

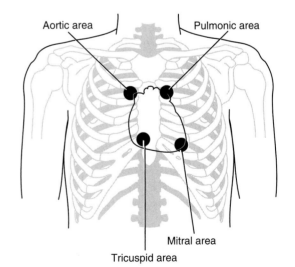

**Figure 16-17** Areas to auscultate for sounds generated from the aortic, pulmonary (pulmonic), tricuspid, and mitral valves. In the normal heart, the mitral area is the apical pulse point and the point of maximal impulse. (Redrawn from Leatham A. Introduction to the Examination of the Cardiovascular System. 2nd ed. Oxford, Oxford University Press, 1979.)

- The tricuspid area: located at the lower left sternal border, approximately the fourth to fifth intercostal space
- The mitral area (apex of heart): located in the fifth left intercostal space, medial to the midclavicular line

As with breath sounds, auscultation of heart sounds should be performed in a systematic manner, such as by beginning at the aortic area and listening to both the first and second heart sounds. When listening to the sounds, the intensity and timing, as well as any splitting, extra sounds, or murmurs should be noted. The intensity varies according to the proximity to the valve and chest wall.

The first heart sound, S1 (the lub of the lub-dub), is associated with the closure of the mitral and tricuspid valves and corresponds with the onset of ventricular systole. The S1 sound is normally louder and longer and lower pitched when auscultated at the apex or even in the tricuspid region.

The second heart sound, S2 (the dub of lub-dub), is associated with the closure of the aortic and pulmonary valves and corresponds with the start of ventricular diastole. The S2 sound has greatest intensity when auscultated at the aortic or pulmonary regions.

Transient splitting of the first or second sound may be noted during inspiration. Splitting of the S1 is best heard over the tricuspid region, whereas splitting of the S2 is heard more readily over the pulmonary region. Both splitting sounds are considered to be normal and are indicative of slight timing differences between closure of the left heart valves and the right heart valves.

## Abnormal Heart Sounds

### Third Heart Sound

A third heart sound (S3) occurs early in diastole while the ventricle is rapidly filling (immediately following S2 and sounding like lub-dub-dub). The S3 sound is low pitched and must be auscultated with the bell of the stethoscope. Auscultation is often best performed with the patient lying on the left side so that the apex of the heart is closest to the chest wall. When an S3 is heard in healthy children or young adults, it is considered to be normal and is called a physiologic third heart sound. When an S3 is auscultated in an older, physically inactive person or in the presence of heart disease, it typically indicates a loss of ventricular compliance (failure), often called a ventricular gallop. In patients with suspected ventricular dysfunction, the clinician should search carefully for the presence of a ventricular gallop because it is a key diagnostic sign for congestive heart failure.

### Fourth Heart Sound

The fourth heart sound (S4) occurs late in diastole (just before S1 and sounding like la-lub-dub) and is associated with atrial contraction. S4 is also a low-pitched sound best heard with the bell of the stethoscope. S4, otherwise known as the atrial gallop sound, is not normal and is associated with an increased resistance to ventricular filling. An S4 is commonly heard in individuals with hypertensive cardiac disease, coronary artery disease, or pulmonary disease and is also commonly found in individuals with a history of myocardial infarction or coronary artery bypass surgery.

### Murmurs

Murmurs can be very complex and difficult to understand for the entry-level practitioner. However, there are three broad classifications of murmurs that can help one understand the mechanism of the murmurs:

- Murmurs caused by high rates of flow either through normal or abnormal valves
- Murmurs caused by forward flow through a constricted (stenotic) or deformed valve or by flow into a dilated vessel or chamber
- Murmurs caused by backward flow through a valve (regurgitation).[18]

Murmurs are classified according to their timing, quality, intensity, pitch, location, and radiation. In addition, murmurs are classified by the position of the patient in which the murmur is best heard and by the part of the respiratory cycle in which it is best heard.

**Systolic and diastolic murmurs.** Systolic murmurs are the most common and may be caused by either ejection or regurgitation. These murmurs are heard between S1 and S2 and are best described as a "swishing" sound associated with S1 (instead of hearing lub-dub, one usually hears "lush-dub"). One of the most classic systolic murmurs is associated with aortic stenosis. The murmur heard is a high-pitched murmur, best heard at the right sternal border, second intercostal space, frequently radiating to the neck and the carotid arteries.

Systolic murmurs may be produced from other forms of valvular dysfunction, including congenital defects of the atria and ventricles. In addition, diastolic murmurs, although uncommon, may occur. These murmurs are heard immediately following the S2 and diminish in intensity quickly. Pathologic conditions associated with these murmurs include aortic and pulmonary regurgitation and mitral stenosis.

Another common murmur is associated with mitral valve dysfunction and is called mitral valve prolapse. Mitral valve prolapse is a common and benign valvular dysfunction often found in females. When abnormalities exist with the chordae tendineae (as with papillary muscle rupture after a myocardial infarction or with mitral valve prolapse), clicking sounds in the middle of ventricular systole may be heard. These are referred to as midsystolic clicks.[19] Further discussion of murmurs is beyond the scope of this text because it is beyond the level of the entry-level practitioner.

### Pericardial Friction Rub

An abnormal sound associated with each beat of the heart is known as a pericardial friction rub. It is the sign of pericardial inflammation (pericarditis). Auscultation for a pericardial friction rub is best performed with the patient in the supine position, with the therapist listening over the third or fourth intercostal space along the anterior axillary line. The pericardial friction rub sounds like a "creak" with each beat and has

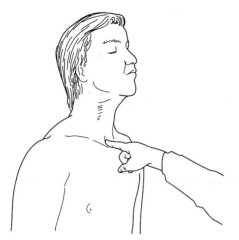

**Figure 16-18** Palpation for position of the mediastinum to evaluate for tracheal deviation.

also been described as a "leathery" sound, as if two pieces of leather were being rubbed together.[19]

## Palpation

Palpation is an assessment technique employed to refine the information previously gathered from the chart review, inspection, and auscultation. The purpose of palpation is to evaluate the mediastinum (for tracheal shift), chest motion, chest wall pain, fremitus, muscle activity of the chest wall and diaphragm, and circulatory status.

### The Mediastinum (Tracheal Position)

Evaluation of the mediastinum assesses tracheal shift that is due to disproportionate intrathoracic pressures or lung volumes between the two sides of the thorax. The contents of the thorax may shift toward the affected side when the lung volume or intrathoracic pressure on that side is decreased. This can happen following a lobectomy or pneumonectomy or a large degree of atelectasis. The content of the thorax may shift to the unaffected side (the contralateral side) when there is increased pressure on the same side, as happens in a pleural effusion, a tumor, or an untreated pneumothorax.

Palpation for such shifts is performed while the patient is sitting upright with the neck flexed slightly to allow relaxation of the sternocleidomastoid muscles, and the chin should be positioned in the midline. Palpation proceeds with the tip of the index finger being placed in the suprasternal notch, first medially to the left sternoclavicular joint and pushed inward toward the cervical spine. Then the index finger is placed medial to the right sternoclavicular joint and pushed inward toward the cervical spine (Fig. 16-18).

When a significant shift to the unaffected side occurs, aggressive treatment is usually indicated. If the shift is due to a pneumothorax, a chest tube is usually inserted immediately. In the case of the large pleural effusion, a thoracentesis may be performed to drain the fluid or to evaluate the contents of the fluid or both. When the shift goes to the affected side in the patient after a lobectomy or pneumonectomy, the patient

should be cautioned against lying on the affected side, because this would only increase the mediastinal shift.

### Chest Motion

Palpation is performed segmentally to compare the chest wall motion over the upper, middle, and lower lobes while the patient is breathing quietly and while breathing deeply. The important components of the evaluation include the amount of movement of the hands, the presence or absence of symmetry of movement, and the timing of the movement (Fig. 16-19).

The upper chest wall expansion is evaluated by the therapist placing the palms of the hands anteriorly over the chest wall from the fourth rib upward. The fingers should be stretched upward and over the trapezius, and the thumbs should be placed together along the midline of the chest. The skin on the patient's chest may need to be mobilized to position the palms down with the thumbs touching. The patient should be asked to take a maximal inspiration, and the therapist's hands should be relaxed so that they move with the chest wall. Notation of the extent of movement and the symmetry of the movement is important (see Fig. 16-19). Chest wall motion over the right middle lobe and lingula segments of the left upper lobe is evaluated by the therapist placing the fingers laterally and over posterior axillary folds, with the palms pressed firmly on the anterior chest wall. The skin is then drawn medially until the thumbs meet at the midline. The patient should take a maximal inspiration with the therapist's hands gliding with the movement of the lobes underneath. Again, extent of movement and symmetry of movement should be documented (see Fig. 16-19B).

The lower chest wall expansion is evaluated with the patient's back toward the therapist, and the therapist's fingers wrapped around the anterior axillary fold. The skin is then drawn medially until the tips of the thumbs meet at the spinal column. While a maximal inspiration is performed by the patient, the therapist should allow the hands to glide with the movement of the rib cage, and the extent of the movement as well as the symmetry should be documented (see Fig. 16-19C).

### Evaluation of Fremitus

Fremitus is defined as the vibration that is produced by the voice or by the presence of secretions in the airways and is transmitted to the chest wall and palpated by the hand. Palpation of fremitus is performed with the palms of the hands placed lightly on the chest wall while the patient repeats some word, such as "99," to distinguish normal vocal fremitus from the abnormal fremitus produced by secretions. Normally palpation reveals a uniform vibration throughout the entire chest wall. Increased fremitus is palpated in the presence of an increase in secretions in a particular area. Decreased fremitus indicates an increase in air in the particular area. Palpation of fremitus is especially important when auscultation has defined an area of decreased breath sounds that may be an area of consolidation resulting from secretions. When fremitus is increased, the suspicion of consolidation is supported.

Rest                    Inspiration

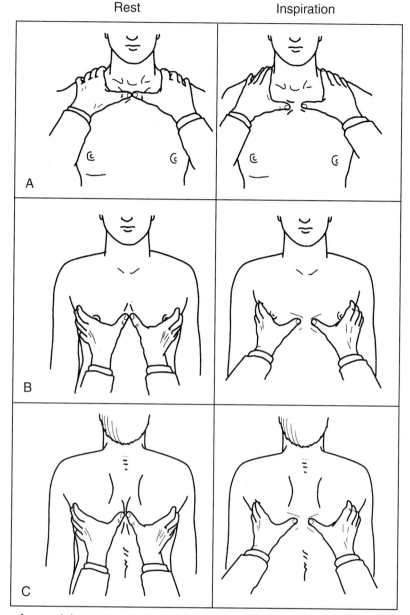

**Figure 16-19 A,** Palpation of upper lobe motion. **B,** Palpation of right middle and left lingula lobe motion. **C,** Palpation of lower lobe motion. (Redrawn from Cherniack RM, Cherniack L. Respiration in Health and Disease. 2nd ed. Philadelphia, WB Saunders, 1972.)

## Evaluation of Muscle Activity of Chest Wall and Diaphragm

Palpation is an excellent tool to evaluate the amount of accessory muscle activity used during quiet breathing. By palpating the accessory muscles, in particular the scalenes and the trapezii, an assessment of the amount of work of breathing may be made (Fig. 16-20). In addition, the extent of the diaphragmatic contribution can be assessed with the patient in the supine position (Fig. 16-21). Normal quiet breathing is mostly performed by the diaphragm, with equal and upward motion of the lower rib cage. Palpation of the anterior chest wall with the thumbs over the costal margins and thumb tips meeting at the xiphoid gives the most accurate assessment of the extent of diaphragmatic activity. With a deep inspiration, the hands should travel equally apart, total

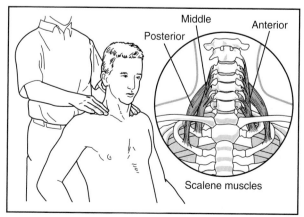

**Figure 16-20** Palpation of the activity of the scalene muscles during quiet breathing.

circumferential diameter increasing by at least 2 to 3 inches. The extent of movement is an important part of the assessment of diaphragmatic excursion. For example, an individual with significant chronic obstructive lung disease might exhibit increased muscle activity of the respiratory accessory muscles and decreased diaphragmatic contribution to quiet breathing.

## Chest Wall Pain or Discomfort

Palpation may also be performed to evaluate chest wall discomfort and should include all areas of the chest wall: anterior, posterior, and lateral regions of the thorax. Patients may often develop musculoskeletal pain from bedrest and inactivity, which are frequently associated with diseases of the cardiopulmonary system. Musculoskeletal pain must be differentiated from anginal pain; palpation is an extremely useful tool to distinguish between the two. If chest pain is increased with deep inspiration or if it is increased or reproduced by direct point palpation, it is less likely to be of cardiac origin than of skeletal muscle origin. If a patient reports chest pain during the patient interview and can point to the exact area of pain, then palpation should be done to assess whether this pain is of musculoskeletal origin.

## Evaluation of Circulation

Pulses throughout the extremities should be palpated during the initial evaluation because of the diffuse nature of atherosclerotic disease (see Chapter 3) (Fig. 16-22). Identification of the risk factors and symptoms of arterial disease is a component of the history that assists in the assessment of arterial disease. Ischemic pain appears in the soft tissue served by the artery that is diseased. In addition to history taking, visual inspection for trophic changes (hair loss, muscle

atrophy, dry skin, and in some cases dry gangrene or ulcers) is a valuable evaluation tool, particularly for examining individuals with moderate to severe arterial occlusion. Blood flow tests provide additional information about the degree of occlusion in the extremities. A reactive hyperemia test may be performed by sharply elevating the limbs to produce blanching. Blanching is more rapid in the partially or severely occluded extremity than in the normal extremity. In addition, palpation of pulses and skin temperature can be performed to assess perfusion of the extremities and the head and neck. Patients with diabetes or peripheral vascular disease often have diminished pulses, particularly in the hands and feet. In addition, individuals with right-sided heart failure and bilateral peripheral edema demonstrate

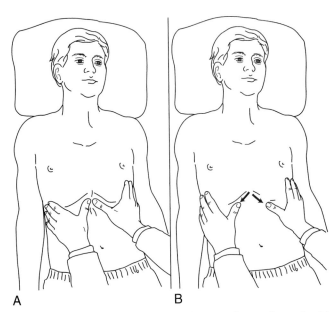

**Figure 16-21** Palpation of diaphragmatic motion. **A,** At rest. **B,** At the end of a normal inspiration. (Redrawn from Cherniack RM, Cherniack L. Respiration in Health and Disease. 2nd ed. Philadelphia, WB Saunders, 1972.)

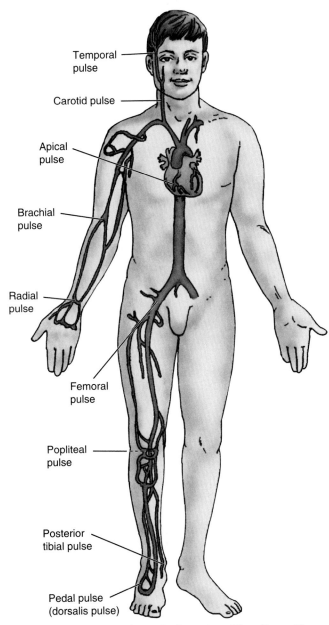

Temporal pulse

Carotid pulse

Apical pulse

Brachial pulse

Radial pulse

Femoral pulse

Popliteal pulse

Posterior tibial pulse

Pedal pulse (dorsalis pulse)

**Figure 16-22** Pulses through the extremities. (From Pierson FM. Principles & Techniques of Patient Care. 4th ed. St. Louis, MO, Saunders, 2008.)

diminished pulses in the foot and ankle. The following is a list of locations for pulse palpation:

- Brachial artery
- Radial artery
- Carotid artery
- Femoral artery
- Popliteal artery (palpated using the fingers of both hands)
- Posterior tibial artery
- Dorsalis pedis artery

The quality of the pulse should be noted, and a comparison should be made to the pulses of the opposite extremity to determine unilateral or individual differences. Pulse palpation may be difficult to quantify and does have a degree of unreliability from one clinician to the next. As a result, pulse palpation is now often supplemented by noninvasive techniques to measure blood flow such as Doppler velocimetry. Doppler velocimetry is particularly useful in identifying individuals with asymptomatic arterial disease or those whose pulses are severely obliterated.[20]

## Mediate Percussion

Mediate percussion is the final component of the chest examination and is performed to further evaluate any abnormal findings, especially changes in lung density. In addition, percussion is also useful to evaluate the extent of diaphragmatic excursion.

Percussion is performed with the middle finger of one hand placed flat on the chest wall along the intercostal space between two ribs (usually the nondominant hand), while all other fingers are lifted off the chest wall. The other hand is positioned with the wrist in dorsiflexion, acting like a fulcrum, and the hand moving forward and back in rapid succession with the tip of the middle finger striking the nondominant middle finger on the chest wall (Fig. 16-23). Percussion usually proceeds in a cephalocaudal direction and back and forth between the left and right sides, anteriorly and posteriorly.

Three types of sounds are typically produced with percussion. A normal sound is when normal lung tissue is percussed and normal resonance is produced. A dull sound is produced with percussion over the liver or other dense tissue (as occurs with consolidation or tumors) and is described as a "thud." The student can reproduce the dull sound by percussing on a bare thigh. A tympanic sound is loud, long, and hollow and may be heard over an empty stomach or a hyperinflated chest. Figure 16-24 shows the areas of normal, tympanic, and dull sounds on a chest. Figure 16-25 demonstrates the systematic technique for evaluation of lung density.

Diaphragmatic excursion can also be assessed by percussion. The patient must be in a seated position with the back exposed to evaluate diaphragmatic excursion. Percussion from the apex of the lungs to the bases of the lungs is performed while a patient is quietly breathing and a line measuring the point of demarcation between resonance to dullness is drawn on the left side and the right. After these lines are drawn, the therapist asks the patient to take a maximal inspiration and to hold this breath. At this time, the therapist continues percussion from the line downward to determine where the new point of dullness to resonance is located and draws a second line. The distance between the lines is the distance of diaphragmatic excursion. Normal

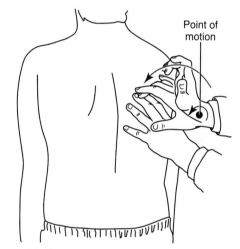

**Figure 16-23** The technique for mediate percussion.

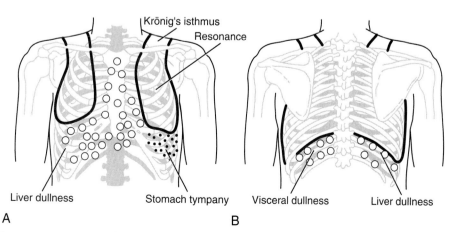

**Figure 16-24** Normal resonance pattern of the chest. **A,** Anteriorly. **B,** Posteriorly. Also shown are areas of dullness (*circles*) and tympanic areas (*small dots*). (Redrawn from Irwin SI, Techlin JS. Cardiopulmonary Physical Therapy. 2nd ed. St. Louis, Mosby, 1990.)

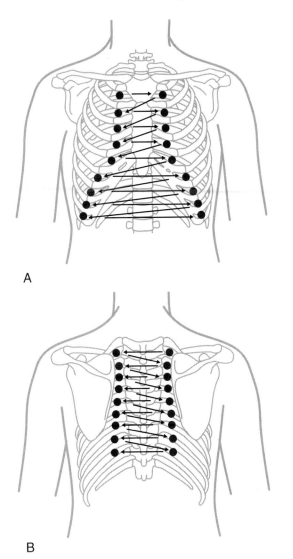

A

B

**Figure 16-25** The systematic technique for evaluation of lung density anteriorly (**A**) and posteriorly (**B**).

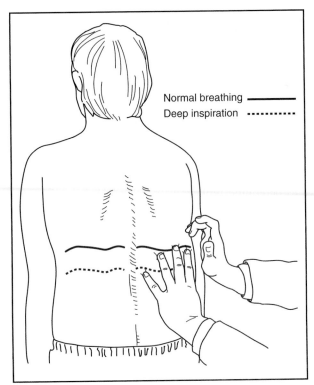

Normal breathing ————
Deep inspiration ----------

**Figure 16-26** Evaluation of diaphragmatic excursion (normal, 3 to 5 cm); normal breathing (*solid line*), deep inspiration (*broken line*).

excursion is 3 to 5 cm but may be extremely decreased in the patient with chronic obstructive lung disease because of hyperinflation of the chest and a flattened diaphragm (Fig. 16-26).

## Activity Evaluation

Following the chest wall examination, the therapist is ready to perform an initial evaluation of the patient's responses to exercise. The activity evaluation is an assessment of the patient's responses to the following situations: rest (supine), sitting, standing, some type of activity of daily living (e.g., dressing lower or upper extremities, combing hair, brushing teeth), and ambulation of some distance; in some cases, Valsalva's maneuver is also performed.

For patients recently recovering from a myocardial infarction, the evaluation discussed previously should be performed as soon as the patient is able to get out of bed. This often occurs as early as 1 to 2 days after an uncomplicated myocardial infarction. If the patient has not experienced a

myocardial infarction but has some sort of cardiovascular or pulmonary dysfunction, this assessment is made as soon as the patient is considered stable. Patients receiving mechanical ventilatory assistance can perform these activities while still on the ventilator.

During the activity evaluation, the patient's heart rate and rhythm (via ECG telemetry if possible), blood pressure, and symptoms should be monitored with all activities (and $O_2$ saturation, if applicable). Heart and lung sounds should be assessed before each activity and immediately following the last activity. The responses should be recorded and interpreted throughout the entire evaluation. The evaluation is terminated at any time during the assessment that an abnormal response is identified if such response makes continuing the evaluation inappropriate or unsafe. On conclusion of the activities evaluation, an individualized program of progressive monitored increased activity is initiated if the responses were assessed as safe and appropriate. Studies have shown that the heart rate, blood pressure, and ECG responses with ambulation during the activities evaluation strongly correlate with the responses that occur with the patient's daily monitored ambulation program.[21]

---

**Clinical Tip**
Activity evaluation is a key assessment of the patient's ability to perform activities of daily living (ADLs). This assessment should include an evaluation of what the patient was doing prior to hospital admission, as well as the patient's goal on discharge.

### Table 16-8 Normative Values for Resting HR

| Age | Low (Beats/Minute) | High (Beats/Minute) |
| --- | --- | --- |
| Infant: Birth-1 year | 100 | 160 |
| Toddler 1–3 years | 90 | 150 |
| Preschooler 3–6 years | 80 | 140 |
| Elementary school age 6–12 years | 70 | 120 |
| Adolescent 12–18 years | 60 | 100 |
| Adult 18+ years | 60 | 100 |

> **Clinical Tip**
> Heart rate can also be measured with a pulse oximeter that can provide information on a patient's $O_2$ saturation of the blood. However, this equipment may be inaccurate when there is poor peripheral circulation, when heart rhythm is not regular, or with mishandling of the equipment. Verify accuracy by checking the pulse manually.

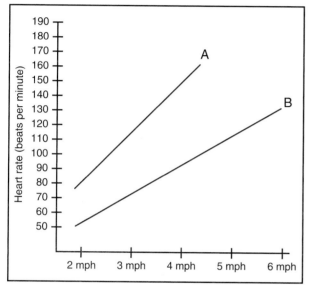

**Figure 16-27** Heart rate response to increased workload in a normal sedentary individual (**A**) versus a trained individual (**B**).

and lower peak) heart rate response to exercise is anticipated and considered normal. The slower rate of rise aspect of the response is similar to that exhibited by highly trained individuals who also demonstrate a very gradual rate of rise in heart rate with increased work.

In addition, the heart rate achieved with activity should be compared with the predicted maximal heart rate. The predicted maximal heart rate of an individual is related to age. One method of determining the predicted maximal rate is to subtract the patient's age from 220 (220 – age). However, this method is known to underestimate the maximal heart rate in well-trained and in elderly persons. For these patients, the following two formulas are recommended: for males, 205 – 1/2 age; for females, 225 – age.[22] Therefore, if an individual were performing near maximal capacity, it is reasonable to expect the measured maximal heart rate to approximate predicted maximal heart rate. Normally, in the acute care setting, patients should not be working anywhere near maximal heart rate.

> **Clinical Tip**
> If a decrease in heart rate is palpated with activity, this may be due to an increase in arrhythmias that are palpated as pauses. Check telemetry recordings for arrhythmias. An increase in PVCs with activity is an abnormal response to activity.

### Heart Rate Measurement

The heart rate can be measured via palpation and is usually done via the radial pulse; it can also be measured from the ECG, either directly from a digital reading or from a recording of a 6-second ECG strip. See Table 16-8 for normal resting HR (heart rate) values. Although an ECG recording may be more accurate, the palpation method may be more common in the clinic owing to the lack of availability of ECG equipment. Heart rhythm (the presence or absence of rhythm disturbances) can also be evaluated if palpated continuously for at least 1 minute but is more accurately recorded via the ECG. See Chapter 9 for heart rate measurement on ECG and arrhythmia definitions.

The heart rate should be recorded with all activity, but the important factor is the heart rate response to activity. The normal heart rate response to any exertion is a gradual rise with an increase in work. If the individual is well trained (participates regularly in an aerobic exercise activity), the rate of heart rate rise is much more blunted (Fig. 16-27).

In a patient taking certain cardiac medications, specifically β-blocking medications, a blunted (slower rate of rise

Abnormal heart rate responses are of three types:
- A very rapid rise in heart rate with increased workload
- A very flat rate of rise (bradycardic response)
- A decrease in palpated heart rate

Patients who demonstrate a rapid rise in heart rate generally have one of two problems: severe deconditioning or a cardiovascular condition that is limiting the stroke volume. Patients who are not taking cardiac medications and who demonstrate a very flat rate of rise in heart rate are believed to have underlying cardiovascular disease. Also, individuals who have a decrease in palpated heart rate are not actually showing a true decreased heart rate but rather a decrease in palpable heart rate. If an ECG telemetry unit were available, these individuals should be monitored, because the palpable decrease in heart rate indicates an increase in arrhythmias (probably ventricular). When premature ectopic beats arise in the heart, they can often be palpated as a skip or pause in the pulse. When an increased number of pauses are palpated, it might appear to the therapist palpating the pulse that the heart rate actually decreased with exercise, when in reality the number of arrhythmias increased. If the pauses as well as the palpable beats were counted, one might not see a decrease in heart rate with exercise but rather an increase in heart rate with exercise. So, in reality, the heart rate does not decrease with exercise, but the palpated heart rate may appear to decrease if the number of arrhythmias increase. An increase in arrhythmias with exercise is also considered to be an abnormal response to exercise (see Heart Rhythm).

## Heart Rhythm

Heart rhythm can be palpated to assess regularity during exercise, but the interpretation of any specific rhythm disturbance cannot be made without ECG monitoring. Numerous patients, with and without cardiopulmonary dysfunction, have arrhythmias, so physical therapists must be able to identify commonly observed basic and life-threatening arrhythmias as well as be able to assess the severity of these arrhythmias to make appropriate clinical decisions. Arrhythmias are discussed in Chapter 9.

Heart rhythm should remain regular with exercise; however, if an individual has arrhythmias at rest, the normal response would be a lack of change in the frequency or type of arrhythmia with an increase in activity. If a change occurs with increased activity, four factors should be considered in the clinical decision-making process: (1) whether the arrhythmias represent a new finding, (2) whether the arrhythmias are benign or life-threatening, (3) whether the patient's pharmacologic regimen may be producing the arrhythmias, and (4) the severity of the symptoms associated with the arrhythmias.

Clinically, patients with occasional arrhythmias may not demonstrate serious arrhythmias with increased activity; in fact, arrhythmias may decrease or disappear with activity (as in sinus arrhythmia). In addition, arrhythmias may be well controlled by medication when the patient is at rest but not when the patient becomes active. A serious problem exists when a patient develops symptoms because of an arrhythmia or when the arrhythmia changes in character to become life threatening. Individuals who demonstrate an increasing frequency of premature ventricular ectopy with activity have been shown to have more serious coronary artery disease (two- and three-vessel disease) than individuals who do not.[23] In addition, patients who demonstrate premature ventricular ectopy at rest that disappears with activity have also been shown to have an increased incidence of coronary disease.[24]

Clinically, disturbances in heart rhythm should, at least, be monitored during an initial evaluation by means of direct palpation. When patients are known to have rhythm disturbances (either by direct palpation or history), further efforts should include ECG monitoring during activity and evaluating symptoms with the arrhythmias.

## Blood Pressure Measurement

Arterial blood pressure is a general indicator of the function of the heart as a pump. The arterial blood pressure is defined as the systolic pressure (pressure exerted against the arteries during the ejection cycle) and diastolic pressure (pressure exerted against the arteries during rest). Factors affecting blood pressure include cardiac output, peripheral resistance, distensibility of the arteries (vasomotor tone), volume of blood in the system, viscosity of the blood, and neural input.

Normal blood pressure in the aorta and arteries is defined as less than 120 mm Hg. Table 16-9 includes guidelines from the National Heart Lung Blood Institute for normal, prehypertension, and stage I and II hypertension. Pediatric values are found in Table 16-10. In addition, recommendations for treatment are included in Table 16-11. Blood pressure can be measured directly by means of indwelling arterial catheterization using a catheter inserted into an artery (as done in laboratory or critical care situations) or indirectly using a sphygmomanometer. Blood pressures are usually taken on the upper arm with the distal margin of the cuff approximately 3 cm above the antecubital fossa. Palpation is performed to locate the brachial artery pulse. This is the location for auscultation of the blood pressure. Following inflation of the cuff, auscultation of the first audible sound designates the systolic pressure, whereas the diastolic pressure is the value when the sounds become muffled.

The blood pressure may vary between extremities, with change of position, and with any type of activity. The changes between like extremities may reflect uneven peripheral resistance due to either differences in vasomotor tone or arterial occlusion. Changes in blood pressure with body position may reflect the influences of the vasomotor tone, the venous return, or the hydrostatic effects of gravity, or a combination of all three. Blood pressure changes associated with activity typically reflect the amount of work the heart must do to meet the metabolic demands of the activity.

> **Clinical Tip**
> Portable automatic blood pressure cuffs are often used in the hospital. This equipment is not always accurate with multiple uses.

Accuracy in measurement is critical to the correct interpretation of the blood pressure. Problems arise in the accurate measurement of blood pressure with activity when a therapist is not using good technique. When a patient stops performing

## Table 16-9 NHLBI Guidelines to Resting Blood Pressure Definitions (Adults)

|  | Normal | Prehypertension | Stage I Hypertension | Stage II Hypertension |
|---|---|---|---|---|
| Systolic (mm Hg) | <120 | 120–139 | 140–159 | >159 |
| Diastolic (mm Hg) | <80 | 80–89 | 90–99 | >99 |

*NHLBI, National Heart, Lung and Blood Institute.*

## Table 16-10 Pediatric Low-Normal Systolic Pressure Values

| Age | Low Normal (mm Hg) |
| --- | --- |
| Infant (birth-1 year) | >60[a] |
| Toddler (1–3 years) | >70[a] |
| Preschooler (3–6 years) | >75 |
| Elementary school age (6–12 years) | >80 |
| Adolescent (12–18 year) | >90 |

[a]*Infants and children age 3 years or younger: substitute strong central pulse for blood pressure reading from NY State Dept of Health.*

## Table 16-11 Treatment Guidelines for Hypertension (NHLBI 2003)

| Type of Hypertension | Treatment Guidelines |
| --- | --- |
| Prehypertension<br>120–139 systolic<br>80–89 diastolic | Lifestyle modification |
| Stage 1 hypertension<br>140–159 systolic<br>90–99 diastolic | Thiazide diuretics<br>May consider ACE inhibitor<br>β-Blocker, calcium-channel blocker |
| Stage 2 hypertension<br>≥160 systolic<br>≥100 diastolic | Two-drug combination<br>Thiazide and ACE or other |

*ACE, angiotensin-converting enzyme; NHLBI, National Heart, Lung and Blood Institute.*

an activity, the direct metabolic demands decrease while the muscle activity that assists in the return of the venous blood stops. As a result, the blood pressure may drop rapidly (within 15 seconds).[24] Therefore, it is essential that the physical therapist be competent in blood pressure measurement and knowledgeable regarding normal blood pressure responses to exertion in addition to being able to identify and react to abnormal responses.

> **Clinical Tip**
> It is essential to monitor both blood pressure and heart rate during activity rather than making these assessments after activity because blood pressure can drop within 15 seconds of stopping the activity. Heart rate and systolic blood pressure are the key determinants of myocardial oxygen demand.

### Evaluation of Oxygen Saturation

Patients with heart failure, pulmonary hypertension, or pulmonary disease should be evaluated for activity tolerance by monitoring heart rate, blood pressure, symptoms, and oxygen

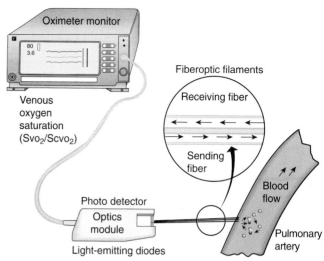

**Figure 16-28** Principles of reflectance spectrophotometry. Fiberoptics transmit two or three wavelengths of light from light-emitting diodes. Another fiberoptic bundle sends information back to the photodetector about the amount of light reflected by the oxygenated and deoxygenated hemoglobin. The microprocessor then calculates the percentage of hemoglobin saturated with oxygen. (Courtesy Edwards Lifesciences, Irvine, CA.)

saturation. A pulse oximeter (Fig. 16-28) is used to assess oxygen saturation of hemoglobin, which has a normal range of 98 to 100% (saturation of Hb). The portable pulse oximeter compares the signals received and calculates the degree of oxyhemoglobin saturation based on the intensity of the signal received. Normal response to activity is for the $O_2$ saturation to remain in the normal range. However, patients with chronic pulmonary dysfunction or congestive heart failure often desaturate their oxygen from hemoglobin with activity. Caution should be taken with patients who desaturate with activity below 90%. Exercise should not be continued if oxygen saturation drops to 88% or below (unless otherwise noted in the facility policy and approved by the medical director). See Chapter 10 for further information.

### Normal Responses

To understand normal responses to exercise, it is important to recognize that two key factors affect the blood pressure response: cardiac output and peripheral vascular resistance. Generally, with increased work, the cardiac output increases and the peripheral vascular resistance decreases as a result of (1) the hypothalamic response to increased body temperature and (2) the local effects of hydrogen ions, heat, decreased availability of oxygen, and increased carbon dioxide production on the arterioles. Thus, there is a normal increase in systolic blood pressure with increasing levels of exertion (Fig. 16-29). It is important to note that adult females tend to demonstrate a slower rate of rise in the systolic pressure during exertion in contrast to adult males.

The normal diastolic response is a maximum of 10 mm Hg increase or decrease from the resting value because of the adaptive dilation of the peripheral vascular bed that occurs with exercise. Younger persons and trained athletes may

### Table 16-12 Summary of Normal Responses to Activity

| Physiological Variable | Response to Increased Work | Response to Endurance Activity |
|---|---|---|
| Heart rate | Gradual rate of rise with increase in workload | Remains the same with continuation of the activity past steady state (first few minutes) |
| Systolic blood pressure | Gradual rate of rise with increase in workload | Remains the same with continuation of the activity past steady state (first few min) |
| Diastolic blood pressure | ±10 mm Hg with any activity | ±10 mm Hg with any activity |
| SpO₂ | Stays the same or increases | Stays the same or increases |
| Respiratory rate | Gradual increase with workload, rapid rate of rise after anaerobic threshold | Stays the same |

*SpO₂, pulse oximeter oxygen saturation.*

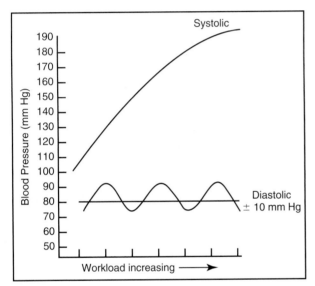

**Figure 16-29** The systolic blood pressure gradually rises with a gradual increase in workload. The diastolic blood pressure should change very little (±10 mm Hg) with an increase in workload. (Redrawn from Scully R, Barnes ML. Physical Therapy. Philadelphia, JB Lippincott, 1989.)

demonstrate a progressive decrease in diastolic pressure during exercise as a result of the increased peripheral vasodilation. Therefore, a fall in diastolic pressure greater than the 10 mm Hg can be considered a normal response in this population but not in older, untrained individuals.

The normal systolic and diastolic blood pressure responses to endurance activity (when an individual maintains a constant submaximal workload) are to remain constant or even to decrease slightly. This indicates that the body has achieved a steady-state condition and that the central and peripheral mechanisms that adjust the blood pressure (e.g., cardiac output and peripheral vascular resistance) have accommodated to the workload. See Table 16-12 for a summary of normal responses to activity.

### Abnormal Responses

If one knows and understands the normal blood pressure responses to exercise, then identifying abnormal responses is simplified. Abnormalities can exist with the systolic or diastolic response or both. The abnormal responses are first defined, and then the mechanism of action and clinical implications are described.

#### Abnormal Systolic Responses

There are three abnormal systolic blood pressure responses to activity that are described in the literature: hypertensive, hypotensive, and blunted or flat. A hypertensive blood pressure response is one in which an individual who is normotensive at rest exhibits an abnormally high systolic blood pressure for a given level of exertion. This type of response has been associated with an increased risk for the future development of hypertension at rest. Furthermore, this response should be distinguished from that found in an individual who is hypertensive at rest yet exhibits a normally increasing systolic blood pressure during increasing levels of exertion.[25] Although the mechanism for the hypertensive blood pressure response is not fully understood, it may be related to the following: an increased plasma concentration of catecholamines, an increased resistance to blood flow arising from peripheral vascular occlusive disease, or an abnormal centrally mediated resting vasomotor tone.

Exertional systolic hypotension is described as a normally rising systolic pressure at submaximal levels, followed by a sudden progressive decrease in systolic blood pressure in the face of increasing workload (Fig. 16-30); it has been highly correlated with pathologic cardiac conditions.[26] Individuals with exertional hypotension often demonstrate coronary perfusion defects on exercise thallium tests and severe coronary disease, poor ventricular function, or both as documented by coronary angiography.[25]

A blunted blood pressure response is defined as a slight increase in systolic blood pressure at low levels of exertion with a failure to rise with increasing levels of work. This definition applies only to those individuals who are not receiving pharmacologic intervention that might affect blood pressure. Failure to reach a systolic blood pressure in excess of 130 mm Hg at maximal effort in the absence of any medication that restricts the blood pressure is associated with a high risk for future sudden death.[27] However, this is equivalent to the

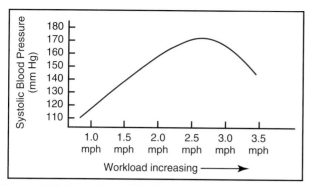

**Figure 16-30** An abnormal blood pressure response to an increase in workload. Greater than 2.5 mph workload caused the systolic blood pressure to decrease continually, demonstrating a failure of the heart muscle to meet the demands. (Redrawn from Scully R, Barnes ML. Physical Therapy. Philadelphia, JB Lippincott, 1989.)

blunted response that is seen in individuals who are receiving β-adrenergic antagonists as part of a therapeutic pharmacologic regimen. When these medications are prescribed, the blunted blood pressure response is expected and considered normal.

A hypotensive or blunted blood pressure response indicates that either the cardiac output is failing to meet the demands of the body or that the peripheral vascular resistance is rapidly decreasing. Evidence in the literature suggests that hypotensive or blunted blood pressure responses are most often due to a failing cardiac output.[28,29] Because the cardiac output is directly dependent on stroke volume and heart rate, if the stroke volume is unable to increase appropriately for a given level of work, any increase in cardiac output arises solely as the result of an increase in the heart rate. In this situation, the blood pressure may rise slightly or may remain flat. Unfortunately, because of the concomitant increase in myocardial oxygen demand that accompanies an increase in heart rate, the heart is unable to maintain an increased cardiac output for any significant period of time, which results in a falling blood pressure.

When an individual is performing endurance exercise (of greater than 3 to 5 minutes in duration), a continuous rise in systolic blood pressure is considered an abnormal response. Persons who demonstrate an abnormal blood pressure response during endurance exercise typically have one of two conditions: either a high degree of ventricular wall dysfunction or a dysfunction in the ability of myocardial tissue to extract oxygen from the circulatory system.

### Clinical Implications

Patients who demonstrate abnormal blood pressure responses during exercise typically suffer from coronary artery disease (e.g., have a history of angioplasty, angina, coronary bypass surgery, or myocardial infarction), moderate to severe aortic valvular stenosis, or other cardiac muscle dysfunction.[30,31]

The assessment of peak blood pressure as well as the interpretation of the blood pressure response during activity is an essential component of the initial and continuing

evaluation of every patient. Although restrictions on any activity might be unnecessary, patients with abnormal systolic blood pressure responses should be monitored closely during typical activities and especially during new exertional activities. In addition, the treatment or exercise prescription may require alterations in duration, intensity, or both. Some activities may require supervision so that the patient can perform the activity safely. Also, the patients themselves should be educated regarding their specific limitations and the signs and symptoms of overexertion when performing any activities.

### Abnormal Diastolic Responses

As stated previously, a normal diastolic blood pressure response is one in which a change is no greater than 10 mm Hg: an abnormal diastolic blood pressure response would be either an increase or decrease of more than 10 mm Hg (in an untrained or older population). In addition, a sustained elevation of the diastolic blood pressure during the recovery phase of activity is considered to be abnormal.[32]

The mechanism behind the progressive rise in diastolic blood pressure is thought to be a response to the need for an increased driving pressure in the coronary arteries, which is necessary to overcome the increased resistance to flow within the coronary arteries. When blood flow through the coronary arteries is decreased below the level needed to meet the demand of the myocardium as a result of either increased vascular tone or vascular occlusion, a stimulus is created for an increased driving pressure to make the blood flow through the resistant arteries.[32] Despite the lack of research-based documentation regarding this abnormality, the physical therapist should be aware of the normal anticipated physiologic response and therefore be very sensitive to a progressive rise in diastolic pressure, interpreting this as an abnormal response. Patients who demonstrate a progressive rise in diastolic pressure usually have numerous risk factors for heart disease, are deemed high risk for or already have coronary artery disease, or have a previous history of coronary angioplasty or bypass surgery. Patients with hypertensive heart disease and compensated heart failure may also demonstrate this abnormal response. See Table 16-13 for a summary of abnormal responses to activity.

## Other Symptoms of Cardiovascular Inadequacy

The other symptoms associated with cardiovascular inadequacy are more difficult to interpret and therefore more difficult to treat. Angina, shortness of breath, and palpitations are the most common symptoms of patients with cardiopulmonary dysfunction. The other classic symptoms to be aware of are dizziness, pallor, and fatigue. The therapist, therefore, must have a thorough understanding of how to assess these symptoms.

### Angina

Angina is a discomfort found anywhere above the waist but more likely in the chest, neck, or jaw and is typically described using terms such as dull ache, tightness, fullness, burning,

**Table 16-13 Summary of Abnormal Responses to Activity**

| Physiological Variable | Response to Increased Work | Response to Endurance Activity |
|---|---|---|
| Heart Rate | Rapid rate of rise | Progressively increasing HR |
| | Blunted rate of rise and NOT on medications to affect HR | Significant drop in HR |
| | Drop in HR | |
| Heart Rhythm | Starts regular, becomes irregular | Starts regular, becomes irregular |
| | More than 6 'skips' per minute or documentced PVCs above resting amount | More than 6 'skips' per minute or documented PVCs above resting amount |
| Systolic blood pressure | Rapid rate of rise | Progressive rise |
| | Blunted rise not on beta blockers | Decrease and symptomatic with decrease |
| | Decrease with increase work | |
| Diastolic blood pressure | > 10 mm rise | > 10 mm rise |
| SpO$_2$ | Decrease with increase work | Decrease |

pressure, indigestion, or neck or jaw discomfort. Classic (or stable) angina is brought on by exertion or emotional upset and at times by eating; it is relieved by either rest or nitroglycerin. Angina and other chest wall or neurologic complaints are differentiated by the activity that reproduces the discomfort. Angina is reproducible only by increasing myocardial oxygen consumption (as in activity or emotion), whereas musculoskeletal pain can be reproduced by palpation or deep inspiration and expiration, and neurologic pain may follow a dermatome and exist all the time.

Men and women often present with different symptom complaints of angina. Men classically complain of substernal or chest tightness or indigestion that radiates, sometimes into the arm or into the jaw or neck. Women on the other hand complain of tightness or discomfort posteriorly between the scapula, or they present with symptoms of indigestion, nausea, shortness of breath or even simply excessive fatigue. Because of the different symptoms that women experience, their symptoms are not assessed as cardiovascular in nature and are often ignored by the medical community. Should either men or women present with these symptoms, risk factor analysis for cardiovascular disease should be performed and in the event of moderate to high risk for disease, these symptoms should be considered to be of good probability to be related to cardiovascular disease.

There are six types of "chest pain" that make the differential diagnosis of angina difficult, however. Two of these situations relate to angina and include variant angina (as found in the pure form called Prinzmetal's angina) and preinfarction angina.

**Variant angina.** Variant angina, defined as angina produced from vasospasm of the coronary arteries in the absence of occlusive disease (i.e., the arteries are free of disease), is called Prinzmetal's angina. Individuals who experience vasospasm often develop resting chest pain, making the classic definition of angina inappropriate.[33] In the case of variant angina, an individual is more likely to have discomfort that is due to emotional upset or inspiration of cold air.

Variant angina usually responds to nitroglycerin and is typically diagnosed when nitroglycerin is found to be effective or when other long-term pharmacologic therapy is found effective. Calcium-channel blockers are typically the long-term pharmacologic choice for the treatment of variant angina. These drugs retard the uptake of the calcium in the cells and therefore inhibit smooth muscle contraction of the arterial walls (see Chapters 2 and 14).

> **Clinical Tip**
> Women and diabetic patients with coronary artery disease do not complain of the typical chest tightness with exertion, but rather shortness of breath. This shortness of breath goes away slowly (or "eases") with rest. Therefore, shortness of breath in these patient groups should be assessed in great detail to rule out that the shortness of breath is not an angina equivalent. Assess risk for coronary disease in these patients.

**Preinfarction angina.** Preinfarction angina is defined as unstable angina; it occurs at rest and worsens with activity. An individual may or may not have had symptoms of classic angina before experiencing the intense and constant pain of preinfarction angina. This condition is one that requires immediate medical treatment to prevent full transmural infarction.

Although the description of angina may vary from individual to individual, the description remains constant for each individual. Therefore, once the therapist concludes that the symptoms being described constitute angina, then the patient's terms used to describe the angina should be remembered and used in all future assessments of symptoms. The other four types of chest pain in addition to angina are pericarditis, mitral valve dysfunction, bronchospasm, and esophageal spasm.

*Pericarditis*

Pericarditis is an inflammation of the pericardial sac that surrounds the heart and may actually result in a restriction of cardiac output. Patients who are suspected of having pericardial pain should be referred for immediate medical treatment and discontinued from exertional activities until the pericarditis subsides. Pericarditis produces a chest pain symptom that is constant and sharp and is described as intense and "stabbing." Pericarditis pain *usually* does not increase with activity (however, in some cases it may increase with activity) and often remains constant 24 hours per day and is very intense. Associated fever and fatigue may also occur with the stabbing pain, as well as ECG changes.[34] Pericardial pain is a common symptom following coronary artery bypass surgery and occurs occasionally in the early phase following a myocardial infarction. Pericardial pain is also more common in some of the inflammatory diseases such as systemic lupus erythematosus. Treatment usually includes anti-inflammatory medications.

### Mitral Valve Dysfunction
Individuals with mitral valve dysfunction (mitral valve prolapse or mitral valve regurgitation) may demonstrate classic angina with exertion yet lack a suspicious risk factor profile. They tend to be younger and are free of cardiovascular occlusive disease. Auscultation of heart sounds usually reveals a systolic murmur or click. Echocardiography usually identifies mitral valve dysfunction. The angina pain from mitral valve dysfunction arises from the diminished blood flow resulting from the subsequent decreased cardiac output.[35]

### Bronchospasm
Some patients experience exercise-induced bronchospasm, which can manifest itself as chest wall tightness or discomfort, or both, with exertion. Differentiation of exercise-induced bronchospasm from exertional angina is performed by assessing the individual's degree of difficulty in breathing. An individual experiencing exercise-induced bronchospasm usually demonstrates a greatly increased work of breathing as well as an extreme effort to take the next breath. The chest wall pain or tightness often changes with breathing, which is a sign that it is not angina.

### Esophageal Spasm
Esophageal spasm or inflammation may produce a midsternal pain that is mistaken for angina.[36] Diffuse esophageal spasm is usually idiopathic and produces a chest pain with dysphagia. Esophageal spasm is suspected when the chest discomfort develops with eating and can be diagnosed with esophageal manometry or with barium swallow. Treatment for this type of chest pain includes medication to decrease the acid reflux into the esophagus, sublingual nitroglycerin, and calcium-channel blockers.[37]

### Shortness of Breath
Shortness of breath is one of the other common symptoms found in patients with cardiopulmonary dysfunction. Shortness of breath may be due to several different physiologic mechanisms, including the equivalent of angina in individuals who cannot perceive chest pain or discomfort, as in the diabetic with peripheral neuropathy. Shortness of breath may also be due to limited cardiovascular reserve in patients with coronary disease or cardiac muscle dysfunction; pulmonary disease with limited ventilatory reserve, diffusion, or arterial oxygen-carrying capacity; and finally physiologic limitations in an individual's oxygen transport system when shortness of breath occurs during exercise. When shortness of breath does develop during the assessment, these mechanisms need to be evaluated to determine the cause of the shortness of breath and to make appropriate clinical decisions regarding progression of activity.

### Palpitations
Palpitations are a common complaint of patients with cardiopulmonary dysfunction. Palpitations usually indicate arrhythmias.[38] Palpitations must be evaluated to determine the seriousness of any rhythm disturbances as well as the cause of any symptoms. If telemetry is available, the patient should be connected to telemetry for any activity assessment. Formal assessment usually involves 24-hour Holter monitoring.

### Dizziness
Dizziness can have several origins, including the vestibular system, vision, medications, blood pressure, and cardiac output. Dizziness is a symptom that must be evaluated with reference to the activity that produces it and then compared with the blood pressure response. If an individual becomes dizzy on standing and a blood pressure drop is noted, the condition is described as orthostatic hypotension. However, if the patient complains of dizziness with an increase in activity and a blood pressure drop is noted, this patient is defined as having exertional hypotension. Clinical decision making therefore depends on the constellation of symptoms presented by the patient and the effect the associated dizziness has on his or her activity.

### Fatigue
Fatigue may also have several origins, including depression, general deconditioning, pharmacologic management and side effects, and physiologic limitation, as seen in the individual with cardiac muscle dysfunction. Therefore, fatigue should never be the only symptom the therapist uses to make a clinical decision regarding exercise prescription or progression. The cause of the fatigue may need to be investigated further if it is the only symptom-limiting activity and all other responses are normal.

## Evaluation

On completion of the full cardiopulmonary examination (assessment), including chest examination and activity evaluation, the physical therapist develops a clinical judgment (evaluation) based on the data gathered and formulates a decision regarding interventions to be used. Acute care interventions are discussed in Chapter 17, cardiac interventions in Chapter 18, pulmonary rehabilitation in 19, and pediatric interventions in 20. However, the therapist must always remember that each treatment session becomes an assessment, particularly of responses to the treatment. Therefore, each treatment session is, in essence, a monitored activity session, requiring constant reevaluation and assessment as to the significance of the clinical findings.

Evaluation includes the development of a diagnosis or diagnoses based on the clinical findings and includes the impact of the findings or problems, otherwise known as functional limitations and disability. With the development of a diagnosis, the therapist is guided to a classification scheme that involves placing the patient *based on primary dysfunction* into a diagnostic grouping or practice pattern. This allows the therapist to select from available interventions a plan of care for the patient that will optimally achieve the expected outcomes in the documented amount of time described in the

prognosis associated with the practice pattern. See Table 16-1 for the list of cardiovascular and pulmonary practice patterns that are described in great detail in the *Guide to Physical Therapist Practice.*[1]

---

**Clinical Tip**

Physical therapists develop a diagnosis which is a *physical therapy* diagnosis not a medical diagnosis.

---

A re-examination is the formal process of selecting tests and measures to evaluate progress and modify or redirect the interventions. Indications for a reexamination include a failure of the patient to respond the interventions, or when new clinical findings or problems develop.

---

## CASE STUDY 16-1

A 72-year-old woman who contracted poliomyelitis in 1948 fell in her retirement home apartment, fracturing the proximal left femur. She was found immediately because she used her emergency call cord in her apartment.

The patient underwent open reduction internal fixation with spinal anesthesia 3 days earlier, and the physician has just ordered physical therapy for out-of-bed activities and ambulation with a walker.

The chart review revealed the following:

- A 54-year history of smoking approximately 1.5 to 2 packs per day
- No history of hypertension, family history of heart disease, or other major medical problems (patient had been ambulatory with wheeled tripod walker and lives alone)
- Laboratory study results within normal limits
- Chest radiograph demonstrates hyperinflated chest with few patchy areas of infiltrate in both bases

In the interview, the patient reported that she is in a lot of pain. She plans to return to extended care at the retirement home until she is able to take care of herself.

The physical examination revealed the following:

- General appearance: slight grayish color; thin, slightly underweight
- Neck: observation of hypertrophy of sternocleidomastoid muscles bilaterally; forward head, and sits in bed with the head of the bed elevated to 60 degrees
- Chest: Upward movement of chest with every breath; patient is observed to have increased accessory muscle use, increased AP diameter, and increased respiratory rate

- Phonation, cough, and cough production: patient is observed to have moist, nonproductive, ineffective cough; phonation requires breaths between words in sentence; extremities have mild clubbing, gray-blue color with tobacco stains
- Auscultation: decreased breath sounds auscultated with coarse wheezing and wet crackles on expiration in bilateral bases but slightly cleared with a cough; auscultation of the heart demonstrates loud atrial gallop with rapid heartbeat
- Palpation: decreased chest wall motion palpated throughout, with palpable fremitus in bilateral bases; increased accessory muscle use including sternocleidomastoid and scalenes, with decreased diaphragmatic excursion; good pulses throughout, except bilateral dorsalis pedis
- Percussion: mild dullness to percussion noted in bases
- Activity evaluation: patient was evaluated in supine-to-sit position only; patient could not tolerate standing owing to increased pain in left lower extremity and dizziness
- Vital signs: heart rate 100 (supine), 120 (sitting); blood pressure 110/70 (supine), 90/66 (sitting)

These findings from the cardiopulmonary assessment demonstrate an elderly female with a long-term history of smoking and signs of chronic obstructive pulmonary disease in addition to the hip fracture. She is at extreme risk for pneumonia. Also, the patient has a problem with orthostatic hypotension as evidenced by her vital signs. The chronic obstructive pulmonary disease and the present pulmonary condition (e.g., infiltrates in bases, retained secretions), as well as the orthostatic hypotension, will affect her activity progression. These need to be addressed.

---

## Summary

- A thorough examination of the patient is essential for optimal treatment.
- Included in the cardiopulmonary examination (assessment) is a thorough chart review to identify past medical history, diagnostic studies, and current medical status.
- The physical therapist must remember that although the chart should have all the necessary information about the

patient, the optimal situation is one that allows the acquisition of pertinent information directly from the patient.
- The patient interview can shed new light on the chart information, or it can provide a completely different picture.
- Performing a physical examination of the patient provides the most accurate information regarding the patient's current cardiopulmonary status.

- The physical examination includes a thorough inspection, auscultation, palpation, percussion, and activity assessment.
- Based on the initial assessment, a plan of treatment or exercise prescription can be developed for optimal rehabilitation.
- The assessment must be ongoing, and components of the physical examination need to be performed on a daily basis to assess the patient's status with increased activity.

## References

1. American Physical Therapy Association. Guide to Physical Therapist Practice. 2nd ed. Baltimore, APTA, 2003.
2. Walter SD, Cook RJ. A PC Program for Analysis of Observer Variation. Department of Clinical Epidemiology and Biostatistics, McMaster University Medical Center, Hamilton, Ontario, Canada, 1988.
3. Kannel WB, Castelli WP, Gordon T, et al. Serum cholesterol, lipoproteins, and the risk of coronary heart disease: the Framingham study. Ann Intern Med 24:1, 1971.
4. Laposata EA. Cocaine induced heart disease: mechanisms and pathology. J Thorac Imaging 6(1):68–75, 1991.
5. Rezkalla SH, Hale S, Kloner RA. Cocaine induced heart diseases. Am Heart J 120(6):1403–8, 1990.
6. Morris DC. Cocaine heart disease. Hosp Pract [Off] 26(9):83–92, 1991.
7. McNeer JF, Wallace AG, Wagner GS, et al. The course of acute myocardial infarction. Circulation 51:410, 1975.
8. Steinhart MJ. Depression and chronic fatigue in the patient with heart disease. Prim Care 18(2):309–25, 1991.
9. Wilkins RL, Dexter JR, Murphy RL Jr, DelBono EA. Lung sound nomenclature survey. Chest 98(4):886–9, 1990.
10. Kramin SS. Determination of the site of production of respiratory sounds by subtraction phonopneumography. Am Rev Respir Dis 122:303, 1980.
11. American College of CP & ATS Joint Committee on Pulmonary Nomenclature: Pulmonary Terms and Symbols. Chest 67:583, 1975.
12. Wilkins RL, Hodgkin JE, Lopez B. Lung Sounds: A Practical Guide. St. Louis, Mosby, 1988.
13. Piirila P, Sovijarvi AR, Kaisla T, et al. Crackles in patients with fibrosing alveolitis, bronchiectasis, COPD and heart failure. Chest 99(5):1076–83, 1991.
14. Nath AR, Capel LH. Inspiratory crackles and the mechanical events of breathing. Thorax 29:695, 1974.
15. Forgacs P. The functional basis of pulmonary sounds. Chest 73:399, 1978.
16. Nath AR, Capel LH. Inspiratory crackles—Early and late. Thorax 29:223, 1974.
17. Murphy RLH. Discontinuous adventitious lung sounds. Semin Respir Med 6:210, 1985.
18. Ravin A. In Auscultation of the Heart. Chicago, Year Book Medical Publishers, 1968.
19. Luisada AA, Portaluppi F. In The Heart Sounds: New Facts and Their Clinical Applications. New York, Praeger Publishers, 1982.
20. Criqui MH, Fronek A, Klauber MR. The sensitivity, specificity and predictive value of traditional clinical evidence of peripheral arterial disease: Results from noninvasive testing in a defined population. Circulation 71(3):516–22, 1985.
21. Butler SM. Phase one cardiac rehabilitation: The role of functional evaluation in patient progression. Master's thesis, Atlanta, Emory University, 1983.
22. Cooper KH. The Aerobics Way. New York, Bantam Books, 1981.
23. Pleskot M, Pidrman V, Tilser P, et al. Programmed ventricular stimulation in the evaluation of the clinical significance of premature ventricular contractions. Vnitr Lek 37(6):548–56, 1991.
24. Henachel A, De La Vega F, Taylor HL. Simultaneous direct and indirect blood pressure measurements in man at rest and work. J Appl Physiol 6:506, 1954.
25. Dlin RA, Hanne N, Silverberg DS, et al. Follow-up of normotensive men with exaggerated blood pressure response to exercise. Am Heart J 106(2):316, 1983.
26. Hakki A, Munley BM, Hadjimiltiades J. Determinants, of abnormal blood pressure response to exercise in coronary artery disease. Am J Cardiol 57:71, 1986.
27. Bruce RA, DeRouen T, Peterson DR, et al. Noninvasive predictors of sudden death in men with coronary heart disease. Am J Cardiol 39:833, 1977.
28. Frenneaux MP, Counihan PJ, Caforior AL, et al. Abnormal blood pressure response during exercise in hypertrophic cardiomyopathy. Circulation 82(6):1995–2002, 1990.
29. Pavlovic M. [Decrease in systolic blood pressure during physical exertion in stress tests]. Srp Arh Celok Lek 117(11–12):777–86, 1989. [In Serbian]
30. Cavan D, O'Donnell MJ, Parkes A, et al. Abnormal blood pressure response to exercise in normoalbuminuric insulin dependent diabetic patients. J Hum Hypertens 5(1):21–6, 1991.
31. Guerrera G, Melina D, Colivicchi F, et al. Abnormal blood pressure response to exercise in borderline hypertension. A two year follow-up study. Am J Hypertens 4(3Pt 1):271–3, 1991.
32. Guyton AC, Jones CE, Coleman TG. Circulatory Physiology: Cardiac Output and Its Regulation. Philadelphia, WB Saunders, 1973.
33. Maseri A, Crea F, Kaski JC, et al. Mechanisms of angina pectoris in syndrome X. Am Coll Cardiol 17:499, 1991.
34. Phillips RE, Feeney MK. The Cardiac Rhythms: A Systematic Approach to Interpretation. Philadelphia, WB Saunders, 1990.
35. Albert MA, Mukerji V, Sabeti M, et al. Mitral valve prolapse, panic disorder, and chest pain. Med Clin North Am 75(5):1119–33, 1991.
36. Rakel RE. Conn's Current Therapy. Philadelphia, WB Saunders, 1991:424–5.
37. Nevens F, Janssens J, Piessens J, et al. Prospective study on prevalence of esophageal chest pain in patients referred on an elective basis to a cardiac unit for suspected myocardial ischemia. Dig Dis Sci 36(2):229, 1991.
38. Cohen M, Michel TH. Cardiopulmonary Symptoms in Physical Therapy Practice. New York, Churchill Livingstone, 1988.

## CHAPTER 17

# Interventions for Acute Cardiopulmonary Conditions

*Alexandra Sciaky, Amy Pawlik*

## Chapter Outline

In the United States, more than 5 million patients survive an episode of critical illness in an acute care hospital each year.[1] Some of these patients return to their former level of function relatively quickly. A significant number of them, however, experience life-altering changes in their physical, cognitive, and emotional functioning. A variety of factors, specific to hospitalized patients, contribute to these functional losses, including acute inflammation, severity of illness, marginal baseline function, exposure to corticosteroids and neuromuscular blockers, and prolonged immobilization (bed rest) and length of stay. Physical therapists providing therapeutic interventions for patients with acute cardiopulmonary conditions must appreciate the unique circumstances and patient responses that occur in the hospital environment. These circumstances include working with patients in intensive care units who usually require continuous monitoring in conjunction with medical interventions such as the use of vasoactive medications, sedation, circulatory assist devices, and mechanical ventilation through artificial airways. Psychological stresses are common in these patients and their families and can include powerlessness, vulnerability, fear, anxiety, isolation, and spiritual distress.[2]

Acute cardiopulmonary conditions can be defined as diseases or states in which the patient's oxygen transport system fails to meet the immediate demands placed on it.[3] Such failure may result in significant periods of bed rest for the patient and the associated adverse effects (Table 17-1). The loss of muscle strength and endurance for such patients with low-level baseline functional mobility can have significant consequences. For them, the loss of even a small amount of functional mobility may mean the difference between going home and going to a nursing home.[1] Ischemic cardiovascular diseases, chronic obstructive pulmonary diseases, postoperative pulmonary complications, and complications of hypertension, diabetes, and obesity are perhaps the most common conditions associated with acute cardiopulmonary dysfunction and seen by physical therapists in the hospital setting. See Table 17-2 for a more complete list that is cross-referenced with the APTA Guide's Cardiopulmonary Practice Patterns.[4]

The overall objective of this chapter is to provide the clinician with physical therapy interventions and evidence for hospitalized, acutely ill patients with primary or secondary cardiopulmonary conditions and the associated functional

### Table 17-1 Clinical Systemic Effects of Immobilization

| System | Effects |
|---|---|
| Cardiovascular system | Increased basal heart rate |
| | Decreased maximal heart rate |
| | Decreased maximal oxygen uptake |
| | Orthostatic hypotension |
| | Increased venous thrombosis risk |
| | Decreased total blood volume |
| | Decreased hemoglobin concentration |
| Respiratory system | Decreased vital capacity |
| | Decreased residual volume |
| | Decreased $PaO_2$ |
| | Impaired ability to clear secretions |
| | Increased ventilation–perfusion mismatch |
| Musculoskeletal system | Decreased strength |
| | Decreased girth |
| | Decreased efficiency of contraction |
| | Joint contractures |
| | Decubitus ulcers |
| Central nervous system | Emotional and behavioral disturbances |
| | Intellectual deficit |
| | Altered sensation |
| Metabolic system | Hypercalcemia |
| | Osteoporosis |

impairments described by the Practice Patterns in Table 17-2. For any given patient, addressing the pulmonary needs of the patient is generally the physical therapist's first priority. Once the patient is breathing (or being mechanically ventilated) effectively, additional interventions may be provided. Patient examination, which leads to the physical therapist's evaluation, is covered in Chapter 16. This chapter will discuss clinical decision making relative to choosing and providing cardiopulmonary interventions in the hospital environment and the special considerations that acutely ill patients demand. These interventions include airway clearance techniques, breathing strategies, and monitored exercise progression. Safely mobilizing patients with or without assistive devices in the hospital setting and determining the most appropriate discharge destination (home, nursing home, subacute unit, rehabilitation unit) will also be discussed.

Patients in the acute care setting can present with multiple cardiopulmonary impairments regardless of the primary diagnosis. They may demonstrate difficulty performing effective airway clearance, cough, or achieving enough inspiratory effort to support therapeutic or functional activities. A patient may also demonstrate deconditioning as a result of the primary medical condition, prolonged bedrest, or a combination of both. This physical state can result in a decrease in endurance and activity tolerance and may limit functional mobility. Addressing the patient's cardiopulmonary impairments can result in improved oxygen transport, improving overall health and allowing the patient to progress toward functional goals.

## Airway Clearance Techniques

Airway clearance techniques are defined as manual or mechanical procedures that facilitate mobilization of secretions from the airways. The techniques include postural drainage, percussion, vibration, cough techniques, manual hyperinflation, and airway suctioning. See Table 17-3 for a summary of mechanical devices used for airway clearance. The indications for airway clearance techniques include impaired mucociliary transport, excessive pulmonary secretions, and an ineffective or absent cough. The clinician can facilitate the mobilization of secretions by using one or more airway clearance techniques with acutely ill patients. Consideration of the pathophysiology and symptoms, the stability of the medical status of the patient, and the patient's adherence to the technique(s) are all important factors in choosing an optimal airway clearance plan of care. Adherence to hospital infection control policies and procedures is critical to maintain the safety of caregivers and patients. Body substance precautions such as gowns, masks, gloves, and goggles apply to the performance of airway clearance techniques.

Patient examination before, during, and after treatment provides the clinician with important information by which to judge the patient's tolerance and the treatment's effectiveness. In addition to gathering the necessary equipment and assistance to perform the intervention(s), airway clearance techniques should be performed before or at least 30 minutes following the end of a meal or tube feeding. Continuous tube feedings should be interrupted and the patient's stomach checked for residual feeding that might be aspirated during the treatment.[5] Optimal pain control allows the patient to have the greatest comfort and offer fullest cooperation during the procedure. Inhaled bronchodilator medications given prior to airway clearance procedure enhance the overall intervention outcome. Inhaled antibiotic medications, however, will have better deposition into the lung if they are given following the airway clearance procedure. The clinician should also take care to observe proper body mechanics while performing airway clearance techniques to avoid self-injury. In the hospital setting, monitoring vital signs is important in determining the patient's response to therapeutic interventions.

**Table 17-2   Conditions Associated with Acute Cardiopulmonary Dysfunction and Associated Preferred Practice Patterns**

| Conditions | Practice Pattern | Associated Clinical Findings |
|---|---|---|
| Obesity, cigarette smoking, hypertension, hyperlipidemia Diabetes type II | 6A: Primary prevention/risk reduction for cardiovascular/ pulmonary disorders | Hypoventilation, atelectasis, $CO_2$ retention, resting SBP >140 mm Hg, |
| Prolonged immobilization, sedentary lifestyle | 6B: Impaired aerobic capacity/ endurance associated with deconditioning | Elevated resting heart rate, early fatigue, dyspnea on exertion |
| Cystic fibrosis, bronchiectasis, acute bronchitis, pneumonia, lung abscess, asbestosis, inhalation burns, asthma, pulmonary fibrosis | 6C: Impaired ventilation, respiration/ gas exchange, and aerobic capacity/endurance associated with airway clearance dysfunction | Cough productive of more than 30 mL of secretions per 24 hours, fever, shortness of breath, hypoxemia, $CO_2$ retention, respiratory acidosis, decreased FEV1 |
| Congestive heart failure, coronary artery disease, diseases of aortic and mitral valves, cardiomyopathy, endocarditis, shock, peripheral arterial disease, congenital heart anomalies | 6D: Impaired aerobic capacity/ endurance associated with cardiovascular pump dysfunction or failure | Shortness of breath, jugular venous distension, S3 heart sound, crackles on auscultation, decreased ejection fraction, cyanosis, dependent edema, claudication |
| Chest trauma, Guillain–Barré syndrome, spinal cord injury, multiple sclerosis, muscular dystrophy, post–polio syndrome, emphysema, burns to upper body, Parkinson disease | 6E: Impaired ventilation and respiration/gas exchange associated with ventilatory pump dysfunction or failure | Paradoxical breathing, inability to cough, dyspnea, reduced peak expiratory flow rate, reduced tidal volume and peak inspiratory pressure |
| Acute respiratory distress syndrome, pneumonia, pulmonary edema, sepsis | 6F: Impaired ventilation and respiration/gas exchange associated with respiratory failure | Hypoxemia, abnormal chest radiograph, increased resting respiratory rate, mechanical ventilation required, fever, hypoxemia |
| Bronchopulmonary dysplasia, CMV pneumonia, asthma, meconium aspiration | 6G: Impaired ventilation, respiration/ gas exchange, and aerobic capacity/endurance associated with respiratory failure in the neonate | Intercostal retraction, stridor, wheezing, physiological intolerance of routine care, impaired airway clearance |
| Lymphedema | 6H: Impaired circulation and anthropometric dimensions associated with lymphatic system disorders | Edema (nondependent), difficulty moving, impaired skin integrity, peau d'orange |

The goals of airway clearance techniques are to optimize airway patency, increase ventilation and perfusion matching, promote alveolar expansion and ventilation, and increase gas exchange.[6–8] Duration and frequency of the techniques are based on pulmonary reevaluation at each session. Often family members or other caregivers will be trained to continue the airway clearance techniques following hospital discharge. In this case, the clinician should provide written instructions including techniques, duration, frequency, and precautions as well as personal demonstration of the desired techniques. Intervention is discontinued when the goals have been met or the patient can independently perform his or her own airway clearance techniques.

## Postural Drainage

Postural drainage (PD) is the assumption of one or more body positions that allow gravity to assist with draining secretions from each of the patient's lung segments.[9] In each position, the segmental bronchus of the area to be drained is arranged perpendicular to the floor (Fig. 17-1). These positions can be modified when a patient presents with a condition that qualifies as a precaution or relative contraindication to PD (Box 17-1). For example, a modified position to treat the lateral segment of the right lower lobe would be the left side-lying position with the bed flat rather than in the Trendelenburg position.

## Table 17-3 Summary of Devices Used for Airway Clearance

| Device | Example | Common Indications | Advantages | Disadvantages | Home Unit Available? |
|---|---|---|---|---|---|
| High frequency chest wall oscillation (HFCWO) | The Vest | Cystic fibrosis | Unassisted use is possible, can be used in any position, can be passive, percusses all sides of chest, not recommended for intubated patients | Expensive, bulky, not appropriate for postoperative patients | Yes |
| Positive expiratory pressure (PEP) | TheraPEP | Bronchiectasis, cystic fibrosis, pneumonia | Portable, inexpensive, quiet, simple to operate | Requires patient effort | Yes |
| Vibratory positive expiratory pressure | Acapella,[a] Flutter[b] | acute bronchitis, cystic fibrosis, pneumonia | Portable, inexpensive, simple to operate | Requires patient effort | Yes |
| Mechanical percussor | Pneumopulse | Pneumonia including intubated patients, aspiration pneumonia | Can be passive, low caregiver effort, can be used postoperatively | Can be painful, not appropriate for patients with low bone density or platelets, not effective with obese patients | Yes |
| Mechanical vibrator | Flimm Fighter | Postoperative pneumonia, chest trauma | Can be passive, low caregiver effort, can be used postoperatively, can be used with low bone density or platelets, has accessory strap to use for posterior lung fields | Not effective for obese patients | Yes |
| Insufflator–exsufflator | CoughAssist | Guillain–Barré, spinal cord injury, muscular dystrophy, multiple sclerosis | Noninvasive, easy to operate, reduces the need for airway suctioning | Expensive, cannot be used with patients with pneumothorax or at risk for pneumothorax | Yes |
| Bed percussor | Hill ROM bed | Unstable ICU patients with excess pulmonary secretions | | | |

[a]*AxcanScandipharm, Birmingham, AL.*
[b]*DHD healthcare, Wampsville, NY.*

Positioning the patient requires the use of an adjustable bed, pillows or blanket rolls, and enough personnel to assist in moving the patient safely. Tissues, a sputum cup, airway suctioning equipment, and body substance barriers should be available to safely collect any secretions that are produced. The patient's face should always be in view to be able to monitor tolerance to treatment. Postural drainage may be used exclusively or in combination with other airway clearance techniques. If PD is used exclusively, each position should be maintained for 5 to 10 minutes or longer, if tolerated.[10] The clinical approach to adding additional airway clearance maneuvers such as percussion and vibration during postural drainage includes reexamination and utilization of the techniques until the secretions clear.[11] Precautions and

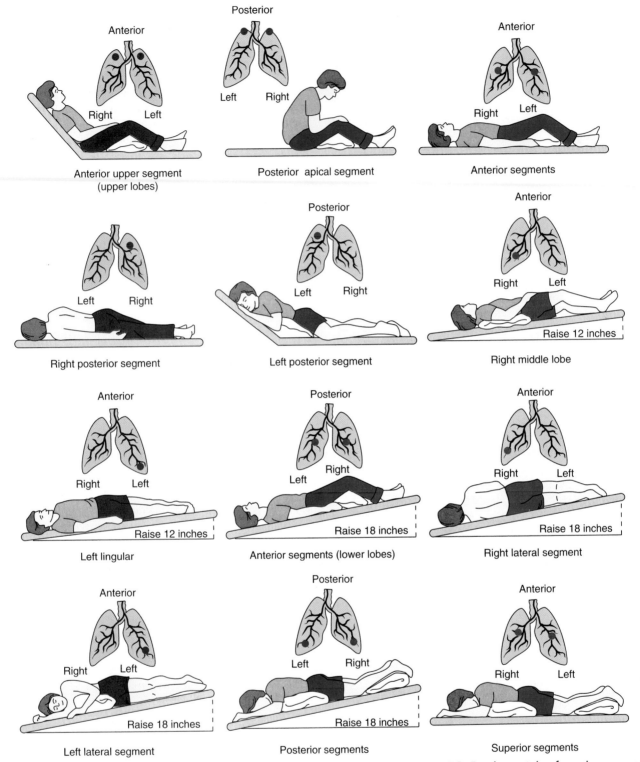

**Figure 17-1** Patient positions for postural drainage. (Modified from Potter PA, Perry AG: Fundamentals of nursing: concepts, process and practice, ed 4, St Louis, 1997, Mosby. In Wilkins RL. Egan's Fundamentals of Respiratory Care, ed 9. St. Louis, 2009, Mosby).

relative contraindications for percussion and vibration may be found in Box 17-2.

Priority should be given to treating the most affected lung segments first, and the patient should be encouraged to take deep breaths in the PD position and cough (or be suctioned)

between positions as secretions mobilize. The number of PD positions tolerated per treatment session will vary with each patient. If the patient can tolerate only two or three positions in a session, it is recommended that the clinician vary the PD positions in subsequent sessions in order to drain all

## Box 17-1

### Precautions and Relative Contraindications for Postural Drainage

| Precautions | Relative Contraindications |
|---|---|
| • Pulmonary edema<br>• Hemoptysis<br>• Massive obesity<br>• Large pleural effusion<br>• Massive ascites | • Increased intracranial pressure<br>• Hemodynamically unstable<br>• Recent esophageal anastomosis<br>• Recent spinal fusion or injury<br>• Recent head trauma<br>• Diaphragmatic hernia<br>• Recent eye surgery |

## Box 17-2

### Precautions and Relative Contraindications for Percussion and Vibration

| Precautions | Relative Contraindications |
|---|---|
| • Uncontrolled bronchospasm<br>• Osteoporosis<br>• Rib fractures<br>• Metastatic cancer to ribs<br>• Tumor obstruction of airway<br>• Anxiety<br>• Coagulopathy<br>• Convulsive or seizure disorder<br>• Recent pacemaker placement | • Hemoptysis<br>• Untreated tension pneumothorax<br>• Platelet count below 20,000 per mm³<br>• Unstable hemodynamic status<br>• Open wounds, burns in the thoracic area<br>• Pulmonary embolism<br>• Subcutaneous emphysema<br>• Recent skin grafts or flaps on thorax |

affected lung segments. PD positioning may also be coordinated with other procedures such as bathing, turning schedules for skin protection, or changing the bed linen. Signs of treatment intolerance include increased shortness of breath, anxiety, nausea, dizziness, hypertension, and bronchospasm.

### Percussion

Chest percussion aimed at loosening retained secretions can be performed manually or with a mechanical device (see Table 17-3). Care should be taken during percussion to apply the device to the affected lung segments individually and not just generally on the lungs. Manual percussion consists of a rhythmical clapping with cupped hands over the affected lung segment (Fig. 17-2, A).[12] Air is trapped between each cupped hand and the patient's chest with each clap. A hollow thumping sound should be produced. Slapping sounds indicate poor technique and may cause discomfort or injury to the patient. For caregivers unable to cup their hands, soft plastic percussor cups are available to be held in the hands and tapped over the patient's chest. Caregivers may also reduce their own fatigue by using a mechanical percussor. Mechanical percussion has been found to be similar in effectiveness to manual percussion.[13] Electrically or pneumatically powered percussion devices (Fig. 17-2, B) can enable patients to treat themselves independently as their medical condition improves. Patients may need assistance with treating the posterior lung fields; however, some mechanical percussor devices do percuss the posterior lung fields (see Table 17-3).

According to Downs, during manual percussion the hand is cupped with the fingers and thumb adducted.[14] The hands are clapped over the thorax while the wrists and elbows remain relaxed.[14] Percussion is performed during inspiration and expiration. The hands essentially "fall" on the chest in an even, steady rhythm between 100 and 480 times per minute. The amount of force need not be excessive and should be adjusted to promote patient comfort. Clapping on bony prominences such as the spinous processes of the vertebrae and the clavicles as well as surgical incisions and medical appliances should be avoided while performing percussion. Precautions and relative contraindications for percussion and vibration are listed in Box 17-2.

### Vibration

Vibration is an airway clearance technique that can be performed manually or with a mechanical device (see Table 17-3). As with percussion, vibration is utilized in postural drainage positions to clear secretions from the affected lung segments. To perform vibration, the palmar aspect of the clinician's hands are in full contact with the patient's chest wall, or one hand may be partially or fully overlapping the other (Fig. 17-3). At the end of a deep inspiration, the clinician exerts pressure on the patient's chest wall and gently oscillates it through the end of expiration. Manual vibration frequency has been reported to be 12 to 20 Hz.[15] This sequence is repeated until secretions are mobilized. Vibration may be a useful alternative to percussion in acutely ill patients with chest wall discomfort or pain. The clinician may assess depth and pattern of breathing during manual vibration. The pressure on the thorax exerted during vibration on expiration often causes a volume of air to be expired that is greater than what is expired during tidal breathing. This may encourage a deeper than tidal inspiration to follow and support a more effective cough. Mechanical vibration devices are also available for use; however, they may be more difficult to coordinate with the patient's breathing pattern.

### Cough Techniques and Assists

In the acute care setting, patients generally initiate a cough one of two ways: voluntarily or reflexively. Either way, an

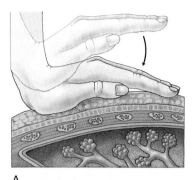

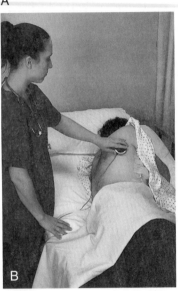

**Figure 17-2 A,** Percussion is performed with "cupped" hands. The chest is protected with a towel while the hands rhythmically clap the chest wall. Using the wrist to control the motion ensures a gentle clapping motion. **B,** Use of a vibrator for chest percussion. (**A** from Linton AD. Introduction to Medical-Surgical Nursing, ed 4. St. Louis, 2008, Saunders. **B** from Harkreader H, Hogan MA, Thobaben M. Fundamentals of Nursing: Caring and Clinical Judgment. 3rd ed. St. Louis, 2008, Saunders.)

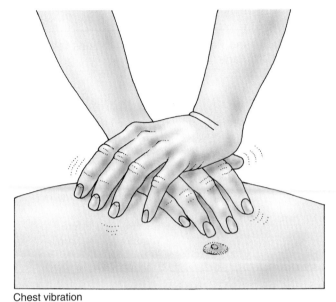

Chest vibration

**Figure 17-3** Hand placement for chest vibration. (From Linton. Linton AD. Introduction to Medical-Surgical Nursing, ed 4. St. Louis, 2008, Saunders.)

effective cough consists of four stages. The first stage entails an inspiration greater than tidal volume. Adequate inspiratory volumes for an effective cough are noted to be at least 60% of the patient's predicted vital capacity.[11] The second stage is the closure of the glottis. In the third stage, the abdominal and intercostal muscles contract, producing positive intrathoracic pressure. The fourth stage consists of the sudden opening of the glottis and the forceful expulsion of the inspired air. This forceful airstream is designed to carry any materials in its path up and out through the trachea to the mouth for expectoration.

---

**Clinical Tip**

In acutely ill patients with limited ability to follow instruction (i.e., "take a deep breath"), vibration may help facilitate deep breathing and huffing.

---

Successful intervention for the acutely ill patient with excessive bronchial secretions includes mobilization and removal of the secretions. Examination of cough effectiveness by the physical therapist is vital in determining the amount and type of intervention the patient will need for adequate removal of secretions. According to Massery, an effective cough should maximize the function of each of the preceding four stages.[11] Therefore, the patient should exhibit a deep inspiration combined with trunk extension, a momentary hold, and then a series of sharp expirations while the trunk moves into flexion. Any absence or deficiency in this sequence of events is likely to result in an ineffective cough. This condition can lead to retained secretions and, if left untreated, can progress to atelectasis, hypoxemia, pneumonia, and potentially respiratory failure. For acutely ill patients with reduced cough effectiveness and the ability to follow instructions, the first line of intervention is positioning and teaching proper coughing technique. Massery[11] recommends the following:

- Position the patient to allow for trunk extension and flexion.
- Maximize the inspiratory phase via verbal cues, positioning, and active arm movements.
- Improve the inspiratory hold by giving verbal cues and by positioning.
- Maximize intrathoracic and intraabdominal pressures with muscle contractions or trunk movement.
- Orient the patient to respective timing and trunk movements for expulsion.

Surgical patients will need to be instructed in how to splint their incision by applying pressure over it with a pillow or blanket roll during the expiratory phase of the cough. If pain is inhibiting the patient's ability to perform proper coughing techniques, pain medication should be administered in time for it to be effective during the patient's session with the physical therapist.

As an alternative to coughing, therapists can employ huffing to afford the most desirable result. Huffing is a deep inspiration followed by a forced expiration without glottal closure. It is often used in postoperative patients who find coughing to be too painful.

## Active Cycle of Breathing

The active cycle of breathing (ACB) consists of a series of maneuvers performed by the patient to emphasize independence in secretion clearance and thoracic expansion. Pryor[16] showed that this forced expiratory technique is as effective as airway clearance techniques performed by a therapist or caregiver. The cycle is as follows:

1. Breathing control: The patient performs diaphragmatic breathing at normal tidal volume for 5 to 10 seconds.
2. Thoracic expansion exercises: In a postural drainage position the patient performs deep inhalation with relaxed exhalation at vital capacity range. This inhalation can be coupled with or without percussion during exhalation.
3. Breathing control for 5 to 10 seconds.
4. Thoracic expansion exercises repeated three to four times.
5. Breathing control for 5 to 10 seconds.
6. Forced expiratory technique: The patient performs one to two huffs at mid to low lung volumes. The patient is to concentrate on abdominal contraction to help force the air out. The glottis should remain open during the huffing.
7. Breathing control for 5 to 10 seconds.

Precaution for this technique includes splinting for postoperative incisions. Hyperactive airways may become irritated with the deep breathing and huffing. Administration of inhaled bronchodilators prior to ACB may be helpful.

## Mechanical Aids for Coughing

Inspiratory and expiratory mechanical aids are devices and techniques that involve the manual or mechanical application of forces to the body or intermittent pressure changes to the airway to assist inspiratory or expiratory muscle function (Fig 17-4). The use of an inspiratory aid provides air under pressure during attempts to inhale (intermittent positive-pressure ventilation [IPPV]). The use of an expiratory aid provides a negative pressure (vacuum) to the airway via the nose and mouth during the patient's attempt to cough along with a manual thrust to the abdomen to further increase cough flows. Peak cough flows (PCF) most often exceed 160 liters per minute to be effective for coughing up secretions. PCF are increased by manually assisted coughing. If the vital capacity is less than 1.5 liters, insufflating or air

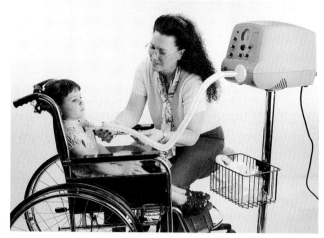

**Figure 17-4** Cough assist machine (see also Fig. 20-16). (From Frownfelter D, Dean E. Cardiovascular and Pulmonary Physical Therapy: Evidence and Practice. 4th ed. St. Louis, Mosby, 2006.)

stacking to the maximum insufflation capacity (MIC) becomes crucial to optimize cough flows. Once the person is insufflated to the MIC, an abdominal thrust is timed to the cough to increase the flow.[17]

Mechanical cough assist devices (J. H. Emerson Co., Cambridge, MA) deliver deep insufflations followed immediately by deep exsufflations. The insufflation and exsufflation pressures and delivery times are independently adjustable. An abdominal thrust can be applied in conjunction with the exsufflation. Maximal insufflation-exsufflation (MI-E) can be provided via an oral–nasal interface, a simple mouthpiece, or via an invasive airway tube such as a tracheostomy tube with an inflated cuff. One session consists of one or more sets of five cycles of MI-E followed by a short period of normal breathing or ventilator use to avoid hyperventilation. Insufflation and exsufflation pressures are almost always from +35 to +60 cm $H_2O$ to −35 to −60 cm $H_2O$. MI-E often eliminates the need for deep airway suctioning.

## Manual Hyperinflation and Airway Suctioning

Airway suctioning is performed routinely for intubated patients to facilitate the removal of secretions and to stimulate the cough reflex. Airway suctioning is indicated for patients with artificial airways who have excess pulmonary secretions and the inability to clear the secretions from the airway. If physical therapists reserve airway suctioning for those secretions that the patient is unable to clear from the airway independently or with assists, rehabilitation of cough effectiveness can be initiated prior to extubation. Patients with artificial airways can be instructed in huffing and cough assist techniques to enable them to progress to an effective cough, with the exception of glottal closure. Endotracheal and tracheal tubes prevent glottal closure from contributing to the intubated patient's attempts to clear secretions. Deep inspiration may be difficult for the intubated patient, in which case lung inflation by means of a manual resuscitator bag may be used.

The frequency of suctioning is determined by the amount of secretions produced in the airway. It is important to remember that the suction catheter can reach only to the level of the mainstem bronchi. Therefore, when lung secretions are retained in the small airways, postural drainage with percussion and/or vibration should be utilized to mobilize the secretions centrally, prior to suctioning. The fundamental steps of the suctioning procedure are as follows:

1. Administer supplemental oxygen to the patient via manual resuscitator bag or mechanical ventilator to increase arterial oxygenation (Fig. 17-5, A).
2. Monitor oxygen saturation with a pulse oximeter. Document drops in oxygen saturation below 90% and continue bagging with 100% $O_2$ until saturation is above 90% before continuing.
3. Adjust the pressure on the suction apparatus to 100 to 150 mm Hg, as needed.
4. Connect the vent end of the catheter to the suction tubing.
5. Don sterile gloves. Remove the catheter packaging without causing contamination; maintain sterility of any part of the catheter that will touch the patient's trachea.

6. Disconnect the patient from the ventilator or oxygen source.
7. Give five to ten breaths via manual resuscitator bag.
8. Quickly and gently insert the catheter into the tracheal tube without applying suction (Fig. 17-5, B). The diameter of the catheter should be no larger than one half of the diameter of the airway.
9. Stop advancing the catheter once gentle resistance is met at the level of the carina or one of the mainstem bronchi. Apply suction by placing a finger over the catheter vent.
10. Then, while applying suction, withdraw the catheter slowly, rotating the catheter to optimize the exposure of the side holes to the secretions.
11. Reconnect the patient to the oxygen source and reinflate the patient's lungs with the manual resuscitator bag or the ventilator for five to ten breaths.
12. Repeat Steps 6 through 9 until the airway is cleared of secretions, the patient is too fatigued to continue, or intolerance develops.

> **Clinical Tip**
>
> For patients who are able to exhale forcefully, the least invasive method of assisted airway clearance is preferable, with suctioning to be reserved as a last resort. To stimulate a cough, first attempt positioning, then active coughing or huffing. If this is not effective, attempt inspiratory facilitation with chest wall stretching or manual bagging. Lavage, or instillation of sterile saline solution to the airway, can be used in an attempt to stimulate a reflexive cough. MI-E with a cough assist device is another noninvasive technique to be tried, if available. If none of these less-invasive techniques is effective, then suctioning is indicated to clear the airway of secretions.

## Breathing Strategies, Positioning, and Facilitation

### Therapeutic Positioning Techniques and Ventilatory Movement Strategies

Employing therapeutic positioning techniques and ventilatory movement strategies can assist with the progression from dependence to independence in mobility and breathing.[18] The techniques involve selecting positions to assist the patient with efficient, diaphragmatic breathing patterns. The techniques are indicated for patients who have weakness of the diaphragm, are unable to correctly use the diaphragm for efficient inspiration, or who have inhibition of the diaphragm muscle due to pain. The training can begin in the intensive care unit during range-of-motion (ROM) activities. To facilitate inspiratory effort, the therapist instructs the patient to breathe in during shoulder flexion, abduction, and external rotation along with an upward eye gaze. The opposite is true during exhalation; the therapist uses shoulder extension, adduction, and internal rotation with downward eye gaze. In

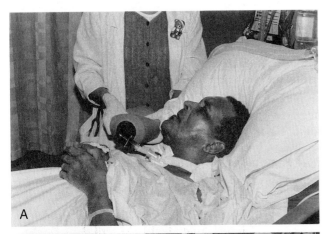

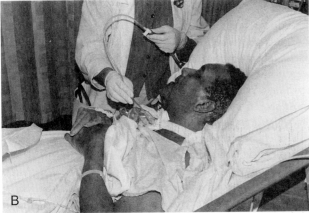

**Figure 17-5** Suctioning procedure. **A,** Administration of supplemental oxygen via manual resuscitator bag. **B,** Insertion of sterile catheter into tracheal tube.

addition, a posterior pelvic tilt position will encourage a diaphragmatic breathing pattern and optimize the length–tension relationship of the diaphragm. The patient should be encouraged to progress this technique to active shoulder ROM coupled with the breathing patterns previously described.

As the patient progresses from partial to full participation in therapy sessions, the therapist can use these positioning concepts during functional mobility activities (ventilatory movement strategies). While performing bed mobility, the patient is instructed to breathe out during rolling, and inhale as he or she extends the trunk to sit. This breathing pattern is used because trunk extension coincides with inspiration as trunk flexion does with exhalation. The progression of these techniques can be applied to transfers, ambulation, and stair climbing. The patient is instructed to breathe out when leaning forward to stand, and then to inhale when extending into the standing position. Orthopedic (fractures or dislocations) and vascular (deep-vein thrombosis, presence of invasive lines and monitors) dysfunctions require precautionary measures. If the patient has a central intravenous line, a peripheral intravenous line directly over a joint surface, or an intraaortic balloon pump, then extreme ROM positions are to be avoided in the joint beneath the catheters.

---

**Clinical Tip**
Range-of-motion activities are tailored to the patient's level of participation. If a patient cannot participate, then passive range of motion is performed. As the patient's ability to participate improves, then active-assisted range of motion is used and progressed to active range of motion. The last step is to add resistance, either manually or with small weights.

---

The position of the body greatly influences ventilation and respiration. As an acutely ill patient lies supine in a hospital bed, gravity will cause secretions to pool in the posterior aspects of the lungs. The supine position can reduce functional residual volume by up to 50%.[19,20] Positioning the patient in side-lying can reduce the pressure on the sacrum and other posterior bony prominences as well as assist in lung expansion and secretion removal. The therapist can perform this activity with the help of another person, or independently if necessary, depending on the size and the participation level of the patient. The therapist needs to use correct body mechanics during positioning of the patient. The following are step-by-step instructions for turning an intensive care patient onto the left side.

1. Vital signs are monitored continuously during patient positioning.
2. While the patient is still in the supine position, move the patient to the right side of the bed. It is advisable to use a draw sheet to avoid shearing forces on the patient's skin.

3. Arrange all tubes, lines, and cords so they will not be kinked or pulled during the rolling. Allow for adequate length.
4. If the patient is requiring the use of a ventilator, make sure that the endotracheal tube is secured with tape or the tracheostomy in held in place with cloth ties. The ventilator tubing should be emptied of residual water to prevent accidental lavage.
5. Place the patient's right foot over the left (unless orthopedic precautions dictate otherwise), and place a pillow between the knees.
6. Gently roll the patient onto the left side using the draw sheet. This will distribute the force more evenly against the patient's body. If two people are performing the positioning, then one person controls the head and upper trunk while the other person controls the lower trunk and the legs.
7. As the person at the head and trunk continues to hold the patient in the side-lying position with the draw sheet, the other person should place pillows and wedges behind the patient to keep the patient in this side-lying position. If the patient is alert and is strong enough, he or she can hold onto the bedrail while one person adds the external support.
8. If the patient is not alert, gently pull the left scapula out once the support has been added. This will prevent the patient from lying on the shoulder and potentially developing skin breakdown.

After the patient is positioned, the therapist can perform airway clearance techniques if indicated. Prone positioning has been shown to assist in mobilizing secretions, and allowing greater volumes of ventilation and increased $PaO_2$ for the patient with acute respiratory distress syndrome (ARDS).[21] This procedure requires the use of three people. The same first five steps for side-lying positioning are used, with the addition of placing a towel roll for forehead support and a pillow for chest support to where the patient's positioning end point will be. Then, the therapist continues with positioning using these steps.

- One person is positioned at the patient's head, another at the shoulders, and the third at the hip level. The person at the head should coordinate the timing for the roll.
- As the patient is rolled to the prone position, the person at the head is responsible for the integrity of the artificial airway and ventilator tubing, if applicable. If the patient can tolerate 10 to 20 seconds without mechanical ventilation, disconnection of the ventilator tubing can be made. If this is contraindicated (see Box 17-5), then

---

**Clinical Tip**
Before the therapist leaves the room, he or she should check all lines, tubes, and wires to make sure all are functioning as they were prior to the treatment session. All alarms need to be reset if they were silenced during the treatment session.

the person at the patient's head makes sure that no torque is placed on the trachea.[22]

Trendelenburg positioning is optimal for facilitating secretion drainage from the lower lobes of the lungs (Fig. 17-6). It can also be used to increase the blood pressure of a hypotensive patient, but is contraindicated for patients with congestive heart failure or cardiomyopathy. Reverse Trendelenburg position helps reduce hypertension and facilitate the movement of the diaphragm by using gravity to decrease the weight of the abdominal contents against it.

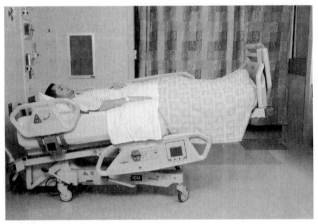

**Figure 17-6** Trendelenburg position. (From Perry AG. Clinical Nursing Skills & Techniques. 7th ed. St. Louis, Mosby, 2010.)

## Positioning for Dyspnea Relief

Dyspnea is defined as the sensation of difficult or labored breathing.[23] The patient may experience dyspnea at rest or after a period of activity. The therapist needs to be aware of other potential causes of dyspnea in addition to pulmonary dysfunction. These causes include myocardial ischemia, heart failure, and left ventricular hypertrophy.[23] The therapist should monitor for other signs and symptoms of intolerance to exercise with the occurrence of dyspnea (see Box 17-4). When dyspnea is caused by pulmonary dysfunction, a patient may inherently find a position that allows for easier ventilation. With the arms supported, the accessory breathing muscles can act on the rib cage and the thorax, allowing more expansion for inspiration. The accessory muscles are the sternocleidomastoid, the levators, the scalenes, and the pectoralis major muscles. When the patient leans forward on supported hands, the intraabdominal pressure rises and thus pushes the diaphragm up in a lengthened position. In view of the improved length–tension relationship, the diaphragm has an increased strength of contraction (Fig. 17-7). The patient often experiences relief of the dyspnea in this position.

## Breathing Exercises

A number of breathing strategies can be incorporated into treatment of a patient with cardiopulmonary impairments

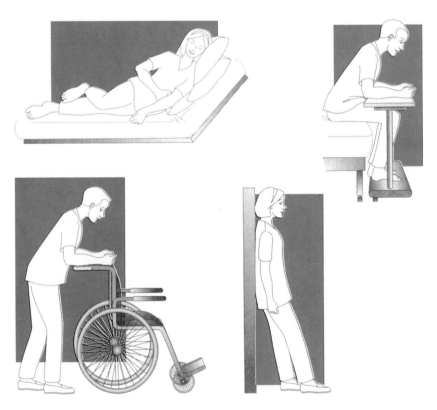

**Figure 17-7** Positioning for relief of dyspnea.

## Table 17-4 Indications and Outcomes for Breathing Strategies

| Strategies | Indications | Desired Outcome |
|---|---|---|
| Pursed lip breathing | Dyspnea at rest and/or with exertion, wheezing | Relief of dyspnea, improved activity tolerance, reduced wheezing |
| Diaphragmatic breathing | Hypoxemia, tachypnea, atelectasis, anxiety, excess pulmonary secretions | Eupnea, improved oxygen saturation, resolution of atelectasis, lower anxiety, mobilization of secretions |
| Lateral costal breathing | Asymmetrical chest wall expansion, localized lung consolidation or secretions, asymmetrical posture | Symmetrical chest wall expansion, mobilization of secretions, proper posture |
| Inspiratory hold technique | Hypoventilation, atelectasis, ineffective cough | Improved ventilation and perfusion matching, resolution of atelectasis, improved cough effectiveness |
| Stacked breathing | Hypoventilation, atelectasis, ineffective cough, pain, uncoordinated breathing pattern | Improved ventilation and perfusion matching, resolution of atelectasis, reduced pain, improved cough effectiveness |
| Paced breathing | Low endurance (especially with activities of daily livings and ambulation distance/stairs), dyspnea on exertion, fatigue, anxiety, tachypnea | Increased activity tolerance, reduced dyspnea, reduced fatigue, lower anxiety, eupnea |
| Upper chest inhibiting technique | Excessive use of accessory muscles during breathing | Reduced use of accessory muscles during breathing |
| Trunk counter rotation techniques | Impaired chest wall mobility, hypoventilation, impaired trunk muscle performance or tightness, ineffective cough | Increased chest wall mobility, increased ventilation and perfusion matching, improved trunk muscle length, improved cough effectiveness |
| Butterfly techniques | Impaired chest wall mobility, hypoventilation, impaired trunk muscle performance or tightness, ineffective cough | Increased chest wall mobility, increased ventilation and perfusion matching, improved trunk muscle length, improved cough effectiveness |
| Chest wall stretching | Impaired chest wall mobility, hypoventilation, Cheyne–Stokes breathing, paradoxical breathing, impaired trunk muscle performance or tightness, ineffective cough | Increased chest wall mobility, increased ventilation and perfusion matching, improved trunk muscle length, improved cough effectiveness |

(Table 17-4). Traditionally, the following techniques have been described for use in rehabilitation and outpatient settings; however, they can be useful in the acute care setting as well.

### Pursed-Lip Breathing

Pursed-lip breathing is used to decrease a patient's symptoms of dyspnea. It has been shown to slow a patient's respiratory rate, decreasing the resistive pressure drop across the airways, thus decreasing airway collapse during expiration.[24] Airway collapse during exhalation presents in the advanced stages of COPD. To employ pursed-lip breathing, a patient is instructed to inhale through the nose for several seconds with the mouth closed and then exhale slowly over 4 to 6

seconds through lips held in a whistling or kissing position. This can be done with or without abdominal muscle contraction.[25]

### Paced Breathing

Paced breathing is defined as "volitional coordination of breathing during activity." During rhythmic activities, breathing can be coordinated with the rhythm of the activity. During nonrhythmic activities, the patient can be instructed to breathe in at the beginning of the activity and out during the activity. This can be combined with pursed-lip breathing or diaphragmatic breathing. In the acute care setting, this technique can help the patient control his or her respiratory rate and associated feelings of dyspnea.[26]

## Inspiratory Hold Technique

An inspiratory hold technique involves prolonged holding of the breath at maximum inspiration. It can be used in conjunction with vibration techniques to aid in airway clearance.[27] It can also improve the flow of air into poorly ventilated regions of the lungs.[27] The patient is instructed to hold his or her breath (without using a valsalva maneuver) at the height of inspiration for 2 to 3 seconds[28] followed by a relaxed exhalation.

## Stacked Breathing

Stacked breathing is a series of deep breaths that build on top of the previous breath without expiration until a maximal volume tolerated by the patient is reached. Each inspiration is accompanied by a brief inspiratory hold.[29]

## Diaphragmatic Controlled Breathing

Diaphragmatic controlled breathing (with or without manual facilitation) can be used to manage a patient's dyspnea, reduce atelectasis, and increase oxygenation. This technique has been described as "facilitating outward motion of the abdominal wall while reducing upper rib cage motion during inspiration."[18] The physical therapist can assess a patient's skill with this technique by observation or measuring abdominal excursion. Patients should be instructed in diaphragmatic breathing in all positions as there is not necessarily carryover from one position to the next.[30] It is often easiest for patients to achieve a diaphragmatic breathing pattern while in the supine position. Once the patient has mastered the breathing pattern in supine, it can be attempted in sitting, then standing, then during activity.

Diaphragmatic breathing can be achieved through a series of activities designed to decrease accessory muscle use and increase recruitment of the diaphragm. The first consideration is positioning. Positioning the patient with a posterior pelvic tilt can help facilitate use of the diaphragm. In the acute care setting, simply placing a towel roll under the patient's ischial tuberosities can help achieve this position. Next, it is important to help the patient relax the accessory muscles by verbal and tactile cuing. It may also be helpful to use a contract-relax technique.

If the desired breathing pattern is not achieved using the above techniques, *sniffing* can be added to help engage the diaphragm. The patient is positioned to eliminate gravity, either in the side-lying or semi-Fowler position. The pelvis is positioned with a posterior tilt. The patient's hands are positioned on his or her abdomen for proprioceptive feedback and the patient is asked to sniff three times and then exhale slowly. The therapist notes whether the patient is demonstrating an abdominal rise or rise in the area of the accessory muscles and gives this feedback to the patient. Next, ask the patient to sniff twice and then progress to one slow sniff. If this technique is successful, the therapist focuses on instructing the patient to perform sniffing more slowly and quietly

until the patient is breathing in a relaxed manner. The patient is instructed to continue this technique independently. It may be useful as a relaxation technique or to control breathing during an activity such as ambulation.

In the acute care setting, the presence of incisions, lines, and drains may prohibit the use of manual facilitation techniques. If this is the case, the techniques listed above can be used to help improve a patient's breathing pattern and manage symptoms. If the patient's medical management does not contraindicate the use of manual facilitation, techniques such as diaphragmatic scoop, lateral costal breathing, upper chest inhibiting technique, thoracic mobilization techniques, and chest wall stretches can be used.

Another technique to help facilitate diaphragmatic breathing is the *scoop technique*. Again, the patient is positioned in either side-lying or the semi-Fowler position and with a posterior pelvic tilt. The therapist places his hand on the patient's abdomen and allows two to three breathing cycles to occur to become familiar with the patient's breathing pattern. Following exhalation, the therapist scoops his hand up and under the anterior thorax giving a slow stretch and subsequently instructs the patient to "breathe into my hand." The scoop stretch is repeated with each breath at the end of exhalation and the patient is instructed to "breathe into my hand" during inhalation. As this improves the patient's use of the diaphragm, the therapist's hand can be removed. To progress the technique, it can be done in supine, then sitting, then standing, then with activity. The therapist can use the scoop technique at the beginning of each new position and then remove his hand as the patient becomes proficient in the breathing pattern in that position.

## Lateral Costal Breathing

Unilateral costal expansion or bilateral costal exercises address one side or both sides, respectively, of the rib cage and corresponding intercostal muscles. Unilateral costal expansion exercises may be more useful in the treatment session with a patient who has a large incision from surgery on one side of the thorax. Splinting is a common reaction to incisional and postoperative pain. However, this may lead to decreased expansion on the respective side and prevent full alveolar ventilation. In addition, as incisions heal, they can bind to the underlying tissue and further limit chest wall expansion. Active range-of-motion (AROM) exercises mobilize the rib cage performed in conjunction with a variety of breathing techniques help prevent scar immobility. This exercise is most efficiently performed in a side-lying position with the uninvolved side against the bed. The patient brings the arm on the involved side into an abducted position to the level of the head. The therapist gives a stretch before inspiration and continues giving resistance through the inspiratory phase (Fig. 17-8). Any contraindications to lying on a particular side need to be acknowledged before using unilateral costal expansion. For example, a patient who has undergone a left partial or whole lung removal may have precautions against lying on the left side. Unilateral costal expansion

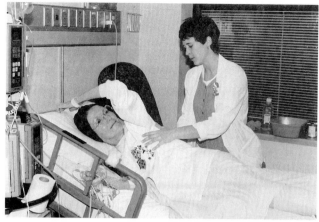

**Figure 17-8** Positioning for application of lateral costal breathing and chest wall stretching.

with resistance is also useful for the patients in the intensive care unit (ICU). These patients are often positioned in side-lying for respiratory and integumentary considerations. Bilateral costal expansion is performed with the patient in a semireclined or sitting position. In this technique, the therapist places both hands on the lateral aspects of the rib cage and gently applies pressure against the ribs during inspiration. The patient can also be taught to perform this exercise independently.

### Upper Chest Inhibiting Technique

Inhibiting the upper chest can help a patient recruit the diaphragm during inhalation. This technique should be used only after other techniques have been attempted. The patient is positioned in side-lying, three quarter supine or supine. A diaphragm scoop is used to facilitate the diaphragm while the therapist's other hand rests on the upper chest and moves with inhalation and exhalation. After assessing the patient's chest movement through a respiratory cycle, the therapist's arm follows the upper chest to the resting position on exhalation. When the patient inhales, the therapist's arm position does not move, thus applying pressure to the upper chest and resisting expansion. Add more pressure after each expiratory cycle until the patient increases lower chest breathing. When this occurs, encourage the patient to reproduce this breathing pattern and progressively release pressure on the upper chest with each breathing cycle while continuing to facilitate diaphragm movement with the other arm.[30]

### Thoracic Mobilization Techniques

If mobility of the thorax is restricted, it may be difficult for a patient to improve his or her breathing pattern through controlled breathing alone. It may be necessary to incorporate simple thoracic mobilization techniques to increase the ability of the thorax to expand during breathing. Simple positioning can be used to increase thoracic mobility. Placing a towel roll vertically down the thoracic spine while the patient is in a supine position can improve anterior chest wall mobility. Similarly, placing the patient in side-lying over a towel roll can increase lateral chest wall mobility. Upper extremity movement can be paired with each position to increase mobility. The upper extremity is either actively or passively elevated to further stretch the affected areas. This technique can be progressed to sitting or standing positions.

### Counterrotation

Counterrotation technique can increase tidal volume and decrease respiratory rate by reducing neuromuscular tone and increasing thoracic mobility. It is effective for (1) patients with impaired cognitive functioning following neurological insult, (2) young children who are unable to follow verbal cues, and (3) patients with high neuromuscular tone.[30] Briefly, this technique incorporates rotating the upper trunk to one side while the lower trunk is rotated in the opposite direction.[31] The patient is positioned in side-lying with knees bent and arms resting in front. The patient should be in a comfortable position to facilitate relaxation. The therapist stands behind the patient, perpendicular to the patient's trunk. With one hand on the patient's shoulder and one hand on the patient's hip, the therapist assesses the patient's breathing cycle. Next, the patient is log-rolled gently from the side-lying position toward prone. At the same time, the therapist is audibly breathing with the patient. As the technique progresses, the therapist gradually slows audible cuing for a decreased respiratory rate.

In phase two, the therapist moves to stand behind the patient near his or her hips and faces the patient's head, and then the therapist changes his hand position. If the patient is lying on the left side, the therapist slides his left hand to the patient's shoulder and his right hand to the patient's right gluteal fossa at the beginning of expiration. Then, the therapist can facilitate more complete exhalation, compressing the rib cage manually at the end of exhalation by pulling the shoulder back and down and the hip up and forward.

The opposite occurs during inhalation. The therapist slides his left hand to the patient's right scapula and his left hand to the patient's right iliac crest. During inhalation, the therapist stretches the chest by pulling the pelvis back and down and the scapula up and away from the spine.

Initially, this is done along with the patient's breathing cycle and respiratory rate but slows as the treatment progresses. Audible breathing cues slow along with the manual facilitation. The technique progresses by gradually decreasing manual input and then by eliminating verbal cues.[30]

### Butterfly

The butterfly technique is an upright version of the counterrotation technique and can be used if the patient has good motor control. The patient sits unsupported and the therapist stands either in front of or behind the patient. The therapist assists the patient with bringing his or her arms up into a butterfly position. The therapist breathes audibly with the patient. With inhalation, the therapist brings the patient's arms into increased shoulder flexion and lowers the arms during exhalation. The therapist then slows the audible breathing pattern and the facilitation of shoulder movement to encourage an increased tidal volume and decrease respiratory rate. The therapist can incorporate diagonal movement into the technique to facilitate increased intercostal and oblique abdominal muscle contractions.[30]

## Inspiratory Muscle Training

Inspiratory muscle training (IMT) is indicated for patients who exhibit signs and symptoms of decreased strength or endurance of the diaphragm and intercostal muscles. Signs and symptoms include, but are not limited to, decreased chest expansion, decreased breath sounds, shortness of breath, uncoordinated breathing patterns, bradypnea, and decreased tidal volumes.[32,33] Patients with respiratory muscle weakness or fatigue may have such diagnoses as COPD, acute spinal cord injury, Guillain–Barré syndrome, amyotrophic lateral sclerosis, poliomyelitis, multiple sclerosis, muscular dystrophy, myasthenia gravis, or ankylosing spondylitis.[33] In addition, IMT may be indicated for patients on mechanical ventilation to improve weaning from ventilation.

The goal of IMT is to increase the ventilatory capacity and decrease dyspnea. An IMT program has two parts: strengthening and endurance training. Each part will have increased or decreased priority according to the needs and medical condition of the patient. Concepts of ventilatory muscle training are the same as those for other skeletal muscle training, incorporating the concepts of overload, specificity, and reversibility.[34] The overload principle applied to endurance muscle training requires low load imposed over longer periods of time. Specificity refers to training the muscles for the function they are to perform, for example, resistance applied to inspiratory versus expiratory muscles. Training effects may be lost over time if training is discontinued.

The first step in any program is to teach the patient (if alert and oriented) the correct way to use the inspiratory muscles to ensure efficient inhalation. Including family members and support system members in the teaching can reinforce the program.

Weakness of a muscle is the inability to generate force against resistance. The length of the muscle affects the force output, as demonstrated in the length–tension curve. In the respiratory system, the strength of the diaphragm and other inspiratory muscles is measured as a function of standard pressure–volume curves.[35] Weakness of the diaphragm will decrease the negative inspiratory pressure generated by the patient, and thereby decrease the volume of air inhaled. Patients with COPD have hyperinflated lungs and a flattening of the diaphragm, which alters the length–tension relationship of this muscle. Fatigue of the inspiratory muscles, particularly of the diaphragm, will result in the failure to meet the demand for adequate alveolar ventilation. Hypoventilation will decrease the arterial partial pressure of oxygen

($PaO_2$) and increase the arterial partial pressure of carbon dioxide ($PaCO_2$), and can lead to acute respiratory failure.

The diaphragm is made up of all three types of muscle fibers, including slow-twitch oxidative (SO), fast-twitch oxidative glycolytic (FOG), and fast-twitch glycolytic (FG).[36–38] The adult diaphragm is approximately 55% slow-twitch fibers, compared with about 10% in the infant.[39] Fatigue is related to the SO fibers, whereas weakness is attributed to the FG fibers. When initiating physical therapy treatment, the therapist should realize that all fibers need to be addressed in the cardiopulmonary treatment program. While mechanically supported on a ventilator, the diaphragm can lose 5% of its strength per day.[40] When the patient begins the weaning process, the inspiratory muscles will gain endurance while performing inhalations without the assistance of the ventilator. Endurance training of the diaphragm will increase capillary density, myoglobin content, mitochondrial enzymes, and the concentration of glycogen. Overall, it will increase the proportion of fatigue-resistant slow-twitch fibers.[41,42] The recommendations include two to three daily sessions of 30 to 60 minutes of deep breathing concentrating on using a diaphragmatic breathing pattern.[18]

An early-stage IMT technique is sniffing. Sniffing naturally enlists the diaphragm. With the patient in a comfortable position such as side-lying or reclined, the therapist may assist the patient in placing both hands on the abdominal area to provide proprioceptive feedback. Then, in a relaxed tone of voice, the therapist instructs the patient to sniff quickly through the nose three times with slow, relaxed exhalations. The therapist gives feedback throughout this technique on the quality of sniffing, assessing whether the patient is showing a diaphragmatic breathing pattern. If the patient is able to perform this effectively, the progression of this technique is to reduce the number of sniffs from three down to one at an increasingly slower pace. The goal of this technique is to increase the awareness of correct use of the diaphragm. The technique progression continues until the patient shows the diaphragmatic breathing pattern at a normal rate and depth for all levels of functioning. According to Massery and Frownfelter, there is an 80% success rate, with patients affected by primary pulmonary pathologies or neurologic impairments.[18,43]

Strength training can be performed in a number of different ways, depending on the initial strength of the diaphragm. One method that can be utilized easily for the patient achieving tidal volumes of 500 mL or better is resisted inhalation. This can be performed manually by the therapist. The therapist has the patient assume a comfortable position as described earlier to promote diaphragmatic excursion. The therapist gently places the hands just below the rib cage on both sides of the patient's thorax. Before the patient initiates an inspiration, the therapist gives a small amount of resistance to the diaphragm by pushing gently up and in, and continues this pressure through the inspiratory phase. No resistance is given during exhalation. The therapist may also use weights for diaphragmatic strengthening. To evaluate if this is an appropriate method, the therapist first observes to determine if normal diaphragmatic excursion occurs at rest and then, with the addition of weights. The patient should be able to breathe comfortably and without accessory muscles for 15 minutes; if the amount of weight is excessive, the pattern of inspiration will become uncoordinated.[44] Several authors suggest that strength training in this manner should include two or three sets of 10 repetitions once or twice a day.[9] However, with either the manual or the weights method, the quality of the contraction needs to be monitored. The patient should not be "pushing" with the abdominal muscles against the resistance, which enhances the exhalation phase of breathing rather than the muscles of inspiration. For a patient with "fair or reduced" diaphragmatic strength (tidal volume less than 500 mL), active breathing exercises are indicated without resistance. A patient with poor strength will find it difficult to exercise with the head of the bed elevated; a supine position will prevent the abdominal contents from pushing up on the diaphragm and limiting its excursion.

Another form of resistive training utilizes specific hand-held training devices, such as the P-flex, DHD device, Threshold, or the Peace Pipe. The resistance is increased by decreasing the radius of the device's airway. The patient inhales through the device at a level that does not cause adverse effects, such as dyspnea or a drop in oxygen saturation, for a 15- to 30-minute session twice per day.[45] When this level is comfortable for the patient, then the resistance is gradually increased.

Much controversy has surfaced regarding the efficacy of IMT since its introduction into clinical practice. Evidence has been presented both supporting and dismissing IMT as a reliable treatment method. The major discrepancy may exist in the diagnosis for which this treatment is prescribed. A patient with insult to the lung tissue itself—for example, chronic obstructive pulmonary disease (COPD) or adult respiratory distress syndrome (ARDS)—may not tolerate IMT. IMT, which is a strengthening exercise, would increase the demand for oxygen delivery in the diseased lungs. However, a patient with a neuromuscular disease and intact lungs may be more likely to tolerate the increased oxygen demand and derive a benefit, as would the patient on mechanical ventilation who is trying to be weaned from the ventilator.

Deep breathing exercises are indicated for the patient with atelectasis, which is caused by hypoventilation and the collapse of alveoli in the lungs.[18] The use of an incentive spirometer is an effective way to practice diaphragmatic breathing and prevent or reverse atelectasis, and stimulate a cough (Fig. 17-9). Often, it is given to the patient preoperatively so he or she can practice deep breathing. Then after surgery, the patient may be able to perform this technique from memory as the effects of anesthesia start to diminish. The patient is instructed to perform deep breathing exercises with the incentive spirometer 10 times every hour to replenish surfactant, which is lost in the presence of atelectasis.[32] The patient needs to be instructed to perform a slow, relaxed breath through the mouthpiece. It is often helpful to have

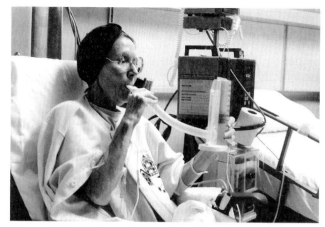

**Figure 17-9** Patient using an incentive spirometer.

the patient place a hand on the abdominal area to feel the diaphragm working in the correct way. If the patient is having a difficult time performing this technique, the therapist may place a hand over the patient's hand to facilitate the proper technique. Then the therapist should instruct the patient to perform the breathing slowly, with the abdomen rising out during inspiration. The goal is for the patient to be able to use the incentive spirometer independently without proprioceptive or verbal feedback. Alternatively, early mobilization has been shown to be as effective as deep breathing exercises after gallbladder and cardiac bypass surgery.[46–48]

Endurance training of the extremities is another technique that has been explored in an effort to increase ventilatory muscle endurance. Keens[48] studied pediatric patients with cystic fibrosis and found that upper extremity endurance training did increase the endurance of the ventilatory muscles. However, Belman and Kendregan examined the effects of upper and lower extremity training on ventilatory muscle endurance with adult patients with COPD and found no correlation.[49]

> **Clinical Tip**
> Surfactant production is reduced postoperatively, making patients at risk for serious pulmonary complications such as pneumonia and respiratory failure. Surfactants' role is to reduce surface tension and prevent alveolar collapse (atelectasis). Surfactant is produced by the type II pneumocytes in the alveoli of the lungs. By expanding the alveoli and stretching the type II pneumocytes with deep breaths, surfactant production is stimulated. Deep breathing is the most effective way to prevent alveolar collapse that, without intervention, can lead to more serious postoperative pulmonary complications.

## Special Considerations for Mechanically Ventilated Patients

Intubation and mechanical ventilation are required for most patients with acute respiratory failure. One of the main goals for these patients is to return to spontaneous breathing. The process of discontinuing mechanical ventilation is called weaning. Mechanical ventilation is a means of ensuring adequate gas exchange in a patient who is unable to do so without external support.[50] The benefits of weaning from mechanical ventilation in an expedient manner include minimizing iatrogenic complications, minimizing the duration of ICU stay, and preventing atrophy of the inspiratory muscles.[51] From the physical therapist's perspective, a mechanical ventilator is an assistive device capable of performing a wide range of support for the act of breathing. Acutely ill ventilated patients are typically seen with volume-cycled, positive-pressure ventilators although pressure-cycled ventilators may be used for patients at risk for barotrauma. Coordinating physical therapy interventions with the weaning process is critical for the patient to receive optimal benefit and successfully progress toward the goal of continuous spontaneous breathing.

Patients who are critically ill and mechanically ventilated often required sedative and analgesic drugs. The effects of these medications and the associated period of immobility can lead to complications including neuromuscular weakness, delirium, and impaired physical function. Studies in which intravenous sedation was stopped for a period each day to allow the patient to become alert showed a reduction in duration of mechanical ventilation, a reduction in ICU length of stay, and a reduction in complications associated with prolonged intubation and mechanical ventilation.[52,53] Pairing periods of sedation interruption with physical and occupational therapy has been shown to improve functional outcomes, reduce ICU-acquired delirium, and reduce duration of mechanical ventilation.[54]

## Weaning Criteria

The process of weaning begins with determining whether or not the patient meets a set of criteria. The factors listed in this section have been shown to indicate that the patient is a candidate to begin the weaning process.[55] The primary consideration for beginning the weaning process is resolution or relative resolution of the initial event or disease that led to acute respiratory failure. The patient's status should be maximized in regard to nutrition, metabolic stability, fluid and electrolyte balance, hemodynamic stability, and cardiac function. The patient should be afebrile and must demonstrate an improving or stable chest x-ray, and respiratory secretions should be manageable. Preferably the patient is alert and cooperative, but at the minimum he or she should be initiating breaths spontaneously. The patient should be psychologically ready for the weaning process. Specific respiratory parameters include the following:

- Adequate gas exchange with $FIO_2$ less than 50% and $SaO_2$ greater than 90% with a positive end-expiratory pressure (PEEP) of less than 5 cm $H_2O$.
- Negative inspiratory force of 20 to 30 cm $H_2O$.
- The ratio of respiratory rate to tidal volume (RR/VT) less than 105, with respiratory rate less than 35 breaths per minute. This ratio is an indicator of rapid shallow breathing and has been found to be the most accurate predictor of weaning failure.[56]

- Minute ventilation (VE = respiratory rate × tidal volume) less than 15 L/minute.
- During the wean, the patient will be monitored for respiratory rate, depth and pattern, ABG (arterial blood gas) values, pulse oximetry, cardiac rate and rhythm, and mental status changes.

The wean attempt will be terminated with any of the following signs of respiratory distress[51,52,56]:
- Respiratory rate greater than 35 breaths per minute
- Appearance of paradoxical breathing pattern, use of accessory muscles of respiration, or dyspnea
- Desaturation with $SaO_2$ less than 90%, any decrease of $PaO_2$, or increase in $PaCO_2$ of 5 mm Hg as monitored by ABG values, especially in the presence of acidosis with a pH less than 7.30
- Change in heart rate greater than 20 beats per minute, a change in blood pressure more than 20 mm Hg, angina, cyanosis, or cardiac arrhythmias
- Change in level of consciousness

## Methods of Weaning

Common methods of weaning currently utilized include intermittent mandatory ventilation (IMV), timed spontaneous breathing periods using a T-piece, and pressure support ventilation (PSV). Dries indicated superior outcomes with pressure support and T-piece weans in comparison to IMV weans.[57] With IMV, weaning is gradually achieved as the number of ventilator preset breaths is gradually decreased and the patient is progressively more responsible for breathing spontaneously. With a T-piece wean, the patient breathes spontaneously on supplemental $O_2$ for progressively longer periods of time. PSV augments the patient's inspiratory effort with pressure assistance. Weaning using this method gradually reduces the amount of pressure provided to assist the patient during spontaneous breathing.

## Intervention Considerations

Physical therapy interventions facilitate the weaning process by optimizing airway clearance and pulmonary function. Balancing the patient's energy expenditure during the weaning process with the added energy required for performing functional mobility activities or exercise is a challenge for the physical therapist. Communication between therapist, patient, and clinical care team is critical to the success of the weaning process for patients requiring prolonged mechanical ventilation (more than 5 days).

Developing a communication system with the patient is usually difficult, as most often mechanical ventilation interrupts the patient's verbal communication. In addition, many ICU patients have weakness and decreased coordination associated with critical illness which precludes the use of written communication. Further impairing communication is the presence of an oral endotracheal tube which interferes with lip reading. Simple means of communication such as eye blinks or head nods for answering to yes–no questions may be utilized, or available gestures and facial expressions can be a way for the patient to communicate needs. Whatever methods are deemed effective must be utilized consistently to further enhance reliability of communication, and they must be reinforced by all staff. Speech–language pathologists may evaluate swallowing and speech functions and provide treatment.

Once communication is established, tools for assessing dyspnea can be utilized. The simplest method for assessment is a yes–no question: Are you short of breath? This can be further qualified by using a numerical scale, similar to a pain scale, rating dyspnea from 0 to 10, with 0 indicating no shortness of breath and 10 indicating the worst imaginable shortness of breath.[58] Dyspnea is a clinical manifestation of work of breathing. Although dyspnea during the weaning process may not necessarily be correlated with decreasing respiratory function, it can be directly related to anxiety experienced by the patient, which in itself may lead to weaning failure.[59,60] The importance of emotional support and calm reassurance combined with positive feedback in facilitating the weaning process cannot be overemphasized.[51]

Airway clearance techniques discussed earlier in this chapter are also an important part of the weaning process. These techniques should be employed prior to the patient's specific weaning trials if presence of excessive secretions are impeding a successful wean. During weaning, these techniques remain a priority to assist in continued success with spontaneous breathing.

Biofeedback for increasing tidal volume and relaxation have been shown to reduce weaning time.[61] Breathing strategies, including manual hand placement on the abdomen for recruitment of the diaphragm, can be utilized in conjunction with watching the tidal volume monitor on the ventilator. The biofeedback screen can be positioned to give the patient visual feedback from inspiratory efforts. Breathing exercises with encouragement of slow, deep breaths and positioning can be used to normalize the breathing pattern and to keep the respiratory rate within preset limits.

Inspiratory resistance training has been demonstrated to improve respiratory muscle strength and endurance in patients with respiratory failure and has facilitated increased weaning success. Adrich demonstrated substantially lower mortality rates in the group weaned from mechanical ventilation.[62]

Mechanical advantage of the diaphragm muscle can be optimized by attention to positioning.[63] Creating a more normal length–tension relationship may be useful and can be achieved with manual facilitation of the diaphragm. This positioning will decrease the work of breathing and facilitate an efficient breathing pattern. Optimal positioning for the patient will vary with different individuals, with options including dangling at the edge of the bed, sitting in a chair, reverse Trendelenburg position and semi- to high Fowler position (see following discussion under Positioning).[54]

Optimizing communication with other health care professionals—namely, the nurse, respiratory therapist, and physician—during the weaning process is imperative for coordination of care. Timing of the physical therapy treatment is essential for optimizing patient success and meeting functional goals. This may mean that physical therapy is not indicated just prior to, during, or after a wean attempt in order to allow rest and minimal environmental stimuli. In contrast, the therapist may be urgently contacted to assist with positioning just prior to weaning, relaxation, or breathing exercises during a wean, or airway clearance techniques before, during, or after a wean to facilitate management of secretions.

---

**Clinical Tip**

Specific strategies may be discussed to help the patient realistically fit the exercise routine into a personal schedule. For example, range-of-motion exercises to regain full mobility can be incorporated into function. To ensure functional shoulder range of motion postoperatively, the patient can be encouraged to emphasize a stretch each time during the day when reaching, such as into a high cabinet. A stretch can also be incorporated when brushing his hair, while also utilizing the mirror for visual feedback. For another example, a postural drainage program can be done while reading, studying, or watching a favorite television program.

---

Special attention can be focused on preoperative teaching for prevention of pulmonary complications after major surgeries of the thoracic or abdominal cavity.[64-68] The benefits of teaching deep breathing and coughing exercises preoperatively include an increased level of alertness compared with postoperative status, and absence of pain. It is an opportune time to gather baseline data on functional level, discharge options, and social support. However, preoperatively, anxiety levels may be high, which could be a barrier to learning. An example preoperative session is provided here.

## Exercise

In the acute care setting, patients often have limitations in strength and endurance that prevent optimal functional mobility and efficient breathing patterns. Critical illness neuromyopathy is the most common peripheral neuromuscular disorder seen in the ICU[69] and often presents as profound extremity and respiratory muscle weakness.[69,70] Neuromuscular weakness can result from systemic inflammation, hyperglycemia, corticosteroid use and deconditioning associated with prolonged bedrest.[69,70] Survivors of critical illness have been shown to have persistent functional limitations 1 year after being discharged from the ICU.[71] Exercise, in the form of both endurance and strength training, in the acute care setting should be used to in an effort to both prevent and treat the negative neuromuscular sequelae of critical illness.

The goal of endurance training in acute care is to maximize the independence and efficiency by which the patient performs ADLs and functional mobility. The indications for mobilization and exercise are listed in Box 17-3. As a patient begins the functional mobility progression, the therapist must

---

**Box 17-3**

### Acute Conditions That Are Indications for Mobilization and Exercise

- Alveolar hypoventilation
- Pulmonary consolidation
- Pulmonary infiltrates
- Inflammation of bronchioles and alveoli
- Pleural effusions
- Acute lung injury and pulmonary edema
- Systemic effects of immobilization (see Table 17-1)

From Dean E. Mobilization and exercise. In Frown-felter D, Dean E (eds.). Principles and Practice of Cardiopulmonary Physical Therapy. 3rd ed. St. Louis, Mosby-Year Book, 1996.

---

### Table 17-5 Normal Adult Ranges for Cardiopulmonary Values at Rest

| Value | Normal Range |
| --- | --- |
| Heart rate | 50–100 beats per minute |
| Systolic blood pressure | 85–140 mm Hg |
| Diastolic blood pressure | 40–90 mm Hg |
| Respiratory rate | 12–20 breaths per minute |
| Oxygen saturation | >95% on $FIO_2$ |

---

**Box 17-4**

### Abnormal Responses to Exercise

- Heart rate increases more than 20 to 30 bpm above resting heart rate
- Heart rate decreases below resting heart rate
- Systolic blood pressure increases more than 20 to 30 mm Hg above resting level
- Systolic blood pressure decreases more than 10 mm Hg below resting level
- Oxygen saturation drops below prescribed level
- Patient becomes short of breath or respiratory rate increases to a level not tolerated by the patient
- ECG changes
- Nonverbal/nonvital signs of possible exercise intolerance:
  - Color changes
  - Diaphoresis
  - Increased accessory mm use
  - Agitation, nonverbal signs of pain

---

remember that the smallest amount of effort by the patient can cause an abnormal exercise response in some cases, thereby stressing the cardiopulmonary system. Using such parameters as heart rate (HR), systolic and diastolic blood pressure (SBP, DBP), oxygen saturation ($SaO_2$), respiratory rate (RR), and electrocardiograms (ECG) gives the therapist important information on how the patient is tolerating the activity. Normal ranges for these physiologic parameters are listed in Table 17-5.

## Components of Exercise: Intensity, Duration, Frequency, and Modes

The acute care patient's response to activity or exercise is dependent on the body's ability to meet the oxygen transport demand. Monitoring cardiopulmonary parameters before, during, and after activity allows the therapist to provide the safest and most effective treatment intervention. In addition to these parameters, signs and symptoms of exercise intolerance that occur during physical therapy treatment indicate that the intervention needs to be stopped or modified. Signs and symptoms of exercise intolerance are listed in Box 17-4. The therapist also needs to be aware of the patient's current medications and their effect on exercise response. A β-adrenergic blocker medication, for example, suppresses the expected heart rate increase with exercise (see Chapters 14 and 15 on medications).

Heart rate is most commonly measured at the radial artery in the wrist. However, this may be hard to detect in patients with cardiopulmonary disease, so the carotid or brachial artery can be used, or the therapist can use a stethoscope over the heart. The heart rate should be measured for 30 seconds to 1 minute. Level I cardiac rehabilitation exercise heart rate guidelines are 12 to 24 bpm above the resting heart rate, unless the patient is taking β-adrenergic blocking medications.[72] With these medications, heart rates do not increase as expected during exercise. Monitoring the rate of perceived exertion (see Box 17-4) or level of dyspnea would be an acceptable alternative in this case. If the patient cannot report RPE, look for symptoms of fatigue and intolerance of activity and other nonverbal indications (other than vitals) of activity intolerance.

Blood pressure is measured at the brachial artery with a sphygmomanometer, with the cuff placed $2\frac{1}{2}$ inches above the antecubital space. The bladder of the cuff is placed over the brachial artery and should cover approximately 80% of the patient's upper arm. If the cuff is too narrow, then the blood pressure will read high, and if the cuff is too wide, the blood pressure will read low. The cuff should be at the level of the heart, and the patient's arm should be relaxed.

Systolic blood pressure is expected to rise in direct proportion to the level of exertion performed. A hypertensive response to low-level exercise (over 160/90 mm Hg) in the patient who is at least 3 days post–myocardial infarction may be indicative of cardiac ischemia.[73] There should be an increase of 7 to 10 mm Hg for each metabolic equivalent of energy expenditure (MET). Level I cardiac rehabilitation remains in the 1 to 3.5 MET range.[73] The failure of the SBP to rise (when individuals are NOT on β-blockers) is a sign of a severe pathologic condition, such as aortic stenosis or poor left ventricular function.[9,74] Patients with recent coronary artery bypass surgery may also show an abnormal BP response to activity.[74] Diastolic BP should not change significantly with activity.[75]

Respiratory rate should be measured at rest and during activity. It is best if the patient is not aware of the therapist taking this vital sign. Otherwise, the therapist may not obtain a true reading; the patient may subconsciously or consciously alter the breathing pattern and rate. The respiratory rate should rise proportionally to the workload.

Oxygen saturation ($SaO_2$) is measured with a pulse oximeter. The physician should determine a minimum acceptable saturation level that the therapist then uses to determine exercise or functional mobility training and provide titration guidelines, should the patient's $SpO_2$ level decrease with activity. Typically, the saturation level is to remain between 90 and 94% for acute respiratory problems, with higher minimum levels (96% to 97%) set for acute cardiac conditions. If a patient has supplemental oxygen, the amount of oxygen given must be adequate to keep the saturation at the prescribed minimum level (usually ≥90%). The physical therapist has the responsibility to monitor this level during activity when oxygen consumption rises (Fig. 17-10). If the $SpO_2$ drops below the minimum threshold, the therapist increases the amount of oxygen to keep the saturation in the prescribed range. However, in a very small subset of patients with COPD, oxygen may reduce the hypoxic drive in patients and the $PCO_2$ may increase. If the patient is having difficulty maintaining appropriate saturation levels, the therapist should have the patient rest or reduce the intensity or duration of the exercise first and communicate these findings with the patient's physician.

> **Clinical Tip**
>
> By law in many states, oxygen is considered a drug that must be prescribed by a physician (or practitioner licensed to prescribe it). Accordingly, changes in the amount of $O_2$ a patient receives should also be directed by the physician. However, often, a prescription will read "Titrate $O_2$ to maintain $SpO_2$ >90%," in which case the physical therapist could adjust the $O_2$ according to the patient's need. Consult with the referring physician if you think a similar order might be appropriate for your patient.

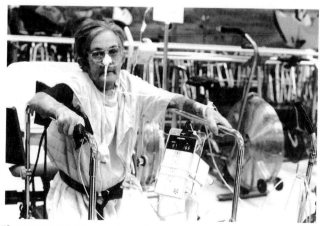

**Figure 17-10** Monitoring of oxygen saturation during activity. (monitor hangs from walker).

## Intensity

Acute care patients' responses to exercise intensity can be measured in several ways. One subjective scale that is used to monitor intensity is the Borg rate of perceived exertion (RPE).[74] The therapist can monitor exercise intensity by asking the patient to rate the intensity of the activity using the Borg scale. Warm-up and cool-down should remain in the 9 to 11 range, whereas peak activity should be within the 13 to 15 range. An RPE level of 12 to 13 equals approximately 60% of maximum heart rate and a level of 16 equals about 85%.[9] A strong correlation exists between RPE, heart rate, and work rate among patients taking β-adrenergic blockers; this group of medications can reduce the maximum heart rate by 20% to 30%, making traditional objective methods of interpretation of exercise response ineffective in this patient population.[76]

Another method of determining intensity of exercise is by monitoring levels of shortness of breath using the dyspnea index (DI).[9] The following is a description of implementation of the DI. A patient takes a deep breath and then counts to 15 slowly. The number of breaths the patient requires to count to 15 is the dyspnea index. During warm-up and cool-down, it should take the patient with normal lung function 1 to 2 breaths to reach 15, with that rate going up to 3 breaths for the peak activity.

Monitoring the acute care patient for subjective complaints of angina during treatment is important. Angina correlates with ECG changes, including ST-segment depression or elevation. Table 17-6 lists the stages of stable angina. Stable angina appears to occur at a consistent rate pressure product (RPP) during exercise.[75]

## Duration

Duration is the amount of time that a patient can tolerate performing a certain activity. The patient's cardiovascular response will help determine the desired duration of activity during the inpatient exercise or mobility session. The therapist may progress a patient from 5 minutes on a lower extremity ergometer to 15 minutes at a time within 3 or 4 days, for example. This can be repeated 2 or 3 times per day as tolerated and should be performed six or seven times per

### Table 17-6 Stages of Stable Angina

| Stage | Description |
|-------|-------------|
| 1 | Initial perception of discomfort |
| 2 | Increase in the intensity of Level 1 or the radiation of pain to other areas (jaw, throat, shoulders, arms, or other body parts) |
| 3 | Relief is obtained only through cessation of activity |
| 4 | Infarction pain |

*From Atwood JA, Nielsen DH. Scope of cardiac rehabilitation. Phys Ther 65:1812–1819, 1985.*

week.[72] Patient education is vital in this stage, so that the patient can begin to self-monitor HR, RR, RPE, and DI. Approximately 3 to 4 days after admission for an acute asthma attack, young patients were able to exercise for 5 minutes at 50% $VO_2$ without a significant change in peak expiratory flow, mean arterial oxygen tension, and mean alveolar–arterial oxygen difference.[77] For acute patients nearing the end of their hospital stay, a 6-minute walk test may be performed. Progress is measured by increases in the distance walked. The patient can also perform this test at home, or possibly at a mall or fitness center, to further assess progress and increase motivation in complying with a home exercise program.

## Frequency

Usually, in the acute care patient population, multiple short intervals of exercise followed by rest periods are tolerated better than one long session of exercise on a given day. The therapist may accomplish this by performing airway clearance techniques first in the morning and then using the afternoon treatment session for functional mobility or other exercises.

## Modes of Exercise

Mode refers to the method of exercise or technique that is to be used for training. In the acute care setting, most patients have limited exercise capacities because of their medical or surgical conditions. Therefore, in order to maximize independence, physical therapists often choose functional activities as the preferred mode of exercise for patients in acute care. Examples of activities that could be performed in the hospital are bed mobility, standing, transfers, ambulation, stairs, stationary bike, pedal exerciser or restorator, recumbent bike, upper body ergometer, and treadmill.

In the acute care setting, a patient may not be able to complete a 6-minute walk test. A 3-minute walk test may be used[78] instead, or any period of time can be used, as long as it is used consistently. The objective measure is the distance walked in a specified time, which can then be used to show progress in a patient's level of endurance.[78]

> **Clinical Tip**
> A patient with decreased venous return, as in congestive heart failure, may need to start an exercise program in a semi-Fowler position so that venous return is not compromised further by gravity and blood pooling in the lower extremities.

## Functional Mobility Training

Functional mobility training may be initiated as soon as the patient can roll bilaterally in the bed and maintain blood pressure and oxygenation parameters. Before the treatment of a patient in the ICU, however, the therapist should become familiar with the emergency procedures of each individual unit in addition to alarms from ventilators and monitoring devices. A check of the patient's medical status, including laboratory values, x-ray reports, vital signs, last dosage of medications, and past medical/surgical history, is warranted. It has been found that 75% of patients admitted for cerebrovascular disease also have coronary artery disease (CAD), but only 25% to 48% of these patients have a history or prior diagnosis of CAD.[9] On entering the patient's room, the therapist should look at positioning and lengths of lines, tubes, and catheters so they can be monitored and protected. Optimally, the therapist will coordinate activities with other disciplines involved with the care of the patient. This arrangement could mean that the therapist will set up a time with the nursing staff the day prior to the start of physical therapy, so that the patient is ready to start at the predetermined time. The goal of functional mobility progression is to have the patient perform as much of the activity as he or she can for as long as possible. The clinical decision making for activity progression is based on the patient's response.

## Bed Mobility

Beginning an exercise program often starts at the patient's bedside with the first level of functional mobility, bed mobility. One of the first activities that should be emphasized is bridging. The act of bridging helps with placement and removal of the bedpan, linen changes, and positioning in bed. This activity can be a first step of independence for the patient.

Next, the therapist can have the patient actively assist with rolling. If the therapist is using airway clearance techniques, the therapist can instruct the patient in rolling to position for this technique. Mechanically ventilated, critically ill patients show a 40% to 50% increase in oxygen consumption during chest physical therapy combined with rolling.[79-81] The therapist should bring the bedrail to the most upright position so the patient can use it to assist with the activity.

The patient may then be progressed to sitting at the edge of the bed, or dangling. The therapist should be mindful of proper body mechanics during this stage of functional mobility. The therapist may want the assistance of other staff or may raise the bed up to a level that prevents a forward flexed posture. As the patient is sitting on the edge of the bed, the thorax can move in all planes and the patient has the opportunity to stretch the muscles of the thorax. The patient's tidal volume increases, as well as respiratory rate. Again, the patient's vital signs and response to the activities need continuous monitoring throughout each stage of functional mobility progression.

## Transfers and Ambulation

Once the patient is able to sit at the edge of the bed unsupported for 5 minutes and can perform full knee extensions bilaterally for at least 3 minutes with acceptable responses in vital signs, the patient may progress to standing and ambulating. The use of the four-wheeled walker (Fig. 17-11) allows the patient to walk with support and the availability of a fold-down seat if it is needed. The patient does not need to

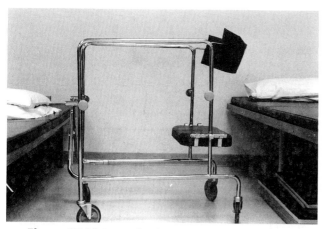

**Figure 17-11** Four-wheeled walker for ambulation.

---

**Box 17-5**

**Contraindications or Precautions for Advancing Functional Mobility**

- Untreated deep-vein thrombosis
- Unstable vital signs
- Patient not able to follow commands
- High ventilatory support (for removing the patient from the ventilator for mobility)
  - Contraindication: PEEP or CPAP > 10 cm $H_2O$
  - Precautions: PEEP or CPAP > 5 cm $H_2O$ PAP > 50 cm $H_2O$ minute ventilation > 15 L/min
- Other orthopedic, vascular, or neurologic injury that requires alternative bed activities

---

be extubated to start ambulation training. Contraindications or precautions for advancing functional mobility are listed in Box 17-5.

If needed, the patient should be educated on how to use the walker, complete with verbal and visual instructions, as well as demonstration. After the decision has been made that an intubated patient is ready to use the walker, the therapist must arrange for sufficient amounts of assistance. One person needs to assist the patient physically during ambulation while another is responsible for bagging the patient with a self-inflating bag connected to supplemental oxygen. A portable ventilator may also be used, if available. A third person is recommended for pushing intravenous poles and watching for adequate slack on IV lines. A gait belt is warranted for the patient's and the therapist's safety. The therapist should note resting vital signs, including oxygen saturation. Vital signs are monitored frequently, with cessation of activity if warranted by abnormal responses to heart rate, blood pressure, $SpO_2$, or fatigue by the patient. The progression of this activity is based on the patient's response.

Once the patient is extubated, the therapist may continue with the wheeled walker or progress the patient to the next least restrictive assistive device as indicated. The therapist continues to use other personnel according to the level of

independence of the patient and the amount of additional IV poles that need to be advanced with the patient. If a patient depends on supplemental oxygen during rest, then oxygen saturation levels need continued monitoring before, during, and after ambulation, with oxygen titration to keep $SpO_2$ within the recommended range. All vital signs should be monitored before, during, and after ambulation.

As a patient progresses in ambulation, the therapist and the patient work toward goals of increasing ambulation distance and decreasing the levels of assistance. It may be the goal of the patient to ambulate independently without an assistive device or oxygen. The therapist needs to assess whether this is an attainable goal within the acute hospital setting and must determine the patient's course of action to attain these goals.

## Injury Prevention and Equipment Provision

Patient safety is paramount in all areas of physical therapy. Physical therapists and physical therapist assistants working in acute care with patients who have cardiovascular and pulmonary impairments must monitor patients closely to determine how the patient is responding to physical therapy interventions. Failure to monitor relevant parameters such as heart rate, electrocardiograph, blood pressure, respiratory rate, oxygen saturation, and pain level could result in serious injury or worsening of the patient's condition. Signs and symptoms such as shortness of breath, chest pain, dizziness, lightheadedness, cyanosis, pallor, diaphoresis, nausea, and headache in response to interventions are all cause for concern as well as modification or cessation of the intervention. Level of patient acuity can vary from day to day or hour to hour in the hospital setting. Therefore, it is important for clinicians to choose to monitor one or more relevant parameters and note any signs or symptoms before, during, and after providing interventions.

Acutely ill patients with cardiovascular and/or pulmonary impairments often have multiple comorbidities. Determining the exercise progression for a patient with a recent stroke recovering from acute pneumonia can be a challenge. Published guides that provide a classification system of standardized MET (metabolic equivalent of task) may form a basis for estimating energy cost of physical activity in individuals but are not intended to determine precise energy cost in ways that account for differences in body mass, age, efficiency of movement, and environmental conditions.[82] By starting at a low level of exercise, progressing slowly, and monitoring the patient's response, the clinician can progress the patient safely and effectively. Use of assistive devices such as a wheeled walker with a seat and oxygen tank holder provides the patient with balance support as well as energy conservation. Other devices that may provide reduced energy demand and safety include canes, front-wheeled walkers, dynamic orthoses, sliding boards, mechanical lifts, and power wheelchairs.

## Patient Education

Patient and caregiver education is an important physical therapy intervention in the acute care setting. Patient education has been shown to decrease length of stay,[83] decrease patient anxiety,[84,85] increase quality of life,[86] increase adherence with medical advice,[87] and increase the patient's participation as an active member of the health care team.[88]

Patient education has been defined as cognitive improvement that results in a positive change in health behavior.[89] This can begin by setting educational goals with the patient or caregivers, and documenting these goals in an objective, measurable, and functional manner. The therapist should discuss these goals with the patient and caregiver to ensure they are realistic and applicable. A sample goal for an airway clearance program for a cystic fibrosis patient may be, "Patient's caregiver independently completes percussion and postural drainage to assist in airway clearance." The caregiver's independence with the specific techniques can then be observed by the therapist and documented, or verbally assessed if demonstration is not possible. An example of a functional educational goal for exercise with a cardiopulmonary patient might be, "Patient independently monitors self with exercise by accurately taking heart rate and stating his functional heart rate limits for rest (70 to 90 beats per minute) and exercise (80 to 120 beats per minute)." If a patient is unable to accurately take his own heart rate, the goal may be, "Patient independently monitors self with exercise using the RPE scale and is able to maintain an exertion level of 13 to 15 during the peak activity period." The accuracy of the patient's reported RPE level can be assessed by correlation with the heart rate taken by the therapist during the peak activity period.

When preparing to teach a patient or caregiver, the physical therapist must assess the learner to determine areas of knowledge to avoid unnecessary duplication and areas where further education is needed. The learning style should be taken into account, whether it is visual, auditory, or kinesthetic or a combination of styles. The therapist should inquire about the patient and caregiver expectations for learning and tailor the education to the learner's needs and abilities in several domains.[89] These domains include the following:

- Perceptual. The learner's perceptual needs must be considered in order to ensure the ability to receive input and comprehend the material presented. This would include speaking of adequate volume and clarity for learners that are hard of hearing, or providing visual aids such as larger print or personal prescription glasses for visual information.
- Cognitive. If the patient is unable to cognitively comprehend the educational material because of memory deficits, then using repetition or providing written material as a backup of information may help to compensate. If the patient is still unable to comprehend, then the material should be taught to a caregiver. In general, materials should be written at an eighth-grade reading level.

- Motor. If the motor skills are deficient, practice and continued coaching with intrinsic and extrinsic feedback can contribute to motor learning.
- Affective. The affective domain includes a patient or caregiver's attitudes, belief system, and motivation levels. It is more difficult for a patient to learn when not motivated to do so. If teachings threaten cultural or religious beliefs, this conflict may be a detriment to learning.
- Environment. Environmental factors should also be taken into consideration, as it may be difficult for a patient to learn in a noisy environment or while in a position that is uncomfortable or painful.

It is advisable to invest time in planning the implementation of the educational program. Does the patient population or material to be covered lend itself to a group teaching and learning situation? Is it cost effective and practical to do a group teaching? Does the patient or caregiver learn best by reading, watching a demonstration, physically performing the task, or a combination of methods? Make sure to have written and teaching demonstration materials immediately available, if used.

Facilitating patient adherence to exercise programs can create a challenge for the physical therapist. Sluijs, Kok, and van der Zee have suggested that the three main factors contributing to noncompliance are the barriers that patients perceive, lack of positive feedback, and perceived helplessness.[85] Barriers often reported are lack of time, fatigue, pain, lack of motivation, or difficulty fitting exercise into a daily routine. These issues need to be discussed at length with the patient during development of the program so that adjustments can be made to adapt the program to each individual, eliminating as many barriers as possible.[90] This may require compromising, with prescribed frequency from three times per day to one time per day to minimize fatigue and time commitment required. The patient should not feel pain during exercise; if pain is experienced, modification of the program is necessary to eliminate this barrier to adherence. A family member may be recruited as a coach or a partner to help keep the patient motivated to complete the exercise program, or a more structured program such as cardiac or pulmonary rehabilitation programs (see Chapters 18 and 19) can be utilized to promote adherence.

Finally, the therapist should evaluate the effectiveness of the education program.[89] This may be done formally by written or verbal testing, or informally by discussion or observation (Box 17-6). If postdischarge teaching is indicated, the physical therapist can refer the patient to other health care professionals, to community organizations, or other resources.

## Discharge Planning

With length of hospital stays decreasing dramatically, discharge planning has become a crucial part of the physical therapist's role in the acute care setting.[91,92] This role is shifting and expanding from providing interventions to acting as

## Box 17-6

### Sample Preoperative Session

"Hello, Mrs. Hunt, I am Erica, from Physical Therapy. I am here to talk with you about your upcoming surgery. First of all, what do you prefer that I call you? Have you ever had physical therapy before?" Here I offer a general overview of physical therapy and the purpose of this education session. "I am here to teach you a little bit about what to expect after your surgery and to teach you your responsibilities and expectations of you after the surgery to help prevent postoperative complications. Your main responsibility after the surgery is to do a lot of deep breathing and coughing to keep your lungs healthy. The deep breathing makes sure air is getting to all parts of your lung to prevent collapse and to make it easier to clear secretions. General anesthesia has a depressant effect on your body and makes your respirations slower and more shallow. As soon as you can, begin taking deep breaths." Specific techniques for breathing can be discussed, including diaphragmatic breathing, lateral costal expansion, unilateral expansion, and use of an inspirometer (see Fig. 17-9). Mention to the patient that a written handout that explains these techniques in detail will be provided. "Coughing to clear your lungs is another very important responsibility to prevent the opportunity for pneumonia to develop. The anesthesia has a dehydrating effect, making the mucus thicker and harder to clear. You will also have an abdominal incision, which may make it uncomfortable to cough. Utilize available pain medication and support your incision site with a pillow." Effective technique for coughing can be demonstrated, followed by having the patient demonstrate the technique (Fig. 17-12). This is an excellent opportunity to assess cough strength. "In addition to deep breathing and coughing, it is also important to learn a few simple exercises for your legs to help maintain muscle tone and circulation." Ankle pumps, quadriceps sets, and gluteal sets can then be taught. "The first day after your surgery we will work together to regain your full range of motion, check your posture, develop a walking program that you can continue at home for fitness, and return to activities of daily living."

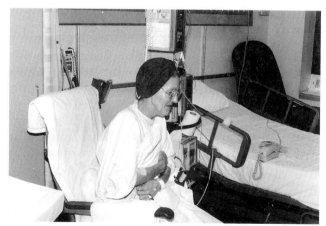

**Figure 17-12** Patient supporting incision site with a pillow to maximize comfort.

a consultant, offering recommendations on the patient's current status and rehabilitation potential, discharge destination, activity tolerance, and equipment needs. Anticipating the patient's discharge needs must often be included in the initial physical therapy visit. Because of the increased acuity level of patients being discharged from the acute care setting, an increasing involvement of family members is needed in determining the site for the next level of care. The therapist is often responsible for interpreting information from the patient's performance and the family support system as part of the discharge plan.

During the initial physical therapy evaluation, the patient's current level of function is evaluated and a prognosis is made regarding his or her potential abilities. Determination of the patient's rehabilitation potential has a large bearing on the discharge disposition. This may include preparing the patient for discharge home or for the next level of care, whether that level is acute rehabilitation, subacute rehabilitation, or long-term care. Fig 17-13 offers an example of a decision-making tree for determining discharge destination, taking into consideration accessibility of the home (including number of stairs, presence or absence of a railing, location of bedroom and bathroom, and wheelchair accessibility) and family or social support available. There must be precision in aligning the amount of realistic family or social support available with the amount of assistance the patient requires. This amount of assistance can vary from weekly help with shopping and laundry to 24-hour maximal assistance. Family members will need to be instructed in the level of assistance required by the patient for specific activities of daily living and the home physical therapy program, if needed.

In many acute care settings a discharge planner, often a nurse or a social worker, has the role of arranging a variety of health support services needed after discharge and coordinating the discharge process. This role may include services over a broad spectrum, such as home physical or occupational therapy, home skilled nursing service, home health aides to provide basic care such as bathing, community support services (i.e., meal delivery), and emergency monitoring services for safety checks.

Physical therapists are also involved in securing durable medical equipment to meet a patient's needs. This may include recommending equipment that is ordered by another health care professional, issuing the equipment from department supplies, or contacting a vendor to supply and deliver needed equipment. Insurance coverage is often an integral part of decision making, as is discussion with the patient on what items will be most appropriate.

Because a patient's status may change on a daily basis, this discharge plan must be frequently reassessed and modified according to the patient's improvement or lack thereof. As a result of this ongoing assessment, a crucial responsibility of the therapist is to communicate these updated recommendations to other members of the health care team. It must be remembered at this point that the most important member of the health care team is the patient. The therapist's professional opinions must be discussed with the patient and

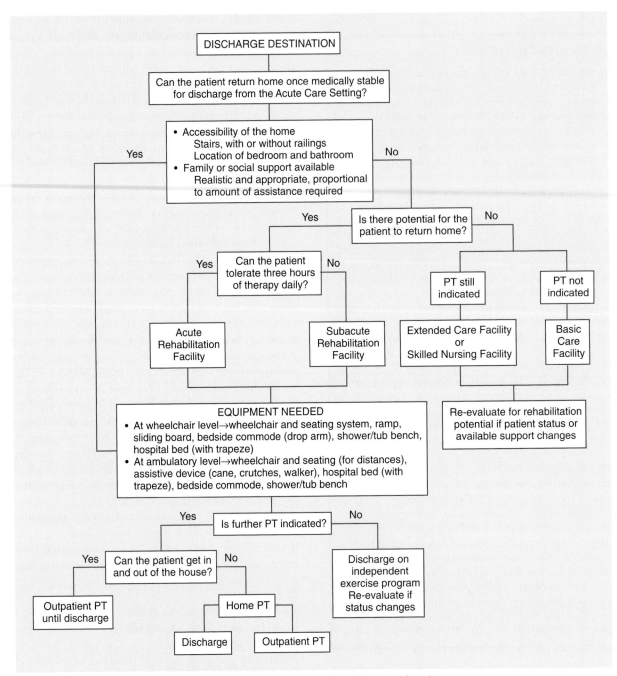

**Figure 17-13** Decision tree for discharge planning.

caregivers, decisions reached, then shared with other members of the health care team.

## Pediatric Considerations

Whether a physical therapist is providing direct cardiopulmonary care to acutely ill pediatric (neonates, infants, and children) patients or incorporating cardiopulmonary techniques into developmental therapy, a knowledge of cardiopulmonary development and congenital pathology is essential. Treatment in the pediatric population is directed at problems that arise from developmental abnormalities, prematurity,

infection, immunologic deficiencies, trauma, and diseases associated with childhood. Cystic fibrosis, a genetic exocrine gland involvement affecting the pulmonary system, is discussed in Chapter 6. Pediatric conditions are discussed in more detail in Chapter 20. Provision of cardiopulmonary physical therapy in the pediatric population may require postgraduate or specialized training of the physical therapist.

Interventions for pediatric patients with cardiopulmonary dysfunction are not the same as for adults because of body size and physiologic differences. Pediatric patients also require very close monitoring because of their decreased tolerance for hemodynamic changes and limitations in communicating distress. The purpose of this section is to briefly describe the intervention considerations that are indicated in pediatrics because of body size, physiologic differences, and level of psychological and communicative development. Moerchen and Crane offer a more detailed description of pediatric cardiopulmonary care.[93]

Cardiac dysfunction in pediatric patients is often related to congenital heart anomalies, whereas in adults coronary artery disease is most often the source. Surgical intervention in both populations is common. Postoperative physical therapy aims to increase respiration, mobilize secretions, and progress functional mobility.[94] It is important to prevent the deconditioning effects of bed rest postoperatively in children as with adults and to try to mobilize the patient out of bed by the second postoperative day. For children who were able to walk preoperatively, ambulation is possible following extubation once arterial and groin lines have been removed.

Modification of airway clearance techniques for pediatric patients involves positioning the child or infant on the therapist's lap or on pillows and conforming the therapist's hand to the patient's chest. Small handheld percussors and vibrators are also available. In caring for premature infants, careful evaluation of the risks and benefits of treatment is required owing to the infant's limited tolerance to handling. The therapist can minimize stimulation to the infant by coordinating position changes for bronchial drainage with other patient care procedures. The bronchial drainage positions for infants are the same as for adults because fetal development of the bronchial tree is complete at the end of 16 weeks of gestation. The bronchial drainage positions may need to be approximated if the infant becomes hemodynamically unstable. The head-down positions should be avoided if intracranial bleeding is suspected. Infants and small children often need assistance in clearing secretions loosened by bronchial drainage, percussion, or vibration. If the patient is unable to cough effectively, the nasal and oropharyngeal areas can be suctioned while using supplemental oxygen to prevent desaturation. Older children can be encouraged to huff or cough using toys or games that involve forceful breathing (i.e., pinwheels, blowing bubbles). When working with children in general, the therapist can reduce patient anxiety, generate interest, and build rapport by being creative and making treatment sessions as playful as possible.

A child's acute illness ultimately has an impact on the child's parents, siblings, and extended family. The physical therapist can be helpful in instructing family members about the illness as well as the pertinent physical therapy interventions. Parents and others may feel particularly supported when they are encouraged to learn treatment techniques, such as percussion and bronchial drainage, and to perform them as the patient's medical condition stabilizes. In the case of a child with asthma, for example, family members can become familiar with the signs of an impending asthma attack and help the child minimize its effects. They can do this by calming the child, providing medication (as prescribed), and helping with relaxation and breathing exercises. They can also learn to monitor the child for changes in respiratory rate, intercostal retractions, and cyanosis.[95] Family members can also be helpful to the physical therapist, who is trying to understand the child's nonverbal or preverbal communications. Certain facial expressions or gestures may have specific meanings for the child. By sharing this information with the therapist, the family can facilitate better communication between the therapist and the patient.

---

## CASE STUDY 17-1

Patient Name: Charles Brown
Referral Type: MD
Inpatient/Outpatient: IP
Informed Consent: by daughter
Living Will: no
Code Status: full
Precaution Orders: none specified
Length of Physical Therapy Episode of Care: 3 days

History of Present Illness: 53-year-old African American man admitted to an acute care hospital via the emergency room with crushing chest pain and shortness of breath on May 10. Mr. Brown was diagnosed with an acute anterior wall myocardial infarction (MI). He was taken to the cardiac catheterization lab and received a percutaneous transluminal coronary angioplasty (PTCA). On May 12, his condition stabilized and he was transferred to a monitored bed on the cardiac floor. Soon after, he developed swelling in his ankles, rales in the bases of his lungs and an S3 heart sound. His ECG showed sinus bradycardia with heart rate of 50. On May 15, a DDD pacemaker (permanent) with rate modulation (upper heart

rate [HR] limit = 120 bpm) was placed. On May 16, he is referred to physical therapy by the cardiologist.

PMH/PSH: Depression, deep-vein thrombosis (1 year ago), hypertension (diagnosed 1 year ago, has not taken Inderal, which was prescribed to treat HTN), moderate emphysema

Medications: Procardia, Bumex, Lanoxin, Aspirin, K Lor

SH/Mental Health Issues: Mr. Brown is a divorced autoworker who lives alone in a middle-class neighborhood. He has a 12th-grade education. He has three adult children. He is estranged from his two sons but stays in touch with his daughter, who brought him to the emergency room. He has suffered from depression for years and has been prescribed Wellbutrin but does not feel he needs it. "I get by with a few beers every night," he says. Mr. Brown also smokes 1.5 packs of cigarettes a day. He is 6' tall and weighs 232 lbs. He states he grew up Baptist but does not attend church now.

Living Environment/Equipment: Lives in two-story house, 6 steps to enter, 14 steps to bedroom on second floor. Railings at both. Was independent with ambulation, stairs, and activities of

*Continued*

## CASE STUDY 17-1—cont'd

daily living (ADLs) prior to admission. Occupation involves lifting 20-pound loads several times per day. Used no assistive devices prior to admission.

Functional Status/Activity Level: Rolls bilaterally in bed independently. Supine to sit independent. Sit to stand with contact guard, complains of feeling light-headed. Pivots to a chair with contact guard for balance. Able to ambulate 100 ft with contact guard, then fatigues and needs to rest. Independent with personal-care ADLs.

Systems Review: HR = 70 bpm, regular. Blood pressure (BP) = 90/60 in supine. Respiratory rate (RR) = 18. Temperature = 98.6° F. Skin: 3+ edema bilateral ankles, pacer incision clean and dry. Musculoskeletal: L shoulder flexion limited to 90 degrees for 24 hours post pacer placement. Able to move all four extremities against gravity. Neuro: Sensation to proprioception, pain/light touch intact throughout. Alert and oriented X 3.

Medical Tests and Procedures: Chest X ray (CXR): increased density in pulmonary vasculature markings. Serum sodium (Na): 120 mEq/L. CBC: RBC 4.0 million/$\mu$L, WBC 5000, WBC differential—neutrophils 60%, lymphocytes 30%, monocytes 5%, eosinophils 1%, basophils 0.50%; hematocrit 30%, hemoglobin 10 g/100mL, platelets 300K/$\mu$L.

Physical Therapy (PT) Tests and Measures (initial evaluation): Resting values—ECG paced rhythm, HR = 72. BP = 95/60 supine, 90/60 sitting, 90/60 standing. $SaO_2$ on 2 L/min $O_2$ per nasal cannula—94% at rest. RR = 18, no accessory muscle use. Cough strong, dry and nonproductive. Temperature = 98.7° F. Inspection—increased A-P diameter of chest, 4 cm incision under L clavicle, clean and dry, 2+ pedal edema. Palpation—no fremitus, pacer battery palpated under L clavicle, expansion is symmetrical. Mediate percussion—hyperresonant bilaterally. Auscultation—

lungs with crackles (rales), bilateral bases, heart S1, S2. Functional capacity via 3-minute walk test—patient achieved 325 ft on 2 L/min $O_2$, $SaO_2$ 90%, RPE 12-15, dyspnea scale +1 to +3, max HR = 84, BP = 124/62 mm Hg.

PT Diagnosis/Evaluation: 53-year-old man with impaired endurance related to impaired cardiovascular pump function and resulting in impaired ability to transfer, ambulate. He also has impaired gas exchange as evidenced by desaturation on supplemental $O_2$ during the 3-minute walk test. Recommend physical therapy for monitored therapeutic exercise progression, functional mobility training, ambulation, and patient education.

PT Goals: Patient able to transfer independently. Pt able to ambulate 300 ft on room air and maintain $PO_2$ >92%. Patient able to ambulate 300 ft independently on room air with acceptable hemodynamic response to exercise. Patient able to ambulate up and down 14 steps independently. Patient is independent with home exercise program. Patient is able to identify his risk factors for coronary artery disease. Patient is able to identify lifestyle modifications to lower his risk for coronary artery disease progression.

PT Plan of Care/Interventions: Inpatient monitored therapeutic exercise progression, functional mobility training, ambulation, and patient education, one to two times daily for 3 days.

PT Prognosis/Expected Outcomes: Patient is expected to reach PT goals above. Symptom-limited stress test results (just prior to discharge): Patient achieved 6 METs on modified Bruce protocol, stopped as a result of shortness of breath. No ST changes noted. Max HR was 120 bpm, BP 145/64 mm Hg.

Discharge Plan: Home with outpatient cardiac rehabilitation program for 6 to 8 weeks, two to three times per week.

## Summary

In acute care settings, physical therapy interventions for patients at any age, with primary or secondary cardiopulmonary dysfunction, is aimed at optimizing the patient's oxygen transport system. Therapeutic interventions designed to meet this goal include airway clearance techniques, therapeutic positioning, breathing and chest wall exercises, patient education, and functional mobility exercises. Interventions in the pediatric population require modifications based on body size, physiologic differences, and level of psychological and communicative development. Physical therapists working in acute care have a unique challenge in that they must recognize dynamic pathophysiologic changes in their patients and adapt interventions and activity progressions accordingly. This chapter describes the therapeutic interventions, identifies their indications and precautions, and emphasizes the importance of monitoring acutely ill patients during treatment. Issues pertinent to prioritizing patient care and planning hospital discharge were also discussed.

- Cardiopulmonary physical therapy treatment in the acute care setting is aimed at correcting or improving the function of the patient's oxygen transport system.
- Physical therapy interventions for acutely ill patients with cardiopulmonary dysfunction include airway clearance techniques, therapeutic positioning, breathing strategies and exercises, patient education, and functional mobility exercise.
- Patients with multiple medical problems and acute respiratory failure may require prolonged periods of mechanical ventilation. Physical therapy interventions for these patients need to be coordinated with the weaning process in order to balance the patient's energy expenditure for breathing with that which would be required for participation in therapy activities.
- Therapeutic positioning techniques are indicated for patients with diaphragmatic weakness or inefficiency. These techniques facilitate inspiratory effort and assist in ventilation and perfusion matching.

- Monitoring patient tolerance to physical therapy treatment using parameters such as HR, BP, SpO$_2$, RR, and ECG is crucial to safe and effective activity progression for acutely ill patients.
- The primary role of the acute care physical therapist is shifting from providing treatment to acting as a consultant, offering recommendations based on the patient's functional status and rehabilitation potential, and assisting with determining discharge destination and equipment needs.
- Therapeutic interventions in the pediatric population with acute cardiopulmonary dysfunction are directed at problems that arise from developmental abnormalities, prematurity, infection, immunologic deficiencies, trauma, and diseases associated with childhood.

## References

1. Milbrandt EB. Use it or lose it. Crit Care Med 36(8):2444–5, 2008.
2. Urban N. Patient and family responses to the critical care environment. In Kinney MR, Brooks-Brunn JA, Molter N, et al. (eds.): AACN's Clinical Reference for Critical Care Nursing. 4th ed. St. Louis, Mosby, 1998:145–62.
3. Dean E. Oxygen transport: the basis for cardiopulmonary physical therapy. In Frownfelter D, Dean E (eds.): Principles and Practice of Cardiopulmonary Physical Therapy. 3rd ed. St. Louis, Mosby-Year Book, 1996:3.
4. American Physical Therapy Association. Guide to Physical Therapy Practice. 2nd ed. Baltimore, APTA, 2003.
5. Ciesla N. Postural drainage, positioning, and breathing exercises. In Mackenzie CF (ed.): Chest Physiotherapy in the Intensive Care Unit. 2nd ed. Baltimore, Williams & Wilkins, 1989:102.
6. Ciesla ND, Klemic N, Imle PC. Chest physical therapy to the patient with multiple trauma: Two case studies. Phys Ther 61:202–5, 1981.
7. Hammon WE, Martin RJ. Chest physical therapy for acute atelectasis. Phys Ther 61:217–20, 1981.
8. Sutton PP, Pavia D, Bateman JRM, Clarke SW. Chest physiotherapy: a review. Eur J Respir Dis 63:188–201, 1982.
9. Watchie J. In Cardiopulmonary Physical Therapy: A Clinical Manual. Philadelphia, WB Saunders, 1995:212–14.
10. Downs AM. Clinical application of airway clearance techniques. In Frownfelter D, Dean E (eds.): Principles and Practice of Cardiopulmonary Physical Therapy. 3rd ed. St. Louis, Mosby-Year Book, 1996:343.
11. Massery M, Frownfelter D. Facilitating airway clearance with coughing techniques. In Frownfelter D, Dean E (eds.): Principles and Practice of Cardiopulmonary Physical Therapy. 3rd ed. St. Louis, Mosby-Year Book, 1996:369.
12. Imle PC. Physical therapy for patients with cardiac, thoracic, or abdominal conditions following surgery or trauma. In Irwin T, Tecklin J (eds.): Cardiopulmonary Physical Therapy. 3rd ed. St. Louis, Mosby-Year Book, 1995:380.
13. Maxwell M, Redmond A. Comparative trial of manual and mechanical percussion technique with gravity assisted bronchial drainage in patients with cystic fibrosis. Arch Dis Childhood 54:542–4, 1979.
14. Downs AM. Clinical application of airway clearance techniques. In Frownfelter D, Dean E (eds.): Principles and Practice of Cardiopulmonary Physical Therapy. 3rd ed. St. Louis, Mosby-Year Book, 1996:345.
15. Sutton PP, Lopez-Vidriero MT, Pavia D, et al. Assessment of percussion, vibratory-shaking, and breathing exercises in chest physiotherapy. Eur J Respir Dis 66:147–52, 1985.
16. Pryor JA, Webber BA, Hodson ME, Batten JC. Evaluation of the forced expiration technique as an adjunct to postural drainage in treatment of cystic fibrosis. Br J Med 18:417–18, 1979.
17. Expiratory Aids. http://theuniversityhospital.com/ventilation/html/howitworks/ex.htm (accessed April 26, 2009)
18. Massery M, Frownfelter D. Facilitating ventilation pattern and breathing strategies. In Frownfelter D, Dean E (eds.): Principles and Practice of Cardiopulmonary Physical Therapy. 3rd ed. St. Louis, Mosby-Year Book, 1996:387–8.
19. Craig DB. Postoperative recovery of pulmonary function. Anesth Analg 60:46–52, 1981.
20. Ray JF, Yost L, Moallem S, et al. Immobility, hypoxemia, and pulmonary arteriovenous shunting. Arch Surg 109:537–41, 1974.
21. Langer M, Mascheroni D, Marcolin R, et al. The prone position in ARDS patients. Chest 94:103–7, 1988.
22. Sciaky A. Mobilizing the intensive care unit patient: pathophysiology and treatment. Phys Ther Pract 3:69–80, 1994.
23. Peel C. The cardiopulmonary system and movement dysfunction. Phys Ther 76:448–55, 1996.
24. Dechman G, Wilson CR. Evidence underlying breathing retraining in people with stable chronic obstructive pulmonary disease. Phys Ther 84(12):1189–97, 2004.
25. Faling LJ. Pulmonary rehabilitation: physical modalities. Clin Chest Med 7(4):599–618, 1986.
26. Dechman G, Wilson CR. Evidence underlying cardiopulmonary physical therapy in stable COPD. Cardiopulm Phys Ther J 13:20–2, 2002.
27. Porter S (ed): Tidy's Physiotherapy, ed 14. London, 2009, Churchill Livingstone.
28. Baker WL, Lamb VJ, Marini JJ. Breath-stacking increases the depth and duration of chest expansion by incentive spirometry. Am Rev Respir Dis 141:343–6, 1990.
29. Gosselink RA, Wegenaar RC, Rijswijk H, et al. Diaphragmatic breathing reduces efficiency of breathing in patients with advanced chronic obstructive pulmonary disease. Am J Respir Crit Care Med 151:1136–42, 1995.
30. Tecklin JS. Pediatric Physical Therapy. 4th ed. Philadelphia, PA, Lippincott, Williams & Williams, 2007:36.
31. Shekleton M, Berry JK, Covey MK. Respiratory muscle weakness and training. In Frownfelter D, Dean E (eds.): Principles and Practice of Cardiopulmonary Physical Therapy. 3rd ed. St. Louis, Mosby-Year Book, 1996:447.
32. Wolfson MR, Bhutani VK, Shaffer TH. Respiratory muscles. In Irwin S, Tecklin JS (eds.): Cardiopulmonary Physical Therapy. St. Louis, CV Mosby, 1985:386–9.
33. Faulkner JA. New perspectives in training for maximum performance. JAMA 205:741–6, 1968.
34. West JB. In Respiratory Physiology. 4th ed. Baltimore, Williams & Wilkins, 1990:87–113.
35. Peter JB, Bernard RJ, Edgerton VR, et al. Metabolic profiles of three fiber types of skeletal muscle in guinea pigs and rabbits. Biochemistry 11:2627–34, 1972.
36. Gesell R, Atkinson AK, Brown RC. The gradation of the intensity of inspiratory contractions. Am J Physiol 131:659–73, 1941.

37. Iscoe S, Dankoff J, Migicovsky R, Polosa C. Recruitment and discharge frequency of phrenic motoneurons during inspiration. Resp Phys 26:113–28, 1975.

38. Keens TG, Bryan AC, Levison H, Ianuzzo CD. Developmental pattern of muscle fiber types in human ventilatory muscles. J Appl Physiol 44:909–13, 1978.

39. Dantzker DR. Respiratory muscle function. In Bone RC, George RB, Hudson LD (eds.): Acute Respiratory Failure. New York, Churchill Livingstone, 1987:49.

40. Gollnick PD, Armstrong RB, Saltin B, et al. Effect of training on enzyme activity and fiber composition of human skeletal muscle. J Appl Physiol 34:107–11, 1973.

41. Holloszy JO, Booth FW. Biochemical adaptations to endurance exercise in muscle. Annu Rev Physiol 38:273–91, 1976.

42. Barach AL. Breathing exercises in pulmonary emphysema and allied chronic respiratory disease. Arch Phys Med Rehab 36:379–90, 1955.

43. Adkins HV. Improvement of breathing ability in children with respiratory muscle paralysis. Phys Ther 48:577, 1968.

44. Holtackers TR. Physical rehabilitation of the ventilator-dependent patient. In Irwin S, Tecklin JS (eds.): Cardiopulmonary Physical Therapy. 3rd ed. St. Louis, Mosby-Year Book, 1995:480.

45. Jenkins S, Soutar SA, Loukota JM, et al. Physiotherapy after coronary artery surgery: are breathing exercises necessary? Thorax 44:634–9, 1989.

46. Dull JI, Dull WL. Are maximal inspiratory breathing exercises or incentive spirometry better than early mobilization after cardiac surgery? Phys Ther 63:655–9, 1983.

47. Hallbook T, Lindblad B, Lindroth B, et al. Prophylaxis against pulmonary complications in patients undergoing gallbladder surgery: a comparison between early mobilization, physiotherapy with and without bronchodilation. Ann Chir Gynaecol 73:55–8, 1984.

48. Keens TG, Krastin IRB, Wannamaker EM, et al. Ventilatory muscle endurance training in normal subjects and patients with cystic fibrosis. Am Rev Respir Dis 116:853–60, 1977.

49. Belman MJ, Kendregan BA. Physical training fails to improve ventilatory muscle endurance in patients with chronic obstructive pulmonary disease. Chest 81:440–3, 1982.

50. Henneman EA. The art and science of weaning from mechanical ventilation. Focus Crit Care 18:490–501, 1991.

51. Calhoun CJ, Specht NL. Standardizing the weaning process. ACCN Clin Issues Crit Care Nurs 2:398–404, 1991.

52. Kress JP, Pohlman A, O'Connor MF, et al. Daily interruption of sedative infusions in critically ill patients undergoing mechanical ventilation. N Engl J Med 342:1471–7, 2000.

53. Schweickert WD, Gehlbach B, Pohlman AS, Hall JB, Kress JP. Daily interruption of sedative infusions and complications of critical illness in mechanically ventilated patients. Crit Care Med 32(6):1272–6, 2004.

54. Schweickert WD, Pohlman MC, Pohlman AS, et al. A randomized trial of early physical and occupational therapy in mechanically ventilated, critically ill patients. Lancet 373(9678):1874–82, 2009.

55. Folk L, Kewman S. CCMU Protocol for Weaning from Mechanical Ventilation. 1997, Policy per Critical Care Medicine Unit, University of Michigan Health Systems, Ann Arbor.

56. Yang KL, Tobin MJ. A prospective study of indexes predicting the outcome of trials of weaning from mechanical ventilation. N Engl J Med 324:1446–95, 1991.

57. Dries DJ. Weaning from mechanical ventilation. J Trauma 43:372–84, 1997.

58. Carrieri-Kohlman V. Dyspnea in the weaning patient: assessment and intervention. AACN Clin Issues Crit Care Nurs 2:462–73, 1991.

59. Gift AC, Plant SM, Jacox A. Psychologic and physiologic factors related to dyspnea in subjects with chronic obstructive pulmonary disease. Heart Lung 15:595–601, 1986.

60. Knebel A. Describing mood state and dyspnea in mechanically ventilated patients prior to weaning (abstract). Am Rev Respir Dis 141:A412, 1990.

61. Holliday JE, Hyers TM. The reduction of weaning time from mechanical ventilation using tidal volume and relaxation biofeedback. Am Rev Respir Dis 141:1214–20, 1990.

62. Aldrich TK, Darpel JP, Uhrlass RM, et al. Weaning from mechanical ventilation: adjunctive use of inspiratory muscle resistive training. Crit Care Med 17:143–7, 1989.

63. Shekleton ME. Respiratory muscle conditioning and the work of breathing: a critical balance in the weaning patient. AACN Clin Issues Crit Care Nurs 2:405–14, 1991.

64. Dean E, Perlstein MF, Mathews M. Acute surgical conditions. In Frownfelter D, Dean E (eds.): Principles and Practice of Cardiopulmonary Physical Therapy. 3rd ed. St. Louis, Mosby-Year Book, 1996:498–9.

65. Stein M, Cassara EL. Preoperative pulmonary evaluation and therapy for surgery patients. JAMA 211:787–90, 1970.

66. Vraciu JK, Vraciu RA. Effectiveness of breathing exercises in preventing pulmonary complications following open heart surgery. Phys Ther 57:1367–71, 1977.

67. Kigin CM. Chest physical therapy for the postoperative or traumatic injury patient. Phys Ther 61:1724–36, 1981.

68. Dean E. Mobilization and exercise. In Frownfelter D, Dean E (eds.): Principles and Practice of Cardiopulmonary Physical Therapy. 3rd ed. St. Louis, Mosby-Year Book, 1996:271.

69. DeJonghe B, Lacherade JC, Durand MC, Sharshar T. Critical illness neuromuscular syndromes. Crit Care Clin 23:55–69, 2007.

70. Schweickert WD, Hall J. ICU-acquired weakness. Chest 131:1541–9, 2007.

71. Herridge MS, Cheung AM, Tansey CM, et al. One-year outcomes in survivors of the acute respiratory distress syndrome. N Engl J Med 348:683–93, 2003.

72. Atwood JA, Nielsen DH. Scope of cardiac rehabilitation. Phys Ther 65:1812–19, 1985.

73. Irwin S. Clinical manifestations and assessment of ischemic heart disease. Phys Ther 65:1806–11, 1985.

74. Borg G. Perceived exertion as an indicator of somatic stress. J Rehab Med 2:92–8, 1970.

75. ACSM's Guidelines for Exercise Testing and Prescription. 7th ed. Baltimore, Lippincott Williams & Wilkins, 2006:119.

76. Eston RG, Thompson M. Use of ratings of perceived exertion for predicting maximal work rate prescribing exercise intensity in patients taking atenolol. Br J Sports Med 31:114–19, 1997.

77. Packe GE, Freeman W, Cayton RM. Effects of exercise on gas exchange in patients recovering from acute severe asthma. Thorax 45:262–6, 1990.

78. Leerar PJ, Miller EW. Concurrent validity of distance-walks and timed-walks in the well-elderly. J Geriatr Phys Ther 25:3–7, 2002.

79. Weissman C, Kemper M. Stressing the critically ill patient: the cardiopulmonary and metabolic responses to an acute increase in oxygen consumption. J Crit Care 8:100–8, 1993.

80. Weissman C, Kemper M, Damask MC, et al. Effect of routine intensive care interaction on metabolic rate. Chest 86:815–19, 1984.

81. Weissman C, Kemper M. The oxygen uptake-oxygen delivery relationship during ICU interventions. Chest 99:430–5, 1991.

82. Byrne NM, Hills AP, Hunter GR, Weinsier RL, Schutz Y. Metabolic equivalent: one size does not fit all. J Appl Physiol 99:1112–19, 2005.

83. Devine E, Cook T. A meta-analysis of effects of psychoeducational interventions on length of post surgical hospital stay. Nurs Res 32:267–74, 1983.

84. O'Rourke A, Lewin B, Whitcross S, Pacey W. The effects of physical exercise training and cardiac education on levels of anxiety and depression in the rehabilitation of CABG patients. Int Disability Stud 12:104–6, 1990.

85. Sluijs EM, Kok GJ, van der Zee J. Correlates of exercise compliance in physical therapy. Phys Ther 73:771–86, 1993.

86. Manzetti JD, Goffman LA, Serreida SM, et al. Exercise, education, and quality of life in lung transplant candidates. J Heart Lung Transplant 13:297–305, 1994.

87. Mazzuca SA. Does patient education in chronic disease have therapeutic value? J Chron Dis 35(7):521–9, 1982.

88. Smith CE. Nurse's increasing responsibility for patient education. In Smith CE (ed.): Patient Education. Nurses in Partnership with Other Health Professionals. Orlando, Grune & Stratton, 1987.

89. Sciaky AJ. Patient education. In Frownfelter D, Dean E (eds.): Principles and Practice of Cardiopulmonary Physical Therapy. 3rd ed. St. Louis, Mosby-Year Book, 1996:453–65.

90. Chase L, Elkins JA, Readinger J, Shepard KF. Perceptions of physical therapists toward patient education. Phys Ther 73:787–96, 1993.

91. Reynolds JP. LOS: SOS? You could say that managed care is about one thing: discharge planning. PT Magazine 4:38–46, 1996.

92. Lopopolo RB. The effect of hospital restructuring on the role of physical therapists in acute care. Phys Ther 77:918–36, 1997.

93. Moerchen VA, Crane LD. The neonatal and pediatric patient. In Frownfelter D, Dean E (eds.): Principles and Practice of Cardiopulmonary Physical Therapy. 3rd ed. St. Louis, Mosby-Year Book, 1996:635–67.

94. Johnson B. Postoperative physical therapy in the pediatric cardiac surgery patient. Pediatr Phys Ther 3(1):14–22, 1991.

95. Magee CL. Physical therapy for the child with asthma. Pediatr Phys Ther 3(1):23–8, 1991.

## CHAPTER 18

# Interventions and Prevention Measures for Individuals with Cardiovascular Disease, or Risk of Disease

*Ellen Hillegass, William Temes*

## Chapter Outline

Therapeutic interventions for individuals with cardiovascular disease will be presented in this chapter and will also include therapeutic interventions to prevent cardiovascular disease (primary prevention). Information will be presented on the appropriate patient groups including the special considerations for each patient group, the settings where rehabilitation may be provided, the components and goals that should be considered in rehabilitation as well as the outcomes that should be measured, the administrative concerns involved in specific cardiac rehabilitation programs, and the justification for rehabilitation of these individuals. An important distinction needs to be made between "rehabilitation of the patient with cardiovascular disorders" and "cardiac rehabilitation" and a "cardiac rehabilitation program": As there is a distinct difference in billing and reimbursement for cardiac

rehabilitation programs in the outpatient setting. Cardiac rehabilitation and rehabilitation of the patient with cardiovascular disorders are synonymous and used in this chapter to discuss the interventions used for individuals with cardiac disease and dysfunction. A *cardiac rehabilitation program* in the outpatient setting is defined as a multidiscipline program of exercise, education, and lifestyle modification and is a covered service under the Centers for Medicare and Medicaid (CMS) and outlined in a National Coverage Determination (NCD), including a description of patient diagnoses, program components, etc. (see the CMS page on the website of the U.S. Department of Health & Human Services for NCD information).[10] Individuals with cardiovascular disorders may be seen in a variety of outpatient settings for rehabilitation; however, if individuals are referred specifically for a cardiac rehabilitation program there are specific guidelines set that must be followed and specific billing practices that are implemented because of the standards set by the CMS National coverage. Therefore, to prevent confusion in this chapter, *cardiac rehabilitation programs* will be the term used for the multidiscipline program and discussed later in this chapter. Interventions for individuals with cardiovascular disorders will be the main focus of this chapter.

## Primary Prevention

Therapeutic interventions, including cardiac rehabilitation for individuals with cardiovascular disease, might not be necessary for many individuals if primary prevention of the disease existed (active intervention for risk factors that cause cardiovascular disease). Therefore, primary prevention is an important component of wellness and rehabilitation programs that should be incorporated in all programs. Candidates for a primary prevention are those individuals who are at moderate or high risk of developing cardiovascular disease (prior to manifestation of the disease) and those with family histories of cardiovascular disease.

When presenting the need for primary prevention programs, one needs only to look at the statistics regarding the prevalence of modifiable risk factors in the current population.[1-4] Cigarette smoking is the number one most preventable cause of disease, disability, and death in the United States today.[1] More than half of all adult Americans have a blood cholesterol level higher than 200 mg/dL.[4] One in four adult Americans has hypertension.[2] In addition, there is a large proportion of the population in the United States that leads a sedentary lifestyle, despite the fact that epidemiologic studies have demonstrated that regular physical activity protects against the development and progression of several chronic diseases. Obesity, identified as an important risk factor for both men and women, appears to interact with or amplify the effects of other risk factors, although the mechanisms are unknown. Obesity has increased during the past 20 years, and statistics state that 47 million adult Americans are overweight, thereby making this risk factor a serious health problem.[3] Primary prevention programs therefore have a large target audience.

Two major problems inherent in a primary prevention program are compliance (especially long term) and lack of payment for services by medical insurance companies. Also, the expected outcome of a primary prevention program is a lack of manifestation of the disease, which is a difficult outcome to measure for an individual. This often creates a situation of denial or "it won't happen to me" attitude, which interferes with continual motivation and subsequently compliance. In addition, when medical insurance companies do not reimburse payment for services, individuals are less likely to continue to pay for services. Therefore, similar statistics as reported in the fitness literature regarding compliance and long-term commitment to diet, exercise training, and behavior modification would be applicable to this population.[4]

Although research is somewhat limited in long-term outcomes of primary prevention programs, scientific literature does support the reduction of risk factors as a result of a primary prevention program.[1-4] Risk factors that are affected by a primary prevention program include reduction of total cholesterol to (high-density lipoprotein (HDL) ratio, reduction in low-density lipoprotein (LDL) cholesterol, improvement in aerobic capacity and exercise tolerance, reduction in weight, reduction in resting blood pressure in hypertensive individuals, improved glucose tolerance and insulin sensitivity, improved feeling of well-being, and improved tolerance to stressful situations. Box 18-1 presents the guidelines for risk assessment as determined by the American Heart Association's guidelines for primary prevention of cardiovascular disease.[5,6] The specific components of a primary prevention program should include the following:

- Therapeutic exercise to include development of an aerobic exercise prescription and possibly a resistance training exercise prescription
- Dietary counseling for those with diabetes, weight management problems, and elevated cholesterol
- Stress management or biofeedback
- Smoking cessation
- Pharmacologic management for blood pressure, diabetes, or hypercholesterolemia (Box 18-2 presents the goals for interventions as identified by the American Heart Association [AHA] guidelines[5])
- Education and self-management techniques

The *Guide to Physical Therapist Practice* describes the patient group appropriate for primary intervention/risk reduction for cardiovascular and pulmonary disorders in the Practice Pattern 6A and includes detailed interventions to achieve the expected outcomes that will assist the individual in lowering his or her risk for cardiovascular and pulmonary disorders.[7]

Primary prevention programs should be implemented at the work site, fitness centers, senior citizen centers, and primary physician's offices as well as in outpatient physical therapy clinics and cardiac rehabilitation centers. As most primary prevention programs are not reimbursed from medical insurance, individual fee for service or monthly payment plans may motivate more participation in these programs. Until the time that scientific and clinical outcomes demonstrate the efficacy of such programs, primary prevention probably will not be reimbursed under health care plans. Encouragement by primary physicians also increases involvement in a program. Centers that provide these services should therefore be documenting both short-term and long-term (morbidity, mortality rates) outcomes for possible inclusion in medical insurance reimbursement plans in the future.

## Rehabilitation of Patients with Documented Cardiovascular Disease

Individuals with documented cardiovascular disease benefit from therapeutic interventions to improve their aerobic

---

**Box 18-1**

## Guidelines for Risk Assessment

### Hypertension

- Known high blood pressure prior to hospitalization
- Taking antihypertension medicines prior to hospitalization
- Unknown prior to hospitalization
- History of normal BP

### Physical Activity

- Not participated in >3 exercise sessions/week
- Regularly exercises 3/week

### Family History

- Father and mother with CAD
- Father or mother with CAD
- Grandparents or uncles/aunts with CAD
- No family hx of CAD

### Alcohol or Substance Use

- Self-reports hx of alcohol substance abuse
- Presentation suggests hx of substance abuse
- No evidence of abuse

### Smoking History

- Current smoker (>9 cigarettes/day)
- Quit at time of hospitalization
- Former smoker
- Never smoked

### Stress: Hostility, Anger

- Self-reports hx of high stress levels
- Self-reports no hx
- Others report hx
- Demonstrates hostility, anger

### Diabetes

- Hx of elevated blood sugar or diabetes
- Hx of normal blood sugar

### Hypercholesterolemia

- Known elevated cholesterol
- Elevated at time of hospitalization
- Unknown
- Hx of normal cholesterol

### Weight

- >15 lb overweight
- Within normal weight

### Other

- Age
- Male sex
- Menopausal female

CAD, coronary artery disease

---

**Box 18-2**

## Goals for Intervention for Primary Prevention

- To prevent the harmful effects of prolonged bedrest when a patient is hospitalized with heart disease.
- To develop cardiovascular fitness after acute illness, with an emphasis on optimal ability for employment and leisure.
- To identify patients whose psychological response to cardiac disease may require extra support and additional measures for successful rehabilitation.
- To initiate a program of secondary prevention of cardiovascular disease aimed at reducing the risks of illness and death as well as improving function and quality of life.
- To accomplish the preceding goals through interdisciplinary efforts directed at discovering each patient's optimal activity level, diet, and ability to improve unfavorable risk factors.

capacity, functional mobility or any other impairments, as well as to prevent progression of the disease (secondary prevention) or progression of impairments. The actual interventions used for their rehabilitation depend upon their specific impairments that are determined based upon the thorough examination of the patient using tests and measures, the prognosis, and the plan of care previously discussed in Chapter 16. The interventions used include coordination and communication with other members of the patient's health care team, education/instruction, and procedural interventions (Fig 18-1).

## Patient Populations

Populations appropriate for rehabilitation may have a primary cardiovascular disorder (such as acute coronary syndrome [ACS], myocardial infarction [MI], coronary artery bypass graft [CABG] surgery, heart or heart–lung transplant, heart valve repair or replacement surgery, congestive heart failure [CHF], etc.) or a secondary cardiovascular disorder (such as history of coronary artery disease, CHF, MI, etc.) and the therapeutic interventions used in their rehabilitation will be based upon impairments identified in the initial examination. Therefore, history taking via medical chart or interview with the patient is extremely important to uncover the secondary diagnoses of cardiovascular disease if the patient presents to the clinic with a primary neuromuscular, musculoskeletal, or integumentary disorder. Rehabilitation of the heart and heart–lung transplant patients is discussed in great detail in Chapter 12 and therefore will not be discussed in this chapter. Specific patient populations appropriate for cardiac rehabilitation outpatient programs will be discussed later in this chapter.

## Rehabilitation Programs

Rehabilitation of the patient with cardiovascular disease should be a multidisciplinary program of education, exercise, and behavioral change to assist individuals with cardiovascular disease in achieving optimal physical, psychological, and functional status within the limits of their disease. This type of rehabilitation includes the following:

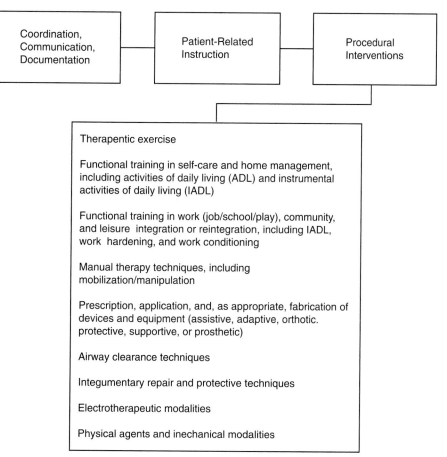

**Figure 18-1** The three components of physical therapy intervention.

- Education of the patient and family in the recognition, prevention, and treatment of cardiovascular disease
- Amelioration or reduction of risk factors
- Dealing with the psychological factors that influence recovery from heart disease
- Structured, progressive physical activity either in a rehabilitation setting or home program
- Vocational or return to leisure activities counseling
- Activity of daily living (ADL) and functional training

Cardiac rehabilitation is typically organized in progressive phases of programming to meet the specific needs of individuals and their families in their stages of recovery. The acute or in-hospital phase has been referred to as Phase I, the early outpatient or intensive monitoring has been referred to as Phase II, the training and maintenance phase has been known as Phase III, and Phase IV has been reserved for the high-risk patients in a disease prevention program (Table 18-1).

## The Beginning in Acute Care

In 1952, Levine and Lown demonstrated that early mobilization of the acute coronary patient to activity reduced complications and improved the mortality rate.[8] Since then, physicians have increasingly realized the benefits of early rehabilitative measures. Physical conditioning can improve heart rate response, arterial blood pressure response in hypertensive individuals, myocardial oxygen uptake, and maximum cardiac output.[9] In addition, improvements in the peripheral circulation, the pulmonary ventilation, and the autonomic nervous system benefit one's tolerance for work. Accompanying these physical improvements are greater emotional stability and self-esteem.

Early mobilization of stable individuals after a cardiac event has become a well-established practice. The time course of care for coronary disease is changing dramatically owing to early diagnostic testing, new interventions, and the current managed care environment. Although rest is important to the impaired myocardium, optimal improvement of the patient requires redefinition of the degree and duration of rest. No longer is the patient lying in bed for weeks at a time. The average patient who undergoes coronary artery bypass surgery is ambulating on the unit by Day 2 at the latest. After MI, patients are usually moved out of the intensive care unit and into the step-down (or telemetry) unit within 24 to 48 hours and if uncomplicated, are often discharged 1 to 2 days later. Patients are no longer encouraged to seek alternative lifestyles or contemplate early retirement as a result of coronary disease. They are no longer spectators, but rather active participants, and many become more active and healthier in life after a cardiac event than they were before.

Individuals who are not considered to be good candidates for rehabilitation are usually unstable and include the following:

**Table 18-1 Phases of Cardiac Rehabilitation**

|  | Phase | Description |
|---|---|---|
| Phase I | Acute phase or monitoring phase | Begins when patient medically stable following a MI, CABG, PTCA, valve repair, heart transplantation, or CHF |
| Phase II | Subacute phase of rehab or conditioning phase | Begins as early as 24 hours after discharge, and lasts up to 6 weeks. Frequency of visits depend on the patient's clinical needs. Initiate secondary prevention of disease. |
| Phase III | Training or intensive rehabilitation | Begins at end of Phase II and extends indefinitely. Patients exercise in larger groups and continue to progress in their exercise program. Resistance training often begins in this phase. |
| Phase IV | Ongoing conditioning (maintenance) phase or prevention program | Candidates are individuals who are at high risk for infarction because of their risk factor profile, as well as those who want to continue to be followed by supervision of trained personnel. |

*CABG, coronary artery bypass graft surgery; CHF, congestive heart failure; MI, myocardial infarction; PTCA, percutaneous transluminal coronary angioplasty.*

- Patients who have overt CHF (see Chapter 4), unstable angina pectoris (chest pain at rest), hemodynamic instability (falling blood pressure with exercise), serious arrhythmias, conduction defects, or impaired function of other organ systems
- Patients who have uncontrolled hypertension
- Patients who have other disease or illness that precludes exercise
- Apparently healthy individuals (mixing healthy individuals with persons who have heart disease may inhibit the former and frustrate the latter)

## Management and Evaluation of Patients during the Acute Phase

Inpatient cardiac rehabilitation begins when a patient arrives in the telemetry unit, but it may commence at the bedside in the intensive or coronary care unit, especially if the individual has had to remain there for an extended period of time. Overall, the goals of inpatient cardiac rehabilitation are to assess for safety to perform activities in the home or the alternative care site after discharge from the hospital, and to increase knowledge of the disease and the management of the disease. In addition, the team members must function cohesively in preparing the patient for discharge so as not to make the instructions too complicated or too simple. Specific goals of inpatient cardiac rehabilitation are as follows:

- Evaluation of individual physiologic responses to self-care and ambulation activities. In the telemetry or step-down unit, patients are usually closely monitored by electrocardiogram (ECG) while at rest. However, the hemodynamic changes that can take place with position change, self-care activities, toileting, and the like are potentially dangerous and usually go unobserved or are not closely monitored.

- Provision of feedback to physicians and nurses regarding the patient's response to activity so that recommendations for activity can be made. The cardiac rehabilitation assessment is worthless unless the results can be applied practically while the patient is in the hospital or preparing for discharge. Information should be shared with all team members.
- Provision of safe guidelines for progression of activity throughout convalescence. A day-to-day reassessment of function, as well as hemodynamic and ECG responses to progressive activity provides further information to the physician. This is especially important because it relates to decisions on medication adjustments and on preparation for discharge. To facilitate the team's effectiveness, an overall activity plan can be used for progression in Phase I.
- Provision of patient and family education with reference to disease entity, risk factors and appropriate modification, self-monitoring techniques, and general activity guidelines. It is most important to instill a sense of confidence about what the patient can do safely and what rate of recovery to expect regarding activity. Because patients stay in the acute care phase for limited time, and the patient may not be ready to learn, this step may actually occur during outpatient rehabilitation, but at least some written materials should be provided to the patient and family to assist them in understanding the disease and modifications to reduce impairment, disability, and progression of the disease/dysfunction.

### Initial Assessment/Examination

The initial assessment is conducted as soon as the patient is considered stable by each team member involved in the patient's care, usually within a few hours of referral. A quick response is important to the patient who is anticipating resuming activity, as well as to the medical and health care team who have only a short amount of time to work with the patient and family during the inpatient stay. The assessment should include a thorough chart review, patient-family interview, physical examination, and activity (self-care) and ambulation assessment or screening.

- Chart review—to obtain information, a review of pertinent medical history; physician admission report and subsequent chart notes; surgical report, including cardiac catheterization data; medications; laboratory studies (e.g., cardiac enzymes, hemoglobin/hematocrit, lipid analysis, brain natriuretic peptide [BNP]); noninvasive studies (e.g., echocardiography, ECG, exercise tests, nuclear studies); nurses' notes; physician orders, including those for activity and special instructions for cardiac rehabilitation; and any other pertinent data (e.g., age, hometown, insurance provider, height, weight).
- Patient-family interview—to gain a subjective description of symptoms and other problems; to assess the risk factor profile (see Box 18-1), diet profile, and patient-family goals; and to guide discharge disposition.
- Physical examination—to include assessment of vital signs (e.g., heart rate, blood pressure), auscultation of lung and heart sounds, chest wall inspection and palpation, examination of extremities (peripheral pulses, edema), and gross range of motion and strength.
- Activity (self-care) and ambulation evaluation (ADL monitor)—to monitor the patient's hemodynamic, symptomatic, and ECG response to typical self-care activities. This evaluation is performed one-on-one with a physical therapist and involves the use of a portable ECG monitor so the therapist can observe ECG changes as they occur when the patient becomes mobile (Fig. 18-2). Another option is to have a second person stationed at the central ECG monitors to observe any changes; however, a direct method of communication between therapist and observer must be available. Parameters to be measured during the evaluation include heart rate, blood pressure, ECG, and signs and symptoms. Each parameter is recorded at rest, with activity, immediately after the activity, and 1 to 3 minutes after the activity. Activities may include resting supine, sitting, standing, hygiene and grooming, Valsalva's maneuver (with nonsurgical patients), and lower and upper extremity dressing.
- Ambulation activity—to determine, in addition to the physiologic parameters, the patient's balance and coordination, level of independence, and distance traveled relative to normal ambulation velocity. Response to stair climbing should be evaluated before discharge if the patient must negotiate stairs at home and is considered well enough to do so; however, this is not an activity to be performed early in the recovery phase.

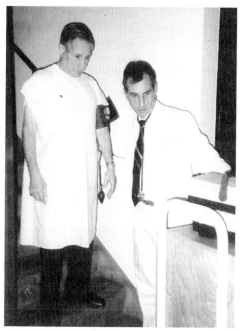

**Figure 18-2** Monitoring the electrocardiogram and blood pressure during stair climbing.

## Activity Program Guidelines

### Indications for an Unmodified Program

Patients who demonstrate appropriate hemodynamic, ECG, and symptomatic responses to the self-care and ambulation evaluation can have their activity levels increased. The rate of progression is individualized and adjusted to each patient's particular limitation, depending on many clinical and functional factors (e.g., complicated versus uncomplicated course, ventricular function, premorbid functional level, number of days on bedrest, philosophy of the referring physician). The physiologic parameters of heart rate, blood pressure, signs and symptoms, ECG findings, and heart sounds continue to be monitored each session, with the results communicated when possible to the patient's nurse and always documented in the chart. Exercise periods are usually conducted at least once daily, lasting approximately 10 minutes for patients on modified programs and 15 minutes for patients who have no limitations. Intensity of activity should be gauged by more than just heart rate limits and should be based on the patient's clinical status and medication regimen. Historically, heart rate levels up to 120 beats per minute (bpm) or 20 to 30 bpm above the resting rate have been used as guidelines; however, with the wide variety of rate-limiting medications, this method is not appropriate. It is the combination of all factors (hemodynamic, symptoms, and ECG findings) that must be considered in determining specific intensity parameters.

### Indications for a Modified Program

Program parameters are modified for persons designated as "complicated" for one or more of the following reasons:

- Large infarction clinically, although stable after 2 to 3 days

**Box 18-3**

**McNeer Criteria for Complicated Myocardial Infarction**

- Poor ventricular function
- Significant ischemia with low-level activity
- Cardiogenic shock
- Ventricular tachycardia and/or fibrillation
- Atrial flutter or fibrillation
- Second- or third-degree atrioventricular (AV) block
- Persistent sinus tachycardia (HR > 100 at rest)
- Persistent systolic hypotension (systolic BP <90 mm Hg at rest)
- Pulmonary edema

Data from McNeer JF, Wallace AG, Wagner GS, et al. The course of acute myocardial infarction: Feasibility of early discharge of the uncomplicated patient. Circulation 51:410, 1975.

- Resting tachycardia (100 bpm) or inappropriate heart rate increase with self-care activities
- Blood pressure failing to rise or decreasing with self-care activities
- The ECG revealing more than six to eight premature ventricular complexes per minute or progressive heart block with self-care activities
- Angina or undue fatigue with self-care activities
- Need for prolonged bedrest (more than 4 days)
- In addition, if an individual is considered to have experienced complications with their acute MI per McNeer Criteria (Box 18-3)

### Indications for Withholding a Program

The following are criteria to exclude patients from participation in the activity program (until instability improves):
- Severe pump failure (as evidenced by shortness of breath, peripheral edema, diaphoresis, or chest x-ray *and* falling blood pressure response to activity).
- Classification in a high-risk subset, described by
  - Recurrent malignant arrhythmias (ventricular tachycardia, four premature ventricular complexes in a row, ventricular fibrillation)
  - Angina at rest
  - Second- or third-degree heart block
  - Persistent hypotension (less than 90 mm Hg)
  - Rapid atrial rhythm
  - Unstable angina pectoris or change in symptoms in the preceding 24 hours

### General Precautions

Before initiating each activity session, the patient's status should be reassessed. There must be a review of the patient's chart. The ECG monitor should be checked for any new changes and vital signs; cardiac rhythm, symptoms, and heart and lung sounds need to be rechecked. Activity sessions should not be initiated within 1 hour after meals. This delay

**Table 18-2 Progressive Activity for 5-Day Length of Stay**

| Day | MET Level | Activity |
|---|---|---|
| Day 1, CCU | 1–2 | Bedrest until stable, use of bedside commode, out of bed to chair if stable |
| Day 2, step-down unit | 2–3 | Sitting warm-ups, walking in room, self-care activities |
| Days 3–5 | 2–3 | Out of bed as tolerated if stable, walk 5–10 minutes in hall (supervised as needed) |
|  | 3–4 | Shower with seat, walk 5–10 minutes 2–3 times/day, up/down one half flight of stairs |

*CCU, critical care unit.*

allows adequate digestion to occur without increased myocardial oxygen demand. It is also important to avoid isometric exercise, specifically breath holding with exercise, because it may produce dramatic changes in blood pressure and arrhythmias. Table 18-2 provides a sample progressive activity plan for a typical length of stay.

### Relative Contraindications to Continuing Exercise

Whenever one of the following occurs, the event should be documented appropriately and the patient's nurse, physician, or both should be contacted immediately.
- Unusual heart rate increase—greater than 50 bpm increase with low-level activity
- Blood pressure indicative of hypertension—abnormally high systolic (greater than 210 mm Hg) or diastolic (greater than 110 mm Hg) pressure
- Drop in systolic blood pressure (greater than 10 mm Hg) with low-level exercise (not just a drop in systolic blood pressure with standing)
- Symptoms with activity:
  - Angina (Level 1 of 4)—see index of angina levels (see Table 18-12)
  - Excessive dyspnea (Level 2+/4+)—see dyspnea index (see Table 18-12)
  - Excessive fatigue
  - Mental confusion or dizziness
  - Severe leg claudication—Level 8/10 on a pain scale of 10
- Signs of pallor, cold sweat, ataxia
- Changing heart sounds with activity—new murmur or ventricular gallop

- Changing lung sounds with activity—increase in level of rales with symptoms of shortness of breath (SOB)
- An ECG abnormality, including marked ST-segment changes (may be only a single event that requires notification, as well as a sustained event) or serious arrhythmias (development of coupled premature ventricular complexes or three in a row, second- or third-degree atrioventricular block, or intermittent rate-dependent conduction disturbance).

## Other Components of the Acute Phase

The amount and type of information provided to patients and their families depend on a variety of factors, which include ability to follow directions, emotional stability after the cardiac event, patient and family's readiness to learn, and basic level of understanding and education. Considering the wealth of information they receive and the usual emotional fragility of the participants, it is best to keep information that patients and their families should retain in a neatly organized packet to which they can refer in the future. The instructions should be kept as simple as possible. It is particularly helpful to have the various team members coordinate their educational materials in one packet. Table 18-3 gives a sample clinical pathway for rehabilitation services.

Any education plan should be specific to the individual's needs and particular risk factors. Almost all patients, and especially family members, are concerned about the prognosis of the disease, the foods they can or cannot eat, what to do in an emergency or if chest pain recurs, and what they can or cannot do physically when they get home. Concerns about acceptable activity usually include sexual activity, although many individuals do not verbalize this concern.

It is no one person's responsibility to provide all the information, but rather that of each team member within the particular specialty area. The educational component should include, but not be limited to, discussions about the following:

- The particular disease process and prognosis—usually discussed by the patient's physician and reinforced by nursing and other allied health team members
- The individual's risk factors and recommendations for behavior modification—usually performed by team members relative to their impact on the problem
- General activity guidelines and home exercise prescription—performed by the physical therapist with specific input from the physician
- The role of exercise—performed by the physical therapist and reinforced by other team members
- Medications (especially the use of nitroglycerin)—performed by the physician, nurse, or pharmacist and reinforced by other team members
- Nutrition and prescribed diet—performed by the physician and dietitian
- Self-monitoring techniques—according to the patient's ability (usually based on symptom-limited response because heart rate may be difficult or inappropriate for

### Table 18-3 Rehabilitation Services in Typical Clinical Pathway for Uncomplicated Myocardial Infarction*

| Day | Activity | Education |
|---|---|---|
| Day 2 | Up in chair Assessment | Explanation of event |
| | Bedside commode | Treatment plan |
| Day 3 | Walk 5–10 min in hall | Assess readiness to learn |
| | Self-care activities | Teach signs/ symptoms |
| | | Nitroglycerin use |
| | | Emergency response to symptoms |
| Day 4 | Walk in hall 5–10 min, 3–4/ day, assess stairs | Safety factors |
| | | Do's and don'ts for home activity |
| | | Introduce Phase II: secondary prevention |
| Discharge planning | | |

*Indications for variations in pathway: frailty, orthopedic problems, cognitive impairment, cerebrovascular accident, renal insufficiency, postoperative bleeding, serious arrhythmias, pulmonary complications, severely impaired left ventricular function

patients to learn to monitor at this time) and performed by the physician, nurse, and physical therapist
- What to do in an emergency

Audiovisual aids (e.g., videos, books) are helpful for patients and family and may be left with them for a time when they are most alert, rested, and prepared to hear the message being presented. This level of readiness is not always present at the time a team member visits.

### Diet and Nutrition

Individual counseling by the dietitian with input from the attending physician usually begins during the inpatient stay. Specific problem areas such as hyperlipidemia, obesity, diabetes, and sodium restriction need to be addressed on an individual basis. Usually the person who prepares the meals at home wants to spend as much time as possible learning what he or she should or should not prepare. More specifics on this topic are discussed later in this chapter in the section on outpatient settings.

### Psychological and Behavioral Rehabilitation

Most patients experience some degree of fear, anxiety, depression, and/or anger that should be monitored. Psychologists,

**Table 18-4 Optimal Outcomes for Patients with Cardiovascular Pump Dysfunction or Failure per APTA Guide to Physical Therapist Practice**

| Functional Limitation/Disability | Patient Satisfaction | Secondary Prevention |
|---|---|---|
| Health-related quality of life is improved | Access, availability, and services provided are acceptable to patient/family, others | Risk of functional decline is reduced |
| Optimal return to role function (worker, student, spouse, grandparent) is achieved | Administrative management of practice is acceptable to patient, family, others | Risk of impairment or of impairment progression is reduced |
| Risk of disability associated with cardiovascular pump dysfunction is reduced | Clinical proficiency of physical therapist is acceptable to patient, family, others | Need for additional physical therapist intervention is decreased |
| Safety of patient and caregivers is increased | Coordination and conformity of care acceptable to patient, family, others | Level of patient adherence to the intervention program is maximized |
| Self-care and home management activities, including ADLs and work/leisure activities, including IADLs are performed safely, efficiently, and at a maximal level of independence with or without devices and equipment | Interpersonal skills of physical therapist are acceptable to patient, family, significant others, and caregivers | Need for reexamination or a new episode of care understood, including changes in: caregiver status, community adaptation, leisure activities, living environment, disease, or impairment |
| Understanding of personal and environmental factors that promote optimal health status is demonstrated | | Professional recommendations are integrated into home, community, work, or leisure |
| Understanding of strategies to prevent further functional limitation and disability is demonstrated | | Utilization and cost of health care services are decreased |

*From American Physical Therapy Association. Guide to physical therapist practice. Phys Ther 77:1163–1650, 1997.*
*ADLs, activities of daily living; IADLs, instrumental ADLs.*

specialized clinical nurse practitioners, social workers, and others are often available to help patients deal with these problems. However, in day-to-day interactions with therapists, dietitians, and other cardiac rehabilitation team members, patients often more readily trust and look to these individuals for support in dealing with their disability. Patients need to be observed by all team members for any degree of denial or anxiety, which may be demonstrated in a variety of ways, such as anger, irritability, or conflict with different team members. Team members should be alert for patients and family members who have a need for psychological intervention.

## Outcome Measures

Because of the limitation of time that a patient stays in the hospital, the acute phase of cardiac rehabilitation is limited. Therefore, the outcomes expected are based upon the functional limitations or disabilities of the patient as assessed upon the initial assessment and any subsequent examinations

made by the therapist. The *Guide to Physical Therapist Practice* provides guidelines on optimal outcomes for patients as well as appropriate terminology for documentation based upon the severity of their cardiovascular pump dysfunction.[7] Table 18-4 provides overall outcomes for patients with cardiovascular pump dysfunction and pump failure. Specific outcome measures for the acute phase are given in Box 18-4 and outcomes are discussed in great detail in Chapter 22.

## Discharge Planning

Patients and their families usually have little time to prepare for discharge, although discussions typically begin as soon as the patient is stabilized in the intensive care unit. Cardiac rehabilitation team members begin presenting discharge information early rather than waiting until the day of discharge. The planning should include the following:
1. A review of general activity guidelines, exercise prescription, dietary regimen, medications (indications, when to take them, and when to contact the physician),

and symptoms to observe with actions to take if they occur.

2. A referral to outpatient rehabilitation for continued treatment and lifestyle modification, to begin as early as 2 to 3 days after discharge. Patients who are not referred immediately and are not given a date or time for return before discharge are less likely to return. Therefore, optimally this referral is a standing order for all patients with cardiac dysfunction or disease upon discharge.

3. A low-level, symptom-limited exercise test for the patient before discharge is preferred; however, some patients return to their physician's office after discharge and have an exercise test performed in the office at that time. The test provides valuable information to the rehabilitation team in establishing discharge activity guidelines and prescriptions for exercise on return to the outpatient program, although some programs accept patients who are unable to perform an exercise test. If a patient has been able to tolerate ambulation in the acute phase and is not referred for a formal exercise test, a 6-minute walk test should be performed to provide the outpatient program a baseline.

## Post Acute Phase Rehabilitation

Cardiac rehabilitation is defined in a CMS NCD and reads as follows: Cardiac rehabilitation is described as consisting of "comprehensive, long-term programs involving medical evaluation, prescribed exercise, cardiac risk factor modification, education, and counseling." These programs "are designed to limit the physiologic and psychological effects of cardiac illness, reduce the risk of sudden death or reinfarction, control cardiac symptoms, stabilize or reverse the atherosclerotic process, and enhance the psychosocial and vocational status of selected patients." In addition, cardiac rehabilitation programs aim to reduce subsequent cardiovascular-related morbidity and mortality.[10]

The NCD 20-10 provides the coverage guidelines for Medicare beneficiaries but many private payers follow this model, including the diagnoses covered for cardiac rehabilitation as well as the amount of coverage. In the prior NCD for cardiac rehabilitation, rewritten in 2006, there was extensive language regarding the use of psychotherapy, psychological testing, and physical and occupational therapy. According to the changed NCD in 2006 (20-10), "the discussion of those services in an NCD for cardiac rehabilitation is inappropriate as the language states that all other payment and coverage rules regarding those services apply regardless of the patient's participation in a cardiac rehabilitation program. Therefore, language regarding psychotherapy, psychological testing, and physical and occupational therapy is removed."[10]

Therefore, according to the NCD, individuals who are beneficiaries of Medicare are candidates for a cardiac rehabilitation program if they have any of the diagnoses described in the clinical box; however, if they do not have access to cardiac rehabilitation or if they do not have a diagnosis covered by the NCD for cardiac rehabilitation (such as CHF) then they still are eligible for rehabilitation in the post–acute care phase and may receive benefits from physical and occupational therapy for identified functional impairments.

Many patients are not of Medicare age, and many other individuals may not have access to a formal cardiac rehabilitation program; therefore, they may still benefit from post–acute phase rehabilitation in the outpatient rehabilitation setting. The following sections help to guide individuals in interventions for patients with primary and secondary cardiovascular disease or dysfunction. The American Association of Cardiovascular and Pulmonary Rehabilitation also publishes guidelines for Cardiac Rehabilitation and Secondary Prevention programs, which includes other program information including documentation and billing that is a great resource for the practitioner.[11]

## Candidacy

Traditionally the patient groups referred to cardiac rehabilitation included patients with complicated and uncomplicated MI, heart failure, angioplasty, heart transplant, and stable angina and postbypass or valve replacement.

Beyond the typical postinfarction and coronary bypass groups, the population base for cardiac rehabilitation has grown to include individuals who at one time were thought not to be good candidates for rehabilitation (including individuals with comorbid conditions, poor ejection fraction, cardiomyopathy, and serious arrhythmias). Therapists must be flexible in program planning, must address each patient's needs on an individual basis, and must provide services through a patient-oriented rather than a program-oriented approach.

In fact, patients with low functional capacity may show significant changes in both physical and functional work capacity (perhaps more than other groups) because they usually function at such a low level.[12-15] Lee and colleagues reported improvement in mean functional aerobic impairment (decreased from 32% to 24%) along with significantly lower ($p < .01$ and $< .05$, respectively) resting and submaximal heart rates in 25 men with ejection fractions less than 40% who were followed for an average of 18.5 months.[14] Coates and associates demonstrated similar improvement in physical work capacity, rate pressure product, and symptom scores in a group of 11 coronary patients who had very low ejection fractions (mean ejection fraction of 19%).[15] Neither of these studies found that exercise was detrimental to cardiovascular health.

Currently under the CMS NCD for cardiac rehabilitation programs (in the outpatient setting), the specific diagnoses that are included are as follows:

- MI within the past 12 months
- CABG surgery
- Stable angina
- Percutaneous transluminal coronary angioplasty (PTCA)
- Heart or heart–lung transplantation
- Heart valve repair or replacement surgery

Congestive heart failure is *not* a diagnosis that is covered in the NCD for cardiac rehabilitation, but individuals who have CHF are excellent candidates for outpatient rehabilitation in a physical therapy setting.

Also, individuals with the above diagnoses who do *not* attend cardiac rehabilitation programs (because of distance to rehab program, etc.) are eligible for outpatient rehabilitation with physical and occupational therapy as part of their Medicare benefit or possibly as part of their insurance benefit using not only their ICD9/10 medical diagnostic code but also an ICD9/10 code indicating their treatment diagnosis.

## Home-Based Cardiac Rehabilitation

Patients with heart disease who have had an uncomplicated hospital course (low-risk) and are considered to be candidates for cardiac rehabilitation but are unable to attend the outpatient program on a regular basis owing to the travel distance may be considered for a home-based program. For this group of patients, a different approach should be considered so that they benefit from the structure and support of a regular rehabilitation program. During the inpatient interview process, the therapist can determine whether at-home therapy could be safely performed. Patients considered candidates for the program are given more extensive discharge instructions regarding self-monitoring techniques, exercise guidelines, dietary management, medications, and the like, and are taught to keep an accurate daily activity log. A weekly telephone call is made by a member of the rehabilitation team to the patient to discuss progress or problems and to provide additional information or materials for program progression. Some programs also have the capability of having ECG information transmitted over the telephone lines while the patient exercises at home. When the patient returns for follow-up care with the physician or for exercise testing (usually performed 3 to 6 weeks after discharge), a 2- to 3-hour follow-up session is arranged with cardiac rehabilitation team members to review the individual's program. Follow-up telephone calls continue weekly for the next month, and activity logs are sent by the patient every 2 weeks; thereafter, monthly contacts are maintained for up to 6 to 12 months. Studies on this form of rehabilitation versus no program versus supervised exercise programs have been favorable; however, physical work capacity improves most significantly in supervised programs.[16,17]

## Rehabilitation/Secondary Prevention in the Outpatient Setting

### The Rehabilitation Team

Successful rehabilitation programs emphasize an interdisciplinary approach, with team members contributing to all phases of patient assessment and direct patient care. The number of team members, as well as the role and function of each, may vary from center to center. Some facilities may have one person performing more than one function. In all cases, primary patient care remains the responsibility of the referring physician. Typical members of the cardiac rehabilitation program are found in Table 18-5. In addition, core competencies for cardiac rehabilitation professionals were published by the American Association of Cardiovascular and Pulmonary Rehabilitation as well as roles and responsibilities of the medical director and should be reviewed.[18,19]

### Program Components

Because cardiac rehabilitation involves more than exercise, the components of a cardiac rehabilitation program should include all aspects of secondary prevention of cardiovascular disease.[20] Exercise training has long been the center of cardiac rehabilitation, yet is only one of several components aimed at reducing risk of illness and death as well as improving function and quality of life. Actual behavior change is necessary for cardiac rehabilitation to be successful. Therefore, because cardiovascular disease involves many factors, a program that assesses the many factors and develops intervention strategies for each one is necessary. Program outcomes are individualized based upon the applicable risk factors that require monitoring and intervention and should be assessed in short-term and long-term follow-up of the patients who have entered the program. See Table 18-6 for program components.

If the cardiac rehabilitation program does not have certain program components on site, a system of referral and follow-up is necessary. This should include a system of assessing goal achievement of desired outcomes for each component and for each participant.

### Efficacy of Cardiac Rehabilitation

Medically prescribed and supervised exercise as part of a comprehensive rehabilitation program is a well-accepted

## Table 18-5 Members of the Cardiac Rehabilitation Team

| Member | Role |
|---|---|
| Medical director | A physician responsible for overall effectiveness and safety of the program. The medical director works closely with the program coordinator and other members of the team, being available for consultation. |
| Program coordinator | Individual skilled in personnel and team management who oversees all team personnel and facilities. Responsible for developing and revising policy, procedures, and budgets; selects needed equipment; and responsible for coordinating and supervising staff. Evaluates program needs. May be a physical therapist, registered nurse, or exercise physiologist. |
| Exercise training professional | A professional who is knowledgeable in exercise physiology, pathology, exercise training techniques, monitoring equipment, arrhythmia recognition, cardiopulmonary resuscitation, and advanced cardiac life support (including defibrillation). Committed to a healthy lifestyle .The preparation and training of physical therapists make them the ideal professional group for this position. Registered nurses and exercise physiologists fill this role in many programs. |
| Dietitian | A professional knowledgeable in nutrition assessment and counseling and experienced in dietary planning and modification |
| Behavior specialist | A professional skilled in behavioral evaluation and counseling techniques who is familiar with coping mechanisms, family patterns of interaction, and available community resources. A psychologist or medical social worker usually fits this position. |
| Vocational counselor | A referral source to the program to assist the individual in a return to work, or in counseling and referral for training for a different career. |

## Table 18-6 Cardiac Rehabilitation Program Components

| Risk Factor | Assessment | Intervention |
|---|---|---|
| Smoking | Current and past smoking habits | Referral to smoking cessation |
| Exercise | Exercise habits, weekly calorie expenditure, maximal functional capacity | Exercise prescription for supervised or individual exercise training |
| Nutrition/lipids | Weight, body fat (body mass index), cholesterol, LDL, and HDL | Nutritional counseling, medical management for elevated cholesterol, weight management |
| Psychosocial | Stress, hostility, depression | Referral for counseling, group support |
| Hypertension | Blood pressure, vascular status (pulses, bruits) | Diet, exercise, counseling, and medication, if necessary |
| Diabetes | Blood glucose fasting blood sugars, urine testing | Diet, exercise, medication (insulin) and diabetic education regarding multisystem dysfunction |
| Menopausal females | Estrogen status, possibly bone density | Dietary evaluation and counseling, estrogen replacement, calcium and other bone-building supplements |

*HDL, high-density lipoprotein; LDL, low-density lipoprotein.*

standard of care throughout the world for cardiac patients, particularly following an acute MI or coronary revascularization procedure. The degree of benefit from cardiac rehabilitation programs as documented in the literature varies considerably. However, exercise rehabilitation has made a positive impact on several risk factors, functional capacity, cardiovascular efficiency, and to some degree on cardiac mortality rate.[21]

Risk factors have been shown to be favorably affected by exercise training in individuals with and without cardiac conditions.[22-25] The benefits of exercise training include the following:

- Loss of excess weight or body fat
- Lowering of lipid levels, including total cholesterol and triglycerides
- Elevation of levels of HDLs

- Reduction of elevated blood pressure levels
- Improvement in glucose insulin dynamics

Heart rate, systolic blood pressure, and the rate–pressure product are generally lower during submaximal efforts following exercise conditioning, resulting in reduced myocardial oxygen demand.[26,27] This is particularly important to patients with exertional ischemia. Reported improvements in symptom-limited, maximal oxygen consumption for patients with angina pectoris ranged from 32% to 56%.[26]

Reduction of physical work capacity is thought to be the result of the degree of myocardial damage, myocardial ischemia, or both. Patients with acute MI and coronary bypass surgery have been shown to demonstrate significant improvement in aerobic capacity following exercise conditioning, on the order of 11% to 66%. The greatest improvements were found in patients with the lowest initial maximum oxygen consumption levels.[26,28,29] The specific cardiovascular adaptations that occur in coronary patients vary depending on the training stimulus and the duration of the program. Eshani and colleagues demonstrated an increase in ejection fraction, stroke volume, and rate–pressure product during maximal exercise in post-MI patients who were trained at intensities of at least 85% of maximal heart rate for at least 1 year in duration.[30] However, no matter what mechanism or physiologic adaptation takes place in trained coronary patients, an increase of aerobic capacity means increased tolerance for daily-life activities consisting of repeated submaximal physical exertion. This translates into a potential for an improved quality of life.

A definitive randomized clinical trial on the independent effect of exercise in prevention of recurrent coronary events in patients recovering from MI, coronary bypass surgery, or angina pectoris has not been conducted. The ability of a single study to test the hypothesis that exercise reduces the mortality rate from coronary heart disease would require a randomized trial of more than 4000 patients. The ability to control all the variables in a single study is nearly impossible and certainly improbable. Nonetheless, several reports have attempted to demonstrate a reduced cardiac mortality rate based on combined data from several larger studies (meta-analysis) and have, in fact, shown some interesting trends and statistical significance with a reduction in mortality rate similar to the salvage rate attributed to β-blocking drugs in clinical trials following an MI.[31]

Unfortunately, many individuals with coronary disease and heart failure are not referred to or do not attend cardiac rehabilitation in the outpatient environment even though it would be extremely beneficial. According to the Agency for Health Care Policy and Research (AHCPR) clinical practice guidelines on cardiac rehabilitation, "of the several million patients with coronary disease who are candidates for cardiac rehabilitation services, only 11 to 38% of patients typically participate in cardiac rehabilitation programs."[32] In addition, "an estimated 4.7 million patients with heart failure may also be eligible, but few such patients participate in cardiac rehabilitation."[32] As a result of the low referral rate to cardiac rehabilitation and the scientific evidence demonstrating

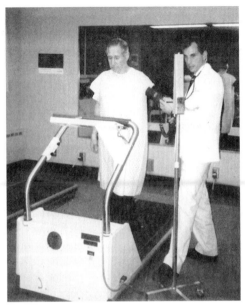

**Figure 18-3** A physical therapist conducting a low-level exercise test.

efficacy of cardiac rehabilitation, the American Association of Cardiovascular and Pulmonary Rehabilitation (AACVPR) and AHA recommended referral to cardiac rehabilitation as performance measures demonstrating quality performance, and these performance measures are outlined in a published joint statement that will hopefully increase appropriate referrals to cardiac rehabilitation.[33]

## Initial Assessment

The objective of the physical evaluation is to assess ventricular function (myocardial reserve, infarct size, or both; presence and severity of ischemia or serious arrhythmia, or both) as it relates to the ramifications of the disease state on the functional abilities of the patient. Components of the initial assessment include the following:

- A thorough medical history
- A patient-family interview
- A physical examination
- An exercise test (Fig. 18-3) or a 6-minute walk test
- A blood chemistry panel

However, as sometimes patients are referred to outpatient rehabilitation without undergoing an inpatient assessment and Phase I rehabilitation or have been referred because of a diagnosis of stable angina or who have undergone angioplasty, all patients should undergo an initial assessment on entry into outpatient rehabilitation. This assessment is discussed in detail in Chapter 16.

## General Management Strategies

The maintenance of a safe and effective risk reduction program is paramount in establishing treatment-monitoring guidelines. The frequency of monitoring and the degree of

## Table 18-7 Stratification for Risk of Event (Not Specific Solely to Exercise)

| Lowest Risk | Moderate Risk | Highest Risk |
|---|---|---|
| No significant LV dysfunction (EF > 50%) | Moderately impaired LV function (EF = 40%-49%) | Decreased LV function (EF < 40%) |
| No resting or exercise-induced complex dysrhythmia | Signs/symptoms including angina at moderate levels of exercise (5-6.9 METs) or in recovery | Survivor of cardiac arrest or sudden death |
| Uncomplicated MI, CABG, angioplasty, atherectomy, or stent | Moderate risk is assumed for patients who do not meet the classification of either highest risk or lowest risk. | Complex ventricular dysrhythmia at rest or with exercise |
| Absence of CHF or signs/symptoms indicating postevent ischemia | | MI or cardiac surgery complicated by cardiogenic shock, CHF, and/or signs/symptoms of postprocedure ischemia |
| Normal hemodynamics with exercise or recovery | | Abnormal hemodynamics with exercise (especially flat or decreasing systolic blood pressure or chronotropic incompetence with increasing workload) |
| Asymptomatic, including absence of angina with exertion or recovery | | Signs/symptoms including angina pectoris at low levels of exercise (<5.0 METs) or in recovery |
| Functional capacity <7.0 METs* | | Functional capacity <5.0 METs* |
| Absence of clinical depression | | Clinically significant depression |
| Lowest risk classification is assumed when each of the risk factors in the category is present. | | Highest risk classification is assumed with the presence of any one of the risk factors included in this category. |

*If measured functional capacity is not available, this variable is not considered in the risk stratification process.
CABG, coronary artery bypass graft; CHF, congestive heart failure; EF, ejection fraction; LV, left ventricle; METs, metabolic equivalent table; MI, myocardial infarction.
Adapted from American Association of Cardiovascular and Pulmonary Rehabilitation. Guidelines for Cardiac Rehabilitation and Secondary Prevention Programs. 4th ed. Champaign, IL, Human Kinetics, 2004, Figure 5-1, p. 63.

direct supervision of an exercise treatment program must be determined for each patient based on prior clinical course (complicated or uncomplicated), exercise test results, degree of ventricular impairment, initial assessment, and risk stratification (Tables 18-7 and 18-8). For some patients, direct monitoring and close supervision of each exercise session may be required and entirely appropriate for the first several weeks (Box 18-5). However, for the majority of patients who have had a clinically uncomplicated course and an exercise test that was uneventful, or that produced no negative findings, such close supervision and monitoring at each session can be counterproductive, implying more risk than is warranted. A number of studies have shown that the incidence of serious complications in the latter group is quite low. For such patients, an effective risk reduction program must concern itself with the development of self-confidence, the motivation for change, the sense of direct involvement of the patient with the management

### Box 18-5

**Recommended Methods and Tools for Daily Assessment of Risk for Exercise**

Pre-exercise assessment should include patient interview regarding recent signs/symptoms and medication adherence. Risk also is assessed with following clinical measures:
- Continuous or intermittent ECG monitoring
  - Telemetry or hardwire monitoring
  - Quick look using defibrillator paddles
  - Periodic rhythm strips
- BP
- HR (palpated)
- Symptoms and evidence of effort intolerance
- Rating of perceived exertion (RPE)

From American Association of Cardiovascular and Pulmonary Rehabilitation: Guidelines for Cardiac Rehabilitation and Secondary Prevention Programs. 4th ed. Champaign, IL, Human Kinetics, 2004.

## Table 18-8  Additional Medical Therapy to Be Considered in Assessing Level of Risk for Subsequent Events

| | |
|---|---|
| Lipids | A. If LDL > 100, consider pharmacologic intervention; if HDL < 35, emphasize weight loss and exercise |
| Antiplatelet | A. Start ASA 80–325 mg qd if not contraindicated |
| | B. Manage warfarin to international normalized ratio = 2.0-3.5 for post-MI patients |
| ACE inhibitors | A. Start early post-MI in stable, high-risk patients (anterior MI, Killip class II (S3 gallop, rales, radiographic CHF) |
| | B. Continue indefinitely for all with LV dysfunction (EF < 40%) or symptoms of failure |
| | C. Use as needed to manage blood pressure or symptoms in all other patients |
| β-Blockers | A. Consider starting in all post-MI patients except those with acute symptomatic heart failure or other contraindications |
| | B. Use as needed to manage angina, rhythm, or blood pressure in all other patients |
| Estrogen replacement | A. Consider estrogen replacement in all postmenopausal women |
| | B. Individualize recommendation consistent with other health risks |

*Adapted from American Association of Cardiovascular and Pulmonary Rehabilitation. Guidelines for Cardiac Rehabilitation and Secondary Prevention Programs. 4th ed. Champaign, IL, Human Kinetics, 2004.*
*ACE, angiotensin-converting enzyme; ASA, acetylsalicylic acid; CHF, congestive heart failure; EF, ejection fraction; HDL, high-density lipoprotein; LDL, low-density lipoprotein; LV, left ventricle; MI, myocardial infarction.*

of the exercise program, and the development of skill in self-monitoring.

Some conditions should limit participation in an exercise program. Patients are not considered candidates for a cardiac rehabilitation program when they have one of the following:

- Unstable status—for example, recurrent ischemic pain, uncompensated CHF, resting tachycardia (greater than 100 bpm; slightly higher for postoperative patients), severe bradycardia (less than 50 bpm)
- Uncontrolled hypertension

- Other illness or disease that precludes exercise
- Apparently good health (low risk for cardiac disease; these individuals should be in a primary prevention program)

Many approaches to outpatient cardiac rehabilitation exist, from large, multidisciplinary team approaches to smaller programs in which one person performs multiple functions. Although there are philosophic differences regarding frequency of activity, mode of exercise, monitoring, and the like, the goals are generally the same. Ideally, the program begins within 48 to 72 hours following discharge from the hospital. Thus, problems that arise early after discharge can be sorted out, questions about care can be answered, and, most important, patients and their families can receive support from the staff and other patients. The goals of outpatient cardiac rehabilitation programs include the following:

- Provision of a flexible, individualized exercise program of the proper intensity to elicit improvement in the patient's cardiovascular fitness without exceeding the safe limits of exercise
- Provision of a program that emphasizes patient education so that the individual can begin to understand the disease and to implement lifestyle changes
- Provision of a program to enhance the confidence of patients with ischemic heart disease or other cardiovascular disorders in their ability to work at safe, functional levels of activity
- Provision of a program to aid the patient in personal risk factor reduction (secondary prevention) to help prevent new or recurrent cardiovascular complications
- Provision of a program that assists in and accelerates the return to work (most patients who have had an uncomplicated course should be able to return to work within 2 months)
- Promotion of psychological, behavioral, and educational improvement

### Interventions

Three interventions are used in the rehabilitation of the patient with cardiovascular disorders in the outpatient setting, including

- Therapeutic exercise
- Patient instruction
- Coordination/communication

### Therapeutic Exercise

A patient's exercise plan should be determined by objective assessment of clinical status, functional capacity, and personal need. What may be good for one person may prove to be detrimental to another. In addition to making a clinical evaluation, the therapist must determine the patient's exercise needs, interests, abilities, and previous habits. The exercise plan should also consider the facilities and equipment that are available as well as the climate and environmental factors that may affect whether the program can be carried out conveniently. These considerations are important in

## Table 18-9 Summary of Individualized Exercise Plan

| Components | Specifics |
|---|---|
| Specificity of exercise | Specific exercise related to patient's regular daily needs and interests |
| Aerobic exercise prescription including: | |
| Mode | Functional, large muscle mass, something fun |
| Intensity | May use target HR |
| | Perceived exertion |
| | Perceived dyspnea |
| Duration | Start with short intervals of 2–5 min; build to 20–30 min |
| Frequency | Short intervals for impaired patient: multiple times/day |
| | Individuals who exercise 20–30 minutes: 5–7 times/week |
| Resistance training | Avoid straining, exhale during exertion |
| | Weight should be 30%-50% 1RM |
| | Perform 8-10 repetitions of each muscle group |
| Flexibility | Assess for any limitations in flexibility |
| | Minimal flexibility exercises: upper extremities, lower extremities—hamstrings and gastrocnemius |
| Build in ability to self-manage symptoms | Instruct in self heart rate monitoring |
| | Weigh self daily if diagnosed with CHF |
| | Instruct in differentiating between chest wall pain, angina and pleuritic pain |

*CHF, congestive heart failure; HR, heart rate.*

motivating the patient to be compliant with the program. The therapeutic exercise program should consist of aerobic exercise training, resistance training, and flexibility exercises (Table 18-9).

## Exercise Training and Effects of Training

The specific demand of habitual physical exercise produces a biochemical change that ultimately enhances the functioning of skeletal muscle and the cardiovascular system. To a large degree, the improvement made by the cardiac patient depends on the degree of ventricular impairment and function. Several studies have demonstrated that some coronary patients can, in fact, improve not only the maximal aerobic capacity but the cardiac output as well.[34-37] Even patients with clinically large infarctions and poor ventricular function demonstrated significant improvement with regard to physical work capacity.[35] There are perhaps even greater functional consequences for them because their reserve is usually so low initially that simple, light household and ADL tasks are very difficult to perform. Persons with less-impaired ventricular function (ejection fraction greater than 50%) often do not notice a very substantial difference in exercise tolerance with usual activities unless they are stressed significantly (at which point they would probably slow down or stop).

Exercise training creates change specifically in the muscle groups that are challenged (a principle that is known as specificity of exercise). This fact becomes important in selecting the most appropriate activity to produce the greatest functional gain. Nearly everyone needs to walk some distance. In addition, we all need to use our arms to some degree, some of us more than others. Why is it then that so many cardiac patients ride stationary bicycles? The exercise program should produce changes specific to the functional needs of the patient, especially those who have upper extremity demands. Upper extremity testing and training must be incorporated into the patients' plans, particularly if they will be returning to a vocation that requires a significant amount of arm work (e.g., maintenance workers, loggers, carpenters, plumbers). The specific testing and training should be specific for the type of work or leisure the individual wishes to return to performing.

The effects of conditioning last only as long as the individual continues to exercise. Cardiac patients must understand that exercise must be included as a lifetime process for the results to be lasting.

### Components of the Exercise Prescription for Aerobic Training

Aerobic exercise involving moving large muscle groups in a dynamic manner has been shown to produce a substantial benefit in cardiorespiratory endurance. The components of the exercise intervention include (see Table 18-9 for a summary) mode, intensity, frequency, duration or frequency, intensity, type, and time.

**Mode.** The mode of exercise should include muscles that perform the regular activity the patient is used to. Therefore, aerobic exercise training of leg muscles should be performed to improve aerobic capacity of patient with walking. Upper extremity exercise training (aerobic and strength) should be included as an intervention, but specific training may be limited in individuals with recent MI or CABG surgery with sternal incisions until the tissues have healed (6–12 weeks, depending on the injury, procedure, and physician's guidelines). Static or isometric (anaerobic) exercise involving the development of tension but little or no change in muscle length or movement for short periods of time may improve strength but may also produce undesirable responses in the cardiac patient. Isometric exercise may, in fact, impose a

## Table 18-10 Abnormal Responses to Exercise

| Response | Description |
|---|---|
| Exercise hypertension | Systolic: > 240 mm Hg |
| | Diastolic: > 110 mm Hg, or until controlled |
| Systolic hypotension | >20 mm Hg drop from upright resting blood pressure) |
| Unusual heart rate response | Too rapid an increase, failure to increase, or a decrease with exercise |
| Symptoms | Significant anginal response |
| | Undue dyspnea |
| | Excessive fatigue |
| | Mental confusion or dizziness |
| | Severe leg claudication |
| Signs | Pallor |
| | Cold sweat |
| | Ataxia |
| | New murmur |
| | Pulmonary rales |
| | Onset of significant third heart sound |
| ECG abnormalities | Serious arrhythmias |
| | Second- or third-degree heart block |
| | Onset of right or left bundle branch block |
| | Acute ST changes |

## Box 18-6

### Upper Limits (Signs and Symptoms) for Exercise Intensity

Peak exercise training heart rate should be set below the heart rate that occurred at the onset of any of the following:

- Angina or other symptoms of cardiovascular insufficiency
- Plateau or decrease in systolic blood pressure (SBP)
- SBP > 240 mm Hg or diastolic BP > 110 mm Hg
- Electrocardiographic evidence of ischemia (ST-segment depression)
- Increased frequency of ventricular arrhythmias
- Ventricular arrhythmias of >6/minute
- Exercise electrocardiographic evidence of left ventricular dysfunction
- Other significant ECG disturbances (e.g., second- or third-degree AV block, supraventricular tachycardia, exercise-induced atrial fibrillation)
- Level 3–4 dyspnea
- Other clear signs or symptoms of exertional intolerance

Adapted from ACSM's Guidelines for Graded Exercise Testing and Prescription. 5th ed. Baltimore, Williams & Wilkins, 1995.

## Table 18-11 Formulas for Calculating Predicted and Target Heart Rates*

| A | General population | 220 − age = PMHR |
|---|---|---|
| B | Fit individuals older than 40 | 205 − age = PMHR |
| C | Karvonen method | ([MHR − RHR] × training %) + RHR = Target HR |

*Formulas A and B should not be used when the true maximal heart rate can be determined or the patient is taking medications that would affect the resting and exercise heart rate (e.g., β-blocking medications).
HR, heart rate; MHR, maximum heart rate; PMHR, predicted maximal heart rate; RHR, resting heart rate.

pressure load on the left ventricle that is not tolerated well, increasing myocardial demand, especially in patients who have poor ventricular function.[38,39] Examples of isometrics includes intensive weight bearing on upper extremities while using a walker, as well as static lifting.

**Intensity.** Training intensity is the key element in the exercise prescription for an individual starting an aerobic exercise program because if exertion is too intense, training can be compromised, hazardous, or both (Table 18-10 and Box 18-6). Heart rate is often a reliable indicator of myocardial and total oxygen requirement during exercise if the patient is not on β-blocking medications (see Chapter 14). Heart rate responses are commonly used to quantify and monitor endurance training. Aerobic forms of exercise can be performed continuously and can produce a training effect on the central mechanisms (changes in resting heart rate and stroke volume) at workload intensities of 70% to 85% of maximal heart rate (as low as 40% to 50% in the elderly or in individuals with severe ventricular dysfunction) or 50% to 85% of maximal oxygen consumption.[21] However, training intensity may be kept lower than 40% to 50% of maximal

heart rate in the severely endurance-impaired individual or individuals with impaired ventricular performance.[40,41]

Formulas used to predict appropriate training heart rates have been used in planning exercise programs for healthy individuals and for some patient groups, including those with coronary artery disease (Table 18-11). The commonly accepted range of training heart rate is 70% to 85% of maximal heart rate or 50% to 85% of maximal oxygen consumption.[42,43] The effects of β-blockers, calcium-channel blockers, surgical intervention, and pacemakers, among others, make it improbable that these methods would be accurate for cardiac patients who need more precise and effective measurements. β-Blockers and some calcium-channel blockers decrease resting and exercising heart rate response. However, neither β- nor calcium-blocking medications alter the relationship between the percentage of heart rate and the percentage of oxygen consumption.[44] The important implication is that, when exercise-testing an individual before beginning exercise training, the individual should be taking the medication that will be used during the training program. The medication should not be discontinued for the exercise test. If medication that affects heart rate is started or discontinued, or if the dosage is significantly altered after the initial test, a repeat exercise test should be performed to define the training heart rate. The key principle in determining a safe and appropriate intensity of exercise for individuals with heart disease is individualizing the prescription of exercise. In the event an exercise test has not been performed on patients referred for outpatient rehabilitation, then a 6-minute walk test should be performed prior to developing an exercise prescription in view of the fact that formulas are inaccurate.

The importance of ventilatory threshold in exercise prescription has begun to be examined. This measurement, which is determined during metabolic exercise testing, is the level of exercise at which there is a nonlinear increase in the ventilation in relation to oxygen uptake. It is the estimated upper limit of aerobic exercise. Comparing heart rate relationships with the measured oxygen consumption and the ventilatory threshold provides a much more exact measurement of exertion levels and is a preferred noninvasive method of assessing training limitations. This method is particularly helpful in patients who have multisystem dysfunction, such as coronary artery disease with chronic obstructive pulmonary disease, coronary artery disease and diabetes, and ventricular pump dysfunction. In particular, patients on β-blockers and calcium-channel blockers and those with pacemakers would benefit most from this type of assessment. Most testing, however, is done *without* metabolic analysis of exercise (because of cost and availability of equipment); therefore, a combination of other intensity parameters should be examined in establishing a training heart rate.

Establishing a Training Heart Rate by Rating of Perceived Exertion. This method of measuring heart rate was first introduced in 1962 by Gunnar Borg.[45] It is a scale of subjective levels of exertion beginning with "very, very light level" and advancing to "very, very hard level." This scale has been adapted several times to make it more easily understood. It has been shown to be a fairly accurate marker in some studies relating it to ventilatory threshold (a perceived exertion score of 13 is equivalent to the ventilatory/anaerobic threshold). Using it in conjunction with other markers of ischemia and arrhythmias and relative to maximal heart rate makes this a very valuable tool, especially for the individual who has difficulty in accurately measuring a pulse, such as in the presence of atrial fibrillation or the patient on β-blockers.

Establishing Training Heart Rates Using Signs and Symptoms. Patients may initially demonstrate symptoms of ischemia in the form of angina pectoris, dyspnea, or both. This should always be documented in relation to ECG changes and levels of myocardial oxygen consumption (heart rate times blood pressure at time of initiation of symptoms). Usually this response has made itself evident in the testing laboratory, and precautions or limitations are documented before exercise training begins. However, changes can occur rapidly in this patient population, and it is often the therapist in the exercise area who first identifies this change (see Box 18-6). Levels of angina should be discussed with all patients before beginning exercise, with instructions as to appropriate responses. Stable cardiac patients are often allowed and even encouraged to exercise up to level 1 (Table 18-12) as long as they are comfortable and recover well when they cool down. Some patients prefer to use nitroglycerin during exercise when symptoms begin or even during warm-up to prevent the onset of angina. Taking nitroglycerin often allows them to exercise at higher levels of intensity. Heart rate, blood pressure, and ECG changes must be monitored in these patients.[46]

## Table 18-12 Angina and Dyspnea Rating Scales

| 5-Grade Angina Scale | 5-Grade Dyspnea Scale | 10-Grade Angina/ Dyspnea Scale |
|---|---|---|
| 0 = No angina | 0 = No dyspnea | 0 = Nothing |
| 1 = Light, barely noticeable | 1 = Mild, noticeable | 1 = Very slight |
| 2 = Moderate, bothersome | 2 = Mild, some difficulty | 2 = Slight |
| 3 = Severe, very uncomfortable: preinfarction pain | 3 = Moderate difficulty, but can continue | 3 = Moderate |
| 4 = Most pain ever experienced: infarction pain | 4 = Severe difficulty, cannot continue | 4 = Somewhat severe |
| | | 5 = Severe |
| | | 6 |
| | | 7 = Very severe |
| | | 8 |
| | | 9 |
| | | 10 = Very, very severe; maximal |

Dyspnea is often another indication of exercise intolerance and may be used as a guide to limit intensity. Coronary patients with a smoking history and perhaps some degree of chronic obstructive pulmonary disease may find this a particularly useful tool to determine intensity (see Table 18-12).

**Continuous aerobic training.** Aerobic training involves three phases of exercise: a warm-up phase, a peak interval phase, and a cool-down phase. Each phase is important in the cardiac patient population because it allows certain physiologic adaptations to occur for the patient to exercise safely. The warm-up phase usually lasts 5 to 10 minutes and involves a form of stretching routine of the exercising muscles and a period of slower performance of the aerobic activity (e.g., walking before a walk/jog or before jogging). This allows time for the exercising muscles to achieve adequate stretch to the length they will be used during peak exercise, as well as time for the peripheral vasculature and coronary arteries to dilate and carry larger volumes of arterial blood.

The peak interval usually lasts 15 to 45 minutes, depending on the level of conditioning, and is the period when the individual works at training intensity levels. Established parameters should be checked every 10 minutes or less to determine if the individual is exercising at, above, or below expected levels. The cool-down is a period of 5 to 15 minutes after the peak interval, during which time the exercising muscles are slowly brought to rest. Too abrupt an end or a cessation of exercise can reduce the return of blood to the myocardium, creating irritation and increased arrhythmia. Included in the cool-down period should be some stretching exercises for individuals who are extremely deconditioned or who have notable muscular inflexibility.

Patients with limited exercise tolerance may not be able to tolerate even 10 minutes of exercise, so that the warm-up, peak interval and cool down are all condensed into one. These individuals will require a longer time (weeks/months) of exercise training, and should be exercised to their tolerance and then insert a rest. Interval training is the best method of improving exercise tolerance in these severely limited individuals. Frequent bouts of exercise are important for these individuals, but not increased intensity. The goal should be to increase the number of bouts to try to increase endurance.

**Four- versus two-extremity exercise.** Most exercise programs with coronary patients have emphasized dynamic leg exercise; however, activity patterns during daily life are more varied. Many tasks require static or isometric efforts, sometimes in combination with dynamic exercise and often involving more upper than lower extremity efforts. In prescribing exercises for conditioning, it is desirable to impose a large metabolic load on the individual without causing cardiovascular or subjective strain. Spreading the work over greater muscle mass by using arms and legs together may allow a greater load to be tolerated with similar cardiac and subjective strain; however, the ability of the individual with left ventricular dysfunction to tolerate and benefit from this mode of training may vary. Combining upper and lower

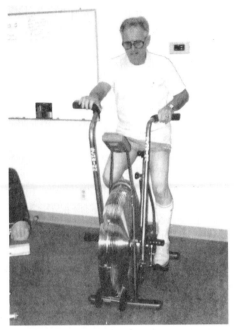

**Figure 18-4** A patient performing a four-extremity exercise.

extremity exercise can produce a higher maximal oxygen consumption than that produced by either body segment alone.[47] A larger actively exercising skeletal muscle mass may explain this finding (Fig. 18-4).

Gutin and colleagues have examined the physiologic response to arm and leg work with special attention to oxygen consumption and ventilatory threshold.[48] They found maximal oxygen consumption and heart rate significantly lower for exercise with arms alone but not for arms and legs combined or legs alone. The ventilatory threshold was significantly higher for arms alone than for legs alone, and even though adding arms to legs did not increase peak physiologic measures, it did not result in the ventilatory threshold occurring at a higher percentage of oxygen consumption. The rate pressure product and rating of perceived exertion were similar for all of these modes.

**Frequency and duration of exercise.** Just as there is no best method to determine training heart rate, there is no standard exercise duration for all coronary patients. Exercise duration should be individualized and based on several factors:
- Length of disability
- Reduced activity as a result of the acute event
- Premorbid activity level and neuromuscular capability

Individuals who were quite active and who had good to moderate ventricular function usually can tolerate 20 to 30 minutes of exercise within 1 to 2 weeks of beginning the outpatient program, whereas individuals who have sustained considerable ventricular impairment or have a long-standing illness may have difficulty exercising for more than a few minutes before fatigue sets in. These patients usually do best with an intermittent activity program of low intensity, short duration, frequent rest periods, and progressing by systematically reducing periods of rest and increasing periods of exercise. In either case, it is important to remember that the exercising muscle needs time to recover before further activity can be tolerated comfortably.

Understanding the way the body recovers from exercise and the need for modified activity patterns and rest periods, especially in Phase II, is of utmost importance. Patients should learn that they are just beginning a process that, it is hoped, will last a lifetime and that a slow, systematic approach is not only safer but more enjoyable. The goal is to have the patient reach 45 minutes of continuous aerobic activity, including a warm-up and cool-down period, as soon as the patient can adjust and without exercising beyond the symptom limit. This may take 3 to 6 weeks or longer.

Most patients should be able to tolerate daily exercise. Some patients may find it difficult to maintain the same intensity or duration every day; however, they should be encouraged to work to their prescribed levels at least four times a week for the best conditioning effect. Initially, some patients with less than 20 minutes of exercise tolerance will be asked to work out two times per day and perhaps three times a day if tolerance is 10 minutes or less. Unless a patient is on bed rest or is hospitalized with restricted activity, independent exercise should be possible, even for most high-risk patients, as long as the patient understands how to monitor signs and symptoms and control activity levels. This should be an early lesson to enhance a patient's psychological outlook.

**Resistance exercise training.** The previous perception of muscle resistance exercise was that it was harmful or of no benefit to cardiac patients; however, the scientific literature did not support this perception. Instead, muscle-strengthening programs using resistive weight exercises have become an acceptable component of cardiac rehabilitation for many patients. As resistive exercises improve muscle strength and endurance, these exercises may improve exercise tolerance as well.[49-51] Muscle strengthening and endurance may be important for the return to activities of daily living and leisure and vocational activities in many patients.

Muscle resistive exercises of low weight (approximately 40% of one repetition maximum) and high repetitions have demonstrated lower myocardial oxygen consumption as compared to dynamic exercise and have proven to be safe and efficacious.[52,53] Careful selection of candidates is imperative. The AACVPR provides guidelines on patient selection for resistive training (Box 18-7).[54] Once a patient is cleared as a candidate, the patient needs to be monitored (including HR, BP, ECG, and symptoms) during the initial assessment. The initial assessment may involve a one–repetition maximum lift (1-RM), a modified 1-RM (90% of expected repetition maximum), isokinetic testing, or a progressive increase in weight loads to tolerance. After the initial assessment, the resistive program should be performed approximately two to three times/week. The AHA and the AACVPR have developed guidelines based upon current literature that recommend a low-intensity program of resistance training for cardiac and older patients (Box 18-8).[54,55]

---

> ### Clinical Tip
>
> A one–repetition max strength test as an initial assessment of strength should be recorded and used as an outcome measure in the rehabilitation program rather than the manual muscle test traditionally used by therapists. The one repetition max or modified 1-RM is measurable and is a better test to demonstrate change in this population than a manual muscle test. Another option is a multiple repetition maximal test.

---

### Box 18-7

#### Patient Considerations for Resistance Exercise Programming*

Although there are no data documenting safety of resistance training after myocardial infarction (MI), coronary artery bypass graft (CABG), or percutaneous transluminal coronary angioplasty (PTCA), certain precautions should be taken. Care must be taken to avoid problems associated with sternal wound healing (CABG) and femoral arterial puncture site (PTCA). In addition, avoidance of excessive myocardial work early after MI is essential.

- For all cardiac patients, there must be no evidence of
  - Symptomatic congestive heart failure
  - Uncontrolled arrhythmias
  - Severe valvular disease
  - Unstable symptoms
  - Uncontrolled hypertension
- Patients with moderate hypertension (systolic BP ≥ 160 mm Hg or diastolic BP ≥ 100 mm Hg) should be referred to appropriate management, but it is not an absolute contraindication for participation in a resistance training program.
- Participation in resistance training may begin following:
  - A minimum of 5 weeks post-MI including 4 weeks of continuous program participation
  - A minimum of 8 weeks post CABG including 3 weeks of continuous program participation
  - A minimum of 2 weeks of consistent participation post PTCA

*A resistance exercise program, for the purposes of this table, is defined as one in which patients lift weights 50% or greater than 1-RM. The use of elastic bands, 1-to 3-lb hand weights and light free weights may be initiated in a progressive fashion at immediate outpatient program entry, provided there are no other contraindications.
Data from American Association of Cardiovascular and Pulmonary Rehabilitation. Guidelines for Cardiac Rehabilitation and Secondary Prevention Programs. 4th ed. Champaign, IL, Human Kinetics, 2004.

---

Resistive exercise programs can include a variety of options including elastic bands, light hand or cuff weights, free weights or dumbbells, wall pulleys, or weight machines (Fig 18-5). Table 18-13 lists progressive resistance options.

As the outcome of the resistance program is to return the individual to work, recreational, or daily living activities with less fatigue and less risk of injury, outcome measures should be based upon the limitation assessed. Muscle strength, endurance, and hemodynamic and symptomatic responses to activities should be measured and recorded before and after resistance training sessions.

## Box 18-8

### Recommendations for Resistance Training

Pretest: To identify the load that should be performed, a 1 repetition maximum (1-RM) should be performed.

Training: Weights should be set at approximately 30%-50% of the 1-RM.

Perform one set of 8–10 repetitions for each major muscle group 2–3 times/week with a day of rest between each workout.

Specific considerations during resistance training:

1. Exercise large muscle groups before small muscle groups.
2. Raise weights slowly with controlled movements, and return weights slowly with controlled movements.
3. Exhale during the exertion phase of the lift, inhale during the return to rest position.
4. Increase loads by 5–10 lb when 12–15 repetitions can be performed comfortably.
5. Minimize rest periods between exercises if trying to maximize endurance of muscles.
6. Avoid straining; avoid sustained tight gripping; rating of perceived exertion (RPE) should be between 11 and 13 (on scale of 20).
7. Stop exercise in event of warning signs or symptoms such as dizziness, palpitations, unusual shortness of breath, or angina.

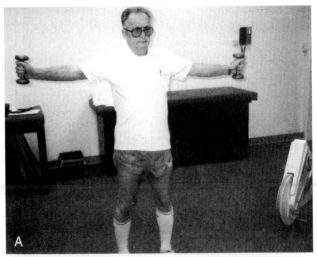

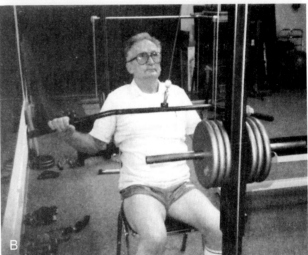

**Figure 18-5 A,** A patient using weights to perform upper extremity exercises. **B,** A patient performing a resistance workout as part of a comprehensive cardiac rehabilitation program.

### Circuit Training

Circuit training entails performing a series of activities one after another while keeping the heart rate elevated. At the end of the last activity, one starts at the beginning again and carries on until the entire series has been repeated several times. The advantage is that every individual undergoes a program adjusted to a personal level of fitness. Circuit training can also be performed in a limited space and produces a high degree of motivation, yet the improvements seen in circuit training is only related to the muscle groups that are used in the exercises, thus improving endurance in the muscles but no appreciable improvement in aerobic capacity.

### Flexibility Programs

Activities of daily living, leisure activities, and occupational activities all require an optimal range of motion of joints involved in work; therefore, maintaining or improving range of motion may be an important component of the cardiac rehabilitation program. Rehabilitation programs should emphasize proper stretching as part of a warm-up and cooldown, especially of upper and lower trunk, neck, and low back and hip regions. Flexibility exercises should be performed in a slow, controlled manner after the muscle has had an increase in circulation (Fig. 18-6).

### Program Progression

Patients should be taught to pay attention to their bodies' responses to increasing activity and to progress in an orderly fashion based on acceptable evidence of tolerance of the activity (Fig. 18-7). Patients should have their program goals reviewed on a regular basis (at least every 2 weeks initially) to reestablish guidelines for their exercise program (including contraindications to exercise), and for risk reduction in general. Program progression can take several forms:

- Increasing the duration of exercise (increase duration first until one reaches 20 to 30 minutes)
- Increasing the intensity of exercise
- Changing the mode of exercise (e.g., including upper or combined upper and lower extremity exercise)

Many patients in Phase II can progress to 85% to 95% or greater of the initial exercise test results, especially if the test was low level and was stopped before any limiting symptoms appeared. A determination of the patient's safety of progression should be based on a daily observation and reassessment by the therapist. Cardiac bypass patients are often quite limited during the initial few weeks of the program owing to various medical factors, such as a low hemoglobin level and a healing sternum, but they demonstrate a rather quick turnaround and begin to work at much higher levels when these conditions normalize. Upper

## Table 18-13   Options for Progressive Resistance Exercise

| Option | Pros and Cons |
| --- | --- |
| Elastic bands (sometimes referred to as Thera-Band) | Inexpensive |
| | Variable thickness makes it variable in resistance (different colors are used for different thickness and resistance) |
| | Progressive resistance can be performed throughout entire range of motion |
| | Portable; can be carried anywhere |
| Cuff and hand weights | Inexpensive |
| | Variable weight ranges from $\frac{1}{2}$ lb |
| | Portable |
| | Add to energy cost of activity of walking or other aerobic activity |
| | Used for progressive resistive exercise as well as increasing energy cost |
| Free weights: dumbbells and barbells | Inexpensive |
| | Variable weights ranging from 1 lb with increments of 1–5 lb |
| | Dumbbells are handheld; free weight plates are attached on the ends of a barbell |
| | Used for progressive resistance exercises |
| | Light dumbbells are portable; heavier weights are not practical to be carried outside rehabilitation center |
| Wall pulleys | Relatively inexpensive |
| | Require little space |
| | Require some instruction for correct use |
| Weight machines | Expensive, requires substantial space |
| | Used for circuit training or multistation format |

extremity stretching and strengthening are important with this population in particular and should be included in the exercise program when the sternum is well healed at approximately 6 weeks. Some patients may also develop complications or problems that force them to discontinue their program for a period of time. When they resume, they must be cautioned about trying to catch up and progress too quickly. In general, if the individual becomes better conditioned, exercise intensity can be increased without significant increase in heart rate response, symptoms, or ECG changes. Most patients can be expected to increase the peak interval period of exercise by at least 5 minutes a week barring medical complications.

### Other Considerations in Planning Exercise Programs

**Altitude.** At 3000 feet above sea level and less, most patients find little discomfort exercising; however, above this level, and certainly above 5000 feet, the atmospheric pressure begins to drop, and the body adapts to achieve the same cardiac output by increasing the heart rate. Angina levels may be reached sooner in terms of exercise intensity and physically demanding activity that may not be a problem at sea level. Patients who enjoy skiing (especially cross-country) or who travel to destinations with an elevation above 3500 feet (e.g., Denver, Mexico City) should be counseled about activity guidelines at these levels.

**Cold.** Cold temperatures cause an increase in peripheral resistance at rest and with exercise. This peripheral vasoconstriction can subsequently cause an increase in arterial blood pressure and possibly create a situation for earlier ischemic changes with increased myocardial oxygen demands as well as cold-induced vasospasm. Patients exercising outdoors in cold weather should be counseled about the importance of wearing layers of clothing, a wool hat and gloves for body heat retention; and a scarf around the mouth to warm the air; and taking in an adequate amount of fluid despite the lack of noticeable perspiration.

**Heat and humidity.** In response to higher temperatures and dilation of peripheral vasculature, heart rate increases to maintain adequate cardiac output. The ability of an individual to perform successfully in hot environments depends on the magnitude of heat, the existing humidity, the movement of air, and the intensity and duration of exercise. The amount of direct exposure as opposed to shade or cloud cover is also a critical factor. One of the primary concerns when exercising in the heat is dehydration. With high sweat rates, the body loses a large volume of water. Because a major portion of the water comes from blood volume, a serious condition exists unless rehydration is accomplished by consuming appropriate fluids (preferably water), both during and after exercise. Again, early symptoms of angina may occur. Avoidance of vigorous exercise or activity in temperatures

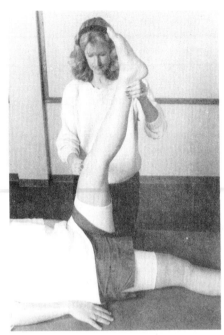

**Figure 18-6** Incorporating flexibility exercises into an exercise prescription is important in cardiac rehabilitation. One of the key flexibility exercises involves stretching the hamstring muscle. Hamstring stretching is optimally performed with one leg flat on the table, while the opposite hip is flexed to 90 degrees, starting with the knee bent at 90 degrees. The lower leg (knee to foot) is then passively extended to the end of the passive range while maintaining the pelvis in neutral position.

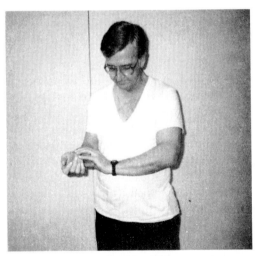

**Figure 18-7** This patient is taking his own pulse as part of a self-monitoring instructional session. Patients learn self-monitoring in order to assess the intensity of their exercise session and to be able to progress their activity on their own.

above 75°F or humidity greater than 65% to 70% is usually recommended. Wearing looser fitting and fewer clothes, protecting the skin by applying a sun screen, exercising at cooler times of the day, and staying in shaded areas as much as possible are recommended. Patients should consult with their physicians before using a steam bath or sauna.

## Secondary Prevention: Management of Risk Factors

### Early Intervention

Educating the individual with heart disease about the problem of CAD plays a significant role in preventing further cardiovascular disease and in the rehabilitation process as a whole. Patients and their families must be informed about how to make lifestyle changes and kept up to date on current medical information as it pertains to the disease process. Many changes have occurred in the past 10 years that have had a profound effect on the management of cardiovascular disease, including exercise interventions, dietary modifications, and other lifestyle changes. Once through the crisis stage, and perhaps as early as the first or second day after the event (MI, CABG surgery, or other cardiovascular disorder), patients and their families are most receptive to learning about what they can do to reduce the risk of disease progression. It is at this time that, in addition to being supportive, the health care team (including the physician, nurse, physical therapist, and dietitian) should begin the process of presenting specific information relating to the individual's particular risk factor profile. As patients progress through the hospitalization, small amounts of information in various forms prepare them to make educated choices about their cardiac health.

### The Outpatient Setting

A patient's educational background should not be a limiting or predisposing factor in achieving an understanding of the disease and rehabilitative process or risk factor modification. There is no limit to the number of health care professionals, including physicians and nurses, whose level of understanding falls far short of what is necessary to make appropriate "heart healthy" choices. These individuals often need the most guidance and supervision because of the preconceived expectation that they will make all the correct decisions.

Basic education should be provided in both an individual encounter and in a group format. Initially, the patient and the family must understand their particular requirements regarding lifestyle modifications and a specific plan of action. The core components of secondary prevention have been outlined in a scientific statement by the AHA and AACVPR and are a resource for the cardiac rehabilitation professional.[20] The need to establish a specific time for follow-up should not be overlooked. Frequent checks of the level of understanding and progress being made should be performed by all team members with each visit. If a patient or family member seems to be having difficulty with the plan, for whatever reason, a team member should intervene to determine if goals were set too high, if certain points need to be clarified, or if some other problem mandates attention and program modification (e.g., problems related to the side effect of medications, new symptoms, or psychological problems).

Participation in group education programs is an excellent source of support for patients with similar cardiac diagnoses.

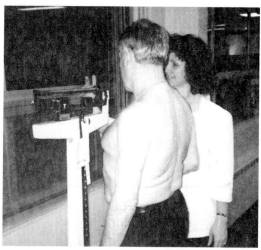

**Figure 18-8** The dietitian checks a patient's weight during a cardiac rehabilitation treatment session.

**Table 18-14 Lipid Values Indicative of Higher Risk**

| | | |
|---|---|---|
| Total cholesterol (mg/dL) (>75th percentile) | >220 | 20–29 years old |
| | >220 | 30–39 years old |
| | >240 | 40 years or older |
| Low-density lipoprotein (LDL) (mg/dL) | >100 | |
| | >175 | Extremely high risk |
| High-density lipoprotein (HDL) (mg/dL) | <35 | |
| LDL:HDL | 3:1 | |
| Triglycerides (mg/dL) | >200 | |

*Adapted from the National Cholesterol Education Program (NCEP) Executive summary of the third report of the Expert Panel on Detection, Evaluation and Treatment of High Blood Cholesterol in Adults (Adult Treatment Panel III). JAMA 285:2486–2497, 2001.*

Most programs include, and should encourage, spousal or family participation because their concerns and level of understanding play a vital role in the patient's rehabilitation process. Sharing their cardiac experiences helps individuals adjust to their feelings and fears about the present and the future. Skilled, knowledgeable leaders are required for these education programs and should encompass a variety of disciplines because no single individual can address all aspects of care in the depth of expertise required.

## Diet and Nutrition

Dietary management for the cardiac outpatient should be designed to fit that person's specific lipid abnormality, cultural background, and lifestyle. To determine specific needs for intervention, a nutritional assessment should be performed by a dietitian or physical therapist that includes the following anthropometric, biochemical, dietetic, and clinical parameters. Anthropometric parameters include height, weight, weight history, and skinfold measurements (when capable) to help determine the appropriate percentage of body fat. This information is useful in determining ideal weight and may show tendencies of the patient for weight gain or loss (Fig. 18-8). A biochemical analysis includes the following:

- Lipid profile (total serum cholesterol, HDL cholesterol, LDL cholesterol, very-low-density lipoprotein [VLDL] cholesterol, and triglycerides)
- Electrolyte panel ($Na^+$ and $K^+$)
- Complete blood cell count (hemoglobin, hematocrit, white blood cells, and platelets)
- Blood urea nitrogen, creatinine, prealbumin, and serum albumin

The lipid profile is helpful when the ratio of total cholesterol to HDL cholesterol is calculated and compared with the data collected in the Framingham study.[56] Total cholesterol values should be evaluated as well as values for LDL and HDL cholesterol, total cholesterol to HDL cholesterol, LDL to HDL cholesterol ratio, apolipoproteins, and triglycerides

(Tables 18-14 and 18-15). Optimal values for apolipoproteins are still under investigation. Even with an established normal cholesterol level, the validity of the values obtained during the analysis of lipids is questionable.[57] Much discrepancy has been observed among laboratories when lipids are analyzed.[58]

To decrease the risk of coronary artery disease and its progression, it is necessary to increase levels of HDL and decrease levels of LDL cholesterol, total cholesterol, and triglycerides. Studies indicate that for each 1% decrease in total cholesterol there is a corresponding 2% decrease in the risk of developing coronary disease.[59,60] Lipids may be altered through many methods, some of which offer better results than others (Table 18-16). There are many causes of hyperlipidemia, each of which must be identified and treated. If one method to alter lipids fails, other methods are available. Family members should also be screened because of the genetic link between lipids and coronary artery disease.

A complete blood cell count helps to identify patients, especially postoperative patients, who may be limited functionally because of poor oxygen-carrying capacity of the blood cells. Electrolyte panels determine deficiencies or abnormalities in other systems or organs.

## Weight Loss

Obesity is a significant risk factor for coronary artery disease, and one reason is the effect that it has on serum lipid levels. Weight loss has been shown to reduce total cholesterol, LDL cholesterol, and triglycerides and to increase HDL cholesterol.[61,62]

A dietetic or clinical analysis should include a 24-hour recall of food eaten or a 3- to 7-day food diary, and a nutritional history specific for coronary heart disease, including information on the use of fat, types of oils, cholesterol-rich foods, alcohol, caffeine, sucrose, sodium, and fiber. An individual diet prescription can be outlined, using the patient's

## Table 18-15 Lipid Management and Recommendations for Intervention

| Intervention | Recommendations |
|---|---|
| Primary goal:<br>LDL < 100 mg/dL | Start AHA Step II Diet in all patients: <30% fat, <7% saturated fat, <200 mg/dL cholesterol |
| Secondary goals:<br>HDL > 35 mg/dL<br>TG < 200 mg/dL | Assess fasting lipid profile. In post-MI patients, lipid profile may take 4–6 weeks to stabilize. Add drug therapy according to following guide:<br>LDL < 100 mg/dL: no drug therapy<br>LDL 100–130 mg/dL: consider adding drug therapy to diet listed below<br>LDL > 130 mg/dL: add drug therapy to diet as listed here:<br>When TG < 200 mg/dL: use statin, resin, niacin<br>When TG 200–400 mg/dL: use statin or niacin<br>When TG > 400 mg/dL: use combined drug therapy of niacin, fibrate, statin<br>If LDL goal not achieved: use combination drug therapy<br>HDL < 35 mg/dL<br>Emphasize weight management and physical activity<br>Advise smoking cessation, if needed, to achieve LDL goals; consider niacin, statin, fibrate |

*Adapted from the National Cholesterol Education Program (NCEP) Executive summary of the third report of the Expert Panel on Detection, Evaluation and Treatment of High Blood Cholesterol in Adults (Adult Treatment Panel III). JAMA 285:2486–2497, 2001.*
*HDL, high-density lipoproteins; LDL, low-density lipoproteins; TG, triglycerides.*

## Table 18-16 A Comparison of the Various Methods to Alter Lipids Effects

| Methods | Total Cholesterol | LDL | HDL | Triglycerides |
|---|---|---|---|---|
| Diet low in cholesterol and saturated fat, high in polyunsaturated fat | −16 to −30%<br>(−27 to −58 mg/dL)<br>(−12 mg/dL per 100 mg/dL decrease in dietary cholesterol) | −38%<br>(−45 mg/dL) | 0 to −33%<br>(−6 mg/dL) | −13% |
| Fish consumption | −8 to −57%<br>(88 mg/dL) | −15%<br>(−17 to −26 mg/dL) | +4 to +18% | −35 to −79%<br>(−237 mg/dL) |
| Monounsaturated fats | −13 to 18% | −21% | − | − |
| Increased intake of beans, wheat, oats, and other grains | −10 to −30% | −14 to −24% | −5.6 to −12.7% | −8 to −41% |
| Vegetarian or modified vegetarian diet | −30 to −58 mg/dL | −20 to −45 mg/dL | −4 to −7 mg/dL | −27 mg/dL |
| Weight loss | −5.5 to −57 mg/dL | −11.1 to −13 mg/dL | +2.3 to +5 mg/dL | −21.5 to −503 mg/dL |
| ≤ Two cups of coffee/day | −20 mg/dL | −20 mg/dL | − | −10 to −20% |
| Exercise | −10 to −39.2 mg/dL<br>(−16.4%) | −5 to −8 mg/dL<br>(−13%) | +1.2 to +14 mg/dL<br>(0 to +25%) | −15.8 to −131 mg/dL<br>(−45%) |
| Smoking cessation | −3.45 to −23 mg/dL | − | +2 to +6 mg/dL | − |
| Stress reduction | −29 to −47 mg/dL<br>(−4 to −35%) | − | −8 mg/dL | −29 mg/dL |
| Lipid-lowering drugs | −28 to −48% | −24 to −42% | −9 to +21% | −5.8 to −18.4% |

*From Cahalin LP. A comparison of various methods to alter lipids. Cardiopulm Phys Ther 1:5, 1990.*
*HDL, high-density lipoproteins; LDL, low-density lipoproteins.*

nutritional history and food preferences as well as estimating caloric needs by considering activity level and basal energy requirements.

## Psychosocial Recovery

Readjustment after a cardiac event can be influenced by the degree of anxiety, depression, or denial each patient manifests on recovery from the acute stage. The more pronounced the symptoms at this point, the poorer the rehabilitation potential. Some of the scientific literature discusses the detrimental effects of depression, hopelessness, social isolation, and acute mental stress on the recovery process and risk of progression of disease.[63-68] The patients' perceptions of their health status are also influenced by previous experience, premorbid health misconceptions, and body concerns, especially an increased awareness of the chest region. According to the AACVPR guidelines, several risk factors for psychosocial adjustment following a cardiac event have been identified (Box 18-9).

The support of the cardiac rehabilitation team and other patients can be a significant factor in reversing this state. Some patients need extra support and education, but exaggerated attention to the disease may be harmful to others. Fostering adequate communication and good relationships with patients promotes recovery by precluding misunderstandings and correcting patients' misperceptions of their state of health. Relatives, neighbors, and friends should be made aware of the goals of the active rehabilitation program. Information must be provided to counteract restrictive attitudes that can lead to psychological invalidism.

During this readjustment period, the patient increases self-confidence and improves self-image while learning an individual response to increasing levels of activity. Sexual activity is still of great interest in the age groups in which heart disease is prevalent. There may be problems due to physical load, effect of medications, or even fear of performance. It is therefore worthwhile to focus on this point in discussions with both the patient and the partner.

It has been suggested that adequate social support is an important ingredient in recovery from the crisis of acute illness. Mumford and colleagues found that informational and emotional support to hospitalized heart patients can reduce their length of stay.[69] Successful rehabilitation and return to a productive lifestyle are of interest from the standpoint of both economic benefit and improved quality of life. Another study addresses problems and interventions germane to heart patients. In a controlled study of 46 patients who had experienced an MI, researchers found that educational and counseling interventions produced better outcomes in measures of psychological dysfunction, unhealthy lifestyle, and dependence on health care than did educational interventions alone.[70] Successful adjustment has been shown to have a positive impact on medical recommendations, return to work, and morbidity and mortality rates.[71-74] Social support literature is often vague about what specific ingredients or processes within supportive relationships lead to positive health outcomes. In a study of disaster survivors, Murphy addresses this issue and proposes that self-efficacy may be a key variable.[75] Self-efficacy is defined as the individual's expectation of capability to execute a specific behavior. The presence of supportive others seems to increase self-confidence in one's ability to carry out specific behavior. Self-efficacy theory also suggests that levels of self-efficacy can be enhanced by increasing social support generally and by breaking down the specific denied behavior into small manageable steps, which is referred to as goal scaling.[76] According to Southard, the majority of patients recovering from cardiac events have not had their psychosocial needs addressed or optimally treated in both the inpatient and outpatient settings.[77] Therefore, the AACVPR recommends certain guidelines (Table 18-17) in regard to psychosocial concerns of the cardiac rehabilitation patient.[78] In addition, the recommendations from the AACVPR guidelines on depression screening include identifying a uniform measurement tool and routine screening of all patients.[78]

## Compliance

A major problem in all cardiac rehabilitation programs regardless of type or structure is compliance. Although the data are variable, only 20% to 50% of participants continue to exercise after 1 year.[79] The factors that promote poor compliance are rather complex and may include duration of rehabilitation, regimen complexity, nature of side effects, presence of symptoms, and social and environmental factors, as well as factors related to the therapist, such as patient–therapist interaction. Another key factor is physician encouragement, support, and effectiveness in the role of cardiac rehabilitation team leader.

---

### Box 18-9

#### Risk Factors for Adjustment Difficulties in Cardiac Patients

Patients with a combination of the following characteristics should be considered at higher risk for adjustment difficulties necessitating additional evaluation and support:

- Patients who live alone
- Patients who are not married and do not have a confidant
- Patients who are recently divorced or widowed
- Patients who are socially isolated
- Patients from multiproblem families
- Patients with low incomes
- Patients who smoke
- Patients who are obese
- Patients who have multiple chronic illnesses
- Patients without spiritual or religious comfort
- Patients who have impaired cognitive functioning
- Patients with a history of mental health difficulties
- Patients who have cultural or religious values that conflict with a philosophy of self-reliance and optimism

## Table 18-17 Assessment and Outcomes Related to Psychosocial Concerns

| Assessment | Outcomes | |
|---|---|---|
| Staff should identify clinical significant levels of psychosocial distress using a combination of clinical interview and psychosocial screening instruments at program entry, exit, and periodic follow-up. | *Clinical:*<br>The patient should experience emotional well-being as evidenced by the absence of:<br>1. Psychosocial distress indicated by clinically significant levels of depression, social isolation, anxiety, anger, hostility<br>2. Drug dependency<br>3. Excessive psychophysiologic arousal | *Behavioral:*<br>Program services should enhance the patient's ability to<br>1. Describe the recovery and rehabilitation process<br>2. Develop realistic health-related expectations<br>3. Assume responsibility for behavior change<br>4. Demonstrate problem-solving capabilities<br>5. Engage in physical exercise, meditation, and other relaxation techniques<br>6. Demonstrate effective use of other cognitive–behavioral stress management skills<br>7. Obtain effective social support<br>8. Comply with psychotropic medications if prescribed<br>9. Reduce or eliminate alcohol, tobacco, caffeine usage, or other nonprescription psychoactive drugs<br>10. Return to meaningful social, vocational, and avocational roles |

*From American Association of Cardiovascular and Pulmonary Rehabilitation. Guidelines for Cardiac Rehabilitation and Secondary Prevention Programs. 4th ed. Champaign, IL, Human Kinetics, 2004, Guideline 8.6, p. 123.*

Programs should include mechanisms to combat recidivism. Strategies generally involve education and behavioral measures, as well as attempts to remove barriers to participation. Such barriers begin with the convenience factor. Location, time of day, and facility amenities are among the determinants of convenience to the patient. Few patients will travel more than 10 miles to participate in an exercise program, especially if it is not in the same geographic area as their work. Programs should be scheduled to be convenient for employed and retired persons. Facilities and amenities, particularly parking and locker rooms, are other factors in the perception of convenience to the patient.[80]

The rehabilitation team plays a vital role in the long-term compliance of the patient. Strong leadership, enthusiasm, and development of a good relationship between therapist and patient can reinforce and motivate appropriate lifestyle change. The process begins with obtaining a history of the patient's previous exercise habits, health beliefs, and perceptions of the need to make lifestyle changes. This helps in setting reasonable goals and in identifying potential problems. Special efforts should be made to improve patients' satisfaction with the care and attention they receive. At the same time, their concept of self-management should be reinforced by encouraging them to take responsibility for their own health actions and providing techniques for self-monitoring, such as the rating of perceived exertion and heart rate limits. Patients can thus obtain more immediate feedback, which, in turn, becomes a powerful source of

### Box 18-10

**Substantial Benefits of Cardiac Rehabilitation**

- Improvement in exercise tolerance
- Improvement in symptoms
- Improvement in blood lipids
- Reduction in cigarette smoking
- Improvement in psychosocial well-being and reduction of stress
- Reduction in mortality rate

reinforcement for maintaining the exercise habit. Involving the family as much as possible, including allowing spouses to exercise with patients, is encouraged.

## Outcome Measurement

Outcome evaluation permits assessment of effectiveness in providing patient care and the subsequent improvement in quality of care. According to the AHCPR's summary of the scientific literature on cardiac rehabilitation, the most substantial results of cardiac rehabilitation services are identified in Box 18-10. In addition, the measures that were not strongly affected by cardiac rehabilitation, and in particular the exercise training, include those factors in Box 18-11. Therefore, specific outcome measures that can be used in a

## Box 18-11

### Factors Not Affected by Cardiac Rehabilitation Exercise Training Alone

- Body weight (when exercise training was a sole intervention)
- Rates of nonfatal reinfarction
- Development of coronary collateral circulation
- Regression or limitation of progression of angiographically documented coronary atherosclerosis (when exercise training was a sole intervention)
- Ventricular ejection fraction and regional wall motion abnormalities
- Occurrence of cardiac arrhythmias

multidiscipline outpatient cardiac rehabilitation include the following:

- Lipid changes
- Smoking cessation
- Body weight
- Blood pressure (at rest and with activity)
- Exercise tolerance
- Symptoms (at rest and with various activities)
- Psychological well-being
- Quality of life
- Morbidity
- Mortality

Table 18-18 provides the four outcome domains that should be monitored (health, clinical, behavioral, and service) as well as examples of specific measures for each domain. The AACVPR also provides resources on outcome tools as well as references in their document on outcome assessment for cardiac rehabilitation programs.[81]

### Follow-Up Assessment

Routine follow-up assessment by each team member should be performed and discussed with the patient at least twice a month during the subacute and intensive rehabilitation phases. At this time each team member should review the progress made by the patient since entering the program and any problems (risk factors) that still need to be modified. New short-term goals and changes in the program should be established as patients increase their exercise performance and are cleared to resume various activities, for example, returning to work. A copy of these assessments must be forwarded to the attending physician, who remains the primary physician throughout.

### Criteria for Discharge

When to discharge a patient from any program is a difficult decision to make, probably more so for cardiac patients because they are making lifelong changes, some of which require long-term support mechanisms from the appropriate

## Table 18-18 Outcomes: Four Domains with Their Corresponding Categories

| Domains | Outcome Categories |
|---|---|
| Behavioral | Diet |
| | Weight management |
| | Exercise |
| | Smoking cessation |
| | Stress reduction |
| | Recognition of signs/symptoms |
| | Medical management |
| Clinical | Physical |
| | Weight |
| | Blood pressure |
| | Lipids |
| | Functional capacity |
| | Blood nicotine levels |
| | Oxygenation, $O_2$ saturation |
| | Symptom management |
| | Psychosocial |
| | Return to vocation/leisure |
| | Psychological status |
| | Medical utilization |
| | Hospitalizations |
| | Medication |
| | Physician/ER visits |
| Health | Morbidity |
| | Future events |
| | MI |
| | CABG |
| | Angioplasty |
| | New angina |
| | Serious arrhythmias |
| | Mortality |
| | Quality of life |
| | Functional |
| | Social |
| | Vocational status |
| | Independent living status |
| Service | Patient Satisfaction |
| | Re: care received |
| | Financial and economic |
| | Reimbursement |
| | Deductibles |

*CABG, coronary artery bypass graft; MI, myocardial infarction.*

sources. It is not easy for the patient and spouse to maintain a continuous awareness of the requirements of the program, and self-motivation is often hard. However, reimbursement agencies are requesting definitions of discharge criteria, and perhaps they are correct in trying to identify the point at which the individual is considered to have completed the rehabilitation phase of recovery. Therefore, rehabilitation goals and plans must be outcome-oriented. Some key points for discharge (adapted from the *Guide to Physical Therapist Practice*)[7] include the following:

- The anticipated goals and the desired outcomes have been achieved.
- Patient declines to continue intervention.
- Patient is unable to continue to progress toward goals because of medical or psychosocial complications.
- Failure to make reasonable progress toward goals, owing to nonadherence to the home program
- Failure to attend scheduled appointments
- Lack of willingness or ability to participate in the program

## Special Patient Populations

The prescription of exercise for special patient populations requires the integration of clinical information and exercise physiology. The need for an appropriate exercise prescription in patients with noncardiac disease has been documented; however, patients with multiple system dysfunction may require special attention and an individualized approach. The more we learn about exercise and disease, the more we find an influence of one on the other. Women, children, and the elderly are distinct groups that also may require a different approach with therapeutic interventions and rehabilitation. Therefore, the following sections provide additional information to consider when working with these populations See Table 18-19 for summary of special considerations with these patient populations.

## Patients with Peripheral Arterial Disease

Peripheral arterial disease (PAD) is a fairly common disorder among individuals with coronary artery disease. The limiting factor to exercise is claudication—angina-like pain usually in the buttocks, the calf of one or both lower extremities, or both. Much like angina, claudication is related to exertional level. Exercise training has demonstrated significant functional improvement with reduction of symptoms at equivalent workloads.[82-84] Patients must be tolerant of working to various levels of discomfort, and the supervising therapist should use a symptom-limited approach with varying modes of exercise. One mode should include walking because it is the most functional and usually limited activity for the individual to perform. Patients should be encouraged to walk to leg pain, rest and resume walking. Cigarette smokers must also agree to a smoking cessation program if they are serious about reducing their risk of disease progression. In addition, all other risk factors for atherosclerosis should be addressed in this population.[84]

## Patients with Chronic Obstructive Pulmonary Disease

Many patients with coronary disease have a long-standing history of cigarette smoking with some degree of obstructive airway disease; therefore, both the cardiovascular system and pulmonary system impairments need to be addressed in the rehabilitation. Some individuals may be taking medications (e.g., theophylline) that are known to induce supraventricular arrhythmia with activity. Considerations with exercise prescription in this population include the following:

- Dyspnea levels, discussed earlier in this chapter (see Intensity), are most effective for determining an appropriate exercise intensity level.
- For patients with chronic obstructive pulmonary disease, pursed-lip breathing may enhance exercise performance because it helps control ventilation and oxygenation by reducing respiratory rate, increasing tidal volume and improving gas exchange, and improving ventilation of previously underventilated areas.
- Use of upper extremity support with exercise, such as holding the bars of treadmills, stationary bikes, and rolling walkers, may assist the patient in stabilizing accessory muscles for improved ventilation.
- In more severe cases, supplemental oxygen may be of benefit. Blood saturation levels with exercise should be monitored, but preferably with arterial blood gases. Pulse oximetry is the minimal amount of monitoring. The supervising therapist should pay close attention to clinical signs of desaturation (e.g., blue nail beds and overall change in coloration). Additional information on pulmonary rehabilitation is found in Chapter 19.

> **Clinical Tip**
> Caution should be taken with patients who have COPD and who are taking β-blocking medications, specifically nonselective β-blockers (e.g., Inderal). These medications block sympathetic stimulation to the $\beta_1$ receptors in the heart as well as the $\beta_2$ receptors found in the smooth muscles of the bronchi. The result of blocked $\beta_2$ receptors can be bronchoconstriction, resulting in an increase in dyspnea. Because this increase in dyspnea may occur with some $\beta_1$-selective drugs, evaluation of dyspnea is a critical component *during* exercise (particularly auscultation for wheezing with exercise).

## Patients with Diabetes Mellitus

Diabetes is a risk factor for coronary disease, and diabetes patients are three times more likely to have coronary artery disease than those without diabetes.[85] In addition, type II diabetes (non–insulin-dependent type, which includes 80% to 90% of all diabetes patients) is associated with obesity. Research on the effect of exercise on the lives of patients with type II diabetes has been promising, demonstrating improvements in insulin activity and glucose tolerance, potential reductions in dosage and need of insulin or oral hypoglycemic medications, and reduction of body fat.[86] Patients should be cautious and aware of signs and symptoms of hypoglycemic

**Table 18-19 Special Patient Populations Requiring Special Considerations with Exercise Prescription and Supervision**

| Patient Population | Special Considerations |
|---|---|
| PAD with claudication | Claudication is related to exertional level |
| | Evaluate responses on all modalities and assess symptom onset and pain scales with activities[84] |
| COPD | Monitor $O_2$ saturation and watch for desaturation with exercise |
| | May have to titrate supplemental $O_2$ and instruct in pursed-lip breathing exercises |
| | Utilize level of dyspnea scale for monitoring intensity of exercise |
| Diabetes | Monitor glucose pre and post exercise |
| | When BG levels are elevated prior to therapy, adjustments in treatment may be indicated |
| | If BG is ≥250 mg/dL and the patient is on insulin, she or he should check for ketosis (via urine dip stick or BG meter that measures ketones) and, if present, *no* exercise, at least until more insulin is administered and hyperglycemia and ketosis resolve. |
| | Know the insulin patient is taking, and peak effect of insulin ... avoid exercising during peak effect |
| | SOB may be an angina equivalent |
| | Watch for S/S of hypoglycemia: be prepared with glucose tablets and protein food for long-term management of hypoglycemia |
| | Be careful if patient taking β-blockers—will not perceive hypoglycemia |
| CVA | May tolerate bicycle or four-extremity modality for aerobic exercise |
| | TMs have been shown to improve gait speed in this population |
| | Remember these are high-risk patients for CAD |
| Renal disease | Overall this group has *low* exercise tolerance |
| | Schedule exercise sessions around dialysis |
| Women | Angina symptoms are *different* watch for SOB, fatigue, scapular discomfort, and indigestion |
| Elderly | May have multiple joint and musculoskeletal limitations; modify program based upon limitations |
| | Start and progress exercise program *slowly* in those who have not been regular exercisers. |
| Obese | With ↑ in BMI; ↓ max $VO_2$, ↑ thermoregulation |
| | Will have ↑ HR response with activity |
| | Build in multiple bouts of short duration activity, add resistive exercise |
| Arthritis | Limit excessive joint stress |
| ICDs | Need to know the threshold for discharge |
| Heart transplant | Patients will have altered HR response—need longer warm-up and cool-down |
| | Address potential steroid myopathy by adding resistive ex. |
| CHF | Have patients weigh daily in am and monitor SOB daily |
| | Multiple bouts of short duration activity to begin.[40,41] |

*BG, blood glucose; BMI, body mass index; CHF, congestive heart failure; COPD, chronic obstructive pulmonary disease; CVA, cerebrovascular accident; ICD, international classification of disease; PAD, peripheral arterial disease; SOB, shortness of breath.*

episodes that can occur during or after the exercise session and for 24 hours after as well:

Just before starting an exercise session each day, the patient should obtain a pre-exercise blood glucose (BG) reading. This reading is in addition to that for the daily fasting BG value. If BG levels are low (70 to 100 mg/dL) prior to therapy, the individual should be given a 10- to 15-g carbohydrate snack and exercise should be postponed until hypoglycemia is corrected (typically about 20 to 30 minutes). If marked

hypoglycemia is present (<70 mg/dL), exercise is contraindicated and a snack should be ingested.[87]

If the pre-exercise BG value is between 100 and 250 mg/dL, the person can engage in exercise. Because of the enhancement of insulin sensitivity with exercise, persons with diabetes should abstain from exercise during the peak activity of their insulin. If the pre-exercise value is equal to or greater than 250 mg/dL, exercise may induce a rise in BG rather than a decline. If BG is ≥250 mg/dL and the patient is on insulin, that individual should check for ketosis (via urine dip stick or BG meter that measures ketones) and, if present, should not perform any exercise, at least until more insulin is administered and hyperglycemia and ketosis resolve. Because of the major role of glucose as a fuel for exercise, there may not be enough energy to sustain the exercise if the pre-exercise BG level is equal to or less than 100 mg/dL.

- If a hyperglycemic patient feels well, is adequately hydrated, and is on oral medications or urine and/or blood ketones are negative, she or he can perform low- to moderate-intensity exercise for 10 to 15 minutes and then BG should be rechecked. If BG rises, exercise should be terminated, and if it drops exercise can be continued with BG monitoring every 15 minutes.[87]
- Some form of simple carbohydrate (e.g., juice, sugar, glucose) should be kept in the exercise area in case of such an emergency, as well as a long-term solution to blood sugar maintenance (protein and/or fat like peanut butter and complex carbohydrate).
- As with anyone who exercises, persons with diabetes should begin the session with a 5- to 10-minute warm-up, which includes stretching and light calisthenics.
- At the end of the session, time must be allotted for a cool-down session. The exercise prescription for a person with diabetes is similar to the nondiabetic.
- Because of the postexercise recovery phase, a person may have a decrease in BG values for up to 24 hours. Persons with diabetes must be told that on days they do not engage in exercise their BG values may be higher. See Chapter 7 for more information on diabetes.

---

> **Clinical Tip**
> Similarly, individuals who are diabetic and on β-blocking medications should be monitored closely when initiating or progressing their exercise prescription. When an individual becomes hypoglycemic the sympathetic nervous system produces a systemic response, including tremors, rapid heart rate, and lightheadedness, which are warning signs to increase sugar intake immediately. β-Blocking medications block the sympathetic response to hypoglycemia, thereby blocking all the warning signs as well.

---

## Patients Who Have Had a Cerebrovascular Accident

Some individuals present to the rehabilitation program with impaired cardiac dysfunction as well as having previously sustained a cerebrovascular accident. They therefore have special medical and physical needs[88]:

- Common sequelae of cerebrovascular accidents include weakness or neglect of one or more extremities, problems in communication, cognitive–perceptual dysfunction, and dysphagia.[89]
- Inability to exercise weakened muscles or ones with excessive tone for prolonged periods may necessitate exercise of short duration.

- Despite unilateral limb dysfunction, the use of four-extremity ergometers such as the Schwinn Airdyne may allow for greater intensity of exercise. Blood pressure and heart rate responses to isometric and to upper and lower extremity ergometry have been found to be no greater in those who have had cerebrovascular accidents than in an age-matched control group[90]; however, with four-extremity ergometry and impaired ventricular function, these patients are extremely important to monitor.
- The supervising therapist should be attuned especially to symptoms that exercising patients may have but cannot easily express because of a communication disorder.

## Patients with Renal Disease

Patients with end-stage renal disease can benefit significantly from regular exercise training, although they may not exhibit the same responses to exercise as the patients usually seen in the cardiac rehabilitation program. Exercise tolerance in patients on hemodialysis has been found to be significantly below normal.[91,92] This low tolerance is probably due to lower arterial oxygen content because of the following:

- Lower hematocrit and hemoglobin values for oxygen transport
- Altered stroke volume affected by the disease or its treatment
- Peripheral factors as a result of autonomic dysfunction and metabolic acidosis

Exercise training has been found to increase physical work capacity, increase HDL cholesterol levels, and increase hematocrit values in this group. Improvements in glucose tolerance, blood pressure control, and physiologic profiles—important risk factors for heart disease—also result from exercise training.[93]

- Exercise sessions should be scheduled according to the patient's condition before and after dialysis and the time requirements of the treatment. Often the day before and the day of dialysis are the patient's weakest days.
- Intermittent exercise, with work-to-rest ratios of 1:2 or 1:1, may be appropriate initially, although most patients can gradually increase to 30 to 45 minutes of continuous exercise over time.
- Training heart rates are difficult to use because of variable heart rate response, medication schedule, and physiologic changes that occur in these patients from day to day depending on their dialysis schedule. The Borg perceived exertion scale works well in evaluating these patients.

## Heart Disease and Women

Coronary artery disease is the leading killer of women and kills more women than all cancers combined.[94] Studies report that coronary artery disease is underdiagnosed and undertreated in women as compared to men.[95,96] This finding is related to the fact that women present a different clinical picture (different symptoms) and therefore present a different challenge to both primary and secondary prevention programs. Women are usually older (an average of 10 years older) than men when first presentation of the disease occurs and present with different symptoms; they are more likely to complain of abdominal pain, nausea, excessive fatigue, or shortness of breath.[96-98] Women also are less likely than men to be referred for diagnostic tests and intervention. The sensitivity and specificity of diagnostic testing for coronary artery disease differ in women, especially in exercise testing.[97,99] Certain diagnostic tests, particularly exercise echocardiography and exercise thallium sestamibi testing, offer more prognostic information than exercise testing alone.[100,101] Long-term survival rates are similar for men and women after coronary artery disease procedures (angioplasty and CABG surgery); however, the mortality rate is higher in women at the time of the actual procedure.[97,102-104]

Certainly rehabilitation is a recommended treatment following any cardiac procedure or acute injury, but limited information exists on compliance with rehabilitation in women.[96,105] Studies including women have shown improvements after cardiac rehabilitation similar to those in men with regard to risk factor modification, exercise training, and psychosocial and vocational counseling.[96,106-109] However, women are less likely than men to enroll in cardiac rehabilitation,[110] and their drop-out rates are higher than men.[111] In programs in which women are brought together for exercise and education sessions separately from the men, compliance to rehabilitation has not been a problem. Therefore, separate times for women may be a recommendation to encourage compliance. For further information on cardiovascular disease prevention and women, see the American Heart Association evidence-based guidelines published in 2007.[96]

## Pediatric Programs

As children with congenital cardiovascular disorders survive into their adult years, it becomes increasingly important to evaluate, train, and advise them and their families in activity and exercise prescription guidelines. Cardiac rehabilitation for children after cardiac surgery is emerging as an area of considerable interest. The Children's Hospital National Medical Center in Washington, D.C., has established a 12-week training program focusing on this specialty in an environment similar to that used in an elementary and secondary physical education class.[112] It is led by experienced physical education teachers who have expertise in current methodology and techniques of physical education and by other staff members, including exercise specialists and a pediatric cardiologist. Parents and siblings are encouraged to participate in the activity component of the program. These programs have demonstrated significant improvement in the child's physical work capacity as well as improved social interactions.

Cardiac rehabilitation in children should be provided to patients with repaired complex congenital diseases who have functional or psychosocial problems with the disease. The purpose of these programs is to improve exercise efficiency, aerobic capacity, and quality of life, as well as to reduce the incidence of sudden death and enable young individuals to participate safely and effectively in sports. On survey of international centers, very few actually treat pediatric cases. Of those who were surveyed, the chief outcome of these programs demonstrated increased exercise capacity, increased cardiac output at rest and with peak exercise, increased $O_2$ uptake, increased exercise test duration, and improved quality of life.[113] See Chapter 20 for more information on pediatrics.

Screening of children for cardiovascular risk has become a topic of interest and some controversy. The American Academy of Pediatrics recommends screening children with a family history of premature coronary artery disease or hyperlipidemia; others support mass screenings of all children because some research has shown that as many as two thirds of the children with elevated cholesterol levels would go undetected by use of the Academy's recommendations.[114,115] Several studies have noted a stronger relationship between several risk factors such as exercise and serum lipids and glucose intolerance and weight–height and skinfold thickness.[116] Advocates of mass screening also encourage aggressive early management of hyperlipidemia in this population and point to school-based interventions as the best means of reaching the greatest number of children.[117]

## The Elderly Coronary Patient

Most elderly cardiac patients who have not exercised in their recent past probably have low expectations and possibly negative attitudes toward the rehabilitation process, participating only because their physicians told them they should. These same individuals may show the most improvement functionally. Exercise can promote a sense of well-being and heighten self-esteem, both of which are essential to independent living.

Regular physical activity can modify known coronary risk factors in the elderly. In a study of elderly Japanese men in Hawaii, higher levels of physical activity were associated with higher serum HDL and lower triglyceride levels.[118] Likewise, athletic elderly men have been shown to have higher HDL levels and lower total cholesterol to HDL ratios than sedentary elderly men.[119]

Many elderly patients present with multiple joint and musculoskeletal limitations. Therefore, a thorough mechanical assessment should be performed before initiating any exercise program. To achieve the greatest success early in the program and to diminish patient discouragement because "it hurts too much," light calisthenics and stretching exercises should be employed. Jarring activities such as jogging should be minimized to avoid musculoskeletal injury. Swimming is an excellent exercise; however, some weight-bearing activity should be encouraged, especially for women, to forestall the adverse effects of osteoporosis. A cool-down period is especially important for the elderly following aerobic activity and should actually be of slightly longer duration for adequate recovery. Frequency of exercise may need to be limited to every other day to give the musculoskeletal system a chance to rest.

## Administrative Considerations

### Safety in the Outpatient Cardiac Rehabilitation Setting

Safety in the outpatient cardiac rehabilitation exercise setting must be the top priority for any program. Even with the best precautions, major cardiovascular events may occur, the most frequent of which is sudden cardiac arrest.[21] Selection of appropriate patients who are adequately evaluated and deemed appropriate candidates for training (e.g., under medical supervision outside the program, screened via exercise test before entry to the program); who are cooperative, especially in understanding and use of heart rate and symptoms as limitations in exercise; and who are willing to follow the prescribed medical regimen is of critical importance.

The ability to deal with cardiac arrest and other medical emergencies depends on the immediate response of trained personnel in the exercise area, available emergency equipment, and availability of trained physicians. All professional exercise personnel must be trained to perform immediate basic cardiac life support in accordance with American Heart Association standards (advanced cardiac life support preferred), including defibrillation. All persons involved with the cardiac rehabilitation program must know their roles and have practice in the various emergency procedures (Box 18-12).

---

### Box 18-12

#### Emergency Procedures for Cardiac Rehabilitation

The following is instituted for persons who demonstrate cardiopulmonary distress and require emergency procedures during cardiac rehabilitation.

- Nonmonitored patient: Individual who is found unconscious or loses consciousness with no respiration or palpable pulse.
  - Person discovering victim:
    Assess situation, determine need for CPR
    Call for help
    Initiate CPR
    Remain with patient until relieved
  - Second person to respond:
    Call for assistance
    Activate the EMS (call 911)
    Alert facility, front desk of emergency department, and person to inform medical director
    Obtain AED or defibrillator, Assist with CPR
  - Third person to respond:
    Delivers crash cart to scene of code
  - Exercise assistants:
    Assist with CPR
    Escort other patients from the area and remain with them
    Direct ambulance personnel
- If a code is called during cardiac rehabilitation, the cardiac rehabilitation coordinator is in charge of the code procedure. In the coordinator's absence, designated ACLS personnel will assume charge role and initiate ACLS standards of care until the emergency department personnel arrive or the paramedics, if program is held out of hospital.
- Monitored arrest: The first available staff member who observes the emergency should immediately assess the patient's status and respond by performing the specific procedure that that staff member is authorized to deliver.
- The second available staff member activates the emergency medical system and returns to assist the first rescuer. The third staff member delivers the crash cart to the code site and prepares it for use.

- Ventricular tachycardia (losing or lost consciousness), ventricular fibrillation
  If no change in rhythm, defibrillate at 360 Watts/sec
  Wait 10 seconds, check rhythm
  If no change, defibrillate again at 360 Watts/sec
  If no response, initiate CPR
- Severe bradycardia, asystole, or other pulmonary emergency—initiate CPR and continue until directed to stop by physician
- Severe myocardial ischemia (with persistent symptoms and signs)
  Sitting or supine posture, check ECG
  Give oxygen and nitroglycerin and aspirin
  Evaluate blood pressure and symptoms
  Notify the cardiologist covering the exercise class or the patient's attending physician

Emergency procedures vary according to established hospital and community standards.

Basic equipment:
- Blood pressure cuffs and mercury sphygmomanometers (mercury sphygmomanometers are preferred owing to ease of calibration, accuracy, and long-lasting components)
- Dual-head (bell and diaphragm) stethoscopes
- Telemetry monitoring with strip chart recorder
- Exercise equipment—bicycle ergometers, treadmills, arm ergometers, rowing machines, pulleys, free weights, track, four-extremity ergometers
- Wall clock with second hand
  Emergency equipment:
- Defibrillator with monitor or AED
- Emergency medications, airway maintenance supplies, artificial respirator, suction machine, and the like (see American Heart Association, Advanced Cardiac Life Support, American College of Sports Medicine Guidelines)
- Oxygen and supplies for oxygen administration
- First aid equipment
- Communication system (telephone)

ACLS, advanced cardiac life support; AED, automated external defibrillator; CPR, cardiopulmonary resuscitation; EMS, emergency medical service.

Most data available demonstrate a relatively low rate for cardiovascular complications during supervised cardiac rehabilitation programs. Van Camp and Peterson's survey of 167 cardiac rehabilitation programs suggests an incidence rate of 8 to 9 per 1 million patient hours of exercise for cardiac arrest, 3 to 4 per 1 million patient hours of exercise for MI, and 1.3 per 1 million patient hours for fatalities.[120]

Other precautions with regard to safety in the cardiac rehabilitation setting include the following:

- Avoidance of exercise within 1 to 2 hours after meals
- Avoidance of isometrics and breath holding with exercise
- Adding warm-up and extended cool-off periods of 15 minutes or more with strenuous exercise
- Keeping showers brief and not at a hot or cold temperature (keep legs active)

## Facility Concerns

The cardiac rehabilitation center is the facility in which an interdisciplinary team provides the planned and monitored program to promote physical, psychological, educational, and vocational improvement of the cardiac patient. Ideally, the center has classroom space for group patient education, private counseling facilities, and a library for educational materials. Exercise space should allow freedom of movement for warm-up and cool-down exercises and perhaps should have cameras to monitor patients in hallways and around blind corners. The facility should be easily accessible, pleasant, and clean—qualities that are important to boost morale and to support patient compliance. The facility may also be combined with a sports medicine, pulmonary rehabilitation, or fitness facility to increase use and decrease costs. Phases II and III are often based in a hospital or satellite setting because of the likelihood of dealing with higher-risk patients and the potential need for emergency medical services; however, these services can be performed in independent practice settings with appropriate medical support systems. Reimbursement issues may dictate where these programs are carried out. Phase IV or prevention and maintenance programs are often held outside the hospital setting in local YMCAs, or community colleges. Recommendations are made regarding the usual length of time in each phase, but programs should last as long as the patient's symptoms indicate. Often patients terminate the programs as a result of the termination of the reimbursement.

## Records and Documentation

Records provide a method of retrieving information, evaluating the value and validity of the rehabilitation process, and analyzing cost effectiveness and quality assurance. Records should be kept thoroughly and accurately, subject to periodic analysis, and include the following:

- Attending physician referral and authorization for treatment
- Copies of pertinent medical data: results of ECG, echocardiogram, exercise tests, other noninvasive tests, cardiac catheterization report, results of cardiac surgery, and report from attending physician
- Initial cardiac rehabilitation evaluation summary and goals listed by team members
- Regular progress notes from each session that summarize the patient's performance, including resting and exercise heart rates, resting and exercise blood pressures, signs and symptoms, workload, peak interval time, ECG results, and any other pertinent data (e.g., medication changes, physician appointments, environmental conditions)
- Monthly reports to attending physician as summarized by the medical director, program coordinator, and staff
- Monthly log records—copies of patient's home records (e.g., exercise log, weight record, diet diary)
- Discharge summary, including progress the patient has made regarding functional changes; physiologic and psychological changes; risk factor modifications achieved and those still needing further attention; compliance with home program; reasons for limited change, if that is the case; recommendations for follow-up testing or counseling; and reason the patient is being discharged

## Medical and Legal Considerations

At times, certain legal and insurance considerations assume a very significant role in the rehabilitation of the cardiac patient. Possible legal problems stem from two aspects of this program:

- Adverse effects of medically prescribed exercise testing and fitness conditioning
- Consideration of disability pension and insurance benefits that may influence the patient's motivation to return to work and may affect the attitude of an employer toward a person with "a heart problem"

Exercise testing and recommendations to patients in the conditioning program by a physician constitute medical treatment. All medical personnel must be continuously alert to those aspects of testing and training that are eventually dangerous to each individual. They must pay special attention to recognize indications and contraindications to be sure that a thorough pre-exercise screening examination has been performed, that the exercise sessions are properly supervised and monitored, and that exercise is terminated when potentially dangerous situations arise. There must be adequate advance preparation for and training in emergency procedures in accordance with generally accepted medical standards. Patients also must be fully informed of the potential benefits, risks, and hazards associated with exercise conditioning programs and be given an opportunity to ask questions and withdraw from treatment without jeopardy of future medical care so that the informed consent document can be classified as legally valid. In addition, when a physician authorizes a return to work for the patient, the physician must understand the duties and potential hazards of the work for which clearance is being given.

## Charges to Patients and Third-Party Carriers

Cardiac rehabilitation is not a major income producer in most facilities. In fact, cardiac rehabilitation often has difficulty breaking even in many settings in which both direct and indirect costs are factored, the latter being difficult to budget. Cardiac rehabilitation is considered by many administrations to be part of the total picture of cardiology care (product line) and can, to some degree, be carried by other subdepartments, given the positive influence a quality cardiac care program can have on the hospital and the community. The business structure and nature of each program and the overhead expenses dictate how fees are established. During the 1990s, dramatic changes in health care management and subsequently health care reimbursement took place. As a result of a changing health care environment, personnel in the program should stay current with changes in health care costs and health care reimbursement. Specifically, personnel should verify each individual's policy, level of reimbursement, and number of rehabilitation sessions covered by each plan. Private health care plans change regularly as they are being bought and sold by other agencies; therefore, each enrollee should be assessed for health care plan, and a telephone number to contact the insurance company to verify cardiac rehabilitation reimbursement. Some health maintenance organizations (HMOs) have contracts with specific institutions and may cover only six sessions of outpatient rehabilitation, whereas all inpatient care is covered. Sometimes these organizations require a letter to the medical director of the HMO to explain the seriousness of the patient's condition asking for greater than six sessions to be covered.

As of 2006, Medicare provided for cardiac rehabilitation for up to 12 weeks or 36 visits of an approved outpatient cardiac rehabilitation program for individuals with a diagnosis of acute MI (within the preceding 12 months), who have undergone coronary bypass surgery, have undergone percutaneous translumina coronary angioplasty (PTCA), or valve surgery or heart transplantation, or who have stable angina pectoris and are considered to have a medical need for cardiac rehabilitation and up to 72 sessions in an evidence-based documented intensive cardiac rehabilitation program ((ICR) or Ornish Lifestyle program or similar). Because a growing percentage of the cardiac patient population is covered by Medicare, it is important to have the program certified by Medicare. Many other insurance carriers follow Medicare's lead in coverage and, as Medicare changes, they will probably follow.

Medicare's additional requirements include that a physician be directly supervising the program with cardiopulmonary emergency equipment readily available, and that staffing must consist of qualified personnel. Box 18-13 gives Medicare guidelines for obtaining reimbursement. Blue Cross-Blue Shield coverage varies considerably from state to state; however, the national policy is to support and provide some degree of coverage.

Patient education is felt to be the role of the physician and is not reimbursed. State-aid agencies rarely cover cardiac

---

### Box 18-13

### Medicare Guidelines for Reimbursement and Fee-for-Services Payment

Professional staff should:
- Obtain a signed physician order from the referring physician with appropriate Medicare diagnosis code for establishing medical necessity.
- Obtain the Physician's Current Procedural Terminology (known as the CPT-4 Code Book), which is a listing of all outpatient procedures applied within the services of medicine. Review the established numerical code for each procedure. As part of the 2009 CPT-4 Code Book, the following two codes are appropriate to the program:
  - 93797—physician services for outpatient program without continuous ECG monitoring (The 93797 code is subject to regional interpretation and is not accepted by all intermediaries.)
  - 93798—physician services for outpatient program with continuous ECG monitoring
- Identify the appropriate diagnosis code that must accompany the procedure charge. The diagnosis code is obtained in two steps: (1) the physician must denote the diagnosis on referral, and (2) the diagnosis is coded using the International Classification of Diseases also called the ICD-9 Code Book. Current acceptable diagnoses and codes for reimbursement are as follows:
  - Stable angina—413.9
  - CABG—414 and then V45.81
  - Anterolateral MI—410.02
  - Anterior AMI—410.12
  - Inferior lateral AMI—410.22
  - Inferior AMI—410.42
  - Lateral AMI—410.52
  - Unspecified AMI site—410.92
  - Heart or heart–lung transplant—V42.1 or V42.1 &V42.6
  - Heart valve repair or replacement—394, 395, 396 (V42.2, V43.3 or V45.8)
  - PTCA—V45.82
- Where required, obtain preadmission or precertification for services, recording insurance policy, managed care plan, and coverage benefits
- Appropriate contact person
- Precertification confirmation, notation of number of visits, time of service, copayments, and amount of reimbursement

Adapted from American Association of Cardiovascular and Pulmonary Rehabilitation. Guidelines for Cardiac Rehabilitation and Secondary Prevention Programs. 4th ed. Champaign, IL, Human Kinetics, 2004.

---

rehabilitation services. Nutrition counseling is rarely reimbursed as a separate service. Reimbursement for exercise testing depends on the policy; however, it is usually reimbursed as a procedure when ordered by the physician before commencing rehabilitation. When working in a cardiac rehabilitation program, it is extremely necessary to be familiar with the NCD policy (20-10) and for physical therapists practicing in the outpatient setting to be familiar with their local coverage policy under their Medicare Administrative Coverage (MAC).

It is important to the financial success of the program to be familiar with reimbursement rates, company policies, and limitations in coverage of insurance companies in the area for inpatient and outpatient cardiac rehabilitation. Policies regarding treatment of uninsured or uncovered services must be established and understood by all team members and

explained to the patient and family before commencing the rehabilitation program. Each individual should also be familiar with the program charges for each phase. Some programs take the position that it is the patient's responsibility to find out whether a particular insurance company covers cardiac rehabilitation. Having someone who can answer basic questions about insurance coverage can be helpful when the patient and family are going through a stressful time.

---

## CASE STUDY 18-1

A.L. is a 52-year-old male who presented to the emergency room with a 1-week history or worsening dyspnea, lower extremity edema, and paroxysmal nocturnal dyspnea. Patient reported a history of weight gain (of 8 lbs) over the past week. Patient denied any fever, chills, anorexia, change in diet, abdominal pain, problems with urination, or chest pain. Patient has a long history of dilated cardiomyopathy. He was assessed to be in right and left heart failure and admitted for diuresis

> Edema, +3 in bilateral ankles, + edema in abdomen, +3 in hands and fingers
> Bilaterally (impaired)
> Scar : 2 – abdominal incision from previous aortic/femoral bypass, and AAA
> Height: 5'10"
> Weight: 180 lbs
> BMI: 25.8

Past medical history includes a diagnosis of dilated cardiomyopathy in 1997, with a functional classification of heart failure as New York Class III (see Table 4-12). Patient has history of an inferior myocardial infarction detected on ECG and followed by cardiac catheterization in 2000 demonstrating a 100% blockage of the right coronary artery. Patient underwent bilateral aortic–femoral bypass surgery in April 2003 for long history of claudication, and an infrarenal aortic abdominal aneurysm repair in April 2002. Patient has a long-standing history of hypertension, gastroesophageal reflux disease (GERD), and alcohol use. Patient used to smoke 3 packs per day (ppd), but currently only smokes ½ ppd, drinks two to six beers/day, and works as a manager of a hotel. No family history of heart disease is reported. He was started on IV diuretics and IV dobutamine and scheduled for pre-transplant workup. Patient remained on bedrest during the first 5 days of hospitaliza-

tion, at which time physical therapy was ordered to increase mobility and assess functional activities.

During the hospitalization, he was evaluated for possible heart transplant and was determined to be placed lower on priority transplant list. He was referred for outpatient rehabilitation.

Initial rehabilitation:

Problem list:

Impaired aerobic capacity

Abnormal lipids

Impaired ADLs

205 ft walk distance on 6-minute walk

Impaired quality of life

Poor dietary intake

Poor knowledge of disease and no self-monitoring

Referred to smoking cessation program and recommended to refrain from alcohol intake

Risk for serious arrhythmias: referred for ICD evaluation

Initial Interventions:

1. Aerobic exercise prescription: frequent short intervals (2 to 3 minutes) followed by rest with goal of 20 to 30 minutes continuous exercise
2. Functional training to improve ADLs
3. Dietary instruction
4. Instruction in self-management of CHF, diabetes, lifestyle modifications
5. Smoking cessation program
6. Monitoring of all activities with ECG, HR, SpO$_2$, BP, and symptoms
7. Referral to psychosocial
8. Education regarding knowledge of disease

---

## Summary

- Individuals with cardiovascular disorders may be seen in a variety of outpatient settings for rehabilitation; however, if individuals are referred specifically for a cardiac rehabilitation program, there are specific guidelines set that must be followed, and specific billing practices that are implemented as a result of standards set by the CMS National coverage.

- Cardiac rehabilitation is described as consisting of "comprehensive, long-term programs involving medical evaluation, prescribed exercise, cardiac risk factor modification, education, and counseling." These programs "are designed to limit the physiologic and psychological effects of cardiac illness, reduce the risk of sudden death or reinfarction, control cardiac symptoms, stabilize or reverse the atherosclerotic process, and enhance the psychosocial and vocational status of selected patients."

- Stratification of patients as low, moderate, and high risk is an important element in the rehabilitation process to maintain a safe environment for all patients and to assist individuals who need a higher degree of support.
- Physical therapists should be acutely aware of the cardiovascular implications of the problems of all patient populations, especially when treating the elderly.
- A growing number of patient populations are identified as appropriate candidates for exercise training.
- A patient's exercise plan should be determined by objective assessment of clinical status, functional capacity, and personal need.
- Longer duration and higher levels of intensity may produce the greatest change in exercise performance and risk factors across all patient populations.
- One future problem to be confronted in cardiac rehabilitation is that of ensuring adequate reimbursement for all patients who choose to participate. This may in turn help to improve long-term patient compliance.

## References

1. US Government Printing Office. Reducing the Health Consequences of Smoking: 25 Years of Progress. Washington, DC, Government Printing Office, 1989.
2. National High Blood Pressure Education Program of the National Institutes of Health, National Heart Lung and Blood Institute. The Sixth Report of the Joint National Committee on Detection, Evaluation, and Treatment of High Blood Pressure. NIH Publication 98-1080. Bethesda, MD: NHLBI, 1997.
3. St. Jeor ST, Brownell KD, Atkinson RL. American Heart Association Prevention Conference III: Obesity. Circulation 88:1392–7, 1993.
4. Gotto AM. Lipid lowering, regression, and coronary events. Circulation 92:646–56, 1995.
5. Pearson TA, Blair SN, Daniels SR, et al. Adult patients without coronary or other atherosclerotic vascular diseases: 2002 update: Consensus panel guide to comprehensive risk reduction for AHA guidelines for primary prevention of cardiovascular disease and stroke. Circulation 106:388–91, 2002.
6. American Heart Association Nutrition Committee, Lichtenstein AH, Appel LJ, et al. Diet and lifestyle recommendations revision 2006: A scientific statement from the American Heart Association Nutrition Committee. Circulation 114:82–96, 2006.
7. American Physical Therapy Association. Guide to Physical Therapist Practice, 2nd ed. Phys Ther 81:9–744, 2001.
8. Levine SA, Lown B. "Armchair" treatment of acute coronary thrombosis. JAMA 148:1365–9, 1952.
9. Leon AS, Certo C, Comoss P, et al. Position paper of the American Association of Cardiovascular and Pulmonary Rehabilitation: Scientific evidence of the value of cardiac rehabilitation services with emphasis on patients following myocardial infarction—section I: Exercise conditioning component. J Cardiopulm Rehabil 10:79–87, 1990.
10. Statement from CMS National coverage determination 20-10 found: http://www.cms.hhs.gov/mcd/viewdecisionmemo.asp
11. AACVPR guidelines.
12. McNeer JF, Wallace AG, Wagner GS, et al. The course of acute myocardial infarction: Feasibility of early discharge of the uncomplicated patient. Circulation 51:410, 1975.
13. Maskin C, Reddy H, Gulanick M, Perez L. Exercise training in chronic heart failure: Improvement in cardiac performance and maximum oxygen uptake. Circulation 74(Suppl II):310, 1986.
14. Lee AP, Ice R, Blessey R, San Marco ME. Long-term effects of physical training on coronary patients with impaired ventricular function. Circulation 60:1519–26, 1979.
15. Coates AJ, Adamopoulos S, Meyer TE, et al. Effects of physical training in chronic heart failure. Lancet 335(8681):63–6, 1990.
16. Heath GW, Malorey PM, Fure CW. Group exercise versus home exercise in coronary artery bypass graft patients: Effects on physical activity. J Cardiopulm Rehabil 7:190–5, 1987.
17. DeBusk RF, Haskell WL, Miller NH, et al. Medically directed at-home rehabilitation soon after clinically uncomplicated acute myocardial infarction. A new model for patient care. Am J Cardiol 55:251–7, 1985.
18. Southard DR, Certo C, Comoss P, et al. Core competencies for cardiac rehabilitation professionals. J Cardiopulm Rehabil 14:87–92, 1994.
19. King ML, Williams MA, Fletcher GF, et al. Medical director responsibilities for outpatient cardiac rehabilitation/secondary prevention programs: A scientific statement from the American Heart Association/American Association for Cardiovascular and Pulmonary Rehabilitation. Circulation 112:3354–60, 2005.
20. Balady G, Fletcher BJ, Froelicher EF, et al. Core components of cardiac rehabilitation/secondary prevention programs: 2007 update: A scientific statement from the American Heart Association and AACVPR. J Cardiopulm Rehabil Prev 27:121–9, 2007.
21. Wenger NK, Hellerstein HK. In Rehabilitation of the Coronary Patient. New York, Wiley, 1984.
22. Garrow JS. Effects of exercise on obesity. Acta Med Scand 711(Suppl):67–74, 1986.
23. Haskell WL. The influence of exercise training on plasma lipids and lipoproteins in health and disease. Acta Med Scand 711(Suppl):25–38, 1986.
24. Hagberg JM, Seals DR. Exercise training and hypertension. Acta Med Scand 711(Suppl):131–6, 1986.
25. Holloszy JO, Schultz J, Kusnierkiewicz J, et al. Glucose tolerance and insulin resistance. Acta Med Scand 711(Suppl):67–73, 1986.
26. Clausen JP. Circulatory adjustments to dynamic exercise and physical training in normal subjects and in patients with coronary artery disease. In Sonnenblick EH, Lesch M (eds.): Exercise and the Heart. New York, Grune & Stratum, 1977: 39–75.
27. Detry J-MR, Rousseau M, Vandenbroucke G, et al. Increased arteriovenous oxygen difference after physical training in coronary heart disease. Circulation 64:109–18, 1971.
28. Pollack ML, Wilmore JH. In Exercise in Health and Disease: Evaluation and Prescription for Prevention and Rehabilitation. 2nd ed. Philadelphia, WB Saunders, 1990: 1–750.
29. Thompson PD. The benefits and risks of exercise training in patients with chronic coronary artery disease. JAMA 259:1537–40, 1988.

30. Ehsani AA, Biello DR, Schultz J, et al. Improvement of left ventricular contractile function in patients with coronary artery disease. Circulation 74:350–88, 1986.

31. May GS, Eberlein KA, Furberg CD, et al. Secondary prevention after myocardial infarction: A review of long term trials. Prog Cardiovasc Dis 24:331–62, 1982.

32. Wenger NK, Froelicher ES, Smith LK, et al. Cardiac Rehabilitation. Clinical Practice Guideline No. 17. AHCPR Publication No. 96-0672. Rockville, MD: US Department of Health and Human Services, Public Health Service, Agency for Health Care Policy and Research, and the National Heart, Lung and Blood Institute, 1995.

33. Thomas RJ, King M, Lui K, et al. AACVPR/ACC/AHA 2007 performance measures on cardiac rehabilitation for referral to and delivery of cardiac rehabilitation/secondary prevention services. J Cardiopulm Rehabil Prev 27:260–90, 2007.

34. Froelicher V, Jensen D, Genter F, et al. A randomized trial of exercise training in patients with coronary heart disease. JAMA 252:1291–7, 1984.

35. Conn EH, Williams RS, Wallace AG. Exercise responses before and after physical conditioning in patients with severely depressed left ventricular function. Am J Cardiol 49:296–300, 1982.

36. Arvan S. Exercise performance of the high risk acute myocardial infarction patient after cardiac rehabilitation. Am J Cardiol 62(4):197–201, 1988.

37. Sullivan MJ, Cobb FR. The anaerobic threshold in chronic heart failure. Relation to blood lactate, ventilatory basis, reproducibility and response to exercise training. Circulation 81(Suppl 2):47–58, II, 1990.

38. Naughton JP, Hellerstein HK. In Exercise Testing and Exercise Training in Coronary Heart Disease. New York, Academic Press, 1973.

39. American College of Sports Medicine. In ACSM's Guidelines for Exercise Testing and Prescription. 5th ed. Baltimore, Williams & Wilkins, 1995.

40. O'Connor CM, Whellan DJ, Lee KL, et al. Efficacy and safety of exercise training in patients with chronic heart failure: HF-ACTION randomized controlled trial. JAMA 301(14):1439–50, 2009.

41. Flynn KE, Piña IL, Whellan DJ, et al. Effects of exercise training on health status in patients with chronic heart failure: HF-ACTION randomized controlled trial. JAMA 301(14):1451–9, 2009.

42. Goldberg L, Elliott DL, Kuehl KS. Assessment of exercise intensity formulas by use of ventilatory threshold. Chest 94:95–8, 1988.

43. Gibbons E. The influence of anaerobic threshold in exercise prescription. Sports Med 27:357–61, 1987.

44. Dwyer J, Bybee R. Heart rate indices of the anaerobic threshold. Med Sci Sports Exerc 15:72–6, 1983.

45. Borg G, Linderholm H. Perceived exertion and pulse rate during graded exercise in various age groups. Acta Med Scand (Suppl) 472:194–206, 1967.

46. Ades PA, Grunvald MH, Weiss RM, Hanson JS. Usefulness of myocardial ischemia as a predictor of training effect with cardiac rehabilitation after acute myocardial infarction or coronary artery bypass graft. Am J Cardiol 63(15):1032–6, 1989.

47. Bergh V, Kamstrup L, Ekblom B. Maximal oxygen uptake during exercise with various combinations of arm and leg work. J Appl Physiol 41:191–6, 1976.

48. Gutin B, Ang EK, Torrey MA. Cardiorespiratory and subjective responses to incremental and constant load ergometry with arms and legs. Arch Phys Med Rehabil 69:510–13, 1988.

49. Keleman MH. Resistance training safety and essential guidelines for cardiac and coronary prone patients. Med Sci Sports Exerc 21:675–7, 1989.

50. McCartney N, McKelvie RS, Haslam DR, Jones NL. Usefulness of weightlifting training in improving strength and maximal power output on coronary artery disease. Am J Cardiol 12:254–60, 1991.

51. Steward KJ. Resistance training effects on strength and cardiovascular endurance in cardiac and coronary prone patients. Med Sci Sports Exerc 21:678–82, 1989.

52. DeBusk RF, Valdez R, Houston N, Haskell W. Cardiovascular responses to dynamic and static effort soon after myocardial infarction: Application to occupational assessment. Circulation 58:368–75, 1978.

53. Sparling P, Cantwell JD. Strength training guidelines for cardiac patients. Phys Sports Med 17:190–6, 1989.

54. American Association of Cardiovascular and Pulmonary Rehabilitation. In Guidelines for Cardiac Rehabilitation and Secondary Prevention Programs. 3rd ed. Champaign, IL, Human Kinetics, 1999.

55. American Heart Association. Exercise standards: A statement for healthcare professionals. Circulation 91:580–615, 1995.

56. Kannel WB, Castelli WP, Gordon T, et al. Serum cholesterol lipoproteins and risk of coronary heart diseases: The Framingham study. Ann Intern Med 74:1–12, 1971.

57. Lowering blood cholesterol to prevent heart disease. JAMA 253:2080–90, 1985.

58. Blank DW, Hoeg JM, Kroll MH, et al. The method of determination must be considered in interpreting blood cholesterol levels. JAMA 256:2867–70, 1986.

59. Lipid Research Clinics Program. The Lipid Research Clinics Coronary Primary Prevention Trial Results I. Reduction in incidence of coronary heart disease. JAMA 251:351–64, 1984.

60. Lipid Research Clinics Program. The Lipid Research Clinics Coronary Primary Prevention Trial Results II. The relationship of reduction in incidence of coronary heart disease to cholesterol lowering. JAMA 251:365–74, 1984.

61. Wood PD, Stefanick ML, Dreon DM, et al. Changes in plasma lipoproteins in overweight men during weight loss through dieting as compared with exercise. N Engl J Med 319:1173–9, 1988.

62. Tran ZV, Weltman A. Differential effects of exercise on serum lipid and lipoprotein levels seen with changes in body weight. A meta-analysis. JAMA 254:919–24, 1985.

63. Allison TG, Williams DE, Miller TD, et al. Medical and economic costs of psychologic distress in patients with coronary artery disease. Mayo Clinic Proc 70:734–42, 1995.

64. Case RB, Moss AJ, Case N, et al. Living alone after myocardial infarction: Impact of prognosis. JAMA 117:1003–9, 1992.

65. Everson SA, Goldberg DE, Kaplan GA, et al. Hopelessness and risk of mortality and incidence of myocardial infarction and cancer. Psychosom Med 58:113–21, 1996.

66. Frasure-Smith N, Lesperance F, Talajic M. Depression and 18-month prognosis after myocardial infarction. Circulation 91:999–1005, 1995.

67. Rozanski A, Bairey CN, Krantz DS, et al. Mental stress and the induction of silent myocardial ischemia in patients with coronary artery disease. N Engl J Med 311:552–9, 1984.

68. Wenger NK. In hospital exercise rehabilitation after myocardial infarction and myocardial revascularization: Physiologic basis, methodology, and results. In Wenger NK, Hellerstein HK (eds.): Rehabilitation of the Coronary Patient. 3rd ed. New York, Churchill Livingstone, 1992.

69. Mumford E, Schlessinger H, Glass G. The effects of psychological intervention on recovery from surgery and heart attacks: An analysis of the literature. Am J Public Health 72(2):141–51, 1982.

70. Oldenburg B, Perkins R, Andrews G. Controlled trial of psychological intervention in myocardial infarction. J Consult Clin Psychol 53:852–9, 1985.

71. Amery A, Birkenhager W, Brixko P, et al. Mortality and morbidity results from the European Working Party on high blood pressure in the elderly trial. Lancet 1:1349–54, 1985.

72. Berkman L, Syme SL. Social networks, host resistance and mortality: A nine-year follow-up study of Alameda County residents. Am J Epidemiol 109:186–204, 1979.

73. Cooper CL, Faragher ED, Bray CL, Ramsdale DR. The significance of psychosocial factors in predicting coronary disease in patients with valvular heart disease. Soc Sci Med 20:315–18, 1985.

74. Oldridge NB, Guyatt G, Jones N, et al. Effects on quality of life with comprehensive rehabilitation after acute myocardial infarction. Am J Cardiol, 67:1084–9, 1991.

75. Murphy S. Self efficacy and social support-mediators of stress on mental health following a natural disorder. West J Nurs Res 9(1):58–87, 1987.

76. Strecher V, McEvoy B, Becker M, Rosenstock I. The role of self efficacy in achieving behavior changes. Health Educ Q 13(1):73–91, 1986.

77. Southard DR, Broyden R. Psychosocial services in cardiac rehabilitation: A status report. J Cardiopulm Rehabil 10:255–63, 1990.

78. Herridge ML, Stimler CE, Southard DR, King ML; AACVPR Task Force. Depression screening in cardiac rehabilitation: AACVPR Task Force Report. J Cardiopulm Rehabil 25:11–13, 2005.

79. Oldridge NB. Cardiac rehabilitation exercise programme. Compliance and compliance-enhancing strategies. Sports Med 6(1):42–55, 1988.

80. Pashkow F, Pashkow P, Schafer M, Ferguson C. Successful Cardiac Rehabilitation. Loveland, CO, The Heartwatchers Press, 1988.

81. Sanderson BK, Southard D, Oldridge N; Writing Group. AACVPR consensus statement: Outcomes evaluation in cardiac rehabilitation/secondary prevention programs: Improving patient care and program effectiveness. J Cardiopulm Rehabil 24:68–79, 2004.

82. Mannarino E, Pasqualini L, Menna M, et al. Effects of physical training on peripheral vascular disease: A controlled study. Angiology 40(1):5–10, 1989.

83. Johnson EC, Vogles WF, Atterbom HA, et al. Effects of exercise training on common femoral artery blood flow in patients with intermittent claudication. Circulation 80(5 Pt 2):III59–III72, 1989.

84. ACC/AHA 2005 guidelines for the management of patients with peripheral arterial disease (lower extremity, renal, mesenteric, abdominal aortic). A collaborative report from the American Association for Vascular Surgery/Society for Vascular Surgery, Society for Cardiovascular Angiography and Interventions, Society for Vascular Medicine and Biology, Society of Interventional Radiology, and the ACC/AHA Task Force on Practice Guidelines (Writing Committee to Develop Guidelines for the Management of Patients With Peripheral Arterial Disease). J Am Coll Cardiol 47:e1–192, 2006.

85. Kannel WB, McGee DL. Diabetes and cardiovascular risk factors: The Framingham study. Circulation 59:8, 1979.

86. American Diabetes Association. The Physicians Guide to Type II Diabetes (NIDMM): Diagnosis and Treatment. New York, American Diabetes Association, 1984.

87. Sigal RJ, Kenny GP, Wasserman DH, et al. Physical activity/exercise and type 2 diabetes. Diabetes Care 27:2518–39, 2004.

88. Smith SC Jr, Allen J, Blair SN, et al. AHA/ACC guidelines for secondary prevention for patients with coronary and other atherosclerotic vascular disease: 2006 update: Endorsed by the National Heart, Lung, Blood Institute. Circulation 113:2363–72, 2006.

89. Fowler RS, Fordyce WE. Strokes: Why Do They Behave That Way? Dallas, Texas, American Heart Association, 1974.

90. Monga TN, DeForge DA, Williams J, Wolfe LA. Cardiovascular responses to acute exercise in patients with cerebrovascular accidents. Arch Phys Med Rehabil 69:937–40, 1988.

91. Painter P, Hanson P. A model for clinical exercise prescription: Application to hemodialysis patients. J Cardiopulm Rehabil 7:177–89, 1987.

92. Painter P, Messer-Rehale D, Hanson P, et al. Exercise capacity in hemodialysis, CAPD and renal transplant patients. Nephron 42:47–51, 1986.

93. Christie I, Pewen W. A 12 week trial of exercise training in patients on continuous ambulatory peritoneal dialysis (unpublished manuscript).

94. American Heart Association. In 1992 Heart and Stroke Facts. Washington, DC, American Heart Association, 1997.

95. Redberg RF. Coronary artery disease in women: Understanding the diagnostic and management pitfalls. Medscape Women's Health 3(5):1, 1998.

96. AHA evidence-based guidelines for cardiovascular disease prevention in women. Circulation 115, 2007.

97. Limacher MC. Exercise and rehabilitation in women: Indications and outcomes. Cardiol Clin 16(1):27–36, 1998.

98. Brezinka V, Kitrel F. Psychosocial factors of coronary heart disease in women: A review. Soc Sci Med 42(10):1351–65, 1996.

99. Weiner D, Ryan T, McCabe C, et al. Exercise stress testing: Correlations among history of angina, ST segment response and prevalence of coronary artery disease in the Coronary Artery Surgery Study. N Engl J Med 301:230–5, 1979.

100. Taillefer R, DePuey EG, Udelson JE, et al. Comparative diagnostic accuracy of T1-201 and Tc-99m sestamibi SPECT imaging (perfusion and ECG-gated Spect) in detecting coronary artery disease in women. J Am Coll Cardiol 29(1):69–77, 1997.

101. Sawada S, Ryan T, Fineberg N. Exercise echocardiographic detection of coronary artery disease in women. J Am Coll Cardiol 14:1440–7, 1989.

102. Fisher L, Kennedy J, Davis K, et al. Association of sex, physical size and operative mortality after coronary artery bypass in the Coronary Artery Surgery Study (CASS). J Thorac Cardiovasc Surg 84:334–41, 1981.

103. Khan SS, Nessim S, Gray R, et al. Increased mortality of women in coronary artery bypass surgery: Evidence for referral bias. Ann Intern Med 112(8):561–7, 1990.

104. Cowley MJ, Mullin SM, Kelsey SF, et al. Sex differences in early and long-term results of coronary angioplasty in the NHLB Registry TCA. Circulation 71:90–7, 1985.

105. Ginzel AR. Women's compliance with cardiac rehabilitation programs. Prog Cardiovasc Nurs 11(1):30–5, 1996.

106. Balady GJ, Fletcher BJ, Froelicher ES, et al. Cardiac rehabilitation programs. A statement for healthcare professionals from the American Heart Association. Circulation 90:1602–10, 1994.

107. Pashkow FJ. Cardiac rehabilitation: Not just exercise anymore. Cleve Clin J Med 63(2):116–23, 1996.

108. Carhart RL Jr, Ades PA. Gender differences in cardiac rehabilitation. Cardiol Clin 116(1):37–43, 1998.

109. Lieberman L, Meana M, Stewart D. Cardiac rehabilitation: Gender differences in factors influencing participation. J Womens Health 7(6):717–23, 1998.

110. Thomas RJ, Miller NH, Lamendola C, et al. National survey on gender differences in cardiac rehabilitation programs: Patient characteristics and enrollment patterns. J Cardiopulm Rehabil 16:402–12, 1996.

111. Cannistra LB, Balady GJ, O'Malley CJ, et al. Comparison of the clinical profile and outcome of women and men in cardiac rehabilitation. Am J Cardiol 69:1274–9, 1992.

112. Tomassoni TL, Galioto FM, Vaccaro P, et al. The pediatric cardiac rehabilitation program at Children's Hospital National Medical Center, Washington DC. J Cardiopulm Rehabil 7:259–62, 1987.

113. Calzori A, Pastore E, Biodi G. Cardiac rehabilitation in children: Interdisciplinary approach. Minerva Pediatr 49(12):559–65, 1997.

114. American Academy of Pediatrics. Position statement on cholesterol screening. Pediatrics 83:141–2, 1989.

115. Blessey R, Blessey S. Hypercholesterolemia in children: Is it a problem requiring intervention? Cardiopulm Phys Ther J 1:10–12, 1990.

116. Srinivasan SR. Biological determinants of serum lipoprotein. In Berenson G (ed.): Causation of Cardiovascular Risk Factors in Children. New York, Raven Press, 1986:83–129.

117. Walter HJ, Hofman A, Vaughan RD, et al. Modification of risk factors for coronary heart disease: Five year results of a school based intervention trial. N Engl J Med 318:1093–100, 1988.

118. Seals DR, Allen WK, Hurley BF, et al. Elevated high density lipoprotein cholesterol levels in older endurance athletes. Am J Cardiol 54:390–3, 1984.

119. Lampman RM. Evaluating and prescribing exercise for elderly patients. Geriatrics 42(8):63–5, 1987.

120. Van Camp SP, Peterson RA. Cardiorespiratory complications of outpatient cardiac rehabilitation programs. JAMA 256(9):1160–3, 1986.

## CHAPTER 19

# Pulmonary Rehabilitation

*Rebecca Crouch*

Rehabilitation programs for patients with chronic obstructive pulmonary disease (COPD) have existed for more than 30 years. The American College of Chest Physicians in 1974 defined pulmonary rehabilitation and described aspects of care for patients with respiratory impairments. The American Thoracic Society incorporated these into an official position statement in 1981.[1] More recently, the 2006 American Thoracic Society and the European Respiratory Society Statement on Pulmonary Rehabilitation stated, "Pulmonary rehabilitation is an evidence-based, multidisciplinary, and comprehensive intervention for patients with chronic respiratory diseases who are symptomatic and often have decreased daily life activities. Integrated into the individualized treatment of the patient, pulmonary rehabilitation is designed to reduce symptoms, optimize functional status, increase participation, and reduce health care costs through stabilizing or reversing systemic manifestations of the disease."[2] Most of the research available has addressed the benefits of rehabilitation for patients with COPD while neglecting rehabilitation outcomes for patients with other chronic respiratory diseases such as restrictive lung diseases, spinal and chest deformities, neuromuscular conditions that lead to respiratory failure, pulmonary vascular diseases, and those that affect the very obese.[3] Early research in the area of pulmonary rehabilitation focused on the lack of improvement, as documented by pulmonary function testing, or the failure to reverse the natural progression of the disease process.

Today, many successful pulmonary rehabilitation programs exist and the need for early detection and treatment of respiratory dysfunction is widely accepted.[4] Rehabilitation research now emphasizes symptom improvement, functional and exercise gains, and health-related quality-of-life outcomes as measures of efficacy instead of changes in pulmonary physiologic parameters. This research supports the benefit of pulmonary rehabilitation.[2,5]

The history of physical therapy involvement in the care of pulmonary patients has roots back to the First World War. A British nurse, Winifred Linton, initially treated traumatic respiratory complications during the war. Following the war, she entered physical therapy training and began to teach localized breathing exercises to other physical therapists (PTs) and surgeons at the Royal Brompton Hospital in London. Her work continued through the 1940s and during the Second World War. A few PTs in the United States were instructed in airway clearance techniques and began to use and teach them to patients during the polio epidemic of the 1940s.[6,7]

The Cardiovascular and Pulmonary Section of the American Physical Therapy Association (APTA) is an organization formed 30 years ago to promote and support the practice of Cardiovascular and Pulmonary Physical Therapy. The organizational website states, "The Cardiovascular and Pulmonary Section will serve its members, the physical therapy profession, and the community, by promoting the development, application and advancement of cardiovascular and pulmonary physical therapy practice, education, and research."[8] All licensed PTs and physical therapy assistants (PTAs) who are members of APTA are eligible to join the section.

A cardiovascular and pulmonary residency was initiated in 2008 by APTA that includes an intensive 1-year plan of didactic, clinical practice, and research study. This residency is intended to expand the physical therapist's knowledge and clinical skill and to prepare those who successfully complete the residency to sit for the Cardiovascular and Pulmonary APTA Board Certification examination.[9,10]

Pulmonary rehabilitation principles can be generalized to many chronic disease patient populations: the need for multidisciplinary programming; individualized goals aimed at restoring optimal physical and psychological functioning; and adding components of exercise, education, and counseling. Disease-specific aspects of rehabilitation include the following:

- Patient assessment and goal-setting
- Exercise training
- Self-management education
- Nutritional intervention
- Psychosocial support

In this chapter, goals for rehabilitation of the pulmonary patient, the structure of pulmonary rehabilitation programs, and physical therapy strategies are presented.

## Choosing Goals and Outcomes in Pulmonary Rehabilitation

The goals for an individual pulmonary patient must be very specific and pertinent to his or her lifestyle, needs, and personal interests. This is possible only after a thorough evaluation of the patient's disease state and clinical course, physical examination, and possibly a patient-family interview.

The rehabilitation personnel should assist the patient in identifying realistic goals that can be described in behavioral terms and measured as outcomes for rehabilitation. They should be goals that can make the most impact on daily function as well as be realistic and life enhancing. Examples of unrealistic goals are to eliminate dyspnea, to have a normal lifestyle, or to discontinue supplemental oxygen use. Examples of more realistic goals would be learning and implementing strategies to relieve dyspnea, increasing activity tolerance, and improving oxygen saturation levels during activity.

Pulmonary rehabilitation outcomes are measures that generally assess the success of set goals. Outcome assessments are usually a combination of objective and subjective measures. Three essential areas that require outcome measurements in pulmonary rehabilitation include the following:

- Exercise capacity
- Symptoms (dyspnea and fatigue)
- Health-related quality of life

These domains have been supported by various national and international organizations as key areas for outcome assessment in pulmonary rehabilitation.[2,5,11-20]

- Improvement in exercise capacity. The patient will (1) gain sufficient strength, flexibility, and endurance to accomplish identified activities of daily living (ADLs) and requirements of employment and recreational tasks and (2) learn to employ strategies to manipulate the environment to maximize physical functioning. Outcome measures related to this area of improvement include

graded exercise tests, timed distance walk tests, incremental or endurance shuttle walk tests, and timed ADL tests.[21-35]

- Improvement in clinical symptoms. For example, the patient will (1) be able to effectively mobilize respiratory secretions, (2) employ strategies to relieve symptoms of dyspnea and cough, (3) recognize early signs of the need for medical intervention, (4) decrease the frequency and severity of respiratory exacerbations, and (5) obtain optimal oxygen saturation throughout the day and night. Outcome measures for this area may include the use of a Borg or visual analog scale to measure dyspnea or fatigue, dyspnea questionnaires to measure the impact of dyspnea on ADLs, the distress of dyspnea, the influence of dyspnea on quality of life (QOL), and the evaluation of fatigue.[2,5,11,16-19]

- Improvement in health-related behaviors. For example, the patient will (1) stop tobacco use and drug or alcohol misuse, (2) comply with medical and rehabilitation treatments, (3) improve coping skills, and (4) improve psychosocial function. Outcome measures for this area of change include behavioral surveys, patient diaries, and other self-report tools, as well as carbon monoxide levels for tobacco use.[2,5,11,16,18,19,36-38]

Other outcome assessments such as functional performance, home-based activity, psychosocial outcomes (anxiety and depression), adherence (dropout or attendance rate), knowledge and self-efficacy, smoking cessation, nutrition/weight, healthcare utilization, mortality and morbidity, and patient satisfaction may also be of interest and some pulmonary rehabilitation programs may choose to measure these parameters (Table 19-1).[36-39]

## Structure of the Pulmonary Rehabilitation Program

Pulmonary rehabilitation programs vary widely in their overall structure and settings. Programs are offered in an inpatient rehabilitation or subacute facility, as an outpatient program in a hospital or freestanding clinic, or in the patient's home. Each setting has its advantages and disadvantages in terms of convenience for patients, cost of delivering services, resources available, and socialization opportunities. Benefits associated with pulmonary rehabilitation have been demonstrated in each setting.[40]

In some cases, pulmonary rehabilitation begins during an acute hospitalization, at which time appropriate candidates for outpatient rehabilitation can be identified, patient education and support can be initiated, and the response to activity and exercise can be evaluated. Treatment is aimed at reducing immobility and maintaining function during the hospitalization. All components of pulmonary rehabilitation can begin during the acute inpatient program, within the limits of patient tolerance and medical condition.[41,42]

Despite the variability in the structure of pulmonary rehabilitation programs, there are some accepted

## Table 19-1 Pulmonary Rehabilitation Outcome Measures

| Domain | | | Outcome Measurement |
|---|---|---|---|
| Exercise capacity and function | | | Symptom-limited graded exercise test |
| | | | Submaximal exercise test |
| | | | 6-minute walk test |
| | | | Shuttle walk tests (incremental or endurance) |
| Symptoms | | | |
| Dyspnea | Borg Scale | | Visual Analogue Scale (VAS) |
| | | | Baseline (BDI) and Transitional (TDI) Dyspnea Indexes |
| | | | Medical Research Council (MRC) |
| | | | University of California San Diego (UCSD) Shortness of Breath Questionnaire |
| | | | Pulmonary Functional Status and Dyspnea Questionnaire (PFSDQ or PFSDQ-M) |
| | | | Pulmonary Function Status Scale (PFSS) |
| | | | Symptom domain of the St. George Respiratory Questionnaire (SGRQ)—evaluates dyspnea, cough, sputum, and wheeze |
| | | | Activity domain of SGRQ—evaluates activity limitation resulting from dyspnea |
| | | | Dyspnea Domain of the Chronic Respiratory Disease Questionnaire (CRQ) |
| Fatigue | | | Borg scale (substitute the word *dyspnea* with a comparable word of fatigue (e.g., tired, exhausted) |
| | | | Visual Analogue Scale (VAS) (with word substitution) |
| | | | Multidimensional Fatigue Inventory (MFI) |
| | | | Multidimensional Assessment of Fatigue (MAF) |
| | | | Vitality dimension of the Short-Form 36 (SF-36) |
| | | | Fatigue dimension of the CRQ or PFSDQ-M |
| | | | Fatigue/inertia and vigor/activity subscales of the Profile of Mood States (POMS) |
| Health-related quality of life | | | Medical Outcomes Study (MOS)—Commonly called the SF-36 |
| | | | St. George Respiratory Questionnaire (SGRQ) |
| | | | Chronic Respiratory Disease Questionnaire (CRQ) |
| | | | Seattle Obstructive Lung Questionnaire (SOLQ) |

recommendations for the qualifications of personnel, program components, and patient candidacy.[2,5,40]

### The Pulmonary Rehabilitation Team

The specific professionals involved in pulmonary rehabilitation vary from program to program. Optimally, the core of the pulmonary rehabilitation program team consists of at least three to four rehabilitation specialists who have experience and varied academic backgrounds. Additional professionals may consult with patients on an as-needed basis or serve as program advisers to meet the needs of a diverse patient population.[40]

### The Patient and Family

The patient with pulmonary disease participating in the pulmonary rehabilitation program, the patient's spouse or family, and the primary care provider play a central role on the team.

The patient must be empowered to lead the rehabilitation process with the assistance and guidance of the rehabilitation professionals and family. This may be difficult for some patients who have taken a passive role in their own treatment, and for families who have become caretakers. Individualized and family counseling may be indicated for those who are unable to assume the responsibility of this role.

### The Medical Director

The medical director should be a physician who has interest and expertise in pulmonary diseases. He or she directs the rehabilitation program in matters of overall policy, procedures, and medical care, including specialized diagnostic tests and medical treatments for pulmonary diseases.

### The Program Director

The program director is the administrator or coordinator of services. This person is the team leader, directing day-to-day functions of the pulmonary rehabilitation program according to established policies and procedures. A diverse background in pulmonary care, education, and administration are necessary for this individual. In most programs, the program director also provides direct patient care services.

## Other Team Members

Other team members may include a variety of specialists who can assume leadership in the areas of exercise, breathing re-training, respiratory care, education, counseling or behavior management, pharmacology, and nutrition.

## Program Components

A comprehensive pulmonary rehabilitation program should incorporate the following components:[2,5,40]
- Patient assessment and goal-setting
- Exercise and functional training
- Self-management education
- Nutritional intervention
- Psychosocial management

A physical therapist may participate in any or all of these pulmonary rehabilitation program components, but makes their greatest contributions in the areas of pulmonary care, exercise and functional training, and education.

## Patient Assessment and Goal Setting

The patient evaluation is the foundation for an individualized program design and measurement of outcomes. Each patient is different and each will have a distinctive plan of care. Components of the initial patient assessment include the following:
- Patient interview
- Medical history
- Physical assessment
- Review of diagnostic tests
- Symptom assessment

The patient interview can set the stage for ongoing communication, trust, and a healthy rapport between the patient and rehabilitation team. Establishing a comfortable atmosphere during the initial interview will facilitate a feeling of ease with the staff and rehabilitation setting, decrease anxiety or fear associated with therapy, and allow the patient to ask any questions he or she may have concerning rehabilitation.

A thorough review of the medical history by reading the patient's medical records and personal communication will offer a snapshot into the history of the patient's disease course and comorbidities. Items to be noted include surgical procedures, family history, use of medical resources (e.g., hospitalizations, emergency department visits), medications, oxygen use, allergies, smoking/alcohol/other substance abuse history, occupational and environmental exposures, social support, and prior level of function.

An overall physical evaluation gives the physical therapist a baseline pathophysiological assessment of the patient upon which specific musculoskeletal and functional parameters

may be observed. Basic components of the physical evaluation include vital signs (e.g., blood pressure, heart rate, oxygen saturation, respiratory rate), height, weight, body mass index, breathing pattern including use of accessory breathing muscles, chest examination (e.g., auscultation of lung and heart sounds, inspection, palpation, symmetry), presence of clubbing of distal digits (see Fig 16-12), vascular integrity (e.g., edema, skin coloration, hair growth), and skin integrity (e.g., bruising, skin tears). A review of diagnostic tests will offer additional information to accurately plan the treatment regime and adjuncts to treatment (e.g., need for oxygen use, exercise tolerance and fatigue, special precautions with exercise, such as negative bone density scores).

Finally, asking specific questions and observing the patient during the interview will provide added information related to symptom assessment. Those may include dyspnea, fatigue, cough and sputum production, wheezing, hemoptysis, chest pain, gastroesophageal reflux, dysphasia, pain and/or weakness, feelings of anxiety/panic/fear/isolation, and depression.[43]

## Exercise and Functional Training

The determination of safe and appropriate exercise should be preceded by a thorough musculoskeletal assessment by the physical therapist. The assessment should begin with a gross manual muscle test of the upper and lower extremities and the trunk. A range-of-motion (ROM) and flexibility examination must focus on specific areas such as the rib cage, shoulders, cervical/thoracic/lumbar spine, hamstrings, and gastrocnemius/soleus muscles. The rib cage, shoulders and spine lose ROM as a result of progressive lung disease, poor posture, and accessory breathing muscle use. The lower extremity musculature typically loses flexibility because of disuse.

Poor posture also develops simultaneously as lung disease progresses, activity levels decrease, and metabolic changes effect bone density. Furthermore, postural changes continue to occur with the loss of chest mobility, the adoption of propping postures, and the use of accessory breathing muscles of the shoulders, cervical and thoracic spine (see Fig 16-3). Poor postural habits further inhibit breathing mechanics, and particular attention should be given to chest wall mobility within the treatment plan.

Many patients with chronic respiratory disease simultaneously suffer from musculoskeletal abnormalities, for instance, pulmonary diagnoses of restrictive lung disease (e.g., scleroderma, pulmonary fibrosis due to unspecified connective tissue disease, rheumatoid arthritis, spinal cord injury, and scoliosis). Elderly chronic respiratory disease patients often experience osteoarthritis of the shoulders, spine, hips, knees, and feet. Those who have used systemic corticosteroids for prolonged periods of time and in higher doses may experience pain and functional disabilities due to osteoporosis, vertebral compression fractures, or loss of peripheral joint and neurological integrity.

Instruction in posture, balance, gait, strengthening, flexibility, energy conservation/pacing, and the use of adaptive equipment may be necessary to optimize the patient's ability to carry out usual daily activities for home, work, community mobility, and recreation. Exercise to improve cardiopulmonary endurance and breathing mechanics are a major component of rehabilitation.[43] Specific guidelines for exercise for the pulmonary patient are addressed later in this chapter.

---

**Clinical tip**

The physical therapist is instrumental in the instruction of pulmonary patients in body mechanics, posture correction, use of ambulatory assistive devices, energy conservation/pacing, and balance.

---

## Self-Management Education

An educational assessment is helpful to determine how well the patient understands and manages his or her disease. This information allows the physical therapist to design an educational plan and evaluate change following intervention. The educational focus in pulmonary rehabilitation has transitioned from only didactic lectures in a group setting to instruction in self-management in collaboration with the health care provider.[38] For example, the chronic respiratory disease patient should be able to recognize an early acute exacerbation of his or her disease; when/how to initiate or increase specific therapy such as antibiotics, steroids, and bronchodilators; and when to contact their health care provider. Other areas to note are the patient's ability to read, write, hear, and see. Physical therapists should also be aware of cognitive impairments, language barriers, and cultural diversity issues.

Educational topics may include anatomy and pathophysiology of chronic respiratory diseases, use and misuse of oxygen, and practical solutions to incorporate activity into daily lives. Self-management education involves the transfer of knowledge and skill in performing self-care techniques. Other topics include airway clearance and relieving dyspnea, breathing techniques, cough facilitation, postures to improve breathing, and relaxation techniques.

It is important to try a variety of procedures while the patient is in the rehabilitation setting and evaluate which are most effective for the patient in the home environment. Patients whose production of mucus is copious may require two to three airway clearance sessions each day, whereas other patients may require treatment only during an acute illness. These procedures are described in more detail in Chapter 17 and later in this chapter under Physical Therapy Management.

## Nutritional Assessment and Intervention

Patients with respiratory disease frequently have alterations of their nutritional status and body mass index (BMI). Chronic respiratory disease patients such as those with COPD or cystic fibrosis experience malabsorption, decreased body mass with muscle mass depletion, and high energy costs as a result of an increased work of breathing.[44-46] Obesity associated with respiratory disease may be related to hypercarbia due to obesity-hypoventilation syndrome, a decreased activity level due to dyspnea and fatigue, and comorbidities such as cardiac disease.[44]

Accordingly, the nutritional assessment should include at least the measurement of height, weight, calculation of BMI (Weight [kg]/Height$^2$ [m$^2$]),[47] and documentation of a recent and significant (>3 lbs.) weight change.[48] Additional notations regarding nutrition may include dysphasia, dentition, mastication problems, gastroesophageal reflux, change of the taste of food due to oxygen use, dyspnea while eating, fluid intake, person responsible for buying and cooking food, alcohol consumption, caffeine consumption, laboratory values for serum albumin and prealbumin, drug–food interactions, and use of nutritional or herbal supplements.

## Psychosocial Evaluation and Plan of Care

Screening questionnaires are useful in assessing the psychosocial symptoms of anxiety and depression. Moreover, a psychosocial assessment should address motivational level, emotional distress, family and home environment, substance abuse, cognitive impairment, conflict and/abuse, coping strategies, sexual dysfunction, and neuropsychological impairments (e.g., memory, attention, concentration).

It is important to assess the patient's psychosocial status in order to tailor the educational and exercise intervention accordingly. Patients with significant psychosocial problems should be referred to appropriate professionals, in particular, social workers, a psychiatric nurse, licensed counselor, psychologist, or psychiatrist. Failure to do so may lead to poor outcomes following rehabilitation.[36]

## Patient Candidacy

Most of the research devoted to pulmonary rehabilitation has addressed the benefit to COPD patients.[2,5,40] The basic components of pulmonary rehabilitation may, however, be applied to a variety of chronic disease patients such as those with restrictive lung disease, pulmonary hypertension, significant musculoskeletal disease (e.g., arthritis), heart failure, and other stable cardiovascular diseases (e.g., peripheral vascular disease and stroke).

Pulmonary function test data are not exclusively considered when determining candidacy for pulmonary rehabilitation. Most patients are referred and seek rehabilitation as a result of disabling symptoms of dyspnea, inability to perform everyday household activities such as dressing and climbing steps, or a decreased ability to perform job responsibilities. These disabilities may not have a strong correlation to pulmonary function test results.

Patients who continue to smoke, yet have lung disease, may have a significant need for pulmonary rehabilitation and may demonstrate adequate motivation and adherence to therapy. Smoking cessation counseling should be included as part of the therapy and considered a rehabilitation goal. Similarly, a lack of motivation perceived by health care professionals may reverse during and following participation once the patient begins to understand his or her disease and begins to feel better.

Additional issues to consider in patient candidacy include the patient's financial ability and transportation to rehabilitation. Personal out-of-pocket expense must be clearly defined. Third-party payers should be contacted to verify coverage and co-pays. Financial and insurance counselors are helpful in this respect. Discussing transportation with the patient and providing a list of local transportation options are helpful to facilitate regular attendance.

Generally, candidates for pulmonary rehabilitation have a diagnosed pulmonary disease and functional limitation. Because of legislation passed by Congress in July 2008, via the Medicare improvements for Patients and Providers Act (MIPPA), pulmonary rehabilitation benefits for COPD patients insured by Medicare will change. Those COPD patients, referred by a physician, with moderate to very severe disease (GOLD classification II, III, and IV) will be covered for pulmonary rehabilitation under a bundled billing code. Comprehensive Medicare Services (CMS) will cover 36 one-hour sessions, with a maximum of 2 sessions per day. Each session must include a form of aerobic exercise. Physician supervision is required during the pulmonary rehabilitation session(s) and no component services may be billed separately (e.g., evaluation, 6-minute walk test).[49]

Other patients with risk factors (Box 19-1) for the development of pulmonary disease, mild or very advanced disease, chronic respiratory diseases other than COPD, pre–post pulmonary surgical, and others who are limited by respiratory symptoms can demonstrate important functional gains and should not be excluded from rehabilitation programs.[3,7,35,47]

## Physical Therapy Management

Because of regional differences in practice patterns, the role of the physical therapist in pulmonary rehabilitation varies widely among programs. Some programs do not have a physical therapist at all, whereas others consult with a physical therapist only for patients with certain diagnoses, such as those who have musculoskeletal or neuromuscular conditions in addition to pulmonary disease.

Optimally, the physical therapist has expertise in evaluating and treating patients with a wide variety of pulmonary conditions, and is involved in all components of the program. In addition to evaluating each patient and leading exercise sessions, the physical therapist may provide educational sessions, smoking cessation programs, stress management, and relaxation training. The physical therapist also re-evaluates the patient's response to activity, guides exercise progression, assesses outcomes, and provides individualized home exercise programs.

## Patient Evaluation Procedures

Information on patient evaluation, treatment, and follow-up are reviewed in this section to facilitate the development of the physical therapist in assuming a significant role in pulmonary rehabilitation. A more comprehensive guide for examination, evaluation, intervention, and outcomes is described in "The Cardiopulmonary Preferred Practice Patterns" in the *Guide to Physical Therapist Practice* (Table 19-2).[43] A patient referred to a pulmonary rehabilitation program should be receiving regular medical care from a personal physician and should have seen a physician within the last 30 days. Diagnostic testing should be completed and all medical conditions must be considered stable prior to beginning the rehabilitation program.

The physical therapist should evaluate each pulmonary rehabilitation candidate by completing a chart review of medical conditions, laboratory and other test results, interviewing the patient, and performing a physical examination, including an assessment of activity tolerance.

---

### Box 19-1

#### Risk Factors for the Development of Obstructive Pulmonary Disease

- Smoking: cigarette, pipe, cigar, environmental tobacco smoke
- Environmental exposures: air pollution, cooking over an open fire in enclosed spaces
- Occupational dusts and chemicals: asbestos, grain farmers, furnace workers, vapors, irritants, and fumes
- Family history (genetic): $\alpha_1$-antitrypsin, cystic fibrosis
- Allergies and asthma
- Dietary: poor nutrition (e.g., low levels of vitamins A, C, and E)
- Gestational and childhood factors: low birth weight, respiratory infections
- Periodontal disease

Simon H (ed.). COPD Risk Factors. http://www.healthcentral.com/copd/

---

### Table 19-2 Practice Patterns for Patients with Pulmonary Diseases

| | |
|---|---|
| 6A | Primary prevention/risk reduction for cardiovascular/pulmonary disorders |
| 6B | Impaired aerobic capacity/endurance associated with deconditioning |
| 6C | Impaired ventilation, respiration/gas exchange, and aerobic capacity/endurance associated with airway clearance dysfunction |
| 6E | Impaired ventilation and respiration/gas exchange associated with ventilatory pump dysfunction or failure |
| 6F | Impaired ventilation and respiration/gas exchange associated with respiratory failure |

## Chart Review

The chart should be reviewed for the current pulmonary diagnosis and all diagnostic and laboratory testing that has established the diagnosis, prognosis, and stage of disease. This may include, but is not limited to, pulmonary function testing, chest x-ray, arterial blood gas analysis, electrocardiogram, blood counts, and blood chemistry. In addition, all treatments related to the disease should be identified, such as surgical interventions, medication, oxygen therapy, and assisted ventilation therapy.

Equally important to pulmonary conditions, the chart must be reviewed for other medical diagnoses that should be addressed during rehabilitation. These diagnoses include cardiac disease, diabetes, hypertension, peripheral vascular disease, lipid disorders, arthritis, and cancer, or any chronic condition that may interfere with activity tolerance and function. Pertinent family history may indicate the patient's risk for developing some chronic conditions such as hypertension, diabetes, and cardiac disease.

The information obtained in the chart review will assist the physical therapist in setting individualized goals and treatments, monitoring for adverse responses, providing appropriate education and counseling, or initiating referrals to other professionals.

## Patient Interview

The physical therapist can gather additional information from the patient and family during the interview. To prompt the therapist and make this process efficient, interview questions may be standardized for all participants.

The physical therapist should make sure to ask about the following:
- Use of tobacco, alcohol, and nonprescription drugs
- Usual activity level, including employment, recreation, and home
- Regularity of exercise, including availability of equipment at home
- Two to three activities that the patient names as the most difficult to perform because of his or her pulmonary disease
- Compliance with prescribed medication and treatments
- Pain levels
- Support from family and friends
- History of environmental exposures and sensitivities (including passive smoke)
- Goals for participating in the rehabilitation program

As discussed earlier in this chapter, outcomes questionnaires related to quality of life and function may be used to further assess the patient's current status.

## Patient Examination

The patient examination should include tests and measurements that yield a description of function and physical capabilities. The initial physical therapy evaluation will lead to the formation of patient-specific rehabilitation goals and treatments and provide a baseline measurement for re-evaluation and documentation of change as a result of rehabilitation.

The nutritional evaluation should include the following:
- Weight
- Height
- Calculation of BMI
- Documentation of recent weight change

Patients with respiratory disease often have significant alterations in nutritional status and body composition. Excess weight contributes to higher energy demands and work of breathing. Patients who are underweight must have adequate nutrition and calorie intake to build strength and endurance. Poor nutritional status is a significant and independent predictor of mortality among chronic respiratory patients.[44-46]

Chest evaluation should include the following:
- Auscultation of lung and heart sounds
- Cough assessment
- Inspection of breathing pattern

Patients who demonstrate lung secretion retention or an ineffective cough may benefit from airway clearance techniques. Those who demonstrate bronchial wheezing may benefit from a trial of bronchodilator therapy. All patients with atypical use of respiratory accessory muscles at rest or with activity will benefit from instruction in breathing re-training, relaxed, and paced breathing techniques.

Musculoskeletal and integumentary evaluation should include the following:
- Joint range of motion
- Gross strength assessment of extremities and trunk
- Posture
- Gait
- Skin inspection
- Edema inspection

Patients undergoing pulmonary rehabilitation may have a multitude of joint abnormalities, pain, postural deviations, gait, and strength deficiencies—often because of inactivity.[50] Indeed, it is not unusual for this population to experience musculoskeletal anomalies due to nutritional deficits, systemic inflammation, or as a result of medication side effects.[51] Furthermore, the frequent existence of cardiac and endocrine comorbidities add to the likelihood of integumentary disorders that the physical therapist must consider when developing the treatment plan.

Functional evaluation should include the following:
- ADLs
- Balance and gait assessment
- Prior level of function
- Need for adaptive equipment
- Fall risk
- Leisure, social and family activity

Shortness of breath, muscle weakness, and poor stamina frequently lead to a diminished ability and desire to perform ADLs among respiratory disease patients. Even individuals who were previously gainfully employed and involved in community, family, and recreational activities may have to face severe limitations in mobility. Even basic self-care such as taking a shower or getting dressed may be overwhelmingly difficult. For these reasons, the physical therapist must assess the respiratory patient's ability to perform everyday tasks.

Various questionnaires and functional tests are available to evaluate occupational performance and ADLs; specifically, the Functional Independence Measure (FIM), the Assessment of Motor and Process Skills (AMPS), and a Functional Capacity Evaluation (FCE).[52] Occasionally, metabolic equivalent values (METs) may be used to gauge the endurance and performance levels of patients (1 MET = 3.5 mL $O_2$/kg/min) (Table 19-3).[34] Knowing these values will assist the therapist to determine the need for adaptive equipment and set realistic performance expectations and goals. If specific functional abnormalities are observed in conjunction with muscle weakness or gait disturbances, it may be necessary to perform additional testing such as balance and/or sit-to-stand tests.[53]

As is the case in standard physical therapy practice, following evaluation of the respiratory disease patient, the PT must synthesize the assessment findings and transition them to a reasonable treatment plan. The treatment plan should be designed to improve the patient's deficits and progress them toward their expressed goals. The physical therapist functions as the navigator, allowing the patient to move forward toward achieving success.

## Treatment Intervention

### Airway Clearance

The physiologic basis for treatment and descriptions of airway clearance techniques are reviewed in Chapter 17. The main emphasis of airway clearance in the rehabilitation setting is the removal of excessive secretions that obstruct airways, to improve cough, and decrease the incidence of respiratory infections and deterioration of lung function.[54-56] This is especially important for patients who have chronic, copious, or thick pulmonary secretions, such as those with cystic fibrosis, bronchiectasis, and chronic bronchitis.[55] Patients with severe neuromuscular weakness of the respiratory muscles may also benefit from airway clearance techniques because acute pulmonary infections often cause respiratory failure in this patient group.[56]

Following a thorough evaluation, the physical therapist should employ treatment techniques that offer the best therapeutic results and are most convenient for the patient to continue at home. It is essential to offer the patient and family a variety of treatment options to enhance compliance and encourage self-management. Treatment modifications may be necessary if the patient does not have assistance at home. Modifications that may allow for self-treatment include the following:

- Percussion and/or vibration may be necessary under certain circumstances. If assistance is not available, palm cups, or a self-administered, high-frequency chest compression system can be used.[35]

**Table 19-3 Calculation of MET and Metabolic Costs of Certain Activities**

| Intensity | MET Level | Activity |
|---|---|---|
| Very light activity | 1 MET | Resting |
| | | Eating |
| | | Writing |
| | | Knitting |
| | 2 METs | Light calisthenics |
| | | Driving (nonstressful conditions) |
| | | Light housework (sweeping, ironing, dusting) |
| | | Walking (2.2 mph) |
| Light activity | 3 METs | Self-care (washing, dressing) |
| | 4 METs | Gardening (weeding) |
| | | Ballroom dancing |
| | | Canoeing, golf |
| | | Bed-making |
| | | Woodworking (drilling, sawing) |
| | | Walking on level ground (4 mph) |
| Moderate to heavy activity | 5 METs | |
| | 6 METs | Shovelling snow |
| | | Digging vigorously |
| | | Tennis |
| | | Downhill skiing (slow) |
| | | Walking on level ground (5 mph) |
| | 7 METs | |
| | 8 METs | Cycling (13 mph) |
| | | Swimming (40+ yard/min) |
| | | Cross-country skiing (4 mph) |
| | | Running |
| | | Walking on level ground (5-6 mph) |
| Very heavy activity | 9 METs | |
| | 10+ METs | Swimming (crawl, 55 yards/min) |
| | | Downhill skiing (fast) |
| | | Walking uphill (5 mph) |

*Adapted from Woods SL. Cardiac Nursing. 5th ed. Philadelphia, Lippincott, Williams & Wilkins, 2004.*

- Postural drainage positions in conjunction with the performance of a series of deep breathing exercises, forced expirations, and coughing or use of devices that provide intermittent positive expiratory pressure are effective to mobilize secretions.[56] Breathing and coughing exercises may be done after bronchodilator treatments to remove the secretions that have accumulated overnight, or before and after each exercise session.
- Sustained exercise, if tolerated by the patient, can have very beneficial airway-clearing effects.[54,56]

Pulmonary rehabilitation should include an assessment of the patient's ability to perform treatments independently and effectively. The short-term effects or outcomes of these treatments, such as improved breath sounds, decreased atelectasis, increased tissue perfusion and oxygenation, and subjective improvements in shortness of breath, are important to monitor immediately after treatments.

Long-term benefits or outcomes of airway clearance that are monitored over the rehabilitation period may include the following[43]:

- Ability to perform physical actions, tasks, or activities related to self-management, home management, work (job/school/play), community, and leisure is improved.
- Performance of and independence in ADLs with or without devices, equipment, and assistance, are increased.
- Health status is improved.
- Cost of health care services is decreased.
- Sense of well-being is improved.

## Functional Training

Functional training is especially important for patients who have symptoms of weakness, fatigue, or dyspnea that limit activities. Essential to rehabilitation is the reversal of deconditioning to improve the patient's ability to do work.[52]

Treatment goals include the following:

- Adapting the environment to improve the ease of performing ADLs
- Altering the performance of tasks to decrease energy costs
- Incorporating methods to relieve symptoms associated with activity

## Energy Conservation

Identification of the ADLs that are most problematic for the patient is the first step to modify the environment. Once identified, the areas in the home in which these activities are performed should be evaluated for modification. Adaptations are usually necessary in the bathroom, bedroom, and kitchen. Basic concepts include the following:

- Providing work areas with supported seating of appropriate height for tasks done on a counter or table
- Placing equipment that is used most often in convenient locations so that bending, reaching, and lifting are minimized

- Locating a table or counter at work stations on which one can slide heavy items instead of lifting and carrying them
- Locating chairs at appropriate places when rests are needed, such as on the landing of stairs or beside the bathtub
- Using adaptive equipment to simplify tasks and improve comfort, for instance, a bath seat and hand-held shower head, a wheeled cart for transporting laundry or items for the dinner table, a set of grab bars or booster seats to get up from a toilet or a low chair, a wheeled walker and hospital bed if necessary
- Improving ventilation for the bathroom, kitchen, or other areas in which fumes, dust, smoke, or steam may cause respiratory symptoms

Including energy conservation techniques to modify tasks allow the patient to complete work that might otherwise be impossible. Each activity can be broken down into smaller tasks and analyzed with regard to the most energy-efficient method of work.[52] Basic concepts include the following:

- Instruct in paced breathing techniques
- Slow down the pace
- Setting priorities and organizing activities to minimize wasted movement
- Planning appropriate amounts of time to complete the task, including rest breaks

---

### Clinical tip

The basic concepts of paced breathing/activity are inhale with rest/exhale with work, slow down, set priorities, get organized, and take rest breaks along the way toward task completion. Instructions can include examples such as "Exhale during the hardest part of an activity and inhale during the rest phase"; "When you stand up from a chair, take a breath *in* before you stand, and then exhale *as* you stand"; and "Blow yourself out of the chair."

---

## Relief of Dyspnea

Simple procedures to minimize and relieve shortness of breath during ADLs can become incorporated into the functional training. Controlling the breathing pattern with paced breathing and movement, altering postures to improve respiratory muscle function, and using relaxation techniques are some key principles of treatment.[52] Bending over at the waist, from either a standing or a sitting position, should be limited because a Valsalva maneuver actually occurs, making the patient more breathless and raising the blood pressure. It is more work efficient to bring work closer; for example, when donning/doffing socks and shoes, have the patient cross their leg over the opposite leg, or place their foot onto an ottoman so that the bend is modified.

It may also be beneficial for the patient to learn dyspnea monitoring with functional training. Patients should become aware of their dyspnea level with all tasks. Instruction in methods to decrease dyspnea with activity and manage symptoms by using paced breathing and pursed-lip breathing are

**Table 19-4 Dyspnea Scale**

| Grade | | Degree |
|---|---|---|
| None | 0 | Not troubled with breathlessness except with strenuous exercise |
| Slight | 1 | Troubled by shortness of breath when hurrying on the level or walking up a slight hill |
| Moderate | 2 | Walks slower than people of the same age on the level because of breathlessness, or has to stop for breath when walking at own pace on the level |
| Severe | 3 | Stops for breath after walking about 100 yards or after a few minutes on the level |
| Very severe | 4 | Too breathless to leave the house or breathless when dressing or undressing |

Brooks SM. Surveillance for respiratory hazards. ATS News 8:12-16, 1982.

frequently helpful. Using a dyspnea scale may help make symptoms objective for evaluation (Table 19-4).[57-59]

## Breathing Re-Training

An important principle in relieving dyspnea is to avoid breath holding, Valsalva maneuver, or unnecessary talking during the task. Pursed-lip breathing is useful for patients whenever an increase in breathing effort is noticed or to facilitate a paced breathing pattern. This naturally slows down respirations and decreases minute ventilation, relieving dyspnea in some patients.[60-62] Exhalations through pursed lips during walking, lifting, pushing, or pulling activities prevents breath holding and straining. Physiologically, pursed-lip breathing decreases premature airway closure/trapping thereby decreasing residual volume (see Fig 16-7).[60]

Patients with restrictive lung disease experience greater work of breathing as a result of progressive stiffness, increased compliance, and scarring of lung tissue. At rest and more dramatically during effort, these patients may demonstrate a rapid, shallow breathing pattern and dry cough. Typically, interstitial lung disease patients have low lung volumes and reduced diffusing capacity; thus the need for increased amounts of supplemental oxygen during activity. They have difficulty pacing their breathing and often have increased accessory muscle use.[3] Breathing re-training or teaching the patient to use a specific breathing strategy is not always easy. When successfully re-trained in a new breathing pattern, the patient is likely to resume his inherent breathing pattern when attention is diverted to a task and away from breathing. This is normal behavior; the patient should still be encouraged to use daily "practice sessions" of breathing re-training using newly learned mechanics.[62]

Many patients with severe COPD have diaphragms flattened by lung hyperinflation. A leaning-forward position (see Fig. 16-4) may offer postural relief from dyspnea by improving the function of a flattened diaphragm.[35,61,63] This position increases the intraabdominal pressure and pushes the diaphragm up into the thorax and into a better position for contraction. Leaning forward with upper extremity support has the additional benefit of fixing the proximal muscle attachments of respiratory accessory muscles (e.g., pectoralis major or sternocleidomastoid) and allowing the thoracic attachments to pull the chest into inspiration. Supported leaning-forward postures, along with a comfortable, controlled breathing pattern may be used when experiencing dyspnea with activity to help relieve shortness of breath.

Relaxation techniques may decrease energy consumption and hasten relief of dyspnea. Contraction–relaxation techniques or autogenic (mental imaging) relaxation may be used for this purpose. In some cases, biofeedback may help the patient learn to relax specific muscle groups. By teaching the patient control of the relaxation response and breathing pattern, the anxiety associated with dyspnea can be reduced.

More recently, the conventional medical community has shown an increased interest in complementary and alternative therapies for a wide range of common diagnoses. There have been a few studies to look at the effect of yoga postures and breathing within the pulmonary population. By far, the majority of yoga studies have been conducted with the asthmatic population.[64] However, Behera conducted a preliminary study by instructing a small group of chronic bronchitis patients in yoga therapy consisting of 8 asans (postures) and pranayamas (breathing control) over a 4-week period. The results were a perceptible improvement in dyspnea measured by a visual analog scale and an improvement in selected lung function parameters.[65]

Three additional small studies instructed patients with COPD in asans and pranayamas with improvements, including lower dyspnea-related distress with activity, decreased breathing rate, greater breathing depth, and improved 6-minute walk test distances.[66-68]

## Oxygen Evaluation and Use

Physiologic monitoring during functional training should be employed to ensure the safety and appropriateness of exercises. Pulse oximetry, dyspnea and effort scales such as the Borg and Visual analog scales, respiratory rate, heart rate, and blood pressure are typically monitored.[58] Among lung disease patients, it is imperative that physical therapists understand the proper use of oxygen, be able to accurately monitor its use, and appreciate the logistics regarding the operation of oxygen equipment.

The APTA recognizes the role physical therapists have in the administration and adjustment of oxygen while treating various patient populations.[43] The APTA's *Guide to Physical Therapist Practice*, second edition, delineates the physical therapist's scope of practice in the management of patients who require oxygen to improve ventilation and respiration/gas exchange. The APTA is unaware of any regulations that prohibit the use of oxygen for patient management if it is prescribed and if parameters set by the physician are maintained.[69] Physicians specify oxygen flow rates in their orders, and any deviation in the prescribed dosage requires an updated order from the physician. The Food and Drug Administration of the United States Department of Health and Human Services states that "medical oxygen is defined as a prescription drug which requires a prescription in order to be dispensed except ... for emergency use."[70]

Within the APTA's Guide, supplemental oxygen is listed as a procedural intervention within the scope of physical therapist practice under Prescription, Application, and, as appropriate, Fabrication of Devices and Equipment (supportive device) to improve ventilation and respiration/gas exchange.[43] The APTA has a position statement adopted by the House of Delegates that states:

*PT patient/client management integrates an understanding of a patient's/client's prescription and nonprescription medication regimen with consideration of its impact upon health, impairments, functional limitations, and disabilities. The administration and storage of medications used for physical therapy interventions is also a component of patient/client management and thus within the scope of PT practice. Physical therapy interventions that may require the concomitant use of medications include, but are not limited to, agents that facilitate airway clearance and/or ventilation and respiration.[71]*

There are no official statements or opinions in any individual state Board of Physical Therapy regarding the administration of oxygen at this time.

A thorough knowledge of oxygen equipment is imperative for the physical therapist. Pulse oximetry is a noninvasive method of photoelectrically determining the oxyhemoglobin saturation of arterial blood.[72] A sensor is placed on a thin part of the patient's anatomy such as a fingertip or earlobe and a light containing both red and infrared wavelengths is passed through the skin to the small arteries. A microprocessor compares the signals received and calculates the degree of oxyhemoglobin saturation based on the intensity of transmitted light.[72] Larger, stationery oximetry monitors are typically used in intensive care units. Small, hand-held, portable monitors are easily clipped to the distal end of a finger or attached to the earlobe by an earlobe clip.

A variety of oxygen delivery devices may be used to administer oxygen to the patient. The most common is the nasal cannula, which can provide oxygen flows from 0.25 to 6 L/min. An Oxymizer delivery device is a nasal cannula with a reservoir incorporated into the tubing mechanism.[73] During exhalation, the reservoir fills with oxygen and is available to the patient upon the next inhalation, essentially providing equivalent saturations at lower flow rates. Manufacturers state that an oxygen savings of approximately 75% may be obtained by using the Oxymizer, and lower flow rates provide greater patient comfort.[73]

In addition, oxygen masks are used to deliver even higher concentrations of supplemental oxygen. When pulmonary patients exercise, higher percentages of oxygen are needed to meet the demand of working muscles and to maintain oxygen saturation levels within prescribed limits (usually 88% to 90%).[72] Two types of oxygen masks may be used during exercise with pulmonary patients. The venturi mask uses a mechanical opening that increases the rate at which the oxygen flows into the mask (commonly 24% to 50%). A partial rebreather mask has a reservoir bag attached and delivers between 70% and >80% of oxygen. A non-rebreather mask also incorporates a reservoir bag, but can deliver up to 100% oxygen. Flows between 7 and 10 L/min are required to keep the reservoir bag inflated at all times.[74] See Chapter 13 for pictures of oxygen devices. Less conspicuous forms of oxygen delivery are available for low to moderate oxygen flow patients. Transtracheal oxygen delivery consists of a small catheter being surgically placed into the trachea through the second and third tracheal rings. Transtracheal is well accepted by patients and delivers oxygen more efficiently than a nasal cannula. Because oxygen is delivered directly into the trachea, approximately 50% less oxygen is needed.[74] Other more aesthetically appealing methods of oxygen delivery exist such as small oxygen tubes being imbedded into eyeglass frames.[75]

Physical therapists must be well informed about the varied pathologies that may lead to the need for supplemental oxygen. A spectrum of lung, heart, and blood abnormalities warrants the use of supplemental oxygen. Accordingly, PTs should be able to choose the proper equipment for individual patients with various diagnoses by using cardiopulmonary evaluation techniques, monitoring equipment, and evidence-based practice. Oxygen flow rates may require titration depending on the level of physical activity (rest vs. exercise vs. sleep). In addition, different diagnoses, because of their pathophysiology, require lower or higher oxygen flow rates depending on the patient's activity level.

The physician normally sets the flow rate for sleep and rest, but with exercise, the PT is instrumental in determining the proper oxygen flow rate needed. The indications for supplemental oxygen use are as follows:

- Arterial partial pressure of oxygen ($PO_2$) $\leq$ to 55 mm Hg or $SpO_2 \leq 88\%$
- Arterial $PO_2 \leq 59$ mm Hg or $SpO_2 \leq 89\%$ if evidence of cor pulmonale, right heart failure, or erythrocytosis[76,77]

It is important to communicate with the physician about oxygen requirements during exercise. Specifically, it is important to request an oxygen prescription by a saturation level, for example, 88% to 90%, rather than by a specific oxygen liter flow, or fraction of inspired oxygen ($FiO_2$). To determine $FiO_2$, for every 1 L/min of oxygen, add 3% to the room air $FiO_2$ of 21%. For example: 4 L/min = ~33% $FiO_2$ (21 + 12) (Fig 19-1).[77] With this knowledge, the physician can make crucial decisions concerning the patient's medication effectiveness, dosage, stability of the disease, and surgical options.

A few basic concepts of oxygen delivery, functional ability, and biomechanics are necessary to guide the patient, physician, and oxygen vendor in meeting a patient's specific

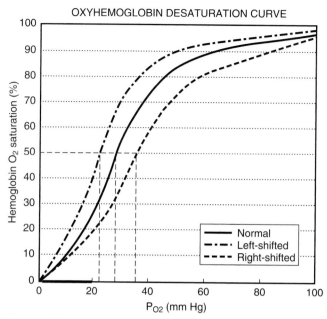

**Figure 19-1** Oxyhemoglobin saturation-desaturation curve. The normal curve for adult hemoglobin is depicted, as are examples of left-shifted (poor tissue $O_2$ unloading) and right-shifted (improved tissue $O_2$ unloading) curves. The curve is shifted to the left by alkalemia, carboxyhemoglobinemia, hypocarbia, hypothermia, methemoglobinemia, a high fetal hemoglobin content, and low 2,3-diphosphoglycerate (2,3-DPG). The curve is shifted to the right by acidemia, hypercarbia, hyperthermia, sulfhemoglobinemia, and high levels of 2,3-DPG, an end product of red cell metabolism. Note the $PO_2$ at which 50% of the $O_2$ is unloaded for each curve and the range of tissue $PO_2$ (*thick bar from 3 to 20*). (From Zaoutis LB, Chiang VW. Comprehensive Pediatric Hospital Medicine. Philadelphia, Mosby, 2007.)

equipment needs. There are essentially three types of oxygen delivery systems. First, an oxygen concentrator has the ability to deliver oxygen up to a level of 5 L/min. It is a device that separates oxygen from room air. There are stationary models, under electrical power, that are suitable to use around the house and during sleep. Different lengths of oxygen tubing are available to accommodate movement from room to room. More recently, portable oxygen concentrators have become available that allow a patient to move in and out of the house and community under battery power. These units are much smaller, sit in a small two-wheeled stroller, and are pulled along behind the patient similar to a rolling suitcase. These units are appropriate for patients on oxygen flows, at rest and with exercise, between 1 and 5 L/min. The oxygen production is only limited by the life of the portable battery charge when away from an electrical outlet.[78]

Second, compressed gas oxygen tanks are available in a range of sizes for portable use. These are also mobile on a two-wheeled stroller or in a pack that can be supported over the shoulder. More recently, these tanks are being manufactured from aluminum rather than iron or other heavy metals, which is much lighter-weight and manageable for small-frame individuals. These tanks are used with an oxygen flow

regulator that attaches to the top of the cylinder. The regulator must be manually changed to a full tank once the tank is emptied. There are two types of regulators: continuous-flow and pulsed-dose oxygen conservers. The continuous flow delivers oxygen during the full respiratory cycle (inspiration and expiration). Variations of these regulators will allow flow rates between 0.25 and 25 L/min. At a flow rate of 2 L/min, one E cylinder tank will last approximately 4 to 5 hours.[78] The oxygen conserver regulator delivers oxygen during inhalation only (demand system), or at preset intervals (pulsed system), thus saving on the amount of oxygen used over time.[79] These regulators are typically used with smaller compressed gas tanks and last various amounts of time depending on the interval and volume of oxygen puffs and the size of the tank. An E cylinder tank with an oxygen conserver regulator can last >15 hours at a flow rate of 2 L/min.[78] Depending on the pathology and the individual oxygen requirements, the PT must decide which compressed gas oxygen tank and regulator will best meet the patient's needs. Ambulatory oxygen systems are defined as those weighing less than 10 lbs. Many patients find 8.5 lbs a practical weight to carry, but smaller-framed patients may be better served with a unit in the ≤5 lb. range.[80] Biomechanical and psychomotor factors to be considered are that some patients have difficulty with the manual task of changing regulators because of weakness of the hands, joint deformities, pain, or cognitive deficits. Other patients who have osteoporosis or back pain may have difficulty lifting compressed gas tanks in and out of a car because of their weight and awkward shape. Still other patients with gait abnormalities have difficulty maneuvering tanks in strollers over curbs, steps, and through doors.[81]

A third type of oxygen delivery is a liquid-oxygen system. A large stationary tank is typically delivered to the patient's home. The patient is also provided with a portable tank that is refilled off of the stationary tank. Portable liquid tanks come in a variety of sizes and weights. The largest liquid system has the capability of a 15 L/min flow rate and can be carried either on the shoulder, in a backpack, or in a two-wheeled stroller. One of the smallest units has a maximum of 4 L/min flow rate, pulsed or continuous, and may be carried by the small handle on the unit or worn around the waist in a waist pack.[78]

For Medicare Part B patients, a Durable Medical Equipment (DME) carrier supplies supplemental oxygen. The physician must complete and sign a certificate of medical necessity (CMN) describing the patient's need for oxygen, arterial blood gases or oxygen saturation levels, prescribed flow rate, and medical diagnosis. If a specific type of portable system or flow rate is required for a patient to participate in a full range of physical activities, it must be noted on the CMN. Otherwise, because DME suppliers are reimbursed at a fixed rate, regardless of the oxygen system they provide the patient, suppliers realize a larger profit by providing less costly systems. A supplier cannot change a physician's prescription; therefore, it must be filled as written.[82]

It is not uncommon for PTs to treat a variety of patients who require supplemental oxygen, either on an inpatient or outpatient basis. It is within the physical therapy scope of practice to administer and adjust oxygen according to the physician's prescription. The physical therapist must have a thorough knowledge of oxygen equipment and how to use various devices to meet the physiological and biomechanical needs of the patient.

---

**Clinical tip**
It is within the physical therapy scope of practice to administer and adjust oxygen according to the physician's prescription. The prescription should be written based upon $SpO_2$ (e.g., keep $SpO_2 > 90$).

---

## Physical Conditioning

Activity can be described in terms of intensity, workloads, duration (minutes of continuous or intermittent work), and frequency or number of repetitions of the activity carried out. Symptoms (e.g., significant shortness of breath, fatigue, palpitations, chest discomfort) and musculoskeletal discomfort should be noted. Caution should be taken with all patients who have coexisting conditions, especially when the coexisting illness is cardiovascular disease. (See Chapter 3 for additional information.)

The physical therapist may advance functional training by the following:

- Increasing repetitions using lower weights and proper technique for strength training
- Encouraging a higher/level of work within a given time: bike, ambulation
- Encouraging fewer rest periods during task performance
- Decreasing the dependence on adaptive equipment: wheelchairs, motorized carts, ambulatory assistive devices

The ultimate goal is for the patient to be able to perform necessary functional activities with as much independence as possible, and without desaturation, or undue fatigue, and shortness of breath.

Progress in rehabilitation can be documented using a variety of measures, such as the quantity of work performed or the decrease in perceived exertion, symptoms, and heart rate during performance of the functional task. Such changes indicate that the patient is more efficient at performing the task. Improvement can also be documented by observing the patient apply the treatment concepts to new tasks or environments. As discussed earlier in the chapter, standardized timed walking tests or questionnaires that focus on functional abilities and quality of life offer outcome measures for functional training.

The goals of physical conditioning exercises are aimed at increasing cardiorespiratory endurance, maximizing work capacity, and improving strength, flexibility, and respiratory muscle function. Priorities should be set for individualized goals based on the needs and desires of the patient. It is optimal to prescribe exercises that accomplish more than one goal at a time and emphasize functional gains, such as increasing cardiorespiratory endurance for walking.

## Endurance Training

Aerobic endurance training may be performed at high or low intensity. High-intensity training (e.g., 70% to 85% of maximal work rate) must be undertaken to gain maximal physiologic improvements in aerobic fitness such as increased $VO_2max$, delayed anaerobic threshold, decreased heart rate for a given work rate, increased oxidative enzyme capacity, and capillarization of muscle.[51,83-86] High-intensity training is associated with substantial gains in exercise endurance.[83]

---

**Clinical tip**
Endurance training for the pulmonary patient should include components of frequency, duration, mode, and intensity of exercise for the upper and lower extremities.

---

Not all patients can tolerate sustained high-intensity exercise training. However, these patients, working at their maximal tolerated exercise level, will achieve gains over time.[85] Interval training, alternating periods of high and low intensity (or rest), is an effective training option for persons who cannot sustain extended continuous periods of high-intensity exercise.[87-89] This less-intense aerobic exercise training does lead to significant improvements in exercise endurance, even in the absence of measured gains in aerobic fitness.[16,90] In addition, lower-intensity training may be more readily incorporated into the patients' daily activities, although this has not been demonstrated in clinical trials.

Transcutaneous neuromuscular electrical stimulation can improve lower extremity muscle strength and exercise endurance even in the absence of traditional cardiovascular exercise training.[91-93] Although no large trials are available, this may be an option for patients with very severe diseases who are bed-bound or wheelchair-bound and are unable to participate in a conventional exercise training program.

### Frequency and Duration of Exercise
In general, the frequency and duration of the supervised exercise component during a pulmonary rehabilitation program may vary from 3 to 5 times per week,[2,11,51,83,94-97] 60 to 120 minutes per session,[2,34,97,98] and extend over a period of 4 to 72 weeks.[5,11,18,19,33,34] If program constraints will not allow for supervised exercise at least 3 days per week, one or more unsupervised sessions per week in the home with specific guidelines and instruction may be an effective alternative. If the patient is very debilitated, the duration of the initial exercise sessions can be shorter, with more frequent rest breaks; however, the ultimate goal is to achieve fewer or no rest breaks and at least 30 minutes of endurance exercise within the first few weeks of rehabilitation.

### Modes of Exercise
Many different modes of exercise training have been used successfully with pulmonary patients, including walking (e.g., treadmill, track, supported walking via walker or wheelchair),

cycling, stationary bicycling, arm ergometry, arm lifting exercises with or without weights, step exercise, rowing, water exercises, swimming, modified aerobic dance, and seated aerobics. Warm-up and cool-down periods must be included in each exercise session. Warm-up exercise allows for gradual increases in heart rate, blood pressure, ventilation, and blood flow to the exercising muscles. Cool-down reduces the risk of arrhythmias, orthostatic hypotension, and bronchospasm.

## Intensity of Exercise

Because exercise training is in many ways a tool to help patients learn to cope with the frightening and disabling sensation of breathlessness that often limits their exercise capacity, almost any type of exercise that the patient enjoys or is willing to do can be helpful. When developing the exercise prescription, the rehabilitation team must incorporate the patient's activity goals into the training plan. For example, if the patient wants to be able to walk the dog for 30 minutes each day at a relatively slow but steady pace without rest stops, the intensity of training should be designed to accomplish that goal.

The intensity of exercise should be related to time, workload, and physiological responses. The rehabilitation team may choose to have the patient work up to a selected level on the perceived exertion scale. Similarly, the team may instruct the patient to work up to a certain number on the dyspnea scale or to a predetermined MET level. A target heart rate is not always used during exercise training. It is important, however, to be aware of the patient's heart rate at rest and with exercise, keeping in mind the age-predicted maximum heart rate, the upper limits achieved on the exercise test, and other factors that influence heart rate, such as medications and deconditioning.

In exercising patients with chronic lung disease, it is important to evaluate and monitor oxyhemoglobin saturation to determine the need for supplemental oxygen and the appropriate levels to use with various activities. While attending rehabilitation, patients should be tested during the maximal intensity level exercise they may undertake at home or in the community while using the type of portable oxygen system they will use outside the program.

It is important to optimize bronchodilator and other pharmacologic therapy before and during an exercise program. This includes not only ensuring that maintenance bronchodilators are taken but also that short-acting bronchodilators are used when necessary before exercise and kept with the patients at all times.[2] Optimization of respiratory medication status allows for exercise training at higher intensities and for longer periods of time.

## Upper and Lower Extremity Training

It is most beneficial to direct exercise training to those muscles involved in functional living. This typically includes training the muscles of both the lower and upper extremities and the trunk. Exercise that improves neuromuscular ability, such as balance and coordination to decrease fall risk, are

equally important with the pulmonary population, particularly as the general population ages.[99]

Lower extremity training involves large muscle groups; this modality can improve ambulatory stamina, balance, and performance in ADLs.[83] Types of lower extremity training include the following:

- Walking
- Stationary cycling
- Bicycling
- Stair climbing
- Swimming

Exercise training of the lower extremities often results in dramatic increases in exercise tolerance of patients with COPD and other respiratory diseases.[2,3,5,11,16,18,33,50]

Exercise training of the arms is also beneficial in patients with chronic lung disease, although virtually all of the evidence comes from patients with COPD. Patients with moderate to severe COPD, especially those with mechanical disadvantage of the diaphragm due to lung hyperinflation, have difficulty performing ADLs that involve use of the upper extremities. Arm elevation is associated with high metabolic and ventilatory demand, and activities involving the arms can lead to irregular or dyssynchronous breathing. This is because some arm muscles are also accessory muscles of inspiration.[100-102]

Benefits of upper extremity training in COPD include improved arm muscle endurance and strength, reduced metabolic demand associated with arm exercise, and increased sense of well-being. In general, benefits of upper extremity training are task-specific. Because of its benefits, upper extremity training is recommended in conjunction with lower extremity training as a routine component of pulmonary rehabilitation.[2,5,100,101] Alternative types of upper extremity endurance training, other than arm ergometry, must be used in those patients with osteoporosis or under post–surgical incisional precautions (Table 19-5).[35,103]

## Strength Training

In addition to endurance training, strength training is beneficial for patients with chronic lung disease. Weight lifting may lead to improvements in muscle strength, increased exercise endurance, and fewer symptoms during ADLs.[2,5,103,104] Lower extremity strengthening may be augmented through aerobic training such as cycling, stair climbing, bench stepping, and walking. Strength training should be started with low resistance and progressed first by increasing repetitions, for example, 10 to 20 repetitions, before adding additional weight.

Upper body (trunk and upper extremity) training requires more ventilatory work, and patients are more likely to hold their breath, develop asynchronous breathing patterns, and become dyspneic. However, clinical studies have demonstrated that patients with respiratory disorders can train successfully with upper body resistive work, which produces improvements in dyspnea, fatigue, and respiratory muscle function.[2,5,18,99,100,105,106] The strengthening program should

**Table 19-5 Movement/Exercise Precautions**

| Condition | Precautions |
|---|---|
| Incisional | Perform bilateral arm movement rather than unilateral arm movement for 6 weeks |
| | Avoid driving for 6 weeks, unless physician gives permission |
| | Upper extremity lifting should be <5-10 lbs. |
| | Avoid arm ergometry for 6 weeks |
| | Avoid significant trunk twisting for 6 weeks |
| Osteoporosis | Avoid arm ergometry |
| | Avoid trunk flexion/twisting |
| | Avoid biceps weight machine for strength training (dumbbells with attention to posture is permitted) |
| Pulmonary arterial hypertension | Avoid Valsalva maneuver |
| | Avoid weight lifting >2 lbs. |
| | Avoid high workloads on stationary bicycle (increase time instead) |
| | Avoid desaturation <92% |

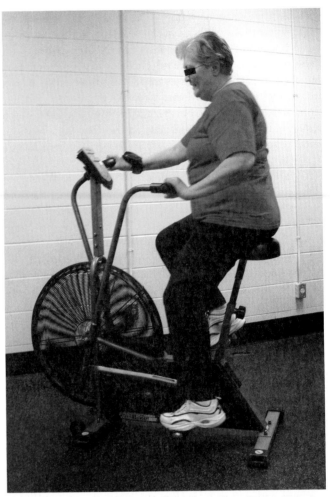

**Figure 19-2** Combined arm and leg cycling. (From Cameron MH, Monroe LG. Physical Rehabilitation: Evidence-Based Examination, Evaluation, and Intervention. St Louis, Saunders, 2008.)

start with light weights (dumbbells, pulleys, elastic bands, weighted wands) and, again, advance first by increasing the number of repetitions. For stronger patients or patients not on special exercise precautions, weight machines can be used. Rotating days between machines for upper extremity and lower extremity exercise may also improve tolerance for the strengthening program. Aerobic training modes of arm cranking and leg cycles that include arm work, rowing machines, or cross-country ski machines can also promote upper body strengthening and endurance (Fig 19-2).

> **Clinical tip**
> Evidence indicates that strength training may lead to improvements in muscle strength, increased exercise endurance, and fewer symptoms during ADLs.

During resistive work, the physical therapist should monitor the breathing pattern and pulse oximetry. If the patient has a history of hypertension, blood pressure should be intermittently monitored during weight training.[101]

The results of standardized lifting tests or dynamometry or records of the resistive loads tolerated during training are objective ways to demonstrate the outcomes of a strengthening program. Recording the increase in repetitions of an

exercise can show improvement in muscle endurance. Lastly, the measured or reported ability of the patient to carry out employment-specific, recreational, or daily activities should be documented.[103]

## Flexibility

Most patients with chronic respiratory disease have significant changes in posture and reduced mobility. These changes can be a result of inactivity or structural changes of the chest wall, with hyperinflation and hypertrophy of the accessory respiratory muscles. Flexibility exercises should be included to improve posture, increase joint range of motion, decrease stiffness, and prevent injury.

Gentle stretching with full body movements, as occurs with yoga, are appropriate for the pulmonary rehabilitation patient, especially if breathing exercises are coordinated with the movements.[53,63,107] For instance, movements that bring full shoulder flexion, back extension, and inspiration can be performed together to increase trunk flexibility and facilitate breathing. Exercises with forward-reaching and trunk flexion or with unilateral or bilateral hip and lower trunk flexion may be combined with expiration.

The purpose of combined flexibility and breathing exercises is to teach the patient how body movements can influence and assist or resist ventilation. The flexibility or mobility exercises can be used as a warm-up or cool-down activity for aerobic conditioning or at any time to relieve muscle tension or anxiety.

Monitoring changes in posture, range of motion, and subjective ratings of stiffness can be used to document the effects of a flexibility program. Long-term outcomes of the program may be documented from a reduced incidence of back pain or joint injuries.

## Respiratory Muscle Exercise

Exercises for improving respiratory muscle awareness and function are usually included in a pulmonary rehabilitation program. The increased work of breathing and chest wall changes that occur with chronic lung disease and poor breathing habits make abnormal breathing patterns more likely to occur.[108-110] Respiratory muscle dysfunction and fatigue is common and may be related to symptoms of shortness of breath. An approach for improving respiratory muscle function is to improve the performance of the respiratory muscles through exercise training.[2,5] This type of respiratory muscle training can take several forms.

First, the work of breathing is increased with most exercise or activity. Both tidal volume and respiratory rate increase during exercise, thus increasing the minute ventilation (TV $\times$ RR = $V_E$). Similarly, the respiratory muscles must increase their work to allow the minute ventilation to increase. Aerobic exercise training of the upper or lower extremities or both, that is moderate to high intensity, may be an adequate stimulus to improve respiratory muscle endurance and strength.

Second, instruction in breathing re-training exercise, such as diaphragmatic breathing, may improve the strength, awareness, and coordination of the diaphragm muscle. It is not clear which chronic lung disease patients may benefit from diaphragmatic breathing. It has been suggested that patients with COPD who have elevated respiratory rates, low tidal volumes that increase during diaphragmatic breathing, and abnormal arterial blood gases with adequate diaphragmatic movement may benefit from instruction.[61]

Last, instruction in pursed-lip breathing improves $SpO_2$ by increasing alveolar ventilation, increases tidal volume, reduces respiratory rate, slows expiratory flow, and improves $CO_2$ removal.[60] An emphysema patient often discovers this method of breathing that speeds postexertion breathlessness and accelerates recovery, on their own accord.

Training respiratory muscles with a resistive breathing device may be beneficial in patients who have decreased inspiratory muscle strength and breathlessness despite receiving optimal medical therapy. Recent studies have shown consistent improvements in inspiratory muscle function, increases

in exercise performance, and reductions in dyspnea related to ADLs. Note that when a patient stops an inspiratory muscle training (IMT) program, clinically the benefit of inspiratory muscle training stops as well, similar to when individuals stop skeletal muscle training. Therefore, inspiratory muscle training needs to be a lifelong training program, or the benefits are diminished.

Although most of the clinical studies on the efficacy of inspiratory muscle training have included only patients with COPD or quadriplegia as subjects, the treatment may be applicable to other patient groups in whom respiratory muscle weakness or fatigability is demonstrated: those who have neuromuscular syndromes, those who have been on mechanical ventilation for extended time periods, those with thoracic wall deformities such as kyphoscoliosis, and those who are morbidly obese. Even though more recent studies provide further support for the efficacy of inspiratory muscle training, the ACCP/AACVPR guidelines do not support the routine use of IMT as an essential component of pulmonary rehabilitation.[5]

Outcomes of respiratory muscle training can be documented by recording increases in the training resistance and maximal inspiratory pressures. Reported improvements in dyspnea and the ability to carry out ADLs are also potential outcomes of respiratory muscle training

## Exercise Considerations for Different Stages of Lung Diseases

Because exercise performance varies with the severity of disease, a discussion of the patient with mild, moderate, and severe respiratory disease is presented. Several classifications for describing clinical status are available, most of which use a combination of pulmonary function tests, symptoms, and exercise tolerance.[49,103,104]

One of the best resources for identifying the stages of obstructive lung disease is the Global Initiative for Chronic Obstructive Lung Disease (or GOLD) guidelines. These guidelines were updated in 2008 and were created to increase awareness of COPD among health professionals, public health authorities, and the general public and to improve prevention and management of COPD.[4]

### Patients with Mild Lung Disease

Spirometry testing of the patient with mild disease shows values $\geq$80% of predicted values for forced expiratory volume in 1 second ($FEV_1$). Ventilatory responses to exercise are normal, with sufficient ventilatory reserves during maximum effort. Arterial blood gas values are normal or have slight reductions in arterial oxygen levels.

Patients with mild lung disease usually have shortness of breath only with relatively heavy exercise, such as climbing hills and stairs, but may be asymptomatic with usual daily activities. Because respiratory symptoms are very mild, they do not often present to the physician for treatment of lung disease. The only indicating signs of mild disease may be symptoms with extreme effort, a chronic cough or sputum production, or a history of smoking or occupational exposure. Identifying the presence of lung disease at this early stage may be possible through routine employment screenings and annual physical examinations.

Exercise for patients with mild disease can be recommended using testing and training protocols that would be used for a normal population. Pulmonary rehabilitation is usually not recommended for this stage of obstructive lung disease.[4] Because exercise intensities associated with physiologic conditioning of the aerobic system are easily attainable, the patient should do very well on an independent training program following consultation with the physical therapist.

## Patients with Moderate Lung Disease

The patient with moderate lung disease has an $FEV_1$ <80% of predicted values and an exercise tolerance that is limited by ventilation.[4] That is, the ventilatory reserves are exhausted at peak exercise loads. The patient becomes short of breath with usual ADLs and with a moderate to fast walking pace (approximately 3 to 4 METs). Mild to moderate hypoxemia may be present at rest and may either improve or worsen with exercise.

Patients with moderate lung disease may present with an acute exacerbation of their disease or worsening symptoms of shortness of breath with normal daily activities. These patients may describe a pattern of restricting or modifying their activity level to prevent respiratory symptoms. Still, they may attribute their symptoms to normal aging, to being out of shape or overweight, or to a smoking habit. Many believe that their symptoms could be resolved with simple changes in lifestyle.

An episode of acute pneumonia or pulmonary complications following an elective surgery may be the time the patient is identified with moderate lung disease and treatment initiated.[4] Rehabilitation at this stage of the disease can modify risk factors and decrease the likelihood of future pulmonary complications.

Exercise tolerance assessments for patients with moderate lung disease can be performed using progressive exercise protocols. An electrocardiogram (ECG) should be taken and the blood pressure, heart rate, and pulse oximetry should be monitored continuously during the test. Alternatively, a functional 6-minute walking test with vital sign measurement can be used.[7,35,40,43,50] (See Chapter 16 for more information on assessment.)

The aim of the exercise prescription is to increase the duration of a workload that is sufficient to cause physiologic adaptation to effort. An initial training workload can be estimated from the data gathered during the Graded Exercise Test (GXT). Supplemental oxygen may be needed to maintain $SpO_2$ levels ≥88%. The patient should first work to maintain this work level for 20 to 30 minutes. Intermittent short bouts of slightly higher workloads can then be introduced through interval training. As rating of perceived exertion (RPE) and HRs go down and exercise time is maintained at a satisfactory work level without rest breaks, workloads can be gradually advanced by the therapist.

The patient should exercise at least three to seven times per week. The total dosage of the exercise stimulus will bring about modest increases in the symptom-limited maximum $O_2$ and a decrease in the heart rate and minute ventilation response during submaximum workloads.[2,5,11,16]

If the patient demonstrates arterial desaturation by pulse oximetry during exercise, supplemental oxygen will improve performance.[111] It is unlikely that the majority of patients who require supplemental oxygen during exercise will be able to discontinue its' use due to physiological and anatomical lung tissue alterations.

## Patients with Severe Lung Disease

Patients with severe lung disease may be restricted by symptoms of shortness of breath during most daily activities. Even walking at a slow pace may be limited. With spirometric testing, patients with severe lung disease demonstrate an $FEV_1$ below 50% of predicted values. The patient may require intermittent or continuous oxygen at rest and with activity and may have elevated arterial carbon dioxide levels, for example, carbon dioxide ($CO_2$) retainer. Some patients with severe disease show signs of right ventricular dysfunction during exercise, which is related to oxygen desaturation. This may improve with supplemental oxygen during exercise.[2,111]

In some cases, patients with severe lung disease require a modified approach to exercise testing. Lower workloads and interval training will facilitate improved tolerance to longer bouts of endurance exercise. A 6-minute walk test should be utilized as part of the evaluation process to determine functional levels and exercise tolerance. Monitoring the patient closely for desaturation and exercise-induced arrhythmias is important during testing procedures. Supplemental oxygen dosages that maintain a saturation level higher than 88% should be identified and prescribed for patients who reach desaturation levels during exercise.[76,77]

The exercise prescription for patients with severe lung disease should be based on the exercise test. Interval training programs may be best to use with initially short exercise bouts and rests. The prescription may be advanced gradually by increasing the number of bouts, lengthening the bouts, or decreasing the length of the rest periods. Because the initial training prescription (intensity and duration) is low, the patient should exercise a minimum of one time per day. As the total exercise duration increases to 20 minutes continuously, the frequency may be reduced to five to seven times per week. Even very small gains in exercise tolerance for the patient with severe lung disease can be significant for functional improvements and quality of life.[16-18]

Patients in each lung disease category must be monitored using pulse oximetry, dyspnea and exertion scales, and heart rate with intermittent determinations of resting and exercise blood pressure. All patients should gradually require less supervision and monitoring as rehabilitation goals are met, and the patient develops independence in self-regulation and monitoring of the exercise intensity, duration, and frequency. When this occurs, the patient is ready for discharge from supervised therapy to an independent exercise regime.

**CASE STUDY 19-1**

For a detailed case study examining the pre- and postoperative pulmonary rehabilitation for a COPD patient undergoing lung transplantation, please see Evolve.

## Summary

- "Pulmonary rehabilitation is an evidence-based, multidisciplinary, and comprehensive intervention for patients with chronic respiratory diseases who are symptomatic and often have decreased daily life activities. Integrated into the individualized treatment of the patient, pulmonary rehabilitation is designed to reduce symptoms, optimize functional status, increase participation, and reduce health care costs through stabilizing or reversing systemic manifestations of the disease."

- Rehabilitation research now emphasizes symptom improvement, functional and exercise gains, and health-related quality-of-life outcomes as measures of efficacy instead of changes in pulmonary physiologic parameters.

- Three essential areas that require outcome measurements in pulmonary rehabilitation include exercise capacity, symptoms (dyspnea and fatigue), and health-related quality of life.

- A comprehensive pulmonary rehabilitation program should incorporate the following components: patient assessment and goal-setting, exercise and functional training, self-management education, nutritional intervention, and psychosocial management.

- Many patients with chronic respiratory disease simultaneously suffer from musculoskeletal abnormalities, for instance, pulmonary diagnoses of restrictive lung disease (e.g., scleroderma, pulmonary fibrosis due to unspecified connective tissue disease, rheumatoid arthritis, spinal cord injury, and scoliosis).

- The chronic respiratory disease patient should be able to recognize an early acute exacerbation of his or her disease; when and how to initiate or increase specific therapy such as antibiotics, steroids, and bronchodilators; and when to contact their health care provider.

- Patients with respiratory disease frequently have alterations of their nutritional status and body mass index (BMI).

- A psychosocial assessment should address motivational level, emotional distress, family and home environment, substance abuse, cognitive impairment, conflict and/or abuse, coping strategies, sexual dysfunction, and neuropsychological impairments (e.g., memory, attention, concentration).

- The basic components of pulmonary rehabilitation, may, however, be applied to a variety of chronic disease patients such as those with restrictive lung disease, pulmonary hypertension, significant musculoskeletal disease (e.g., arthritis), heart failure, and other stable cardiovascular diseases (e.g., peripheral vascular disease and stroke).

- Most patients are referred and seek rehabilitation as a result of disabling symptoms of dyspnea, inability to perform everyday household activities such as dressing and climbing steps, or a decreased ability to perform job responsibilities.

- Patients with respiratory disease often have significant alterations in nutritional status and body composition. Excess weight contributes to higher energy demands and work of breathing. Patients who are underweight must have adequate nutrition and calorie intake to build strength and endurance. Poor nutritional status is a significant and independent predictor of mortality among chronic respiratory patients.

- Patients undergoing pulmonary rehabilitation may have a multitude of joint abnormalities, pain, postural deviations, gait, and strength deficiencies—often due to inactivity.

- The main emphasis of airway clearance in the rehabilitation setting is the removal of excessive secretions that obstruct airways, improve cough, and decrease the incidence of respiratory infections and deterioration of lung function.

- Including energy conservation techniques to modify tasks allow the patient to complete work that might otherwise be impossible. Each activity can be broken down into smaller tasks and analyzed with regard to the most energy-efficient method of work.

- Simple procedures to minimize and relieve shortness of breath during activities of daily living can become incorporated into the functional training. Controlling the breathing pattern with paced breathing and movement, altering postures to improve respiratory muscle function, and using relaxation techniques are some key principles of treatment.

- Patients with restrictive lung disease experience greater work of breathing due to progressive stiffness, increased compliance, and scarring of lung tissue.

- A variety of oxygen delivery devices may be used to administer oxygen to the patient. The most common is the nasal cannula, which can provide oxygen flows from 0.25 to 6 L/minute.

- The Oxymizer delivery device is a nasal cannula with a reservoir incorporated into the tubing mechanism.

- It is important to request an oxygen prescription by a saturation level, for example, 88% to 90%, rather than by a specific oxygen liter flow, or, fraction of inspired oxygen ($FiO_2$).

- Endurance training for the pulmonary patient should include components of frequency, duration, mode, and intensity of exercise for the upper and lower extremities.

- Evidence indicates that strength training may lead to improvements in muscle strength, increased exercise endurance, and fewer symptoms during ADLs.

- Training respiratory muscles with a resistive breathing device may be beneficial in patients who have decreased inspiratory muscle strength and breathlessness despite receiving optimal medical therapy.

## References

1. American Thoracic Society. Pulmonary rehabilitation: Official American Thoracic Society position statement. Am Rev Respir Dis 124:663–16; 1981.

2. Nici L, Donner C, Wouters E, et al. American Thoracic Society/European Respiratory Society statement on pulmonary rehabilitation. Am J Respir Crit Care Med 173:1390–413, 2006.

3. Disease-specific approaches in pulmonary rehabilitation. In Crouch R, ZuWallack R (eds.): American Association of Cardiovascular and Pulmonary Rehabilitation: Guidelines for Pulmonary Rehabilitation Programs. 3rd ed. Champaign, IL, Human Kinetics, 2004:67–92.

4. Global Initiative for Chronic Obstructive Lung Disease. Global strategy for the diagnosis, management, and prevention of chronic obstructive pulmonary disease: GOLD executive summary. www.goldcopd.com.

5. Ries AL, Bauldoff GS, Carlin BW, et al. Pulmonary rehabilitation: Joint ACCP/AACVPR evidence-based clinical practice guidelines. Chest 131:4–42, 2007.

6. Harken DE, Carter BN, DeBakey ME. Reconditioning and rehabilitation. In U.S. Army Medical Department, Office of Medical History.

7. Crouch R, Ryan K. Physical therapy and respiratory care: Integration as a team in pulmonary rehabilitation. In Hodgkin JE, Celli BR, Connors GL (eds.): Pulmonary Rehabilitation: Guidelines to Success. 3rd ed. Philadelphia, Lippincott Williams & Wilkins, 2000:173–211.

8. American Physical Therapy Association. Cardiovascular and pulmonary section. http://www.cardiopt.org/about.cfm.

9. Duke University Department of Physical and Occupational Therapy. Cardiovascular and pulmonary residency. http://ptot.duhs.duke.edu/modules/ptot_residencies.

10. American Physical Therapy Association. Credentialed clinical residency and fellowship programs. http://www.apta.org/AM/Template.cfm.

11. Ries AL, Make BJ, Lee SM, et al. The effects of pulmonary rehabilitation in the National Emphysema Treatment Trial. Chest 128(6):3799–809, 2005.

12. Guell R, Casan P, Belda J, et al. Long-term effects of outpatient rehabilitation of COPD: A randomized trial. Chest 117:976–83, 2000.

13. Man WD, Polkey MI, Donaldson N, et al. Community pulmonary rehabilitation after hospitalization for acute exacerbations of chronic obstructive pulmonary disease: Randomised controlled study. BMJ 329:1209, 2004.

14. Griffiths TL, Burr ML, Campbell IA, et al. Results at 1 year of outpatient multidisciplinary pulmonary rehabilitation: A randomized controlled trial. Lancet 355:362–8, 2000.

15. Salman GF, Mosier MC, Beasley BW, et al. Rehabilitation for patients with chronic obstructive pulmonary disease: Meta-analysis of randomized controlled trials. J Gen Intern Med 18(3):213–21, 2003.

16. Ries AL, Kaplan RM, Limberg TM, et al. Effects of pulmonary rehabilitation on physiologic and psychosocial outcomes in patients with chronic obstructive pulmonary disease. Ann Intern Med 122(11):823–32, 1995.

17. Strijbos JH, Postma DS, van Altena R, et al. A comparison between an outpatient hospital-based pulmonary rehabilitation program and a home-care pulmonary rehabilitation program in patients with COPD: A follow-up of 18 months. Chest 109:366–72, 1996.

18. Lacasse Y, Martin S, Lasserson TJ, et al. Meta-analysis of respiratory rehabilitation in chronic obstructive pulmonary disease: A Cochrane systematic review. Eura Medicophys 43:475–85, 2007.

19. Plankeel JF, McMullen B, MacIntyre NR. Exercise outcomes after pulmonary rehabilitation depend on the initial mechanism of exercise limitation among non-oxygen-dependent COPD patients. Chest 127:110–16, 2005.

20. ZuWallack RL, Haggerty MC. Clinically meaningful outcomes in patients with chronic obstructive pulmonary disease. Am J Med 117(12A):49S–59S, 2004.

21. Hirayama F, Lee AH, Binns CW, et al. Physical activity of patients with chronic obstructive pulmonary disease: Implications for pulmonary rehabilitation. J Cardiopulm Rehabil Prev 28:330–4, 2008.

22. American Thoracic Society. ATS statement: Guidelines for the six-minute walk test. Am J Respir Crit Care Med 166:111–17, 2002.

23. Spencer LM, Alison JA, McKeough ZJ. Six-minute walk test as an outcome measure: Are two six-minute walk tests necessary immediately after pulmonary rehabilitation and at three-month follow-up? Am J Phys Med Rehabil 87(3):224–8, 2007.

24. Enright PL. The six-minute walk test. Respir Care 48(8):783–5, 2003.

25. Sciurba F, Criner GJ, Lee SM, et al. Six-minute walk distance in chronic obstructive pulmonary disease: Reproducibility and effect of walking course layout and length. Am J Respir Crit Care Med 167:1522–7, 2003.

26. Six-minute walk test. Pulmonary rehabilitation tool kit. Available at: http://www.pulmonaryrehab.com.au.

27. Redelmeier DA, Bayoumi AM, Goldstein RS, et al. Interpreting small differences in functional status: The six-minute walk test in chronic lung disease patients. Am J Respir Crit Care Med 155:1278–82, 1997.

28. Puhan M, Mador MJ, Held U, et al. Interpretation of treatment changes in 6-minute walk distance in patients with COPD. Eur Respir J 32:637–43, 2008.

29. Revill SM, Morgan MDL, Singh SJ, et al. The endurance shuttle walk: A new field test for the assessment of endurance capacity in chronic obstructive pulmonary disease. Thorax 54:213–22, 1999.

30. Eaton T, Young P, Nicol K, et al. The endurance shuttle walking test: A responsive measure in pulmonary rehabilitation for COPD Patients. Chron Respir Dis 3(1):3–9, 2006.

31. Singh SJ, Morgan MDL, Hardman AE, et al. Comparison of oxygen uptake during a conventional treadmill test and the shuttle walking test in chronic airflow limitation. Eur Respir J 7:2016–20, 1994.

32. Win T, Jackson A, Groves AM, et al. Relationship of shuttle walk test and lung cancer surgical outcome. Eur J Cardio-Thoracic Surg 26:1216–19, 2004.

33. Bailey SP, Brown L, Bailey EK. Lack of relationship between functional and perceived quality of life outcomes following pulmonary rehabilitation. Cardiopulm Phys Ther J 19(1):3–10, 2008.

34. ACSM's Guidelines for Exercise Testing and Prescription. 8th ed. Philadelphia: Wolters Kluwer/Lippincott Williams & Wilkins, 2010.

35. Crouch R. Physical and respiratory therapy for the medical and surgical patient. In Hodgkin JE, Celli BR, Connors GL (eds.): Pulmonary Rehabilitation: Guidelines to Success. 4th ed. St. Louis: Mosby/Elsevier, 2009:154–79.

36. Emery C, Hauck E, Schein R, et al. Psychological and cognitive outcomes of a randomized trial of exercise among patients with COPD. Health Psychol 17:232–40, 1998.

37. Steele BG, Belza B, Cain KC, et al. A randomized clinical trial of an activity and exercise adherence intervention in chronic pulmonary disease. Arch Phys Med Rehabil 89:404–12, 2008.

38. Bourbeau J, Julien M, Maltais F, et al. Reduction of hospital utilization in patients with chronic obstructive pulmonary disease: A disease-specific self management intervention. Arch Intern Med 163:585–91, 2003.

39. Paz-Diaz H, Montes de Oca M, Lopez JM, et al. Pulmonary rehabilitation improves depression, anxiety, dyspnea and health status in patients with COPD. Am J Phys Med Rehabil 86:30–6, 2007.

40. Crouch R, ZuWallack R (eds.). American Association of Cardiovascular and Pulmonary Rehabilitation: Guidelines for Pulmonary Rehabilitation Programs. 3rd ed. Champaign, IL, Human Kinetics, 2004.

41. Herridge MS, Cheung AM, Tansey CM, et al. One-year outcomes in survivors of the acute respiratory distress syndrome. N Engl J Med 348:683–93, 2003.

42. Bailey P, Thomsen GE, Spuhler VJ, et al. Early activity is feasible and safe in respiratory failure patients. Crit Care Med 35:139–45, 2007.

43. American Physical Therapy Association: Guide to Physical Therapist Practice. 2nd ed. Alexandria, VA: APTA, 2003.

44. Nazir SA, Erbland ML. Chronic obstructive pulmonary disease: An update on diagnosis and management issues in older adults. Drugs Aging 26:813–31, 2009.

45. Weekes CE, Emery PW, Elia M. Dietary counseling and food fortification in stable COPD: A randomised trial. Thorax 64:326–31, 2009.

46. Clini EM, Ambrosino N. Nonpharmacological treatment and relief of symptoms in COPD. Eur Respir J 32:218–28, 2008.

47. American College of Sports Medicine (ed.). Pathophysiology and treatment of pulmonary disease. In ACSM's Resource Manual for Guidelines for Exercise Testing and Prescription. 6th ed. Philadelphia: Wolters Kluwer/Lippincott Williams & Wilkins, 2010:119–38.

48. Goodman CC, Snyder TK. Screening for endocrine and metabolic disease. In Differential Diagnosis for Physical Therapists: Screening for Referral. St. Louis, Saunders, 2007.

49. American Physical Therapy Association, Cardiovascular and Pulmonary Section. Reimbursement update July 21, 2009. www.cardiopt.org.

50. Troosters T, Gosselink R, Langer D, et al. Pulmonary rehabilitation in chronic obstructive pulmonary disease. Respir Med: COPD Update 3(2):57–64, 2007.

51. Vogiatzis I, Terzis G, Nanas S, et al. Skeletal muscle adaptations to interval training in patients with advanced COPD. Chest 128:3838–45, 2005.

52. Coppola S, Wood W. Occupational therapy to promote function and health-related quality of life. In Hodgkin JE, Celli BR, Connors GL (eds.): Pulmonary Rehabilitation: Guidelines to Success. 4th ed. St. Louis, Mosby, 2009.

53. Hillegass EA, Temes WC. Therapeutic interventions in cardiac rehabilitation and prevention. In Essentials of Cardiopulmonary Physical Therapy. 2nd ed. Philadelphia, W. B. Saunders, 2001:676–726.

54. Lee A, Button B, Denehy L. Current Australian and New Zealand physiotherapy practice in the management of patients with bronchiectasis and chronic obstructive pulmonary disease. NZ J Physiother 36:49–58, 2008.

55. Gibson RL, Burns JL, Ramsey BW. State of the art. Pathophysiology and management of pulmonary infections in cystic fibrosis. Am J Respir Crit Care Med 168:918–51, 2003.

56. Langer D, Hendriks EJM, Burtin C, et al. A clinical practice guideline for physiotherapists treating patients with chronic obstructive pulmonary disease based on a systematic review of available evidence. Clin Rehabil 23:445–62, 2009.

57. Borg GAV. Psychophysical bases of perceived exertion. Med Sci Sports Exer 14:377–81, 1982.

58. Mahler DA, Horowitz MB. Perception of breathlessness during exercise in patients with respiratory disease. Med Sci Sports Exer 26:1078–81, 1994.

59. Horowitz MB, Littenberg B, Mahler DA. Dyspnea ratings for prescribing exercise intensity in patients with COPD. Chest 109:1169–75, 1996.

60. Tiep BL. Pursed lips breathing—Easing does it. J Cardiopulm Rehabil Prev 27:245–6, 2007.

61. Cahalin LP, Braga M, Matsuo Y, et al. Efficacy of diaphragmatic breathing in persons with chronic obstructive pulmonary disease: A review of the literature. J Cardiopulm Rehabil 22:7–21, 2002.

62. Nield MA, Soo Hoo GW, Roper JM, et al. Efficacy of pursed-lip breathing: A breathing pattern retraining strategy for dyspnea reduction. J Cardiopulm Rehabil Prev 27:237–44, 2007.

63. Dias CS, Kirkwood RN, Parreira VF, et al. Orientation and position of the scapula, head and kyphosis thoracic in male patients with COPD. Can J Respir Ther 45:30–4, 2009.

64. Raub JA. Psychophysiologic effects of hatha yoga on musculoskeletal and cardiopulmonary function: A literature review. J Altern Complement Med 8:797–812, 2002.

65. Behera D. Yoga therapy in chronic bronchitis. J Assoc Physicians India 46:207–8, 1998.

66. Donesky-Cuenco D, Nguyen HQ, Paul S, et al. Yoga therapy decreases dyspnea-related distress and improves functional performance in people with chronic obstructive pulmonary disease: A pilot study. J Altern Complement Med 15:225–34, 2009.

67. Tandon MK. Adjunct treatment with yoga in chronic severe airways obstruction. Thorax 33:514–7, 1978.

68. Pomidori L, Campigotto F, Amatya TM, et al. Efficacy and tolerability of yoga breathing in patients with chronic obstructive pulmonary disease: A pilot study. J Cardiopulm Rehabil Prev 29(2):133–7, 2009.

69. American Physical Therapy Association. Oxygen administration during physical therapy. www.apta.org.

70. Human drug CGMP Notes. 4(4), December 1996. www.fda.gov.

71. Pharmacology in physical therapist practice. HOD P06-04-14-14 (Program 32). www.apta.org.

72. Sadowsky HS. Pulmonary diagnostic tests and procedures. In Hillegass EA, Sadowsky HS (eds.): Essentials of Cardiopulmonary Physical Therapy. 2nd ed. Philadelphia, W. B. Saunders, 2001:421–49.

73. Oxymizer disposable oxygen-conserving devices. www.chadtherapeutics.com.

74. Frownfelter D, Baskin MW. Respiratory care practice review. In Frownfelter D, Dean E (eds.): Cardiovascular and Pulmonary Physical Therapy: Evidence and Practice. 4th ed. St. Louis, Mosby, 2006:759–71.

658 SECTION 6 Cardiopulmonary Assessment and Intervention

75. Hoffman LA, Wesmiller SW. Home oxygen: Transtracheal and other options. Am J Nurs (JSTOR) 88(4):464–9, 1988.

76. Medical Research Council Working Party. Long term domiciliary oxygen therapy in chronic hypoxic cor pulmonale complicating chronic bronchitis and emphysema. Lancet 1:681–6, 1981.

77. Calculating $FiO_2$. http://forums.studentdoctor.net.

78. Petty TL. Guide to prescribing home oxygen: Types of home oxygen systems. National Lung Health Education Program (NLHEP). www.nlhep.org.

79. NLHEP. Conserving device technology. www.nlhep.org.

80. NLHEP. Keys to successful treatment. www.nlhep.org.

81. NLHEP. Patient considerations in selecting equipment. www.nlhep.org.

82. NLHEP. Costs and reimbursement. www.nlhep.org.

83. Gimenez M, Servera E, Vergara P, et al. Endurance training in patients with chronic obstructive pulmonary disease: A comparison of high versus moderate intensity. Arch Phys Med Rehabil 81:102–9, 2000.

84. Maltais F, LeBlanc P, Jobin J, et al. Intensity of training and physiologic adaptation in patient with chronic obstructive pulmonary disease. Am J Respir Crit Care Med 155:555–61, 1997.

85. Casaburi R, Patessio A, Ioli F, et al. Reductions in exercise lactic acidosis and ventilation as a result of exercise training in patients with obstructive lung disease. Am Rev Respir Dis 143:9–18, 1991.

86. Vogiatzis I, Nanas S, Roussos C. Interval training as an alternative modality to continuous exercise in patients with COPD. Eur Respir J 15:517–25, 2002.

87. Coppoolse R, Schols AM, Baarends EM, et al. Interval versus continuous training in patients with severe COPD: A randomized clinical trial. Eur Respir J 14:258–63, 1999.

88. American Thoracic Society Committee on Pulmonary Function Standards. Guidelines for methacholine and exercise challenge testing—1999. Am J Resp Crit Care Med 161:309–29, 2000.

89. Datta D, ZuWallack R. High versus low intensity exercise training in pulmonary rehabilitation: Is more better? Chron Respir Dis 1:143–9, 2004.

90. Neder JA, Sword D, Ward SA, et al. Home based neuromuscular electrical stimulation as a new rehabilitative strategy for severely disabled patients with chronic obstructive pulmonary disease (COPD). Thorax 57:333–7, 2002.

91. Sillen MJ, Speksnijder CM, Eterman RM, et al. Effects of neuromuscular electrical stimulation of muscles of ambulation in patients with chronic heart failure or COPD: A systematic review of the English-language literature. Chest 136:44–61, 2009.

92. Vivodtzev I, Lacasse Y, Maltais F. Neuromuscular electrical stimulation of the lower limbs in patients with chronic obstructive pulmonary disease. J Cardiopulm Rehabil Prev 28:79–91, 2008.

93. Ringbaek TJ, Broendum E, Hemmingsen L, et al. Rehabilitation of patients with chronic obstructive pulmonary disease: Exercise twice a week is not sufficient! Respir Med 94:150–4, 2000.

94. Puente-Maestu L, Sanz ML, Sanz P, et al. Comparison of effects of supervised versus self-monitored training programs in patients with chronic obstructive pulmonary disease. Eur Respir J 15:517–25, 2000.

95. Exercise Prescription in Patients with Pulmonary Disease. In Ehrman JK (ed.): ACSM's Resource Manual for Guidelines for Exercise Testing and Prescription. 6th ed. Philadelphia, Wolters Kluwer/Lippincott Williams & Wilkins, 2009: 575–99.

96. Endurance Training. Pulmonary rehabilitation tool kit. www.pulmonaryrehab.com.au.

97. Hassanein SE, Narsavage GL. The dose effect of pulmonary rehabilitation on physical activity, perceived exertion, and quality of life. J Cardiopulm Rehabil Prev 29:255–60, 2009.

98. Falls among older adults: An overview. Centers for Disease Control and Prevention. http://www.cdc.gov/Homeand RecreationalSafety/Falls/adultfalls.html.

99. Holland AE, Hill CJ, Nehez E, et al. Does unsupported upper limb exercise training improve symptoms and quality of life for patients with chronic obstructive pulmonary disease? J Cardiopulm Rehabil 24:422–7, 2004.

100. Costi S, Crisafulli E, Antoni FD, et al. Effects of unsupported upper extremity exercise training in patients with COPD: A randomized clinical trial. Chest 136:387–95, 2009.

101. Porto EF, Castro AA, Velloso M, et al. Exercises using the upper limbs hyperinflate COPD patients more than exercises using the lower limbs at the same metabolic demand. Monaldi Arch Chest Dis 71:21–6, 2009.

102. Biskobing DM. COPD and osteoporosis. Chest 12:609–20, 2002.

103. O'Shea SD, Taylor NF, Paratz JD. Progressive resistance exercise improves muscle strength and may improve elements of performance of daily activities for people with COPD: A systematic review. Chest 136:1269–83, 2009.

104. Houchen L, Steiner MC, Singh SJ. How sustainable is strength training in chronic obstructive pulmonary disease? Physiotherapy 95:1–7, 2009.

105. Spruit MA, Wouters EFM. New modalities of pulmonary rehabilitation in patients with chronic obstructive pulmonary disease. Sports Med 37(6):501–18, 2007.

106. Serres I, Gautier V, Varray A, et al. Impaired skeletal muscle endurance related to physical inactivity and altered lung function in COPD patients. Chest 113:900–5, 1998.

107. Greendale GA, Huang M, Karlamangla AS, et al. Yoga decreases kyphosis in senior women and men with adult-onset hyperkyphosis: Results of a randomized controlled trial. J Am Geriatr Soc 57:1569–79, 2009.

108. Reid DC, Bowden J, Lynne-Davies P. Role of selected muscles of respiration as influenced by posture and tidal volume. Chest 70:636–40, 1976.

109. Weiner P, Magadle R, Beckerman M, et al. Maintenance of inspiratory muscle training in COPD patients: One year follow-up. Eur Respir J 23:61–5, 2004.

110. Geddes EL, O'Brien K, Reid WD, et al. Inspiratory muscle training in adults with chronic obstructive pulmonary disease: An update of a systematic review. Respir Med 102:1715–29, 2008.

111. Nici L, Raskin J, Rochester CL, et al. Pulmonary rehabilitation: What we know and what we need to know. J Cardiopulm Rehabil Prev 29:141–51, 2009.

## CHAPTER 20

# Pediatric Cardiopulmonary Physical Therapy

*Jennifer Edelschick, Debra Seal*

## Chapter Outline

This chapter presents a basic review of cardiopulmonary development, as well as application of interventions in all treatment settings, from the special care nursery to the outpatient pediatric clinic. Knowledge of the development of the cardiovascular and pulmonary systems is essential to the understanding of the physical therapist's role in the treatment of the pediatric patient. As a detailed embryologic review is beyond the scope of this chapter, please refer to other texts such as Moore, *The Developing Human*, or Beachey, *Respiratory Care Anatomy and Physiology*.

## Respiratory System Development

Development of the respiratory system begins during the fourth week of gestation (Fig. 20-1).[1] At approximately 28 days' gestation, an outgrowth develops from the primordial pharynx called the *laryngotracheal groove*. The endodermal tissue lining of the laryngotracheal groove gives rise to the epithelium and glands of the trachea, larynx, bronchi, and pulmonary epithelium.[2] The laryngotracheal groove then gives rise to the lung bud (aka respiratory diverticulum) through invagination. The lung bud differentiates into two bronchial buds, which give rise to the bronchi and lungs. The maturation of the lungs can be divided into four periods: pseudoglandular period (weeks 6 to 16), canalicular period (weeks 16 to 26), terminal saccular period (week 26 to birth), and alveolar period (32 weeks to 8 years).[2] The lung buds grow and subdivide into smaller airways during weeks 5 through 16. All the major elements of the lung have formed during this pseudoglandular period except the elements involved with gas exchange. The diaphragm also begins to form by the end of the pseudoglandular period. It should be noted that a fetus who is born during this period cannot survive.

A critical event occurs during weeks 16 through 26 (canalicular period), which is the appearance of pulmonary

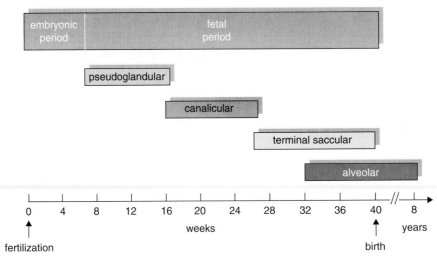

**Figure 20-1** The major phases of respiratory development. (From Wilkins RL, Stoller JK, Kacmarek RM. Egan's Fundamentals of Respiratory Care. 9th ed. St. Louis, Mosby, 2009.)

capillaries. Terminal bronchioles give rise to respiratory bronchioles, which, in turn, give rise to alveolar ducts. Some *terminal saccules* develop at the ends of the respiratory bronchioles. Lung tissue becomes vascularized, making it possible for a fetus born at the end of this period to survive as gas exchange can now take place. In the terminal saccular period, more terminal saccules develop. These cells become lined by type I alveolar cells, which is where gas exchange occurs.

Surfactant, which is a complex mixture of phospholipids, forms over the internal walls of the terminal saccules. It is secreted by type II alveolar cells, and it aids respiration by decreasing the surface tension within the alveolus. Surfactant production increases during the terminal stages of pregnancy, notably the final 2 weeks.[2] Although surfactant production begins around 20 weeks' gestation, it does not reach a mature level to allow maintenance of continuous respiration until approximately 34 weeks' gestation. After birth, the surface area and the volume of lung tissue for gas exchange grow rapidly as a result of multiplication of alveoli and capillaries. The alveolar period is marked by the increase in alveoli to their adult number. Approximately 95% of mature alveoli develop after birth. Between the time of birth and the eighth year of life, the alveoli increase from 50 million to 300 million.[2]

---

**Clinical Tip**
When working with the pediatric population, ensure thorough history taking, which includes the child's gestational age at birth. Knowing the child's gestational age helps the therapist understand potential developmental problem's in the child's cardiopulmonary system.

---

## Cardiac Development

The earliest semblance of a heart is a pair of endothelial strands (angioblastic cords) that appear in the third week of gestation. These cords form the heart tubes, which develop

by day 21 (Fig. 20-2), and the tubes then fuse to form a single heart tube. The heart beats by day 22 to 23,[2] and it is circulating blood from the heart to the rest of the embryo by the twenty-seventh day. At about the twenty-third day of gestation, the surrounding pericardial cavity elongates, and the truncus arteriosus, bulbus cordis, ventricle, atrium, and sinus venosus can be distinguished within the heart tube (see Fig. 20-2). The truncus arteriosus divides into the pulmonary artery and aorta during week 6. Simultaneously, a myoepicardial mantle is formed from a thickening of the splanchnic mesenchyme around the heart tube. This myoepicardial mantle differentiates into the myocardium and the epicardium of the heart. The inner endocardial tube becomes the epithelial lining of the heart, called the *endocardium* (see Fig. 1-17). The heart bends or loops upon itself, thereby forming the bulboventricular loop, which evolves into the ventricle and the bulbus cordis. The pericardial cavity is formed as the heart elongates and bends.

During the middle of the gestational week 4, the atrium begins to separate into right and left atria with the sequential growth of two septa (see Fig. 20-2). A crescent-shaped membrane grows from the dorsocranial wall of the primitive atrium toward the endocardial cushions, which forms the septum primum. As the septum primum advances, the two atria communicate through a diminishing foramen primum.

By gestational week 5, the dorsal part of the septum deteriorates, thereby forming a new right-to-left shunt, through the foramen secundum. Near the end of the eighth gestational week, the septum secundum grows from the ventrocranial wall of the atrium on the right side of the septum primum. This septum eventually covers the foramen secundum; the opening in the septum secundum is called the *foramen ovale*. The septum primum forms a valve for the foramen ovale. Before birth, the foramen ovale permits most of the blood entering the right atrium to pass into the left atrium. After birth, the foramen ovale normally closes, and the septum becomes a complete partition. The ventricles divide equally by gestational week 7 (Fig. 20-3). Blood flow in the womb

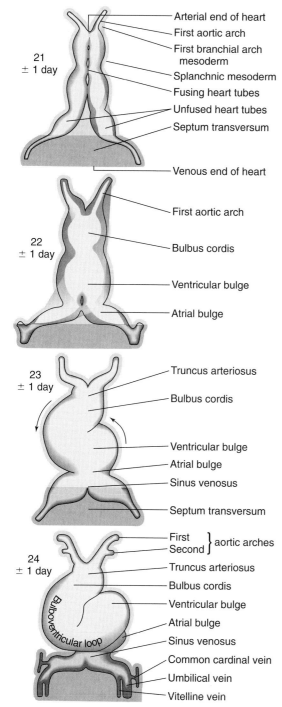

**Figure 20-2** Formation of the primordial heart chambers following fusion of the heart tubes at 3 weeks' gestational age. (From Moore KL, editor: The developing human: clinically oriented embryology, ed 3. Philadelphia, 1982, Saunders.)

---

**Box 20-1**

**Categories of Acyanotic and Cyanotic Lesions**

| Common Acyanotic lesions | Common Cyanotic lesions |
|---|---|
| Atrial septal defects (ASDs) | Tetralogy of Fallot |
| Ventricular septal defects (VSDs) | Transposition of the great arteries |
| Atrioventricular septal defects (AVSDs) | Tricuspid atresia |
| | Pulmonary atresia |
| Patent ductus arteriosus (PDA) | Truncus arteriosus |
| | Total anomalous pulmonary venous return |
| Coarctation of the aorta | Hypoplastic left-sided heart |
| Pulmonary stenosis | syndrome |
| Aortic stenosis | |

the lung tissue (as opposed to gas exchange in normal, post-natal circulation). See Chapter 1 for details of cardiovascular anatomy and normal, postnatal circulation.

By the tenth week of gestation, cardiac development is primarily complete.

## Congenital Heart Defects

The incidence of congenital heart defects (CHDs) is reported as 6 to 8 per 1000 livebirths.[3] Congenital heart disease accounts for 3% of all infant deaths and 46% of death from congenital malformations.[3]

Approximately 10% of children with CHDs also have other physical malformations.[4] Diagnosis of cardiac dysfunction may be made prenatally, at birth, and through childhood as late as adolescence. Cardiac defects are typically described as *cyanotic* (arterial oxygen saturation is decreased) or *acyanotic* (normal oxygen saturation). Box 20-1 lists the categories of cyanotic versus acyanotic CHDs. Figure 20-4 depicts various CHDs. Although not all conditions could be covered in this chapter, some more commonly observed conditions by pediatric clinicians were selected for further description.

### Acyanotic Lesions

Acyanotic lesions increase pulmonary blood flow, and fully oxygenated blood is shunted back into the lungs as well as to the body. This flow is also known as left-to-right shunting. Symptoms can include sweating, increased respiratory rate, and heart failure.

The most common problem these individuals have is low partial pressure of oxygen ($PO_2$) to periphery, low systemic stroke volume, and increased work on the heart.

### Atrial Septal Defects

Atrial septal defects (ASDs) are most commonly caused by a patent foramen ovale. This hole in the atrial wall usually closes after birth. Without closure of the foramen ovale, symptoms such as heart murmur and an enlarged pulmonary

---

(fetal circulation) is different from postnatal circulation. In fetal circulation, most of the blood bypasses the lungs and reaches the left ventricle via the foramen ovale or ductus arteriosus (vessel connecting the aorta with the pulmonary artery). The fetus uses the placenta to obtain oxygen and to get rid of $CO_2$. The blood vessels of pulmonary circulation are vasoconstricted in the fetus, and the blood travelling to and through the lungs is primarily used to nourish and develop

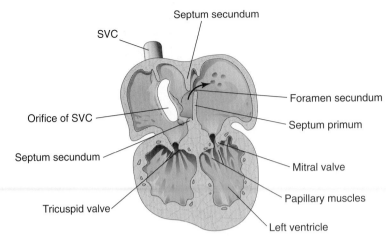

**Figure 20-3** Frontal section of the heart (about 8 weeks) showing the heart after it is partitioned into four chambers. The *arrow* indicates the flow of well-oxygenated blood (from the placenta) moving from the right to the left atrium. SVC, superior vena cava. (From Moore KL. The Developing Human: Clinically Oriented Embryology. 7th ed. Philadelphia, Saunders, 2003.)

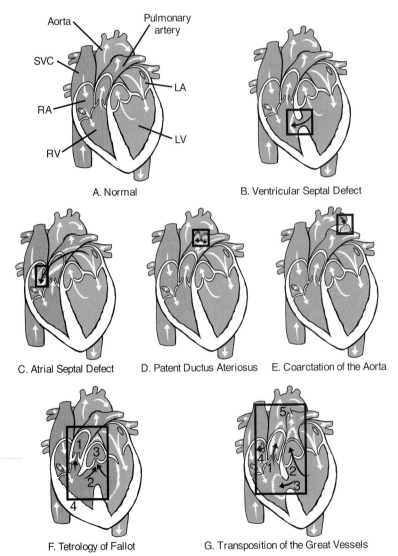

**Figure 20-4** Various types of CHDs. (From Goodman CC. Differential Diagnosis for Physical Therapists: Screening for Referral. 4th ed. Philadelphia, Saunders, 2006.)

artery could develop after many years. Surgery is typically performed if the hole has not closed by 2 to 3 years of age. Anticoagulation therapy may be involved postoperatively.

## Patent Ductus Arteriosus

Patent ductus arteriosus (PDA) is often associated with prematurity or Down syndrome. The ductus arteriosus is the normal circulatory pathway between the descending aorta and the pulmonary artery in the fetus. Prostaglandin $E_1$ is involved in maintaining an open (patent) ductus arteriosus. As the oxygen level in the body increases after birth, the prostaglandin production is signaled to decrease, thereby closing the PDA within 5 to 14 days after birth. When the ductus arteriosus does not close, too much blood may enter the lungs. A high incidence of patency is found in premature infants because of respiratory distress syndrome and the resulting hypoxia. The degree of symptoms associated with the PDA varies based on the size of the opening, gestational age, and the presence of lung disease. Symptoms of a very large opening can include tachycardia, increased respiratory distress, and poor weight gain. Treatment for the PDA can include minimally invasive surgical closure (ligation) or medical management with intravenous indomethacin (which decreases the prostaglandin production).

## Ventricular Septal Defect

Ventricular septal defect (VSD) is characterized by one or more small openings in the wall separating the ventricles (ventricular septum) (see Fig. 20-4B). Small defects may spontaneously close, and the child may be asymptomatic. Large defects may lead to bacterial endocarditis, pulmonary vascular obstructive disease, aortic regurgitation, increased incidence of lower respiratory tract infections, or congestive heart failure (CHF). Symptoms of the large defects could include feeding problems, poor weight gain, restlessness, rapid breathing, and irritability. Treatment may involve surgery; however, the VSD may close within the first 5 months to 6 years of life without treatment. Children with a VSD must be carefully monitored to avoid the life-threatening condition known as *Eisenmenger complex*, which leads to CHF.[5] Eisenmenger complex is characterized by a defect of the ventricular septum, a malpositioned aortic root that overrides the interventricular septum, and a dilated pulmonary artery.[6]

## Atrioventricular Septal Defects

Atrioventricular septal defects (AVSDs; see Fig. 20-4) are also known as atrioventricular canal defects or endocardial cushion defects (because of abnormalities in endocardial cushion formation). The endocardial cushions complete the separation of the mitral and tricuspid valves by dividing the single valve between the embryonic atria and ventricles. An AVSD may involve failure of formation of any or all of these structures. AVSDs are cited as occurring in 15% to 40% of children with Down syndrome. Symptoms in *complete* ASVDs include pulmonary hypertension, lung congestion, and heart failure. Surgery is usually required within the first few months of life.

> **Clinical Tip**
> Be aware that CHDs may accompany other genetic disorders, causing developmental delays.

## Coarctation of Aorta

Coarctation of aorta (see Fig. 20-4) involves obstruction of left ventricular outflow as a consequence of a narrowing of the aorta. The pressure proximal to the constriction of the aorta is increased, and the pressure distal to the constriction is decreased. In turn, this causes hypertension in the upper body (above the level of the coarctation) and normal to low blood pressure in the lower extremities, as some of the blood flows around the coarctation through small collateral arteries. Coarctation of the aorta is also known as a condition causing secondary hypertension. Surgery is performed to remove the constriction of the aorta; however, recoarctation may occur.

## Cyanotic Lesions

Cyanotic lesions of the heart involve right-to-left shunting, where most of the blood bypasses the lungs. Decreased arterial oxygen saturation occurs as unoxygenated blood is returned to the body. The body signals increased red blood cell formation as a result of the decreased arterial oxygen saturation levels, and polycythemia results. With increased blood viscosity because of an excess of red blood cells, the body is at risk for cerebrovascular insult. Cyanosis may be present.

## Tetralogy of Fallot

Tetralogy of Fallot (see Fig. 20-4) is named for its tetrad of defects: (1) pulmonary stenosis, (2) VSD, (3) overriding aorta, and (4) right ventricular hypertrophy. The pulmonary stenosis causes obstruction to right ventricular outflow. The VSD allows blood between the two ventricles to mix freely. The overriding aorta means that the position of the aorta is above the VSD. The hypertrophy of the right ventricle is cause by the obstruction to the right ventricular outflow. Low oxygen levels throughout the body result. The degree of the cyanosis depends largely on the degree of the pulmonary stenosis. Surgery is usually required.

## Hypoplastic Left-Heart Syndrome

The hypoplastic left-heart syndrome (HLHS; Fig. 20-5) includes (1) hypoplastic (underdeveloped) left ventricle, (2) aortic and mitral valve stenosis (narrowing) or atresia (complete closure), and, often, (3) coarctation of the aorta. Symptoms of this condition may be minimal until closure of the ductus arteriosus. Because systemic blood supply is dependent on the PDA, the child may develop severe CHF upon closure of the ductus arteriosus. Prostaglandin $E_1$ may be required so as to maintain the ductus arteriosus open and mechanical ventilation may be required until surgery or heart transplantation can occur. Surgical intervention or heart transplantation is required in order for a child with HLHS to survive.

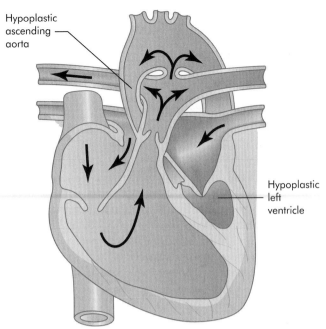

**Figure 20-5** Hypoplastic left heart syndrome (HLHS). (Redrawn from Hockenberry MJ et al: Wong's nursing care of infants and children, ed 8, St Louis, 2007, Mosby. In Huether SE. Understanding Pathophysiology, ed 4. St. Louis, 2008, Mosby.)

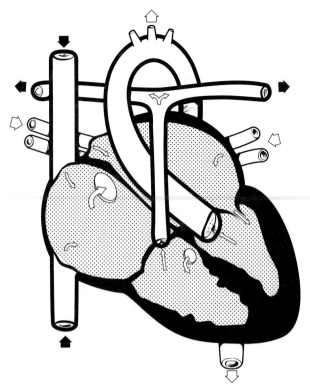

**Figure 20-6** Tricuspid atresia. (From Campbell SK. Physical Therapy for Children. 3rd ed. Philadelphia, Saunders, 2006.)

### Transposition of the Great Arteries

Transposition of the great arteries involves the pulmonary artery leaving the left ventricle and the aorta exiting the right ventricle with no communication between the systemic and pulmonary circulations. In other words, the positions of the aorta and pulmonary artery are reversed. The severity of the condition depends on the amount of blood mixing that occurs between the two sides. Severe cyanosis is observed in the absence of a PDA, VSD, or ASD to allow the blood to mix and allow some blood to be delivered to the tissue. This condition is not compatible with life. Prostaglandin $E_1$ may be given to maintain a PDA until surgery is successfully completed. The treatment for transposition of the great arteries is surgery. Arrhythmias or ventricular dysfunctions may develop later in life.

### Tricuspid Atresia

In tricuspid atresia (Fig. 20-6), the tricuspid valve between the right atrium and right ventricle is either not patent or absent. This results in obstruction of blood flow into the right ventricle, and the right ventricle is frequently underdeveloped. Other cardiac defects such as ASDs or VSDs may be present, with some degree of shunting into the lungs. Symptoms can include anoxia, signs of right-sided heart failure, severe cyanosis, and dyspnea.[6] Surgical repair is required.

### Pulmonary Atresia

In pulmonary atresia, the pulmonary valve fails to develop, therefore there is an obstruction of blood from the right side of the heart to the lungs. Blood flow to the lungs is initially dependent on a PDA. The presence of other cardiac defects, such as the ASDs and the VSDs, would allow right-to-left shunting, and thereby blood flow to the rest of the body.

### Truncus Arteriosus

When normal separation of the aorta and main pulmonary artery do not occur during fetal development, both the right and left ventricles empty into a single large vessel (Fig. 20-7). A single great artery arises from the ventricles, which carries both pulmonary and systemic blood flow. A VSD is always present, and the heart functions practically as a single ventricle. Surgical repair is required for correction this defect.

### Total Anomalous Pulmonary Venous Return

In total anomalous pulmonary venous return (Fig. 20-8), the pulmonary veins attach to the right atrium or to other veins that drain into the right atrium. Symptoms can include pulmonary congestion, cyanosis, and heart failure. An ASD may also be present, which will aid right-atrium decompression. Anastomosis (surgical joining) of the pulmonary veins to the left atrium is usually performed as early as possible.[7]

## Respiratory Conditions of Infancy

### Prematurity (Born <37 Weeks' Gestation)

There are additional anatomic and physiologic challenges to consider with respiration of the premature infant (Table 20-1). Premature infants may demonstrate *periodic breathing* patterns, where they take 5- to 10-second pauses in breathing.

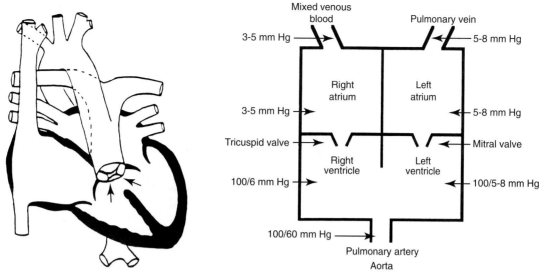

**Figure 20-7** Truncus arteriosus. A single great artery arises from the ventricles carrying both pulmonary and systemic blood flow. (From Mullin CE, Mayer DC. Congenital Heart Disease: a Diagrammatic Atlas. New York, John Wiley, 1988.)

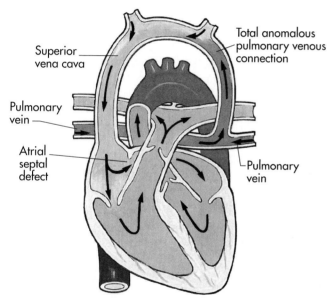

**Figure 20-8** Total anomalous venous return. From Hockenberry MJ. Wong's Nursing Care of Infants and Children, ed 8. St. Louis, 2007, Mosby.

This type of breathing is not to be confused with apnea of prematurity, which lasts longer than premature periodic breathing patterns and is associated with bradycardia and hypoxemia (deficiency in arterial blood oxygen concentration). Apnea of prematurity is a relatively common and controllable disorder in premature infants. It is defined as cessation of breathing for 20 seconds or longer in an infant born less than 37 weeks' gestation, and causes bradycardia, cyanosis, or both.[8]

## Persistent Pulmonary Hypertension

Prematurity is also commonly associated with PDA. Recall from the earlier section of this chapter, that the PDA is

## Table 20-1 Anatomic and Physiologic Challenges in the Premature Infant

| Anatomic | Physiologic |
|---|---|
| Capillary beds not well developed before 26 weeks of gestation | Increased pulmonary vascular resistance leading to right-to-left shunting |
| Type II alveolar cells and surfactant production not mature until 35 weeks of gestation | Decreased lung compliance |
| Elastic properties of lung not well developed | |
| Lung "space" decreased by relative size of the heart and abdominal distension | |
| Type I, high-oxidative fibers compose only 10% to 20% of diaphragm muscle | Diaphragmatic fatigue; respiratory failure |
| Highly vascular subependymal germinal matrix not resorbed until 35 weeks of gestation, increasing the vulnerability of the infant to hemorrhage | Decreased or absent cough and gag reflexes; apnea |
| Lack of fatty insulation and high surface area-to-body weight ratio | Hypothermia and increased oxygen consumption |

*From Irwin S. Cardiopulmonary Physical Therapy: A Guide to Practice. 4th ed. St. Louis, Mosby, 2004.*

normal anatomy as a fetus. Within hours to days of birth, the PDA spontaneously closes in response to prostaglandin $E_1$ levels dropping after birth. When it remains open (patent), persistent pulmonary hypertension (PPHN) of the newborn can result. PPHN is a syndrome observed in infants shortly after birth, and it is characterized by increased pulmonary vascular resistance. PPHN usually appears within the first 12 hours of life and can be associated with cyanosis, tachypnea, intercostal retractions, nasal flaring, or grunting.[8]

---

**Clinical Tip**
PPHN can also be seen in infants with *infant respiratory distress syndrome* and meconium aspiration syndrome.

---

### Respiratory Distress Syndrome

The most common respiratory disorder in premature infants is *hyaline membrane disease* or infant respiratory distress syndrome (RDS). It is caused by a deficient amount of pulmonary surfactant. Because surfactant decreases surface tension, the alveoli involved in RDS have increased surface tension and collapse. Underdeveloped alveoli and pulmonary capillary beds further compromise gas exchange. RDS (Fig. 20-9) is characterized by airless alveoli, inelastic lungs, a respiration rate greater than 60 breaths per minute, nasal flaring, intercostal and subcostal retractions, grunting on expiration, and peripheral edema.[6] The incidence of RDS increases with decreasing gestational age. Continuous positive airway pressure will aid in preventing alveolar collapse.

A cross-sectional study of 126 children with a mean age of 10 years old whose mean gestational ages at birth were 27 weeks was published in 2008.[9] The children in the study had birth weights less than 1000 g, and they were born 1992 through 1994. The study compared term-born children with the group of children described above. They examined the lung function of each group, using spirometry, as well as the fitness level, which they determined by using the 6-minute walk test and the 20-m shuttle run test. The data demonstrated no difference between the two groups in the distance walked on the 6-minute walk test. The two groups did, however, demonstrate significant difference in spirometry. The preterm group showed exercise capacity of approximately half that of the control group. The authors concluded that although exercise capacity was reduced, it is unknown if training can change that finding. This study is an excellent example of using information that exists about the children we treat to motivate us to learn more.

### Sudden Infant Death Syndrome

Sudden infant death syndrome (SIDS) is the sudden, unexpected death during sleep of an otherwise healthy infant. SIDS may be linked with respiration; the mechanism of SIDS, however, is still largely unknown. The "Back to Sleep" campaign was launched by National Institute of Child Health and Human Development (NICHD) at the National Institutes of Health in 1994 in order to decrease the incidence of SIDS. The campaign initially promoted infants sleeping on their backs or sides. The campaign later revised its message to encourage putting infants to sleep *only in the supine position*. SIDS incidence has declined by greater than 50% since launching the "Back to Sleep" campaign. Physical therapists should be aware of the "Back to Sleep" campaign and the American Academy of Pediatrics recommendations in regard to sleeping position. Given that, physical therapists should

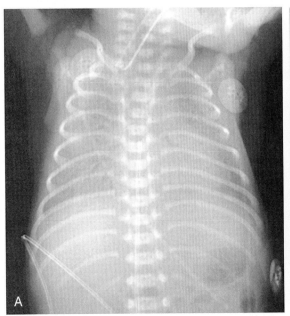 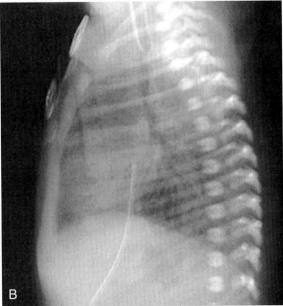

**Figure 20-9** Anteroposterior **(A)** and lateral **(B)** chest radiographs of a preterm infant with respiratory distress syndrome. Both views show diffuse hazy, ground-glass appearance, air bronchograms, and low lung volumes. (From Wilkins RL. Clinical Assessment in Respiratory Care. 5th ed. St. Louis, Mosby, 2005.)

also be aware of the importance of educating families about intermittent periods of prone play while the baby is awake and under direct observation. The pediatric physical therapist plays a key role in encouraging compliance with sleeping recommendations in supine for safety, as well as encouraging supervised prone activities when the baby is awake, for optimal development.

> **Clinical Tip**
> "Tummy time" promotes optimal development of the trunk flexors and extensors. The position allows babies the opportunity to bear weight through their forearms and later, their hands. Babies who do not spend time in the prone position for play may be at risk for other developmental issues.

## Meconium Aspiration Syndrome

Meconium is the fecal matter that is normally present in the fetal colon in late gestation. It consists of mucopolysaccharides, cholesterol, bile acids and salts, intestinal enzymes, and other substances. Vagal stimulation and hypoxic stress caused by various factors, including cord compression, may cause fetal rectal sphincter muscles to relax, resulting in release of *meconium* into the amniotic fluid. Deep gasping movements of a distressed fetus can cause amniotic fluid and meconium to be aspirated into the infant's lung. Meconium aspiration can lead to respiratory distress after birth as a consequence of airway obstruction or chemical irritation. Air trapping may occur on expiration, as the particulate lodges in the lungs. Mechanical ventilation or supplemental oxygen may be required to treat meconium aspiration syndrome (MAS), and extracorporeal membrane oxygenation (ECMO) may be required to manage severe MAS.

## Bronchopulmonary Dysplasia

Bronchopulmonary dysplasia (BPD) is a chronic respiratory disorder characterized by scarring of lung tissue, thickened pulmonary arterial walls, and mismatch between lung ventilation and perfusion (Fig. 20-10).[6] Infants with severe respiratory failure during the first few weeks of life may develop the chronic condition of BPD. Persistence of respiratory symptoms after 1 month of life, abnormal radiographic findings, and dependence on supplemental oxygen characterize BPD.[10] Mechanical ventilation is considered to be an etiologic factor in BPD. It should be noted that BPD predicts poor developmental outcomes in infants whose birthweight was less than 1500 g.[11] Because children with severe BPD demonstrate higher incidences of developmental delays,[11] the physical therapist should be acutely aware of the need for early referral to multidisciplinary therapeutic services in the hospital, home, and/or school settings.

## Cystic Fibrosis

This chapter presents a brief overview of cystic fibrosis. For a more in depth description, see Chapter 6. Cystic fibrosis (CF)

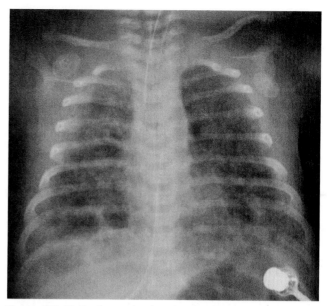

**Figure 20-10** Radiograph of patient with bronchopulmonary dysplasia. Anteroposterior radiograph shows areas of scarring, atelectasis, emphysema, and cysts. This film is consistent with severe bronchopulmonary dysplasia. (From Wilkins RL, Stoller JK, Kacmarek RM. Egan's Fundamentals of Respiratory Care. 9th ed. St. Louis, Mosby, 2009.)

is a genetic, autosomal recessive disease that affects exocrine gland function. Approximately 1000 new diagnoses are made each year. The median age of survival has increased dramatically over the years with advancements in treatment. Fifty years ago, children were not expected to live to school age. Now, the median age of survival is 37 years and more than 40% of people living with CF are adults.

As stated in Chapter 6, 90% of CF-related deaths are caused by pulmonary compromise. Consequently, the physical therapist has an important role in the treatment of these patients. Treatment methods must include airway clearance, rib cage mobility, postural training, and exercise. Various pulmonary treatment techniques are discussed in detail later in this chapter. Specific considerations for the treatment of children with CF, however, include time required daily for treatment of their disease, nutrition, and risk for pulmonary infection.

When treating a child with CF, the therapist must be sure to take into account the already demanding home treatment program. Typically, a child with CF will need to use nebulizer treatments (bronchodilators, mucolytics, and/or inhaled antibiotics) followed by airway clearance twice a day. They also must take various oral medications (vitamins A, D, E, and K, oral antibiotics, and/or reflux medication) as well as enzymes with all meals and snacks that they eat. This must all be done in addition to other activities of daily living, school, and entertainment. The therapist must work with each child and family to determine how best to fit airway clearance and exercise into the patient and family's busy schedules. Exercise needs to be fun and preferably a family activity in order for the child to consistently make it a priority. Airway clearance may be done while watching TV, listening to music, doing homework, or playing video games. It also has been shown that playing recorded music during Chest Physical Therapy (CPT) with infants assists in their enjoyment of CPT and establishes a positive routine.[12]

Other factors to consider when treating a child with CF include nutrition, electrolyte replacement, and infection control. As explained in Chapter 6, children with CF have malabsorption of nutrients and thus require additional caloric intake. Because the children will burn more calories with exercise, a plan should be made in conjunction with the nutritionist to replace expended calories. In the event that the child sweats during exercise, rehydration should focus on electrolyte and fluid replacement as the concentration of sodium chloride in the child's sweat will be increased. If the child has diabetes, the therapist needs to be aware of recent blood sugar readings. Juice or other sugary products should be available in the event that the child becomes hypoglycemic. In the hospital setting, care must be taken to thoroughly clean all equipment used by patients with CF so as to prevent the spread of dangerous bacteria. Each facility treating patients with CF may have its own specific protocol regarding cleaning equipment that has been used by children with CF. The Cystic Fibrosis Foundation recommends that all patients with CF maintain a distance of at least 3 feet from one another and wear a mask when in the same room. This limits the ability of the therapist to have interactive exercise groups involving multiple children with CF at one time.

## Primary Ciliary Dyskinesia

Primary ciliary dyskinesia is a rare disease in which mucociliary clearance is impaired because of a defective motility of the cilia.[13] Without the forward thrust of the cilia and coordinated ciliary beating, mucus transport is slowed. There is a subsequent accumulation of particles, secretions, and bacteria in the dependent portions of the lungs. These patients are treated much like patients with CF, as the outcome of decreased mucus motility is similar in both conditions.

# Pediatric Conditions with Secondary Cardiopulmonary Issues

The following section presents cardiopulmonary implications of commonly treated pediatric conditions. For more a more detailed description of any of these conditions (beyond the scope of the cardiopulmonary aspects), the reader is referred to other sources.[7]

## Down Syndrome

Down syndrome is associated with endocardial cushion defect, VSD, ASD, and tetralogy of Fallot.[14] Cardiac defects and sleep apnea are more common in persons with Down syndrome than the general population.[15] As lower fitness levels are reported in individuals with Down syndrome, exercise throughout their life span is critical to their health.[16] Identifying the contributing factors to a child's decreased fitness level is important. Factors could include poor eating habits, lack of opportunity for recreational activities, poor coordination, and poor motivation for physical activity.

## DiGeorge Syndrome

DiGeorge syndrome is a primary immunodeficiency disease, which in most cases is caused by deletion of chromosome 22 (at position 22q11.2). The disease has been termed the chromosome 22q11.2 deletion syndrome. Individuals with DiGeorge syndrome vary greatly in their clinical presentation. The variation in symptoms of this disease tends to be related to the amount of genetic material lost in the deletion. Cardiac anomalies, abnormal facial features, thymic hypoplasia, cleft palate, and hypocalcemia are often observed with DiGeorge syndrome. The cardiac anomalies can include tetralogy of Fallot, truncus arteriosus, interrupted aortic arch, VSD, and pulmonary atresia. Less commonly associated cardiac anomalies include vascular ring anomaly, transposition of the great arteries with VSD, coarctation of the aorta, ASD, pulmonary stenosis, hypoplastic left heart, and PDA. Cardiac surgery or medications may be necessary. Thymus transplantation is the typical medical treatment for DiGeorge syndrome.

## VATER Association

*VATER* (*v*ertebral defects, imperforate *a*nus, *t*racheoesophageal fistula, and radial and *r*enal dysplasia) or *VACTERL* association is a nonrandom association of symptoms, including vertebral anomalies, imperforate anus, tracheoesophageal fistula, and renal or radial anomalies. In VACTERL, cardiac anomalies are added, and renal and limb anomalies replace renal or radial anomalies in the acronym.

## Marfan Syndrome

Marfan syndrome is a connective tissue disease that is commonly associated with aortic aneurysm and aortic/mitral insufficiency.[14] The connective tissue of the cardiac valves and great arteries are affected. The skeletal system and the skin are affected. For example, there may be excessive growth at the epiphyseal plates. Striated muscles tend to be poorly developed. The patient with Marfan syndrome can have minimal to severe cardiovascular impact.

## Williams Syndrome

Williams syndrome involves deletion of the long arm of chromosome 7 (7q1). It is associated with supravalvular aortic stenosis[6] and supravalvular pulmonary stenosis[14] caused by changes in elastin production. Transient hypercalcemia might also been seen in infancy.[6]

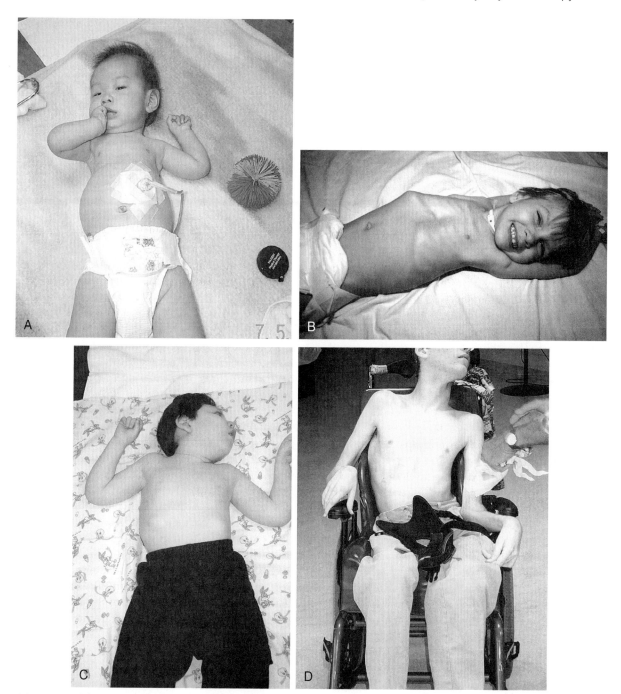

**Figure 20-11 A,** Caitlin, 6 months of age. Caitlin has spinal muscle atrophy, type I. Note persistent immature triangular shaping of chest wall secondary to pronounced muscle weakness and an inability to counteract gravity effectively. **B,** Melissa, 3.5 years of age. Melissa has a C5 complete spinal cord injury as a consequence of birth trauma. Melissa's chest wall has become more deformed than Caitlin's chest as a result of the prolonged exposure to the severe muscle imbalance of the respiratory muscles within gravity's constant influence. Note the marked pectus excavatum and anteriorly flared ribs in supine. **C,** Carlos, 5 years of age and **D,** Kevin, 17 years of age. Both have spastic cerebral palsy. Note the lateral flaring of the lower ribcage, the asymmetry of the trunk, and the flattening of the entire anterior ribcage, all of which are more noticeable in the older child. (From Frownfelter D. Cardiovascular and Pulmonary Physical Therapy: Evidence and Practice. 4th ed. St. Louis, Mosby, 2005.)

## Fetal Alcohol Syndrome

Fetal alcohol syndrome results from chronic alcohol exposure *in utero*; it has multiple clinical features, including facial dysmorphology. Fetal alcohol syndrome is commonly associated with the cardiac anomalies of VSD, tetralogy of Fallot, pulmonary value stenosis, and PDA.[14]

## Pediatric Conditions with Decreased Activity Levels

A child's decreased activity level or impairments to breathing mechanics may be caused by muscle weakness, muscle tone problems such as hypertonicity or hypotonicity, motor planning deficits, motor learning deficits, and medical fragility (Fig. 20-11). Muscle weakness or fatigue of the trunk muscles is not only caused by neuromuscular diseases but can also result from conditions arising outside of the neuromuscular system. For example, oxygen transport deficits from BPD, CHDs, nutritional deficits such as gastroesophageal reflux, or absorption problems can lead to weakness in the trunk.

## Cerebral Palsy

Cerebral palsy is a disorder caused by a nonprogressive but permanent lesion of the brain, occurring *in utero*, during birth, or immediately after birth.[6] The degree of neurologic involvement varies, depending on the degree, location, and nature of the lesion. Cognitive and language impairments may or may not be present. Cerebral palsy causes disturbances of voluntary muscle control. Muscle tone is commonly affected in children with cerebral palsy in the form of hypertonicity or spasticity. Oxygen demands are increased as a result of increased basal and exercise oxygen consumption. Muscle spasms, altered breathing patterns, poor saliva control, and poor gag reflexes can decrease the ability to effectively cough and increase the risk of pulmonary infection.

## Spina Bifida

Spina bifida is a term referring to various types of myelodysplasia, ranging from lack of posterior vertebral arch fusion (occulta) to open spinal defects (myelomeningocele). For information regarding spinal cord injuries and their implications on the cardiopulmonary system, refer to Chapter 7. Spina bifida is a diagnosis that physical therapists commonly equate with issues of mobility; however, ventilatory dysfunction can be involved with children who also have an associated Arnold-Chiari type II malformation.[17-19] The Arnold-Chiari type II malformation, which occurs in 90% of infants with myelomeningocele, is a hindbrain malformation consisting of a caudal herniation of the cerebellum and brain stem into the cervical canal.[20] Ventilatory problems associated with a symptomatic Arnold-Chiari type II malformation include inspiratory stridor (vocal cord paralysis), central apnea, and respiratory distress.[17,21,22]

> **Clinical Tip**
> Also of clinical significance is the tendency for children with spina bifida to be allergic to latex.

## Duchenne Muscular Dystrophy

Duchenne muscular dystrophy is a condition characterized by progressive, symmetrical wasting of the musculature. Proximal musculature tends to be most severely affected. There is progressive weakening of the pelvic musculature and cardiac musculature, the gag reflex may be depressed, and ventilatory contraction and relaxation can be impaired. Respiratory weakness occurs as muscle wasting progresses.

## Spinal Muscular Atrophy

Spinal muscular atrophy (SMA), a lower motor neuron condition, is another instance where severe weakness, muscle atrophy, and contractures, can result in progressive respiratory failure.[7] There are three major types of SMAs. Type I SMA (Werdnig-Hoffman disease) is the most severe form, and respiratory failure can lead to death within the first year of life.[10] The only treatment for SMA type I is supportive care.

## Physical Therapy Examination

The examination of children with cardiac and pulmonary disorders begins with a thorough history, as all good examinations do. The history should be obtained from the medical record and the family. If the child is old enough to answer questions, the child will be a good source of information. As part of the history, the therapist should document the type of disorder the patient presents with as well as prior surgeries, current medications, relevant lab values, therapies the child has had in the past, and prior level of function if the child is not a newborn. For a description of possible effects of various medications, refer to Chapters 14 and 15.

Upon completing a thorough history, the therapist must pause to observe the child and his or her environment. It is important to document the child's resting vital signs and the support equipment that is required to maintain the child in his/her current state. Refer to Table 20-2 for pediatric vital sign norms. The pediatric clinician should consider these questions: Is the child on ECMO), a ventilator (nasal intubation, oral intubation, or tracheotomy), or on oxygen via face mask or nasal cannula? What is the child's mode of meeting nutritional demands? Does the child have a gastrostomy tube or a nasogastric tube for nutrition? Does the child have an IV, central line, femoral line, chest tube, Foley catheter, ECG leads, or pulse oximeter? Recording this information will give a complete picture of the patient to anyone who reads the document.

ECMO involves the use of a device that is external to the body so as to directly oxygenate the blood, assist with the removal of carbon dioxide, or both (Fig. 20-12). The primary indication for ECMO is for cardiac or respiratory failure that is not responding to either maximal medical therapy or traditional mechanical ventilation.

The child's resting position should be observed before a hands-on assessment takes place. In the acute care setting, children are often in a gravity-dependent position (Fig. 20-13). However, positioning with hip flexion, abduction, and external rotation; knee flexion, ankle plantarflexion, and shoulder abduction; external rotation; and retraction is not an organizing position. This position also leads to decreased extensibility and range of motion in the extremities, which, in turn, may slow the return to age-appropriate functional activities as the child's medical condition improves. Patients who have a midline scar or who use accessory muscles

### Table 20-2  Pediatric Vital Sign Norms

| Age | Weight (kg) | Heart Rate (average/min) | Respiratory Rate (average/min) | BP (Systolic) (mm Hg) |
|---|---|---|---|---|
| Premature | 1 | 100–180 | <40 | 42 ± 10 |
| Newborn | 2–3 | 100–180 | <40 | 60 ± 10 |
| 1 mo | 4 | 80–180 | 24–35 | 80 ± 16 |
| 6 mo | 7 | 70–150 | 24–35 | 89 ± 29 |
| 1 yr | 10 | 70–150 | 20–30 | 96 ± 30 |
| 2–3 yr | 12–14 | 70–120 | 20–30 | 99 ± 25 |
| 4–5 yr | 16–18 | 70–110 | 20–30 | 99 ± 20 |
| 6–8 yr | 20–46 | 60–110 | 12–25 | 105 ± 13 |
| 10–12 yr | 32–42 | 55–90 | 12–20 | 112 ± 19 |
| >14 yr | >50 | 55–90 | 12–18 | 120 ± 20 |

*From Mosby's Dictionary of Medicine, Nursing & Health Professions. 8th ed. St. Louis, Mosby, 2008.*

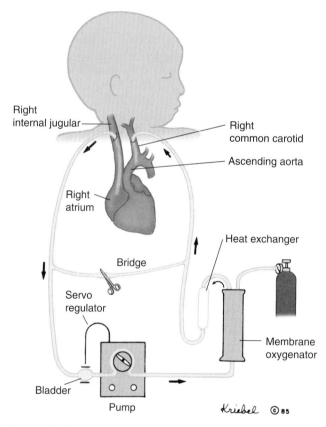

**Figure 20-12** Venoarterial ECMO circuit. Venous blood is removed from the right atrium, oxygenated by passage thru a diffusing membrane, and then returned to the patient. (Modified from O'Rourke PP. Respiratory care of infants and children. Part II. Respir Care 36:7, 1991; Wilkins RL, Stoller JK, Kacmarek RM. Egan's Fundamentals of Respiratory Care. 9th ed. St. Louis, Mosby, 2009.)

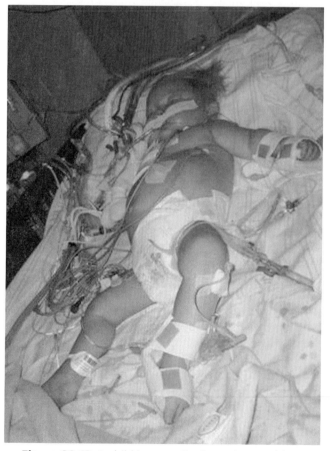

**Figure 20-13** A child in a gravity-dependent position.

excessively, often have increased thoracic kyphosis with shoulder protraction and elevation. In the home or outpatient setting, the therapist can observe the child in his or her crib, stroller, chair, or other resting position. The child often continues to prefer a position that is similar to the one that the child had in the hospital with hip and shoulder abduction and external rotation. Box 20-2 lists other observations that the therapist should document.

Examination of the thorax includes the general shape and mobility of the rib cage. This examination is complicated in the infant by the vast changes in both the shape and mobility that take place during the first year of life. Table 20-3 identifies the normal development of the rib cage.[23]

**Table 20-3  Normal Development of the Rib Cage**

| Age | Shape of the Thorax | Direction of Ribs | Primary Muscles Used for Inspiration |
|---|---|---|---|
| 0–3 months | Triangular | Horizontal | Diaphragm |
| 3–6 months | Rectangular | Horizontal | Diaphragm and accessory muscles |
| 6–12 months | Rectangular | Angled downward | Diaphragm and intercostals |

---

**Box 20-2**

**Components of the Pediatric Cardiopulmonary Examination**

| Observations | Measurements |
|---|---|
| Environment that child is in | Mobility of ribcage |
| Resting position | Thoracic expansion |
| Vital signs (heart rate, oxygen saturation, blood pressure) | Range of motion of extremities |
| Pattern of breathing | Flexibility of extremities |
| Shape of ribcage | Strength |
| Integument (bruising, scar tissue, edema, coloring, clubbing) | Functional mobility (assistance needed, objective measures of distance, time, etc.) |
| Posture | Aerobic capacity (step test or walk test) |

---

The ribs and spine of the child with cardiac or pulmonary disorders can often lose mobility secondary to prolonged immobility, guarding of the postural muscles, overuse of accessory muscles during breathing, scar tissue formation, or shallow breathing. A measurement of thoracic expansion with inhalation can be made by placing a tape measure around the rib cage and measuring the distance the tape moves with inhalation. No normative values for thoracic expansion have been published. However, the mobility should increase as the tape measure is moved further down the rib cage. The presence of increased thoracic kyphosis or scoliosis should also be noted as they will affect the overall size of the thoracic cavity and thus the ventilatory capacity of the child.

The examination of the child, as described thus far, could be completed on a child of any age and of any level on consciousness. However, to assess strength, functional mobility, and aerobic capacity, the child must be awake. Manual muscle testing is a reliable way to assess strength in children who are able to understand instructions and follow commands. However, the therapist must assess strength by observation of functional movement for younger children or children with cognitive impairments. A grade of fair (3/5 on manual muscle testing) can be assessed relatively easily by positioning the infant or child appropriately and watching him/her move against gravity. In an infant, strength may be assessed by the child's ability to hold his/her head upright against gravity, reach for a toy while supine, or lift lower extremities off the

surface. In a toddler, strength measurements greater than fair (>3/5 on manual muscle testing) may be estimated by observing ambulation, ascending/descending stairs, squat to stand, sitting on the floor to stand, and reaching overhead for a toy. Standardized testing, such as the Alberta Infant Motor Scales (AIMS), Gross Motor Function Measurement (GMFM), and Peabody Developmental Motor Scales (PDMS), can also be used to document baseline function and/or developmental age equivalency in children. When deciding which testing instrument to use, consider the following:

- Your goals for testing. Ask yourself what information you need to glean by completing the test. Do you need to document a baseline in function for future comparison? Do you need to establish a gross motor age equivalency to provide to other health professionals or a third-party payer?
- The time and space available to test the child. Some tests may be more appropriate to complete in one setting compared to another, based on time and space available to the therapist and child.
- The age of the child. Each test has a specific age range for which it has been demonstrated or proven reliable.
- Availability of testing materials in your setting.
- Your estimation of the child's developmental age. For example, you are treating a child who is 5 years old; however, the child is not yet ambulating or crawling. A test that tests skills prior to crawling and ambulation would be more appropriate than a test that covers the typical skills of a 5-year-old.

Assessing functional mobility at any age may be difficult depending on how many pieces of supportive equipment the patient has attached to his or her body. However, most of the equipment in the hospital and virtually all of the equipment at home or in the outpatient setting is portable, and with assistance from a parent or nurse, the child will likely be able to attempt mobility. The therapist should take caution when getting the child out of bed in the acute care setting because the child could have significant muscle atrophy, orthostatic hypotension, emesis, or increased pain with standing. In an infant, the therapist should arrange the environment to allow the child to roll, creep, sit, and transition throughout positions. Regardless of the child's age, the amount of assistance the child needs during movement, as well as the quality of movement, should be documented. Objective measures, such as distance ambulated and amount of time the child is able to sit upright, and subjective measures, such as rating of perceived exertion and dyspnea on exertion (see Table 18-12),

## Table 20-4  Practice Patterns for the Pediatric Cardiopulmonary Patient

| Practice patterns | Impairment/limitation |
| --- | --- |
| 6A | **Risk reduction/prevention**<br>Children with neuromuscular impairments are at risk for cardiopulmonary problems secondary to poor breathing mechanics, altered alignment of the thoracic musculoskeletal system, and inactivity. The physical therapist should attempt to prevent or delay cardiopulmonary impairments by treating the root cause. |
| 6B | **Deconditioning**<br>Many children with cardiopulmonary impairments are deconditioned. They have limited functional mobility secondary to their primary diagnosis or general inactivity. |
| 6C | **Airway clearance dysfunction**<br>Children may have difficulty with airway clearance secondary to increased mucus production, decreased clearance secondary to muscle weakness, or decreased clearance secondary to inactivity (such as a patient status postcardiac surgery who is unable to get out of bed for weeks). |
| 6D | **Cardiovascular pump dysfunction or failure**<br>Many children with congenital heart disease will fall into this category. |
| 6G | **Impaired ventilation, respiration/gas exchange, and aerobic capacity/endurance associated with respiratory failure in the neonate.**<br>Any child born at less than 27 weeks' gestation is at significant risk for respiratory failure. |

*In addition to cardiopulmonary practice patterns, children with cerebral palsy, muscular dystrophy, spinal cord injury, or other neuromuscular impairments will also be appropriate for neuromuscular practice patterns. For instance, a child with cerebral palsy may also be placed in practice pattern 5D (impaired motor function associated with a nonprogressive disorder of the central nervous system). Please refer to further neuromuscular practice patterns in Chapter 5.*
*Adapted from The Guide to Physical Therapist Practice, ed 2. Baltimore, 2001, American Physical Therapy Association.*

should also be recorded. Vital signs should be taken during and after mobility. The therapist should also note any changes in the child, such as diaphoresis or pallor.

It is also important to consider the patient's family situation during examination. There may be many additional stressors to the family that will affect the child's experiences during therapy. The family may be from out of town (or out of the country) and staying in a hotel; a parent may have to quit his/her job in order to care for the child; there may be other children who require the parent's attention; or perhaps the family does not speak English. The potential stressors for the family that are not related to the condition of the child are numerous. The therapist must be aware of these stressors so that therapy sessions and home programs accommodate the unique needs of the child and family.

## Physical Therapy Evaluation, Diagnosis, and Prognosis

Once the examination is complete, the therapist must then synthesize all of the information learned about the child to develop a physical therapy diagnosis. Table 20-4 provides appropriate practice patterns from the *Guide to Physical Therapist Practice*. With experience, the therapist is able to determine a likely prognosis for the child's diagnosis and individual circumstances. This allows the therapist to write short-term and long-term goals for therapy. Goals should address the impairments and functional limitations in the areas of rib cage mobility, posture, flexibility, strength, functional mobility, breathing pattern, airway clearance and vital signs that were identified during the examination. Once the prognosis and goals are determined, the therapist must begin discharge planning (for acute care patients). The therapist must address the setting that is most appropriate for discharge (home, inpatient rehabilitation, skilled facility) and the type of services that may be needed (early intervention, home health, outpatient, or inpatient rehabilitation). Discharge equipment should also be considered, including ambulation devices and a wheelchair as needed.

## Physical Therapy Intervention

Physical therapy interventions should address the impairments and functional limitations identified during the examination. They should also be related to the short- and long-term goals that were established. The interventions must address rib cage mobility, flexibility, strength, posture, breathing pattern, airway clearance, functional mobility, and endurance.

### Rib Cage Mobility

Gentle rib cage mobilizations may be performed with the child in supine, prone, or side-lying position.[24] The therapist

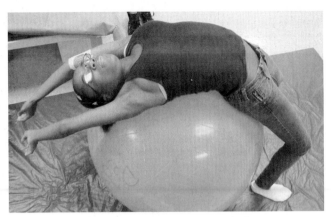

**Figure 20-14** Supine over a ball.

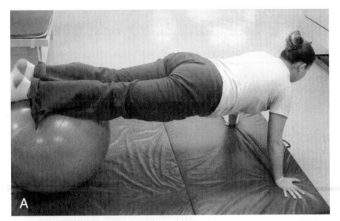

must be very cautious with rib mobilizations on children who have osteopenia. It may also be beneficial to perform manual release techniques over the intercostals to gain extensibility. If there is a scar from a thoracic incision, scar tissue massage should be performed after the incision is completely closed. Several techniques for scar tissue massage may be used including friction massage perpendicular to the scar, plucking the scar to loosen its attachment to the underlying fascia, or stretching the scar with two fingers at each end of the scar and opposing forces applied. Another method involves kneading the tissue proximal to the scar tissue in a circular manner.

### Flexibility

The therapist should assist the child in performing exercises to elongate all musculature that was found to have decreased extensibility during the examination. Most children with cardiac or pulmonary disorders will benefit from side-lying trunk rotation to elongate the intercostals. Lying supine over a ball will also elongate rib cage musculature and assist with decreasing thoracic kyphosis and shoulder protraction (Fig. 20-14). A corner stretch to elongate the pectoralis major is often indicated. Stretches to target the quadratus lumborum, latissimus dorsi, and rectus abdominis may also be indicated. The therapist must not forget to address the lower-extremity muscles that have attachments into the pelvis. The position of the pelvis will affect the thoracic muscles that have attachments on the pelvis and will thus affect posture and breathing. For example, decreased extensibility in the hamstrings may lead to a posterior pelvic tilt which will increase kyphosis.

### Strength

In pediatrics, strengthening exercises should utilize the child's own body and gravity for resistance. To target muscles noted to be weak during the examination, play games that involve upper-extremity weight bearing (e.g., wheelbarrow walking or crab walking), lower-extremity weight bearing (e.g., squat to stand to retrieve toys, hopping, jumping), and dynamic trunk stabilization (e.g., reaching for toys while seated on a

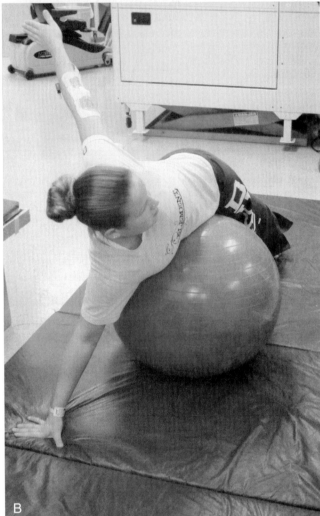

**Figure 20-15 A,** Core stabilization exercise with legs supported by ball. **B,** Trunk rotation over a ball (can reach for toys).

therapy ball, prone on therapy ball and walking hands out until only feet are on the ball [Fig. 20-15A]). Spinal extension exercises should also be included to strengthen the spinal extensors and scapular retractors. These muscles are often in an overlengthened, and thus weakened, position in the child with cardiac or pulmonary disorders. Traditional Thera-Band and prone activities can easily be modified by using prone-over-a-therapy-ball and reaching activities to achieve spinal extension and shoulder retraction (Fig. 20-15B).

The therapist should also remember to strengthen the muscles of inspiration. An inspiratory muscle trainer may be used in pediatric patients that are able to follow directions. This is a device with variable resistance to inspiration. There are many different treatment protocols suggested in the literature for inspiratory muscle training. One study found that an effective treatment protocol for adults with chronic obstructive pulmonary disease is to use an inspiratory muscle trainer at 40% to 50% of their maximal inspiratory pressure for 30 minutes per day, 5 times a week, for 5 consecutive weeks.[25] However, no studies have determined the best treatment protocol for children. The therapist should evaluate each child individually to determine if inspiratory muscle training may benefit him/her.

## Posture

A child's posture is affected by the child's muscle flexibility, strength, and thoracic mobility. Therefore, addressing the items discussed earlier in this chapter will have an indirect effect on the child's posture. In addition to these techniques, the therapist can use a mirror during therapy to provide visual feedback to the child regarding his/her posture. Manual facilitation of the spinal extensors during standing and sitting are also effective. Postural training should be incorporated into the child's daily activities so that there is greater carryover of the postural changes when the child is not in therapy.

For the child with neuromuscular weakness, one must also consider the child's posture in the stroller, car seat, or wheelchair. It is important to make sure that the child is supported in proper alignment so as to prevent or delay the onset of scoliosis or other thoracic deformities. Temporarily, blanket rolls and pillows can be used to aid in supporting the child. However, if there is weakness or increased tone that is expected to be long standing, adaptive equipment may be necessary.

## Breathing Pattern

As stated previously, the child (beginning around age 2 years) should demonstrate little to no activation of accessory muscles during quiet breathing. Children who have had difficulty breathing for a long time have learned to overuse their accessory muscles. Some children also learn to breathe shallowly and use accessory muscles to decrease thoracic expansion secondary to pain from an incision. In both instances, the therapist has a responsibility to train the diaphragm and intercostals to be the prime muscles of inspiration.

In young children who have not practiced their inefficient breathing pattern for very long, visual cueing may be enough to encourage diaphragmatic breathing. With the child supine, place a stuffed animal on the child's abdomen. Tell the child to take the animal for a ride by making it go up every time the child takes a breath in. In the older child, manual facilitation techniques, such as a quick stretch and tactile cueing of

the diaphragm and intercostal muscles, may be necessary. Another technique is to inhibit the accessory muscles during inhalation. This should be attempted last as it is a more uncomfortable technique for the child.

Once the proper breathing pattern is obtained in supine, the child should attempt to maintain this pattern while transitioning to sitting. Once the child can maintain the pattern in sitting, attempt it in standing. With each of these progressively harder positions, the child may require repetition of the facilitation techniques. It is important to then incorporate the desired breathing pattern into functional activities. When performing range of motion or strengthening exercises, add breathing as a component to these exercises. Inhalation should be pared with extension and exhalation pared with flexion.

## Airway Clearance Techniques

CPT is otherwise known as bronchial hygiene. CPT traditionally consists of postural drainage, percussion, and vibration. For an in-depth description of all airway clearance techniques and modalities, including postural drainage positions and devices used to provide percussion, refer to Chapter 17. The postural drainage component allows gravity to assist with moving mucus up to larger airways. This typically involves putting the patient in a Trendelenburg position (the head is lower than the hips). In pediatrics, however, Trendelenburg position is not always an appropriate position. The lower esophageal sphincter is not strong enough until 2 years of age to prevent reflux in this position.[26] Therefore, the therapist should never use or recommend Trendelenburg position in children who is younger than 2 years old. Additionally, it has been shown that older children with CF may reflux and silently aspirate with no observable signs.[27] Although other studies show that modified postural drainage positioning (Trendelenburg position with only 20 degrees of head down) is safe to perform with children who have CF, many CF centers in North America and Europe continue to discourage this practice. However, if the child with CF has an intact Nissen fundoplication (thus preventing stomach contents from entering the esophagus) Trendelenburg position in fact may be a safe position.

When performing CPT with infants or young children, the child is often more comfortable receiving CPT in the therapist's or parent's arms. Singing songs or reading books during CPT can also improve the child's tolerance of the procedure. This population is also likely to fall asleep during CPT if it is time for a nap. It is preferable for the child to stay awake and perform movement after CPT so as to facilitate a cough or sneeze to clear the airway. However, the sleeping baby does not need to be awakened to attempt facilitating coughing.

## High-Frequency Chest Wall Oscillation

High-frequency chest wall oscillation (HFCWO) is a technique for airway clearance that has been in use since 1988. For this technique, the patient dons a vest that contains an air bladder. There is a generator that attaches to the vest via 1 or 2 hoses, depending on the model used. The generator uses air to inflate the vest and then provides high-frequency bursts of air into the vest. These bursts create shear forces on the chest wall and into the lungs that decrease the viscosity of the mucus and aid in mobilizing the secretions up to larger airways.

There are no guidelines for patient age at initiation of vest use. The vest companies have made very small vests to fit even a 1-year-old with CF. Many CF centers in the United States will wait until a child is closer to 2 years old to begin using the vest. Absolute contraindications for usage of HFCWO include an unstable head, neck, rib cage, or back injury, or an active hemorrhage. Relative contraindications for usage of HFCWO include the following:

- Subcutaneous emphysema
- Recent epidural spinal infusion or spinal anesthesia
- Recent skin grafts, or flaps, on the thorax
- Burns, open wounds, and skin infections of the thorax
- Recently placed transvenous pacemaker or subcutaneous pacemaker
- Suspected pulmonary tuberculosis
- Lung contusion
- Bronchospasm
- Complaint of chest wall pain

### Positive Expiratory Pressure

Positive expiratory pressure (PEP) devices provide a resistance to exhalation. This pressure during exhalation splints open the airways and facilitates mobility of the mucus through the open airways. There are PEP devices that are sold that provide only PEP. However, there are also devices that provide oscillations with the PEP (oscillatory positive expiratory pressure). The Acapella and Flutter are two of these devices. The Flutter uses a steel ball that vibrates inside a cone to provide the oscillations. It requires that the device be held parallel to the floor in order for gravity to apply correct forces on the ball. The Acapella provides oscillations as air passes over a pair of magnets. This device is not gravity dependent and can be performed in any position. Although they produce similar levels of PEP and oscillations, the Acapella may be more effective clinically secondary to ease of use.[28]

For younger children, therapy is always more effective when it is fun or incorporated into a game. Bubble PEP is a method of providing PEP with some oscillations. A container is filled with water to the level of the desired pressure (e.g., 10 cm of water). Suction tubing is cut to place into the container as a straw. The child then blows into the straw and creates bubbles. The water provides the PEP and the bubbles provide the oscillations. If soap is placed in the water, the child will attempt to make the bubbles come out of the top of the container. This provides an incentive to continue to blow. Once the bubbles come out of the container, the child can play with the bubbles and then try to make more bubbles once those are gone.

### Blow Toys

Adults are able to use an incentive spirometer 10 times every hour in order to take deep breaths and keep their lungs clear after surgery or when laying in bed for prolonged periods of time. Children are often not as cooperative with the incentive spirometer. However, there are many toys for children that encourage deep breathing (kazoo, party blower, noisemakers, pinwheels, bubbles). Giving a child a couple of toys to work on blowing can be as effective at encouraging deeper breathing as an incentive spirometer. Playing any blowing games can also be effective. For instance, place a cotton ball in the middle of a table. The child stands on one side and the therapist stands on the other. The person to blow the cotton ball off the table on their opponent's side wins.

### Huffing

Huffing is also referred to as a forced expiratory technique. The child uses low to mid lung volumes to force the mucus into larger airways. As the mucus moves up the airway, the huff becomes more forceful. This technique is designed to move the mucus with less risk of dynamic airway collapse than deep, strong coughing. Huffing should be performed after any airway clearance technique to aid in expectoration of mucus.

### Assisted Cough

When a child does not have a strong cough (common in cases of neuromuscular weakness such as in SMA or muscular dystrophy), secretions may build up in the child's lungs. Parents or caregivers may be instructed in how to assist their child with coughing to increase the force generation. To perform an assisted cough, the therapist places his or her hand on the child's abdomen (just below the diaphragm). The child takes a large breath in and holds it for 1 to 3 seconds. The child then attempts to cough as hard as the child can while the therapist provides compression with an upward thrust in the direction of the diaphragm.

When manually assisted coughing is no longer enough to clear mucus secretions, the therapist may try a cough assist machine (Fig. 20-16). It gradually applies a positive pressure to the airway, then rapidly shifts to negative pressure. The rapid shift in pressure produces a high expiratory flow, simulating a natural cough. The cough assist machine can be used in isolation when a child has mucus to clear in the trachea. Or, it can be used after another form of airway clearance to assist in clearing the loosened mucus.

### Choosing the Most Appropriate Airway Clearance Technique

New therapists are often overwhelmed with the options for airway clearance. The best choice for airway clearance varies on the individual patient circumstances. For instance, if the child has a floppy or reactive airway, a form of PEP may aide

## Table 20-5 Guidelines to Aid in Choosing an Airway Clearance Technique That is Right for a Particular Patient

| Technique | Appropriate Age Groups | Chronic Respiratory Diagnosis | Acute Respiratory Diagnosis | Able To Target One Specific Lobe | Amount of Patient Participation | Ease of Parental Education | Patient Expense |
|---|---|---|---|---|---|---|---|
| CPT | All | Not as only method | X | Yes | None | Moderate | 0 |
| Acapella/ Flutter | ≥6* | X | X | No | Moderate | Moderate | $$ |
| Bubble PEP | ≥3* | | X | No | Moderate | Easy | $ |
| Vest | ≥2* | X | Only in hospital | No | None/ minimal | Easy | $$$$ |
| Autogenic Drainage | ≥12* | X | | No | Max | Hard | 0 |
| Huffing | ≥4* | After an above method | After an above method | No | Moderate | Moderate | 0 |
| Exercise | ≥2* | X | X | No | Max | Mod | 0 |

*These ages are estimates. Every patient will be different and techniques should be tried before including or excluding them from the treatment protocol.*

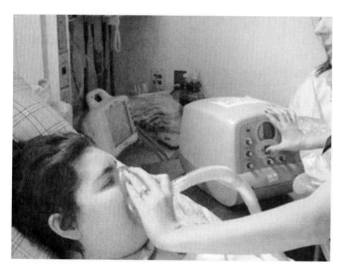

**Figure 20-16** Cough assist.

**Clinical Tip**
When a child presents with increased tone, the muscles of the thorax are also affected. Utilizing methods to reduce tone allows the child to breathe more easily and also allows the therapist to use manual techniques to facilitate proper breathing mechanics. Various tone-inhibiting techniques may be used including positioning the child in flexion in his or her extremities and trunk, rhythmic rocking, dissociating extremities, and decreased external stimulation (loud noises, bright lights, television, siblings, etc.).

in keeping the airway open during mobilization of the mucus. The best plan for home airway clearance is always to give the child and family options. Families should know how to use a few techniques and choose the most appropriate one to fit into their current life situation. For further guidance in choosing the most appropriate airway clearance technique, refer to Table 20-5.

## Functional Mobility

Following surgery (e.g., corrective heart surgery, palliative heart surgery, or a heart or lung transplantation), it is important to get the child out of bed and moving again as quickly as possible. This aids in decreasing cardiopulmonary complications after surgery such as pneumonia and deep vein thrombosis. Children are often afraid to move after surgery. Medical play dolls can help children cope with experiences. It helps many children if they can do the desired activity with a doll first. If the doll has success, they are more willing to try. Rewards are another way to motivate a sick child to move. Have the child walk for a scavenger hunt or to a treasure box. Children also learn to be afraid of medical professionals. It might make them feel better to have a family member assist them in getting out of bed while the therapist directs the transfer from a safe distance away.

Assistive devices should be used as needed to increase mobility. However, attention must be paid to the child's posture during mobility with an assistive device. The tendency is to lean forward with increased kyphosis and protracted shoulders when ambulating with a walker after surgery. If the child has any lifting, pushing, or pulling restrictions after surgery, a walker with upper extremity weight bearing may be contraindicated. The therapist should be aware of each patient's postoperative precautions prior to therapy.

An infant must also return to age appropriate functional activities after surgery. Initially, the therapist needs to focus on helping the infant bring his/her extremities to midline for self calming. If the baby is small enough, the therapist may instruct the family in how to swaddle their child with the baby's hands near the face. If the baby is too large to swaddle, large boundaries may be placed under the upper and lower extremities to facilitate shoulder protraction, hands to midline/mouth, and hip flexion.

Once the baby demonstrates the ability to maintain a quiet alert state, more active developmental activities may be facilitated. Tasks should be geared toward the impairments noted in the examination. With the use of positioning and the support of equipment or the therapist's hands, tasks can be made more or less challenging for the infant. For instance, one child may need full trunk and upper-extremity support from the therapist in order to hold his or her head upright in sitting. Another child may need a large blanket roll or boppy around his or her trunk in order to sit. And another baby may only need occasional tactile cueing of the abdominal muscles to maintain upright sitting balance.

Different surgeons will have different guidelines regarding prone positioning after surgery. The therapist should be familiar with the precautions that the baby's physicians have regarding the appropriate time to resume prone activities. Once the baby has been cleared to be on his or her belly, the baby will tolerate it better if placed prone on the therapist's chest with the therapist sitting upright. As the infant is able to lift his or her head more easily in this position, the therapist can begin to recline gradually. Once the baby tolerates prone on the therapist's (or parent's) chest with the therapist supine, the baby is ready to try prone on a mat. A rolled baby blanket placed under the infant at the level of the axial may also help the baby tolerate being prone more easily.

## Cardiovascular/Endurance Training

The principles of endurance training are the same for children as they are for adults. The therapist should monitor heart rate, oxygen saturation, rating of perceived exertion, and dyspnea on exertion throughout the activity. Activity should be gradually increased over time as the child tolerates it. Box 20-3 lists indications to stop exercise. Patients and their parents should be educated regarding these indications prior to discharge. There are many potential goals for this type of training. The therapist and child may have a goal to increase the distance that the child is able to ambulate without a rest so that the child can go to the mall with his or her friends. Other goals may include increasing the length of time between breaks, increasing the overall time of exercise, decreasing the amount of supplemental oxygen needed for a given activity, decrease rating of perceived exertion for a given task, or increasing the intensity of the task. Once again, performing activities that the child is interested in will

---

> **Box 20-3**
>
> ### When to Stop Exercise
>
> If the child has any of these signs or symptoms, stop exercise and rest. Attempt a lower intensity or duration during the next exercise session.
> - Chest pain or discomfort
> - Rating of perceived exertion greater than 17
> - Dyspnea of 4
> - Dizziness
> - Visual changes
> - Pale or ashen appearance
> - New-onset joint pain
> - Heart rate greater than 80% of maximal heart rate
> - Oxygen saturation fall below 90% (in some cases the physician will indicate that it is OK for the child to exercise with lower oxygen saturation)

---

increase adherence to a home program. Activities to consider for cardiovascular training with the pediatric population include bike riding, Dance Dance Revolution, jumping rope, obstacle courses, and playing tag.

## Treatment in the Early Intervention Setting

Under the *Individuals with Disabilities Education Improvement Act* (IDEIA) of 2004 (Public Law 108–446) Part C, multidisciplinary services including physical therapy are provided to children ages 0 to 3 years old, who are deemed developmentally delayed.[7] The early intervention (EI) physical therapy services are most often provided in the child's "natural environment." Natural environments are defined as settings that are natural or normal for the child's age peers who have no disabilities. There are variations of the implementation of these services from state to state; however, EI physical therapy is typically provided in the child's home or daycare center. Although the model for physical therapy care under IDEIA is educationally based, the physical therapist must be mindful of the cardiopulmonary implications of the child's response to physical therapy intervention as well as the cardiopulmonary aspects of care the child requires.

Special consideration should be made in postoperative cardiac surgical cases, where prone precautions may persist for weeks or months. It is essential to clarify with the child's pediatrician and/or cardiac specialist what positional precautions may exist and their duration. With clearance from the physician, positional education will be of the utmost help to the child and family. Positions should be encouraged that support neutral alignment, comfort, and protection of the medical precautions. Once the child with cardiac involvement is medically cleared for all positions and movements, the child should be gradually introduced to the prone position under supervision. A positive, gradual reentry to prone is critical, as the child may have an aversive response to the position. Because the developmental progression of skills often stems from the prone position, it is ideal for the child to associate prone with positive contributors such as play, mom's face, music, sibling interaction, and the like.

When working children in the EI setting who have a history of cardiopulmonary involvement, it is prudent to take vital signs intermittently so as to monitor their response to physical therapy intervention.

EI therapists often work in settings, such as a child's home, the park, a daycare center, or other community settings, that are nonmedical in nature and not necessarily prepared for cardiovascular-related emergencies. It is prudent to have prepared an action plan in the event of a child having an acute cardiac or pulmonary episode during an EI physical therapy session.

---

## CASE STUDY 20-1

Nate is a 3-year-old boy with a diagnosis of asthma. He has a history of prematurity (born at 26 weeks' gestation) and respiratory distress syndrome. He was on a ventilator for the first 2 weeks of his life and on oxygen via nasal cannula for a week after that. He went to his pediatrician a week ago because of increased work of breathing. At that time, he was prescribed albuterol via a nebulizer twice a day. Two days later, he was admitted to Duke University Medical Center's pediatric intensive care unit (PICU) in severe respiratory distress and placed on continuous albuterol blended with oxygen. He spent 4 days in PICU and was then transferred out to the step down unit on albuterol every 2 hours. His oxygen saturation was 97% on 1 L of oxygen. Physical therapy was then consulted for airway clearance.

- How does asthma affect the lungs (what is the pathophysiology)?

- How will chest physical therapy affect Nate's lungs?
- How does albuterol affect Nate's lungs?
- Why do you think Nate has asthma?
- What other evaluative techniques would you perform?
- What airway clearance techniques and therapeutic procedures would be beneficial for Nate and in what order would you perform them? Why would you choose those treatment interventions?
- What are your short-term and long-term goals for Nate?
- How might your intervention change when Nate is 10 years old? In what ways will it be the same?
- How would your intervention be different if Nate were 10 months old?
- What role should Nate's parents have in his treatments if any? Why? How would you accomplish that?

---

## Summary

Treatment of the child is complex and involves consideration of various systems, including the cardiopulmonary system. Physical therapy management of the child with cardiac and/ or pulmonary disorders uses many of the same guidelines and principles as management of the adult patient. However, there are also many ways in which the care of these children is different and requires specialized knowledge. Below are important points to remember about respiratory and cardiac development and the treatment of children with cardiopulmonary compromise:

- Lung buds are present by week 5, and the heart beats by day 22 to 23 of gestation.
- The cunicular period occurs during the sixteenth to twenty-sixth week of gestation. It is possible for a fetus born at the end of this period to survive because lung tissue is vascularized, and gas exchange can take place.
- Fetal circulation is different than postnatal circulation. In fetal circulation, most of the blood bypasses the lungs and goes directly to the left ventricle via the foramen ovale or ductus arteriosus because oxygenated blood comes from the mother thru the umbilical cord.
- The ductus arteriosus typically closes after birth, once prostaglandin $E_1$ production is signaled to decrease. A

ductus arteriosus that does not close is called a *patent ductus arteriosus*.

- CHDs can be described as cyanotic or acyanotic. Oxygen saturation levels are normal in acyanotic lesions, whereas, arterial oxygen saturation levels are decreased in cyanotic lesions.
- Apnea of prematurity is a relatively common disorder in children born at less than 37 weeks' gestation.
- National Institutes of Health developed a campaign to reduce the occurrence of SIDS in 1994. Their current recommendations include placing babies to sleep only in the supine position (not side lying or prone). It is important to also encourage daily supervised prone time ("tummy time") for optimal development in babies.
- A child's decreased activity level or impairments to breathing mechanics may be caused by muscle weakness, muscle tone problems such as hypertonicity or hypotonicity, motor planning deficits, motor learning deficits, and medical fragility.
- When treating a child with CF, the therapist must be sure to take into account the already demanding home treatment program. The therapist must work with each child and family to determine how best to fit airway clearance and exercise into the patient and family's busy schedules.

- The child's resting position in the acute care setting after a cardiac surgery is typically gravity dependent (hip flexion, abduction, and external rotation; knee flexion, ankle plantarflexion, and shoulder abduction; external rotation; and retraction). This position leads to decreased extensibility and range of motion in the extremities, which, in turn, may slow the return to age-appropriate functional activities as the child's medical condition improves. This position tends to persist in some fashion in the outpatient setting as well.
- The ribs and spine of the child with cardiac or pulmonary disorders can often lose mobility secondary to prolonged immobility, guarding of the postural muscles, overuse of accessory muscles during breathing, scar tissue formation, or shallow breathing.
- Strength may be assessed by the child's ability to hold his or her head upright against gravity, reach for a toy while in supine position, lift lower extremities off the surface, ambulate, ascend/descend stairs, squat to stand, sit on the floor to stand, or reach overhead for a toy.
- Gentle rib cage mobilizations may be performed with the child in supine, prone, or side-lying position. The therapist must be very cautious with rib mobilizations on children who have osteopenia.
- It is important to assess the extensibility of muscles that affect the rib cage such as the intercostals, pectoralis major quadratus lumborum, latissimus dorsi, rectus abdominis, and hamstrings, and elongate any muscles with decreased extensibility.
- Strengthening exercises should utilize the child's own body and gravity for resistance, such as upper-/lower-extremity weight bearing and dynamic trunk stabilization.
- For the child with hypotonia or hypertonia, consider the child's posture in the stroller, car seat, or wheelchair. If the issue with tone is expected to be long standing, adaptive equipment may be necessary.
- The therapist can retrain muscles of inspiration by utilizing manual facilitation techniques, such as a quick stretch and tactile cueing of the diaphragm and intercostal muscles.
- Airway clearance in the child may utilize a variety of techniques, including bronchial hygiene, high-frequency chest wall oscillation, PEP, blowing toys, huffing, and assisted coughing.
- A medical play doll or parents can be helpful when assisting a child with functional mobility after surgery.
- Activities to consider for cardiovascular training with the pediatric population include bike riding, Dance Dance Revolution, jumping rope, obstacle courses, and playing tag.
- EI therapists often work in settings such as a child's home, the park, a daycare center, or other community setting. It is prudent to have prepared an action plan in the event of a child having an acute cardiac or pulmonary episode during an EI physical therapy session.
- When treating a child with cardiopulmonary compromise, it is important to remember to treat the entire child, including the psychosocial aspects and the environment in which the child lives.

## References

1. Moore KL. Before We Are Born: Essentials of Embryology and Birth Defects. 5th ed. Philadelphia, Saunders, 1998.
2. Moore KL, Persaud TVN. The Developing Human. 7th ed. Philadelphia, Saunders, 2003.
3. Sadowski HS. Congenital cardiac disease in the newborn infant: Past, present, and future. Crit Care Nurs Clin North Am 21(1):37–8, 2009.
4. Noonan J. Syndromes Associated with Cardiac Defects. Philadelphia, FA Davis, 1981.
5. Case-Smith J, O'Brien J. Occupational Therapy for Children. 6th ed. St. Louis, Mosby, 2010.
6. Mosby's Dictionary of Medicine, Nursing, and Health Professions. 8th ed. St. Louis, Mosby, 2008.
7. Campbell S, Linden DW, Palisano R. Physical Therapy for Children. 3rd ed. St. Louis, Saunders, 2006.
8. Des Jardins TR, Burton GG. Clinical Manifestations and Assessment of Respiratory Disease. St. Louis, Mosby, 2006.
9. Smith LJ, van Asperen PP, McKay KO, et al. Reduced exercise capacity in children born very preterm. Pediatrics 122:e287–93, 2008.
10. Irwin S, Tecklin J. Cardiopulmonary Physical Therapy. St. Louis, Elsevier, 2004.
11. Jeng SF, Hsu CH, Tsao PN, et al. Bronchopulmonary dysplasia predicts adverse developmental and clinical outcomes in very-low-birthweight infants. Dev Med Child Neurol 50:51–7, 2008.
12. Grasso MC, Button BM, Allison DJ, et al. Benefits of music therapy as an adjunct to chest physiotherapy in infants and toddlers with cystic fibrosis. Pediatr Pulmonol 29(5):371–81, 2000.
13. Montella S, Santamaria F, Salvatore M. Lung disease assessment in primary ciliary dyskinesia: A comparison between chest high-field magnetic resonance imaging and high-resolution computed tomography findings. Ital J Pediatr 35:24, 2009.
14. Frownfelter D, Dean E. Cardiovascular and Pulmonary Physical Therapy: Evidence and Practice. 4th ed. St. Louis, Mosby, 2006.
15. Bosch J. Health maintenance throughout the lifespan for individuals with Down syndrome. J Am Acad Nurse Pract 15:5–17, 2003.
16. Barnhart R, Connolly B. Aging and Down syndrome: Implications for physical therapy. Phys Ther 87(10):1399–406, 2007.
17. Hays RM, Jordan RA, McLaughlin JF, et al. Central ventilatory dysfunction in myelodysplasia: an independent determinant of survival. Dev Med Child Neurol. 1989 Jun;31(3):366–70.
18. Swaminathan S, Paton JY, Ward SL, et al. Abnormal control of ventilation in adolescents with myelodysplasia. J Pediatr. 1989 Dec;115(6):898–903.
19. Ward SL, Jacobs RA, Gates EP, et al. Abnormal ventilatory patterns during sleep in infants with myelomeningocele. J Pediatr. 1986 Oct;109(4):631–4.
20. Charney EB, Rorke LB, Sutton LN, et al. Management of Chiari II complications in infants with myelomeningocele. J Pediatr. 1987 Sep;111(3):364–71.
21. Hesz N, Wolraich M. Vocal-cord paralysis and brainstem dysfunction in children with spina bifida. Dev Med Child Neurol. 1985 Aug;27(4):528–31.

22. Oren J, Kelly DH, Todres ID, et al. Respiratory complications in patients with myelodysplasia and Arnold-Chiari malformation. Am J Dis Child. 1986 Mar;140(3):221–4.

23. Massery MP. Chest development as a component of normal motor development: implications for pediatric physical therapists. Pediatr Phys Ther 3(1):3–8, 1991.

24. Hertling D, Kessler RM. Management of Common Musculoskeletal Disorders, Physical Therapy Principles and Methods. 4th ed. Philadelphia, Lippincott Williams & Wilkins, 2006.

25. Ramírez-Sarmiento A, Orozco-Levi M, Güell R, et al. Inspiratory muscle training in patients with chronic obstructive pulmonary disease. Am J Respir Crit Care Med 166:1491–7, 2002.

26. Button BM, Heine RG, Catto-Smith AG, et al. Postural drainage and gastro-oesophageal reflux in infants with cystic fibrosis. Arch Dis Child 76:148–50, 1997.

27. Lannefors L, Button BM, McIlwaine M. Physiotherapy in infants and young children with cystic fibrosis: Current practice and future developments, J R Soc Med 97(Suppl 44):8–25, 2004.

28. Volsko T, Difiore J, Chatburn R. Performance comparison of two oscillating positive expiratory pressure devices: Acapella versus Flutter. Respir Care 48:124–30, 2003.

## CHAPTER 21

# The Lymphatic System

*Harold Merriman*

The crucial role of the often underappreciated lymphatic system in preserving life and fluid homeostasis is increasingly acknowledged. In recent years, there has been a growing interest concerning the lymphatic system at the clinical and basic science research levels. Physical therapy students are now expected to have a basic understanding of the lymphatic system, and physical therapists are treating an increasing number of patients in the clinic with disorders of the lymphatic system such as lymphedema.

The typical vessel of the lymphatic system is similar to the veins of the venous system in terms of its wall structure, the lack of a thick musculature, and the presence of valves; however, important differences do exist, such as the ability of the lymphatic vessel to contract under the control of the autonomic nervous system. The key functions of the lymphatic system are immune defense and transport and drainage of excess fluids, proteins, and cellular debris from the interstitial spaces that are not reabsorbed by the venous system. One can think of the lymphatic system as the "sanitation system" of the body, similar to the sanitation system of a city. Along with the lymphatic system's key function of "waste material" disposal, it also plays a crucial role in maintaining proper fluid levels in the blood capillaries at the microcirculatory level, as well as facilitating optimal fluid balance in the entire body. If proper fluid balance is not maintained, then chronic impairment of the lymphatic system can lead to pathologies such as lymphedema, or to even more complicated combination forms such as phlebolymphedema (venous insufficiency leading to lymphedema). Finally, another important characteristic of the lymphatic system is that it is a one-way system that drains into the venous system in contrast to the closed cardiovascular system. Specifically, fluid or "lymph" begins its journey in the lymphatic system at blind or dead-end vessels in the connective tissue near blood capillaries and then completes its journey when it is delivered into the venous system at the venous angles located in the upper thorax near the heart.

Although there have been many advances in diverse fields such as cell and molecular biology (better understanding of how the lymphatic system develops), as well as radiology (improved diagnostic imaging methods) and surgery (minimally invasive surgical approaches), the most effective treatment of lymphatic disorders such as lymphedema still involves conservative treatment that can be provided by specially trained physical therapists. This chapter presents the anatomy and physiology of the lymphatic system, including the pathophysiology of this system (with an emphasis on lymphedema), as well as the medical management and physical therapy interventions available for these pathologies.

## Anatomy and Physiology

The lymphatic system is a one-way system designed to transport lymph through a system of superficial and deep lymph vessels and lymph nodes. Lymph originates from blood plasma that leaves the blood capillaries and enters into the interstitium. The portion of interstitial fluid that then enters the lymphatic system is called *lymph*. Lymph matter consists of proteins, water, fatty acids, and cellular components, such as white blood cells, bacteria, viruses, and other cellular debris. Other tissues and organs of the lymphatic system include lymph nodes, the thymus, bone marrow, spleen, tonsils, and Peyer patches of the small intestine that are involved in the production of lymphocytes, which play a key role in the body's immune function.[1–6]

Lymphatic vessel structure varies and depends on the location of the vessel (Fig. 21-1A). The first and smallest vessel of the lymphatic system is called the *initial lymph vessel* or *lymph capillary* (Fig 21-1B). They are blind or dead-end sacs (tubes) of endothelium that lack valves located near blood capillaries just under the epidermis.[1,6] Because the structure of the initial lymph vessel is larger and more permeable than blood capillaries, some experts prefer to use the term "initial lymphatic sinuses" to describe these lymph vessels.[5] It is important to note that the wall of the initial lymph vessels consists of a single layer of endothelial cells. These endothelial cells in the vessel wall can either completely touch adjacent neighboring endothelial cells forming a tight junction or they may overlap creating an opening (open junctions) or inlet valve for larger substances. The initial lymph vessels are secured to the adjacent connective tissues by anchoring filaments that pull open the endothelial cell junctions as the amount of fluid in the interstitial spaces increases (see Fig 21-1B). When the endothelial cell junctions are open, fluid and macromolecules such as proteins, cellular debris and foreign organisms can enter into the initial lymph vessel where macromolecule-laden fluid is now called *lymph*. Interstitial fluid and macromolecules can also enter the initial lymph vessels as a result of movement and tissue pressure changes caused by muscle contraction, respiration, and treatment using manual lymphatic drainage.[4]

The next larger lymphatic vessels are called *precollectors*; they connect the initial lymph vessels to the lymph collectors. The structure of the precollectors is variable in that

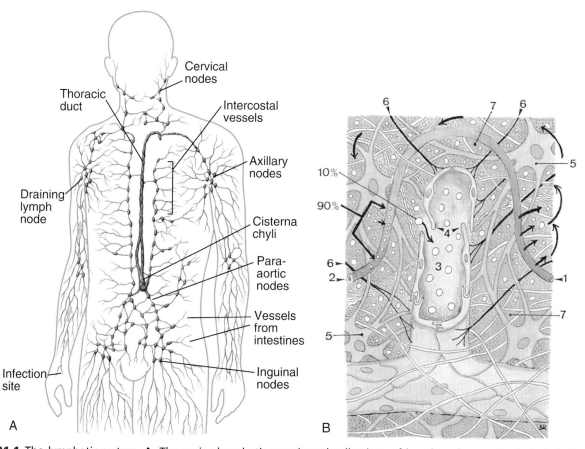

**Figure 21-1** The lymphatic system. **A,** The major lymphatic vessels and collections of lymph nodes are illustrated. Antigens are captured from a site of infection, and the draining lymph node to which these antigens are transported and where the immune response is initiated. From Abbas AK: Cellular and Molecular Immunology, ed 6. Philadelphia, 2010, Saunders. **B,** Incorporation of the lymph capillary into the interstitium. 1, Arterial section of the blood capillary; 2, Venous section of the blood capillary; 3, Lymph capillary; 4, Open intercellular groove-swinging tip; 5, Fibrocyte; 6, Anchor filaments; 7, Intercellular space. Small arrows indicate the direction of blood flow; large arrows indicate the direction of intercellular fluid flow. From Foldi M, Foldi E, Kubik S: Textbook of lymphology for physicians and lymphedema therapists, Munich, 2003, Urban & Fischer Verlag.

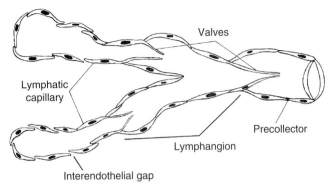

**Figure 21-2** Longitudinal section through an initial lymphatic (lymphatic capillary precollector). Three sets of valves and a lymphangion are shown. Adapted from Guyton AC, Hall JE: Textbook of medical physiology, ed 9, Philadelphia, 1996, WB Saunders, In Irwin S, Tecklin JS. Cardiopulmonary Physical Therapy, ed 4. Philadelphia, 2005, Mosby.

some precollectors are more like the initial lymph vessels, whereas others share properties more characteristic of the larger collectors that have a smooth muscle layer in distinct walls and valves. Precollectors often function as a bridge between the superficial initial lymph vessels and the deeper lymphatic vessels.

Larger lymphatic vessels are called *lymph collectors* or more simply *collectors*. The collectors roughly follow the path of the deep arteries and veins and transport lymph to the lymph nodes and the even larger lymphatic trunks. The diameter of the collectors varies between 0.1 mm and 0.6 mm and contains valves spaced from 0.6 cm to 2.0 cm apart.[3,6] The collector wall resembles the vein wall and is composed of three layers: the inner layer (intima), which consists of endothelial cells anchored to basement membrane, the middle layer (media), which is made up of smooth muscle and elastic tissue, and the outer layer (adventitia), formed by collagen fibers, that is loosely anchored to the extravascular connective tissue.[5] The adventitia also contains the blood vessels and nerves that are important to the function of the collector. The *lymphangion* is the name given to the functional unit of the collectors, which is defined as the part of the collector located between two valves (Fig. 21-2). It is important to note that the lymphangions contract under control of the autonomic nervous system and have a resting frequency of 10 to 12 contractions per minute (lymphangiomotoricity).

The largest lymphatic vessels are called *lymphatic trunks* and have the same wall structure as the collectors, but with a thicker smooth muscle layer. The valves in the trunks can be spaced up to 10 cm apart and the contraction of the lymphatic trunks (like the collectors) is under the control of the sympathetic nervous system. Some of the better known trunks are the lumbar, jugular, supraclavicular, and subclavian trunks. The most important trunks are the right lymphatic duct and the thoracic duct, which drain the lymph into the venous system at the right and left venous angles, respectively. The right lymphatic duct drains approximately

one-fourth of body's lymph, and specifically is responsible for draining mainly the right arm and right head. The thoracic duct is the largest lymph vessel of the body and drains those areas not drained by the right lymphatic duct, namely the left arm, left head, and both legs (Fig. 21-3).

There are approximately 600 to 700 lymph nodes concentrated in the neck, axilla, chest, abdomen, and groin (Fig. 21-4). A group of lymph nodes may drain lymph from several adjacent areas. Lymph nodes range in size (longitudinal diameter) from 0.2 mm to 30 mm. Each lymph node is surrounded by a fibrous capsule consisting of collagen and elastic fibers, which also contains smooth muscle fibers that under certain circumstances can contract under neural stimulation. There is an extensive blood supply present in each lymph node. Lymph nodes have the following functions: (1) filter harmful material such as bacteria, viruses, and cancer cells, (2) being involved in immune surveillance using T and B lymphocytes, and (3) concentrate lymph as lymph enters the lymph node via afferent lymph collectors and exits the lymph node via efferent lymph collectors.[1,5,6]

---

**Clinical Tip**
When treating a patient with manual lymph drainage strokes, the therapist needs to understand which lymph nodes are intact and which ones are impaired or have been removed in order to effectively treat the lymphedema patient.

---

The body is separated into specific regions of lymph drainage called *lymphotomes*, which are separated by watersheds that have relatively few lymph collectors. For example, there is a sagittal watershed that divides the head, neck, and trunk into two equal halves and an upper and lower horizontal watershed that further divides the body into quadrants (Fig. 21-5).[1,6] Because the lymphatic connections are sparse across watersheds, the normal pattern of lymph flow in areas on either side of the watershed is in different directions. For example, because of these watersheds, lymph will normally flow from the right and left breasts to the right and left axillary lymph nodes, respectively. A very important strategy that can be used by the therapist to reduce lymphedema in a particular region is to utilize the few lymph vessels that do cross the watersheds during treatment using manual lymph drainage. This strategy facilitates the movement of lymphedema away from edematous areas, and over time may encourage the formation of new collateral lymph vessels across these watersheds. As the new collateral lymph vessels are formed across the watersheds, further reduction of lymphedema in the affected region can be obtained.[4]

In 1896, the physiologist Ernest Henry Starling formulated a hypothesis describing the various pressures that cause a salt solution to move between a blood capillary and the surrounding tissue. Later, this hypothesis became to be known as the Starling law of capillaries or simply Starling equilibrium or law.[7] The Starling law specifically describes how fluid leaves and enters the semipermeable blood capillaries and

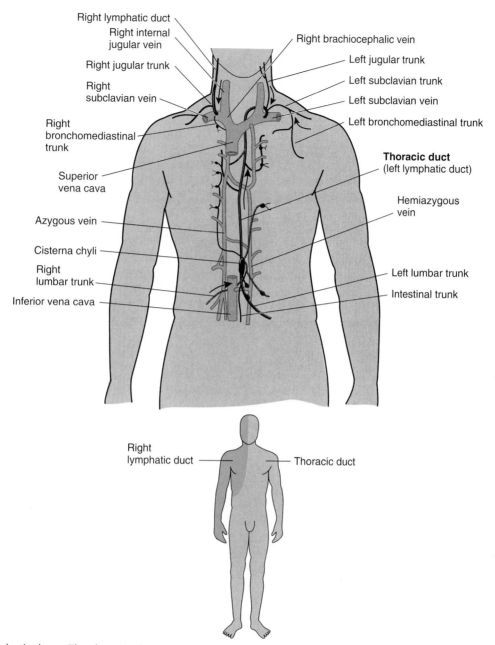

**Figure 21-3** Lymphatic ducts. The thoracic duct (black), leading from the cisterna chyli to discharge into the left subclavian vein, in the neck. (The blood vessels are a lighter shade.) The right lymphatic duct is also shown (see figure on bottom). This carries far less lymph than the thoracic duct, draining mainly the right arm and head, the heart and lungs, and the anterior chest wall. These two main trunks sometimes are linked by large collateral lymphatics. (From Casley-Smith JR, Casley-Smith JR: Modern treatment for lymphoedema, ed 5, Adelaide, Australia, 1997, Lymphoedema Association of Australia.)

surrounding tissues spaces (interstitium). A key principle of the Starling law is osmosis, referring to the net diffusion of water across a semipermeable membrane such as the blood capillary wall.

The four pressures of the Starling law that determine the net flow of fluid into or out of the blood capillaries and interstitium are (1) plasma hydrostatic pressure—the pressure inside the capillaries that is higher on the arterial side and causes fluid to leave the capillary and enter the interstitium (filtration) in contrast to lower pressure on the venous side that causes fluid to leave the interstitium and reenter the capillary (reabsorption); (2) plasma colloidal osmotic pressure—the pressure caused by proteins in the capillaries that results in water being attracted and pulled into the capillary (reabsorption); (3) interstitial fluid hydrostatic pressure—the pressure in the interstitium that can be positive (supports reabsorption of fluid into the blood capillary), negative (less than atmospheric pressure and supports filtration of fluid out of the blood capillary), or near zero; and (4) interstitial colloidal osmotic pressure—the pressure caused by proteins present in the interstitium that results in water being attracted and pulled into the interstitium (filtration).

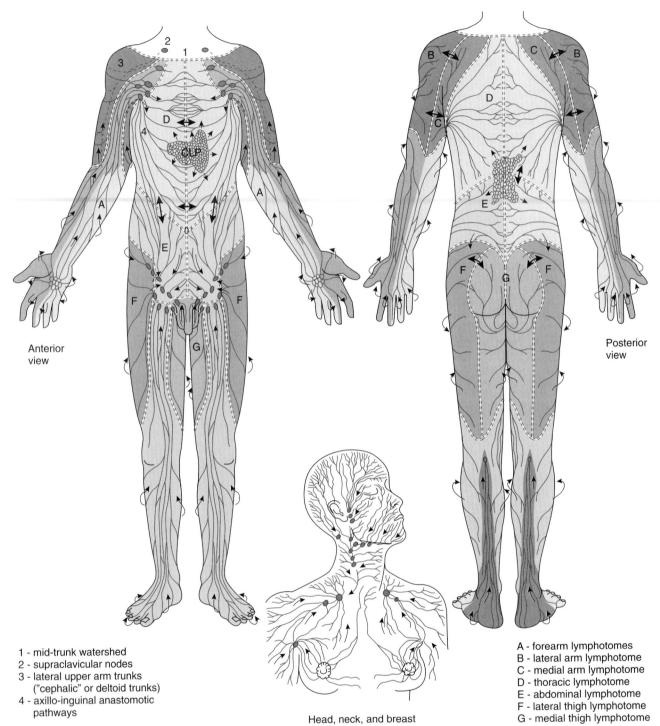

Anterior view

Posterior view

Head, neck, and breast

1 - mid-trunk watershed
2 - supraclavicular nodes
3 - lateral upper arm trunks
    ("cephalic" or deltoid trunks)
4 - axillo-inguinal anastomotic
    pathways

A - forearm lymphotomes
B - lateral arm lymphotome
C - medial arm lymphotome
D - thoracic lymphotome
E - abdominal lymphotome
F - lateral thigh lymphotome
G - medial thigh lymphotome

**Figure 21-4** Regional lymphatic system. The dermal and subcutaneous lymph territories (lymphotomes are indicated by different shadings) of the lymphatic system are separated by watersheds marked by (= = = =). Arrows indicate the direction of the lymph flow. Normal drainage is away from the watershed, but collaterals cross the watershed (thick double arrows). When the main drainage paths from each of these regions are blocked, lymph (thick single arrows) has to be carried across the watersheds via collaterals and the plexuses. The cutaneous lymphatic plexus (CLP) is shown in the center of the chest only. It is filled from the tissues and covers the entire body; this is not shown to avoid confusion. These initial lymphatics fill superficial collectors, which drain into deep ones and then into the lymphatic trunks (small arrows). The lymphotome of the external genitals and perineum is shown but unlabeled. From Casley-Smith JR, Casley-Smith JR: Modern treatment for lymphoedema, ed 5, Adelaide, Australia, 1997, Lymphoedema Association of Australia. Modified from Földi M, Kubik S: Lehrbuch der lymphologie fur mediziner und physiotherapeuter mit anhang: praktische linweise fur die physiotherape, Stuttgart, Germany 1989, Gustav Fischer Verlag.

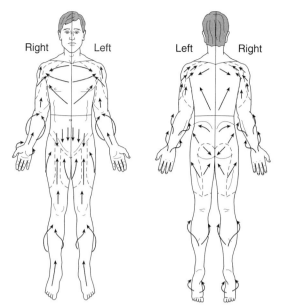

**Figure 21-5** Drawing of body designating lymphotomes, watersheds, and direction of flow. From DeDomenico G: Beard's Massage: Principles and Practice of Soft Tissue Manipulation, ed 5. St Louis, 2008, Saunders.

Right  Left    Left  Right

The combined effect of these four pressures determines how much fluid moves into and stays in the interstitium. Approximately 20 L of fluid (approximately 0.5% of the blood plasma) leaves the nonrenal blood capillaries each day by filtration. Normally, approximately 80% to 90% of this fluid is then reabsorbed back into the blood capillary. With a normally functioning lymphatic system, the rest of the remaining 10% to 20% of fluid (approximately 2 to 4 L/day) is taken up by the lymphatic system and ultimately returned to the venous system.[6]

## Pathophysiology

As already indicated, the lymphatic system is crucial in preserving fluid homeostasis; when fluid homeostasis is disrupted, however, serious complications result. For example, if a person loses blood and is at risk for hypovolemic shock, the lymphatic system (lymphangions) can compensate for up to 25% blood loss by increasing its output (by increasing the amplitude and frequency of lymphangion contraction). Experimental animal models show that if the lymphatic system is blocked and is not allowed to regenerate, the animals will die within a short period of time.[1]

The most common disruption of the lymphatic system is lymphedema. It is estimated that lymphedema affects 140 million to 250 million people worldwide and at least 3 million Americans.[6] In the United States, the highest incidence of lymphedema occurs after breast cancer surgery and treatment, even when using the least-invasive modern treatment techniques. Lymphedema can be described as the inability of the lymphatic system to handle the demands placed on it resulting in an accumulation of protein-rich

edema in the interstitium. The effect of lymphedema is to increase interstitial colloidal osmotic pressure, which results in increased blood capillary filtration and decreased blood capillary reabsorption. If this process is not checked, then the affected body part continues to increase in size. As part of the normal treatment for lymphedema, the external compression provided by compression bandages or garments will reduce an abnormally elevated blood capillary filtration rate and enhance an abnormally low blood capillary reabsorption rate to more normal levels. Thus, external compression is a key factor in restoring out-of-balance microcirculation and helping the affected area(s) return to a more normal size.

To understand how lymphedema develops, it is important to understand how lymph normally flows through a functioning lymphatic system. The maximum ability of the lymphatic system to transport lymph is called the *transport capacity* (TC). Each individual has a defined TC, which can be reduced by factors such as surgery, trauma, infection, or radiation. The amount of lymph that is transported by the lymphatic system is called the *lymphatic load* (LL). In a normal resting situation, the lymphatic system may only be working at approximately 10% of its capacity so that there is an ample functional reserve (FR) to handle the extra demands placed on it. The concept of FR is sometimes also referred to as the "safety valve mechanism."[4]

There are three different types of lymphatic system insufficiences: mechanical, dynamic, and combined (Fig. 21-6).[1,8] Dynamic insufficiency or high-output (volume) insufficiency is the most common insufficiency type and occurs when the LL exceeds the TC, which is functioning at a normal level. This occurs in congestive heart failure, chronic venous insufficiency (stages I and II), immobility, hypoproteinemia, and pregnancy, and results in a pitting edema. It should be stressed that prolonged dynamic insufficiency can damage the lymphatic system, so that the patient with dynamic insufficiency should seek immediate medical help.

Mechanical insufficiency or low-output (volume) insufficiency is caused by an impaired TC. In this case, the LL exceeds the impaired TC, resulting in a protein-rich edema called *lymphedema*. Another possible cause of lymphedema is when the TC is reduced and the LL is abnormally high, resulting in combined insufficiency. This can happen if the patient experiences a prolonged elevated LL, which then damages the lymphatic valves.

As lymphedema develops, the lymphatic vessels dilate making the valves incompetent, resulting in lymphostasis and accumulation of protein-rich edema in the interstitium. The lymphatic system tries to compensate for the increasing protein-rich edema by generating new initial lymphatics, lymph–lymph anastomoses, or collateral lymphatics to bypass the affected edematous areas. If these compensations are unsuccessful, a chronic inflammation develops, leading to a progressive connective tissue fibrosis. The state of chronic infection also leads to a low oxygen state in the lymphedematous areas, thus further compromising the affected tissue.[4]

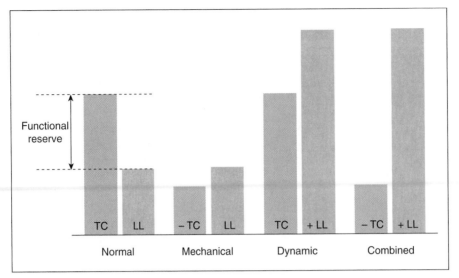

TC, Transport Capacity, LL, Lymphatic Load; –, Decreased; +, Increased

**Figure 21-6** Normal and three types of insufficiencies.

## Excess Weight is Risk Factor for Lymphedema

Another extremely important consideration for the therapist to keep in mind is the connection between excess weight and lymphedema. Not only is obesity and being overweight a risk factor for type 2 diabetes, coronary heart disease, stroke, cancer, and osteoarthritis, but excessive weight is also a consistent risk factor for developing lymphedema in a number of studies.

In a study of stage I and II breast cancer subjects who received radiation and then later developed arm edema (lymphedema), body mass index (BMI) was found to be strongly associated with the frequency of arm edema.[9] Of all of the variables looked at, BMI was also related to increased frequency of severe forms of arm edema. To illustrate this finding, only 2.3% of nonobese subjects, as compared to 9.2% of obese subjects, developed severe arm edema.

Another study looked at the surgical complications associated with sentinel lymph node biopsy in women with early stage breast cancer.[10] The investigators used multivariate logistic analysis with 2904 subjects and found a 7% overall incidence of lymphedema. Although increasing age (grouped by decade) was found to have a positive and significant association with the incidence of lymphedema (p = 0.035), BMI was found to have even a stronger positive association (p < 0.0001). Lymphedema incidence rates were 4.9% for normal subjects (BMI of 18.5 to 24.9), 6.5% for overweight subjects (BMI 25 to 29.9), 9.8% for obese subjects (BMI 30 to 49.9), and 21.7% for morbidly obese subjects (BMI ≥ 50).

Petrek and associates investigated the incidence of lymphedema 20 years after the women had been diagnosed with breast carcinoma and consecutively treated with mastectomy and complete axillary dissection.[11] They looked at 15 potential predictive factors for developing lymphedema and found that only 2 factors were statistically significant for predicting lymphedema: arm infection/injury (p < 0.001) and weight gain since operation (p = 0.02). They also found that women who were overweight when diagnosed with breast carcinoma also had an increased risk of developing lymphedema.

Clearly, the literature supports that being overweight or obese is a risk factor for developing lymphedema in breast cancer patients. Thus, physical therapists should keep in mind that a healthy lifestyle and a normal weight can help to prevent lymphedema in at-risk patients.

## The Role of the Lymphatic System in the Cardiovascular System and in Cardiovascular Disease

The myocardium is populated with a high number of initial lymph vessels that lead to lymph precollectors and collectors. Eventually this lymph is funneled through the cardiac lymph node and enters the thoracic duct. As is true for fluid homeostasis in other body tissues, fluid homeostasis in the intramyocardium is also dependent on a balance of fluid filtration and reabsorption involving the blood vessels, as well as fluid flow into the myocardial lymphatic vessels. In one study using dogs, disruption of the cardiac lymphatic system resulted in electrophysiologic changes in the heart. These changes included decreased impulse conduction and formation that resembled human sick sinus syndrome.[12]

It is important to note that the regular contractions of the heart and the regular extracardiac thoracic movements play a key role in myocardium fluid movement. In fact, the myocardial lymphatic system is the primary pathway for removing excess myocardial interstitial fluid. When a patient's heart is arrested during surgery (such as cardiopulmonary bypass during coronary artery bypass graft [CABG] surgery), myocardial edema results. Thus, a properly functioning myocardial lymphatic system promoted by strong heart contractility is crucial during the postoperative recovery phase of the CABG patient.[13,14]

The role of the lymphatic system in the pathogenesis of cardiovascular disease is becoming better understood. It is well known that inflammation and fibrosis occurs when the lymphatic system is not working properly, but it is a less-appreciated fact that these same processes may play a crucial role during the formation of atherosclerosis in the vascular wall.[15]

The presence of lipoprotein in the vascular wall is now considered to be an independent risk factor of atherosclerosis. One theory is that the lymphatics in the vascular wall help determine the progression of atherosclerosis in that they can regulate the time that the arterial intima is exposed to atherogenic lipoproteins. If the lymphatic system is not working properly, then filtration of lipoproteins will take longer, thus raising the risk of oxidative damage and entrapment within the vessel wall.[16] Another possible key contribution of properly functioning lymphatics is in the epicardial arteries, which in contrast to the heart's intramural arteries, exhibit the highest rates of atherosclerosis. The free flow of lymph in the epicardial lymphatics is particularly dependent on the extracardiac motion of the thoracic cavity as lymph flow in these lymphatics is reduced by regular contractions of the heart. Factors such as a sedentary lifestyle, decreased vital capacity, and obesity reduces this thoracic cavity motion and thus may contribute to the formation of atherosclerosis via reduced lymphatic function.

Animal studies show the crucial nature of myocardial lymph flow during a myocardial infarction (MI). Some enzyme markers of MI (e.g., creatine kinase) are found in higher concentrations in cardiac lymph as opposed to venous serum in the hours after an MI. Despite lymph flow increases of greater than 50%, persistent edema in the interstitial and vascular spaces develops in animal models in which an MI is induced. Studies in both mice and human cadavers show that ischemic injury leads to the development of vascular fibrosis, resulting in obstruction of lymph flow, which then compromises cardiac output.[17,18] Studies in animals and humans indicate that if a MI is treated quickly (within 6 hours of chest pain) with hyaluronidase, an enzyme known to increase the formation and flow of lymph (i.e., lymphagogue), then beneficial results such as a significant increase in cardiac lymph flow and a reduction in cardiac edema are achieved, which can hasten functional recovery.[19-21] Further studies are needed to better define the role of the lymphatic system in the development of cardiovascular disease.

## Medical Management

Along with the many advances made in our understanding of the lymphatic system and lymphedema in the 20th century, much additional progress has been made in recent years concerning the diagnosis and management of disorders of the lymphatic system such as lymphedema. This is evidenced by the preferred practice pattern (6H: Impaired Circulation and

---

**Box 21-1**

### Lymphedema and Preferred Practice Patterns

**7A:** Primary Prevention/Risk Reduction for Integumentary Disorders

**7B:** Impaired Integumentary Integrity Associated with Superficial Skin Involvement

**7C:** Impaired Integumentary Integrity Associated with Partial-Thickness Skin Involvement and Scar Formation

**7D:** Impaired Integumentary Integrity Associated with Full-Thickness Skin Involvement and Scar Formation

**7E:** Impaired Integumentary Integrity Associated with Skin Involvement Extending into Fascia, Muscle, or Bone and Scar Formation

**6H:** Impaired Circulation and Anthropometric Dimensions Associated with Lymphatic System Disorders

**6B:** Impaired Aerobic Capacity/Endurance Associated with Deconditioning

**4B:** Impaired Posture

**4D:** Impaired Joint Mobility, Motor Function, Muscle Performance, and Range of Motion Associated with Connective Tissue Dysfunction

**4E:** Impaired Joint Mobility, Motor Function, Muscle Performance, and Range of Motion Associated with Localized Inflammation

Other practice patterns may be appropriate based on the patient's symptoms and complications.

The lymphatic impairment practice pattern was initially included in the integumentary practice pattern (e.g., 7F: Impaired Anthropometric Dimensions Secondary to Lymphatic System Disorders), but has now been moved to the cardiovascular/pulmonary practice pattern, 6H Impaired Circulation and Anthropometric Dimensions Associated with Lymphatic System Disorders. Although it is true that lymphedema often involves an impaired integumentary system, especially in its combination forms (venous insufficiency and lymphedema, i.e., phlebolymphedema), the lymphatic system structurally has much in common with the cardiovascular system. As mentioned in the main text, obesity (often associated with deconditioning) is a prominent risk factor for lymphedema. Especially in advanced stages of lymphedema, patients often exhibit deficits in posture, functional mobility, joint mobility, motor function, muscle performance, and range of motion.

Adapted from American Physical Therapy Association. Guide to Physical Therapist Practice. 2nd ed. Phys Ther 81:9–744, 2001.

---

Anthropometric Dimensions Associated with Lymphatic System Disorders) according to the *Guide to Physical Therapy Practice.*[22] Box 21-1 provides a more complete discussion of the preferred practice patterns used by physical therapist.

Included among the most notable recent advances made in the area of lymphology are the following:
- Refinements in imaging techniques used to diagnose lymphatic system disorders,
- Molecular and cell biology advances that have identified specific genes involved with lymphatic system development,

- The development of less-invasive surgical techniques, and
- A growing awareness among physicians and therapists of the effectiveness of conservative management techniques.

In this section, both historical and more recent advances that concern the management of the lymphatic with a special emphasis on lymphedema are discussed.

## Diagnosis

Lymphedema is a protein-rich edema that results from a mechanical failure of the lymphatic system. Its major characteristics include nonpitting edema, a positive Stemmer sign in the feet or hands, and occurrence in both sexes. Lymphedema can be divided into two types: primary lymphedema and secondary lymphedema. Although the treatment for both types is very similar, it is important for the therapist to have a thorough understanding of both types because the lymphedema type determines the presentation of the pathology, the needed frequency and duration of treatment, and, often, the treatment prognosis.

Primary lymphedema is believed to result from an abnormally developed lymphatic system that is congenital or heredity although it may take many years to manifest itself. The three types of abnormalities (dysplasia) of the lymphatic systems are (1) hypoplasia—incomplete development (reduced number and size) of lymph vessels, (2) hyperplasia—enlarged diameter of lymph vessels resulting in malfunction of lymph valves, and (3) aplasia—absence of lymph vessels. All three of these dysplasias result in a reduced TC with hypoplasia being the most common form. Primary lymphedema is almost always observed in the lower extremities and involves mostly females, and can be classified based on when in life it is diagnosed. Congenital lymphedema is observed from birth through 2 years. If there is a family history of inheritance it is called *Milroy disease*. The more common form of primary edema manifests itself before age 35 years and is called *lymphedema praecox*, whereas the much rarer form, lymphedema tarda, occurs after the age of 35 years. In many cases there is no known cause for primary lymphedema; however, in some cases heat, puberty, pregnancy, or minor trauma, such as insect bites, infections, sprains, or strains, may be identified.[3,6]

Secondary lymphedema, unlike primary lymphedema, results from a known insult to the lymphatic system that causes a reduced TC. Specific insults to the lymphatic system include surgery, radiation, trauma, tumor growth, infection, chronic venous insufficiency, and artificial (self-induced) lymphedema. The two most common insults to the system include breast cancer surgery and lymphatic filariasis. It should be stressed that the lymphatic system does have some ability to regenerate under certain conditions when it is obstructed or when lymph nodes are surgically removed.[23-25]

Breast cancer surgery is perhaps the best known surgery that involves disruption of the lymph vessels and lymph nodes. The original breast cancer surgery (now rarely performed) is called *radical mastectomy*, which involves removal of the entire breast, the underlying pectoralis major and pectoralis minor muscles, and the axillary lymph nodes. The modified radical mastectomy, which spares the pectoralis muscles and some of the axillary lymph nodes while removing the entire breast, is the preferred form. With the least-invasive form of mastectomy, total (simple) mastectomy, only the breast is removed. Newer techniques such as lumpectomy (removal of only some of the breast and surrounding tissue) and sentinel lymph node biopsy (removal of the first lymph nodes to drain lymph from the breast) reduce, but do not eliminate, the formation of lymphedema.[3,6,10,26]

The most common worldwide nonsurgical cause of lymphedema is lymphatic filariasis, which is a tropical disease. This disease is transmitted by mosquitoes infected by nematode that lives in the lymphatic system and often results in severe forms of lymphedema.

An important concept to understand is the "limb at risk," which is the extremity closest to a disrupted lymph vessel or lymph node. Each person who has a disruption of the lymphatic system is "at risk" for developing lymphedema, although because each person has a unique pattern of lymph vessels in their lymphatic system and some individuals are better able than others to compensate for a given lymphatic system insult, not every person "at risk" will develop lymphedema. However, at present it is not possible to predict in advance who will develop lymphedema. Despite the variability in suggested lymphedema precautions, it is very important that all individuals "at risk" carefully follow these precautions as do those individuals who have lymphedema (Box 21-2).[2,6,27]

Lymphedema is a progressive condition that can be staged according to its severity. Several different scales can be used, but the one developed by Földi is often used (Table 21-1).[28] The timing of each stage varies considerably from patient to patient with lymphedema. Each stage may last many months to years, and initial stage 0 may last a particularly long time. Stage 0 is a clinically edema-free latent stage that can also be called subclinical lymphedema. In this stage there is no swelling and the tissues look "normal," but the TC is reduced. Stage 1, or the reversible stage, is characterized by tissue that has little if any fibrotic changes but does have pitting edema that resolves or is reduced with elevation. Stage 2, or the spontaneously irreversible stage, is characterized by a brawny nonpitting edema that does not reverse with elevation (Fig. 21-7). In this stage, the connective tissue is chronically inflamed and fibrotic. This results in a positive Stemmer sign, which means that the skin present at the dorsal base of the second toe or finger cannot be easily lifted away from the bone (Fig. 21-8).[29] Stage 3, or elephantiasis, is the most severe form of lymphedema and is characterized by extensive amounts of lymphedema and fibrosis along with abnormal skin changes such as papillomas, deep skinfolds, and mycotic infections (Fig. 21-9).

A complete physical examination, including patient history and symptoms, is typically the gold standard for the properly trained examiner to diagnose lymphedema. However,

## Box 21-2

### Lymphedema Prevention (How to Reduce Risk)

These guidelines should be followed by those who have undergone lymph node removal and/or radiation therapy as they are at greater risk for developing lymphedema, which may take months or years to develop. The prevention strategies listed below are designed to keep the lymphatic transport capacity at optimal levels and/or to prevent excessive lymphatic loads. These guidelines refer to the affected extremity(ies) in particular, but depending on the activity, may apply to the whole person.

I. Skin Care—Avoid trauma/injury to reduce infection risk
- Keep a first aid kit with you at all times to treat minor cuts (in particular, alcohol wipes, local antibiotic, and bandages)
- Protect exposed skin with sunscreen and insect repellent
- Keep your extremity clean and dry
- Apply moisturizer daily to prevent chapping/chafing of skin
- Wear gloves while doing activities that may cause skin injury (i.e., washing dishes, gardening, working with tools, using chemicals such as detergent)
- Be meticulous with nail care; do not cut cuticles
- Use care with razors to avoid nicks and skin irritation (use electric razor to remove hair in the axilla)
- Avoid punctures if possible, such as injections and blood draws (may use alternative sites such as buttocks, unaffected extremity)
- If scratches/punctures to skin occur, wash with soap and water, apply antibiotics, and observe for signs of infection (i.e. redness)
- If a rash, itching, redness, pain, increased skin temperature, fever or flulike symptoms occur, contact your physician immediately for early treatment of possible infection
- Be careful when playing with pets to avoid scratches (wear gloves)
- Do not get piercings or tattoos

II. Activity/Lifestyle
- Gradually build up the duration and intensity of any activity or exercise
- Avoid sudden heavy lifting
- Take frequent rest periods during activity to allow for limb recovery

- Monitor the extremity during and after activity for any change in size, shape, tissue, texture, soreness, heaviness, or firmness
- Maintain optimal weight by eating a healthy diet (low salt, low fat, high fiber, lots of fresh fruits and vegetables)

III. Avoid Limb Constriction
- Avoid having blood pressure (BP) taken if possible on the "limb at risk" (if the BP must be taken on the affected limb, have the practitioner take the BP manually to minimize excessive pressure (instead of using an automatic BP device)
- Wear loose-fitting jewelry and clothing

IV. Compression Garments
- Wear garments that fit well
- Support the "limb at risk" with a compression garment for strenuous activity (e.g., weight lifting, prolonged standing, running) except when you have an open wound or have poor circulation in the "limb at risk"
- When flying in an airplane, if you do not have lymphedema, consider wearing a well-fitting compression garment that will cover the entire extremity (including fingers and toes)
- When flying in an airplane, if you do have lymphedema, consider wrapping extra short-stretch bandages over your existing compression garment; also be sure that all exposed areas such as hands (may use a gauntlet or bandages) or fingers/toes (use bandages) are completely covered

V. Extremes of Temperature
- Avoid exposure to extreme cold, which can be associated with rebound swelling, or chapping of skin
- Avoid prolonged (greater than 15 minutes) exposure to heat, particularly hot tubs and saunas
- Avoid placing limb in water temperatures above 102° F (38.9° C)

VI. Additional Practices Specific to Lower-Extremity Lymphedema
- Avoid prolonged standing, sitting or crossing legs
- Wear proper, well-fitting footwear and hosiery

Data from International Society of Lymphology. The diagnosis and treatment of peripheral lymphedema. 2009 Consensus Document of the International Society of Lymphology. Lymphology 42:51–60, 2009; Zuther JE. Lymphedema Management—The Comprehensive Guide for Practitioners. 2nd ed. New York, Thieme, 2009; and Földi E, Földi M, Clodius L. The lymphedema chaos: A lancet. Ann Plast Surg 22:505–515, 1989.

there may be particular circumstances, such as possible malignancy or for research purposes, when it is important to diagnose the exact cause of the lymphedema. A variety of imaging methods can be helpful in these cases (Box 21-3).[1,3,5,6] During the examination, it is extremely important that the therapist take accurate measurements of the affected extremity(ies). A variety of methods have been developed to measure lymphedema, ranging from the inexpensive cloth tape measure or volumeter (water displacement) to the more expensive

infrared laser (perimetry) and devices measuring bioelectrical impedance.[30–33] The therapist needs to carefully monitor and document changes in the size of the affected limb(s) throughout the treatment and on posttreatment followup sessions.

Finally, the fields of molecular and cell biology are providing important insights into lymphatic system development and are assisting in the diagnosis lymphatic system disorders. Although theories concerning lymphatic system development were first proposed more than 100 years ago, many

**Table 21-1 Lymphedema Stages**

| Stages | Characteristics |
| --- | --- |
| Stage 0 (Latency) | No clinical edema |
| | Stemmer sign negative |
| | Tissue and skin appear "normal" |
| | Lymph transport capacity already reduced |
| Stage 1 (Reversible Stage) | Edema present (soft and pitting) |
| | Edema reversible with elevation |
| | Edema increases with standing and activity |
| | Stemmer sign negative |
| | Tissue appears "normal" |
| Stage 2 (Spontaneously Irreversible Stage) | Edema present; initially may still be soft and pitting in early stage 2 but then progresses to nonpitting "brawny" edema |
| | Edema does not reverse with elevation |
| | Stemmer sign positive (although still may be negative at early stage 2) |
| | Tissue appears fibrosclerotic; proliferation of adipose tissue |
| | Frequent infections |
| | Skin changes |
| Stage 3 (Lymphostatic Elephantiasis) | Edema present; severe "brawny" nonpitting edema |
| | Edema does not reverse with elevation |
| | Stemmer sign positive |
| | Tissue appears fibrosclerotic; proliferation of adipose tissue |
| | Frequent infections |
| | Skin changes (papillomas, deep skinfolds, warty protrusions, hyperkeratosis, mycotic infections, etc.) |

*Data from Földi E, Földi M, Strößenreuther RHK, et al. Földi's Textbook of Lymphology for Physicians and Lymphedema Therapists. 2nd ed. Munich, Germany, Elsevier, Urban & Fisher, 2006; Lasinski BB. The Lymphatic System. In Goodman CC, Fuller KS. Pathology: Implications for the Physical Therapist. 3rd ed. St. Louis, Saunders, 2009:642–677; and Zuther JE. Lymphedema Management—The Comprehensive Guide for Practitioners. 2nd ed. New York, Thieme, 2009.*

significant advances have been made concerning this area of scientific inquiry.[34-36] In the early 1900s, Florence Sabin developed a model for the mammalian lymphatic vasculature development that proposed the formation of primitive lymph sacs from venous endothelial cells. The sacs were believed to form the basis for lymphatic endothelial cells that would sprout and form the entire vascular lymphatic system, including the lymph nodes.[37,38] This theory of lymphatic system development was recently confirmed by Wigle and Oliver.[39] Scientists have now identified a number of lymphatic regulators that are crucial for a properly functioning lymphatic system including the homeobox transcription factor, PROX1; the transcription factor, FOXC2; the receptor tyrosine kinase VEGFR-3 and its ligand VEGF-C; and the transcription factor, SOX18 (Box 21-4).[34,39-47]

## Treatment

The scope of treatment is dependent on the type of lymphedema. If the patient has primary lymphedema then the treatment options will be conservative treatment. However, if the patient has secondary lymphedema because of a cancerous tumor, then the appropriate surgical intervention and followup (such as radiation and chemotherapy) needs to be first addressed before proceeding to conservative treatment. Lymphedema should be treated as soon as it is noticed, as untreated lymphedema increases the risk of cellulitis, and in rare cases can even cause cancer, such as the highly lethal angiosarcoma, Stewart-Treves syndrome.[2] A number of treatments options have been tried over the years with mixed results including medications, surgery, intermittent pneumatic compression, thermal therapy, and conservative methods.

## Medications

There is no definitive medication that has been shown to effectively treat lymphedema. As diuretics are typically prescribed to treat patients with high-flow edema such as congestive heart failure, lymphedema patients often are prescribed diuretics, too. However, many experts believe that treating lymphedema with diuretics is ineffective at best and can

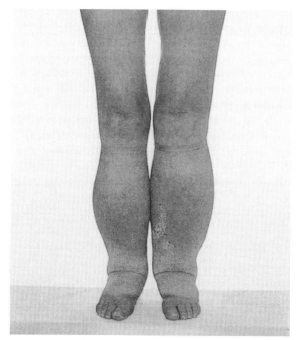

**Figure 21-7** Stage 2 lymphedema. From Browse N, Burnand K, Mortimer P: Diseases of the Lymphatics, London, 2003, Arnold.

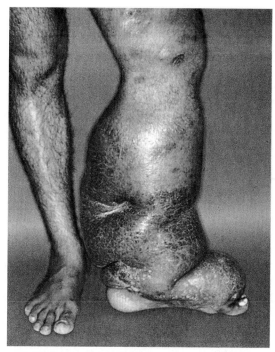

**Figure 21-9** Stage 3 lymphedema. From Goldstein B (ed): Practical dermatology, ed 2, St Louis, 1997, Mosby.

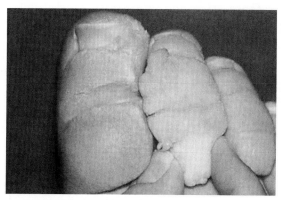

**Figure 21-8** Stemmer sign. (From Browse N, Burnand K, Mortimer P. Diseases of the Lymphatics. London, 2003, Arnold.)

actually lead to fluid and electrolyte imbalances, as well as further concentration of the high-protein edema that may worsen the symptoms of lymphedema.[2,6]

Benzopyrenes such as coumarin and flavonoids stimulate macrophage activity (that is inhibited by the presence of lymphedema), which can degrade the high levels of protein found in lymphedema. These drugs have been prescribed in Australia and Europe; the U.S. Food and Drug Administration (FDA), however, has not approved them. In Australia, oral coumarin has been decertified as a result of increased liver toxicity that resulted in several deaths, although topical coumarin is still available. The use of natural-occurring benzopyrenes, such as bioflavonoids, horse chestnut, and grapeseed extract, is also controversial and should be done with caution.[4,6]

## Surgery

Because the larger lymphatic vessels have valves to prevent backflow and the vessels themselves serve as a pump by contracting at regular intervals under the control of the autonomic nervous system, surgical efforts to simply replace the lymphatic vessels with a synthetic tube have in the past been largely unsuccessful.[6] Newer microsurgical and mapping procedures performed by skilled surgeons well-versed in lymphology such as autologous lymph vessel transplantation, lymphatic-venous anastomoses between lymphatics during axillary dissection, and axillary reverse mapping during sentinel lymph node biopsy do hold promise.[2,48,49]

Debulking (removal of excess skin and subcutaneous tissue) is another surgical method that is sometimes used to treat lymphedema although it does result in the removal of superficial skin lymphatic collaterals. Once a lymphedema patient has been successfully treated using conservative methods, surgical removal of the remaining excess skinfolds can sometimes be helpful. Liposuction (removal of suprafascial fatty tissue) is another surgical procedure performed in some lymphedema patients. Traditional liposuction is likely to further damage the lymphatic vessels that can precipitate the formation of lymphedema or accelerate the progression of existing lymphedema. In contrast, a newer form of liposuction called *tumescent liposuction* is increasingly used worldwide and is less likely to cause damage to the lymphatic system. With this procedure the surgeon injects a vasoconstrictor (epinephrine) and local anesthetic (lidocaine) that makes the fatty areas swollen and firm or "tumescent," which prepares the fatty areas to be surgically removed by small microcannulae.[2,50,51]

---

**Box 21-3**

## Imaging of the Lymphatic System

### Direct Lymphography

This invasive method is rarely used today because of significant complications caused by the contrast medium, such as allergic reaction and damage to the lymphatic vessels. With this method, the examiner injects an oily contrast medium into a lymphatic vessel in the foot or hand, and then serial radiographs are taken of the limb, which allows for mapping of the lymphatic system, including lymph vessels, lymphangions, and lymph nodes. It is still used for more complicated conditions, such as thoracic duct injury and chylous reflux syndrome, and for planning surgery involving the pelvic and retroperitoneal lymphatics.

### Indirect Lymphography (Lymphangiography)

With this method a water-soluble contrast medium is injected subepidermally. Radiographs are then taken to visualize the small superficial lymph vessels (including the initial lymph vessels). It should be pointed out that regional lymph nodes are not observable with this method.

### Lymphoscintigraphy (Lymphangioscintigraphy [LAS])

This is a minimally invasive method that uses a radioactive tracer injected into the back of the hand or foot. The tracer is then assessed using nuclear medical imaging. This method has largely replaced direct lymphography because of its low risk of complications and its ability to visualize lymph vessels and lymph nodes. It can also be used to measure both superficial and deep lymph fluid movement, as well as lymph node uptake speeds, while a patient exercises (e.g., on a treadmill) in what can be called a lymphoscintigraphic function test.

### Magnetic Resonance Imaging (MRI)

This noninvasive, yet costly, method is used primarily to detect and diagnose tumors. The MRI can visualize lymph trunks, lymph nodes, and soft tissues that are located proximal to the sites of lymphatic obstruction, which makes it very useful in combination with the information obtained by lymphoscintigraphy.

### Computed Tomography (CT)

This is a radiologic imaging method that provides cross-sectional views of the body and is typically used to identify tumors.

### Ultrasonography

This method is based on the measured velocity differences using high frequency sound waves in various body tissues. Because of its relative low resolution as compared to other methods, it is used mainly to identify enlarged lymph nodes, lymphoceles, lymphangiomas, and adult filaria in the case of filariasis. A newer technique called color-duplex ultrasonography shows promise as it has a relatively high sensitivity and specificity in identifying abnormal lymph nodes.

### Fluorescent Microlymphography (Microlymphangiography)

This last method is primarily used in research institutions and involves use of a fluorescent tracer that is injected subepidermally in areas such as the medial malleolus or fingers. Diffusion of the tracer is recorded using a video camera and fluorescent microscope system that allows the investigator to study the functional status of the initial lymph vessels.

Data from Data from Földi E, Földi M, Strößenreuther RHK, et al. Földi's Textbook of Lymphology for Physicians and Lymphedema Therapists. 2nd ed. Munich, Germany, Elsevier, Urban & Fisher, 2006; Kelly DG. A Primer on Lymphedema. Upper Saddle River, NJ, Prentice Hall, 2000; Weissleder H, Schuchhardt C (eds.). Lymphedema Diagnosis and Therapy. 4th ed. Essen, Germany, Viavital, 2008; and Zuther JE. Lymphedema Management—The Comprehensive Guide for Practitioners. 2nd ed. New York, Thieme, 2009.

---

## Intermittent Pneumatic Compression

There has been much debate concerning the effectiveness of intermittent pneumatic compression devices (pumps). It should be mentioned that significant technologic advances in compression device design have been made in recent years, such as multichambered compression sleeves that are programmable and controlled by computer. However, in spite of these advances, some experts contend that intermittent pneumatic compression devices should only be used in conjunction with conservative treatment methods if they are used at all.[2,6]

Part of the concern is that the compression pumps may move water but not proteins (as found in lymphedema) from the interstitial spaces. Another problem with intermittent pneumatic compression devices is that the actual pressures applied to the patient may be much greater than the intended pressures selected by the therapist. In one study using a commercially available pump, actual pressures in the

chambers were up to 80% higher than the target pressure. For example, if the target pressure was set at 100 mm Hg, a much higher pressure of 141 mm Hg was actually delivered.[52] High pressures in the 70 to 100 mm Hg range can damage lymphatic vessels in as few as 3 to 5 minutes when applied during forceful massage.[53] Therefore it is very likely that high pump pressures could damage lymphatic vessels.

Another concern is that if pumps are used as the sole method of intervention, the edema is moved proximally, which in the lower extremity can result in genital lymphedema. In fact, one retrospective study found that 43% of lower-limb lymphedema patients using compression devices at a lymphedema treatment facility developed genital edema.[54] In contrast, other studies using subjects with lymphedema report beneficial results using intermittent pneumatic compression alone or as an adjunctive treatment along with conservative treatment methods.[55,56] Newly developed programmable pneumatic compression devices specifically designed to treat lymphedema patients (using lower

**Box 21-4**

### Recent Scientific Evidence: Molecular and Cell Biology Advances in Lymphatic System Development

Molecular and cell biology techniques have greatly expanded our understanding of how the lymphatic system works. The list of known lymphatic regulators is long and growing. This box highlights just a few of the most prominent ones.

One of the most studied regulators is the homeobox transcription factor, PROX1, which plays a key role in lymphangiogenesis. In mice, venous endothelial cells that express PROX1 are found at embryonic day (E) 10 when they migrate to form the first primitive lymph sacs. When scientists inactivate the PROX1 transcription factor in mice, blood vasculature but not lymphatic vasculature is made.[34] In addition, PROX1 heterozygous mice pups die soon after birth and exhibit an abnormal lymphatic system, whereas Prox1 null mouse embryos die around E14.5.[39–41] Other researchers using mouse animal models have found a link between a functionally inactive single allele (haploinsufficiency) of the Prox1 gene and adult-onset obesity.[42]

Lymphedema-distichiasis is a rare autosomal dominant disease characterized by lymphedema that typically develops at or after puberty. Other prominent features of lymphedema-distichiasis include a double row of eyelashes (distichiasis), venous insufficiency, and lymphatic hyperplasia (increased number of lymphatic vessels). Lymphedema-distichiasis is caused by a mutation in the transcription factor FOXC2, which leads to a loss of activity of this transcription factor. Recent evidence suggests that lymphedema-distichiasis may actually be a more frequent cause of adult-onset lymphedema than previously believed.[34,43,44]

Another class of proteins called receptor tyrosine kinases and their ligands (which bind to the receptor) play a key role in the development of the lymphatic system. Specifically, the receptor tyrosine kinase VEGFR-3 and its ligand VEGF-C are essential for lymphatic system development. Mutations in the VEGFR-3 gene can cause Milroy disease (hereditary congenital lymphedema in humans), a rare autosomal dominant lymphedema characterized by hypoplasia of lymphatic vessels and by swelling of one or two legs at birth.[34] Recent studies in mice indicate that even after birth, levels of VEGFR-3 can by influenced by using antilymphangiogenic therapy.[45]

Another form of congenital lymphedema, hypotrichosis-lymphedema-telangiectasia, has been linked to mutations in the transcription factor, SOX18.[46] This disorder is characterized by less than a normal amount of hair (hypotrichosis), lymphedema, and small dilated blood vessels near the skin's surface (telangiectasia). In mouse models, SOX18 has been shown to directly activate Prox1 transcription and in addition, mouse embryos that completely lack the SOX18 gene do not develop lymphatic vessels.[47]

Recent advances made in understanding how the lymphatic system develops, opens the door for genetic testing of affected individuals in the new field called *molecular lymphology*. Advances in this area will not only allow the lymphologist to classify congenital/genetic-dysmorphogenic lymphedema disorders, but will promote potential clinical treatments, such as gene therapy and direct molecular therapy, that are designed to promote lymphangiogenesis. Although these potential treatments are being developed (first in animals then in humans), it should be remembered that the current standard of lymphedema treatment, complete decongestive therapy, has already proved its effectiveness.

---

compression pressures) have also shown promise as an adjunctive treatment.[57–59] Clearly, more research is needed to bring clarity to this controversial method.

### Thermal Therapy

In some regions of the world (Europe and Asia), thermal therapy, such as hot packs and sauna, is advocated as a treatment for lymphedema. However, this contradicts the standard lymphedema prevention recommendations of avoiding prolonged heat for the extremity with lymphedema or the limb at risk (see Box 21-2). Physiologically, heat produces vasodilation of the capillaries which would then increase the demands on the lymphatic system. Thus, one should avoid thermal therapy on the affected limb(s) and adjacent areas of the trunk.[2,6]

### Conservative Methods

Manual techniques to treat lymphedema were first developed in the 1890s by Alexander von Winiwarter, a German surgeon, but afterward were then largely forgotten. Dr. Winiwarter's method included meticulous cleanliness, compression, massage, and exercise.[60] In the 1930s, the Danish couple Emil and Estrid Vodder developed manual techniques called manual lymph drainage (MLD) to treat lymphedema by moving lymph in the desired direction. They named their system of techniques complex decongestive physiotherapy, which is the most common method of conservative lymphedema treatment in North America. In the 1970s, the Hungarian physicians, Michael and Ethel Földi incorporated the Vodder's MLD technique into a comprehensive lymphedema treatment program now called complete decongestive therapy (CDT). CDT occurs in two distinct phases that consist of MLD, compression, exercise, and specific skin care. John and Judith Casley-Smith from Australia and Albert and Oliver Leduc from Belgium have contributed significantly to the development of conservative treatment techniques, as have many others.[3] The nomenclature concerning the naming of the conservative methods for treating lymphedema has varied considerably over the years and in the latest 2009 Consensus Document of the International Society of Lymphology the term combined physical therapy is advocated.[2] However, in North America the term CDT is widely used and is used in this chapter.

## Table 21-2 Educational Resources for the Lymphedema Therapist*

There are a number of excellent organizations that are involved with promoting lymphedema education in general. Some of these organizations have a particular emphasis on breast cancer education and support. The resources listed below may be of interest to both the therapist and to the general public.

| Organization | Additional Notes |
|---|---|
| American Cancer Society (ACS) | |
| American Lymphedema Framework Project (ALFP) | It develops and evaluates appropriate health care services for lymphedema and advances the quality of lymphedema care. |
| American Physical Therapy Association (APTA), Oncology Section | |
| Lymphedema Special Interest Group (SIG) | |
| Breast Cancer Network of Strength | |
| International Society for Lymphology (ISL) | The website lists free of charge the lymphology consensus document—a collaborative document from lymphedema experts around the world. The most recent version was published in 2009. It also publishes the scientific journal *Lymphology*. |
| Living Beyond Breast Cancer (LBBC) | |
| Lymphatic Research Foundation (LRF) | It publishes the scientific journal *Lymphatic Research and Biology*. |
| Lymphoedema Association of Australia (LAA) | |
| Lymphology Association of North America (LANA) | The web site lists LANA-certified therapists, nurses, and physicians who specialize in treating lymphedema. |
| Lymphovenous Canada | |
| National Lymphedema Network (NLN) | The website lists lymphedema centers as well as therapists, nurses, and physicians who specialize in treating lymphedema. It also lists many lymphedema resources available to both patients and medical providers. |
| Susan G. Komen for the Cure | |

*The listing or omission of any particular resource does not denote endorsement or preference for of a particular lymphedema treatment. This resource guide is meant to help the therapist and members of the general public to find additional information concerning lymphedema and related conditions.*

Europe has a number of specialized lymphedema clinics that cater to patients with diseases of the lymphatic system and their insurance plans have historically allowed for twice-daily treatments over a course of 4 to 6 weeks. However, in the United States, most lymphedema patients are seen on an outpatient basis and are limited to once-per-day treatments during the work week because of reimbursement issues. In the United States, patients with lymphedema of the upper extremity are often treated for 3 to 4 weeks, whereas the typical treatment length for lower-extremity lymphedema patients is approximately 4 to 6 weeks. Of course, treatment times are dependent on the number of limbs involved, the severity of lymphedema and the presence of comorbidities such as lipedema and chronic venous insufficiency.

There are many aspects for effective conservative management of the lymphedema patient that the therapist must consider.[60–67] Because treating lymphedema patients with conservative methods is a relatively new area, especially in North America, historically, many physical therapy schools have only covered this topic in a limited manner.

Depending on the physical therapist's preparation in school, the therapist may find it advantageous to seek additional lymphedema education and certification before treating patients with lymphedema. Fortunately, there are many lymphedema schools offering lymphedema certification courses so that obtaining the necessary expertise is not difficult. Table 21-2 provides more detailed information concerning lymphedema schools, lymphedema certification, and lymphedema resources. The Lymphology Association of North America (LANA) and National Lymphedema Network (NLN), in particular, provide the interested therapist with a good overview of lymphedema resources.

### Components of Complete Decongestive Therapy

CDT consists of two phases: phase I is the treatment phase and phase II is the self-management phase. CDT and MLD should only be performed once the patient has been cleared for treatment (Table 21-3).[2,3,6] Phase I consists of MLD, compression (initially is achieved by bandages and then the

## Table 21-3 Precautions and Contraindications for Complete Decongestive Therapy Treatments Including Manual Lymph Drainage and Compression Bandaging

| Condition | Additional Notes |
| --- | --- |
| **Precautions and Relative Contraindications for CDT Treatments*** | |
| Acute infections | Local or systemic, viral, bacterial and fungal: cellulitis, erysipelas, other secondary acute inflammation, note that an acute infection is often a contraindication for CDT depending on the location and severity of the infection |
| Cardiac edema along with lymphedema | Contact referring physician to ensure that the cardiac edema is compensated before proceeding |
| Diabetes | |
| Hypertension | |
| Malignancy | Contact referring physician and discuss potential risks with the patient |
| Renal insufficiency | |
| **Contraindications for MLD Treatments** | |
| *General* | |
| Acute bronchitis | |
| Acute infection | |
| Bronchial asthma | Uncontrolled |
| Cardiac edema | Uncompensated |
| Fever | |
| Renal failure | |
| Pain | Unexplained |
| *Neck* | |
| Cardiac arrhythmia | |
| Hypersensitivity of the carotid sinus | |
| Hyperthyroidism | |
| Patients older than age 60 years | Because of sclerotic arteries and veins |
| *Abdomen* | |
| Abdominal surgery | Recent, contact surgeon; colostomy bag |
| Aortic aneurysm | Also palpation of a strong aortic pulse |
| Menstrual period | Relative contraindication |
| Painful gastrointestinal conditions | Specifically Crohn disease, ileus, diverticulitis, or any type of undiagnosed abdominal pain |
| Pregnancy | |
| Radiation complications | Chronic inflammation, colitis, cystitis, fibrosis |
| *Lower Extremity* | |
| Deep vein thrombosis | Contact physician to determine when MLD is safe to start, newer evidence supports earlier MLD treatment after deep venous thrombosis (as early as 2 weeks) |
| Phlebitis or thrombophlebitis | |
| **Precautions for Compression Bandaging** | |
| Acute infection | Cellulitis |
| Asthma | |
| Cor pulmonale | |
| Diabetes | |

*Continued*

**Table 21-3 Precautions and Contraindications for Complete Decongestive Therapy Treatments Including Manual Lymph Drainage and Compression Bandaging—cont'd**

| Condition | Additional Notes |
|---|---|
| **Precautions for Compression Bandaging (cont'd)** | |
| Hypertension | |
| Malignant lymphedema | |
| Paralysis | |
| | |
| **Contraindications for Compression Bandaging** | |
| Arterial disease of the lower extremity | If ankle-brachial index is <0.8, then bandaging is contraindicated |
| Painful postphlebitic syndrome | |

*Make sure that the physician and patient understand that CDT, and in particular MLD, may very likely cause a temporary increase in circulating blood volume that can put additional stress on the heart, lung, and kidneys. For most patients with the conditions listed, CDT treatment is appropriate but heart, lung, and kidney functions need to be closely monitored. Please contact the referring physician as needed to discuss the appropriateness of CDT before proceeding with treatment.*

patient is transitioned to a compression garment as reductions in limb girth start to plateau), exercise (in bandages), and meticulous skin care. The self-management phase II consists of compression (typically achieved by a garment during the day and bandages at night), exercise (always with the limb compressed in a garment or bandages), meticulous skin care, and MLD as needed. It must be stressed that patient compliance during phase II is a key to successful long-term outcome, and that the most compliant patients are likely to observe further girth reductions during the self-management phase.[62]

## Manual Lymph Drainage

MLD is a gentle manual treatment technique based on a comprehensive knowledge of the anatomy and physiology of the lymphatic system. MLD causes increased lymph flow into desired areas and around blockages, and can even cause lymph to flow superficially in directions that are opposite to its normal direction of flow (i.e., across watersheds). MLD mostly affects the flow of the initial lymph vessels but also can increase the frequency of lymph vessel contraction and as a result, increase the volume of lymph moved.[28,68-72]

To enhance the flow of lymph, the patient should be lying down and further desirable improvements in lymph flow may be obtained if the affected extremity is elevated during MLD treatment. Learning how and when to apply the various types of MLD strokes, as well as the proper order of body regions in which to apply these strokes, is one of the most important components of a lymphedema certification course. To facilitate the maximum reduction in lymphedema, it is critical to first treat the appropriate central areas and uninvolved lymph nodes. In this way, these uninvolved areas are prepared to receive the lymph from the affected extremity(ies). Only then should the involved extremity(ies) be treated. In the self-management phase II, the patient can be taught appropriate manual techniques, which can then be augmented if necessary by MLD in the clinic.

## Compression

External compression is the key component of CDT to preserve and improve on the lymphedema reduction made during MLD. Lymphedema experts believe that at least 50% of the success made during the phase I treatment is a result of compression.[3] Unless compression immediately follows MLD, MLD alone is very unlikely to achieve any long-term progress in lymphedema reduction. Bandages are the key component of compression during phase I, while a combination of compression garments (day) and bandages (night) are the typical means of achieving compression during phase II.

The success of compression in treating lymphedema patients is a result of a number of factors. For example, compression increases the pressure in the bandaged area, including tissues, blood, and lymph vessels. Through a variety of mechanisms including decreasing filtration of fluid into the interstitium and increasing reabsorption into the capillary venules, the amount of lymph needing to be transported by the lymphatics is reduced when the lymphatics are compressed. Bandage or garment compression should be applied using the principle of graded compression—higher compression on the more distal regions of the extremity than on the proximal regions. Graded compression improves venous and lymphatic return away from more distal areas into proximal areas that are more likely to be functioning normally and also improves the efficiency of the muscle pump during contraction of the distal and compressed muscle. In addition, compression provides support for those tissues that have lost their elasticity and can also help soften hardened fibrotic tissue found in the more advanced stages of lymphedema.[3,6]

It is important that the bandages and compression garments are selected carefully so that proper compression levels are achieved. Short-stretch compression bandages (as opposed to elastic "long-stretch" Ace bandages) are the bandage type of choice for treating lymphedema for several different reasons. First, they are textile-elastic (latex free), meaning that their elasticity is a result of the weave of the cotton fibers when they are manufactured and is not because of the presence of latex. When newly made, they stretch approximately 60% more than their original length. Second, the nature of the short-stretch bandage provides for a higher working pressure (temporary resistance to the muscle produced as the muscle contract) than the lower resting pressure (constant pressure of the bandage in the absence of muscle contraction). The amount of resting pressure that is present in a bandaged tissue is dependent on the tension at application. With their high resting pressure, Ace bandages subject the tissue to relatively high pressures at rest that can lead to compression of the more superficial lymphatic and venous

vessels. In contrast, short-stretch bandages allow for the normal flow of fluid in lymphatic and venous vessels at rest and are thus the bandage of choice for effective lymphedema management. Finally, the application of short-stretch bandages is very important. The therapist should apply the bandages with the goal to achieve the desired compression gradient, which is accomplished by applying more layers of the short-stretch bandages distally than proximally instead of increasing the application tension of the bandage. Compression bandages should be secured by tape and not clips (as commonly supplied with the new bandages) to avoid cutting the patient's skin which may lead to an infection (Fig. 21-10).[3,6,66]

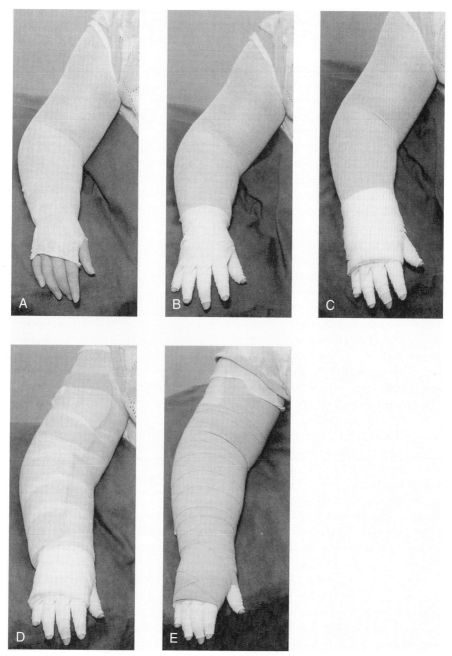

**Figure 21-10** Concentrically-applied bandaging of the upper extremity. (From Browse N, Burnand K, Mortimer P. Diseases of the Lymphatics. London, 2003, Arnold.)

To avoid complications during phase I compression, the therapist should also understand the implications of the Laplace law as it applies to areas of different limb diameters. Simply put, the normal nonlymphedema extremity can be viewed as a cylinder that is larger in diameter at its proximal end than at its distal end. According to the Laplace law, if tension is the same at different parts of the extremity, the pressure is greatest where the radius is the smallest. When bony areas that have a small diameter, such as wrist or ankles, are wrapped with compression bandages, the pressure is highest at these places. Conversely, wrapped areas that are larger in diameter or concave areas (i.e., retromalleolar) have lower pressure and can be refractory to compression therapy. Thus, it is often necessary to add a layer of foam padding in the concave areas under the short-stretch bandage so as to achieve a proper cylinder shape to facilitate the movement of lymphedema away from the distal portions of the lymphedematous extremity.[6]

Phase II of CDT involves the use of both compression garments and short-stretch bandages. Once the reduction of limb girth in lymphedema plateaus, the patient is ready to be fitted for a compression garment that is usually worn during the day. Many different styles and choices of garments exist, and it is extremely important that the patient receives the optimal garment. Garment selection should only be performed by highly trained medical personnel, which in the United States may be the same therapist who provided MLD and CDT. The patient must clearly understand that garments (and bandages) wear out and need to be replaced at regular intervals (often every 6 months). For many patients this can pose a financial hardship as in the United States, compression garments are often not covered by medical insurance. Also, because garments need to be washed at regular intervals, two garments need to be purchased at a time so that the patient can wear one, and dry the other one. At night, many patients find it most comfortable to wrap their affected extremities with short-stretch bandages while their compression garments are drying. However, some patients at nighttime prefer to use a more expensive adjustable compression device that also provides gradient compression, because it can be easier to don and doff.[3,6]

The key components to consider during garment selection are compression level, type of knit, use of custom-made or off-the-shelf garment, and style (Box 21-5).[3,6] All of these factors together are essential in achieving optimal treatment outcomes, as well as producing a comfortable garment that the patient will readily wear. Thus, because this aspect of CDT is of such critical importance, it is important that only highly trained individuals are involved in the garment selection process.

## Exercise

There are many known benefits of general exercise including a more favorable body composition profile (less fat, more muscle, and higher bone mineral density), achieving and maintaining an optimal body weight, improved efficiency in utilizing oxygen, a decrease in resting heart rate, higher

---

### Box 21-5

#### Garment Selection for Lymphedema

Proper garment selection is key not only for effective long-term treatment of lymphedema but to improve patient compliance by making the garment as comfortable to wear as possible. Factors that should be considered during garment selection include compression level, type of knit, use of custom-made or off-the-shelf garment, and style (including body areas to cover).

#### Compression Levels
- Often range from 20 to 60+ mm Hg, with lower extremities typically receiving higher compression levels (e.g., level III: 40 to 50 mm Hg) garments than upper extremities (e.g., level II: 30 to 40 mm Hg).
- The highest listed level of compression for a given garment is found at the most distal segment of the garment as the compression gradient is built into the garment.
- Other factors to consider include the ability of the patient to don and doff the garment, the patient's activity level, and the presence of comorbidities.[3,6]

#### Type of Knit
- Circular knit garments are seamless and are more attractive and cost less.
- Flat-knit garments have a seam, cost more, but allow for higher compression levels (>50 mm Hg) and can be customized to better fit the contours of the patient.

#### Custom Versus Off-the-Shelf Garments
- Standard "off-the-shelf" compression garments come in a variety of sizes and styles and are less expensive than custom garments.
- Custom garments can be fitted to patients of almost any size or shape.
- Flat-knit custom garments can include desirable options, such as zippers, that allow for easier garment donning and doffing, higher compression levels (>50 mm Hg), and garment size adaptability.

#### Style
- Many different styles and types of compression garments are available (such as knee-high or thigh-high garments).
- A number of fastening options are available that can help the compression garment stay in place.[6]

---

cardiac stroke volume at peak exertion, a reduced coronary risk profile, faster nerve conduction velocity, and slower development of disability during aging.[6,73] Specifically, exercise has been documented to positively affect the lymph system by increasing the flow of lymph through increasing lymph vessel contractions (lymphangiomotoricity), increasing the uptake of fluid into the initial lymphatics, increasing muscle contractions that creates tissue pressure differentials that then stimulates lymph flow and prevents additional accumulation of fluid, and by facilitating the flow of lymph

## Box 21-6

### Exercise Principles for the Lymphedema Patient

- Despite the varying opinions concerning the optimal exercise type and intensity, several underlying principles do exist. When the therapist adheres to the following exercise principles, the lymphedema patient will have the best opportunity for success.
- Exercise the lymphedema patient only when the affected extremity(ies) have adequate compression as provided by either compression bandages or garments.
- Gradually progress the exercise or activity type, intensity, frequency, and duration.
- Carefully monitor the size and shape of the affected extremity(ies) as increased demands are placed on the lymphatic system and make appropriate adjustments to the exercise program.

in the thoracic duct by increasing the rate of deep breathing.[1,3,5,6,68]

The two major benefits of exercise in lymphedema patients are to support or improve lymphatic function and to enhance overall functional mobility. Because it is difficult, if not impossible, to predict in advance of treatment which lymphedema patients will react favorably or unfavorably to a given exercise or activity, the therapist must carefully monitor and document the patient's response to a particular exercise or activity. The patient's unique treatment response must be taken into account when developing a highly individualized exercise program and when determining exercise progression (Box 21-6).

When designing an exercise program during phases I and II of CDT, the therapist should carefully consider any limitations found during the examination, such as joint range of motion, muscle strength, posture, and functional mobility. In addition to a more traditional therapy-driven home exercise program, the lymphedema patient should be encouraged to continue activities, if possible, that are enjoyable to that patient. Because exercise is known to produce beneficial psychological effects and lymphedema patients commonly suffer from depression, developing an exercise program that the lymphedema patient can truly enjoy can become a key component to a successful CDT program.[74-76]

Another important exercise consideration is to have the lymphedema patient start or continue with cardiovascular-enhancing low-impact activities (with external compression on the affected extremity[ies]) such as walking, bicycling, and swimming, that are less likely to exacerbate the lymphedema. Simple exercise modifications can be made to decrease the likelihood of developing or exacerbating lymphedema. For example, the upper-extremity lymphedema patient can use a tall walking stick on the affected side(s) to reduce arm swing (and centrifugal forces) that can lead to distal arm edema.[6] Some lymphedema patients have reported adverse affects on their edematous extremity(ies) when they have participated in golf, tennis, cross-country skiing, and ambitious weight

lifting.[3,6] Other studies have shown little or no adverse affects to more strenuous forms of exercise, including supervised resistance training (Box 21-7).[74,77-81] To minimize delayed onset muscle soreness, it is recommended that the patient avoid unaccustomed eccentric exercises, and instead focus on smooth, rhythmic, concentric activities with light resistance.[3] Finally, the exercise program should be adapted to the overall fitness level of the patient. A patient who is used to more rigorous exercise may be able to tolerate more intense exercises without adverse affects to their lymphedema than a more sedentary patient.

### Meticulous Skin Care

Unfortunately, the tissues of lymphedema patients are saturated with protein-rich fluid, which hampers the body's local immune system and also provides ideal conditions for bacterial and fungal infections in the skin and nails. *Streptococcus* bacteria are the most common cause of bacterial infections in lymphedema. If unchecked, these infections can significantly worsen the patient's lymphedema and also cause more serious medical conditions, such as cellulitis, that often require admission to a hospital.[6]

Prevention is key in avoiding skin infections and necessitates daily vigilance in four major areas—inspection, cleansing, moisturizing, and protection. The lymphedema patient should carefully inspect and cleanse the areas affected with lymphedema each day. Also, the lymphedema patient should use suitable skin lotions and moisturizers (e.g., moisturizers for sensitive skin), and when necessary, a mild disinfectant followed by antibiotic–antifungal cream. During phase I of CDT, the therapist should apply moisturizing skin lotions to maintain a normal skin pH of 5.0 before wrapping the patient with compression bandages each day. During phase II, skin lotions should continue to be applied twice a day to the affected areas.[2,6] Activities that might exacerbate lymphedema or cause infection should be avoided in order to protect the affected area(s) (see Table 21-3).

## Lipedema

Lipedema is a frequently overlooked yet fairly common condition. Unlike lymphedema, there is a gradual and progressive symmetrical accumulation of fat in the subcutaneous tissue, typically seen in the buttocks and lower extremities.[1,6,51] Lipedema was first described in 1940 as a condition that only affects women and was differentiated from obesity or lymphedema.[82] Lipedema often appears at puberty, pregnancy, or menopause in women, but in contrast, is now known to be extremely rare in men.[1] It is also believed to be an inherited condition as it often affects more than one woman in a given family.[51]

### Clinical Manifestations and Differential Diagnosis

Although lipedema may be challenging for therapist to identify in its early stages, in later stages, patients with lipedema

## Box 21-7

### Recent Literature on Lymphedema, Exercise Intensity, and Survival Rates

Much debate exists concerning the appropriate level of exercise type, frequency, and intensity for the "limb at risk" or lymphedema patient as such patients respond in an unique way to the additional exercise demands placed on the lymphatic system. If the therapist closely monitors how the affected extremity(ies) responds to the exercise program, such patients can maximize their activity levels while at the same time minimize their risks for developing or exacerbating lymphedema. Highlighted below are a few studies that should help the therapist develop an appropriate exercise program for this patient population.

Although the benefits of physical activity in preventing lymphedema and certain types of cancer such as breast cancer are well known, Holmes and associates[77] investigated the affects of physical activity and survival in nurses after diagnosis of stage I, II, or III breast cancer. They quantified leisure-time physical activity per week according to type, frequency and intensity of physical activity using the metabolic equivalent task (MET) standard. Overall they found the greatest benefit occurred in subjects who performed the equivalent of walking 3 to 5 hours per week at an average pace (equivalent to 9 to 15 MET-hours per week). The relative risk of death was lower in all physical activity groups that were more active than the sedentary group (engaged in less than 3 MET-hours of physical activity per week). They also determined that women who had hormone-receptor-positive tumors for estrogen and progesterone derived a greater benefit from physical activity than did women who had hormone-receptor-negative tumors.

Another study looked at the affects of a weight training program in breast cancer survivors, 15% of whom already had noticeable lymphedema.[78] This supervised weight training program lasted for 6 months and was conducted on women who had already undergone breast cancer treatment 4 to 36 months prior to the study's start. Weight training was performed using a combination of variable-resistance machines and free weights that targeted the muscles of the arms, back, chest, buttocks, and legs. The exercises were slowly progressed only if there were no signs of lymphedema. At the end of 6 months no one in the intervention group had a change in arm girth ≥2.0 cm, nor was there a significant difference between the control and intervention groups concerning self-reported lymphedema symptoms.

There is a growing body of evidence that patients who either are at risk for developing lymphedema or already have lymphedema may engage in a regular exercise program if that program is progressed carefully and the patients are closely monitored.[74,79-81] These newer findings should help resolve the conflict between physical activity recommendations for the "limb at risk" and lymphedema patients that encourage such patients to be physically active while at the same time imposing activity restrictions.

## Table 21-4 Major Characteristics Distinguishing Lipedema from Lymphedema

| Clinical Feature | Lipedema | Lymphedema |
|---|---|---|
| Gender | Almost exclusively in women | Women > men |
| Family history | Common | Rare |
| Distribution | Bilateral lower extremities (rarely UE) symmetric involvement | Unilateral, or bilateral with one leg affected more severely (asymmetric) |
| Cellulitis | Rare | Common |
| Pain on pressure | Present | Absent |
| Easy bruising of affected area (hematoma) | Present | Absent |
| Distal edema in the foot | Absent | Present |
| Stemmer sign | Absent (negative) | Present (positive) |

have characteristic signs that allow for easy differentiation from lymphedema (Table 21-4).[1,6,51]

One of the most important characteristics of lipedema is that it is a bilateral condition affecting the lower but rarely the upper extremities (Fig. 21-11)[83]; consequently, the upper extremities may look quite normal in lipedema patients. Unfortunately, lipedema is often confused with obesity, but there are important differences that exist between the two conditions (Box 21-8).[1,51,82,84] Lipedema typically affects the proximal areas, such as the buttocks and thighs, but not distal areas, such as the feet. That is why a patient with lipedema shows a negative Stemmer sign (thickened skin folds of the toes).[29] Lipedema also affects the skin by reducing the skin's elasticity, which is the ability of the skin to return to its original size and shape, as well as making the skin sensitive to pressure and touch, which makes it bruise easily and be painful.[1,51,82-84] Although the clinical physical presentation can typically determine the diagnosis of lymphedema and lipedema, diagnostic imaging methods such as lymphoscintigraphy and computed tomography can be helpful with the differential diagnosis of lymphedema and lipedema.[5,6]

## Combination Forms of Lipedema and Lymphedema

If untreated, lipedema can cause the formation of lymphedema in what is known as lipolymphedema. It is believed that the abnormal subcutaneous fatty tissue distribution that occurs in lipedema compresses the lymph collectors, thus leading to impaired drainage of the lymphatic system.[6] This combination form of lipedema and lymphedema is frequently

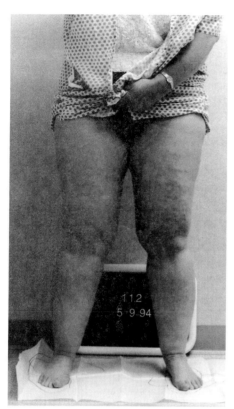

**Figure 21-11** Stage I lipedema. Note that the feet are free of edema and the ankles and lower legs have pitting edema. Fatty nodules are beginning to appear on the distal thighs. (Courtesy Lymphedema Therapy, Woodbury, NY.)

---

**Box 21-8**

**Untangling the Confusion Between Lipedema and Obesity**

Lipedema is not the same as being overweight or obese. Even though a large number of patients with lipedema are overweight, not all are. Frequently, obesity is confused with lipedema but there are several key differences. Fatty tissue in obese patients occurs either in the trunk or over the entire body in normal proportions, is not painful, does not bruise easily, and is present in both men and women.[51,82] Unfortunately with lipedema, diet and exercise are ineffective in reducing the size of the extremity(ies) affected by lipedema (although they can reduce the size of the unaffected extremities), and these women may become emotionally distraught because, despite their best efforts, their affected extremities may remain large and unattractive.[1,51,82,84]

---

seen in lymphedema clinics. One study reported that lipolymphedema occurs on average 17 years after the initial onset of lipedema in patients who do not receive proper treatment for their lipedema.[1] Thus, it is important that the therapist be able to clearly identify lipedema and lymphedema so as to assist in proper patient education and to develop realistic treatment plans and goals.

## Treatment of Lipedema

### Conservative Methods

Physical therapists can treat both patients with lymphedema and lipedema with MLD along with the other components of CDT. However, important differences do exist in the anticipated outcomes for each of these conditions. Typically, a patient who has pure primary lymphedema should respond to CDT faster than one who has a combination of lipolymphedema or pure lipedema.[6] Because patients with lipedema or lipolymphedema usually have pain and hypersensitivity in the areas affected by lipedema, the therapist may need to use less pressure during MLD and bandaging while waiting for the hypersensitivity to resolves, which is usually the case.[6]

### Surgical Methods

There has been considerable discussion concerning the appropriateness of removing the fat deposits in patients with lipedema using liposuction. One of the greatest risks of traditional liposuction is the potential of damaging the lymphatic system, which can develop into lymphedema after the surgical procedure.[1,6] Older techniques of liposuction involved putting the patient under general anesthesia, using a "dry" technique (i.e., the subcutaneous tissue was not infiltrated with fluid) and employing large sharp cannulas that could cause further damage to the lymphatic system.[50]

The newer technique termed *tumescent liposuction* has been developed to reduce the damage to surrounding tissue, including to the lymphatic system.[50,51] Tumescent refers to something, such as tissue, that is abnormally distended, especially by fluids. This newer procedure is performed with a blunt microcannula using a local "wet" anesthetic (combination of lidocaine and prilocaine) to infiltrate and swell up subcutaneous tissue. These refinements allow the skilled surgeon to remove the abnormal fat deposits in a manner that minimizes damage to the lymphatic system. Even though this newer type of liposuction holds promise, the conservative treatment techniques of MLD and CDT still have an important, although reduced role after tumescent liposuction.[50,51]

### Lipedema Education of the Public, Patients, and Healthcare Providers

Compared to lymphedema, much less has been written about lipedema in lymphology textbooks targeting healthcare providers.[85] This has lead to much confusion in the medical establishment, as illustrated by one study in the United States that determined 9 of the 250 patients with a physician diagnosis of "lymphedema" actually had lipedema.[86] Even though lipedema is a little-known disease, it is likely to be widespread. One study conducted in Germany found that 11% of German women have some form of lipedema, which would imply that at a minimum, hundreds of thousands of American women may have lipedema.[1] Given that untreated lymphedema is likely to cause lymphedema as well, proper public and healthcare provider education is key in preventing the progression of lipedema to lipolymphedema.[1]

## CASE STUDY 21-1

JM is a 58-year-old female who comes to your lymphedema clinic with moderate stage 2 lymphedema of the right upper extremity, secondary to sentinel lymph node biopsy (nodes negative) 6 years prior. Last year she got a bad upper-body sunburn while on vacation at Daytona Beach, FL. A few months later her arm started to feel heavy. JM is a computer programmer and works from home. Her two children are grown, and her husband is a truck driver who is home only on the weekend.

Past medical history is significant for diabetes mellitus, high cholesterol, and hypertension. JM has just started an exercise class to help motivate her to lose weight. She is 5'7" in height, weighs 208 pounds (BMI 32.6), and is right-hand dominant.

Assessment found no functional limitations in any extremity concerning range of motion or manual muscle testing. Patient complains of general discomfort in the right upper extremity, but no specific pain. Stemmer sign is positive in the right hand (negative in the left hand), with nonpitting edema present throughout the right upper extremity, most noticeable in the hand dorsum, wrist, and forearm. Initial volume difference between the right and left upper extremities is 2100 mL.

---

### Clinical Tip

This case is a typical secondary lymphedema and the motivated patient should respond well to conservative treatment. Phase I conservative treatment (5 times/week) may last 2 to 3 weeks before progressing to phase II.

---

## Summary

Healthcare workers, including physical therapists, are gaining an increasing appreciation for the important role the lymphatic system plays in sustaining health and quality of life. In recent years, a greater emphasis has been placed in preparing entry-level physical therapists to be able to evaluate and treat disorders of the lymphatic system such as lymphedema. In addition, there are a number of lymphedema certification programs that are available to those postgraduate physical therapists seeking additional expertise.

To effectively evaluate and treat patients with lymphatic system disorders the physical therapist should keep the following key points in mind:

- The lymphatic system is a one-way system that starts with small vessels called *initial lymph vessels* and then progresses to larger vessels called *collectors* and finally ends with larger vessels called *trunks* that drain into the venous system near the heart.
- The unidirectional flow of lymph is assisted by valves found in the larger lymphatic vessels.
- The lymphangion is the functional unit between two valves found in the lymphatic collectors and trunks.
- The frequency of lymphangion contraction (lymphangiomotoricity) can be increased by appropriate and manual techniques.
- Lymph consists of proteins, water, fatty acids, and cellular components (including bacteria and cellular debris).
- The primary function of the lymphatic system is transport and drainage (similar to the sanitation system of a city).
- Lymph nodes are concentrated in the neck, axilla, chest, abdomen, and groin, and drain specific lymph regions called *lymphotomes*.
- Lymphotomes are separated by watersheds that have relatively few lymph collectors.

- The amount of lymph transported by the lymphatic system is called the *lymphatic load*.
- The maximal ability of the lymphatic system to transport lymph is called the *transport capacity*.
- When a normal amount of LL exceeds the TC of the lymphatic system, a mechanical insufficiency results that may lead to a protein-rich edema called *lymphedema*.
- Lymphedema is often staged into four stages (from least to most severe) from the clinically undetectable stage 0 progressing through stages 1 and 2 to the severe form of lymphedema found in stage 3 called *elephantiasis*.
- Lymphedema stages 2 and 3 are characterized by a positive Stemmer sign (thickened skin fold of the digits), fibrosis, chronic inflammation, and skin changes.
- Lymphedema is often categorized into two forms—primary lymphedema (caused by an abnormally developed lymphatic system) and secondary lymphedema (from a known insult to the lymphatic system such as mastectomy).
- Often there is no known cause for primary lymphedema, although sometimes heat, puberty, pregnancy, or minor trauma, such as insect bites, infections, sprains, or strains, may be identified.
- Although surgical advances such as sentinel lymph node biopsy have minimized the damage to the lymphatic system, even the best surgical techniques do damage the lymphatic system and can cause lymphedema.
- People who have had surgical procedures that frequently disrupt the lymphatic system should carefully follow the recommended lymphedema precautions and contraindications so as to decrease the likelihood of developing lymphedema in the "limb at risk."
- Conservative methods of treating lymphedema (as compared to medication or surgery) are still the gold standard for effective lymphedema treatment.
- Conservative methods for treating lymphedema have been called by many different names including complex decongestive physiotherapy, CDT, or combined physical therapy.
- Conservative methods of treating lymphedema consist of two phases: phase I is the treatment phase and phase II is the self-management phase.
- Phase I lymphedema treatments consists of MLD, compression (initially achieved by bandages and then by compression garment), exercise, and meticulous skin care.

- Phase II consists of compression (garment during the day, bandages at night), exercise, meticulous skin care, and MLD as needed.
- MLD is a gentle manual treatment technique based on a comprehensive knowledge of the anatomy and physiology of the lymphatic system and can result in increased lymph flow into desired areas and around blockages.
- Compression is applied using a pressure gradient (higher distally, lower proximally) that uses special short-stretch bandages in phase I and then garments (during the day) in phase II.
- Exercise should only be performed when the affected limb(s) are compressed by bandages or garments so as to facilitate lymphatic flow.
- It is important to differentiate between the conditions of lymphedema and lipedema so as to provide the appropriate treatment.
- Lipedema (in contrast to lymphedema) is a disorder characterized by a gradual symmetrical accumulation of fat in the subcutaneous tissue, typically found only in women where it is located in the buttocks and lower extremities.
- Lipedema can be treated with the conservative methods described above, but with typically slower results.
- The therapist treating lymphedema and lipedema patients should be aware that it is not uncommon for some patients to have both lipedema and lymphedema (called lipolymphedema).
- For conservative treatment to be successful, patients with lymphedema or lipedema must remain highly motivated during the self-management phase II treatment, which lasts for a lifetime.
- In the United States, lymphedema and lipedema patients are most often treated in the outpatient setting, whereas in Europe, specialized inpatient lymphedema clinics do exist.

Successfully treating lymphedema and lipedema patients is one of the most rewarding areas of physical therapy as conservative treatment is still the treatment of choice. In many cases, such patients with long-standing lymphedema have not always previously received the best medical advice or effective treatment for their condition. The properly trained physical therapist often obtains excellent results in the motivated lymphedema or lipedema patient.

## References

1. Földi E, Földi M, Strößenreuther RHK, Kubik S (eds.). Földi's Textbook of Lymphology for Physicians and Lymphedema Therapists. 2nd ed. Munich, Germany: Elsevier, Urban & Fisher, 2006.
2. International Society of Lymphology. The diagnosis and treatment of peripheral lymphedema. 2009, Consensus Document of the International Society of Lymphology. Lymphology 42:51–60, 2009.
3. Kelly DG. A Primer on Lymphedema. Upper Saddle River, NJ: Prentice Hall, 2002.
4. Lasinski BB. The Lymphatic System. In Goodman CC, Fuller KS (eds.). Pathology: Implications for the Physical Therapist. 3rd ed. St. Louis, MO, Saunders Elsevier, 2009:642–77.
5. Weissleder H, Schuchhardt C (eds.). Lymphedema Diagnosis and Therapy. 4th ed. Essen, Germany, Viavital, 2008.
6. Zuther JE. Lymphedema Management—The Comprehensive Guide for Practitioners. 2nd ed. New York, Thieme, 2009.
7. Starling EH. On the absorption of fluids from the connective tissue spaces. J Physiol 19:312–26, 1896.
8. Földi E. Treatment of lymphedema and patient rehabilitation. Anticancer Res 18:2211–12, 1998.
9. Werner RS, McCormick B, Petrek J, et al. Arm edema in conservatively managed breast cancer: obesity is a major predictive factor. Radiology 180:177–84, 1991.
10. Wilke LG, McCall LM, Posther KE, et al. Surgical complications associated with sentinel lymph node biopsy: Results from a prospective international cooperative group trial. Ann Surg Oncol 13:491–500, 2006.
11. Petrek JA, Senie RT, Peters M, Rosen PP. Lymphedema in a cohort of breast carcinoma survivors 20 years after diagnosis. Cancer 92:1368–77, 2001.
12. Gloviczki P, Solti F, Szlavy L, Jellinek H. Ultrastructural and electrophysiologic changes of experimental acute cardiac lymphostasis. Lymphology 16:185–92, 1983.
13. Allen SJ, Geissler HJ, Davis KL, et al. Augmenting cardiac contractility hastens myocardial edema resolution after cardiopulmonary bypass and cardioplegic arrest. Anesth Analg 85:987–92, 1997.
14. Mehlhorn U, Geissler HJ, Laine GA, Allen SJ. Myocardial fluid balance. Eur J Cardiothorac Surg 20:1220–30, 2001.
15. Nakamura K, Rockson SG. The role of the lymphatic circulation in the natural history and expression of cardiovascular disease. Int J Cardiol 129:309–17, 2008.
16. Predescu D, Predescu S, McQuistan T, Palade GE. Transcytosis of $\alpha_1$-acidic glycoprotein in the continuous microvascular endothelium. Proc Natl Acad Sci U S A 95:6175–80, 1998.
17. Ishikawa Y, Akishima-Fukasawa Y, Ito K et al. Lymphangiogenesis in myocardial remodelling after infarction. Histopathology 51:345–53, 2007.
18. Stolyarov VV, Lushnikova EL, Zuevskii VP, Usynin AF. Morphometric analysis of the lymph system in rat heart during myocardial infarction. Bull Exp Biol Med 134:203–5, 2002.
19. Maclean D, Fishbein MC, Maroko PR, Braunwald E. Hyaluronidase-induced reductions in myocardial infarct size. Science 194:199–200, 1976.
20. Maroko PR, Hillis LD, Muller JE, et al. Favorable effects of hyaluronidase on electrocardiographic evidence of necrosis in patients with acute myocardial infarction. N Engl J Med 296:898–903, 1977.
21. Yotsumoto G, Moriyama Y, Yamaoka A, Taira A. Experimental study of cardiac lymph dynamics and edema formation in ischemia/reperfusion injury—With reference to the effect of hyaluronidase. Angiology 49:299–305, 1998.
22. American Physical Therapy Association. Guide to Physical Therapist Practice. 2nd ed. Phys Ther 81:9–744, 2001.
23. Piller NB, Clodius I. Experimental lymphedema: Its applicability and contribution to our clinical understanding. In Johnston M (ed.). Experimental Biology of the Lymphatic Circulation. Amsterdam, Elsevier Science, 1985:189–230.
24. Ryttov N, Holm NV, Qvist N, Blichert-Toft M. Influence of adjuvant irradiation on the development of late arm

lymphedema and impaired shoulder mobility after mastectomy for carcinoma of the breast. Acta Oncol 27:667–70, 1988.

25. Tobbia D, Semple J, Baker A, et al. Lymphedema development and lymphatic function following lymph node excision in sheep. J Vasc Res 46:426–34, 2009.

26. Sener SF, Winchester DJ, Martz CH. Lymphedema after sentinel lymphadenectomy for breast carcinoma. Cancer 92:748–52, 2001.

27. National Lymphedema Network. 18 Steps to Prevention Revised: Lymphedema Risk-Reduction Practices. Available at: http://www.lymphnet.org/lymphedemaFAQs/riskReduction/riskReduction.htm. Accessed September 24, 2009.

28. Földi E, Földi M, Clodius L. The lymphedema chaos: A lancet. Ann Plast Surg 22:505–15, 1989.

29. Stemmer RA. Ein klinisches Zeichen zur Fruh—und Differential—diagnose des Lymphödems. Vasa 5:261–2, 1976.

30. Armer J. The problem of post-breast cancer lymphedema: impact and measurement issues. Cancer Invest 1:76–83, 2005.

31. Karges JR, Mark BE, Stikeleather SJ, Worrell TW. Concurrent validity of upper-extremity volume estimates: comparison of calculated volume derived from girth measurements and water displacement volume. Phys Ther 83:134–45, 2003.

32. Ridner SH, Montgomery LD, Hepworth JT, et al. Comparison of upper limb volume measurement techniques and arm symptoms between healthy volunteers and individuals with known lymphedema. Lymphology 40:35–46, 2007.

33. Taylor R, Jayasinghe UW, Koelmeyer L, et al. Reliability and validity of arm volume measurements for assessment of lymphedema. Phys Ther 86:205–14, 2006.

34. Mäkinen T, Norrmén C, Petrova TV. Molecular mechanisms of lymphatic vascular development. Cell Mol Life Sci 64:1915–29, 2007.

35. Rockson SG. Diagnosis and management of lymphatic vascular disease. J Am Coll Cardiol 52:799–806, 2008.

36. Rockson SG. The unique biology of lymphatic edema. Lymphat Res Biol 7:97–100, 2009.

37. Sabin FR. On the origin of the lymphatic system from the veins and the development of the lymph hearts and thoracic duct in the pig. Am J Anat 1:367–89, 1902.

38. Sabin FR. The lymphatic system in human embryos, with a consideration of the morphology of the system as a whole. Am J Anat 9:43–91, 1909.

39. Wigle JT, Oliver G. Prox1 function is required for the development of the murine lymphatic system. Cell 98:769–78, 1999.

40. Hong YK, Harvey N, Noh YH, et al. Prox1 is a master control gene in the program specifying lymphatic endothelial cell fate. Dev Dyn 225:351–7, 2002.

41. Wigle JT, Harvey N, Detmar M et al. An essential role for Prox1 in the induction of the lymphatic endothelial cell phenotype. EMBO J 21:1505–13, 2002.

42. Harvey NL, Srinivasan RS, Dillard ME, et al. Lymphatic vascular defects promoted by Prox1 haploinsufficiency cause adult-onset obesity. Nat Genet 37:1072–81, 2005.

43. Dellinger MT, Thome K, Bernas MJ, et al. Novel FOXC2 missense mutation identified in patient with lymphedema-distichiasis syndrome and review. Lymphology 41:98–102, 2008.

44. Sholto-Douglas-Vernon C, Bell R, Brice G et al. Lymphoedema-distichiasis and FOXC2: Unreported mutations, de novo mutation estimate, families without coding mutations. Hum Genet 117:238–42, 2005.

45. Karpanen T, Wirzenius M, Mäkinen T, et al. Lymphangiogenic growth factor responsiveness is modulated by postnatal lymphatic vessel maturation. Am J Pathol 169:708–18, 2006.

46. Irrthum A, Devriendt K, Chitayat D, et al. Mutations in the transcription factor gene SOX18 underlie recessive and dominant forms of hypotrichosis-lymphedema-telangiectasia. Am J Hum Genet 72:1470–8, 2003.

47. François M, Caprini A, Hosking B, et al. Sox18 induces development of the lymphatic vasculature in mice. Nature 456:643–7, 2008.

48. Boccardo F, Casabona F, De Cian F, et al. Lymphedema microsurgical preventive healing approach: a new technique for primary prevention of arm lymphedema after mastectomy. Ann Surg Oncol 16(3):703–8, 2009.

49. Boneti C, Korourian S, Bland K, et al. Axillary reverse mapping: Mapping and preserving arm lymphatics may be important in preventing lymphedema during sentinel lymph node biopsy. J Am Coll Surg 206:1038–42; discussion 1042–1044, 2008.

50. Schmeller W, Meier-Vollrath I. Tumescent liposuction: A new and successful therapy for lipedema. J Cutan Med Surg 10:7–10, 2006.

51. Schmeller W, Meier-Vollrath I. Lipedema. In Weissleder H, Schuchhardt C (eds.). Lymphedema Diagnosis and Therapy. 4th ed. Essen, Germany, Viavital, 2008:294–323.

52. Segers P, Belgrado J-P, Leduc A, et al. Excessive pressure in multichambered cuffs used for sequential compression therapy. Phys Ther 82:1000–8, 2002.

53. Eliska O, Eliskova M. Are peripheral lymphatics damaged by high pressure manual massage? Lymphology 28:21–30, 1995.

54. Boris M, Weindorf S, Lasinski BB. The risk of genital edema after external pump compression for lower limb lymphedema. Lymphology 31:15–20, 1998.

55. Pilch U, Wozniewski M, Szuba A. Influence of compression cycle time and number of sleeve chambers on upper extremity lymphedema volume reduction during intermittent pneumatic compression. Lymphology 42:26–35, 2009.

56. Szuba A, Achalu R, Rockson SG. Decongestive lymphatic therapy for patients with breast carcinoma-associated lymphedema. A randomized, prospective study of a role for adjunctive intermittent pneumatic compression. Cancer 95:2260–7, 2002.

57. Cannon S. Pneumatic compression devices for in-home management of lymphedema; Two case reports. Cases J 2:6625, 2009.

58. Maul SM, Devine JA, Wincer CR. Development of a framework for pneumatic device selection for lymphedema treatment. Med Devices Evid Res 2:57–65, 2009.

59. Mayrovitz HN. Interface pressures produced by two different types of lymphedema therapy devices. Phys Ther 87:1379–88, 2007.

60. Földi E, Földi M, Weissleder H. Conservative treatment of lymphedema of the limbs. Angiology 36:171–80, 1985.

61. Boris M, Weindorf S, Lasinski B, Boris G. Lymphedema reduction by noninvasive complex lymphedema therapy. Oncology (Williston Park) 8:95–106; discussion 109–110, 1994.

62. Boris M, Weindorf S, Lasinski B. Persistence of lymphedema reduction after noninvasive complex lymphedema therapy. Oncology (Williston Park) 11:99–109; discussion 110, 113–14, 1997.

63. Casley-Smith JR, Boris M, Weindorf S, Lasinski B. Treatment for lymphedema of the arm—The Casley-Smith method: A noninvasive method produces continued reduction. Cancer 83:2843–60, 1998.

64. Cheville AL. Current and future trends in lymphedema management: Implications for women's health. Phys Med Rehabil Clin N Am 18:539–53, 2007.

65. Ko DS, Lerner R, Klose G, Cosimi AB. Effective treatment of lymphedema of the extremities. Arch Surg 133:452–8, 1998.

66. Mayrovitz H. The standard of care for lymphedema: current concept and physiological considerations. Lymphat Res Biol 7:101–8, 2009.

67. Morgan RG, Casley-Smith JR, Mason MR. Complex physical therapy for the lymphoedematous arm. J Hand Surg Br 17:437–41, 1992.

68. Casley-Smith JR. Varying total tissue pressure and the concentration of initial lymphatic lymph. Microvasc Res 25:369–79, 1983.

69. Franzeck UK, Spiegel I, Fischer M, et al. Combined physical therapy for lymphedema evaluated by fluorescence microlymphography and lymph capillary pressure measurements. J Vasc Res 34:306–11, 1997.

70. Hutzschenreuter P, Brümmer H, Ebberfeld K. Experimental and clinical studies of the mechanism of effect of manual lymph drainage therapy [German]. Z Lymphol 13:62–4, 1989.

71. Hwang JH, Kwon JY, Lee KW, et al. Changes in lymphatic function after complex physical therapy for lymphedema. Lymphology 32:15–21, 1999.

72. Olszewski WL, Engeset A. Intrinsic contractility of prenodal lymph vessels and lymph flow in human leg. Am J Physiol 239:H775–83, 1980.

73. Chodzko-Zajko WJ, Proctor DN, Fiatarone Singh MA, et al. American College of Sports Medicine position stand. Exercise and physical activity for older adults. Med Sci Sports Exerc 41:1510–30, 2009.

74. Courneya KS, Segal RJ, Mackey JR, et al. Effects of aerobic and resistance exercise in breast cancer patients receiving adjuvant chemotherapy: A multicenter randomized controlled trial. J Clin Oncol 25:4396–404, 2007.

75. Radina ME, Armer JM. Surviving breast cancer and living with lymphedema: resiliency among women in the context of their families. J Fam Nurs 10:485–505, 2004.

76. Ridner SH. The psycho-social impact of lymphedema. Lymphat Res Biol 7:109–12, 2009.

77. Holmes MD, Chen WY, Feskanich D, et al. Physical activity and survival after breast cancer diagnosis. JAMA 293:2479–86, 2005.

78. Ahmed RL, Thomas W, Yee D, Schmitz KH. Randomized controlled trial of weight training and lymphedema in breast cancer survivors. J Clin Oncol 24:2765–72, 2006.

79. McKenzie DC, Kalda AL. Effect of upper extremity exercise on secondary lymphedema in breast cancer patients: A pilot study. J Clin Oncol 21:463–6, 2003.

80. Sagen Å, Kåresen R, Risberg MA. Physical activity for the affected limb and arm lymphedema after breast cancer surgery: A prospective, randomized controlled trial with two years follow-up. Acta Oncol 48:1102–10, 2009.

81. Sander AP. A safe and effective upper extremity resistive exercise program for women post breast cancer treatment. Rehabil Oncol 26:3–10, 2008.

82. Allen EV, Hines Jr EA. Lipedema of the legs: A syndrome characterized by fat legs and orthostatic edema. Proc Staff Meet Mayo Clinic 15:184–7, 1940.

83. Warren AG, Janz BA, Borud LJ, Slavin SA. Evaluation and management of the fat leg syndrome. Plast Reconstr Surg 119:9e–15e, 2007.

84. Wold LE, Hines Jr EA. Lipedema of the legs: A syndrome characterized by fat legs and edema. Ann Intern Med 34:1243–50, 1951.

85. Fonder MA, Loveless JW, Lazarus GS. Lipedema, a frequently unrecognized problem. J Am Acad Dermatol 57:S1–3, 2007.

86. Rudkin GH, Miller TA. Lipedema: A clinical entity distinct from lymphedema. Plast Reconstr Surg 94:841–7, 1994.

## CHAPTER 22

# Outcome Measures: A Guide for the Evidence-Based Practice of Cardiopulmonary Physical Therapy

*Kristin Lefebvre*

The practice of physical therapy is grounded in meeting the needs of the individual patient by optimizing their overall health. As consistent with the World Health Organization definition of health, physical therapists attempt to achieve for their patients not only the "absence of infirmity and disease, but also a state of physical, mental and social well-being."[1] Thus in addressing the health of their patient, physical therapists consider not only physiologic and biologic wellness, but also acknowledge the importance the variables of functional status and quality of life.

The foundation for evaluation of the patient with cardiopulmonary dysfunction is based upon the collection of subjective and objective data to provide a diagnosis and prognosis, guide evidence-based interventions, and produce measurable and optimal outcomes. This data, primarily collected at the initial evaluation and readdressed at points along the course of care, consistently includes a chart review to evaluate biologic measures such as lab values and to gather medical history, and a systems review that allows for the gathering of data on functional measures such as pain, range of motion, strength/manual muscle testing, and functional mobility. In addition, the collection of physiologic measures, such as blood pressure, heart rate, respiratory rate, oxygen saturation, ankle brachial index, lung and heart sounds, and rate of perceived exertion (RPE/Borg scale), is essential to providing safe and appropriate interventions and quantifying outcomes. Because the outcome of optimal health is not tied solely to any one of these variables, a comprehensive collection of information is necessary to guide and optimize appropriate care.

In addition to the biologic, functional, and physiologic data collected at initial evaluation, health-related quality of life (HRQL) must also be considered as data that is essential to gather during the initial evaluation and the reevaluation of the patient. HRQL is a measure of how biologic and physiologic processes affect perception of symptoms, which then influences function, general health perception, and quality of life (anxiety, depression, perceived disease burden, general health perception).[2] Thus, HRQL encompasses physical, mental, social, and role functioning, and is a method for assessing the impact of the disease on the life of the patient.[3]

Patients with cardiovascular and pulmonary dysfunction are at high risk for decreased exercise capacity, impaired physiologic response to exercise, poorer quality of life, and higher rates of anxiety and depression. For example, dyspnea and angina are associated with both impaired physical and psychological functioning.[4] In patients undergoing percutaneous coronary intervention, quality of life was found to be decreased 3 months following the intervention.[5] Koch and associates evaluated 6305 patients who underwent coronary artery bypass graft and found a significant association between poor postoperative HRQL during recovery from cardiac surgery and reduced long-term survival.[6] Azevedo and colleagues evaluated 424 adults with heart failure and found that quality-of-life scores significantly lowered as heart failure stages progressed.[7] Finally, depression and anxiety are not only linked to cardiac surgery and coronary artery disease,[8-10] but also predict less compliance during phase II cardiac rehabilitation.[11,12]

Rehabilitation and exercise, however, have been linked with improvements in exercise capacity, physiologic response to exercise, quality of life and decreased symptoms of anxiety and depression among patients with various forms of cardiovascular or pulmonary dysfunction. Theander and associates found improved functional performance and quality of life in a cohort of individuals with chronic obstructive pulmonary disease (COPD) who underwent a pulmonary rehabilitation program.[13] Smart and associates evaluated 51 patients with systolic and diastolic dysfunction and found that exercise training was associated with improved quality of life in both populations.[14] In addition, exercise training has been found to improve quality of life, symptoms, increased physical functioning and self-efficacy for exercise and in individuals with coronary artery disease (CAD) and heart failure.[15,16] Home-based exercise has been shown to improve quality of life and functional capacity in women with heart failure.[17]

Because of the high incidence of anxiety and depression in cardiac populations, the American Association of Cardiovascular and Pulmonary Rehabilitation (AACVPR) recommends screening for depression for all populations. Exercise has been found in some cases to be as beneficial as antidepressant medications in the treatment of symptoms and to provide physiologic changes in the blood that directly impact anxiety.[18–20] In addition, exercise has been found to have an overall positive impact on exercise capacity. For example, Benno and colleagues evaluated 35 randomized controlled trials to evaluate exercise training on cardiac performance, exercise capacity, and quality of life and found exercise was related to significant improvements in blood pressure, end-diastolic volume, heart rate, cardiac output, peak oxygen uptake, anaerobic threshold, and the 6-minute walk test, in addition to improvements in the Minnesota Living with Heart Failure Questionnaire (a measure of health-related quality of life).[21]

For these reasons, it is important for physical therapists to choose methods of quantifying outcomes that address success or achievements in the areas mentioned above. HRQL can also assist the therapist in choosing the most appropriate treatment interventions, modifying those treatment interventions and measuring the results as a reflection of quality of care.

This chapter provides an overview of outcome measures specific to the cardiovascular and pulmonary patient. The outcome measures are addressed from the perspective of physiologic/biologic measures, functional measures, and quality-of-life measures. From a physiologic/biologic perspective, this chapter addresses the importance of gathering and monitoring physiologic data (lab values, blood pressure, heart rate, respiratory rate, $O_2$ saturation, Borg scale, ankle brachial index) and also provides an overview of functional measures that are valid, reliable, and able to detect change in the overall functional status of the cardiovascular patient. Finally, this chapter provides the HRQL measures available for use in the physical therapy practice. The goal is to provide a toolbox of resources for use in the evaluation of patients that will produce optimal and evidence-based outcomes.

## Outcomes Defined

The *Guide to Physical Therapist Practice* defines outcomes as "a systematic examination of patient outcomes in relation to selected patient variables (e.g., age, sex, diagnosis, interventions performed)." Therefore, when measuring outcomes, the therapist must consider the dynamic nature of the evaluation and treatment of the individual patient, as well as the multiple options for outcomes assessment. Box 22-1 lists both clinical and nonclinical factors, which, in addition to the intervention plus random events, results in multiple possible outcomes noted in Box 22-2.

In choosing a comprehensive and sometimes diverse method for outcome measurement, the therapist must be familiar with the psychometric properties of the tool or tools being used for patient assessment. For cross-sectional clinical purposes, it is important to use outcomes not only to inform clinical decision making, but also provide discrimination in treatment decisions that are often subject to time/cost restraints. In addition, the more disease specific the type of measure is, the more likely you are to identify quantifiable changes in your patient population. Consequently, when choosing an appropriate outcome measure, it is necessary to gather certain information about the tools with regard to their psychometric properties as well as their ability to measure change.

---

**Box 22-1**

**Factors Affecting Patient Outcomes**

| Clinical Factors | Nonclinical Factors |
| --- | --- |
| Principal diagnosis, severity | Health-related quality of life |
| Acute clinical stability | Cultural, ethnic, and socioeconomic attributes, beliefs, and behaviors |
| Comorbidity, severity | Patient attitudes and preferences |
| Physical functional status | Psychological, cognitive, and psychosocial functioning |
| Age, sex | |

---

**Box 22-2**

**Diversity of Patient Outcomes**

| Clinical Factors | Nonclinical Factors |
| --- | --- |
| Severity of principal diagnosis | Health-related quality of life |
| Acute clinical stability | Resource utilization |
| Comorbidity, severity | Costs of care |
| Complications, iatrogenic illness | Satisfaction |
| Physical functional status | |
| Survival | |

## Psychometric Properties

As physical therapists, it is important to know whether or not the chosen treatment interventions are providing the highest level of quality care for our patient. In other words, have we chosen and implemented the most appropriate intervention for the patient, based on the evidence, to produce the optimal result. The only method by which to quantify an answer to this question is through use of outcome measures that reflect the highest level of objectivity, the question being: "Are we seeing a clinically significant change and am I able to measure that objectively with the tool I have chosen?"

To answer this question, the therapist must not only be aware of the objective measures available, but also have a good understanding of their psychometric properties. Sherer highlights the various psychometric properties that should be considered when choosing an outcome measure (Table 22-1). The suggested template by Scherer includes considering the intended population; validity; reliability; responsiveness/ sensitivity; minimal detectable change; clinically significant difference or minimally clinically important difference (MCID); and suggested uses in the clinic.[22] This section defines each of these topics and provides examples of each category.

## Intended Population

The more specific the tool is to the population, the more sensitive the tool is toward change. For example, generalized outcomes measures, such as the SF-12 or SF-36 have been found to be reliable and valid across the spectrum of health disorders and chronic diseases, but may not directly, nor in the most sensitive way, measure change in quality of life related to the symptoms of angina, as could be measured with the Seattle Angina Questionnaire (SAQ). Again, when measuring outcomes, it is important to consider the patient population and thus the outcome measure that will be most sensitive to change as a result of the therapist's intervention.

## Validity

An accounting of the validity of the measure being used is usually accessed in the literature. Researchers, who are interested in knowing if the test does in fact measure what it intends to, will evaluate the test by comparing it to a gold standard test or by evaluating it against a theoretical framework (construct validity).[22] A tool with adequate validity will allow for inferences to be made with regard to the results of the outcome measure and provides the assurance that the test

## Table 22-1 Template for Articles Reviewing Outcome Measures

| Topic | Key Aspects to Address |
|---|---|
| 1. Intended population | Identify the purpose of the test. |
| | Describe the patient types on which the test has been used. |
| | Describe patient age, patient characteristics. |
| | Disease characteristics: acute vs. chronic. |
| | Other relevant information. |
| 2. Validity | Describe which constructs or items the test was designed to measure. |
| | Report whether the outcome measure was compared to a "gold standard." |
| 3. Reliability | Provide discussion of tests used to define reliability. |
| | Describe reliability in statistical terms. |
| 4. Responsiveness (sensitivity) to change | Indicate whether test scores change if patient characteristics change. (If patient gets better or worse, do scores also change?) |
| 5. Minimal detectable change (MDC) | Identify the amount of change that exceeds measurement error. |
| | Include how measurement error was determined and report the SEM (standard error of mean). |
| 6. Clinically significant difference (minimally clinically important difference [MCID]) | Describe MCID and how it was determined. |
| | Report the scores in clinical terms, so that clinicians can easily determine what scores indicate change. |
| 7. Suggestions for use in the clinic | Provide suggestions for test administration or interpretation in clinical settings. |
| | What settings are most appropriate for the tool? |
| | How can it be used for groups of patients? |

*From Scherer SA, Wilson CR. Revisiting outcomes assessment. Cardiopulm Phys Ther J 18(1), 21–24, 2007.*

results can discriminate, evaluate change, and make useful and accurate predictions.[23]

## Reliability

Reliability is a measure of the repeatability of a measure through evaluation of its test–retest capability and its internal consistency. The test–retest reliability of the outcome measure refers to the idea that if the measure is given by multiple individuals on various occasions, will the same results be found? Internal consistency, however, refers to the idea that if groups of questions are attempting to measure the same concept (e.g., functional mobility), then consistent answers should be found among these questions.

The test–retest reliability is traditionally measured with the intraclass correlation coefficient (ICC) and the $\kappa$ statistic. The internal consistency is often measured using the Cronbach' $\alpha$ with a value close to 1.0 being of high internal consistency. When selecting an outcome measure, it is important to know that it consistently measures change regardless of the individual using the tool or the patient being measured. Again, the literature is a great place to investigate the reliability of an outcome measure. Reliability scores above 0.70 are considered clinically appropriate.[22]

## Responsiveness/Sensitivity to Change

The sensitivity of a tool refers to its ability to statistically detect change over a period of time in a given patient population and the responsiveness refers to the detection of clinically relevant change.[24] For example, if the patient has made improvements are those improvements consistently and accurately quantified by the chosen outcome tool and does this change make a difference (clinically relevant)?

## Minimal Detectable Change

In considering the type of outcome measure to use with your given patient population, it is important to consider the error measurement of the tool. If the change falls within the error measurement of the tool, as calculated considering the standard deviation of the measurement, then true clinical change has not been achieved. The goal is to use and find outcome measures with low standard error measurements, which will result in an improved ability to measure change and less variability within the tool.

## Minimally Clinically Important Difference

The MCID refers to the amount of change you need to see in an outcome measurement to determine if true clinical change has been attained. A change of the magnitude of the MCID would be considered a significant effect of the chosen intervention thus producing a quantifiable outcome. The MCID can be reported numerically or in percent change. Again this information is available in the literature.

## Importance of Measuring Outcomes

There are a number of important reasons for individual programs to measure outcomes, including to demonstrate accountability, to improve clinical and management decision making for optimal care delivery, for research, and as incentives such as the current physician quality reporting initiative (PQRI). The PQRI is an initiative in which therapists may qualify for bonus payments for using objective measures in practice. Management decision making is enhanced when outcome data lead to the formulation of new protocols, reeducation of practitioners, and redistribution of program resources to improve care delivery. Measuring and sharing outcome information demonstrates accountability to patients, referring physicians, staff, administrators, and payers. Although research has substantiated the efficacy of the intervention in controlled studies, it is the responsibility of individual rehabilitation programs to demonstrate effectiveness in their clinical setting.

Assuring quality of care through measurement of outcomes is of the utmost importance to payers, such as the Center for Medicare and Medicaid Services (CMS), and regulatory agencies, such as the Joint Commission on the Accreditation of Healthcare Organizations (JCAHO). Since 1993, the JCAHO has encouraged outcome measurement as an important form of evaluation leading to continuous improvement, and since 1998, it has been required under the ORYX Initiative (ORYX® is The Joint Commission's performance measurement and improvement initiative, first implemented in 1997).[25] Under the pay-for-performance initiatives, CMS continues to encourage the use of quality measures, with particular focus on health outcomes for the patient, transition of the patient across settings, and resources used to treat the patient, especially in medical settings that include the treatment of patients with heart disease or diabetes. The pay-for-performance initiatives are allowing CMS to transition to a value-based purchasing system, with emphasis placed on evidence-based measures that would have the greatest impact in improving quality and value, and paying based on demonstration of quality, rather than on volume of patients treated.[26]

Physical therapists must be aware that they are not immune to the requirements of value-based purchasing. For example, the 2006 Tax Relief and Health Care Act (TRHCA) (P.L. 109–432) resulted in the establishment of a physician quality reporting system (PQRI), including an incentive payment for eligible professionals who report data on quality measures for covered services furnished to Medicare beneficiaries.[27] Private physical therapists who demonstrate the collection of specific quality data, in the form of at least three specific quality indicators, are eligible for a 2.0% payment bonus from CMS in the year 2009.

Finally, the AACVPR advises that documentation must include records of expected and observed treatment outcomes in cardiac rehabilitation and pulmonary rehabilitation programs. In 1995, the AACVPR Outcome Committee suggested that a minimum of at least one health, one clinical, one behavioral, and one service outcome be measured in all cardiac and pulmonary rehabilitation programs.[6] Outcome measurement is among the requirements for AACVPR program certification. In 2000, the American College of Cardiology (ACC) and the American Heart Association (AHA) spearheaded the formation of quality initiatives to examine the quality of cardiovascular care.[28]

## Selection of Data to Measure

With the dynamic nature of health, it is important that outcomes measures be somewhat individualized to the patient population being evaluated. Guidelines offered by agencies such as the AACVPR and the AHA can give general direction to the selection of such measures. According to the most recent statement on outcomes measures for cardiac rehabilitation programs, the AACVPR recommends use of an outcomes matrix as a conceptual framework for assessing patient and program outcomes that address the behavioral, clinical and health domains.[29]

According to the matrix suggested by AACVPR, clinical factors, such as risk factor profile, symptoms, hemodynamic status, functional capacity, exercise response (heart rate, blood pressure, RPE, $O_2$ saturation), lipid levels, blood pressure, glycosylated hemoglobin (HbA1c) or diabetes management, weight/body mass index (BMI), physical activity, nutrition, psychosocial management, and smoking cessation, should all be considered when measuring patient outcomes (Tables 22-2 and 22-3).[29] These outcomes can all be addressed if measures selected encompass a measurement of biologic/physiologic variables, functional variables, and health-related quality-of-life variables. The remainder of this chapter focuses on appropriate measurements that would fall under each of these categories.

## Biologic/Physiologic Variables

In addition to the collection of demographic data, such as age, gender, race, marital status, primary diagnosis, comorbidities, surgeries, and payer information, data that provides measurement of outcomes should be included at the point of the initial evaluation and should consider the patient from the biologic/physiologic, functional, and quality-of-life perspectives. As the chart review and medical history should provide you with objective information about biologic and physiologic health of your patient, this information should also be considered an outcome measure (as consistent with the AACVPR matrix) and should be monitored and reassessed at points along the continuum of care. Quality of care can be demonstrated when improvements are achieved in areas outlined by the AACVPR outcomes matrix such as blood lipid levels, blood pressure, HbA1c (in patients with diabetes), BMI, hemodynamic regulation, and risk factor modification. Figure 22-1 is a sample form for collection and monitoring of this data.

Rehabilitation and exercise have positive effects on each of the above mentioned biologic/physiologic variables. For example, moderate exercise for at least 30 minutes per day most days of the week, in the form of cardiovascular and resistance training, has been significantly associated with reduction in low-density lipoprotein (LDL) and triglycerides, improvements in high-density lipoprotein (HDL), reduction in C-reactive protein levels, decrease in blood pressure, improvements in insulin sensitivity, reduction in weight, and improvements in hemodynamic regulation.[30–34] Based on recommendations by the AHA and the AACVPR, goals to improve health and reduce mortality include blood pressure < 130/80 mm Hg, HbA1c < 7%, LDL < 100 mg/dL, triglycerides < 150 mg/dL, HDL > 40 mg/dL, and BMI < 25 kg/m².[35,36] These can be followed as outcomes in response to rehabilitation programs for the patient with cardiac and pulmonary risk factors. When physical therapists can demonstrate objective and positive changes in these variables as a result of interventions, they are demonstrating positive outcomes and a high level of quality of care. In all situations where physical therapists are treating individuals with primary or secondary cardiovascular dysfunction, the above variables are appropriate to monitor and document as outcome measures for patients' overall health.

## Ankle Brachial Index

The ankle brachial index (ABI) is a noninvasive, easy, and economical objective outcome measure that can be used to examine perfusion of the lower extremities in individuals who are at high risk of cardiovascular or peripheral arterial disease (PAD). In addition to being highly predictive of CAD, hypertension, acute coronary syndrome, stroke, and overall mortality, low ABI values are associated with physiologic dysfunction such as elevated levels of hemostatic and inflammatory markers, impaired endothelial function, declines in functional mobility, and poorer quality of life.[37–39] Still, lower-extremity ischemia is often underdiagnosed and undertreated.[40]

In a recent study by Cacoub and associates, among 5679 adults age 55 years or older with cardiovascular risk factors, including symptoms of PAD, history of a cardiac event or two or more cardiovascular risk factors (smoking, hypercholesterolemia, diabetes and or hypertension), the prevalence of PAD was more than 26% and as high as 38% in some subgroups.[41] Other programs have also successfully identified significant numbers of individuals with PAD. For example, the Minnesota Regional Peripheral Arterial Disease Screening Program, designed to improve community screening of lower-extremity ischemia, evaluated 347 individuals with a mass media-publicized community screening program. In the screened population, 92 (26.5%) individuals were identified via ABI and questionnaire to have PAD.[42] These individuals had no prior indication of their illness. The Legs for Life National Screening and Awareness Program for PAD involved the evaluation and screening of 700 individuals.[43] A followup survey was given 6 months following the screening program. According to the results, 85% of the individuals identified as having a moderate to high level of PAD had followed up with

**Table 22-2 Summary of Patient Assessment and Outcomes Evaluation in Cardiac Rehabilitation and Secondary Prevention Programs**

| Core Component | Assessment and Outcome Evaluation |
|---|---|
| Patient assessment | Review medical history: diagnoses, interventional procedures, comorbidities, test results, symptoms, risk factors, and medications.<br>Assess: Vital signs, current clinical status, administer a battery of standardized measurement tools to assess status in each component of care.<br>Goal: Develop a goal-directed treatment plan with short- and long-term goals for cardiovascular risk reduction and improvement in health-related quality of life. |
| Lipid management | Assess: Lipid profile; current treatment and compliance.<br>Goal: LDL < 100 mg/dL; secondary goals: HDL > 40 mg/dL, triglycerides < 150 mg/dL. |
| Hypertension management | Assess: Resting blood pressure (BP), current treatment strategies, and patient's adherence.<br>Goal: BP 130 mm Hg systolic and 80 mm Hg diastolic. |
| Diabetes management | Assess: Diabetes present: HbA1C and fasting blood glucose (FBG); current treatment strategies and patient's adherence.<br>Goal: HbA1C < 7.0; FBG 80–110 mg/dL. |
| Weight management | Assess: Weight, height; calculate BMI: determine risk (obese 30 kg/m$^2$; overweight 25–29.9 kg/m$^2$).<br>Goal: If weight risk identified: energy deficit of 500–1000 kcal/day with diet and exercise to reduce weight by at least 10% (1–2 lb/wk). |
| Psychosocial management | Assess: Psychological distress (depression, anxiety, hostility, etc.); refer patients with clinically significant distress to appropriate mental health specialists for further evaluation and treatment.<br>Goal: Reduction of psychological distress; enhance coping and stress management skills. Address issues affecting health-related quality of life. |
| Exercise training | Assess: Functional capacity (maximal or submaximal); physiologic responses to exercise.<br>Goal: Individualized exercise prescription defining frequency (times/week), intensity (THR, RPE, MET levels), duration (minutes), and modality to achieve aerobic, muscular, flexibility, and energy expenditure goals. |
| Physical activity counseling | Assess: Current (past 7 days) physical activity behavior—include leisure and usual activities (occupational, domestic, etc.). Specify: time (min/day) frequency (days/wk) and intensity (e.g., moderate or vigorous).<br>Goal: 30 min/day on most (at least 5) days/wk for moderate (3–5 MET level); 20 min/day for 3–4 days/wk for vigorous (6 MET level). Promote adherence. |
| Nutritional counseling | Assess: Current dietary behavior: dietary content of fat, cholesterol, sodium, caloric intake; eating and drinking habits.<br>Goal: Individualized prescribed diet based on needs assessed. Promote diet adherence. |
| Smoking cessation | Assess: Smoking status: current, recent (quit 6 months), former, never. If current or recent: stage of change, amount of tobacco/day (or other nicotine).<br>Goal: Abstinence from smoking and use of all tobacco products. |

HDL, high-density lipoprotein; LDL, low-density lipoprotein; MET, metabolic equivalent of task; THR, target heart rate.
Data from: AHA/AACVPR Scientific Statement. Core components of cardiac rehabilitation/secondary prevention programs: A statement for healthcare professionals. Circulation 102:1069–1073, 2000; and J Cardiopulm Rehabil 20:310–316, 2000.
From Sanderson BK, Southard D, Oldridge N. Outcomes evaluation in cardiac rehabilitation/secondary prevention programs: Improving patient care and program effectiveness. J Cardiopulm Rehabil 24:68–79, 2004.

a medical physician and were continuing to receive care 6 months after screening.[43] In addition, studies show that PAD can be an indicator of severity of CAD. For example, Moussa and associates studied 800 patients referred for coronary angiography and found that individuals with peripheral arterial disease were significantly more likely to have left main and multivessel CAD.[44]

Patients with claudication in the lower extremity often present to physical therapy with limitation in tolerance for ambulation as a result of ischemic leg pain and cramping.

**Table 22-3 Outcomes Evaluation in Cardiac Rehabilitation/Secondary Prevention Programs: Improving Patient Care and Program Effectiveness**

| Core Components of Care | Health | Clinical | Behavioral | Service |
|---|---|---|---|---|
| Overall management | Health-related quality of life<br>Morbidity<br>Mortality | Risk factor profile<br>Symptoms<br>Hemodynamic regulation<br><br>Untoward events detected during supervised sessions | Improved knowledge and application of self-care actions<br>Appropriate response to symptoms, complications<br>Return to work or desired level of activities<br>Medication adherence<br>Accessing needed resources<br>Session attendance | Patient satisfaction: (e.g., satisfaction with care received, progress toward goals)<br><br>Financial and economic:<br>Patient: healthcare utilization (e.g., clinic, office, emergency visits, hospitalizations, medication use, loss of work days)<br>Access and utilization of service (e.g., referral, enrollment, and completion rates) |
| Exercise training<br>Endurance/aerobic<br>Strength and flexibility | | Functional capacity: maximal and/or submaximal capacity (e.g., walk test)<br>Resting and exercise response: heart rate, blood pressure, rate of perceived effort, rate of perceived breathing, oxygen saturation<br>Measures of strength and flexibility | Physical activity stage of change<br>Energy expenditure: minutes or calories spent in physical activity per week<br>Adherence to exercise prescription | |
| Lipid management | | Lipid levels | Adherence to diet, exercise, and medication<br>Diet and exercise stage of change | |

| | | |
|---|---|---|
| Hypertension | Blood pressure | Adherence to diet, exercise, and medication management |
| | | Diet and exercise stage of change |
| Diabetes management | HbA1c; glucose levels | Adherence to diet, exercise, and medication |
| | | Diet and exercise stage of change |
| | | Self-monitoring behaviors |
| Weight management | Weight, BMI, waist, anthropometric measures | Adherence to diet and exercise |
| | | Diet and exercise stage of change |
| | | Diet/physical activity diaries or logs |
| Psychosocial management | Depression, anxiety, hostility, distress, sexual function | Coping mechanisms |
| | | Stress management and relaxation skills |
| | | Social support network |
| Smoking cessation | | Smoking stage of change |
| | | Number of smokes/day |

Data from: AHA/AACVPR Scientific Statement. Core components of cardiac rehabilitation/secondary prevention programs: A statement for healthcare professionals. Circulation 102:1069–1073, 2000; and J Cardiopulm Rehabil 20:310–316, 2000.
From Sanderson BK, Southard D, Oldridge N. Outcomes evaluation in cardiac rehabilitation/secondary prevention programs: Improving patient care and program effectiveness. J Cardiopulm Rehabil 24:68–79, 2004.

Name: _____ Physician: _____ Date: _____

Diagnosis: _____ Risk Stratification: _____

Comorbidities: _____

| Intervention Needs | Goal | Pre Date | Post Date | % Chg | Treatment Plan |
|---|---|---|---|---|---|

**Behavioral**
- ☐ Physical activity
- ☐ Nutrition
- ☐ Smoking cessation
- ☐ Coping skills
- ☐ Medication adherence

*Behavioral goals are based on measures used.*

Treatment Plan: Education Series (List group classes)

**Clinical**
- ☐ Lipid management — LDL < 100 mg/dL / Trig < 150 mg/dL
- ☐ Hypertension management — SBP < 130 mg/Hg / DBP < 80 mgHg

**Individual Counseling**
- ☐ Diabetes
- ☐ Dietitian
- ☐ Psychosocial
- ☐ Pharmacist
- ☐ Other consults

- ☐ Diabetes management — HbA$_1$C < 7%
- ☐ Weight management (BMI) — Normal < 25 kg/m$^2$
- ☐ Overweight: 25–29.9 kg/m$^2$ — Reduce wgt ≥ 10%
- ☐ Obese; ≥ 30 kg/m$^2$ — Weight goal:
- ☐ Psychosocial management — *Goals are based on measures used.*
- ☐ Exercise training
    Functional capacity

**Exercise Prescription**
- ☐ Aerobic;
- ☐ Muscular/strength
- ☐ Flexibility: (*attach exercise plan*)

**Program**
- ☐ Telemetry monitor
- ☐ Oxygen_____liters/min
- ☐ Pulse oximetry
- Total number of sessions: ___
- Times/week: _____
- Total weeks of program: _____

**Health**
- ☐ Health status or health-related quality of life — *Compare pre/post changes and to reference population.*

Comments: _____

Case Manager _____ Date: _____

Medical Director _____ Date: _____

**Figure 22-1** Sample form of cardiac rehabilitation patient assessment and treatment plan. (From Sanderson BK, Phillips MM, Gerald L, et al. Factors associated with the failure of patients to complete cardiac rehabilitation for medical and nonmedical reasons. J Cardiopulm Rehabil 23:281–289, 2003.)

This pain can be confused with lumbar spine pathology and should be closely monitored and considered in patients with multiple risk factors for cardiovascular disease. Their activity is often limited by the ischemic leg pain brought on during exertion of the peripheral musculature. Evidence supports the fact that physical therapy intervention can make positive physiologic, functional and quality-of-life changes in this patient population. Both resistance and treadmill exercise improves walking distance, walking speed, and lower-extremity endothelial function, and increase life expectancy in those with lower-extremity PAD.[45–47] Screening of lower-extremity ischemia in those at risk for cardiovascular compromise has been found to decrease rates of amputation, decrease cardiovascular morbidity and mortality, reduce the severity of vascular illnesses, and improve quality of life.[48–51]

Consequently, it is essential for physical therapists to understand when and how to use the ABI as an outcome measure in the practice of physical therapy. The ABI should be used in any patient with multiple risk factors for cardiovascular disease (e.g., obesity, diabetes, high LDL, hypertension, past coronary events, smoking, female gender, higher age). The actual measurement of the ABI involves a comparison of an average of the systolic blood pressure of the lower extremity with an average of the systolic blood pressure of the upper extremity (see Chapter 16).

Interpretation of the ABI includes a measurement of 0.90 to 1.10, which is considered a normal finding (Box 22-3). Extremely elevated levels of an ABI (>1.10) can also be indicative of a problem. Patients with an ABI of <0.90 are considered to have PAD, but may be asymptomatic. Most patients with an ABI in the range of >0.50 to 0.90 will typically present with some form of claudication, but can be asymptomatic. ABI values < 0.50 are usually considered to be critical limb ischemia and may be accompanied by rest pain, atrophy, pulselessness, or wounds on the lower extremities. Finally, an ABI of <0.20 is considered severe ischemia. These patients require immediate and emergency medical attention.

The ABI has been found to have high validity, high intra- and interrater reliability, and high sensitivity and specificity for diagnosing lower-extremity ischemia, by using either a stethoscope or hand held Doppler ultrasound unit (Box 22-4).[52,53]

---

**Box 22-3**

### Ranges for Diagnosis and Prevention of Peripheral Arterial Disease

- >1.3 = abnormal
- 1.0 or higher = normal
- 0.8–0.9 = minimal to moderate disease* (not all patients are symptomatic)
- 0.4–0.8 = patients with critical limb ischemia
- 0.4 or less = may indicate tissue necrosis

*Approximately 5% of people with PAD have normal ABI.
Source: Vascular Disease Foundation. 2009.

---

**Box 22-4**

### Instructions for Performing the Ankle Brachial Index

- Place the patient in the supine position.
- Locate the brachial artery in the upper extremity and the dorsalis pedis or posterior tibial artery in the lower extremity (Fig. 22-2A).
- Take an average of three systolic blood pressures from the upper extremity and the lower extremity. A standard stethoscope or hand held Doppler unit can be used to take the measurement (Fig. 22-2B).
- The average of the three systolic measures of blood pressure in the lower extremity is then divided by the average of the three systolic blood pressures taken in the upper extremity, providing you with the ABI.

---

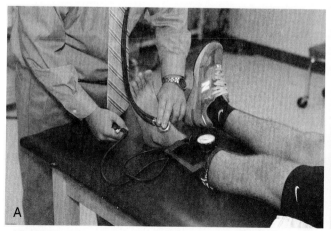 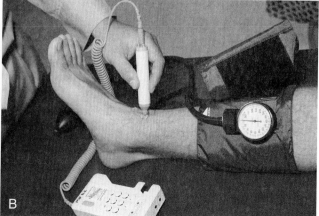

**Figure 22-2** Measuring the ankle brachial index. **A,** Blood pressure measured from the dorsalis pedis artery. **B,** Blood pressure measured using a hand-held Doppler unit.

## Functional Performance

Because physiologic data is not always directly tied to functional performance, as in the case of left ventricular ejection fraction,[54] it is also important to consider functional performance outcome measurement in patient and program assessment. There are many outcome measures available for examination of functional performance and gains in aerobic capacity in the cardiovascular and pulmonary patient population. Although the gold standard for measurement of functional exercise capacity is a measurement of volume oxygen consumption ($VO_2max$), many therapists will not have access to the equipment needed to make $VO_2$ measurements in their day to day treatment environment.

Fortunately, there are many other reliable and valid measures available to evaluate functional performance and outcomes that can be used in the home, outpatient, inpatient acute, rehabilitation, and other treatment environments. A summary of some of these measures include the self-paced walk test, the 2- (2MWT), 3- (3MWT), 6- (6MWT), and 12- (12MWT) minute walk tests, the modified shuffle test, the treadmill endurance test and the 200-meter walk fast test. Although an extended explanation for each of these measures is beyond the scope of this chapter, references for these functional outcomes measures can be found in Table 22-4. This chapter highlights the two measures most often used in research and program outcome assessment, the 6MWT and the modified shuffle test, and provides information and directions you need to perform these tests with your patient populations.

The four walk tests most commonly used in the physical therapy environment for assessment of self-paced functional performance and exercise capacity in the cardiovascular and pulmonary patient population are the 2MWT, 3MWT, 6MWT, and 12MWT. These tests are often used in research, with the 6MWT most recently validated among patients following heart transplantation and patients with cardiac pacemakers, obese patients, poststroke patients, and children with cerebral palsy.[112–116] In addition, the 6MWT shows high test–retest reliability among individuals with chronic heart and lung disease, heart failure, COPD, fibromyalgia, the elderly and PAD, and moderate to high validity when compared to the shuttle walk test, cycle ergometry, physical activity measured with an accelerometer, self-rating of walking ability, and functional status questionnaire scores.

Each of these tests, originally derived from the 12MWT, measure the distance that a patient can walk on a set course, at a self-chosen pace, in the time allotted. The distance of walk test chosen is based on the therapist's assessment of patient tolerance for activity. Although the 2MWT, 3MWT, and 12MWT are valid and reliable for use with the cardiopulmonary population,[117,118] most commonly, the 6MWT, a middle distance, is used for patient examination and objective measurement of outcomes. This section outlines the procedure for using the 6MWT as an examination tool and outcome measure in the cardiovascular

and pulmonary population. The instructions for the 6MWT are based on guidelines created by the American Thoracic Society.[119]

## The Six-Minute Walk Test

The equipment required for performance of the 6MWT is minimal. To effectively perform the test, the examiner needs a 100-foot hallway marked by two cones or a straight path with 50-foot intervals, a clipboard, lap counter, timer, chair, vital signs monitor, Borg scale, oxygen source, and access to emergency assistance as needed. Close monitoring of $SpO_2$ (oxygen saturation measured by pulse oximetry) is vital among patients with pulmonary and cardiac dysfunction to maintain safety during the test period. The use of a treadmill or circular track for this test is *not* recommended. The course should include a 100-foot track that can be marked at the end with two cones on which the patient walks down and back in a straight-line pattern.

Patient preparation includes the following: The patient should wear comfortable clothing and shoes (Fig. 22-3). The patient should use their normal and everyday assistive device, for example, walker, rolling walker, or cane, during the test,

*Text conintued on p. 723*

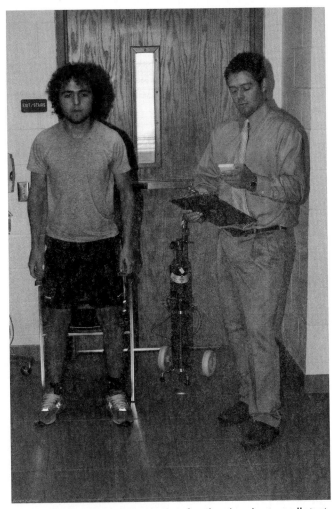

**Figure 22-3** Patient preparation for the six-minute walk test.

**Table 22-4 Comparison of Measurement Instruments**

| Measurement Instrument | Items | Self | Time Per PT (Min) | Time Per Staff (Min) | Parameters Measured |
|---|---|---|---|---|---|
| **General Quality of Life Measures** | | | | | |
| Medical Outcomes Study Short Form (SF-36)[55] | 36 | Yes | 5 to 10 | 5 | Physical, psychological, and social functioning (known as SF-36 or RAND 36) |
| RAND 36-item Health Survey 1.0 (RAND 36) | | | | | |
| Nottingham Health Profile (NHP)[56] | 45 | Yes | 10 | 10 | Energy, pain, emotion, sleep, mobility, social isolation and ADL |
| Sickness Impact Profile (SIP)[57,58] | 136 | Yes | 30 | 20 | Physical, psychosocial, and 5 independent factors |
| Quality of Well-Being Scale (QWB)[59] | 18–62 | No | 10–15 | 20 | Mobility, physical activity, social activity, self care and symptoms |
| Illness Effects Questionnaire (IEQ)[60] | 20 | Yes | 20 | 25 | Biological, psychological and social aspects |
| Dartmouth Primary Care Cooperative Information (COOP)[61] | 9 charts | Yes | 5–7 | 5–7 | Physical, emotional and social role function, pain, overall health, health change and social support |
| DUKE Health Profiles—Revised[62] | 17 | Yes | 2–4 | 3 | Health and dysfunction |
| Multidimensional Health Locus of Control Inventory (MHLOC)[63] | 18 | Yes | 2–4 | Unknown | Perceived control over health and health care |
| Quality of Life Systemic Inventory (QLSI)[64] | 30 | No | 45 | 60 | The gap between patient's condition and goal for 30 life domains prioritized by patient |
| Symptom Questionnaire[65] | 92 | Yes | 2–5 | 10–15 | Depression, anxiety, somatic complaints and anger-hostility |
| **Cardiac-Specific Quality of Life Measures** | | | | | |
| Minnesota Living with Heart Failure Questionnaire (LHFQ)[66] | 21 | Yes | 10–15 | 3–5 | Physical, socioeconomic, and psychological impairment |
| Outcomes Institute Angina Type Specification (MOS-Angina)[67] | 14 | Yes | 2–3 | 5–8 | Patient outcome questions, with additional physician questions based on patient's course of care |
| Quality of Life after Myocardial Infarction (QLMI)[68] | 26 | No | 10 | Trace | Physical limitations (symptoms, restrictions) and emotional function (confidence, self-esteem, and emotions) |

*Continued*

**Table 22-4 Comparison of Measurement Instruments—cont'd**

| Measurement Instrument | Items | Self | Time Per PT (Min) | Time Per Staff (Min) | Parameters Measured |
|---|---|---|---|---|---|
| **Cardiac-Specific Quality of Life Measures (cont'd)** | | | | | |
| MacNew Quality of Life after Myocardial Infarction (MacNew QLMI)[69] | 27 | Yes | | | Physical, emotional, and social domains (modified from QLMI) |
| Ferrans and Powers Quality of Life Index-Version (QLI)[70] | 72 | Yes | 10 | 15–30 | Health and functioning, cardiac, socio-economic, psychological / spiritual, and family |
| Seattle Angina Questionnaire (SAQ)[71] | 19 | Yes | 3–4 | | Physical limitations, angina stability, angina frequency, treatment satisfaction, and disease perception |
| **Pulmonary-Specific Quality of Life Measures** | | | | | |
| Chronic Respiratory Disease Questionnaire (CRQ)[72] | 20 | No | 25–30 | 35 | Dyspnea, fatigue, emotional function, and feeling of mastery over disease |
| St. George's Respiratory Questionnaire (SGRQ)[73] | 76 | Yes | 15 | 10 | Symptoms, activity, and impact of disease |
| Pulmonary Functional Status Scale (PFSS)[74] | 56 | Yes | 15–30 | 10–25 | ADL in respiratory patients |
| Pulmonary Functional Status and Dyspnea Questionnaire (PFSDQ)[75] | 164 | Yes | 15 | 15 | ADL and dyspnea |
| Living with Asthma Questionnaire[76] | 68 | Yes | 20 | 20 | Quality of life in patients with asthma |
| **Functional Activity and Exercise Related Measures** | | | | | |
| The New York Heart Association functional classification (NYHA)[77] | 4 | No | NA | 1 | Physical activity performance |
| The Specific Activity Scale[78] | 5 | No | 5 | 1 | Activities of daily living |
| Baseline Dyspnea Index/Transitional Dyspnea Index[79] | 15 | No | 5–10 | 5–10 | Functional impairment, magnitude of task, magnitude of effort |
| Duke Activity Scale Index[80] | 12 | Yes | 5 | 2 | Functional status |
| Borg Scale[81,82] | NA | No | Seconds | Seconds | Perceived exertion |
| Visual analogue scale[83] | NA | No | Seconds | 1 | Severity of dyspnea during exercise |
| Maximal and Submaximal Progressive Multistage Exercise Test (GXT)[84] | NA | No | 45–60 | 45–60 | Changes in exercise capacity |

## Functional Activity and Exercise Related Measures (cont'd)

| Measure | | | | | |
|---|---|---|---|---|---|
| 6- or 12-minute walk[85,86] | NA | No | 20–30 | 20–30 | Exercise endurance |
| Human Activity Profile (HAP, formerly ADAPT)[87] | 105 | Yes | 15–30 | 20–50 | Activity level (Formerly ADAPT) |
| Functional Status Questionnaire (FSQ)[88] | 34 | Yes | 15 | 3–5 | Physical, psychological, social, and role function in ambulatory patients |

## Psychological Measures

| Measure | | | | | |
|---|---|---|---|---|---|
| Hopkins Symptom Checklist—Revised (SCL-90-R)[89] | 90 | Yes | 20 | 30* | Nine subscales, such as somatization, depression, anxiety, and hostility |
| Minnesota Multiphasic Personality Inventory (MMPI)[90] | 567 | Yes | 180 | 60* | Depression, anxiety, psychosis, personality disorders |
| Cook-Medley Hostility Inventory[91] | 50 | Yes | 15 | 15* | Hostility |
| Buss Durkey Hostility Inventory[92] | | | | | Hostility |
| Beck Depression Inventory (BDI)[93] | 21 | Yes | 5–10 | 15* | Depression, mood state |
| Center for Epidemiological Studies Depression Inventory (CES-D)[94] | 20 | Yes | 10 | 15 | Depression, mood state |
| State-Trait Anxiety Inventory (STAI)[95] | 40 | Yes | 20 | 5* | Anxiety |
| COPD Self Efficacy Scale[96] | 34 | Yes | 5–10 | 30* | Confidence level |
| COPE Inventory (COPE)[97] | 52 | Yes | 20 | 20* | Different ways in which people respond to stress |
| Jenkins Activity Survey (JAS)[98] | 20 | Yes | 20 | 15* | Four common components of type A behavior |
| Profile of Mood States (POMS)[99] | 65 | Yes | 15 | 20* | Various mood states (e.g., tension, anger, depression, confusion) |
| Cardiac Depression Scale (CDS)[100] | 26 | Yes | 10 | 40 | Depression |
| Face Scale[101] | 20 | No | 2 | 2* | Mood |
| Psychological General Well-Being Index (PGWB)[102] | 22 | Yes | 15 | 25* | Both negative (depression, anxiety) and positive (vitality, health) mood states |
| Ways of Coping Questionnaire[103] | NA | Yes | 10 | 20 | Thoughts and actions that people use to handle stressful situations |

Continued

## Table 22-4 Comparison of Measurement Instruments—cont'd

| Measurement Instrument | Items | Self | Time Per PT (Min) | Time Per Staff (Min) | Parameters Measured |
|---|---|---|---|---|---|
| **Sociological Measures** | | | | | |
| Marital Adjustment Scale (MAS)[103] | 16 | Yes | 5 | 5 | Marital adjustment |
| MOS Social Support Survey[104] | 20 | Yes | 10 | 5 | Four functional support scales |
| Psychosocial Adjustment to Illness[105] | 45 | Yes | 15 | 10 | Coping with illness or handicap |
| **Other Health-Related Behavior Measures** | | | | | |
| Harvard-Willett Food Frequency Questionnaire[106] | 116 | Yes | 45–60 | † | Type, quantity, and frequency of food ingested |
| Block Food Questionnaire[107] | 128 | No | 30–45 | 45 | Calories, fat, fiber, protein, carbohydrates, linoleic/oleic acids, vitamins, minerals |
| Diet Habit Survey[108] | 32 | Yes | 30 | 20–30 | Cholesterol, saturated fat intake, complex carbohydrates, salt |
| Quick Check (Quantitative)[109] | 74 | Yes | 15 | 3–5 | Fat, saturated fat, cholesterol |
| Health Knowledge Test[110] | 40 | Yes | 15–20 | 5–10 | Knowledge of disease management skills in pulmonary patients |
| Cardiac Knowledge Questionnaire[111] | 55 | Yes | | | Knowledge of cardiovascular system and coronary heart disease, lifestyle change issues, and perceptions of severity/prognosis |

Key: Under "Self", yes = self-administered, no = structured interview. Under Time per Pt is time in minutes for patient to complete questionnaire. Time per Staff refers to time in minutes for staff to administer, score, and interpret questionnaire.
* Psychologist must interpret.
†Must be mailed out for computer scoring.
Adapted from Pashkow P, Ades PA, Emery CF, et al. Outcome measurement in cardiac and pulmonary rehabilitation. J Cardiopulm Rehabil 15(6):397–398, 1995; with permission from Lippincott-Raven. Adapted from Pashkow P: Outcomes in cardiopulmonary rehabilitation. Phys Ther 76(6):647, 1996.

## Box 22-5

### Patient Instructions for Performing the Six-Minute Walk Test Per the American Thoracic Society

"The object of this test is to walk as far as possible for 6 minutes. You will walk back and forth in this hallway. Six minutes is a long time to walk, so you will be exerting yourself. You will probably get out of breath or become exhausted. You are permitted to slow down, stop, and to rest as necessary. You may lean against the wall while resting, but resume walking as soon as you are able. You will be walking back and forth around the cones. You should pivot briskly around the cones and continue back the other way without hesitation. Now I'm going to show you. Please watch how I turn without hesitation (demonstrate a lap). Are you ready to do that? I am going to use this counter to keep track of the number of laps you complete. I will click it each time you turn around at this starting line. Remember that the object is to walk *as far as possible* for 6 minutes, but don't run or jog. Start now or whenever you are ready."

Singh S, Morgan M, Scott S, et al. Development of a shuttle walking test of disability in patients with chronic airways obstruction. Thorax 47:1019–1024, 1992.

## Box 22-6

### Patient Instructions for Performing the Modified Shuttle Walk Test

"Walk at a steady pace, aiming to turn around when you hear the signal. You should continue to walk until you feel that you are unable to maintain the required speed without becoming unduly breathless."

Singh S, Morgan M, Scott S, et al. Development of a shuttle walking test of disability in patients with chronic airways obstruction. Thorax 47:1019–1024, 1992.

and the patient's normal medical regimen should be continued. Patients should not have exercised vigorously within 2 hours of the exam. The instructions provided to the patient are very explicitly outlined by the American Thoracic Society and are found in Box 22-5.

To prepare for the 6MWT, the patient should be placed in a seated position at the start line and vital sign/Borg scale/contraindication information collected. Once instructions and demonstration of a lap have been provided to the patient, the test begins when the patient starts walking. The examiner should not say "ready, set go!" In addition, it is important that the examiner use limited and neutral encouragement once a minute (giving the patient an update on the time that has passed), in addition to not walking with the patient during the exam. These two errors can affect the validity of the exam.

During the exam, if any rest breaks are taken, vital sign and Borg scale information should be recorded, as long as it does not disrupt possible continuation of the exam. Following the exam or upon termination by the patient, the Borg scale and vital signs should again be recorded and the patient should be questioned as to what, if anything, might have limited them from going further. The total distance should be recorded. Gait speed can also be calculated by taking the distance walked and dividing by time.

The average distance walked can vary based on the patient population, but distances of less than 400 meters are predictive of mortality across various patient populations. The MCID for this test was also found to be approximately 86 meters for an individual patient.[120] In addition to being predictive of mortality, the test is a

good indicator of outcomes from a pulmonary or cardiac rehabilitation program and should be considered across all settings in which therapists see patients with cardiopulmonary dysfunction.

### The Modified Shuttle Test

In contrast to the self paced 2MWT, 3MWT, 6MWT, and 12MWT, Singh and colleagues developed an incremental modified shuttle test that allows for assessment and clinical management of patient performance through evaluation of the patient during incremental and progressive exercise stress. This exam allows for a more specific examination of symptom-limited performance than the self-paced walk tests because of the incremental nature of the assessment, and was found to show a greater cardiovascular response than the 6MWT. The test was originally designed to objectively evaluate symptom-limited disability in individuals with chronic airway obstruction, but has since been validated in individuals with COPD, heart failure, awaiting heart transplantation, cystic fibrosis, rheumatoid arthritis, myocardial infarction, or status after coronary artery bypass graft surgery. It also has high test–retest reliability and moderate to high validity when compared with the 6MWT, Chronic Respiratory Disease Questionnaire, St. Georges Respiratory Questionnaire, SF-36, and the treadmill endurance test.[121]

During the modified shuttle walk test, patients are required to walk up and down a 10-meter course (Box 22-6). The course is set with two cones that are 0.5 meters from the end of the 10-meter course, allowing room for the patient to turn within the 10 meters (Fig. 22-4). The patient's walking speed is dictated with an audio sound played over an audio cassette. During the exam, the patients speed is increased over 12 levels of intensity to place increased cardiovascular demand on the patient as they progress through the exam. At each minute, the walking speed increases in an increment of 0.17 m/sec. During the course of the test, the overall speed will increase from 0.50 m/sec to 2.37 m/sec. With each increase in speed, the increase in the number of shuttles required also increases. Table 22-5 provides the speed and number of shuttles per level of test.

The beginning of the modified shuttle walk test is indicated by a triple beep on the audio recording. This is followed by select and incremental single beeps that come in decreased

### Table 22-5 The Shuttle Walk Protocols

| | DOWNGRADED PROTOCOL | | | MODIFIED PROTOCOL | | |
|---|---|---|---|---|---|---|
| | Speed | | | Speed | | |
| Level | M/Sec | Mph | Shuttles Per Level | M/Sec | Mph | Shuttles Per Level |
| 1 | 0.62 | 1.39 | 3 | 0.50 | 1.12 | 3 |
| 2 | 0.72 | 1.61 | 4 | 0.67 | 1.50 | 4 |
| 3 | 0.82 | 1.83 | 4 | 0.84 | 1.88 | 5 |
| 4 | 0.92 | 2.06 | 5 | 1.01 | 2.26 | 6 |
| 5 | 1.02 | 2.28 | 6 | 1.18 | 2.64 | 7 |
| 6 | 1.12 | 2.51 | 6 | 1.35 | 3.02 | 8 |
| 7 | 1.22 | 2.73 | 7 | 1.52 | 3.40 | 9 |
| 8 | 1.32 | 2.95 | 7 | 1.69 | 3.78 | 10 |
| 9 | 1.42 | 3.18 | 8 | 1.86 | 4.16 | 11 |
| 10 | 1.52 | 3.40 | 9 | 2.03 | 4.54 | 12 |
| 11 | | | | 2.20 | 4.92 | 13 |
| 12 | | | | 2.37 | 5.30 | 14 |

*From Singh S, Morgan M, Scott S, et al. Development of a shuttle walking test of disability in patients with chronic airways obstruction. Thorax 47:1019–1024, 1992.*

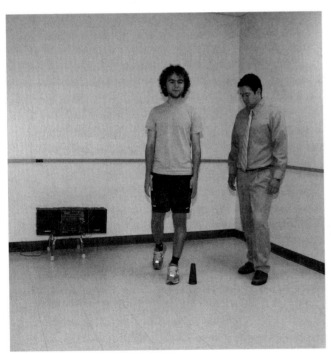

**Figure 22-4** Preparation for the modified shuttle walk test.

time intervals throughout the test. The patient attempts to be at the end of the course or at the opposite cone prior to each single beep on the audio recording. If the patient reaches the opposite end of the course prior to the beep, they are instructed to wait there until the beep and then proceed forward.

To establish the patient's walking speed, the first minute of the test involves accompanying the patient during walking to set the pace. After the first minute, the patient must then pace themselves. Like the 6MWT, encouragement should not be provided to the patient during this test, the only feedback to the patient being the audio beeps from the recording and instructions to the patient to increase walking speed slightly at each minute.

The end of the test is determined by one of three criteria: (1) the patient is too breathless to continue or has desaturated to a level unsafe for continued exertion; (2) the patient failed to complete a shuttle in the given time; or (3) the patient attains 85% of maximal heart rate per the formula $210 - (0.85 \times \text{age})$. Distance walked should be recorded in meters. One practice test may be required in certain patient populations.

### Other Functional Performance Measures

Other functional performance measures are utilized to assess rehabilitation outcomes in different populations and may include those with cardiovascular and pulmonary impairments. The Timed Up and Go test (TUG) is frequently used for assessment of risk of falls in the elderly and may be an appropriate functional outcome tool for heart failure or pulmonary disease patients.[122,123] See Box 22-7 for a description of the TUG.

Gait speed (walking speed) is another functional performance measure that, due to its ease of use and psychometric properties, has been utilized as a predictor and an outcome measure across mutiple diagnoses including older adults, frail elderly, and stroke.[124–128] Measurements of gait speed are

## Box 22-7

### Description of TUG

- Patients are timed (in seconds) when performing the TUG—3 conditions
  - TUG alone-from sitting in a chair, stand up, walk 3 meters, turn around, walk back, and sit down.
  - TUG Cognitive-complete the task while counting backwards from a randomly selected number between 20 and 100.
  - TUG manual-complete the task while carrying a full cup of water.
- The time taken to complete the task is strongly correlated to level of functional mobility, (i.e. the more time taken, the more dependent in activities of daily living).
- The cutoff levels for TUG is 13.5 seconds or longer with an overall correct prediction rate of 90%; for TUG manual is 14.5 seconds or longer with a 90% correct prediction rate; and Tug cognitive is 15 seconds or longer with an overall correct prediction rate of 87%.[122,123]

### Table 22-6 Calculated Gait Speed

| Meters/Second | Miles/Hour |
|---|---|
| 0.4 | 0.9 |
| 0.6 | 1.3 |
| 0.8 | 1.8 |
| 1.0 | 2.2 |
| 1.2 | 2.7 |
| 1.4 | 3.1 |

### Table 22-7 Functional Tasks Related to Gait Speed

| Walking Speed | | | Function that Can Be Performed |
|---|---|---|---|
| *M/Sec* | *Mph* | *METS* | |
| 0.67 | 1.5 | <2 | Self care |
| 0.89 | 2.0 | 2.5 | Household activities |
| 1.11 | 2.5 | 3.0 | Carry groceries, light yard work |
| 1.33 | 3.0 | 3.5 | Climb several flights of stairs |

*From Studenski SA, Duncan PW, Richards L Performance Measures in the Clinical Setting J Am Ger Soc 2003;51:1–10.*

highly reliable regardless of the method of measurement and the patient populations.[129,130] Gait speed has also been determined to predict future health status[124,125] as well as functional decline,[131] and rehospitalization.[132] Low gait speeds also are predictors of the type of location an individual would be optimally functional following hospitalization.[133]

Gait speed measurement is easy and can be performed in any setting. A six meter straight path that is obstacle free is optimal for performing the test. One utilizes a stop watch and distance measurements on the floor to obtain a gait speed. An individual is to walk (using assistive devices and/or oxygen if necessary) at their normal speed, and the speed is measured after the individual crosses the first meter marker on the floor (one meter is used for acceleration and one meter is used for deceleration) and speed measurement is concluded after the patient crosses the 5 meter marker on the floor. The 4 meters walked is then divided by the seconds for the walk and a gait speed is calculated and can be converted to miles/hour (see Table 22-6). Table 22-7 presents functional tasks related to gait speed.[124]

Other functional performance measures are available to utilize in the clinical setting and should be researched beyond this chapter as they may be applicable to the cardiovascular and pulmonary population (Box 22-8).

## Health-Related Quality of Life

Healthcare quality and effectiveness is of the utmost importance to ethically practicing physical therapists. As physiologic parameters and quality of life do not always correlate, as in the case of ejection fraction and quality of life,[134] comprehensive evaluation of outcomes from a HRQL perspective must be considered. In addition, because a goal of cardiopulmonary intervention is secondary prevention, that is, smoking

### Box 22-8

### Other Outcomes that can be Measured in Cardiopulmonary Patients

Activity testing
- Lawton Instrumental ADL scale
- Grocery Shelving Test (upper limb activity)
- Gait Speed Test
- London Handicap Scale
- Short Physical Performance Battery
- Chair Stand Test: number that can be performed in 30 seconds
- Berg Balance test

For reference information and links to the source article abstracts in PubMed, please see Evolve.

cessation, increasing exercise, decreasing stress, and so forth, outcomes associated with HRQL need to be considered because of the relationship between poorer quality of life and maintaining these positive changes in lifestyle.[135-137]

There are many valid and reliable instruments available. Resources for administration, collection, and interpretation of data must be considered when selecting which or how many instruments can be used. Instruments that are easy on the staff in that they can be scored and interpreted quickly and efficiently are best. Standardized, self-report

## Table 22-8 Benefits of Generic and Disease-Specific Instruments

| Generic Quality-of-Life Instruments | Disease-Specific Quality-of-Life Instruments |
|---|---|
| Apply to heterogeneous population | Responsive to a specific population with same disease or condition |
| Allow cross-population comparisons (compare with other chronic diseases) | Focus on problematic areas for a given population |
| Address multiple issues related to limitations in health status (e.g., comorbidities, age) | Address issues related to clinical manifestations of a disorder |

questionnaires are most popular and efficient. Many hospitals administer generic quality-of-life questionnaires to all their patients and have established protocols for administration, scoring, and tracking for comparisons over time. The cardiopulmonary rehabilitation staff should access, review, and utilize this data when available, and then determine whether additional disease-specific quality-of-life information is needed and feasible to obtain. Table 22-8 lists the benefits of both generic and disease-specific quality-of-life instruments.

HRQL measures outcomes from the patient's point of view and provides insight into the patient's perception of his or her illness' impact on activities of daily living. A comprehensive assessment of HRQL encompasses an evaluation of the patient from the perspective of perceived symptoms, functional status, mental well-being, social functioning, satisfaction with treatment protocol, and overall life satisfaction.[138] Although many HRQL assessment measures are available, the more specific the tool to the individual being studied, the more sensitive it will be to change. For that reason, this chapter highlights four different quality-of-life measures: the SAQ, the Kansas City Cardiomyopathy Questionnaire, the Chronic Respiratory Disease Questionnaire, and the Walking Impairment Questionnaire. These measures are designed for and are sensitive and specific to individuals with heart failure, angina, dyspnea, and lower-extremity PAD.

## The Seattle Angina Questionnaire

### Background and Administration
The SAQ is designed to specifically assess the impact of chest pain or angina within the previous 4 weeks on a patient's quality of life. The survey was designed to assess the severity of limitations in everyday life because of angina, chest pain, and discomfort using a series of 11 questions.[139] Time to complete this survey will vary from person to person, but it is expected to only take about 5 minutes per individual.

The questionnaire is divided into two distinct sections. The first section assesses the impact of angina on the individual's activities of daily living. In this section, the patient rates perceived day-to-day limitations in activities of daily living. Limitations are rated on the following scale: severely limited, moderately limited, somewhat limited, a little limited, not limited, or limited and unable to complete the task. The second section includes a series of questions in which is patient must choose the statement that best assesses the patient's health conditions. The statements within this section vary from question to question.[139]

### Purpose
The purpose of the SAQ is to quantify the emotional and physical impact of angina. The patient's satisfaction with physical therapy and outcomes related to angina improvement and quality of life can also be assessed using the SAQ. The intended population is individuals with CAD who have experienced chest pain and tightness in the 4 weeks before the survey was completed. A patient is considered to have CAD if the patient fits into one of the following four categories: a previous myocardial infarction, previous vascularization surgery, chest pain with abnormal results during testing, and acute or chronic disease.[139]

### Reliability and Validity
In the area of physical limitation, moderate to strong correlations were seen between activity time, SAQ scores, Duke Activities Index scores, and Specific Activity Scale scores ($r = 0.43$–$0.84$ and $p < 0.001$). Angina stability was found to be correlated with patients global assessment of change ($r = 0.70$ and $p < 0.0001$), and a correlation was also found between frequency of angina reported and 1-year nitroglycerin refills ($r = 0.31$, $p = 0.0006$, and $p < 0.05$). The disease perception sections of the SAQ were highly correlated with the SF-36 ($r = 0.60$ and $p < 0.001$).

Finally, treatment satisfaction was validated against the Internal Board of Medicine's Patient Satisfaction Survey and a moderately high correlation was found between the two surveys ($r = 0.67$ and $p < 0.0001$).

The SAQ also shows high reproducibility. A paired t-test was completed to determine if statistically significant change existed if the test was administered three months after the initial survey was filled out in a stable population. For the paired t-test, $p = 0.10$ to $0.77$, showing that there was no significant difference between the two episodes of filling out the questionnaires.

Finally, the responsiveness, or whether or not the test was able to pick up changes that may occur as a result of improvements, was evaluated. Spertus' sample population of postopenheart-surgery individuals demonstrated dramatically improved scores on the SAQ.[139]

### Suggested Usage
This survey is most appropriate for patients with active symptoms of angina in the setting of CAD or myocardial infarction. It can be used across settings, including cardiac

rehabilitation; outpatient, subacute, or acute rehabilitation; or in-home care. Because the majority of the population evaluated in creation of this tool was male, the SAQ may be most sensitive among the male population. In addition, the study population's age range was 55 to 70 years.

This survey may be very useful in determining a baseline and outcome measure for cardiovascular and pulmonary patients with active symptoms of angina or chest pain. The main advantages of this survey are that it is disease specific, and that it contains information on activity limitations that are very common with CAD. Based on the research, this test appears reliable and valid for use in the physical therapy setting.

## The Kansas City Cardiomyopathy Questionnaire

### Background and Administration

The Kansas City Cardiomyopathy Questionnaire (KCCQ) is a self-response questionnaire made up of 23 items that quantify specific areas of quality of life related to heart failure. These areas include physical limitations (question 1), symptoms (frequency [questions 3, 5, 7, and 9], severity [questions 4, 6, 8], change over time [question 2]), self-efficacy and knowledge (questions 11, 12), social interference (question 16), and quality of life (questions 13 to 15). It is important to note that question 15 was adapted from the Mental Health Inventory of the SF-36, a general quality-of-life tool, to be used as a marker for depression which is an important prognostic variable among those with cardiovascular disease.[140] There are a total of eight different domains that the test encompasses, including physical symptoms, symptoms stability, social limitation, self-efficacy, quality of life, functional status, and clinical summary. This disease-specific questionnaire is a self-administered questionnaire that requires approximately 4 to 6 minutes for the patient to complete.

The instrument is scored based on a 5-point Likert scale that ranges from "extremely limited" to "not at all limited." Each response that is available corresponds to an ordinal value that ranges from 1 to 5, 1 being the lowest functional level, indicating that a higher score is indicative of a better status of health. The total score can range from 0 to 100. Two summary scores were also developed, including a functional status score and a clinical summary score. The functional status score combines the physical limitation and symptoms domains. The clinical summary score is a combination of the functional status with the quality of life and social limitation domains.[140] A clinically significant change in the total score is defined as greater than or equal to 5 points.[141]

### Purpose

The purpose of the KCCQ is to provide a valid and reliable health status measure that goes beyond a general or generic questionnaire. It provides patients and clinicians with a disease-specific approach to evaluate and appropriately monitor and treat those with heart failure. It targets those patients with advanced symptoms of heart failure.[142] A patient is considered to have heart failure if the patient presents with an ejection fraction of less than 40% as well as other signs/symptoms of a heart failure exacerbation, such as orthopnea, dyspnea on exertion, edema in the lower extremities and/or abdomen, persistent cough, and feelings of extreme fatigue.

### Reliability and Validity

To assess the validity of the KCCQ, the tool was compared to the functional limitation domain of the Minnesota Living with Heart Failure Questionnaire (MLHFQ), 6MWT, The New York Heart Association (NYHA) classification for heart failure, and the physical limitation domain of the SF-36. The KCCQ demonstrated moderate to high correlation with the MLHFQ (0.65), the 6MWT (0.48), the NYHA (−0.65), and the physical limitation domain of the SF-36 (0.84). The results showed that the KCCQ had a high Spearman correlation coefficient with the NYHA class and also correlated significantly with the distance walked during the 6MWT. The KCCQ is much more sensitive to clinical change than the MLHFQ and has a greater sensitivity to clinical change than does the SF-36.[140]

The KCCQ is also highly responsive. Upon evaluation, the KCCQ was significantly more sensitive than either the MLHFQ or the SF-36.[1] The KCCQ scores showed an improvement by between 15.4 and 40.4 points, and its responsiveness to change was summarized using a responsiveness statistic that resulted in a statistic of 1.48 in the physical limitation domain, almost three times larger than the corresponding domains of the MLHFQ (0.52) and SF-36 (0.59).[1] The KCCQ was specifically found to detect clinical changes, particularly in the outpatient population with advanced symptoms of heart failure.

The prognostic value of the KCCQ was assessed in a study of the overall score in 1516 patients with heart failure after a recent acute myocardial infarction. The overall scores of the KCCQ were strongly associated with a 1-year cardiovascular mortality and hospitalization (the higher the score the greater the risk of mortality). The KCCQ is also best at reflecting clinical changes in heart failure with regard to direction (improvement vs. deterioration), and in magnitude of clinical change followed by the 6MWT. The KCCQ summary score is the best at discriminative abilities for each category of change, expressing a high sensitivity. The statistics of clinical change are as follows[142]:

- 0.90 for a large/moderate deterioration
- 0.77 for a small deterioration
- 0.68 for a small improvement
- 0.76 for a large/moderate improvement

### Suggested Usage

Based on the above information, the KCCQ is valid, reliable, and responsive, and could be an important tool for determining a patient's prognosis. The KCCQ may be important for providing a clinically meaningful outcome in cardiovascular research, patient management, and patient treatment, as well as quality-of-life assessment. This tool is significant in quantifying improvements of patients with heart failure and has significant value when assessing a patient's outcomes as well as the patient's overall quality of life.

## The Chronic Respiratory Disease Questionnaire

### Background and Administration

The Chronic Respiratory Disease Questionnaire (CRQ) was once administered by an interviewer but a newer version allows the tool to be self-administered.[143] The questionnaire has 20 questions divided into four domains (dyspnea, fatigue, emotional functioning, and mastery). Patients are allowed to choose five activities that cause them to experience shortness of breath, which lets the questionnaire take a more individualized approach.[143]

### Purpose

The CRQ is an appropriate objective measure to use with patients with respiratory dysfunction. The tool provides quality-of-life information in terms of fatigue, emotion, mastery, and dyspnea. In addition, as a result of the individualization of the dyspnea portion of the questionnaire, dyspnea can be scored on its own with or without reporting an overall score. The dyspnea portion of the questionnaire can be used to track patient outcomes as they pertain to their activities of daily living.

### Reliability and Validity

The CRQ demonstrates high reliability and validity for both COPD and asthma patients. Intraclass correlations at the first and second trials displayed very high Pearson $r$ values for all sections of the questionnaire (symptoms, activity, impacts). The St. Georges Respiratory Questionnaire was also correlated with the SF-36, a very prominent quality-of-life assessment tool, with a correlation between the two tools of a moderate to high −0.75.

The tool has also shown high reliability. Molken established an $\alpha$ value of 0.70 as sufficient and measured the reliability of the CRQ to be 0.84 to 0.87 for the four portions of the questionnaire.[143] Wijkstra found a low internal consistency of the dyspnea measure with $\alpha$ values equaling 0.51 and 0.53.[144] Emotion, fatigue, and mastery, however, displayed high consistency with $\alpha$ ranges 0.71 to 0.88. The test–retest values were also high on these three measures, with the p value ranging 0.90 to 0.93. The dyspnea measure was again lower, with a p value of 0.73.[144] Finally, Molken found that the minimally important difference for the questionnaire to be an improvement or deterioration of 0.5.[143]

### Suggested Usage

The importance of establishing a gold standard for cardiopulmonary evaluation and intervention is crucial in identifying problems that may not have been caught by a general health questionnaire. The CRQ allows respiratory problems such as dyspnea to be evaluated at baseline and readministered throughout treatment to look for possible gains or losses made during the treatment period. With a valid and reliable tool such as the CRQ, clinicians hopefully can identify issues specific to their patients' condition and eliminate any issues that may have been overlooked by a general evaluation tool. In addition, as the measurement of outcomes and the demonstration of effectiveness is now a requirement for reimbursement, the CRQ provides an easy and inexpensive way to demonstrate those outcomes in the respiratory therapy environment.

## The Walking Impairment Questionnaire

### Background and Administration

The Walking Impairment Questionnaire (WIQ) is a survey focusing on the amount of difficulty a person has in walking on a level surface, on the stairs, and at different speeds, and the amount of difficulty a person has with walking because of pain.[145] The questionnaire takes 5 to 10 minutes to complete and may be self-administered, administered over the phone, or administered by another individual. The WIQ is used to estimate functional status and measure ambulatory abilities of patients with peripheral vascular disease.[146] It is administered to patients older than age 55 years with an ABI ≤ 0.90 at rest, and is intended for those with intermittent claudication or other associated problems of peripheral vascular disease.

The WIQ contains questions from four categories[145,146]: pain (two questions), walking distance (seven questions), walking speed (four questions), and stair climbing (three questions). These categories provide an overview of a patient's functional walking ability. A Likert scale from 1 (no difficulty) to 5 (unable to do) is used to measure an individual's abilities through self-assessment.

### Purpose

The purpose of the WIQ is to determine the impact of PAD on function. Because of the relationship between function and quality of life, this measure could be considered an indirect objective measure of the impact of PAD on quality of life. The tool can screen for patients who present with multiple risk factors or as an objective measure that provides solid data on outcomes from physical therapy intervention.

### Reliability and Validity

Several studies have compared WIQ scores to other functional measurements of walking. In a study of 26 patients with intermittent claudication, and no exercise-limiting comorbid diseases, WIQ distance and speed scores significantly correlated with peak treadmill walking time and with time to onset of intermittent claudication on a treadmill.[147] WIQ scores also correlate significantly with existing walking tests, p < 0.001[146]; the WIQ distance score demonstrated moderate correlation with the 6MWT ($r = 0.557$), and the speed score from the WIQ correlated moderately with both the usual-paced 4-meter walk ($r = 0.528$) and the fast-paced 4-meter walk ($r = 0.56$).

The WIQ also shows high reliability. The subscales for distance, speed, and climbing stairs of the modified WIQ show good internal consistency, $\alpha = 0.80$, when the test was administered in person, over the phone, or self-administered.[146] Test–retest reliability is also high when the WIQ is self-administered or telephone administered, with an ICC between 0.68 and 0.88, depending on the subscale.[146]

*Suggested Usage*

PAD can be a debilitating illness, with direct effects on quality of life as a consequence of its impact on walking and activities of daily living. The WIQ is an objective measure that can screen and measure outcomes in patients with PAD across a variety of settings. The WIQ should be considered in any patient with two or more cardiovascular risk factors and in patients who present with peripheral vascular disease or circulatory conditions that compromise their exercising capacity.

## Summary

- This chapter provides an overview of the physiologic, functional, and HRQL measures that are available for assessing outcomes in physical therapy practice. Physical therapists must consider using outcome measures in a specific and comprehensive manner to demonstrate the effectiveness of their interventions in given patient populations. In the future, reimbursement for physical therapy practice will be dependent on therapist knowledge of the objective measures available and their consistent use in physical therapy practice across a variety of settings.
- HRQL is a measure of how biologic and physiologic processes affect perception of symptoms, which influences function, general health perception, and quality of life (anxiety, depression, perceived disease burden, general health perception).
- Patients with cardiovascular and pulmonary dysfunction are at high risk for decreased exercise capacity, impaired physiologic response to exercise, poorer quality of life, and higher rates of anxiety and depression.
- Rehabilitation and exercise are linked to improvements in exercise capacity, physiologic response to exercise, quality of life, and decreased symptoms of anxiety and depression among patients with various forms of cardiovascular or pulmonary dysfunction.
- Because of the high incidence of anxiety and depression in cardiac populations, the AACVPR recommends screening for depression for all population.
- Exercise has been found in some cases to be as beneficial as antidepressant medications in the treatment of anxiety symptoms and has been shown to provide physiologic changes in the blood that directly impact anxiety.
- When choosing a comprehensive and sometimes diverse method for outcome measurement, the therapist must be familiar with the psychometric properties of the tool or tools being used for patient assessment.
- The test–retest reliability is traditionally measured with the ICC and the κ statistic.
- The sensitivity of a tool refers to its ability to statistically detect change over a period of time in a given patient population, and responsiveness refers to the detection of clinically relevant change.
- There are a number of important reasons for individual programs to measure outcomes, including to demonstrate accountability, to improve clinical and management

decision making for optimal care delivery, for research, and as incentives, such as the current PQRI in which therapists may qualify for bonus payments for using objective measures in practice.
- Data that provides measurement of outcomes should be included at the point of the initial evaluation and should consider the patient from the biologic/physiologic, functional, and quality-of-life perspectives.
- The ABI is a noninvasive, easy-to-use, and economical objective outcome measure that can be used to examine perfusion of the lower extremities in individuals who are at high risk of cardiovascular disease or PAD.
- A summary of measures for testing exercise capacity include the self-paced walk test, the 2MWT, 3MWT, 6MWT, and 12MWT, the modified shuffle test, the treadmill endurance test, and the 200-meter walk-fast test.
- The four walk tests most commonly used in the physical therapy environment for assessment of self-paced functional performance and exercise capacity in the cardiovascular and pulmonary patient population are the 2MWT, 3MWT, 6MWT, and 12MWT.
- A modified shuttle test allows for assessment and clinical management of patient performance through evaluation of the patient during incremental and progressive exercise stress.
- HRQL measures outcomes from the patient's point of view and provides insight into a patient's perception of his or her illness' impact on activities of daily living.
- The SAQ is designed to specifically assess the impact of chest pain or angina within the previous 4 weeks on a patient's quality of life.
- The KCCQ is a self-response questionnaire made up of 23 items that quantify specific areas of quality of life related to heart failure.
- The KCCQ provides patients and clinicians with a disease-specific approach used to evaluate and appropriately monitor and treat those with heart failure. It targets those patients with advanced symptoms of heart failure.
- The CRQ is an appropriate objective measure to use with patients with respiratory dysfunction. The tool provides quality-of-life information in terms of fatigue, emotion, mastery, and dyspnea.
- The WIQ is a survey focusing on the amount of difficulty a person has in walking on a level surface, on stairs, and at different speeds, and the amount of difficulty a person has with walking because of pain. The WIQ is used to estimate functional status and measure ambulatory abilities of patients with peripheral vascular disease.

## References

1. World Health Organization. WHO definition of health. 2009. Available at: http://www.who.int/suggestions/faq/en/index.html. Accessed June 15, 2009.
2. Wilson IB, Cleary PD. Linking clinical variables with health related quality of life: A conceptual model of patient outcomes. JAMA 273(1):59–65, 1995.

3. Wood-Dauphinee S. Assessing quality of life in clinical research from where have we come and where are we going. J Clin Epidemiol 52(4):355–63, 1999.

4. Ulvik B, Nygard O, Hanestad B, et al. Associations between disease severity, coping and dimensions of health-related quality of life in patients admitted for elective coronary angiography—A cross sectional study. Health Qual Life Outcomes 6:38, 2008.

5. Wong M, Chair S. Changes in health-related quality of life following percutaneous coronary intervention: A longitudinal study. Int J Nurs Stud 44:1334–42, 2007.

6. Koch C, Li L, Lauer M, et al. Effect of functional health-related quality of life on long-term survival after cardiac surgery. Circulation 115:692–9, 2007.

7. Azevedo A, Bettencourt P, Alvelos M, et al. Health-related quality of life and stages of heart failure. Int J Cardiol 129(2):238–44, 2008.

8. Tully P, Baker R, Turnbull D, Winefield H. The role of depression and anxiety symptoms in hospital readmissions after cardiac surgery. J Behav Med 31:281–90, 2008.

9. Bankier B, Barajas J, Martinez-Rumayor A, et al. Association between anxiety and C-reactive protein levels in stable coronary heart disease patients. Psychosomatics 50(4):347–53, 2009.

10. Pignay-Demaria V, Lespérance F, Demaria RG, et al. Depression and anxiety and outcomes of coronary artery bypass surgery. Ann Thorac Surg 75(1):314–21, 2003.

11. Casey E, Hughes J, Waechter D, et al. Depression predicts failure to complete phase-II cardiac rehabilitation. J Behav Med 31:421–31, 2008.

12. Komorovsky R, Desideri A, Rozbowsky P, et al. Quality of life and behavioral compliance in cardiac rehabilitation patients: a longitudinal survey. Int J Nurs Stud 45(7):979–85, 2008.

13. Theander K, Jakobsson P, Jorgensen N, et al. Effects of pulmonary rehabilitation on fatigue, functional status and health perceptions in patients with chronic obstructive pulmonary disease: A randomized controlled trial. Clin Rehabil 23(2):125–36, 2009.

14. Smart N, Haluska B, Jeffriess L, et al. Exercise training in systolic and diastolic dysfunction effects on cardiac function, functional capacity, and quality of life. Am Heart J 153(4):530–6, 2007.

15. Hung C, Daub B, Black B, et al. Exercise training improves overall physical fitness and quality of life in older women with coronary artery disease. Chest 126(4):1026–31, 2004.

16. Collins E, Langbein W, Dilan-Koetje J, et al. Effects of exercise training on aerobic capacity and quality of life in individuals with heart failure. Clin Rehabil 23(3):207–16, 2009.

17. Gary R, Sueta C, Dougherty M, et al. Home-based exercise improves functional performance and quality of life in woman with diastolic heart failure. Heart Lung 33(4):210–18, 2004.

18. Blumenthal J, Sherwood A, Rogers S, et al. Understanding prognostic benefits of exercise and antidepressant therapy for persons with depression and heart disease: the UPBEAT study rationale, design, and methodological issues. Clin Trials 4:548–59, 2007.

19. Kerse N, Falloon K, Moyes S, et al. DeLLITE Depression in late life: An intervention trial of exercise. Design and recruitment of a randomised controlled trial. BMC Geriatr 8(12):1–7, 2008.

20. Strohle A, Feller C, Strasburger C, et al. Anxiety modulation by the heart? Aerobic exercise and atrial natriuretic peptide. Psychoneuroendocrinology 31:1127–30, 2006.

21. Benno VT, Huijsmans RJ, Krron DW, et al. Effects of exercise training on cardiac performance, exercise capacity and quality of life in patients with heart failure: A meta-analysis. Eur J Heart Fail 8(8):841–50, 2006.

22. Scherer S, Wilson C. Research corner: Revisiting outcomes assessment. Cardiopulm Phys Ther J 18(1):21–6, 2007.

23. Portney LG, Watkins MP. Foundations of Clinical Research: Applications to Practice. 3rd ed. Upper Saddle River, NJ, Prentice Hall, 2008.

24. Corzillius M. Responsiveness and sensitivity to change of SLE disease activity measures. Lupus 8(8):655–9, 1999.

25. NLM Gateway: A service of the U.S. National Institutes of Health. 2009. Progress Report on the Joint Commission's Performance Measurement Requirements: System and Measure Selection. Available at: http://gateway.nlm.nih.gov/MeetingAbstracts/ma?f=102194752.html. Accessed June 2009.

26. Centers for Medicare and Medicaid Services. Roadmap for Quality Measurement in the Traditional Medicare Fee-for-Service Program. Available at: http://www.cms.hhs.gov/QualityInitiativesGenInfo/downloads/QualityMeasurementRoadmap_OEA1–16_508.pdf . Accessed June 2009.

27. Centers for Medicare and Medicaid Services. Overview of Physician Quality Reporting Initiative (PQRI). 2010. Available at: http://www.cms.hhs.gov/pqri/. Accessed February 2010.

28. Thomas R, King M, Lui K, et al. AACVPR/ACC/AHA 2007 performance measures on cardiac rehabilitation for referral to and delivery of cardiac rehabilitation/ secondary prevention services. J Cardiopulm Rehabil 27:260–90, 2007.

29. Sanderson B, Southard D, Oldridge N. Outcomes evaluation in cardiac rehabilitation/secondary prevention programs. J Cardiopulm Rehabil 24:68–79, 2004.

30. Walker AE, Eskurza I, Pierce GL. Modulation of vascular endothelial function by low-density lipoprotein cholesterol with aging: Influence of habitual exercise. Am J Hypertens 22:250–6, 2009.

31. Williams PT. Vigorous exercise, fitness and incident hypertension, high cholesterol, and diabetes. Med Sci Sports Exerc 40(6):998–1006, 2008.

32. Lakka TA, Lakka HM, Rankinen T. Effect of exercise training on plasma levels of C-reactive protein in healthy adults: The HERITAGE Family Study. Eur Heart J 26(19):2018–25, 2005.

33. Kodama S, Tanaka S, Saito K, et al. Effect of aerobic exercise training on serum levels of high-density lipoprotein cholesterol. Arch Intern Med 167:999–1008, 2007.

34. Bordenave S, Brandou F, Manetta J, et al. Effects of acute exercise on insulin sensitivity, glucose effectiveness and disposition index in type 2, diabetes patients. Diabetes Metab 34:250–7, 2008.

35. American Heart Association. What Your Cholesterol Level Means. Available at: http://www.americanheart.org/presenter.jhtml?identifier=183. Accessed February 2010.

36. American Association of Cardiovascular and Pulmonary Rehabilitation (AAVCPR). AACVPR Consensus Statement: Outcomes Evaluation in Cardiac Rehabilitation/Secondary Prevention Programs. Available at: http://www.aacvpr.org/Portals/0/resources/professionals/outcomesconsensus04.pdf. Accessed February 2010.

37. Reich L, Heiss G, Boland L, et al. Ankle-brachial index and hemostatic markers in the atherosclerosis risk in communities (ARIC) study cohort. Vasc Med 12:267–73, 2007.

38. Morillas P, Cordero A, Bertomeu V, et al. Prognostic value of low ankle-brachial index in patients with hypertension and acute coronary syndromes. J Hypertens 27:341–7, 2009.

39. Ovbiagele B. Association of ankle-brachial index level with stroke. J Neurol Sci 276(1–2):14–17, 2009.

40. Mitka M. Diabetes group warns vascular complication is underdiagnosed and undertreated. JAMA 291(7):809–10, 2004.

41. Cacoub PP, Abola MT, Baumgartner I, et al. Cardiovascular risk factor control and outcomes in peripheral artery disease patients in the Reduction of Atherothrombosis for Continued Health (REACH) Registry. Atherosclerosis 204(2):e86–92, 2009.

42. Hirsch AT, Halverson SL, Treat-Jacobson D, et al. The Minnesota Regional Peripheral Arterial Disease Screening Program: Toward a definition of community standards of care. Vasc Med 6(2):87–96, 2001.

43. Johnsen MC, Landow WJ, Sonnefeld J, et al. Evaluation of Legs For Life National Screening and Awareness Program for Peripheral Vascular Disease: Results of a follow-up survey of screening participants. J Vasc Interv Radiol 13(1):25–35, 2002.

44. Moussa ID, Jaff MR, Mehran R, et al. Prevalence and prediction of previously unrecognized peripheral arterial disease in patients with coronary artery disease: The Peripheral Arterial Disease in Interventional Patients Study. Catheter Cardiovasc Interv 73(6):719–24, 2009.

45. Shaffer R, Greene S, Arshi A, et al. Effect of acute exercise on endothelial progenitor cells in patients with peripheral arterial disease. Vasc Med 11:219–26, 2006.

46. Crowther RG, Sprinks WL, Leicht AS, et al. Effects of a long-term exercise program on lower limb mobility, physiological responses, walking performance, and physical activity levels in patients with peripheral arterial disease. J Vasc Surg 47(2):303–9, 2008.

47. McDermott MM, Ades P, Guralnik JM, et al. Treadmill exercise and resistance training in patients with peripheral arterial disease with and without intermittent claudication: A randomized controlled trial. JAMA 301(2):165–74, 2009.

48. Kalra M, Gloviczki P, Bower TC, et al. Limb salvage after successful pedal bypass grafting is associated with improved long term survival. J Vasc Surg 33(1):6–16, 2001.

49. McDermott MM, Greenland P, Liu K, et al. The ankle brachial index is associated with leg function and physical activity: The Walking and Leg Circulation Study. Ann Intern Med 136(12):873–83, 2002.

50. McDermott MM, Guralnik JM, Greenland P, et al. Statin use and leg functioning in patients with and without lower-extremity peripheral arterial disease. Circulation 107(5):757–61, 2003.

51. Rice TW, Lumsden AB. Optimal medical management of peripheral arterial disease. Vasc Endovascular Surg 40(4):312–27, 2006.

52. Carmo GL, Mandill A, Nascimento BR, et al. Can we measure the ankle-brachial index using only a stethoscope? Fam Pract 26:22–6, 2009.

53. Lefebvre KM. Outcomes measures in cardiopulmonary physical therapy: Focus on the ankle brachial index (ABI). Cardiopulm Phys Ther J 17(4):13–15, 2006.

54. Dutcher J, Kahn C, Grines B, et al. Comparison of left ventricular ejection fraction and exercise capacity as predictors of two- and five-year mortality following acute myocardial infarction. Am J Cardiol 99(4):436–41, 2007.

55. Stewart A, Hays R, Ware JJ. The MOS short-form general health survey. Reliability and validity in a patient population. Med Care 26:724–35, 1988.

56. Hunt S, McEwen J, McKenna S. A quantitative approach to perceived health. J Epidemiol Community Health 34:281–95, 1980.

57. Gibson B, Gibson J, Bergner M, et al. The sickness impact profile—Development of an outcome measure of health care. Ann Intern Med 65(12):1304–10, 1975.

58. Bergner M, Bobbitt R, Carter W, et al. The Sickness Impact Profile: Development and final revision of a health status measure. Med Care 19:787–805, 1981.

59. Kaplan R, Atkins C, Timms R. Validity of a quality of well-being scale as an outcome measure in chronic obstructive pulmonary disease. J Chronic Dis 37:85–95, 1984.

60. Greenberg G, Peterson R, Heilbronner R. Illness Effects Questionnaire [unpublished]. Philadelphia, Psychology Department, Children's Rehabilitation Hospital, Thomas Jefferson University Hospital, 1989.

61. Wasson J, Keller A, Rubenstein L, et al. Benefits and obstacles of health status assessment in ambulatory settings. Med Care 30(5):42–9, 1992.

62. Parkerson GJ, Broadhead W, Tse C-K. The Duke Health Profile: A 17-item measure of health and dysfunction. Med Care 28:1056–72, 1990.

63. Wallston K, Wallston B. Health locus of control scales. In Lefcourt H (ed.). Research with the Locus of Control Construct. New York, Academic Press, 1981.

64. Dupuis G, Perrault J, Lambany M, et al. A new tool to assess quality of life: The Quality of Life Systemic Inventory. Qual Life Cardiovasc Care. Spring:36–40, 1989.

65. Kellner R. Manual of the symptom questionnaire [unpublished]. No. 87131. Albuquerque, NM, Department of Psychiatry, School of Medicine, 1987.

66. Rector T, Kubo S, Cohn J. Patients' self-assessment of their congestive heart failure. Heart Fail Oct/Nov:198–209, 1987.

67. Rogers W, Johnstone D, Yusuf S, et al. Quality of life among 5025 patients with left ventricular dysfunction randomized between placebo and enalapril: The study of left ventricular dysfunction. J Am Coll Cardiol 23:393–400, 1994.

68. Oldridge N, Guyatt G, Jones N, et al. Effects on quality of life with comprehensive rehabilitation after acute myocardial infarction. Am J Cardiol 67:1084–9, 1991.

69. Lim L-Y, Valenti L, Knapp J, et al. A self-administered quality of life questionnaire after acute myocardial infarction. J Clin Epidemiol 46:1249–56, 1993.

70. Ferrans C, Powers M. Psychometric assessment of the Quality of Life Index. Res Nurs Health 15:29–38, 1992.

71. Spertus J, Winder J, Dewhurst T, et al. Development and evaluation of the Seattle Angina Questionnaire: A new functional status measure for coronary artery disease. J Am Coll Cardiol 25:333–41, 1995.

72. Guyatt G, Berman L, Townsend M, et al. A measure of quality of life for clinical trials in chronic lung disease. Thorax 42:773–8, 1987.

73. Jones P, Quirk F, Baveystock C, Littlejohn P. A self-complete measure of health status for chronic airflow limitation. Am Rev Respir Dis 145:1321–7, 1992.

74. Weaver T, Narsavage G. Physiological and psychological variables related to functional status in chronic obstructive pulmonary disease. Nurs Res 41:286–91, 1992.

75. Lareau S, Carrieri-Kohlman V, Janson-Bjerklie S, Roos P. Development and testing of the Pulmonary Functional Status and Dyspnea Questionnaire (PFSDQ). Heart Lung 23(3):242–50, 1994.

76. Hyland M. The living with asthma questionnaire. Respir Med 85(Suppl B):13–16, 1991.

77. Harvey R, Doyle E, Ellis K, et al. Major changes made by the Criteria Committee of the New York Heart Association. Circulation 49:390, 1974.

78. Goldman L, Hashimoto B, Cook E, et al. Comparative reproducibility and validity of systems for assessing cardiovascular functional class: Advantages of a new Specific Activity Scale. Circulation 64:1227–34, 1981.

79. Mahler D, Weinberg D, Wells C, Feinstein A. The measurement of dyspnea: Contents, interobserver agreement, and physiologic correlates of two new clinical indexes. Chest 85:751–8, 1984.

80. Hlatky M, Boineau R, Higgenbotham M, et al. A brief self-administered questionnaire to determine functional capacity (The Duke Activity Status Index). Am J Cardiol 64:651–4, 1989.

81. Borg G. Perceived exertion as an indicator of somatic stress. Scand J Rehabil Med 2:92–8, 1970.

82. Borg G. Psychophysical basis of perceived exertion. Med Sci Sports Exerc 14:377–81, 1982.

83. Gift A. Validation of a vertical visual analogue scale as a measure of clinical dyspnea. Rehabil Nurs 14:323–5, 1989.

84. American College of Sports Medicine. Guidelines for Graded Exercise Testing and Exercise Prescription. 4th ed. Philadelphia, Lea & Febiger, 1991.

85. Guyatt G, Sullivan M, Thompson P, et al. The 6-minute walk: A new measure of exercise capacity in patients with chronic heart failure. Can Med Assoc J 132:919–23, 1985.

86. Cipkin D, Scriven J, Crake T, Poole-Wilson P. Six minute walking test for assessing exercise capacity in chronic heart failure. BMJ 292:653–5, 1986.

87. Daughton D, Fix A, Kass I, et al. Maximum oxygen consumption and the ADAPT quality of life scale. Arch Phys Med Rehabil 63:620–2, 1982.

88. Jette A, Davies A, Cleary P, et al. The functional status questionnaire: Reliability and validity when used in primary care. J Gen Intern Med 1:143–9, 1986.

89. Derogatis R, Brand R, Jenkins C, et al. In SCL-90-R: Administration, Scoring and Procedures Manual II for the R (revised) Version and Other Instruments of the Psychopathology Rating Scale Series. 2nd ed. Towson, MD, Clinic Psychometric Research, 1983.

90. Dahlstrom W, Walsh G, Dahlstrom L. MMPI Handbook. Clinical Interpretation. Rev. ed. Minneapolis, University of Minnesota, 1975.

91. Cook W, Medley D. Proposed hostility and pharisaic-virtue scales for the MMPI. J Appl Psychol 38:414–18, 1954.

92. Buss A, Durkee A. An inventory for assessing different kinds of hostility. J Consult Psychol 21:343–9, 1957.

93. Beck A. The Beck Depression Inventory. Philadelphia, Center for Cognitive Therapy, 1978.

94. Radloff L. The CES-D scale: A self-report depression scale for research in the general population. Appl Psychol Meas 1:385–401, 1977.

95. Spielberger C, Gonsuch R, Luschene R. Manual for the State—Trait Anxiety Inventory. Palo Alto, CA, Consulting Psychologist Press, 1970.

96. Wigel J, Creer T, Kotses H. The COPD Self-Efficacy Scale. Chest 99:1193–6, 1991.

97. Carver C, Scheier M, Weintraub J. Assessing coping strategies: A theoretically based approach. J Pers Soc Psychol 56:267–83, 1989.

98. Jenkins C, Rosenman R, Friedman M. Development of an objective psychological test for the determination of the coronary prone behavior pattern in employed men. J Chronic Dis 20:371–9, 1967.

99. McNair D, Lorr M, Droppleman L. Profile of Mood States. San Diego, CA, Educational and Industrial Testing Service, 1971.

100. Hare D, Davis C. Validation of a new depression scale for cardiac patients in quality of life assessment. Aust N Z J Med 23:630, 1993.

101. Lorish C, Maisiak R. The face scale: A brief, nonverbal method for assessing patient mood. Arthritis Rheum 29(7):906–10, 1986.

102. Wenger N, Mattson M, Furberg C. Assessment of Quality of Life in Clinical Trials of Cardiovascular Therapies. New York, Le Jacq Communications, 1984.

103. Folkman S, Lazarus R. Ways of Coping Questionnaire. J Pers Soc Psychol 48:150–70, 1985.

104. Sherbourne C, Stewart A. The MOS social support survey. Soc Sci Med 32(6):705–14, 1991.

105. Morrow G, Chiarello R, Derogatis L. Psychosocial adjustment to illness scale. Psychol Med 8:605–10, 1978.

106. Willett W, Sampson L, Stampfer M, et al. Reproducibility and validity of a semi-quantitative food frequency questionnaire. Am J Epidemiol 122:51, 1985.

107. Block G, Clifford C, Naughton M, et al. A brief dietary screen for high fat intake. J Nutr Educ 21:199–207, 1989.

108. Connor S, Gustafson J, Sexton G, et al. The diet habit survey: A new method of dietary assessment that relates to plasma cholesterol changes. J Am Diet Assoc 92(1):41–7, 1992.

109. Blankenhorn DH, Nessim SA, Johnson RL, et al. Beneficial effects of combined colestipol-niacin therapy on coronary atherosclerosis and coronary venous bypass grafts [published erratum appears in JAMA 259(18): 2698, 1988]. JAMA 257(23):3233–40, 1987.

110. Hopp J, Lee J, Hills R. Development and validation of a pulmonary rehabilitation knowledge test. J Cardiopulm Rehabil 8:15–18, 1989.

111. Maeland J, Havik O. Measuring cardiac health knowledge. Scand J Caring Sci 1:23–31, 1987.

112. Doutreleau S, Di Marco P, Talha S, et al. Can the six-minute walk test predict peak oxygen update in men with heart transplant? Arch Phys Med Rehabil 90(1):51–7, 2009.

113. Pereira de Sousa LA, Britto RR, Riberio AL, et al. Six-minute walk test in patients with permanent cardiac pacemakers. J Cardiopulm Rehabil Prev 28(4):253–7, 2008.

114. Larrson UE, Reynisdottir S. The six-minute walk test in outpatients with obesity: reproducibility and known group validity. Physiother Res Int 13(2):84–93, 2008.

115. Fulk J, Storey K. Evaluation of a brief aerobic exercise intervention for high anxiety sensitivity. Anxiety Stress Coping 21(2):117–28, 2008.

116. Maher CA, Williams MT, Olds TS. The six-minute walk test for children with cerebral palsy. Int J Rehabil Res 31(2):185–8, 2008.

117. Leung AS, Chan KK, Sykes K, et al. Reliability, validity and responsiveness of a two-minute walk test to assess exercise capacity of COPD patients. Chest 130:119–25, 2006.

118. Irriberri M, Galdiz JB, Gorostiza A, et al. American Thoracic Society (ATS): ATS Statement: Guidelines for the six-minute walk test. Am J Respir Crit Care Med 166:111–17, 2002.

119. American Thoracic Society. Guidelines for the six-minute walk test. Am J Respir Crit Care Med 116:111–17, 2002.

120. Wise RA, Brown CD. Minimal clinically important differences in the six-minute walk test and the incremental shuttle walking test. COPD 2(1):125–9, 2005.

121. Singh S, Morgan M, Scott S, et al. Development of a shuttle walking test of disability in patients with chronic airways obstruction. Thorax 47:1019–24, 1992

122. Podsiadlo, D., & Richardson, S. (1991). The timed "up & go": A test of basic functional mobility for frail elderly persons. Journal of the American Geriatrics Society, 39, 142–8.

123. Shumway-Cook, A., Brauer, S., & Woollacott, M. (2000). Predicting the probability for falls in community-dwelling older adults using the timed up & go test. Physical Therapy, 80(9), 896–903.

124. Studenski SA, Duncan PW, Richards L. Performance Measures in the Clinical Setting. J Am Ger Soc 2003;51:1–10.

125. Perera S, Mody SH, Woodman RC, Studenski SA. Meaningful Change and Responsiveness in Common Physical Performance Measures in Older Adults. J Am Geriatr Soc 54:743–9, 2006.

126. Purser JL, Weinberger MW, Cohen HJ, Pieper CF, Morey MC, Li T, Williams GR, Lapuerta P. Walking speed predicts health status and hospital costs for frail elderly male veterans. J Rehabil Res Development, 2005;42(4):535–45.

127. Bowden MG, Balasubramanian CK, Behrman AL, Kautz SA. Validation of a Speed-Based Classification System Using Quantitative Measures of Walking Performance Post-Stroke Neurorehabil Neural Repair. Neurorehabil Neural Repair, 2008; 22(6):672–5.

128. Guralnik JM, Ferrucci L, Pieper CF et al. Lower extremity function and subsequent disability: Consistency across studies, predictive models, and value of gait speed alone compared with the Short Physical Performance Battery. J Gerontol A Biol Sci Med Sci 2000;55A:M221–31.

129. Bohannon RW. Comfortable and maximum walking speed of adults aged 20–79 years: reference values and determinants. 1997 Age and Ageing 1997;26:15–19.

130. Steffen TM, Hacker TA, Mollinger L. Age-and gender-related test performance in community-dwelling elderly people: six-minute walk test, berg balance scale, timed up and go test and gait speeds. Phys Ther Vol. 82, No. 2, February 2002, pp. 128–37.

131. Brach JS, VanSwearingen JM, Newman AB, Kriska AM. Identifying early decline of physical function in community-dwelling older women: performance-based and self-report measures. Phys Ther Vol. 82, No. 4, April 2002, pp. 320–8.

132. Montero-Odasso M, Schapira M, Soriano ER, et al. Gait Velocity as a Single Predictor of Adverse Events in Healthy Seniors Aged 75 Years and Older. J Gerontol Med Sci 2005;60A(10):1304–9.

133. Salbach NM, Mayo NE, Higgins J, et al. Responsiveness and predictability of gait speed and other disability measures in acute stroke. Arch Phys Med Rehabil 82(9):1204–12, 2001.

134. Gorkin, L, Follock MJ, Hamm P, et al. Quality of life among patients post myocardial infarction at baseline in the Survival and Ventricular Enlargement (SAVE) Trial. Qual Life Res 3:111–19, 1994.

135. Anda RF, Williamson DF, Escobedo LG, et al. Depression and the dynamics of smoking. JAMA 284:1541–5, 1990.

136. Arrigo I, Brunner-LaRocca H, Lefkovits M, et al. Comparative outcome one year after formal cardiac rehabilitation: The effects of a randomized intervention to improve exercise adherence. Eur J Cardiovasc Prev Rehabil 15(3):306–11, 2008.

137. Komorovsky R, Desideri A, Rozbowsky P, et al. Quality of life and behavioral compliance in cardiac rehabilitation patients: a longitudinal survey. Int J Nurs Stud 45(7):979–85, 2008.

138. McGee H. Can the measurement of quality of life contribute to evaluation in cardiac rehabilitation services. J Cardiovasc Risk 3:148–53, 1996.

139. Spertus JA, Winder JA, Dewhurst TA, et al. Development and evaluation of the Seattle Angina questionnaire: A new functional status measure for coronary artery disease. J Am Coll Cardiol 25(2):333–41, 1995.

140. Green CP, Porter CB, Bresnahan DR, et al. Development and evaluation of the Kansas City Cardiomyopathy Questionnaire: A new health status measure for heart failure. J Am Coll Cardiol 35:1245–55, 2000.

141. Dekerlegand JL. Research corner outcome measures in cardiopulmonary physical therapy: Focus on the Kansas City Cardiomyopathy Questionnaire. Cardiopulm Phys Ther J 16:17–23, 2005.

142. Spertus JA, Peterson ED, Conard MW, et al. Monitoring clinical changes in patients with heart failure: A comparison of methods. Am Heart J 150:707–15, 2005.

143. Molken MR, Roos B, Van Noord JA. An empirical comparison of the St George's Respiratory Questionnaire (SGRQ) and the Chronic Respiratory Disease Questionnaire (CRQ) in a clinical trial setting. Thorax 54:995–1003, 1999.

144. Wijkstra PJ, TenVergert EM, Van Altena RV. Reliability and validity of the chronic respiratory questionnaire (CRQ). Thorax 49:465–46, 1994.

145. Coyne KS, Margolis MK, Gilchrist KA, et al. Evaluating effects of method of administration on walking impairment questionnaire. J Vasc Surg 38:296–304, 2003.

146. McDermott MM, Liu K, Guralnik JM, et al. Measurement of walking endurance and walking velocity with questionnaire: Validation of the walking impairment questionnaire in men and women with peripheral arterial disease. J Vasc Surg 28:1072–81, 1998.

147. Regensteiner JG, Steiner SF, Panzer RJ, et al. Evaluation of walking impairment by questionnaire in patients with peripheral arterial disease. J Vasc Med Biol 2:142–52, 1990.

# Index